Central Nervous System Infectious Diseases and Therapy

NEUROLOGICAL DISEASE AND THERAPY

Series Editor

William C. Koller

Department of Neurology
University of Kansas Medical Center
Kansas City, Kansas

1. Handbook of Parkinson's Disease, *edited by William C. Koller*
2. Medical Therapy of Acute Stroke, *edited by Mark Fisher*
3. Familial Alzheimer's Disease: Molecular Genetics and Clinical Perspectives, *edited by Gary D. Miner, Ralph W. Richter, John P. Blass, Jimmie L. Valentine, and Linda A. Winters-Miner*
4. Alzheimer's Disease: Treatment and Long-Term Management, *edited by Jeffrey L. Cummings and Bruce L. Miller*
5. Therapy of Parkinson's Disease, *edited by William C. Koller and George Paulson*
6. Handbook of Sleep Disorders, *edited by Michael J. Thorpy*
7. Epilepsy and Sudden Death, *edited by Claire M. Lathers and Paul L. Schraeder*
8. Handbook of Multiple Sclerosis, *edited by Stuart D. Cook*
9. Memory Disorders: Research and Clinical Practice, *edited by Takehiko Yanagihara and Ronald C. Petersen*
10. The Medical Treatment of Epilepsy, *edited by Stanley R. Resor, Jr., and Henn Kutt*
11. Cognitive Disorders: Pathophysiology and Treatment, *edited by Leon J. Thal, Walter H. Moos, and Elkan R. Gamzu*
12. Handbook of Amyotrophic Lateral Sclerosis, *edited by Richard Alan Smith*
13. Handbook of Parkinson's Disease: Second Edition, Revised and Expanded, *edited by William C. Koller*
14. Handbook of Pediatric Epilepsy, *edited by Jerome V. Murphy and Fereydoun Dehkharghani*
15. Handbook of Tourette's Syndrome and Related Tic and Behavioral Disorders, *edited by Roger Kurlan*
16. Handbook of Cerebellar Diseases, *edited by Richard Lechtenberg*
17. Handbook of Cerebrovascular Diseases, *edited by Harold P. Adams, Jr.*
18. Parkinsonian Syndromes, *edited by Matthew B. Stern and William C. Koller*
19. Handbook of Head and Spine Trauma, *edited by Jonathan Greenberg*
20. Brain Tumors: A Comprehensive Text, *edited by Robert A. Morantz and John W. Walsh*
21. Monoamine Oxidase Inhibitors in Neurological Diseases, *edited by Abraham Lieberman, C. Warren Olanow, Moussa B. H. Youdim, and Keith Tipton*
22. Handbook of Dementing Illnesses, *edited by John C. Morris*
23. Handbook of Myasthenia Gravis and Myasthenic Syndromes, *edited by Robert P. Lisak*

24. Handbook of Neurorehabilitation, *edited by David C. Good and James R. Couch, Jr.*
25. Therapy with Botulinum Toxin, *edited by Joseph Jankovic and Mark Hallett*
26. Principles of Neurotoxicology, *edited by Louis W. Chang*
27. Handbook of Neurovirology, *edited by Robert R. McKendall and William G. Stroop*
28. Handbook of Neuro-Urology, *edited by David N. Rushton*
29. Handbook of Neuroepidemiology, *edited by Philip B. Gorelick and Milton Alter*
30. Handbook of Tremor Disorders, *edited by Leslie J. Findley and William C. Koller*
31. Neuro-Ophthalmological Disorders: Diagnostic Work-Up and Management, *edited by Ronald J. Tusa and Steven A. Newman*
32. Handbook of Olfaction and Gustation, *edited by Richard L. Doty*
33. Handbook of Neurological Speech and Language Disorders, *edited by Howard S. Kirshner*
34. Therapy of Parkinson's Disease: Second Edition, Revised and Expanded, *edited by William C. Koller and George Paulson*
35. Evaluation and Management of Gait Disorders, *edited by Barney S. Spivack*
36. Handbook of Neurotoxicology, *edited by Louis W. Chang and Robert S. Dyer*
37. Neurological Complications of Cancer, *edited by Ronald G. Wiley*
38. Handbook of Autonomic Nervous System Dysfunction, *edited by Amos D. Korczyn*
39. Handbook of Dystonia, *edited by Joseph King Ching Tsui and Donald B. Calne*
40. Etiology of Parkinson's Disease, *edited by Jonas H. Ellenberg, William C. Koller, and J. William Langston*
41. Practical Neurology of the Elderly, *edited by Jacob I. Sage and Margery H. Mark*
42. Handbook of Muscle Disease, *edited by Russell J. M. Lane*
43. Handbook of Multiple Sclerosis: Second Edition, Revised and Expanded, *edited by Stuart D. Cook*
44. Central Nervous System Infectious Diseases and Therapy, *edited by Karen L. Roos*

Additional Volumes in Preparation

Neurology Practical Guidelines, *edited by Richard Lechtenberg and Henry Schutta*

Central Nervous System Infectious Diseases and Therapy

edited by
Karen L. Roos
Indiana University School of Medicine
Indianapolis, Indiana

MARCEL DEKKER, INC.   NEW YORK • BASEL • HONG KONG

Library of Congress Cataloging-in-Publication Data

Central nervous system infectious diseases and therapy / edited by Karen L. Roos.
p. cm. — (Neurological disease and therapy ; 44)
Includes index.
ISBN 0-8247-9811-2 (hardcover : alk. paper)
1. Central nervous system—Infections. 2. Central nervous system—Infections—Treatment. I. Roos, Karen L. II. Series.
[DNLM: 1. Central Nervous System Diseases. 2. Infection. 3. Bacterial Infections. W1 NE33LD v.44 1997]
RC361.C455 1997
616.8—dc21
DNLM/DLC
for Library of Congress

97-7153
CIP

The publisher offers discounts on this book when ordered in bulk quantities. For more information, write to Special Sales/Professional Marketing at the address below.

This book is printed on acid-free paper.

Marcel Dekker, Inc.
270 Madison Avenue, New York, New York 10016

Current printing (last digit):
10 9 8 7 6 5 4 3 2 1

PRINTED IN THE UNITED STATES OF AMERICA

This book is dedicated to my husband,
Robert M. Pascuzzi, M.D.
and our daughters,
Annie and Jan

Preface

Central Nervous System Infectious Diseases and Therapy has been written with two purposes in mind: (1) to provide easy access for the busy clinician to the information that is needed for the diagnosis and therapy of central nervous system (CNS) infections; and (2) to provide state-of-the-art management of the neurological complications of CNS infections.

This book can be used in several ways. If the clinician knows the diagnosis and is interested in a broader understanding of, or therapeutic recommendations for, a specific disease, he or she can consult the chapter dealing with that specific disease. In addition, a number of the chapters provide either a table or an algorithm that allows for a straightforward approach to the management of the patient presumed to have that infection. These tables and algorithms simplify the clinician's search, and make information readily available for use in the care of critically ill patients.

Chapters 1–4 deal with infectious diseases of infancy and early childhood, including neonatal meningitis, perinatal viral infections, neurological disorders associated with human immunodeficiency virus in children, and neurological complications of immunization.

Chapters 5–28 focus on all the important CNS infectious diseases of older childhood, adolescence, and adulthood.

Topics such as rabies, neurocysticercosis, and cerebral malaria are included in this book because of their worldwide importance as CNS infectious diseases. It also contains a number of topics that are frequently seen in clinical practice, but rarely covered in textbooks (e.g., infectious etiologies of facial palsy, CNS infections in organ transplant recipients, parainfectious syndromes, and the Guillain-Barré syndrome).

Finally, Chapters 29–33 are dedicated to the diagnosis of central nervous system infections: Chapter 29 (neuroimaging of CNS infections); Chapter 30 (EEG in the diagnosis of CNS infections); Chapter 31 (acute management of the neurological complications of CNS infections);

Chapter 32 (systemic and CNS toxicities of antimicrobial agents), and Chapter 33 (interpretation of cerebrospinal fluid abnormalities).

All of the contributors to this volume are well recognized for their expertise in the pathophysiology, diagnosis, and management of central nervous system infectious diseases. Their time and effort on behalf of this work are greatly appreciated. It is anticipated that this textbook will be invaluable to those in clinical practice.

Karen L. Roos

Contents

Contributors

Allen J. Aksamit, Jr., M.D. Consultant and Associate Professor, Department of Neurology, Mayo Clinic and Mayo Medical School, Rochester, Minnesota

James F. Bale, Jr., M.D. Professor, Departments of Pediatrics and Neurology, University of Iowa College of Medicine, Iowa City, Iowa

Anita L. Belman, M.D. Associate Professor, Departments of Neurology and Pediatrics, State University of New York at Stony Brook, Stony Brook, New York

Thomas P. Bleck, M.D. Louise Nerancy Professor of Neurology and Professor of Neurological Surgery and Medicine, Department of Neurology, University of Virginia School of Medicine, Charlottesville, Virginia

Joel C. Boaz, M.D. Clinical Assistant Professor of Surgery, Department of Pediatric Neurosurgery, Indiana University School of Medicine, Indianapolis, Indiana

Cherylee W. J. Chang, M.D. Fellow, Neuroscience Critical Care, University of Virginia School of Medicine, Charlottesville, Virginia

Laurent Christin, M.D. Fellow, Section of Infectious Diseases, Boston University Medical Center, Boston, Massachusetts

Patricia K. Coyle, M.D. Professor of Neurology and Director, MS Comprehensive Care Center, Department of Neurology, State University of New York at Stony Brook, Stony Brook, New York

Michael Frank, M.D. Clinical Assistant Professor, Department of Medicine, Division of Infectious Diseases, Indiana University School of Medicine, Indianapolis, Indiana

David P. Fritz, M.D. Department of Neurological Surgery, Indiana University School of Medicine, Indianapolis, Indiana

Bhuwan P. Garg, M.B. Professor, Department of Neurology, Section of Pediatric Neurology, Indiana University Medical Center, James Whitcomb Riley Hospital for Children, Indianapolis, Indiana

David A. Glander, M.D. Private Practice, Indianapolis, Indiana

E. Clarke Haley, Jr., M.D. Professor of Neurology and Neurosurgery, Department of Neurology, University of Virginia, Charlottesville, Virginia

Thiravat Hemachudha, M.D. Professor, Department of Medicine, Division of Neurology, Chulalongkorn University Hospital, Bangkok, Thailand

Steven W. Huder, M.D. Department of Neurology, Burns Clinic Medical Center, Petoskey, Michigan

Lauren B. Krupp, M.D. Associate Professor of Neurology, State University of New York at Stony Brook, Stony Brook, New York

Omkar N. Markand, M.D., F.R.C.P.(C) Professor of Neurology and Director of Clinical Neurophysiology, Department of Neurology, Indiana University School of Medicine, Indianapolis, Indiana

Christina M. Marra, M.D. Assistant Professor, Departments of Neurology and Medicine (Infectious Diseases), University of Washington, Seattle, Washington

George H. McCracken, Jr., M.D. Professor of Pediatrics, the Sarah M. and Charles M. Seay Chair in Pediatric Infectious Diseases, University of Texas Southwestern Medical Center, Dallas, Texas

Paul B. Nelson, M.D. Professor and Chairman of Neurosurgery, Indiana University School of Medicine, Indianapolis, Indiana

Robert M. Pascuzzi, M.D. Professor and Vice Chairman, Department of Neurology, Indiana University School of Medicine, Indianapolis, Indiana

Hema Patel, M.D. Assistant Professor of Neurology, Section of Pediatric Neurology, Indiana University Medical Center, James Whitcomb Riley Hospital for Children, Indianapolis, Indiana

Rahman Pourmand, M.D. Associate Professor of Neurology, Department of Neurology, Indiana University School of Medicine, Indianapolis, Indiana

Richard W. Price, M.D. Professor of Neurology, University of California, San Francisco, and Chief, Neurology Service, San Francisco General Hospital, San Francisco, California

Amy A. Pruitt, M.D. Assistant Professor, Department of Neurology, University of Pennsylvania Medical Center, Philadelphia, Pennsylvania

Karen L. Roos, M.D. Professor of Neurology, Department of Neurology, Indiana University School of Medicine, Indianapolis, Indiana

Raymond P. Roos, M.D. Professor, Department of Neurology, University of Chicago School of Medicine, Chicago, Illinois

Walter Royal III, M.D. Assistant Professor, Department of Neurology, Johns Hopkins University School of Medicine, Baltimore, Maryland

Shigeru Sato, M.D. Visiting Scientist, Department of Neurology, University of Chicago School of Medicine, Chicago, Illinois

Scott Shapiro, M.D., F.A.C.S. Associate Professor, Department of Neurosurgery, Indiana University School of Medicine, Indianapolis, Indiana

Richard R. Smith, M.D. Associate Professor of Radiology and Neurology, Department of Radiology, Indiana University School of Medicine, Indianapolis, Indiana

Nina J. Solenski, M.D. Assistant Professor, Department of Neurology, University of Virginia, Charlottesville, Virginia

Julio Sotelo, M.D. Director, Division of Research, National Institute of Neurology and Neurosurgery of Mexico, Mexico City, Mexico

Alan M. Sugar, M.D. Associate Professor, Department of Medicine, Boston University Medical Center, Boston, Massachusetts

Monica Trujillo, M.D. Fellow, Pediatric Infectious Diseases, Department of Pediatrics, University of Texas Southwestern Medical Center, Dallas, Texas

Kara K. Wools, M.D. Clinical Assistant Professor, Division of Infectious Diseases, Department of Medicine, Indiana University School of Medicine, Indianapolis, Indiana

1

Perinatal Viral Infections

James F. Bale, Jr.
University of Iowa College of Medicine, Iowa City, Iowa

INTRODUCTION

Women encounter many different viral pathogens during pregnancy, but the vast majority of these exposures occur innocuously and spare the fetus and the developing central nervous system (CNS). By contrast, certain infectious agents—notably rubella and cytomegalovirus (CMV)—can cross the placenta and potentially disrupt fetal CNS development, and other viruses—such as herpes simplex virus (HSV) type 2—can infect the infant in the perinatal period and may severely damage the CNS. These vertical infections constitute a distressing source of permanent visual, audiological, and neurological disability for thousands of children annually.

Infection with CMV illustrates the pathogenetic events that produce fetal damage during *congenital* (intrauterine) infection. Women who contract primary infection with CMV experience viremia of varying magnitude and duration, and this disseminates the virus to many maternal tissues, including the placenta. The virus infects placental cells and probably replicates there, as evidenced by detection of CMV antigens in the placentas of women who deliver CMV-infected infants (1). The virus next enters the fetal circulation, and fetal viremia distributes the virus to target cells of the reticuloendothelial and central nervous systems. CMV replication at these sites produces tissue dysfunction, usually transient in the case of the reticuloendothelial system, but often permanent when the brain, eye, and ear become infected.

Although the pathogenetic events of human fetal CNS infection have not been determined precisely, CMV apparently replicates in the subependymal-germinal matrix zone of the cerebrum and destroys neuronal cells when infection occurs prior to the twentieth week of gestation. Events other than direct viral replication in fetal neuronal cells, such as alterations in global or regional CNS perfusion, may also contribute to the pathogenesis of the CNS lesions identified in infants with congenital infections (2,3). The CNS lesions induced by CMV and other congenital infections can be classified as encephaloclastic (destructive) or developmental. Lesions of the former category include dystrophic calcifications, periventricular leukomalacia, cystic encephalomalacia, hydranencephaly, and porencephaly, whereas potential developmental abnormalities consist of lissencephaly, pachygyria, polymicrogyria, or delayed myelination (2).

During primary CMV infection the virus reaches the fetus in approximately 40% of the maternal infections, and only 5-10% of fetuses experience severe sequelae (4). The variables that influence the risk and severity of fetal infection are incompletely characterized for many viruses, including CMV, but critical factors include the immune responses of the mother, the timing of infection, and, conceivably, factors intrinsic to virus strains. For certain viruses, such as the rubella virus, the consequences of fetal infection relate directly to the timing of maternal infection, as discussed further below.

In contrast to these events, serious neonatal infections with certain viruses, such as HSV types 1 or 2, usually occur in the *perinatal* period. The infants of women with primary or reactivated genital herpes become colonized with HSV during passage through the infected cervix or vagina. The virus attaches to cells of the infant's skin or mucosal surfaces and replicates initially at the site of inoculation. If replication proceeds unabated, viremia ensues, disseminating the virus hematogenously to distant sites such as the CNS, lung, adrenals, or tissues of the reticuloendothelial system. Less frequently, intrauterine infection with HSV develops as the result of transplacental or ascending infection (5).

Upon reaching the CNS, HSV replicates in neuronal cells, inducing cell dysfunction, mononuclear cell infiltration, hemorrhagic necrosis, and tissue edema. Although viral replication represents the inciting and predominant pathogenetic event, host immune responses, such as cell-mediated immunity and cytokine secretion, contribute to the clinical and neuropathological features of perinatal infection with HSV and other viral pathogens (6).

Human immunodeficiency virus (HIV) type 1 can be transmitted vertically during gestation, at birth, or subsequently during breast feeding (7). Fetal or neonatal viremia, the critical event in the pathogenesis of CNS infection, can develop as a consequence of transplacental infection or perinatal acquisition of HIV via contact with infected maternal blood or secretions. Strategies for preventing vertical transmission of HIV thus involve treatment of the infected mother during gestation and delivery, treatment of the neonate during the first few weeks of life, and avoidance of breast feeding (7–9).

SPECIFIC AGENTS

Cytomegalovirus

In the United States and several other countries 0.4–2.5% of newborns excrete CMV in urine or saliva at birth, making CMV infection the most common congenital viral infection (10–12). Fortunately, the majority of these infected infants have no permanent sequelae attributable to CMV. The risk of severe fetal infection relates directly to the maternal antibody status prior to pregnancy (4). Infants born to seronegative women who experience primary CMV infections during their pregnancies have a 10–20% risk of hearing loss or mental retardation (4), whereas the infants of women who are seropositive prior to their pregnancies are protected from the potentially disabling consequences of congenital CMV infection.

CMV spreads by direct human contact, although the virus is not highly contagious. Children or adults infected with CMV typically exhibit few symptoms but commonly excrete the virus in their saliva, urine, semen, or cervical secretions. Primary replication of CMV eventually ceases, and the virus thereafter resides latently in host cells and reactivates periodically, especially during alterations of cell-mediated immunity. In immunocompetent persons, primary CMV infection occasionally produces a mononucleosislike illness with fatigue, adenopathy, hepatosplenomegaly, and fever (13), whereas recurrent infections are usually silent. By contrast immunocompromised persons, such as those with the acquired immunodeficiency syndrome (AIDS), frequently experience invasive disease with chorioretinitis, encephalitis, pneumonitis, or colitis during either primary or recurrent CMV infection (14).

Virus excretion can be prolonged, even in immunologically competent hosts. Studies at the University of Alabama–Birmingham, as an example, indicated that congenitally infected children commonly excrete CMV in urine for several years (15). Young children with silent congenital or acquired CMV infections thus represent a major reservoir of CMV and commonly infect their parents, adult caretakers, and other children (16,17).

Clinical Manifestations

Approximately 90% of the CMV-excreting newborns exhibit no signs of infection at birth. These children, although silently infected, have a 10–15% subsequent risk of sensorineural hearing loss and a smaller risk of other complications, such as microcephaly or chorioretinitis (4,18). Whether such children are also at risk for behavioral disorders or cognitive dysfunction has been intensely debated (12,18–20). Occasional infected neonates have subtle clinical signs, such as borderline microcephaly or mild intrauterine growth failure, and escape recognition in the perinatal period.

Infants overtly symptomatic at birth exhibit a spectrum of clinical features that includes intrauterine growth retardation, jaundice, hepatosplenomegaly, microcephaly, chorioretinitis, and petechial or purpuric rash (11,12,20) (Table 1). Laboratory features compatible with congenital CMV infection consist of thrombocytopenia, hemolytic anemia, direct hyperbilirubinemia, and elevations of serum transaminases (11,20).

Table 1 Neonatal Signs of Symptomatic Congenital CMV Infection

Clinical feature	Prevalence (%)
Somatic	
Petechiae/purpura	54
Small for gestational age	50
Hepatomegaly	46
Splenomegaly	44
Jaundice at birth	38
Death	10
Pneumonia	8
Neurological/Ophthalmological	
Microcephaly	45
Sensorineural hearing loss	33
Abnormal muscle tone	20
Retinal hemorrhage	13
Chorioretinitis	10
Other ocular abnormalities	10
Seizures	10

Percentages based on data from several studies and the National Congenital Cytomegalovirus Registry.
Source: Ref. 105.

Diagnosis

The diagnosis of congenital CMV infection is established best by detecting the virus in urine or saliva obtained during the first 3 weeks of life (12). Detection of CMV-specific IgM in a blood sample obtained in the neonatal period can also be used to confirm infection. Congenital infection can also be established by detecting CMV in amniotic fluid (21), although detection of infectious virus prenatally does not distinguish symptomatic from asymptomatic fetal infections.

Detecting infectious CMV in urine or saliva obtained later in infancy supports infection, but congenital infection cannot be distinguished unequivocally from infections acquired postnatally via breast feeding or through contact with infected playmates. However, detecting CMV in the urine of an infant with compatible clinical features (e.g., chorioretinitis, intracranial calcifications, or microcephaly) *and* negative studies for toxoplasmosis, rubella, varicella zoster virus, HSV, and rare pathogens (see discussion regarding lymphocytic choriomeningitis virus below) strongly support the diagnosis of congenital CMV infection.

Imaging studies of the CNS frequently reveal abnormalities in infants who exhibit symptoms as neonates. Calcifications can be detected in approximately 25–50% of the CMV-infected infants (Fig. 1), and white matter abnormalities (e.g., periventricular leukomalacia) are also common (11,22). Additional neuroradiographic features of congenital CMV infection include lissencephaly-pachygyria, subependymal cysts, intraparenchymal hemorrhage, and cerebellar hypoplasia (2). Calcifications or white matter lucencies can also be detected in occasional

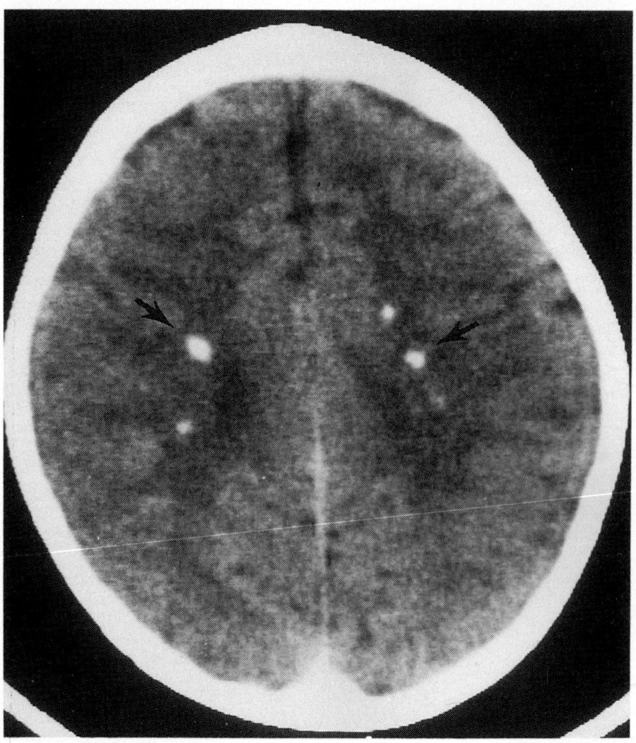

Figure 1 Congenital cytomegalovirus infection: unenhanced CT scans from three different children show intraparenchymal and periventricular calcifications (arrows) and white matter hypodensity (arrowheads) compatible with congenital cytomegalovirus infection.

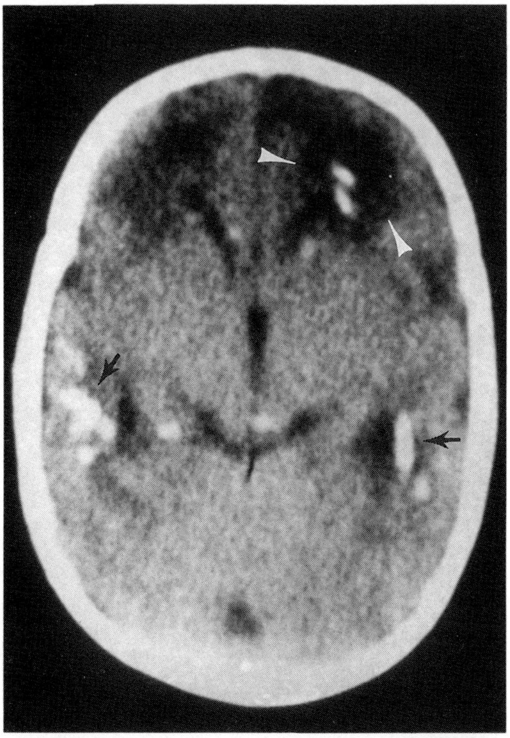

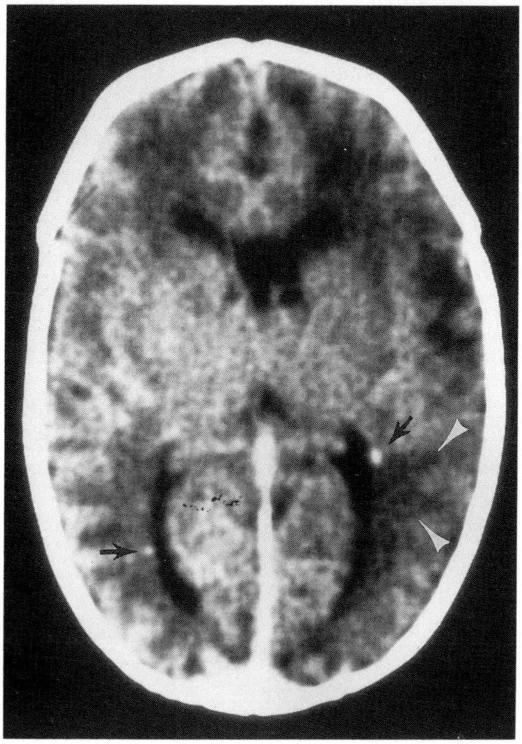

children who are asymptomatic at birth (18), indicating that the absence of systemic reticuloendothelial dysfunction at birth does not preclude the subsequent appearance of neurological sequelae.

Treatment and Prevention

Although vaccine trials have been conducted periodically, no whole virus or subunit vaccine is yet available to prevent congenital CMV infection (23). Certain hygienic measures may diminish the risk of maternal infection, although the ability of these strategies to prevent fetal infection has not been proven. Women can determine their risk of CMV infection *before* pregnancy by assaying their sera for CMV antibodies. If women are seropositive, the risk of contracting CMV and delivering affected infants is exceedingly small.

By contrast, seronegative women are susceptible to CMV. Such women should avoid contact while pregnant with the saliva or urine of young children, including their own, who may be infected silently with CMV. Susceptible women should wash their hands well after contact with urine or saliva and should refrain from kissing or sharing food or eating utensils with young children. Women who work in child care centers or have toddler-aged children who attend child care centers have a very high risk of becoming infected with CMV (16,17). CMV infection is also more likely in women who have multiple sexual partners.

Hospitalized CMV-infected infants require excretion-secretion precautions to prevent inadvertent transmission to seronegative pregnant women. However, many infants and young children excrete CMV asymptomatically, indicating that personnel should wash their hands well after contact with any young child. The risk of CMV infection among health care workers does not exceed that of the general population (24).

The National Institutes of Allergy and Infectious Diseases and the Collaborative Antiviral Study Group have been conducting a prospective, controlled clinical trial of postnatal ganciclovir therapy in symptomatic newborns with evidence of CNS disease or chorioretinitis. Whether postnatal therapy will improve the long-term outcome for CMV-infected infants is not known. Updated information regarding treatment protocols can be obtained from investigators at the University of Alabama–Birmingham.

Infants who survive symptomatic congenital CMV infections have a substantial risk (~ 90%) of having one or more disabling sequelae (Table 2). Predicting accurately the outcome for a symptomatic infant is difficult, and the spectrum ranges from the child who makes little or no developmental progress to one who exhibits only mild cognitive or behavioral deficits (25). Because congenitally infected infants can experience progressive sensorineural hearing loss,

Table 2 Sequelae of Congenital CMV Infection

	Prevalence (%)	
Feature	Symptomatic at birth	Asymptomatic at birth
Sensorineural hearing loss	45	15
Mental retardation	55	Rare
Microcephaly	50	Rare
Visual impairment	59	Rare
Cerebral palsy	41	Rare
Seizures	30	Rare
Developmental concern	80	Up to 34

Source: Ref. 105.

serial audiograms should be obtained biannually for the first 2 years of life and annually thereafter into childhood.

Rubella Virus

The epidemiology of congenital rubella syndrome (CRS), the potential consequence of maternal rubella (German measles), has changed considerably since the disorder was described by Gregg in 1941 (26). In the prevaccine era, epidemics of rubella appeared at 6- to 9-year intervals (27), and the 1964-1965 epidemic in the United States poignantly illustrated the potentially devastating impact of the CRS (28). During the latter epidemic thousands of infants were stillborn or suffered persistent developmental, visual, audiological, and cardiac defects as the result of maternal rubella virus infection (28,29).

After licensure of the rubella vaccine in 1969 and aggressive immunization programs targeting adolescents and adults in the 1980s, the incidence of postnatal rubella and CRS in the United States and other nations with compulsory rubella immunization declined dramatically (30). In the United States, for example, as few as one to three cases of CRS were reported to the Centers for Disease Control (CDC) annually during the mid- to late 1980s, an incidence of <0.1 case of CRS per 100,000 live births. However, in the early 1990s the CDC received reports of 56 cases, corresponding to an incidence of 0.6–0.8 per 100,000 live births (31–35). The reemergence of CRS in the United States reflected rubella outbreaks among unimmunized persons in California, New York, and Pennsylvania as well as sporadic cases in several other locations. As many as 19–20% of adolescents or young adults in some regions of the United States are seronegative for the rubella virus, indicating that the CRS remains a potential threat to the offspring of many women (31,34,35).

Rubella virus infection of children and adults causes a mild syndrome with rash, upper respiratory symptoms, and adenopathy, especially of the occipital and posterior cervical nodes (36). The virus spreads via infected droplets, invades the host through the respiratory mucosa, replicates locally, and disseminates hematogenously. Rash—erythematous, maculopapular—begins 2 weeks after exposure, involving first the face and then the trunk and extremities, and typically lasts fewer than 3 days. Potential complications of acquired rubella include arthropathy, thrombocytopenia, and encephalitis.

Clinical Manifestations

The original report of Gregg linked maternal rubella virus infection to cataracts, hearing loss, and heart disease in young infants (26). Later reports, especially those describing infants infected during the pandemic of the early 1960s, expanded considerably the clinical spectrum of the CRS (28–30). Like several viruses described in this chapter, rubella virus preferentially infects the retina, cochlea, CNS, and reticuloendothelial system. Thus, the neonate with CRS has a spectrum of abnormalities that includes cataracts, retinopathy, microphthalmia, microcephaly, or sensorineural hearing loss, as well as meningoencephalitis, osteopathy, pneumonitis, hepatitis, hepatosplenomegaly, thrombocytopenia, and jaundice. A unique feature of rubella virus, the propensity to infect the heart, produces myocarditis or structural cardiac defects consisting of patent ductus arteriosus, valvular stenosis, or septal defects at the atrial or ventricular level (29).

The fetal consequences of rubella in nonimmune pregnant women relate directly to the timing of infection (28,38,39). Maternal rubella during the initial 8 weeks produces cataracts and congenital heart lesions, and hearing loss correlates with infection during the first 16 weeks (Table 3). Stillbirth or spontaneous abortion can also occur during this time. By contrast, infections after the sixteenth week of gestation typically leave no sequelae, although silently infected infants remain at risk of developing sensorineural hearing loss.

Table 3 Relationship of Gestational Age and the Risk of Congenital Rubella Syndrome

Gestational age at time of maternal infection (weeks)	Incidence of congenital rubella syndrome (%)
<11	100
11–12	50
13–14	17
15–16	50 (hearing loss only)
>17	Negligible

Source: Adapted from Ref. 39.

A review of patients who survived CRS and were evaluated in a single department of ophthalmology provided a relevant perspective regarding the spectrum of sequelae (37). Of 125 patients ranging in age from 1 to 65 years at the time of their last examination, 66, 58, and 42% had sensorineural deafness, cardiac lesions, and mental retardation, respectively. Microcephaly was noted in 42% of the patients, and 18% were labeled hyperactive. Endocrine disorders, consisting of diabetes mellitus or thyroid dysfunction, affected 4–6%.

Diagnosis

The diagnosis of CRS can be confirmed by detecting infectious virus in body fluids (nasal secretions, urine, or CSF) or rubella virus–specific IgM in the infant's serum (40). Postnatal persistence of rubella-specific IgG supports the diagnosis of CRS. Imaging studies of the brain may reveal periventricular calcifications, subependymal cysts, or periventricular leukomalacia (41).

Prevention and Treatment

Because CRS cannot be treated effectively by postnatal antiviral therapy, prevention of maternal infection by vaccination is essential. Serological screening of women can determine the risk of fetal infection and should be performed prior to pregnancy and in pregnant women exposed to rubella (42). The presence of maternal antibody prior to conception or at the time of exposure during pregnancy indicates that the fetus is not at risk.

The Committee on Infectious Diseases of the American Academy of Pediatrics recommends that serological studies in women who are exposed to rubella and initially seronegative be repeated in 3–4 weeks and repeated again 6 weeks after exposure if the second sample was also negative (42). Seroconversion indicates infection and potential risk to the fetus, whereas persistently seronegative samples indicates that maternal infection did not occur. Termination of pregnancy is a consideration for women who have confirmed primary infections early in gestation. When termination is not an option, immune globulin can be considered, although the efficacy of this approach is unproved (42).

The management of an infant with suspected CRS should include (1) an ophthalmologic examination for cataracts or pigmentary retinopathy, (2) audiometry to detect sensorineural hearing loss, and (3) an evaluation for cardiac lesions. Infants with suspected rubella require isolation (private room; masks, gowns, and gloves for persons having patient contact), and infants with confirmed infections should be considered contagious for at least 12 months. Nonimmune pregnant women must not have contact with infants with CRS.

Progressive sensorineural hearing loss can develop in children who survive CRS, indicating the need for serial audiometry, and children with CRS also have an increased risk of growth failure or diabetes mellitus beginning in the second or third decades (43–45). Neurological sequelae, common among infants with CRS, include microcephaly, language delay, autistic features, and developmental or mental retardation (30,38–40). Postrubella panencephalitis, a progressive disorder associated with seizures, ataxia, and dementia, is a rare, potential complication of CRS (46).

Herpes Simplex Virus

Herpes simplex virus types 1 and 2, important potential causes of neonatal morbidity and mortality, affect 1500–2000 infants annually (5). HSV type 2 (HSV-2) causes approximately two thirds of neonatal infections, whereas the remainder are the result of HSV type 1 (HSV-1). Millions of persons in the United States and other regions of the world harbor HSV latently, and many thousands acquire primary HSV-1 or HSV-2 infections annually (47). Although HSV-1 usually causes oral lesions and HSV-2 typically produces genital lesions, either virus type can be found at either site (47).

When primary HSV-2 infection occurs during gestation, pregnant women have an increased risk of spontaneous abortion, stillbirth, or premature labor (5). Women can shed HSV-2 in the cervix asymptomatically after primary or recurrent (reactivated) infections, potentially exposing infants to the virus during passage through infected birth canals. Neonates can acquire HSV-1 during delivery by contact with infected cervical secretions or postnatally by contact with persons with active oral HSV-1 infections (47–50).

Clinical Manifestations

Neonatal HSV infections can be categorized according to three clinical syndromes: (1) mucocutaneous (skin-eye-mouth), (2) disseminated, or (3) encephalitic (48,49). Infants with either mucocutaneous or disseminated infections tend to present at approximately 10 days of age, whereas infants with encephalitis are usually older, averaging 17 days of age (48). However, the symptoms or signs of perinatal HSV infection can develop as early as the first day of life (49).

The early symptoms of HSV infection—poor feeding, irritability, lethargy, or high-pitched cry—are relatively nonspecific and mimic features of enteroviral or bacterial disease (48–51). Systemic signs consist of fever, jaundice, tachypnea, petechiae, or vesicular rash, although the absence of rash or fever does not eliminate HSV from consideration (51). Neurological complications, such as seizures (partial or generalized), hypotonia, hypertonia, or diminished alertness, can be early or late manifestations of HSV disease. HSV-infected infants may also have hepatitis, pneumonitis, adrenalitis, or disseminated intravascular coagulopathy (DIC) (48–52).

Approximately 5% of HSV-infected neonates have acquired the virus, typically HSV-2, as the result of intrauterine infection (5,53,54). These infants, manifesting chorioretinitis, skin lesions at birth, microphthalmia, and microcephaly or hydranencephaly, closely resemble neonates with other congenital infections, especially the fetal varicella syndrome (54). Neuroimaging studies in such infants usually reveal intracranial calcifications and abnormalities of brain parenchyma (Fig. 2).

Diagnosis

Neonatal herpes can be confirmed by isolating HSV-1 or HSV-2 from mucosal surfaces, skin, CSF, or tissues. Infants with suspected HSV infection should be cultured at multiple sites, including the conjunctiva, throat, rectum, circulating leukocytes, CSF, and skin lesions, when present. HSV types 1 and 2 grow rapidly, usually enabling a specific diagnosis within 72–96 h. HSV can be detected in CSF in approximately 50% of the cases of neonatal HSV encephalitis.

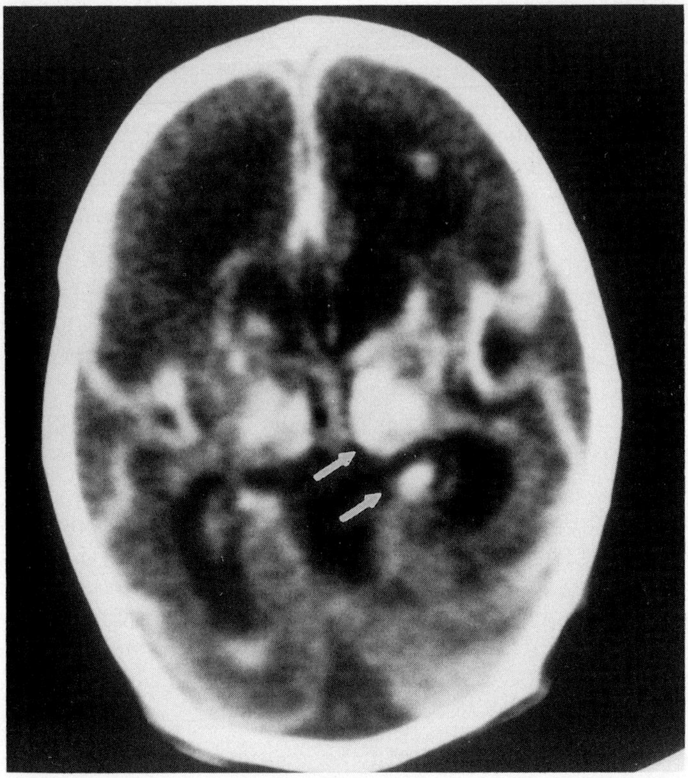

Figure 2 Congenital HSV infection: unenhanced CT shows diffuse encephalomalacia, poorly developed gyri, and periventricular and thalamic calcifications (arrows) in an infant with congenital HSV infection. (From Ref. 54.)

Negative culture results, however, must be interpreted cautiously, since neonates with invasive HSV infections can have negative surface and CSF cultures. The diagnosis of HSV infection can also be established by using the polymerase chain reaction (PCR) (55), as discussed further below.

Infants may also manifest thrombocytopenia, hemolytic anemia, elevated serum transaminases, metabolic acidosis, or CSF abnormalities consisting of a mixed pleocytosis, xanthochromia, modest hypoglycorrachia, and an elevated protein content. Chest radiographs may reveal pneumonitis (52). Because neonatal herpes encephalitis results from hematogenous dissemination of the virus to the brain, neurodiagnostic studies (EEG, CT, or MRI) in affected infants usually reveal diffuse or multifocal abnormalities as opposed to the expected temporal lobe features of postnatal HSV encephalitis (56).

Treatment and Prevention

In two large case series regarding perinatal herpes (48,49), only modest numbers (20–30%) of the mothers reported genital HSV during their pregnancies, and the majority (>75%) of women lacked clinical signs of cervical HSV during labor and delivery. Moreover, neonates have experienced infection after cesarean section in women who had genital herpes and intact amniotic membranes. These observations indicate that preventing neonatal HSV infection remains problematic.

Infants with suspected HSV infection must be managed aggressively and should receive acyclovir at a dosage of 30 mg/kg/day given in evenly divided doses every 8 h (57–59). Therapy should be continued for a minimum of 10 days, and infants with confirmed infections may require up to 21 days of therapy. Complete blood counts, blood urea nitrogen, and serum creatinine should be monitored during therapy with acyclovir since myelosuppression and nephrotoxicity are the major potential side effects.

The prognosis of neonatal HSV infection depends on the extent of organ involvement and the success of antiviral therapy (58). Infants who are recognized early and treated aggressively with acyclovir fare better than infants for whom therapy is delayed. Few treated infants with disease restricted to the skin, eyes, and mucous membranes have adverse sequelae (58). By contrast, infants with CNS or disseminated disease have high rates of mortality and morbidity, and infants with congenital HSV infection uniformly have grim prognoses (53). Mortality in untreated neonatal herpes exceeds 60% (47).

Varicella Zoster Virus

Varicella zoster virus (VZV), the etiological agent of chickenpox (varicella) and shingles (zoster), occasionally causes disease in neonates as a consequence of perinatal or intrauterine transmission (54). Varicella can develop in infants born to mothers who experience varicella peripartum or in nonimmune infants exposed to persons with active chickenpox. Women who experience varicella during pregnancy, especially the first or second trimester, have a 2% risk of delivering an infant with the fetal varicella syndrome (60–63).

Chickenpox in immunocompetent children is usually a mild viral illness with rash, fever, and malaise. The rash, evolving from maculopapular to vesicular, begins on the head or trunk and spreads centrifugally. Potential complications of chickenpox in normal hosts include acute cerebellar ataxia, encephalitis, Reye syndrome, and secondary bacterial infections (64). Severe, potentially fatal varicella, complicated by pneumonitis, hepatitis, coagulopathy, or CNS involvement, can develop in immunocompetent hosts, but persons with immunocompromising conditions, especially AIDS, have an increased potential for severe, fatal varicella (65).

Clinical Manifestations

Although chickenpox is usually a mild illness, the neonate can experience severe, disseminated varicella with pneumonitis, hepatitis, and DIC (60,66). The risk of severe varicella infection is substantial in infants whose mothers have the onset of chickenpox between 5 days before and 2 days after delivery, and neonatal fatalities have occurred after perinatal vertical transmission, particularly in preterm infants. By contrast, term infants exposed postnatally usually have relatively benign illnesses, although such infants must be monitored closely.

Congenitally infected infants with the fetal varicella syndrome exhibit characteristic clinical features (Table 4) that indicate damage to the skin, eye, brain, and spinal cord (54,61,63,67). Manifestations include cicatricial skin lesions, chorioretinitis, microphthalmia, cataracts, limb paralysis, microcephaly, hydrocephalus, congenital Horner syndrome, and limb hypoplasia (54,67). The skin lesion, a pathognomonic feature of congenital varicella infection, consists of scarring and new skin formation (cicatrix) that correspond to a dermatomal distribution. Imaging studies of the CNS may reveal hydranencephaly or cystic encephalomalacia reminiscent of congenital HSV infection. These clinical features reflect the propensity of VZV to infect fetal neuronal tissues (54).

Diagnosis

The clinical features of postnatal varicella or the fetal varicella syndrome are sufficiently characteristic to suggest VZV infection. Infection can be confirmed by detecting VZV-specific

Table 4 Clinical Manifestation of Congenital Varicella Syndrome

Damage to sensory nerves	Damage to the brain (meningoencephalitis)
Cutaneous manifestions	Microcephaly
Zig-zag (cicatricial) skin lesions	Hydrocephalus
Hypopigmentation	Intracranial calcifications
Damage to optic stalk, optic cup, or lens vesicle	Hydranencephaly
Microphthalmia	Damage to the spinal cord
Cataracts	Limb hypoplasia
Chorioretinitis	Motor/sensory deficits
Optic atrophy	Horner syndrome
	Abnormal muscle stretch reflexes
	Anal/vesical sphincter dysfunction

Source: Ref. 54.

IgM in the serum of the fetus or infant (68), VZV antigens or infectious virus in skin lesions, or VZV DNA in amniotic fluid, CSF, or skin lesions (54,61,66,70). Persistence of VZV-specific IgG in the infant's serum postnatally supports congenital varicella infection.

Prevention and Treatment

Although the efficacy of varicella-zoster immune globulin (VZIG) is not absolute, VZIG should be considered for the exposed neonate. According to the 1994 recommendations of the Committee on Infectious Diseases, The American Academy of Pediatrics, VZIG (125 U) should be given as soon as possible to the neonate, term or preterm, whose mother develops chickenpox during the 5 days before or 2 days after delivery of the infant (42). Varicella can develop despite VZIG, although the illness is frequently mild (42,66). Term infants exposed outside the above interval do not require VZIG.

VZIG should also be administered after postnatal VZV exposure to hospitalized preterm infants born before 28 weeks of gestation and/or weighing $\leq$1000 g at birth and hospitalized, more mature preterm infants with negative maternal varicella histories. Screening for VZV antibodies in the infant's serum can determine the risk status of exposed infants (69).

Therapy with acyclovir should be considered for infants in whom chickenpox develops, using 30 mg/kg/day intravenously in divided doses every 8 h (60,66). Therapy should be continued for 7–14 days, during which renal function and hematological parameters should be monitored. Hospitalized infants with varicella should be maintained in strict isolation. Exposed, asymptomatic infants should be discharged, when possible, or cohorted and maintained in strict isolation for 21–28 days (42).

In contrast to the potentially beneficial effects of VZIG or acyclovir for VZV-exposed or infected neonates, infants with the congenital varicella syndrome cannot be treated effectively (54). Fortunately, the risk of symptomatic fetal infection averages 2% or less for pregnant women with varicella, with the risk highest between the thirteenth to twentieth weeks of gestation (61,62). Symptomatic infants who survive uniformly have permanent sequelae affecting visual, motor, or cognitive development (54,67). Infants with congenital varicella syndrome do not require isolation (42).

A varicella vaccine has been developed and licensed recently for use in the United States. This suggests that immunization may prevent cases of congenital varicella. In contrast to the potentially damaging effect of primary VZV infection in pregnant women, reactivated VZV infections (i.e., zoster) appear to pose no risk to the developing fetus (61).

Nonpolio Enteroviruses

Postnatal infections with the nonpolio enteroviruses, a group of more than 60 viral pathogens, cause a diverse spectrum of systemic and neurological disease among humans worldwide. Systemic manifestations can include gastroenteritis, pharyngitis, pneumonia, myocarditis, hepatitis, and febrile illnesses associated with skin rash or oral lesions, whereas potential neurological disorders consist of aseptic meningitis, encephalitis, and strokelike or poliolike paralytic illnesses (71).

Enteroviruses, maintained only in human reservoirs, colonize the upper respiratory and gastrointestinal tracts and spread by direct human contact with infected secretions (71). Infected persons shed enteroviruses for extended periods in oral secretions and feces. The enteroviruses characteristically exhibit seasonal outbreaks (from June to early November in the Northern Hemisphere) suggesting that environmental factors facilitate viral transmission (71). Neonates acquire enterovirus infection vertically from mothers during or after delivery or horizontally from contact with infected persons other than the mother.

Clinical Manifestations

Neonates infected perinatally with the nonpolio enteroviruses usually become symptomatic after the fourth day of life (72–75). The illness begins nonspecifically with fever, poor feeding, jaundice, irritability or lethargy, and thus mimics the early features of bacterial or HSV infections. Although neonatal illnesses with nonpolio enteroviruses can be mild, infected infants may have severe, invasive disease with meningoencephalitis (manifesting as seizures and coma), hepatitis (manifesting as progressive jaundice and hepatic failure), myocarditis (manifesting as shock or congestive heart failure), and disseminated intravascular coagulopathy.

Direct hyperbilirubinemia, metabolic acidosis, thrombocytopenia, and elevated serum transaminases are amoung the potential laboratory correlates of severe disease. The diagnosis of perinatal enteroviral infections can be confirmed by isolating infectious virus from CSF, tissues, or throat or rectal swabs. Enteroviral RNA can be detected by assaying CSF or stool samples by reverse transcription PCR (76).

Treatment and Prevention

At present, neonatal enterovirus infections cannot be prevented by vaccination or treated effectively with specific antiviral chemotherapy. Some horizontally transmitted neonatal enteroviral infections could be prevented, in theory, by discouraging contact postnatally between young infants and persons with viral syndromes, especially during the summer months. Often, however, transmission occurs vertically as a result of maternal infection during the week prior to delivery or horizontally through contact with asymptomatic persons and thus cannot be avoided. Outbreaks amoung hospitalized newborns and hospital personnel emphasize that staff must practice meticulous hygiene (75).

Infants with severe nonpolio enterovirus infections pose complex diagnostic and therapeutic dilemmas since such infants can be difficult to distinguish from those with disseminated HSV or bacterial infections. Consequently, such neonates require comprehensive microbiological evaluations (cultures of blood, urine, and CSF for bacteria, and CSF and swabs of the throat, conjunctivae, and rectum for HSV as well as enteroviruses). Empiric therapy with acyclovir (see discussion regarding HSV) and broad-spectrum antibiotics (e.g., cefotaxime, ampicillin, and an aminoglycoside) is frequently necessary.

Infants with perinatal enterovirus infections require meticulous attention to their fluid and electrolyte status and must be monitored closely for arrhythmias or signs of congestive heart failure. Seizures require therapy with phenobarbital or phenytoin, using standard doses, and severe DIC necessitate transfusions of platelets, fresh frozen plasma, or other blood products. In severe cases, especially those involving echovirus 11, death can result from DIC, hemorrhage, and hepatic failure. Infants who survive perinatal enteroviral infections usually have no long-term neurological sequelae (77,78).

Human Immunodeficiency Virus

Thousands of infants and children worldwide acquire HIV through vertical transmission from infected mothers (7). Although the vast majority of HIV-infected infants do not become symptomatic during the neonatal period, occasional neonates have signs, e.g., hepatosplenomegaly, lymphadenopathy, or meningoencephalitis, that may be attributable to HIV (7,79–81,83). HIV-infected children can present in infancy with opportunistic infections (e.g., CMV, *Pneumocystis carinii*) or with disease caused by co-existing, congenitally acquired pathogens (e.g., syphilis, toxoplasmosis).

Serological studies—enzyme-linked immunosorbent assay and Western blot—can confirm HIV infection in older children and adults. Passive transfer of maternal antibody, however, complicates serodiagnosis in the neonate, indicating that clinicians must employ other methods such as HIV culture, in vitro antibody production, or HIV nucleic acid detection by PCR or similar techniques (7,82,83).

Avoiding maternal infection remains the most effective means to prevent vertical transmission. In HIV-seropositive mothers, the risk of transmitting the virus to the infant averages approximately 30% (7), and transmission can occur in utero, perinatally during delivery, or postnatally via breast feeding. Recent studies indicate that the risk of transmission can be reduced considerably by a combination of prenatal, perinatal, and postnatal therapy with zidovudine (8,9). Currently, women known to be HIV-infected, whether symptomatic or not, should receive zidovudine orally during pregnancy (100 mg five times daily) and intravenously during delivery (2 mg/kg over 1 h, followed by 1 mg/kg/h until delivery). The infant should then receive zidovudine 2 mg/kg orally every 6 h for 6 weeks. This strategy reduced the proportion of infants infected with HIV from 25.5% to 8.3% (9). Breast feeding by HIV-infected women should be avoided, when possible.

Other Viruses

Reports from Europe and the United States indicate that lymphocytic choriomeningitis virus (LCMV), a rodent-borne arenavirus, occasionally causes congenital infection in humans (84,85). Humans acquire LCMV via contact with the stool or urine of infected mice or hamsters. The pathogenesis of human congenital infection has not been determined precisely, although the clinical features suggest fetal infection during midgestation. Infected infants have chorioretinitis and microcephaly or hydrocephalus (Fig. 3) but lack other teratogenic features. The diagnosis can be established by detecting LCMV-specific IgG or IgM in serum obtained in the neonatal period.

Arthropod-borne viruses can cross the placenta during maternal infections and cause fetal or neonatal meningoencephalitis, albeit rarely. Maternal infections with Venezuelan equine encephalitis virus, a South American alphavirus, potentially induce severe encephaloclastic disorders in the fetus, causing hydranencephaly or cystic encephalomalacia (86). Perinatal infections with Western equine encephalitis virus, a North American alphavirus, occasionally produce neonatal meningoencephalitis with fever, irritability, lethargy, bulging fontanelle, or seizures (87).

Adenoviruses occasionally infect the neonate and produce fever, lethargy, hepatosplenomegaly, or coagulopathy (88). Adenoviral infections thus resemble disseminated neonatal infections caused by other viral pathogens, particularly HSV types 1 or 2 or the enteroviruses. The diagnosis can be established by detecting adenoviral antigens in respiratory secretions or infectious virus in urine. Human parvovirus B19, the cause of erythema infectiosum (fifth disease), can infect the fetus and induce red blood cell aplasia, anemia, and cardiac failure (89,90). Severe infections are associated with hydrops fetalis, potentially leading to cerebral hypoperfusion and CNS sequelae. Infection can be determined by detecting parvovirus B19 antigen, DNA, or antiparvovirus B19 IgM in serum (90).

Conditions That Mimic Congenital Viral Infections

Several nonviral and noninfectious disorders (Table 5) produce clinical features that resemble those of the viral infections described above (91). Certain infectious conditions, such as congenital syphilis and toxoplasmosis (92), must be identified and treated appropriately. Furthermore, the clinical features of viral and bacterial sepsis (lethargy, tachypnea, poor feeding, DIC, etc.) often overlap, indicating that certain infants may require empirical therapy with both antiviral and antibacterial agents until culture results become available. Aicardi's syndrome, Warburg syndrome, incontinentia pigmenti, neonatal Graves' disease, and peroxisomal disorders are among the many noninfectious disorders that may be confused with an intrauterine infection (91,93–97).

DIAGNOSIS AND PROGNOSIS

Virological and Serological Studies

The conventional microbiological studies for detecting viral pathogens consist of culture, histological techniques, and serological methods (70,98). Culture provides *direct* evidence of infection by detecting pathogens in body fluids, whereas serological studies provide *indirect* evidence by detecting the presence of antibodies in serum or CSF. Culture diagnosis relies on the clinician's ability to obtain appropriate samples for virus isolation and to ensure proper transport of specimens to the clinical laboratory (98,99). Histologic methods (e.g., Tzanc preparation) also provide direct evidence of infection, although their sensitivity is considerably less than that of culture methods. Serodiagnosis, although useful in many cases, can be confounded by false-negative serological results or complicated by passive transfer of maternal immunoglobulin (Ig) G antibodies. Detecting virus-specific IgM in the infant's serum strongly supports intrauterine or perinatal infection.

The infant's clinical features often allow the clinician to narrow the differential diagnosis and increase the yield of virological investigations (Table 6). When the viral pathogen is unknown, as is frequently the case, infants must undergo a comprehensive evaluation that will consist of serological studies and virological studies. The latter should include cultures of CSF for HSV, rubella, and enteroviruses, urine for CMV and rubella, throat swab for HSV, CMV, rubella, and enteroviruses, rectal swab for enteroviruses and HSV, skin swab (of vesicular lesions) for HSV and VZV, and blood (circulating leukocytes) for CMV, HSV, and, as appropriate, HIV.

Serological studies should include serum samples from the infant for agent-specific IgG and IgM, and concurrent serological studies of the mother may also be useful, especially when HIV is suspected. The diagnosis of certain viral infections, such as lymphocytic choriomeningitis virus, can only be established serologically. TORCH titers alone, however, should *never* be considered a comprehensive evaluation of the infant with a suspected congenital or perinatal infection (100).

Molecular methods enable sensitive and specific detection of virus-specific DNA, RNA, or protein (55,70,76,90,98,101–103). The polymerase chain reaction (PCR), as an example, utilizes heat-stable DNA polymerase and synthetic oligonucleotide fragments ("primers") to recreate multiple copies of viral DNA that can be detected and quantified, if necessary. RNA-containing viruses can be detected, as well, by synthesizing a DNA intermediary (cDNA) by using reverse transcriptase. Because of the remarkable sensitivity of methods such as PCR, however, false-positive results can occur, necessitating meticulous handling of specimens and reagents.

(A)

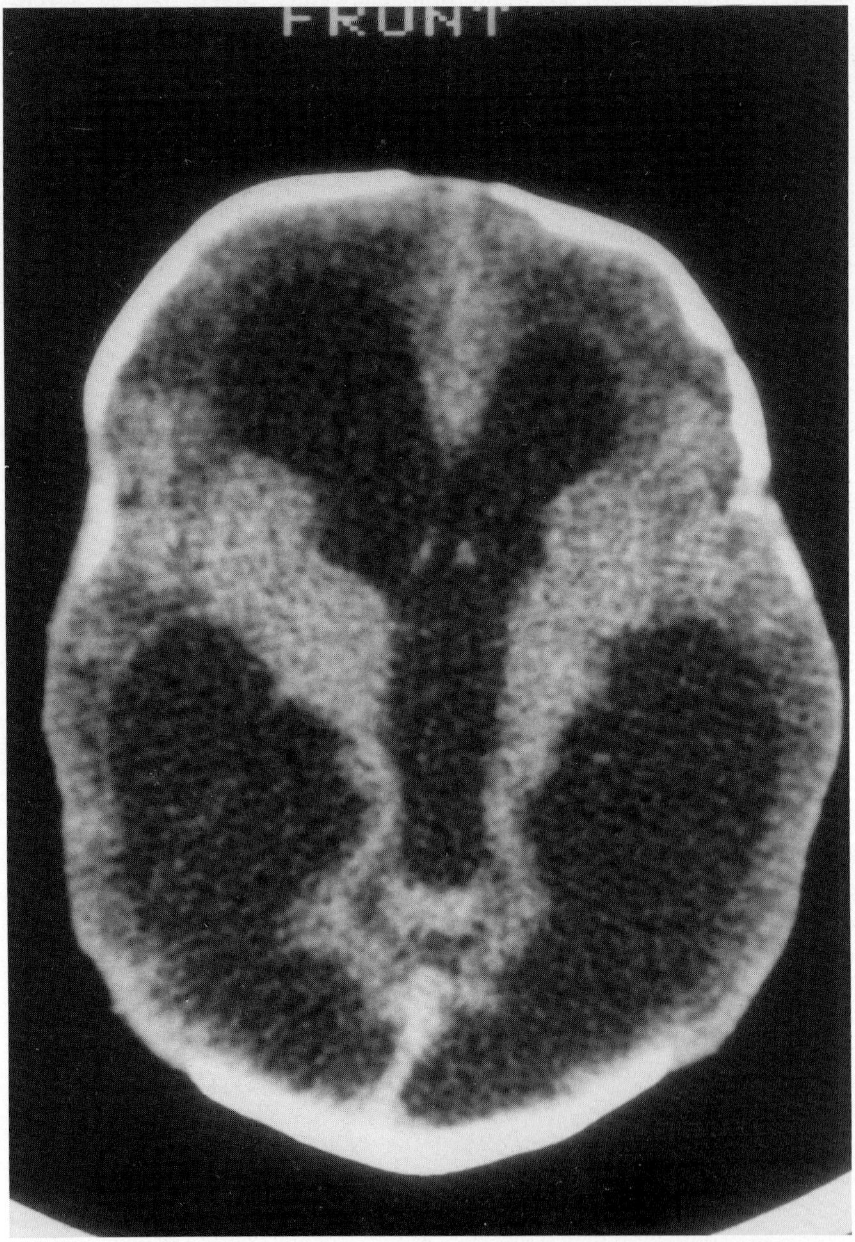

Figure 3 Congenital lymphocytic choriomeningitis virus infection. (A) Unenhanced CT obtained at birth shows markedly enlarged third and lateral ventricles compatible with aqueductal obstruction. (B) Unenhanced CT obtained 8 months after placement of a ventriculoperitoneal shunt shows reduction in the size of the lateral ventricles. Serological studies in the neonatal period revealed marked elevation in LCMV-specific IgG.

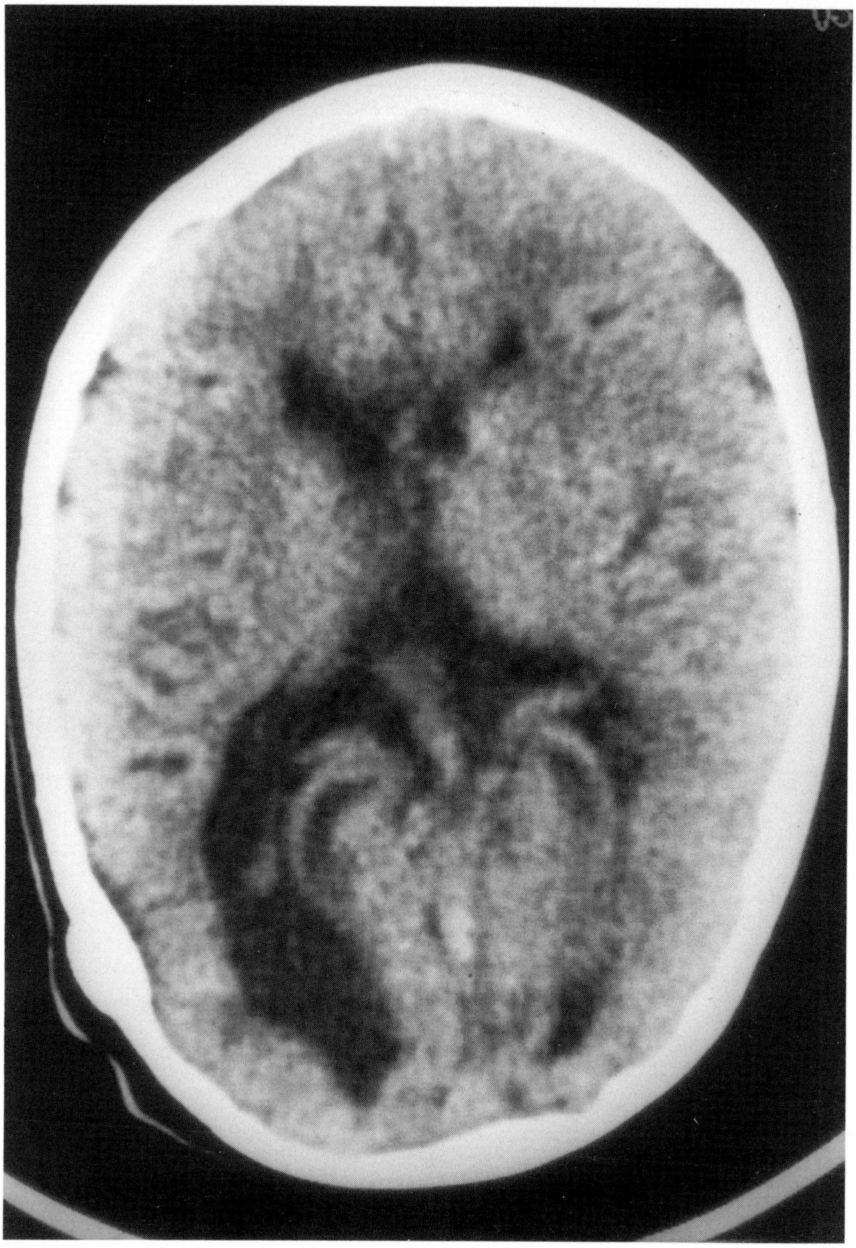

(B)

Table 5 Selected Conditions That Mimic the Clinical Features of Congenital Viral Infections

Infectious diseases	Metabolic conditions
Congenital toxoplasmosis	Neonatal Graves' disease
Congenital syphilis	α_1-antitrypsin deficiency
Neonatal malaria	Galactosemia
Congenital infection with *Trypanosoma cruzi*	Peroxisomal disorders
Genetic disorders	Urea cycle disorders
Aicardi syndrome	Organic acidemias
Warburg syndrome	Drugs or toxins
Lissencephaly syndromes	Fetal isoretinoin syndrome
Tuberous sclerosis	Fetal alcohol syndrome
Incontinentia pigmenti	Fetal cocaine exposure
	Disorders of obscure pathogenesis
	Fetal brain disruption sequence
	NEOMID syndrome

Source: Adapted from Ref. 91.

Neurodiagnostic Studies

Infants with suspected perinatal or congenital infections require an extensive neurodiagnostic evaluation that may include a CSF examination, neuroimaging study, electroencephalogram, and audiogram (104). Because calcifications, a marker for congenital infections, frequently elude detection by MRI, CT is the preferred imaging study in infancy. Infants should also be evaluated by an ophthalmologist since many of the preceding infections have relatively characteristic ophthalmological features. Brain-stem auditory evoked responses may be required to determine precisely the infant's hearing capability.

The CSF may be normal or reveal a mixed pleocytosis and an altered protein or glucose content. The marked variation in the ranges of normal CSF values for preterm and term infants makes interpretation of the CSF difficult in many instances. Neuroimaging studies may reveal a variety of CNS lesions that depend on the offending viral pathogen and the timing of infection (2,10,56). These can include periventricular calcifications (CMV, HSV, VZV, rubella), periventricular leukomalacia (CMV, rubella), hydranencephaly [HSV, VZV, CMV, Venezuelan equine encephalitis virus (VEEV)], lissencephaly-pachygyria (CMV), cystic encephalomalacia (CMV, HSV, VZV, VEEV), basal ganglia and frontal white matter calcifications (HIV), atrophy (many agents), and ex vacuo or obstructive hydrocephalus (CMV, VZV, HSV, lymphocytic choriomeningitis virus).

Prognosis

The prognosis of perinatal viral infections depends on several variables, including the viral agent, maternal immunity, the timing of infection, and the availability of specific antiviral chemotherapy. Mortality rates range from <1% (mucocutaneous HSV infection) to >50% (disseminated HSV infection) or even 100%, if the current outlook for a symptomatic HIV-infected infant is considered. Morbidity varies also, from the 10-15% risk of sensorineural hearing loss in infants with "silent" congenital CMV infections to the 100% risk of disabling sequelae in infants with congenital HSV infection (Table 7).

In general, infants who survive perinatal or congenital viral infections have a substantial risk of cognitive, motor, behavioral, visual, and audiologic sequelae. Thus, these infants should

Table 6 Diagnosis of Perinatal Viral Infections

Pathogen	Clinical features	Microbiological diagnosis
Cytomegalovirus	Hepatosplenomegaly, jaundice, petechiae, microcephaly, chorioretinitis	Culture of urine, saliva; serum for CMV-IgM; PCR of urine, saliva
Rubella	Cataracts, heart disease, microcephaly, retinopathy	Culture of urine, CSF; serum for rubella-IgM
HSV—perinatal	Skin rash, jaundice, hepatomegaly, lethargy, seizures, DIC, fever	Culture of CSF, skin lesions, throat and rectal swabs; PCR of CSF
HSV—congenital	Skin lesions, microcephaly, cataracts	Culture of skin lesions; PCR of CSF
VZV—perinatal	Skin rash, fever, lethargy, DIC, hepatomegaly	Culture of skin lesions; PCR of skin vesicle fluid
VZV—congenital	Cicatricial scars, limb hypoplasia, microcephaly, hydrocephalus, cataracts	Detection of VZV-IgM; postnatal persistence of VZV-IgG
HIV	Hepatosplenomegaly, lymphadenopathy, opportunistic infections	Culture of leukocytes; PCR of leukocytes; in vitro antibody production
Enteroviruses	Fever, lethargy, jaundice, hepatomegaly, myocarditis, DIC, meningoencephalitis	Culture of CSF, throat and rectal swabs; PCR of CSF, stool
Adenoviruses	Fever, pneumonitis, lethargy, hepatosplenomegaly	Culture of urine, respiratory secretions; detection of adenoviral antigens in secretions
Lymphocytic choriomeningitis virus	Chorioretinitis, microcephaly, hydrocephalus	Serum for LCMV-IgM or IgG
Arboviruses	Fever, lethargy, CNS lesions	Culture of CSF; CSF or serum for specific IgM/IgG

Table 7 Outcome of Congenital and Perinatal Viral Infections[a]

Disorder	Mortality (%)	Morbidity (%)
Congenital CMV		
Symptomatic at birth	5–10	~90
Asymptomatic at birth	Negligible	10–15
Perinatal HSV		
Mucocutaneous infection	Negligible	~5
Encephalitis	15	~75
Disseminated infection	50	~40
Congenital HSV	~20	>90
Congenital rubella		
Symptomatic at birth	5–10	>90
Asymptomatic at birth	Negligible	10–15
Perinatal VZV	Up to 30	Low
Congenital VZV	10–20	>90
Perinatal HIV	Up to 100	Up to 100
Perinatal enteroviruses	Up to 30	Low

[a]Assumes appropriate antiviral treatment.

receive periodic assessment by a multidisciplinary team consisting of pediatric neurologists, pediatricians, speech and hearing specialists, physical therapists, and educational psychologists (104). Because progressive or new-onset hearing loss can develop in children with congenital CMV or rubella, such children should undergo frequent audiometry. CMV-infected infants, for example, should be evaluated every 6 months for the first 2 years, and annually thereafter for several years. Because several pathogens also affect physical growth or enhance the risk of endocrinological disorders, growth and pubertal development should be monitored closely.

REFERENCES

1. Sinzger C, Muntefering H, Loning T, et al. Cell types infected in human cytomegalovirus placentitis identified by immunohistochemical double staining. Virchows Archiv A 1993; 423:249–256.
2. Barkovich AJ, Lindan CE. Congenital cytomegalovirus infection of the brain: imaging analysis and embryologic considerations. AJNR 1994; 15:703–715.
3. Dias MJM, Harmant-van Rijckevorsel G, Landrieu P, Lyon G. Prenatal cytomegalovirus disease and cerebral microgyria: evidence for perfusion failure, not disturbance of histogenesis, as the major cause of fetal cytomegalovirus encephalopathy. Neuropediatrics 1984; 15:16–24.
4. Fowler KB, Stagno S, Pass RF, Britt WJ, Boll TJ, Alford CA. The outcome of congenital cytomegalovirus infection in relation to maternal antibody status. N Engl J Med 1992; 326:663–667.
5. Baldwin S, Whitley RJ. Teratogen update: intrauterine herpes simplex virus infection. Teratology 1989; 39:1–10.
6. McKendal RR, Stroop WG, eds. Handbook of Neurovirology. Marcel Dekker, New York, 1994.
7. Falloon J, Eddy J, Wiener L, Pizzo PA. Human immunodeficiency virus infection in children. J Pediatr 1989; 114:1–30.
8. Centers for Disease Control. Recommendations of the U.S. Public Health Service Task Force on the use of zidovudine to reduce perinatal transmission of human immunodeficiency virus. MMWR 1994; 43:1–18.
9. Connor EM, Sperling RS, Gelber R, et al. Reduction of maternal-infant transmission of human immunodeficiency virus type 1 with zidovudine treatment. N Engl J Med 1994; 331:1173–1180.
10. Bale Jr JF, Murph JR. Congenital infections and the nervous system. Pedatr Clin North Am 1992; 39:669–690.
11. Boppana SB, Pass RF, Britt WJ, Stagno S, Alford CA. Symptomatic congenital cytomegalovirus infection: neonatal morbidity and mortality. Pediatr Infect Dis J 1992; 11:93–99.
12. Demmler GJ. Summary of a workshop on surveillance for congenital cytomegalovirus disease. Rev Infect Dis 1991; 13:315–319.
13. Horwitz CA, Henle W, Henlel G, Snover D, Rodnicktt, Balfour Jr HH, Mazur MM, Watson R, Schwartz B, Muller N. Clinical and laboratory evaluation of cytomegalovirus-induced mononucleosis in previously healthy individuals. Report of 82 cases. Medicine 1986; 65:124–134.
14. Tyms AS, Taylor DL, Parkin JM. Cytomegalovirus and the acquired immunodeficiency syndrome. J Antimicrob Chemother 1989; 23(Suppl. A):89–105.
15. Pass RF, Stagno S, Britt WJ, et al. Specific cell-mediated immunity and the natural history of congenital infection with cytomegalovirus. J Infect Dis 1983; 148:953–961.
16. Murph JR, Baron JC, Brown K, Ebelhack CL, Bale Jr JF. The occupational risk of cytomegalovirus infection among day-care providers. JAMA 1991; 265:603–608.
17. Adler S. Cytomegalovirus and child day care. Evidence of an increased infection rate among day-care workers. N Engl J Med 1989; 321:1290–1296.
18. Williamson WD, Percy AK, Yow MD, Gerson P, Catlin FI, Koppelman ML, Thurber S. Asymptomatic congenital cytomegalovirus infection. AJDC 1990; 144:1365–1368.
19. Conboy TJ, Pass RF, Stagno S, Britt WJ, Alford CA, McFarland CE, Boll TJ. Intellectual development in school-aged children with asymptomatic congenital cytomegalovirus infection. Pediatrics 1986; 77:801–806.

20. Alford CA, Britt WJ, Cytomegalovirus. In: Fields BN, Knipe DM, eds. Virology. New York: Raven Press, 1990:1981–2010.
21. Grose C, Meehan T, Weiner CP. Prenatal diagnosis of congenital cytomegalovirus infection by virus isolation after amniocentesis. Pediatr Infect Dis J 1992; 11:605–607.
22. Dobbins JG, Stewart JA, Demmier GJ. Surveillance of congenital cytomegalovirus disease 1990-1991. MMWR 1992; 41:35–39.
23. Yow MD. Congenital cytomegalovirus disease: a now problem. J Infect Dis 1989; 159:163–167.
24. Dworsky ME, Welch K, Cassady G, Stagno S. Occupational risk for primary cytomegalovirus infection among pediatric health-care workers. N Engl J Med 1983; 309:950–953.
25. Pass RF, Stagno S, Myers GJ, Alford CA. Outcome of symptomatic congenital cytomegalovirus infection: results of long-term longitudinal follow-up. Pediatrics 1980; 66:758–762.
26. Gregg NM. Congenital cataract following German measles in the mother. Trans Ophthal Soc Aust 1941; 3:35–41.
27. Witte JJ, Karchmer AW, Case G, et al. Epidemiology of rubella. Am J Dis Child 1969; 118:107–111.
28. Sever JL, Hardy JB, Nelson KB, Gilkeson MR. Rubella in the collaborative perinatal research study. II. Clinical and laboratory findings in children through 3 years of age. Am J Dis Child 1969; 118: 123–132.
29. Dudgeon JA. Congenital rubella. J Pediatr 1975; 87:1078–1086.
30. Cochi SL, Edmonds LE, Dyer K, Greaves WL, Marks JS, Rovira EZ, Preblud SR, Orenstein WA. Congenital rubella syndrome in the United States, 1970–1985. On the verge of elimination. Am J Epidemiol 1989; 129:349–361.
31. Centers for Disease Control. Increase in rubella and congenital rubella syndrome—United States, 1988–1990. MMWR 1991; 40:93–99.
32. Centers for Disease Control. Rubella and congenital rubella syndrome—United States, January 1, 1991–May 7, 1994. MMWR 1994; 43:391–401.
33. Centers for Disease Control. Congenital rubella syndrome among the Amish—Pennsylvania, 1991–1992. MMWR 1992; 41:468–476.
34. Briss PA, Fehrs LJ, Hutcheson RH, Schaffner W. Rubella among the Amish: resurgent disease in a highly susceptible community. Pediatr Infect Dis J 1992; 11:955–959.
35. Herrmann KL. Rubella in the United States: toward a strategy for disease control and elimination. Epidemiol Infect 1991; 107:55–61.
36. Heggie AD, Robbins FC. Natural rubella acquired after birth. Am J Dis Child 1969; 118:12–17.
37. Givens KT, Lee DA, Jones T, Ilstrup DM. Congenital rubella syndrome: ophthalmic manifestations and associated systemic disorders. Br J Ophthalmol 1993; 77:358–363.
38. Ueda K, Nishida Y, Oshmia K, Shepard TH. Congenital rubella syndrome: correlation of gestational age at time of maternal rubella with type of defect. J Pediatr 1979; 94:763–765.
39. Murph JR. Rubella and syphilis: Continuing causes of congenital infection in the 1990's. Sem Pediatr Neurol 1994; 1:26–35.
40. Cradock-Watson JE, Miller E, Ridehalgh MKS, Terry GM, Ho-Terry L. Detection of rubella virus in fetal and placental tissues and in the throats of neonates after serologically confirmed rubella in pregnancy. Prenatal Diagn 1989; 9:91–96.
41. Yamashita Y. Matusuishi T, Murakami Y, et al. Neuroimaging findings (ultrasonography, CT, MRI) in 3 infants with congenital rubella syndrome. Pediatr Radiol 1991; 21:547–549.
42. Committee on Infectious Diseases (American Academy of Pediatrics). 1994 Red Book: Report of the Committee on Infectious Diseases. 23rd ed. Peter G, Halsey NA, Marcue EK, Pickering LK, eds. Elk Grove Village, IL: American Academy of Pediatrics.
43. Wild NJ, Sheppard S, Smithells RW, Holzel H, Jones G. Onset and severity of hearing loss due to congenital rubella infection. Arch Dis Child 1989; 64:1280–1283.
44. Chirboga-Klein S, Oberfield SE, Casullo AM, Holahan N, Fedun B, Cooper LZ, Levine LS. Growth in congenital rubella syndrome and correlation with clinical manifestations. J Pediatr 1989; 115: 251–255.
45. Desmond MM, Fisher ES, Vorderman AL, Schaffer HG, Andrew LP, Zion TE, Catlin FI. The

longitudinal course of congenital rubella encephalitis in nonretarded children. J Pediatr 1978; 93: 584–591.

46. Townsend JJ, Baringer JR, Wolinsky JS, et al. Progressive rubella panencephalitis. Late onset after congenital rubella. N Engl J Med 1975; 292:990–993.
47. Corey L, Spcar PG. Infections with herpes simplex viruses. N Engl J Med 1986; 314:686–691, 749–757.
48. Whitley RJ, Corey L, Arvin A, Lakeman FD, Sumaya CV, Wright PF, Dunkle LM, Steele RW, Soong SJ, Nahmias AJ, Alford CA, Powell DA, San Joaquin V, and the NIAID Collaborative Antiviral Study Group. Changing presentation of herpes simplex virus infection in neonates. J Infect Dis 1988; 158:109–116.
49. Koskiniemi M, Happonen JM, Järvenpää, Pettay O, Vaheri A. Neonatal herpes simplex virus infection: a report of 43 patients. Pediatr Infect Dis J 1989; 8:30–35.
50. Whitley RJ, Nahmias AJ, Visintine AM, Fleming CL, Alford CA. The natural history of herpes simplex virus infection of mother and newborn. Pediatrics 1980; 66:489–494.
51. Arvin AM, Yeager AS, Bruhn FW, Grossman M. Neonatal herpes simplex infection in the absence of mucocutaneous lesions. J Pediatr 1982; 100:715–721.
52. Andersen RD. Herpes simplex virus infection of the neonatal respiratory tract. AJDC 1987; 141: 274–276.
53. Hutto C, Arvin A, Jacobs R, Steele R, Stagno S, Lyrene R, Willett L, Powell D, Andersen R, Werthammer J, Ratcliff G, Nahmias A, Christy C, Whitley R. Intrauterine herpes simplex virus infections. J Pedatr 1987; 110:97–101.
54. Grose C. Congenital infections caused by varicella zoster virus and herpex simplex virus. Sem Pediatr Neurol 1994; 1:43–49.
55. Kimura H, Futamura M, Koto H, Ando T, Goto M, Kuzushima K, Shibata M, Morishima T. Detection of viral DNA in neonatal herpes simplex virus infections: frequent and prolonged presence in serum and cerebrospinal fluid. J Infect Dis 1991; 164:289–293.
56. Smith RR. Neuroadiology of intracranial infection. Pediatr Neurosurg 1992; 18:92–104.
57. Whitley R, Arvin A, Prober C, Burchett S, Corey L, Powell D, Plotkin S, Starr S, Alford C, Connor J, Jacobs R, Nahmias A, Soong SJ, and the National Institute of Allergy and Infectious Diseases Collaborative Antiviral Study Group. A controlled trial comparing Vidarabine with Acyclovir in neonatal herpes simplex virus infection. N Engl J Med 1991; 324:444–449.
58. Whitley R, Arvin A, Prober C, Corey K. Burchett S, Plotkin S, Starr S, Jacobs R, Powell D, Nahmias A, Sumaya C, Edwards K, Alford C, Caddell G, Soong SJ, and the National Institute of Allergy and Infectious Diseases Collaborative Antiviral Study Group. Predictors of morbidity and morality in neonates with herpes simplex virus infections. N Engl J Med 1991; 324:450–454.
59. Whitely RJ, Herpes simplex virus infections of the central nervous system. Encephalitis and neonatal herpes. Drugs 1991; 42:406–427.
60. Brunell PA. Varicella in pregnancy, the fetus, and the newborn: problems in management. J Infect Dis 1992; 166(suppl 1):S42–S47.
61. Enders G, Miller E, Cradock-Watson J, Bolley I, Ridelagh M. Consequences of varicella and herpes zoster in pregnancy: prospective study of 1739 cases. Lancet 1994; 343:1548–1550.
62. Patuszak AL, Levy M, Schick B, Zuber C, Feldkamp M, Gladstone J, Bar-Levy F, Jackson E, Donnenfeld A, Meschino W, Koren G. Outcome after maternal varicella infection in the first 20 weeks of pregnancy. N Engl J Med 1994; 330:901–905.
63. Jones KL, Johnson KA, Chambers CD. Offspring of women infected with varicella during pregnancy: a prospective study. Teratology 1994; 49:29–32.
64. Fleischer G, Henry W, McSorley M, Arbeter A, Plotkin S. Life-threatening complications of varicella. Am J Dis Child 1981; 135:896–899.
65. Gray F, Bélec L, Lescs MC, Chrétien F, Ciardi A, Hassine D, Flament-Sailbour M, Truchis P, Clair B, Scaravilli F. Varicella-zoster virus infection of the central nervous system in the acquired immune deficiency syndrome. Brain 1994; 117:987–999.
66. Friedman CA, Temple DM, Robbins KK, Rawson JE, Wilson JP, Feldman S. Outbreak and control of varicella in a neonatal intensive care unit. Pediatr Infect Dis J 1994; 13:152–154.

67. Alkalay AL, Pomerance JJ, Rimoin DL. Fetal varicella syndrome. J Pediatr 1987; 111:320–323.
68. Cuthbertson G, Weiner CP, Giller RH, Grose C. Prenatal diagnosis of second-trimester congenital varicella syndrome by virus-specific immunoglobulin M. J Pediatr 1987; 111:592–595.
69. Gold WL, Boulton JE, Goldman, Gershon A, Steinberg SP, Chua R, Low DE, McGreer A. Management of varicella exposures in the neonatal intensive care unit. Pediatr Infect Dis J 1993; 12:954–955.
70. Souza IE, Bale Jr JF. The diagnosis of congenital infections: contemporary strategies. J Child Neurol 1995; 10:1–12.
71. Melnick JL. Enteroviruses: Polioviruses, coxsackie viruses, echoviruses, and newer enteroviruses. In: Fields BN, Knipe DM, et al, eds. Virology. New York, Raven Press, 1990:549–605.
72. Lake AM, Lauer BA, Clark JC, Wesenburg RL, McIntosh K. Enterovirus infections in neonates. J Pediatr 1976; 89:787–791.
73. Berry PJ, Nagington J. Fatal infection with echnovirus 11. Arch Dis Child 1982; 57:22–29.
74. Modlin JF. Fatal echovirus 11 disease in premature neonates. Pediatrics 1980; 66:775–780.
75. Mertens T, Hager H, Eggers HJ. Epidemiology of an outbreak in a maternity unit of infections with an antigenic variant of echovirus 11. J Med Virol 1982; 9:81–91.
76. Rotbart HA. Diagnosis of enteroviral meningitis with the polymerase chain reaction. J Pediatr 1990; 117:85–89.
77. Bergman I, Painter MJ, Wald ER, Chiponis D, Holland AL, Taylor HG. Outcome in children with enteroviral meningitis during the first year of life. J Pediatr 1987; 110:705–709.
78. Rorabaugh ML, Berlin LE, Heldrick F, Roberts K, Rosenberg LA, Doran T, Modlin JF. Aseptic meningitis in infants younger than 2 years of age: acute illness and neurologic complications. Pediatrics 1993; 92:206–211.
79. Scott GB, Buck BE, Leterman JG, Bloom FL, Parks W. Acquired immunodeficiency syndrome in infants. N Engl J Med 1984; 310:76–81.
80. Millard DD, Chadwick EG, Yogev R, Modlin JF. Zidovudine treatment of an infant with congenital human immunodeficiency virus infection. Pediatr Infect Dis J 1990; 9:929–931.
81. Srugo I, Wittek AE, Israele V, Brunell PA. Meningoencephalitis in a neonate congenitally infected with human immunodeficiency virus type 1. J Pediatr 1992; 120:93–95.
82. Husson RN, Comeau AM, Hoff R. Diagnosis of human immunodeficiency virus infection in infants and children. Pediatrics 1990; 86:1–10.
83. Rogers MF, Ou CY, Kilbourne B, Schochetman G. Advances and problems in the diagnosis of human immunodeficiency virus infection in infants. Pediatr Infect Dis J 1991; 10:523–531.
84. Sheinbergas MM. Hydrocephalus due to prenatal infection with the lymphocytic choriomeningitis virus. Infection 1976; 4:185–191.
85. Larsen PD, Charatrand SA, Tomashek KM, Hauser LG, Ksiazek TG. Hydrocephalus complicating lymphocytic choriomeningitis virus infection. Pediatr Infect Dis J 1993; 12:528–531.
86. Wenger F. Venezuelan equine encephalitis. Teratology 1977; 16:359–362.
87. Shinefield HR, Townsend TE. Transplacental transmission of Western equine encephalomyelitis. J Pediatr 1953; 43:21–25.
88. Abzug MJ, Levin MJ. Neonatal adenovirus infection: four patients and review of the literature. Pediatrics 1991; 87:890–896.
89. Berry PJ, Gray ES, Porter HJ, Burton PA. Parvovirus infection of the human fetus and newborn. Sem Diagn Pathol 1992; 9:4–12.
90. Rogers BB, Singer DB, Mak SK, Gary GW, Fikrig MK, McMillan PN. Detection of human parvovirus B19 in early spontaneous abortuses using serology, histology, electron microscopy, in situ hybridization, and the polymerase chain reaction. Obstet Gynecol 1993; 81:402–408.
91. Bale Jr JF. Conditions mimicking congenital infections. Sem Pediatr Neurol 1994; 1:63–70.
92. Koskiniemi M, Lappalainen M, Hedman K. Toxoplasmosis needs evaluation. An overview and proposals. AJDC 1989; 143:724–728.
93. Willis J, Rosman NP. The Aicardi syndrome versus congenital infection: diagnostic considerations. J Pediatr 1980; 96:235–239.
94. Bordarier C, Aicardi J, Goutieres F. Congenital hydrocephalus and eye abnormalities with severe developmental brain defects: Warburg's syndrome. Ann Neurol 1984; 16:60–65.

95. Carney Jr RG. Incontinentia pigmenti. A world statistical analysis. Arch Dermatol 1976; 112:535–542.
96. Neal PR, Jansen RD, Lemons JA, Mirkin LD, Schreiner RL. Unusual manifestations of neonatal hyperthyroidism. Am J Perinatol 1985; 2:231–235.
97. Zellweger H. The cerebro-hepato-renal (Zellweger) syndrome and other peroxisomal disorders. Dev Med Child Neurol 1987; 29:821–829.
98. Gleaves CA, Hodinka RL, Johnston SLG, Swierkosz EM. Laboratory diagnosis of viral infections. Cumitech 15A 1994.
99. Johnson FB. Transport of vital specimens. Clin Microbiol Rev 1990; 3:120–131.
100. Garland SM, Gilbert GL, and members of the Pediatric Infectious Diseases Group of the Australasian Society for Infectious Diseases. Investigation of congenital infection—the TORCH screen is not a legitimate test. Med J Aust 1993; 159:346–348.
101. Schlesinger Y, Sawyer MH, Storch GA. Enteroviral meningitis in infancy: potential role for polymerase chain reaction in patient management. Pediatrics 1994; 94:157–162.
102. Naber SP. Molecular pathology—diagnosis of infectious disease. N Engl J Med 1994; 331:1212–1215.
103. Demmler GJ, Buffone GJ, Schimbor CM, May RA. Detection of cytomegalovirus in urine from newborns using polymerase chain reaction DNA amplification. J Infect Dis 1988; 158:1177–1184.
104. Bale Jr JF. Congenital viral infection. In: Johnson RT, ed. Current Therapy in Neurologic Diseases—3. Philadelphia: B.C. Decker, Inc., 1990:111–114.
105. Demmler GJ. Congenital cytomegalovirus infection. Sem Pediatr Neurol 1994; 1:39.

2

Neonatal Meningitis

Monica Trujillo and George H. McCracken, Jr.
University of Texas Southwestern Medical Center, Dallas, Texas

INTRODUCTION

Neonatal sepsis is defined as systemic signs of infection accompanied by bacteremia in the first month of life (1). As many as 20–30% of neonatal sepsis cases are complicated by bacterial meningitis; therefore, a high index of suspicion is required to make a prompt and accurate diagnosis and to institute appropriate therapy in a timely manner.

The etiological agents of neonatal meningitis and sepsis have changed since the early 1900s when *Escherichia coli*, *Staphylococcus aureus*, and group A β-hemolytic streptococci predominated. In the 1940s there was an emergence of coliforms, with *E. coli* being the predominant organism. During the 1960s and 1970s group B *Streptococcus* became the most common etiological agent. Presently group B *Streptococcus* and gram-negative enteric bacilli, especially nosocomial organisms in our neonatal intensive care units, are the most common pathogens (2).

In the preantibiotic era meningitis was almost universally fatal, with mortality rates exceeding 95%. Despite considerable progress in antimicrobial and supportive therapy, meningitis in the newborn period continues to be a life-threatening illness; current case fatality rates are approximately 20–30% (3) and even higher in low-birthweight premature infants. Although antibiotics have had an impact on the number of deaths from this disease, long-term neurological sequelae occur in as many as one third of all survivors.

The purpose of this chapter is to review general aspects concerning meningitis in the neonate and emphasize the characteristics that make this infection unique and challenging in this age group.

EPIDEMIOLOGY

Meningitis is more common in the newborn period (the first 30 days of life) than any other time thereafter (4). The incidence of neonatal meningitis is from 0.3 to 10/1000 live births, depending on the geographic location (3). More than 75% of all cases of neonatal meningitis in developed countries are caused by group B streptococci and gram-negative enteric bacilli, whereas in Latin American countries gram-negative bacilli, mainly *E. coli*, are the predominant pathogens (5–7).

Multiple risk factors predispose the newborn to severe infections. These include maternal, infant, and environmental factors. Among the maternal factors are fever, infections, particularly of the urinary tract, chorioamnionitis, and endometritis with bacteremia (8). Obstetric risk factors such as prolonged rupture of membranes, forceps delivery, and birth trauma can also be important. Factors inherent to the newborn include prematurity, low birthweight, perinatal hypoxia/asphyxia, and congenital anomalies. Environmental factors are invasive procedures related to cardiopulmonary resuscitation and monitoring, prolonged ventilatory support, and intravenous access devices (9).

Of these risk factors the most significant is low birthweight, especially in infants weighing less than 2500 g (10). Louvois et al. (11) reviewed cases of neonatal meningitis in England and Wales and found that 18% had a history of maternal infection or birth asphyxia, 13% had intrauterine growth retardation, and 11% were born prematurely (gestational age <33 weeks) after prolonged rupture of the membranes.

Group B *Streptococcus*

This is the most common etiological agent in neonatal bacterial infections. Approximately 20–25% of parturients have cervicovaginal and/or rectal colonization with group B streptococci (12). Transmission from colonized mothers to their infants during delivery is approximately 50% (13,14). Vertical transmission is responsible for early-onset (<7 days of life) (15) group B streptococcal disease. Neonates can also acquire the disease by nosocomial transmission from hands of nursery personnel or horizontal transmission from family members in cases where the infant presents with disease later in the hospital course or after discharge from the nursery. This explains the increase in colonization rates in infants from 20–25% on the first day of life to 60–65% at 3–7 days of age (16) and the presentation of late-onset (1–6 weeks of age) group B streptococcal disease.

All group B streptococci that cause invasive disease are encapsulated—types Ia, Ib, Ic, II, III, IV, and V—and all are implicated in the etiology of early-onset group B streptococcal disease (17). On the other hand, 90% of the cases with late-onset disease are caused by type III group B *Streptococcus* (18).

Escherichia coli

This is the second most common organism implicated in neonatal bacterial sepsis/meningitis with an incidence rate of approximately 1/1000 live births per year. There are many different antigens that make *E. coli* antigenically complex [i.e., approximately 150 somatic (O), 100 capsular (K), and 50 flagellar (H) antigens]. *E. coli* possessing the K1 antigen cause approximately 75 and 40% of cases of neonatal meningitis and sepsis, respectively, indicating a strong association with invasive disease (19). Approximately 50% of neonates will be colonized at birth following vaginal delivery to women who are colonized rectally by *E. coli* K1 strains (20). Nosocomial transmission from nursery personnel has also been reported in as many as 40% of infants (20). In premature babies colonization occurs around the second or third week of life, and nosocomial transmission (nurse to infant or infant to infant) plays an important epidemiological role.

Listeria monocytogenes

The epidemiology of infections with *Listeria monocytogenes* is not completely understood, but early- and late-onset diseases have been described. In infants with early-onset disease, there is often a history of a flulike syndrome in the mother before delivery (21). *Listeria* is a zoonotic organism that can contaminate milk products that have not been pasteurized (22,23). Several large outbreaks of disease have been associated with maternal consumption of contaminated cheese. The mode of transmission in late-onset disease is less well defined, but there have been cases of nosocomial spread (24).

Fungi

Infants who remain in the hospital for prolonged periods with long-term intravenous access and requiring invasive procedures are at risk for fungal infections such as those caused by *Candida* species, most commonly, *Candida albicans*. Other species causing neonatal disease include *C. tropicalis*, *C. parapsilosis*, and *C. lusitaniae*. Of 51 neonates managed in an intensive care unit for invasive fungal disease reported by Faix (25), 31 had *C. albicans*, 17 *C. parapsilosis*, and 3 *C. tropicalis*. Important factors related to invasive infections with *C. albicans* are of use in broad-spectrum antibiotics, steroids, central hyperalimentation, intravenous lipid emulsions, and use of indwelling venous or umbilical artery catheters, as well as length of stay in the nursery, malnutrition, and prematurity (26,27). *Malassezia furfur* can also cause invasive disease and is associated with administration of lipid emulsions (28).

Viral Pathogens

Although many viruses such as cytomegalovirus, rubella, lymphocytic choriomeningitis virus, and adenovirus can cause infection in newborn infants, we will emphasize the herpes simplex virus and the enteroviruses.

The human enteroviruses (Coxsackie A, Coxsackie B, echovirus, and poliovirus) are ubiquitous, and the majority of cases occur during the summer and fall months (29). Shattuck and Chonmaitree reported that from 1984 to 1988 enteroviruses were the most common cause of meningitis in neonates older than 7 days (30). A predominance of viral etiologies (enteroviruses comprising 63% of cases) was also reported by Dagan et al. (31) in infants hospitalized for suspected sepsis. Transmission from mother to infant can occur in utero, at delivery, or postnatally, the latter being the most common (29). The timing of maternal infection in the perinatal period is critical in determining the outcome of the newborn: maternal infection 5–7 days before delivery will allow for development and passive transplacental transfer of specific IgG antibodies, thus protecting the infant from severe disease, while maternal infection occurring closer to delivery or post partum can be associated with severe neonatal disease due to lack of protective antibodies (32).

The estimated incidence of neonatal herpes simplex virus (HSV) infection is approximately 1 in 2500 to 1 in 30,000 deliveries. Many factors influence transmission to the newborn infant. First, the type of maternal infection at the time of delivery is important; the incidence of neonatal HSV is higher in babies born to women with primary genital infection (33%) compared with those with recurrent infection (3%) (33). Second, the duration of ruptured membranes is directly related to the risk of infection (prolonged rupture of membranes >6 h increases the risk), and cesarean section delivery in women with active HSV genital lesions is believed to reduce the rate of neonatal infection if the membranes have not ruptured (34). Acquisition of HSV infection in the newborn infant can be in utero from transplacental or ascending infection (5%), intrapartum after contact with infected maternal genital secretions (85%), or postnatal, including nosocomial transmission (10%) (33). Of note, 70% of infants who develop HSV infection are born to women who are asymptomatic at delivery and do not provide a history of genital herpes infection or a sexual partner with genital herpes (34,35).

ETIOLOGY

Bacterial infections in neonates that occur during the first 7 days of life are classified as early-onset disease. The usual pathogens responsible for early-onset disease include group B *Streptococcus*, gram-negative enteric organisms such as *E. coli*, *Klebsiella-Enterobacter* species, *L. monocytogenes*, and non–beta-hemolytic streptococci. Late-onset disease occurs most commonly after the first week of life, and the causative agents include those implicated in early-onset disease as well as nosocomially acquired microorganisms such as *S. aureus*, coagulase-negative staphylococci, *Enterococcus*, *Pseudomonas aeruginosa*, and other gram-negative pathogens such as *Klebsiella pneumoniae*, *Enterobacter cloacae*, *Citrobacter diversus*, and *Salmonella* species. Once the infant is discharged from the nursery and exposed to household or outside contacts, infections caused by pathogens commonly seen in older infants (i.e., *Streptococcus pneumoniae*, *Haemophilus influenzae*, and *Neisseria meningitidis*) can develop. Routine immunization with the conjugated *Haemophilus* vaccines has resulted in a sharp decline of *H. influenzae* type b infections in infants and children (36,37).

Fungal infections, mainly with *C. albicans*, occur more frequently in intensive care units as a result of prolonged supportive measures and invasive procedures. Viral meningoencephalitis is caused by many different viruses, as discussed previously.

Table 1 shows the etiological agents of neonatal bacterial meningitis at Parkland Memorial Hospital, Dallas, in 1987–1994. Of 75 cases, 63 (84%) had positive blood cultures with the same etiological agent. Early-onset disease was found in 28 (37%), and males accounted for 39 cases.

Table 1 Etiological Agents of Neonatal Bacterial Meningitis at Parkland Memorial Hospital, Dallas, 1987–1994[a]

Organism	No. (%)	Death (%)
Gram-positive pathogens		
Group B *Streptococcus*	39 (52)	6 (15)
Enterococcus	4 (5)	1 (25)
Group D *Streptococcus*	2 (3)	0
Staphylococcus aureus	6 (8)	1 (50)
Others	2 (2)	0
Gram-negative pathogens		
Escherichia coli	7 (9)	2 (28)
Klebsiella pneumoniae	2 (3)	0
Enterobacter cloacae	2 (3)	0
Serratia marcescens	2 (3)	0
Other gram-negative rods	2 (3)	1 (50)
H. influenzae, nontypeable	2 (3)	1 (50)
Neisseria meningitidis	1 (1)	0
Polymicrobial	3 (4)	0
Fungi		
Candida albicans	1 (1)	0
Total	75	12 (16)

[a]Incidence of all meningitis cases at Parkland Memorial Hospital, 0.67/1000 live births.

Twelve (16%) deaths were reported, 7 of which were associated with early-onset disease. Of note is the absence of *L. monocytogenes* during this period; by contrast, Sáez-Llorens and Siegel (38) reported 17 cases of *L. monocytogenes* meningitis in the first month of life at Parkland Memorial Hospital from 1969 to 1989.

PATHOGENESIS

Although many factors influence the outcome of any particular neonate, it is not fully understood why under similar circumstances some infants develop sepsis or meningitis while others do not.

Under normal circumstances the fetus is protected in a sterile environment as long as the amniotic membranes remain intact and no invasive procedures are performed. Although amniotic fluid has bactericidal activity, after the membranes rupture or when there is contamination with meconium it becomes an excellent medium for growth of the normal maternal flora from the genital or gastrointestinal tracts. Although most infants will become colonized under these circumstances, only a few develop disease. Infectious agents can gain entry through the skin, mucous membranes, lungs, gastrointestinal tract, umbilical cord, nasopharynx, or urinary tract. These barriers may not be sufficient to protect the neonate from infection in cases of congenital anomalies, obstetric trauma, or in association with invasive procedures in the nursery.

The newborn infant has immune deficits that can predispose to infection, especially the premature, low-birthweight infant. These include low concentrations or absence of maternal IgG antibodies to specific pathogens that are passively transferred across the placenta. The premature infant is particularly at risk because of diminished transfer of antibodies early in gestation, especially before 32 weeks of gestation (39). Neonates are also deficient in complement components (C1,C2,C3 proactivator, and C4) that affect the classic and alternate complement pathways and, thus, chemotaxis and opsonization. A reduced bone marrow storage pool results in neutropenia when newborn infants develop systemic bacterial infection because the marrow is unable to produce adequate numbers of polymorphonuclear cells.

Once the microorganisms gain access to the bloodstream, they can avoid phagocytosis because of the presence of a polysaccharide capsule, which renders resistance to the classic complement pathway (40), or of the absence of maternally derived protective antibodies directed against the capsule. When organisms attain a critical concentration in the circulation, they can enter the central nervous system by way of the blood–cerebrospinal fluid (CSF) barrier (i.e., choroid plexus) and blood-brain barrier via the postcapillary venules. Once the bacteria reach the subarachnoid space, host defense mechanisms are inadequate to control the infection (40). The ensuing inflammatory cascade is complex. It involves the production of cytokines such as interleukin-1 (IL-1) and tumor necrosis factor (TNF) (41) by the endothelial cells and monocyte-macrophage equivalent cells in the central nervous system (astroglia) after stimulation by bacterial products (teichoic acid or endotoxin depending on the type of bacteria). The liberation of these bacterial products can increase after treatment with antibiotics due to lysis of the cells, which potentiates the inflammatory response already underway. These cytokines stimulate the production of prostaglandins and platelet-activating factor from the cell membranes of endothelial and polymorphonuclear cells and upregulate adhesion receptors on cerebral vascular endothelial cells resulting in attraction and attachment of leukocytes (42). The leukocytes then traverse the endothelia, and as endothelial injury progresses, the permeability of this membrane increases. Greater numbers of leukocytes enter the perivascular and CSF spaces, resulting in release of more toxic substances causing greater cellular injury. There is also an increase in the concentration of low molecular weight serum proteins in the cerebrospinal fluid secondary to increased permeability of the blood-brain barrier. All of these events have profound effects on the cerebral distribution of intracellular and extracellular fluid, which results in cerebral edema, increased CSF viscosity and intracranial pressure (ICP), and decreased cerebral blood flow (CBF). Decreased cerebral perfusion results in tissue hypoxia and anaerobic conditions leading to hypoglycorrhachia, acidosis, and increasing concentrations of lactate (42). In the presence of increased ICP and a severe inflammatory response, the normal cerebrovascular autoregulatory mechanisms to control intracranial pressure are lost, leaving CBF dependent principally on systemic blood pressure. If systemic hypotension occurs, CBF is jeopardized, resulting in ischemia. Ischemia coupled with vasculitis and thrombosis secondary to the inflammatory response is responsible for irreversible focal or diffuse brain damage (43).

PATHOLOGY

Bacterial Meningitis

In the acute stages of meningeal infection, the macroscopic findings are edema and hyperemia of the brain with congestion of the subarachnoid vessels. The lateral ventricles are small as a result of the surrounding edema. Approximately 24 h after onset of disease there is slight thickening and opacification of the meninges mainly over the base of the brain with exudate in the subarachnoid space along the vessels lining the cerebral convexities and basal cisterns, as depicted in Figure 1. Later it becomes more confluent, involving the cerebrum, cerebellum, brain stem, and occasionally the spinal cord (44). The infection may extend through the foramina of Magendie and Luschka into the ventricles with resulting ventriculitis, most commonly observed with gram-negative organisms. Microscopically, polymorphonuclear leukocytes and fibrin accumulate within the subarachnoid space during the acute phase (up to the end of the first week), and later, toward the end of the second and third weeks, mononuclear and plasma cells appear (45).

Newborns frequently develop vasculitis with arteritis and thrombophlebitis secondary to involvement of the intracranial blood vessels leading to infarcts in as many as 30% of cases (46) and accounting for the high incidence of neurological deficits observed in survivors. The infarcts are usually large and hemorrhagic, involving the cortex and white matter, but can also be periventricular, compromising the basal ganglia. Infection of the infarcted tissue results in abscess formation.

Acute obstructive hydrocephalus may result from occlusion of the aqueduct or foramina of the fourth ventricle with cellular debris or granulation tissue. Communicating hydrocephalus can also be seen as a result of impaired resorption of cerebrospinal fluid at the arachnodonic villi as a result of the inflammatory reaction.

Hemorrhagic meningoencephalitis has been described in cases of gram-negative infection usually from infection with *P. aeruginosa*, *Proteus* species, *Enterobacter sakazakii*, and *Serratia marcescens*. This occurs in association with venous thrombosis. In these cases the features of hemorrhagic necrosis predominate. The brain is swollen with purplish discoloration or areas of hemorrhagic necrosis, with or without the presence of exudate. Microscopic examination reveals extensive necrosis with microorganisms surrounding the vessels and infiltrating the cerebral parenchyma (44).

Fungal Meningitis

Fungal infections of the central nervous system in the newborn period are usually caused by *C. albicans* and present as meningitis with ventriculitis. The exudate contains polymorphonuclear leukocytes, lymphocytes, and pseudohyphi. Hydrocephalus is a common complication. There is invasion of the brain parenchyma with necrotizing encephalitis and granulomatous tissue response (45).

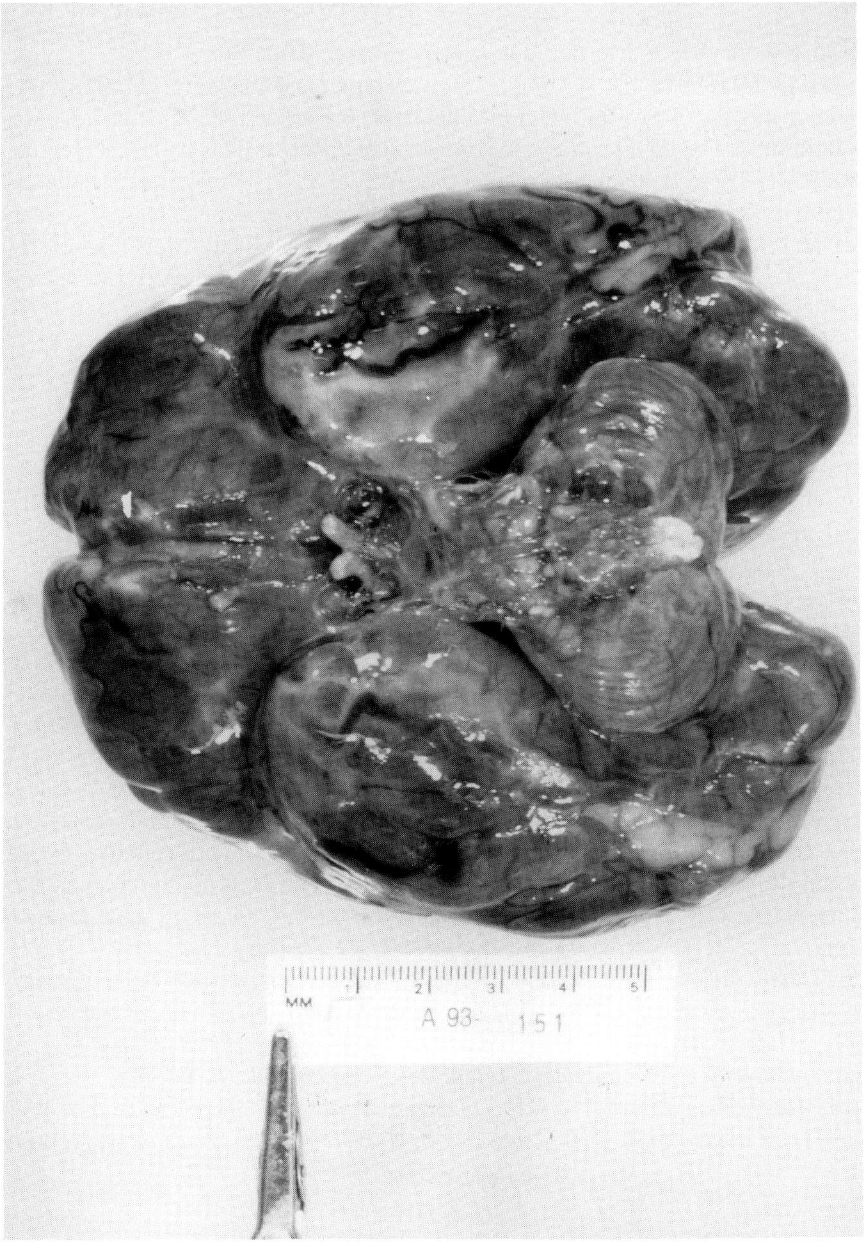

Figure 1 Brain of a 40-week-gestation infant who expired on the third day of life with group B streptococcal sepsis and meningitis. A thick, purulent exudate covers the base of the brain.

Viral Meningitis

During the neonatal period, the central nervous system is one of the target organs of viral infections caused mainly by rubella, herpes simplex viruses type I and II, cytomegalovirus, and Coxsackie and echoviruses. With rubella infection there is a low-grade inflammatory reaction with perivascular infiltration and glial proliferation, which specifically affects the basal ganglia, brain stem, and midbrain. There is frequently resultant microcephaly. The meningoencephalitis seen with cytomegalovirus and herpes simplex viruses is usually more acute and destructive with extensive necrosis and ventriculitis. With cytomegalovirus there is usually development of periventricular calcifications. Herpes simplex virus encephalitis is characterized by unilateral involvement of the temporal lobes (46).

CLINICAL MANIFESTATIONS

Early clinical manifestations of meningitis are frequently nonspecific and indistinguishable from those of septicemia, often overlapping with signs and symptoms of noninfectious diseases and involving many different organs (Table 2). Regardless of the etiological agent (bacteria, fungi, or viruses), the initial presentation in most cases is indistinguishable; the epidemiological and clinical course can be helpful in establishing the diagnosis, but rapid and conventional microbiological techniques are necessary for a definitive diagnosis. Meningitis should always be considered when sepsis is suspected; therefore, the diagnosis of meningitis requires a high index of suspicion and an aggressive approach to avoid misdiagnosis and delay in initiating appropriate therapy. Newborns who present with meningitis have been divided into two groups: those with early-onset disease (i.e., in the first 7 days of life) and those with late-onset disease (i.e., from 8 days to 6 weeks after birth). This designation is important because the etiological agents, clinical presentation, and case-fatality rates are strikingly different between groups. The newborns with early-onset disease usually present with respiratory distress and sepsis, and mortality rates are considerably higher compared with late-onset disease, which can present with central nervous system manifestations (Table 3). The common signs of meningitis observed in older infants and children, such as nuchal rigidity and Kernig and Brudzinski signs, are absent in the neonate.

Among the common pathogens *Listeria* meningitis characteristically has a more benign course. Kessler and Dajani, in a series of 17 cases over a 15-year period, reported no deaths, and only one patient developed complications with seizures and hydrocephalus as a result of *Listeria* meningitis (47).

In disseminated infections with *C. albicans*, meningitis has been found to occur in as many as 44% of infants and usually has a more indolent course than bacterial infections (48). These neonates commonly have infectious complications, such as renal parenchymal infiltration, ab-

Table 2 Clinical Characteristics of Early-Onset and Late-Onset Meningitis

	Early	Late
Age at onset	<7 days	>8 days
Obstetric risks	Frequent	Unusual
Source of infection	Maternal genital tract	Maternal genital tract Environment (nursery)
Clinical presentation	Pneumonia/Sepsis	Meningitis
Mortality (%)	15–70	10–20

Table 3 Signs and Symptoms of Neonatal Meningitis

Temperature instability	Central nervous sytem
Hypothermia	Seizures
Hyperthermia	Lethargy
Respiratory	Irritability
Tachypnea	Bulging fontanelle
Retractions	Cardiovascular
Grunting	Shock
Apnea	Tachycardia
Flaring	Bradycardia
Gastrointestinal	Skin/Mucous membranes
Abdominal distention	Pallor
Vomiting	Cyanosis
Diarrhea	Petechiae
Poor feeding/suck	Rash
Gastric residuals	Jaundice

scesses, endocarditis, pericarditis, ventriculitis with or without hydrocephalus, and rarely skeletal disease or fungus ball uropathy. Failure to recover *C. albicans* from the urine (which can occur in up to 50% of cases) does not exclude renal complications (49). Renal ultrasound, lumbar puncture, and ophthalmological examinations are recommended in all patients with disseminated candidiasis; the yield of these procedures is small but helpful in establishing the diagnosis when cultures are delayed in turning positive or negative. Cardiac and head ultrasound are recommended when clinically indicated (50). The isolation of *C. albicans* from tracheal secretions in the absence of disseminated disease and pulmonary infiltrates usually indicates colonization rather than infection and most often does not require systemic antifungal therapy.

Infection of the central nervous system with HSV can occur as part of disseminated multiorgan infection or as encephalitis alone. HSV I accounts for approximately 30% of neonatal infections, with the genital HSV II strain accounting for the rest (51). Infants usually present at 9–11 days of life with lethargy, irritability, seizures (focal or generalized), or other signs of central nervous system involvement, as described above. Skin lesions are seen in 30% of cases with disseminated disease and encephalitis, whereas as many as 40% of infants with only CNS disease may not have skin lesions, making the diagnosis more difficult (34). Infants with clinical signs suggestive of HSV infection should be completely evaluated even with a negative maternal history of genital HSV lesions or delivery by cesarean section.

Enteroviral infections in the newborn usually present in the first 10 days of life after an incubation period of 2–5 days. It can present as aseptic meningitis or as a component of disseminated infection with myocardial, hepatic, and central nervous system involvement (28). The latter is usually caused by the Coxsackie viruses.

DIAGNOSIS

The diagnosis of meningitis in the newborn infant is confirmed by the finding of organisms on gram-stained smear and isolation from culture of CSF. Cultures of body surfaces (i.e., skin, umbilicus) and mucosal membranes (i.e., nose, throat, or rectum) indicate colonization and are usually not helpful in identifying the etiologic agent (52). Most experience with septic newborn infants occurs in the nursery or intensive care unit, and the diagnostic approach in this setting should include a complete blood cell count with differential, cultures of blood, urine, and CSF (and any other sterile site such as vesicular lesions and peritoneal or pleural fluids). In the outpatient setting the newborn infant who is evaluated for fever (temperature >38.0°C), hypothermia, or is ill-appearing should also be evaluated for central nervous system infection and receive antimicrobial therapy until results of cultures are available.

Routine Laboratory Tests

Tests commonly used in the evaluation of the sick neonate are the complete blood cell count, neutrophil counts, and neutrophil ratios. The leukocyte count in general is considered abnormal if $<5000/mm^3$ or $>15,000/mm^3$ but is of limited value since less than 50% of infants with these values are ultimately diagnosed with invasive infections (53). The neutrophil count is slightly more sensitive than the total leukocyte count and when low ($0–4000/mm^3$) is highly significant, reflecting depletion of the bone marrow reserves and a poor prognosis (54,55). The most extensively studied of the neutrophil ratios is the proportion of immature to total neutrophils (I/T ratio) (56). Bonadio in 1987 (49) reported on the complete blood count differential ratio:

$$\frac{\%\ \text{lymphocytes} + \%\ \text{monocytes}}{\%\ \text{polymorphonuclear leukocytes} + \%\ \text{band forms}}$$

to help in distinguishing neonates with serious infections from those without systemic disease. He found that nearly all (96%) infants in the afebrile group without serious infection had a ratio of more than 1, whereas the majority of febrile infants (87.5%) with serious infections had a ratio of less than 1.

Blood cultures are important adjuvants in establishing the etiology of meningitis and should be obtained on all neonates with suspected meningitis since 70–85% of them will have a concomitant positive blood culture with the same microorganism. The optimal number of blood cultures needed to detect neonatal bacteremia is uncertain, but because the concentration of bacteria in blood is larger in neonates than in other age groups with sepsis and because the total volume of blood is small in neonates, only a single culture is usually obtained.

The urinalysis is of value for diagnosis of urinary tract infection when the leukocytes are greater than 10/hpf and/or the leukocyte esterase is positive (58). Although the yield from urine cultures in newborn infants with early-onset (1.6%) is low compared with that in late-onset (7.4%) disease (59), we recommend obtaining urine samples for culture in all neonates with suspected sepsis/meningitis, because, if positive, it will help in determining the etiology.

Whenever meningitis is suspected, lumbar puncture is the diagnostic procedure of choice, but it is contraindicated in cases with clinical signs of increased ICP and in infants who have hemodynamic or respiratory instability. In these cases it should be deferred until the patient is stable and blood and urine cultures have been obtained before initiation of therapy.

CSF indices differ in newborn infants compared with older infants and children. CSF from normal uninfected neonates can have a total white blood cell count (WBC) as high as 32 cells/mm^3 with 50–60% polymorphonuclear cells, protein concentration as high as 170 mg/dl, and CSF:serum glucose ratio as high as 80% (60–63).

In cases where HSV infection is suspected, viral cultures should be obtained from skin or mucosal lesions, CSF, buffy coat, biopsy samples, if available (such as liver, lung, brain, or gastrointestinal mucosa), and samples of rectal, nasopharyngeal, and conjunctival mucosae. Tzanck preparations of scrapings of the base of skin lesions can also be examined for multinucleated giant cells suggestive of infection with herpes simplex virus or varicella-zoster infection.

With enteroviral infection the virus can be cultured from multiple samples including stool, urine, respiratory secretions, and throat. With the increasing availability of polymerase chain reaction for detection of viral nucleic acids, the diagnosis of enteroviral and herpes simplex virus infections will become more sensitive and rapid, allowing for prompt initiation of specific therapy (56,57).

Acute Phase Reactants

In the context of inflammation secondary to infection, the liver synthesizes certain proteins known as acute phase reactants. Included in this group are the C-reactive protein (CRP), fibrinogen, haptoglobin, and alpha$_1$-acid glycoprotein. Powell and Marcy (66) reviewed the literature and found significant elevation of CRP values at the onset of infection in 50–90% of neonatal cases; CRP concentrations were elevated as early as the first day of infection, peaking at 2–3 days and remaining elevated until the infection was controlled and the inflammatory process was subsiding. Although CRP values cannot be used alone as an early indicator of neonatal bacterial infection and of the need for therapy, they can be of value in following the resolution of infection and response to antimicrobial therapy. Thus, the CRP can be useful in determining duration of therapy and the occurrence of relapse or complications during or following treatment.

The sedimentation rate is influenced by these acute phase reactants, but has little value in evaluating the neonate with bacterial infections because of delayed elevation in response to inflammation. Because normalization of the sedimentation rate can be slow, especially when compared with the CRP, many physicians use this index to determine duration of therapy to be certain that the pathogen has been eradicated.

Rapid Tests

Laboratory techniques have been developed to allow rapid detection of bacterial antigens from body fluid samples. These methods include immunoelectrophoresis, latex agglutination, and radioimmunoassays (66).

Although counterimmunoelectrophoresis (CIE) was the first technique used successfully and extensively for antigen detection, the latex agglutination (LA) test is preferred at present because of its simplicity, greater sensitivity, and speed. The LA test can detect antigens of the most common pathogens in neonatal meningitis, i.e., group B *Streptococcus*, *E. coli* K1 strains, and other less commonly encountered organisms such as *H. influenzae*, *N. meningitidis*, and *S. pneumoniae*. The sensitivity of LA for group B *Streptococcus* varies between 73–100% in CSF and 75–84% in urine (67). False-positive results with LA for group B *Streptococcus* in urine samples can result from contamination of bag specimens of urine with streptococci from rectal or vaginal colonization (68). The LA test is especially useful in patients who have negative gram-stained smears and cultures of CSF such as occurs when therapy is administered before the diagnostic lumbar puncture (69).

Polymerase chain reaction (PCR) has been used to detect specific nucleotide sequences in CSF of patients with infection caused by herpes simplex virus (70,71) and enteroviral (72,73) meningitis. These highly specialized tests are sensitive and highly specific compared with conventional culture techniques.

Radiological Evaluation

Radiological examination is valuable mainly for diagnosis of intracranial complications of meningitis. Ultrasonography has been useful in diagnosis and follow-up of neonates with meningitis, but the introduction of computed tomography (CT) and enhanced magnetic resonance imaging (MRI) provides a more precise definition of the location and extent of infection and complications (74). A CT scan or MRI should be considered in patients with deteriorating neurological examinations, seizures, persistent fevers, enlarging head circumference, persistently elevated protein concentration or polymorphonuclear cells in the CSF, or when brain abscesses or fluid collections are suspected (75). All patients with meningitis caused by *Citrobacter diversus* should have a radiological examination soon after diagnosis to detect brain abscesses that occur in as many as 75% of patients (76).

TREATMENT

Antibacterial Therapy

Initial empiric treatment of neonatal bacterial meningitis should be directed against the most commonly encountered gram-positive and gram-negative pathogens in this age group. A regimen of ampicillin and either cefotaxime or an aminoglycoside, such as gentamicin or amikacin, are recommended (75). Once results of cultures and susceptibility tests are available, the initial antimicrobial regimen can be adjusted accordingly.

For group B streptococcal meningitis the combination of ampicillin or penicillin with an aminoglycoside is preferred for the full course of therapy or until repeat CSF cultures after 48–72 h of therapy are sterile and results of testing demonstrate that the strain is susceptible to ampicillin. It is recommended that the minimum inhibitory concentration (MIC) and minimum bactericidal concentration (MBC) for the organism be determined to be certain that it is not tolerant (i.e., inhibited but not easily killed by usually achieved concentrations of ampicillin in CSF). Treatment is usually given for 10–14 days, depending on the clinical response.

When disease is caused by gram-negative enteric bacilli, we recommend a third-generation cephalosporin, usually cefotaxime, and an aminoglycoside. Because eradication of the organisms from CSF is frequently delayed (average of 3–4 days) and outcome is worse the longer the delay (77,78), we recommend performing daily CSF examinations until sterilization is confirmed. If the organism is susceptible to the cephalosporin and once the CSF culture is sterile, the aminoglycoside can be discontinued provided the patient's condition has improved. Therapy is continued for a minimum of 3 weeks or for 2 weeks after the first negative CSF culture, whichever is longer. If there are any abnormalities in the CSF (e.g., cell count and predominance of neutrophils, hypoglycorrhachia, and elevated protein concentration) at the end of therapy, it is advisable to continue therapy with weekly CSF examinations until these indices have normalized. Administration of an aminoglycoside into the lumbar intrathecal space or intraventricularly is not recommended because the former was shown to be no better than parenteral therapy (78) and the latter resulted in a significantly higher case fatality rate (79).

When nosocomial infection is suspected, knowledge of the common pathogens and their susceptibilities for that neonatal unit is critical for selecting effective antimicrobial therapy. For methicillin-resistant *S. aureus* and for coagulase-negative staphylococci, vancomycin is recommended. For enterococcal meningitis, the combination of ampicillin or vancomycin and an aminoglycoside is preferred. With anaerobic infection, clindamycin or metronidazole is appropriate. The use of chloramphenicol in the newborn infant is not recommended, unless there are no other suitable alternatives, because of the necessity to monitor serum concentrations to avoid potential cardiac (gray baby syndrome) and central nervous system toxicity (80).

Table 4 gives the recommended antimicrobial regimens and durations of treatment for the common neonatal pathogens. The dosages of antibiotics should be individualized according to the chronological age and weight of the infant. Table 5 provides the most commonly used antimicrobials for neonatal infections and the recommended dosages according to weight and age. Additional information about regimens and dosages for treatment of neonatal meningitis is provided in standard texts (81).

Table 4 Recommended Therapy for Most Common Pathogens of Neonatal Meningitis

Organism	Antimicrobial therapy	Minimum duration[a]	Special considerations
Group B *streptococcus*	Ampicillin + aminoglycoside or penicillin + aminoglycoside	10–14 days	Combination therapy is preferred until susceptibilities available and for ampicillin-tolerant strains (i.e., MBC:MIC ratio > 32)
Staphylococcus aureus	Methicillin	21 days	For methicillin-resistant strains vancomycin is indicated
Staphylococcus epidermis	Vancomycin	21 days	Longer duration of therapy depending on clinical response and necessity to remove the indwelling catheter
Listeria monocytogenes	Ampicillin + aminoglycoside	14 days	Combination synergistic in vitro; many physicians discontinue the aminoglycoside after 3–5 days
Gram-negative enteric bacilli	Cefotaxime + aminoglycoside	Minimum 21 days[b]	Cefotaxime preferred over other third-generation cephalosporins because of its renal excretion and greater experience with its use
Candida albicans	Amphotericin B or amphotericin B + flucytosine	30–45 mg/kg total dose	Length of therapy depends on clinical response; monitor renal function closely
Herpes simplex	Acyclovir	14–21 days	Length of therapy depends on clinical response

[a]Duration of therapy depends on clinical and bacteriological response; the numbers given are to be considered as minimum course of therapy.
[b]Eradication of pathogen from CSF is often delayed; therapy should be at least 21 days or 14 days after first negative CSF culture, whichever is longer.

We recommend reexamination and culture of the cerebrospinal fluid at the end of therapy in all cases of neonatal meningitis to confirm eradication of the pathogens and normalization of the CSF indices. If there is evidence of persistent inflammation indicated by elevated WBC, neutrophils, and/or protein concentrations or decreased glucose values, it is recommended to continue therapy until results normalize.

Antivirals

Both vidarabine and acyclovir are effective in treating HSV meningoencephalitis. Because of low toxicity and ease of administration, acyclovir is the preferred treatment (82). Currently, there are no specific antienteroviral agents and the treatment of enteroviral meningitis consists mainly of supportive care.

Antifungals

Antifungal therapy for disseminated infections should be with intravenous amphotericin B, which has been shown to be effective if instituted promptly. Because of the potential for toxicity from amphotericin B, mainly hypokalemia and nephrotoxicity, close monitoring of electrolyte values

Table 5 Recommended Dosages (mg/kg) of the Most Commonly Prescribed Antibiotics for Neonatal Infections and the Intervals for Administration

		Weight < 1200 g	Weight 1200–2000 g		Weight > 2000 g	
Antibiotic	Routes	Age 0–4 wk	Age 0–7 days	Age > 7 days	Age 0–7 days	Age > 7 days
Amikacin	IV, IM	7.5 q18–24h	7.5 q12–18h	7.5 q8–12h	10 q12h	10 q8h
Ampicillin	IV, IM	50 q12h	50 q12h	50 q8h	50 q8h	50 q6h
Cefotaxime	IV, IM	50 q12h	50 q12h	50 q8h	50 q12h	50 q8h
Ceftazidime	IV, IM	50 q12h	50 q12h	50 q8h	50 q12h	50 q8h
Gentamycin	IV, IM	2.5 q18–24h	2.5 q12–18h	2.5 q8–12h	2.5 q12h	2.5 q8h
Methicillin	IV, IM	50 q12h	50 q12h	50 q8h	50 q8h	50 q6h
Metronidazole	IV, PO	7.5 q48h	7.5 q24h	7.5 q12h	7.5 q12h	15 q12h
Penicillin G	IV	50,000U q12h	50,000U q12h	75,000U q8h	50,000U q8h	50,000U q6h
Tobramycin	IV, IM	2.5 q18–24h	2.5 q12–18h	2.5 q8–12h	2.5 q12h	2.5 q8h
Vancomycin	IV	15 q24h	15 q12–18h	15 q8–12h	15 q12h	15 q8h

and renal function is necessary (83). Administration of amphotericin B should start with a dose of 0.25 mg/kg administered over 2–4 h with increments of 0.25 mg/kg every 24 h until a maximum daily dosage of 1 mg/kg is achieved (84). The length of therapy should be adjusted to the clinical and microbiological response; as a rule a total dosage of 30–40 mg/kg is recommended (85). Addition of flucytosine to the amphotericin B regimen has the potential advantage of synergism (86,87), better penetration through the blood-brain barrier, and good activity against *Candida* species that are potentially resistant to amphotericin B such as *C. parapsilosis* (87–90). Liposomal amphotericin B has the advantage over amphotericin B of reduced renal toxicity and the potential of using higher dosages. To date there are no controlled studies in neonates to make definitive recommendations (91).

Drug Monitoring

It is important to monitor peak and trough concentrations of aminoglycosides and vancomycin in order to adjust dosages and dosing intervals to avoid toxicity. Blood samples for drug concentrations should be obtained once the steady state has been achieved (usually after the third to fifth dose).

Adjunctive Therapies

Intravenous human immunoglobulin (IVIG) has been used for treatment of early-onset sepsis in an attempt to provide antibodies against the bacterial pathogens that the neonate usually lacks. On the basis of data derived from animal and human studies, Hill (92) believes a single dose of 750 mg/kg of IVIG can be valuable in treating some neonates with severe early-onset sepsis.

Steroid Therapy

Dexamethasone therapy for *H. influenzae* meningitis in older infants and children has been shown to be beneficial in reducing neurological sequelae (mainly hearing loss) when compared with placebo-treated children (93,94). Although the pathogenesis and molecular pathophysiology of neonatal meningitis is most likely comparable with that found in older children and in experimental meningitis, at present there are no data to recommend the routine use of dexamethasone for the treatment of neonatal meningitis.

COMPLICATIONS AND OUTCOME

Common abnormalities observed during the acute course of meningitis include inappropriate secretion of antidiuretic hormone with ensuing hyponatremia, water retention and risk of seizures secondary to the electrolyte derangements (95), and increased ICP which needs careful monitoring to avoid diminished cerebral perfusion with resulting tissue ischemia.

Subdural effusions are also common in the course of bacterial meningitis in older infants, and most resolve spontaneously. They presumably occur commonly in neonates as well. Drainage is recommended when infection of these fluid collections is suspected (i.e., subdural empyema). Brain abscesses are a common complication of *Citrobacter diversus* meningitis (76,96) and can occur in infants with other causes of meningitis. They are associated with a poor prognosis as indicated by mortality rates as high as 50% and a high incidence of neurological impairment in the survivors (97).

Case fatality rates range from 15–30% depending on the etiology, immaturity of the infant, and experience of the medical staff in managing infants with bacterial meningitis (98,99). Significant neurological sequelae develop in 30–50% of survivors of neonatal meningitis (77,78,100,101).

Sequelae include hearing deficit, hydrocephalus, seizures, motor disabilities, and abnormalities in language skills. Hydrocephalus is common in neonatal meningitis and is usually communicating, resulting from adhesive exudate of the arachnoid membrane around the cisterns in the base of the brain.

Estimates of the frequency of hearing loss vary from 2.4–29% (102,103). Occasionally hearing loss noted at the time therapy is stopped may become less severe on follow-up examinations. Because hearing deficits are common in survivors of bacterial meningitis, a hearing evaluation with evoked response audiometry is recommended at time of discharge from the hospital or soon thereafter. Repeated evaluations are recommended after discharge if the initial examination is abnormal.

PREVENTION

Improving maternal health through appropriate, consistent, and timely prenatal care could have a major impact in decreasing the incidence of invasive neonatal infections by decreasing risk factors that ultimately make the newborn infant more vulnerable to infections, such as prematurity and low birthweight.

Chemoprophylaxis

The American College of Obstetrics and Gynecology and the American Academy of Pediatrics have advised the routine use of intravenous ampicillin during labor in mothers with positive rectal and genital cultures for group B *Streptococcus* and with risk factors for neonatal sepsis (52,104–106). The management of the infants born to these mothers should be individualized.

Immunoprophylaxis

The use of IVIG for prophylaxis of neonatal infections is controversial, although most of the controlled studies have shown no beneficial effect (92). Baker et al. (107) showed significant reduction in the incidence of nosocomial infections mainly with *C. albicans* and coagulase-negative *Staphylococcus* when premature infants (<1750 g) were given IVIG.

REFERENCES

1. Siegel JD, McCracken GH, Jr. Sepsis neonatorum. N Engl J Med 1981; 304:642–647.
2. Wientzen RL, McCracken GH, Jr. Pathogenesis and management of neonatal sepsis and meningitis. Current Problems in Pediatrics VIII. Chicago: Year Book Medical Publishers, 1977:3–61.
3. Sáez-Llorens X, McCracken GH, Jr. Bacterial meningitis in neonates and children. Inf Dis Clin North Am 1990; 4:623–644.
4. Smith ES. Purulent meningitis in infants and children: a review of 409 cases. J Pediatr 1954; 45: 425–436.
5. Umaña MA, Odio CM, Castro E, Salas JL, McCracken GH, Jr. Evaluation of aztreonam and ampicillin vs amikacin and ampicillin for treatment of neonatal bacterial infections. Pediatr Inf Dis J 1990; 9: 175–180.
6. Howard KB, McCracken GH Jr, Trujillo H, Mohs E. Amikacin in newborn infections: Comparative pharmacology with kanamycin and clinical efficacy in 45 neonates with bacterial diseases. Antimicrob Agents Chemother 1976; 10:205–210.
7. Moreno MT, Vargas S, Pareda R, Sáez-Llorens X. Neonatal sepsis and meningitis in a developing Latin American country. Pediatr Inf Dis J 1994; 13:516–520.
8. Sessions CF. Bacterial infections of the newborn. In: Taeusch HW, Ballard RA, Avery ME, eds. Schaffer and Avery's Diseases of the Newborn. Philadelphia: WB Saunders, 1991:350–369.

9. Klein JO, Marcy SM. Bacterial sepsis and meningitis. In: Remington JS, Klein JO, eds. Infectious Diseases of the Fetus and Newborn Infant. Philadelphia: WB Saunders, 1994:835–890.
10. Overall JC. Neonatal bacterial meningitis. J Pediatr 1970; 76:499–511.
11. Louvois J, Blackbourn J, Hurley R, Harvey D. Infantile meningitis in England and Wales: a two year study. Arch Dis Child 1991; 66:603–607.
12. Dillon HC, Gray E, Pass MA, Gray BM. Anorectal and vaginal carriage of group B *Streptococcus* in pregnancy. J Inf Dis 1982; 145:794–799.
13. Baker CJ, Barrett FF. Transmission of group B *Streptococcus* among parturient women and their neonates. J. Pediatr 1973; 83:919–925.
14. Baker CJ, Edwards MS. Group B streptococcal infection. In: Remington JS, Klein O, eds. Infectious Diseases of the Fetus and Newborn Infant. Philadelphia: WB Saunders, 1994:980–1028.
15. Interview with Carol Baker, MD. Prevention of group B streptococcal disease. Pediatr Inf Dis J 1983; 2:1–5.
16. Paredes A, Wong P, Mason EO Jr., Taber LH, Barrett FF. Nosocomial transmission of group B *Streptococcus* in a newborn nursery. Pediatrics 1977; 59:679–682.
17. Rench MA, Baker CJ. Neonatal sepsis caused by a new group B streptococcal serotype. J Pediatr 1993; 122:638–640.
18. Gotoff SD, Kliegman RM. The fetus and the neonatal infant. In: Berhman RE, Kleigman RM, Nelson WE, Vaughan VC, eds. Nelson Textbook of Pediatrics. Philadelphia: WB Saunders, 1992:509–512.
19. Robbins JB, McCracken GH Jr., Gotshlich EC, Orskov F, Orskov I. *Escherichia coli* K1 capsular polysaccharide associated with neonatal meningitis. N Engl J Med 1974; 290:1216–1220.
20. Sarff LD, McCracken GH Jr., Schiffer MI. Epidemiology of *E. coli* K1 in healthy and diseased newborns. Lancet 1975; 1:1099–1104.
21. Svare J, Andersen LF, Langhoff-Roos J, Madsen H, Bruun B. Maternal-fetal listeriosis: two case reports. Gyn Obstet Invest 1991; 3:179–181.
22. Schlech WF, Lavigne PM, Bortolussi RA, et al. Epidemic listeriosis: evidence for transmission by food. N Engl J Med 1983; 308:203–206.
23. Linnan MJ, Mascola L, Lou XD, et al. Epidemic listeriosis associated with Mexican-style cheese. N Engl J Med 1988; 319:823–828.
24. Larsson S, Cederberg A, Ivarsson S, Sranberg L, Cronberg S. *Listeria monocytogenes* causing hospital-acquired enterocolitis and meningitis in newborn infants. Br Med J 1978; 2:473–474.
25. Faix RG. Invasive neonatal meningitis: comparison of *albicans* and *parapsilosis* infection. Pediatr Inf Dis J 1992; 11:88–93.
26. Buchs S. *Candida* meningitis: a growing threat to premature and full term infants. Pediatr Inf Dis J 1985; 4:122–123.
27. Baley JE, Kliegman RM, Fanaroff AA. Disseminated fungal infections in very low-birth-weight infants: clinical manifestations and epidemiology. Pediatrics 1984; 73:144–152.
28. Stuart SM, Lane AT. *Candida* and *Malassezia* as nursery pathogens. Semin Dermatol 1992; 11:19–23.
29. Modlin JF. Perinatal echovirus infections: insights from a literature review of 61 cases of serious infection and 16 reported nursery outbreaks. Rev Inf Dis 1986; 9:918–926.
30. Modlin JF. Neonatal enterovirus infections. Semin Inf Dis 1994; 5:70–77.
31. Dagan R, Hall CB, Powell KR, Menegus MA. Epidemiology and laboratory diagnosis of infections with viral and bacterial pathogens in infants hospitalized for suspected sepsis. J Pediatr 1989; 115:351–356.
32. Modlin JR. Fatal Echovirus 11 disease in premature neonates. Pediatrics 1980; 66:775–780.
33. Brown ZA, Benedetti J, Ashley R, et al. Neonatal herpes simplex virus infection in relation to asymptomatic maternal infection at the time of labor. N Engl J Med 1991; 324:1247–1252.
34. Arvin AM, Prober CG. Herpes simplex virus infections. Pediatr Inf Dis J 1990; 9:765–767.
35. Whitley RJ, Arvin AM. The natural history, pathogenesis and treatment of neonatal herpes simplex virus infections. Semin Pediatr Inf Dis 1994; 5:56–63.
36. Murphy TV, White KE, Pastor P, et al. Declining incidence of *Haemophilus influenzae* Type b disease since introduction of vaccination. JAMA 1993; 269:246–248.
37. Adams WG, Deaver KA, Cochi SL, et al. Decline of childhood *Haemophilus influenzae* type B (Hib) disease in the Hib vaccine era. JAMA 1993; 269:221–226.

38. Sáez-Llorens X, Siegel JD. Neonatal septicemia, meningitis and pneumonia. In: Gellis SS, Kagan BM, eds. Current Pediatric Therapy—14. Philadelphia: WB Saunders, 1993:544–549.
39. Cates KL, Rowe JC, Ballow M. The premature infant as a compromised host. Curr Probl Pediatr 1983; 13:1–63.
40. Tunkel AR, Wispelwey B, Scheld WM. Pathogenesis and pathophysiology of meningitis. Inf Dis Clin North Am 1990; 4:555–581.
41. McCracken GH Jr., Mustafa MM, Ramilo O, Olsen KD, Risser RC. Cerebrospinal fluid interleukin-1 and tumor necrosis factor concentrations and outcome from neonatal gram-negative enteric bacillary meningitis. Pediatr Inf Dis J 1989; 8:155–159.
42. Sáez-Llorens X, Ramilio O, Mustafa MM, Mertsola J, McCracken GH Jr. Molecular pathophysiology of bacterial meningitis: current concepts and therapeutic implications. J Pediatr 1990; 116:671–684.
43. Sáez-Llorens X, McCracken GH Jr. Mediators of meningitis: therapeutic implications. Hosp Pract 1991; 26:68–77.
44. Nelson JS. Pathology of the central nervous system. In: Kissone JM, ed. Anderson's Pathology. St. Louis: Mosby Company, 1990:2154–2155.
45. Friede RL. Purulent leptomeningitis in newborns and infants. In: Friede RL, ed. Developmental Neuropathology. Berlin: Springer-Verlag, 1989: 169–179, 180–181.
46. Wigglesworth JS. Miscellaneous conditions affecting the fetus and neonate. In: Wigglesworth JS, Singer DB, eds. Textbook of Fetal and Perinatal Pathology. Boston: Blackwell Scientific 1991:838–841.
47. Kessler SL, Dajani AS. *Listeria* meningitis in infants and children. Pediatr Inf Dis J 1990; 9:61–63.
48. Faix RG. Systemic *Candida* infections in infants in intensive care nurseries: high incidence of central nervous system involvement. J Pediatr 1984; 105:616–622.
49. Butler CM, Baker CJ. *Candida*: an increasing important pathogen in the nursery. Pediatr Clin North Am 1988; 35:542–563.
50. Bendel CM, Hostetter M. Systemic candidiasis and other fungal infections in the newborn. Semin Pediatr Inf Dis 1994; 5:35–41.
51. Whitley RJ, Lawrence C, Arvin AM, et al. Changing presentation of herpes simplex virus infection in neonates. J Infect Dis 1988; 158:109–116.
52. Klein JO. Neonatal sepsis. Semin Pediatr Inf Dis 1994; 5:3–14.
53. Philip AGS, Hewitt JR. Early diagnosis of neonatal sepsis. Pediatrics 1980; 65:1036–1041.
54. Squire E, Favara B, Todd T. Diagnosis of neonatal bacterial infections: hematologic and pathologic findings in fatal and nonfatal cases. Pediatrics 1979; 64:60–64.
55. Akenzua GI, Hui YT, Milner R, Zipursky A. Neutrophil and band counts in the diagnosis of neonatal infections. Pediatrics 1974; 54:38–42.
56. Manroe BL, Weinberg AG, Rosenfeld CR, Browne R. The neonatal blood count in health and disease. I. Reference values for neutrophilic cells. J Pediatr 1979; 95:89–98.
57. Bonadio WA. Incidence of serious infections in afebrile neonates with history of fever. Pediatr Inf Dis J 1987; 6:911–914.
58. Philip AGS. Detection of neonatal sepsis of late onset. JAMA 1982; 247:489–492.
59. Visser VE, Hall RT. Urine culture in the evaluation of suspected neonatal sepsis. J Pediatr 1979; 94:635–638.
60. Sarff LD, Platt LH, McCracken GH. Cerebrospinal fluid evaluation in neonates: comparison of high risk infants with and without meningitis. J Pediatr 1976; 88:473–477.
61. Rodriguez AF, Kaplan SL, Mason EO. Cerebrospinal fluid values in the very low birth weight infant. J Pediatr 1990; 116:971–974.
62. Naidoo BT. The cerebrospinal fluid in the healthy newborn infant. S Afr Med J 1968; 42: 933–935.
63. Bonadio WA. The cerebrospinal fluid: physiologic aspects and alterations associated with bacterial meningitis. Pediatr Inf Dis J 1992; 11:423–432.
64. Rotbart HA. Diagnosis of enteroviral meningitis with the polymerase chain reaction. J Pediatr 1990; 117:85–89.
65. Schletinger Y, Sawyer MH, Storch GA. Enteroviral meningitis in infancy: potential role for polymerase chain reaction in patient management. Pediatrics 1994; 2:157–162.

66. Powell, KR, March SM. Laboratory aids for diagnosis of neonatal sepsis. In Remington JS, Klein JO, eds. Infectious diseases of the fetus and newborn infant. Philadelphia: WB Saunders, 1994:1223–1239.
67. Fauerborn SA, Capps WI, Jones JC. Use of latex agglutination testing in diagnosing pediatric meningitis. J Fam Pract 1992; 34:176–179.
68. Gray LD, Fedorko DP. Laboratory diagnosis of bacterial meningitis. Clin Microbiol Rev 1992; 5: 130–145.
69. Maxson S, Lewno MJ, Schutze GE. Clinical usefulness of cerebrospinal bacterial antigen studies. J Pediatr 1994; 125:235–238.
70. Troendle-Atkins J, Demmler GJ, Buffone GJ. Rapid diagnosis of herpes simplex virus encephalitis by using the polymerase chain reaction. J Pediatr 1993; 123:376–380.
71. Uren EC, Johnson PD, Montanoro J, Gilbert GL. Herpes simplex virus encephalitis in pediatrics: diagnosis by detection of antibodies and DNA in CSF. Pediatr Inf Dis J 1993; 12:1001–1006.
72. Rotbart HA. Diagnosis of enteroviral meningitis with polymerase chain reaction. J Pediatr 1990; 117:85–89.
73. Schlesinger Y, Sawyer MH, Storch GA. Enteroviral meningitis in infancy: potential role for polymerase chain reaction in patient management. Pediatrics 1994; 94:157–162.
74. Smith RR. Neuroradiology of intracranial infections. Pediatr Neurosurg 1992; 8:92–104.
75. Feigin RD, McCracken GH, Klein JO. Diagnosis and management of meningitis. Pediatr Inf Dis J 1992; 11:785–814.
76. Curless RG. Neonatal intracranial abscess: two cases caused by *Citrobacter* and a literature review. Ann Neurol 1980; 8:269–272.
77. McCracken GH Jr. The rate of bacteriologic response to antimicrobial therapy in neonatal meningitis. Am J Dis Chil 1977; 123:947–953.
78. McCracken GH Jr., Mize SG. A controlled study of intrathecal antibiotic therapy in gram-negative enteric meningitis of infancy. Report of the neonatal meningitis cooperative study group. J Pediatr 1976; 89:66–72.
79. McCracken GH Jr., Mize SG, Threlkeld N. Intraventricular gentamicin therapy in gram-negative bacillary meningitis of infancy. Report of the second neonatal meningitis cooperative study group. Lancet 1980; 1:787–791.
80. Laferriere CI, Marks MI. Chloramphenicol: properties and clinical use. Pediatr Inf Dis J 1982; 1: 257–264.
81. Nelson JD. Therapy for neonatal sepsis. Semin Pediatr Inf Dis 1994; 5:15–19.
82. Whitley RJ, Arvin AM, Prober CG, et al. Predictors of morbidity and mortality in neonatal herpes simplex infection. N Engl J Med 1991; 324:450–454.
83. Baley JE, Kliegman RM, Faranoff AA. Disseminated fungal infection in very low birth weight infants: therapeutic toxicity. Pediatrics 1984; 73:153–157.
84. Nelson JD. Antifungal therapy. In Pine JW, Jr., ed.: Pocketbook of Pediatric Antimicrobial Therapy. Baltimore: Williams & Wilkins, 1995:54–55.
85. Butler KM, Ranch MA, Baker CJ. Amphotericin B as a single agent in the treatment of systemic candidiasis in neonates. Pediatr Inf Dis J 1990; 9:51–56.
86. Montgomerie JZ, Edwards JE, Guze LB. Synergism of amphotericin B and 5-fluorocytosine for *Candida* species. Pediatr Inf Dis J 1975; 132:82–86.
87. Faix RG. *Candida parapsilosis* meningitis in a premature infant. Pediatr Inf Dis J 1983; 2:462–464.
88. Baley JE, Meyers C, Kliegman RM, Jacobs MR, Blumer JL. Pharmacokinetics, outcome of treatment and toxic effects of amphotericin B and 5-fluorocytosine in neonates. J Pediatr 1990; 116:791–797.
89. Johnson DE, Thompson TR, Green TF, Ferrieri P. Systemic candidiasis in very low birth weight infants. Pediatrics 1984; 73:138–143.
90. Sanchez PB, Cooper BH. *Candida lusitaniae*: sepsis and meningitis in a neonate. Pediatr Inf Dis J 1988; 7:758–759.
91. Lackner H, Schwinger W, Urban C. Lyposomal amphotericin B (AmBisome) for treatment of disseminated fungal infection in two infants of very low birth weight. Pediatrics 1992; 89:1259–1262.
92. Hill HR. Intravenous immunoglobulin use in the neonate: role in prophylaxis and therapy of infection. Pediatr Inf Dis J 1993; 12:549–558.

93. Lebel MH, Freij BJ, Syrongiannopoulus GA, et al. Dexamethasone therapy for bacterial meningitis: results of two double-blinded, placebo-controlled trials. N Engl J Med 1988; 319:964–971.
94. Odio CM, Faingezicht I, Paris M, et al. The beneficial effects of early dexamethasone administration in infants and children with bacterial meningitis. N Engl J Med 1991; 324:1525–1531.
95. Kaplan SL, Feigin RD. The syndrome of inappropriate secretion of antidiuretic hormone in children with bacterial meningitis. J Pediatr 1978; 92:758–761.
96. Graham DR, Band JD. *Citrobacter diversus* brain abscess and meningitis in neonates. JAMA 1981; 265:1923–1925.
97. Renier D, Flandin C, Hirsch E, Hirsch JF. Brain abscess in neonates. A study of 30 cases. J Neurosurg 1988; 69:877–882.
98. Ziai M, Haggerty RJ. Neonatal meningitis. N Engl J Med 1958; 259:314.
99. Groover RV, Sutherland JM, Landing BH. Purulent meningitis of newborn infants. N Engl J Med 1961; 264:1115–1121.
100. Sell SHW, Merrill RE, Doyne EO, Zimsky EP. Long-term sequelae of *Haemophilus influenzae* meningitis. Pediatrics 1972; 49:206–211.
101. Sell SHW. Long-term sequelae of bacterial meningitis in children. Pediatr Inf Dis J 1983; 2:90–93.
102. Vienny H, Despland PA, Lutschg J, Deonna T, Dutoit-Marco ML, Gander C. Early diagnosis and evolution of deafness in childhood bacterial meningitis a study using brainstem auditory evoked potentials. Pediatrics 1984; 73:579–586.
103. Kaplan SL, Goddard J, Van Kleeck M, Catlin FI, Feigin RD. Ataxia and deafness in children due to bacterial meningitis. Pediatrics 1981; 68:8–13.
104. American Academy of Pediatrics. Committee on Infectious Diseases and on Fetus and Newborn. Guidelines for prevention of group B Streptococcal infection by chemoprophylaxis. Pediatrics 1992; 90:775–778.
105. Boyer KM, Gotoff SP. Prevention of early-onset neonatal group B streptococcal disease with selective intrapartum chemoprophylaxis. N Engl J Med 1986; 314:1665–1669.
106. Baker CJ. Recommended intrapartum prophylaxis of group B *Streptococcus*. Inf Dis Clin North Am 1992; 6:41–55.
107. Baker CJ, Melish ME, Hall RT, Cast DT, Vasan U, Givner LB. Intravenous immune globulin for the prevention of nosocomial infection in the low-birth-weight neonates. N Engl J Med 1992; 327: 213–219.

3

Neurological Disorders Associated with Human Immunodeficiency Virus Infections in Children

Anita L. Belman
State University of New York at Stony Brook, Stony Brook, New York

HISTORICAL PERSPECTIVE

The first cases of pediatric acquired immunodeficiency syndrome (AIDS) were reported over a decade ago (1–3). Since then, human immunodeficiency virus 1 (HIV-1) infection has become one of the leading causes of morbidity and mortality in children, in this country and worldwide. HIV-1–related neurological disorders are common, add significantly to the morbidity of the disease, and often have devastating complications. This chapter will focus on the neurological and neurobehavioral aspects of pediatric HIV-1 infection. Epidemiological and clinical features of pediatric HIV-1 infection and AIDS will be briefly reviewed.

PEDIATRIC HIV-1 INFECTION

Viral Transmission and Time of Infection

Pediatric HIV-1 infection results from maternal-infant transmission (vertically acquired or congenital HIV-1 infection), from transfusion with contaminated blood or blood products, or, in some cases, from sexual abuse.

Vertically Acquired HIV-1 Infection

Of children born to infected mothers, a 13–45% rate of maternal-fetal transmission has been reported (4–6). Transmission may occur in in utero, during labor and delivery, or by breast feeding (4,7). However, it is not yet certain what proportion of maternal-fetal transmission occurs during gestation, in which trimester (first, second, or third), or what proportion occurs during labor and delivery. Current evidence suggests that, although first trimester in utero transmission is well documented (8–10), transmission during the third trimester and at parturition is probably more common (7,11–24).

Transfusion-Acquired HIV-1 Infection

Prior to HIV-1 blood screening, recipients of HIV-contaminated blood or blood products included individuals with hemophilia or other coagulation defects, children with illnesses that required blood transfusions (e.g., leukemia), and sick neonates. Transfusion-acquired HIV-1 infection was the cause of most teenage AIDS cases.

Nomenclature

For the purposes of epidemiological surveillance, the Centers for Disease Control (CDC) initially defined AIDS in children under age 13 with the same restrictive clinical case definition as adults (i.e., documentation of an opportunistic infection or an AIDS-related malignancy was required). Additionally, primary (congenital) or secondary immunodeficiency disorders and congenital infections had to be excluded. After HIV-1 was identified as the etiological agent, and with the advent of serological testing for the presence of anti–HIV-1 antibodies in 1985, only a small proportion of children with confirmed HIV-1 infection and HIV-1–related disease manifestations were found to fit the case definition criteria for AIDS. Two subsequent revisions by the CDC broadened the case definition criteria. In 1985, biopsy-proven lymphoid interstitial pneumonitis was included as an indicator condition of AIDS in children (25). In 1987, a major revision substantially expanded the criteria (26). This system for classifying children with HIV-1 infection or those born to mothers with HIV-1 infection was based on laboratory evidence of HIV-1 infection, immunological function, and a spectrum of clinical manifestations, further classified as P-2 conditions (Table 1) (27). AIDS-defining conditions are listed in Table 2. The most recent CDC revision (1994) is based on three parameters: (1) infectious status, (2) clinical status, and (3) immunological status (Table 3) (28). The revised classification system reflects the child's disease and establishes mutually exclusive categories.

Epidemiology

Infants and Children

The worldwide increase in the number of AIDS cases in women of childbearing age is paralleled by an increasing number of children with congenital HIV-1 infection. Maternal-infant transmission currently accounts for virtually all reported new cases in the United States (4). The true number of HIV-1–infected children is unknown since surveillance systems have relied on identification of children with clinical manifestations of AIDS. In the United States, it is estimated that there are 15,000–20,000 HIV-1–infected infants and children (4). It is also estimated that since 1988, approximately 6000–7000 HIV-1–infected women have given birth to a live-born infant each year. Assuming a 20% transmission rate of infection from mother to infant, 1200–1400 HIV-1–infected infants will have been born each year. The World Health Organization projects that by the year 2000, 3 million women and children will die from HIV-related disease, and cumulatively 10 million children will be born infected (7,29,30).

Adolescents

Adolescents aged 13–19 comprised less than 1% of total AIDS cases in the United States in 1993. However, statistics show that 20% of total AIDS cases are now in the 13- to 29-year age group. Given that it may take about 10 years between infection with HIV and the onset of symptoms, it can be assumed that many of these young adults were infected as adolescents.

In the past, transfusion-acquired HIV-1 infection had been the most common cause of infection in adolescents. However, with the advent of HIV-1 blood screening, the percentage of all cases that this group represents has declined. Currently the most common risk factors for adolescents

Table 1 CDC Classification System for HIV in Children, 1987

CLASS P-0. INDETERMINATE INFECTION
- Infants < 15 months born to infected mothers but without definitive evidence of HIV infection or AIDS

CLASS P-1. ASYMPTOMATIC INFECTION
- Subclass A. Normal immune function
- Subclass B. Abnormal immune function
  - Hypergammaglobulinemia, T4 lymphopenia, decreased T4-to-T8 ratio, or absolute lymphopenia
- Subclass C. Immune function not tested

CLASS P-2. SYMPTOMATIC INFECTION
- Subclass A. Nonspecific findings (at least two for >2 months)
  - Fever, failure to thrive, generalized lymphadenopathy, hepatomegaly, splenomegaly, enlarged parotid glands, persistent or recurrent diarrhea
- Subclass B. Progressive neurological disease
  - Loss of developmental milestones or intellectual ability, impaired brain growth, or progressive symmetrical motor deficits
- Subclass C. Lymphoid interstitial pneumonitis
- Subclass D. Secondary infectious diseases
  - Category D-1. Opportunitistic infections in CDC case definition
    - Bacterial: mycobacterial infection (noncutaneous, extrapulmonary, or disseminated); nocardiosis
    - Fungal: candidiasis (esophageal, bronchial, or pulmonary), coccidioidomycosis, disseminated histoplasmosis, extrapulmonary cryptococcosis
    - Parasitic: *P. carinii* pneumonia, disseminated toxoplasmosis with onset > 1 month of age, chronic cryptosporidiosis or isosporiasis, extraintestinal stsrongyloidiasis
    - Viral: cytomegalovirus disease (onset > 1 month of age), chronic mucocutaneous/disseminated herpes (onset > 1 month of age), progressive multifocal leukoencephalopathy
  - Category D-2. Unexplained, recurrent, serious bacterial infections (two or more in 2 years)
    - Sepsis, meningitis, pneumonia, abscess of an internal organ, bone/joint infections
  - Category D-3. Other infectious diseases
    - Includes persistent oral candidiasis, recurrent herpes stomatitis (at least two episodes in 1 year), multidermatomal or disseminated herpes zoster
- Subclass E. Secondary cancers
  - Category E-1. Cancers in AIDS case definition
    - Kaposi's sarcoma, B-cell non-Hodgkin's lymphoma, or primary lymphoma of brain
  - Category E-2. Other malignancies possibly associated with HIV
- Subclass F. Other conditions possibly caused by HIV
  - Includes hepatitis, cardiopathy, nephropathy, hematological disorders, dermatological diseases

Source: Refs. 26, 27.

are sexual exposure and intravenous drug use (IVDU). In fact, it is estimated that approximately 65% of adolescents aged 13–19 years and 90% of 20- to 24-year-olds with AIDS were infected through either one of these routes. Unfortunately, the number of new adolescent cases is steadily increasing (4,22,31–33). Adolescents with vertically acquired HIV-1 infection presently comprise a small percentage of adolescent cases. However, as children are living longer, it can be anticipated that this percentage will rise (see below).

Table 2 Diagnoses That Indicate AIDS (1993 CDC Revised Surveillance Definition for AIDS)

Candidiasis of the trachea, bronchi, or lungs[a]
Candidiasis of the esophagus[a,b]
Multiple or recurrent bacterial infections[c]
Invasive cervical cancer[d]
Coccidioidomycosis, disseminated or extrapulmonary[c]
Cryptococcosis, extrapulmonary[a]
Cryptosporidiosis, chronic intestinal[a]
Cytomegalovirus disease (other than liver, spleen, nodes) onset at age > 1 month[a]
Cytomegalovirus retinitis (with loss of vision)[a,b]
HIV encephalopathy[c]
Chronic herpes simplex ulcer (> 1 month duration) or pneumonitis or esophagitis onset at > 1 month of age[a]
Histoplasmosis, disseminated or extrapulmonary[a]
Isopsoriasis, chronic intestinal (> 1 month duration)[c]
Kaposi's sarcoma[a,b]
Lymphoid interstitial pneumonitis[a,b]
Lymphoma, primary brain[a]
Lymphoma (Burkitt's or immunoblastic sarcoma)[c]
Mycobacterium avium complex or *M. kansasii*, disseminated or extrapulmonary[a]
M. tuberculosis or acid-fast infection (species not identified), disseminated or extrapulmonary[c] or pulmonary[d]
Pneumonia, recurrent[d]
P. carinii pneumonia[a,b]
Progressive multifocal leukoencephalopathy[a]
Toxoplasmosis of brain, onset at age > 1 month[a,b]
Wasting syndrome caused by HIV[c]

[a]If indicator disease is diagnosed definitively (e.g., biopsy, culture) and there is no other cause of immunodeficiency, laboratory documentation of HIV infection is not required.
[b]Presumptive diagnosis of indicator disease is accepted, if there is laboratory evidence of HIV infection (1987 addition).
[c]Requires laboratory evidence of HIV infection (1987 addition).
[d]Requires laboratory evidence of HIV infection (1993 addition; adults and adolescents).

PATHOPHYSIOLOGY

The Retrovirus; HIV-1

HIV-1, the etiological agent of AIDS, is an RNA retrovirus that belongs to the lentivirus subfamily of nononcogenic cytopathic retroviruses. The virus, isolated in 1983, was found to replicate in and lyse activated human CD4 cells. Like other retroviruses, HIV-1 contains reverse transcriptase. This makes possible the transcription of DNA from genomic RNA (contrary to the conventional informational flow from DNA to RNA to protein). The provirus, DNA, is integrated into the host cells, where it may replicate, remain latent, and replicate at a restricted rate. Structurally, HIV-1 is similar to other retroviruses. Double-stranded RNA and polymerase (POL) are found in the core. This is surrounded by proteins (GAG) that may have common sequences between related retroviruses. The outer envelope is derived from the host cell lipid bilayer in which viral glycoproteins (ENV) have been inserted. These include the transmembrane protein, gp41, and the external protein, gp120, which contains the ligand to the CD4 receptor and the sequence determining macrophage tropism. The virus matures by budding from the surface of cells or into vacuoles within the cells. The viral genome contains three major segments coding

Table 3 CDC Pediatric Human Immunodeficiency Virus (HIV) Classification, 1994

	Clinical categories			
Immunological categories	N: No signs/ symptoms	A: Mild signs/ symptoms	B: Moderate signs/ symptoms	C: Severe signs/ symptoms
No evidence of suppression	N1	A1	B1	C1
Evidence of moderate suppression	N2	A2	B2	C2
Severe suppression	N3	A3	B3	C3

Source: Ref. 28.

for the structural proteins, which begins with GAG (the core protein), then POL (the polymerase), and ENV (the envelope proteins). In addition, there are several regulatory proteins.

Lentiviruses or "slow viruses" are species specific and have long incubation periods and mechanisms to evade immune clearance and to target specific organs. They cause persistent infection, multisystem disease, and a chronic encephalitis (reviewed in Ref. 34). HIV-1 targets the immune system, the nervous system, and other organ systems, causing a wide spectrum of disease. The most severe form of the disease results in AIDS (see Tables 1 and 2).

Immunodeficiency

The human peripheral blood CD4+ T lymphocyte is a principal target of the retrovirus. There is "tropism" of the viral glycoprotein 160 for the CD4+ molecule on the helper T cell, which results in progressive loss of circulating CD4+ lymphocytes and in the ratio of T4 to T8 cells. (The T8 cell population, a subset of T lymphocytes, is active in cell-mediated cytotoxicity and suppression.) Hypothesized mechanisms for this loss include apoptosis (programmed cell death), antibody and complement-mediated cytolysis, V-B gene deletion of the T-cell receptor due to superantigen activation, CD4+ cell syncytium formation, and autoimmune reactions (35). Several studies also suggest that the pathogenicity of HIV-1 strains increases during the course of infection. This is evidenced by the formation of syncytial cell in vitro (36).

One of the first immunological abnormalities in children may be impairment of B-cell function, manifested by polyclonal hypergammaglobulinemia, spontaneous B-cell proliferation, and increased in vitro spontaneous production of immunoglobulin. Although the quantity of immunoglobulins is elevated, there is a diminished in vivo vaccine response to both T-cell–dependent and independent antigens as well as decreased responses to B-cell mitogens (37,38). In vitro studies demonstrate diminished lymphocyte proliferation to B-cell mitogens. The decreased antibody responses predispose these infants and children to serious bacterial infections (including meningitis), which at times may be overwhelming. The B-cell activation may also result in polyclonal polymorphic B-cell lymphoproliferative disorders, such as lymphoid interstitial pneumonitis, parotitis, and unusual B-cell–related complications such as B-cell lymphomas.

Increased production of autoantibodies may also result from B-cell dysfunction. Circulating immune complexes, antinuclear antibodies, antibody to double-stranded DNA, red cell antibodies, and antiplatelet antibodies have been reported (38). Hypogammaglobulinemia, another manifestion of B-cell dysfunction, has also been noted in some infants with severe advanced disease.

The virus may also exert other direct and indirect effects on the developing infant that, in turn, may have effects that depend on the developmental stage of the specific organ system. It is likely that the developmental maturational stage of the nervous and immune system is an important variable when exposed to the direct or indirect effects of the virus. Fetal thymic abnormalities suggest that an interaction between the virus and the developing fetal immune system may account for the early and severe immune deficiency observed in 15–25% of congenitally infected HIV-1 infants (described below). The pathophysiological mechanism is as yet unclear; both induction of an immune deficiency in utero and a state of immune tolerance have been proposed (39,40).

A large number of peripheral and tissue-based immunocytes are chronically infected, with HIV-1 persisting as a stationary cell intermediate from which HIV may be induced. HIV-1–infected macrophages are also infected with high frequency in brain, spinal cord, lymphatic, and lung tissue; it has been hypothesized that this may parallel organ-specific manifestations of HIV-1 disease. It is unknown whether overall virus burden in peripheral blood reflects the level of compartmentalization of HIV-1 in tissues and whether differences in relative tissue distribution of the retrovirus may contribute to differences in the clinical outcome. It is possible that the subsequent disease course may be determined in part by tissue distribution and by the maturity of CD4 cells and bone marrow–derived myelomonocytic cells in the immature host (41). Additional factors, including differential timing of infection, strain of virus, increased sequence diversity, and the high mutation rate of specific HIV-1 genes, may allow the virus to evade immune surveillance and persist within the host. Emergence of genotypic variants with altered biological activity, such as increased replication rate and cytopathicity, may also increase the pathogenicity of the virus (41,42).

HIV-1–Associated Central Nervous System Disease

Much has been learned about the biology of HIV-1, the cells it infects, and the mechanisms by which viral entry into cells occurs. However, how HIV exerts its effects on the nervous system, i.e. the neuropathophysiological mechanisms is still being elucidated and is the focus of ongoing research (see Chap. 13).

Direct HIV-1 central nervous system (CNS) infection has been confirmed in numerous clinical, neuropathological, and virological studies (Table 4). HIV-1 infects cells of macrophage lineage (macrophages, microglia, perivascular macrophages) and astrocytes. Virus has been demonstrated in the cerebrospinal fluid (CSF) of asymptomatic patients, as well as symptomatic patients (43–45), and in first- and second-trimester fetal brain tissue (8,9,46). The latter suggests that CNS invasion may occur during or soon after maternal-fetal transmission, in at least some patients.

Table 4 Detection of HIV-1 CNS Infection

CSF
Isolation of HIV—co-cultivation techniques
Detection of HIV-1 p24—antigen-capture assay
Anti-HIV-1 antibody—ELISA and Western blot
Intrathecal synthesis of anti-HIV-antibody
Brain
Detection of HIV-1 DNA/RNA—in situ hybridization
Southern blot
Detection of HIV-1 proteins—immunocytochemistry
Visualization of viral particles—electron-microscopy
Increased levels of virus in brain—Southern blot

Source: Refs. 43, 45, 64, 72.

However, despite evidence of early HIV-1 CNS invasion, the development of clinical neurological disease in most patients seems to occur parallel with the development of severe immunodeficiency. As noted below, however, some patients do develop progressive neurological dysfunction as their AIDS indicator condition and in the absence of severe systemic disease.

Localization

HIV-1 is most frequently localized in cells of bone-marrow lineage (see Refs. 47 and 48 for review). These include blood-derived macrophages, intrinsic microglia (the resident mononuclear phagocytic system of the brain), and multinucleated giant cells, formed by the fusion of these cell types (productive infection). Endothelial cell infection has also been reported, but not consistently. In vitro studies show that HIV-1 can infect neuronal and glial cell lines (astrocytes, oligodendrocytes), and there is recent in vivo evidence that glia in children may also be infected (49,50), but this may be restricted infection.

The precise mechanism of HIV-1–mediated neuropathology, features of which are listed in Table 5, is not well understood. In many cases of clinically severe neurological disease, neuropathological findings are relatively mild with little to no evidence of active infection or inflammation. Even in cases with more marked pathological findings, the proportion of infected cells is limited and does not always correlate with the clinical course. This discrepancy has suggested that other factors besides direct cellular damage by HIV-1 may be important in pathogenesis (see Chap. 13) (34). Table 6 lists proposed mechanisms of neural dysfunction.

Experimental studies suggest that products of the immune system, e.g., cytokines, and of the virus may lead to cell dysfunction and to cell death (50–53). Gp120 is toxic to cultured neurons and leads to cell death by causing an increase in cytosolic calcium. This "coat" protein may also sensitize neurons to glutamate-induced cell death mediated at the NMDA receptor (54,55). Neurotoxins such as arachidonic acid metabolites, glutamate, and cytokines released from infected macrophages and astrocytes also lead to activation of the NMDA receptor (50,52,56). It also appears that calcium activation of nitric oxide synthetase and synthesis of nitric oxide may be the final common path to neuronal-excitotoxic cell death.

It is unclear whether one or several neuorpathophysiological processes underlie the clinical diversity described above. It may be that different pathogenetic mechanisms account, at least in part, for different clinical expressions and patterns of pediatric HIV-1–associated CNS disease syndromes. Distinct clinical CNS syndromes may in some subsets of children reflect a continuum of the disease process, with different stages of disease progression. In others, clinical findings may reflect separate and distinct pathophysiological processes. In still other subsets of patients, these processes may coexist or interlink and may be manifested clinically by overlapping signs and symptoms. In other words, it is currently uncertain if there is one or several causes for HIV-1–associated CNS disease(s) syndromes. However, to this investigator, it seems most likely that

Table 5 Neuropathological Findings in Brain

Gross
Cerebral atrophy of variable degrees
Ventricular enlargement
Widening of sulci
Attenuation of deep cerebral white matter
Microscopic
HIV-1 encephalitis
Foci of inflammatory cells, microglia, macrophages, MGC

Table 6 Possible Factors in Pathogenesis of HIV-Associated Disease

Direct effects of infection on neural cells
Cytopathic effects with level virus replication below detection
Defective infection (nef expression in astrocytes)
Soluble factors
Viral proteins
Blocking of transmitters (gp120 homology with VIP)
Toxicity of viral polypeptides (p120, tat, nef in cultures)
Monokines
Direct toxicity (TNF-α on oligodendrocytes)
Indirect stimulating astrocytes (arachidonate metabolites)
Excitotoxins (quinolinic acid)
Autoimmunity
Deregulation and T-cell activation
Molecular mimicry (gp41 and astrocytes)
Opportunistic infections
Transactivation or enhancing effects (CMV, EB, HSV, and HTLV)
Other agents (*Mycobacterium*, *Mycoplasma*, *Rochalimaea henselae*)

Source: Adapted from Ref. 34.

different neuropathophysiological mechanisms account, at least in part, for the different clinical expressions of this syndrome complex.

The route of CNS entry is unclear. The frequent finding of basal ganglia calcification suggests a hematogenous route consistent with early CNS infection. It also points to the vulnerability of the immature vasculature and perhaps to selective tropism for the basal ganglia (and other subcortical structures) and its resident microglia (57).

Developmental-Maturational Considerations

Issues concerning neuropathophysiological mechanisms and clinicopathological correlations are as germane to the understanding of HIV-1–associated CNS disease in children as they are in adults. The study of pediatric HIV-1–associated CNS disease syndromes is even more complex, as developmental-maturational issues must also be considered.

Adult HIV-1 CNS infection and disease occurs in mature, fully developed, and completely myelinated nervous systems. The immune system and CNS elements of the mononuclear phagocyte system (intrinsic microglia) are also fully developed. Vertically transmitted HIV-1 infection occurs in an immature evolving organism. The CNS is probably infected early in the course of infection. The timing of maternal-fetal transmission (i.e., perinatal versus during gestation, and which trimester—early, mid, late?) is likely to be a most important factor. Indeed mother-to-infant transmission may occur during gestation in some patients, while in others, infection may occur during the perinatal period. The developmental stage of the nervous and immune system when exposed to the direct or indirect effects of the virus must be considered. Innumerable dynamic interactions occur between these two systems during development, which will interact in complex ways with HIV-1 variables. The maturational stage of CNS development when exposed to the virus will also vary, and this is likely to manifest as different patterns of HIV-1 CNS disease (58).

In addition, it is also necessary to remember that we are dealing with two different trajectories: the developing brain and a "progressive" neurological disease. During the designated time period of a particular study or observational period, it is not always clinically apparent (1) if the rate of CNS maturation and development is exceeding the slower rate of the ongoing disease process(es), (2) if the disease process is quiescent, or (3) if the disease process has been abated or arrested by therapeutic interventions. Currently there are few prognostic indicators to predict rapidity and severity of CNS disease.

Cerebral atrophy is a common finding in both adults and children. Recent quantitative and morphometric studies in adults have identified loss of neurons with a frontal and temporal predominance and loss of dendritic arborizations (reviewed in Ref. 59) (60–63). Similar studies have not been performed in pediatric AIDS. However, it is tempting to speculate that comparable abnormalities in some subsets of children result in poor brain growth and development of acquired microcephaly. Interference with synaptogenesis could explain in part developmental "delays" and cognitive impairment. Astrogliosis, an extremely common finding in pediatric AIDS, is also noted in the simian immune deficiency virus "model." Of note is a recent report showing the correlation between this pathological finding and functional impairment in juvenile macaques.

CLINICAL PRESENTATION AND CLINICAL COURSE

As the name of the disease implies, HIV-1 infection produces progressive immune dysfunction. Significant immunological abnormalities result in clinically apparent disease. The occurrence of more frequent and more severe infections with common childhood pathogens, the occurrence of opportunistic infections, and the development of progressive neurological dysfunction are clinical manifestations of these abnormalities. In children, both cellular and humoral factors are clearly affected (38).

Natural History of HIV-1 Infection

The natural history of vertically acquired HIV-1 infection differs from that of adults. The adverse effects of HIV-1 on the developing immune and nervous systems often result in more rapid onset of clinical symptoms (development of AIDS) and progression to death. A bimodal evolution of symptomatic HIV-1 disease in children is reported from both clinical and data-modeling studies (4,39,85,86). The first occurs in infancy, and the second later in childhood. In fact, there may actually be a trimodal evolution with the third "hump" (albeit much smaller) occurring later, in the pre- and early adolescent years (4,7,33,87,88). In this older age group of congenitally infected children, the time from infection to onset of symptomatic disease may be as long as 10 or more years.

Infants in the first group generally present between 3 and 8 months of age with symptoms including "HIV encephalopathy," *Pneumocystis carinii* pneumonitis (PCP), cytomegalovirus (CMV) infection, and/or wasting syndrome ("failure-to-thrive") (22). The risk for developing this early and severe form of the disease is highest in infants who as neonates had detectible p24 antigen serum levels and, to a lesser extent, in those who as neonates had positive viral culture or PCR (5,22,23,89).

The second group of children have a more indolent initial course. Lymphoid interstitial pneumonitis (LIP) is their most frequent AIDS indicator disease, and it carries a much better prognosis for survival (4). Evidence of other lymphoproliferative processes characteristic of pediatric HIV-1 infection is frequent and includes lymphadenopathy, hepatosplenomegaly, and parotid gland enlargement. Multiple or recurrent bacterial infections, ranging from otitis media, pneumonia, bone and joint infection, to sepsis and meningitis are common in both groups, as is failure to thrive, persistent oral candidiasis, and chronic or recurrent diarrhea.

Although this second group of congenitally infected children have a form of HIV-1 disease that progresses more slowly, the disease may ultimately involve many organ systems, including the nervous system, heart (cardiomyopathy), and kidneys (nephritis or nephrosis). With progression, T-cell abnormalities develop, including lymphopenia, low absolute numbers of CD4 cells, poor in vitro lymphocyte proliferation to T-cell mitogens, and cutaneous anergy. Children may develop infections indicative of defects in cell-mediated immunity. Pneumocystis pneumonia is the most common opportunistic infection. Disseminated candidiasis, MAI, and disseminated invasive cytomegalovirus are the next most frequent. Cytomegalovirus may produce colitis, pneumonitis, or retinitis. Other infections include disseminated ulcerative herpes simplex infections, cryptosporidiosis, and, more rarely, toxoplasmosis (47).

Neoplasms may also develop and include primary CNS B-cell lymphoma, non-Hodgkin's lymphoma that may metastasize to the CNS, and, less commonly, Kaposi sarcoma. A polyclonal, polymorphic B-cell lymphoproliferative disorder has been described with nodular lymphoid lesions in the lung as well as other organs and with lymphoid infiltrate in both nodal and extranodal sites (90). It is not yet clear whether this associated disorder is a variant of lymphoma.

The difference between these two distinct populations of children with different rates of disease progression and survival does not appear to be related to any difference in PCP prophylaxis, specific AIDS-defining conditions, antiviral therapy, or birthweight (4). Clinical studies do suggest that the stage of maternal HIV-1 illness (viremia) during pregnancy and delivery may be an important factor (11,15,18,23,91). The different rates of disease progression may also relate to viral load, phenotype of the infecting virus, and timing of fetal infection (4).

It is not yet certain if the natural history of HIV-1 infection in adolescents is more similar to that of adults than children. The former appears likely.

Neurological Aspects

HIV-1–Associated CNS Disease

Terminology and Definitions. The pediatric AIDS literature contains many terms pertaining to neurological dysfunction associated with HIV-1 infection. At times these terms are used without accompanying descriptors. This has led to much ambiguity due to the lack of clarity about what deficits, impairments, or disabilities the particular child or cohort of children actually had. A consensus report on nomenclature suggested that the term "HIV-associated progressive encephalopathy (PE) of childhood" replace the various terms found in the literature (92). The well-described "late manifestations" were enumerated (see Table 7). However, early manifestations, rate of CNS disease progression, and stage of CNS disease were not delineated or defined.

Initially, a progressive encephalopathy was described, as were more stable neurological impairments. As children were followed longitudinally several patterns of disease were recognized. Based on progression and severity of neurological deficits, the terms "subacute progressive," "plateau" (with improvement; with deterioration), and "static/stable" were introduced to allow further clinical characterization (73).

During the past several years, continued observations of children in both clinical and research settings suggested that the spectrum and diversity of "HIV-1 encephalopathy" is much wider than previously appreciated (see below). The term HIV-1–associated CNS disease syndromes, as used herein, refers to the CNS disorders (including PE) with a constellation of cognitive, motor, and behavioral manifestations, that are currently believed to be related to the effects of HIV-1 CNS infection. It is anticipated that in the future more precise classification and definitions will evolve as clinical features are further delineated and correlated with underlying neuropathophysiological processes.

Table 7 HIV-1–Associated Progressive Encephalopathy of Childhood

Probable (must have each of the following):
1. Evidence for systemic HIV-1 infection:
   a. Infants and children < 15 months
      i. Virus in blood or tissues, or
      ii. Presence of HIV-1 antibody
         and
         evidence of cellular and humoral immune deficiency
         or
         other conditions meeting CDC case definition for AIDS
   b. Children ⩾ 15 months
      i. Antibody or virus in blood or tissues
2. At least one of the following progressive findings present at least 2 months:
   a. Failure to attain or loss of developmental milestones or loss of intellectual ability, verified by standard developmental scale or neuropsychological tests
   b. Impaired brain growth (acquired microcephaly or brain atrophy demonstrated on serial CT or MRI)
   c. Acquired symmetric motor deficits manifested by *two or more* of the following: paresis, abnormal tone, pathological reflexes, ataxia, or gait disturbance
3. Evidence of another etiology, including active CNS opportunistic infection or malignancy, must be sought from history, physical examination, and appropriate laboratory and radiological investigation (e.g., lumbar puncture, neuroimaging). If another potential etiology is present, it is not thought to be the cause of the above cognitive/motor/behavioral/developmental symptoms and signs.

Possible (must have one of the following):
1. Other potential etiology present (must have each of the following):
   a. As above (see Probable) #1 and 2
   b. Other potential etiology is present, but the cause of #2 is uncertain
2. Incomplete clinical evaluation (must have each of the following):
   a. As above (see Probable) #1 and 2
   b. Etiology cannot be determined (appropriate laboratory or radiological investigations not performed)

Source: Ref. 92.

HIV-1–Associated CNS Disease Syndromes: Clinical Presentation and Clinical Course.

Manifestations. The most frequent signs of HIV-1–associated CNS disease are cognitive impairment, poor brain growth/acquired microcephaly, and abnormalities of tone and motor function (64,73,74,93). Mood and behavioral problems also develop with progressive disease.

Rate and Pattern of Disease Progression. The rate of neurological deterioration, "domains" of function most affected, and severity of neurological deficits differ among patient subsets (73,94). Neurological deterioration in some infants and young children will be rapidly progressive (weeks to months). They develop severe and progressive CNS dysfunction resulting in quadriparesis and mental deficiency. Others have progressive and disabling motor deficits, with relatively stable, though at times, impaired, cognitive function and socially adaptive skills. Other children will have more cognitive than motor impairment, whereas still others will have relatively minor and stable motor and cognitive findings (58,95). Moreover, an individual child may have progressive neurological deterioration that occurs over a period of months followed by a relatively stable period, followed by further deterioration.

Age of Onset and Patterns of Neurological Disease. Because of the considerable clinical diversity, we have more recently adapted a classification based on (1) age of onset of clinically apparent disease, (2) domains of function most affected and severity of deficits, and (3) rate and pattern of disease progression (94–96).

Neonates. The vast majority of congenitally HIV-1–infected neonates are clinically well at birth and are indistinguishable from uninfected newborns. Clinically recognizable neurological features of HIV-1–associated CNS disease are exceedingly rare in newborns. Review of the literature reveals single case reports, e.g., neonatal meningoencephalitis ascribed to HIV-1 (91), an infant with seizures, and cranial ultrasonographic evidence of calcification (97).

However, some HIV-1–infected neonates do have neurological problems due to comorbid conditions associated with disorders of the preterm infant, in utero exposure to drugs, or congenital or acquired infections (see below).

Infants and Young Children. The most severe, devastating, and clearly recognized syndrome is HIV-1–associated PE, "severe infantile" form. Age of onset is usually in the first year of life (3–8 months of age) but may begin in the second year. Neurological deterioration results in spastic quadriparesis and mental deficiency. Characteristic features are (1) progressive corticospinal tract (CST) signs, (2) concomitant loss of previously acquired motor milestones or markedly deviant rate of acquiring motor skills, (3) acquired microcephaly, and (4) marked "delays" in mental development. Opisthotonic posturing and rigidity may develop, and are usually superimposed upon spasticity. Pseudobulbar signs may also develop, and feeding difficulties are frequent. The children develop a characteristic "masklike" facial appearance (58,74). They appear alert and wide-eyed but have a paucity of spontaneous facial expression (manifestations of the basal ganglia and subcortical pathology). Despite these features, there is little facial weakness, evidenced by full movement when crying. Patients are hypophonic with decreased spontaneous and responsive vocalizations. Serial head circumference measurements document poor brain growth (acquired microcephaly). As the CNS disease progresses, play deteriorates and previously acquired language skills and/or adaptive skills are lost. The end-stage picture is an apathetic, withdrawn, quadriparetic child, who has markedly impaired higher cortical function (64,73,74,93).

The rate of neurological deterioration in this "subacute PE" may be slowly progressive, with an insidious decline. Some patients, however, will have rapid deterioration (over weeks), whereas others will have an episodic course. There are periods of deterioration interrupted by periods of relative neurological stability (74).

Psychometric measures document a decline in the composite cognitive score [e.g., Mental Developmental Index (MDI) of the Bayley Scales of Infant Development (BSID)]. The Mental Developmental Age (MDA) may remain stable (no or little gain in "raw" score) (Figs. 1 and 2). With advanced disease it may actually decline (73).

A less severe neurological course may also occur in the first 2 years of life. This has been termed "plateau" (73). Rate of progression and severity of mental and motor deficits differ among subsets of patients. Some infants and young children are hypotonic and have delays in attaining motor milestones. For example, some children will not be able to sit unsupported until 12 months of age and not walk independently until 24 months of age (neurologically "normal" infants sit by 6 months and walk by 12 months). Mental development may also be "delayed," and concomitant expressive language delays and deficiencies are common (64,98–100).

Some of these children will with time develop a "diparesis-type" syndrome. Other children will have even further neurological deterioration (58,73,95).

In the toddler or young child, early signs of motor involvement include a change of gait. Children begin to toe walk and develop increased tone and hyperreflexia in the lower extremities (95). Rate of progression and severity of deficits vary. In some children independent ambulation is maintained for years. They have a mildly spastic gait, or hyperreflexia and clumsiness, often associated with impairment of fine motor ability (94). In others, progression is more rapid, and

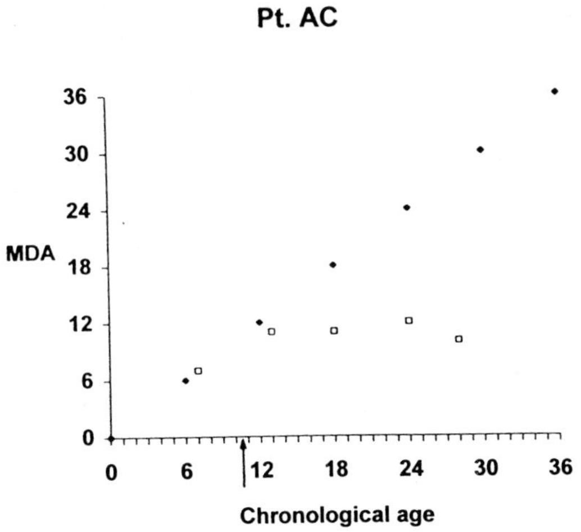

Figure 1 Patient AC. Serial psychometric evaluations [Mental Development Index of Bayley Scales of Infant Development (BSID)] expressed as equivalent mental developmental age (MDA) of a child whose neurological examination (arrow) showed a change at age 10 months, and was considered abnormal. Between ages 12–18 months, long tract signs were slowly progressive. By age 24 months, she could no longer sit unsupported, was quadriplegic, and had severe cognitive impairment. Note her MDA was within the "average" range until age 13 months. Thereafter, she made little mental developmental progress. By age 28 months, formal testing showed loss of previously acquired skills. MDA = Mental developmental age (months); ◆ = MDA normative population; □ = MDA patient.

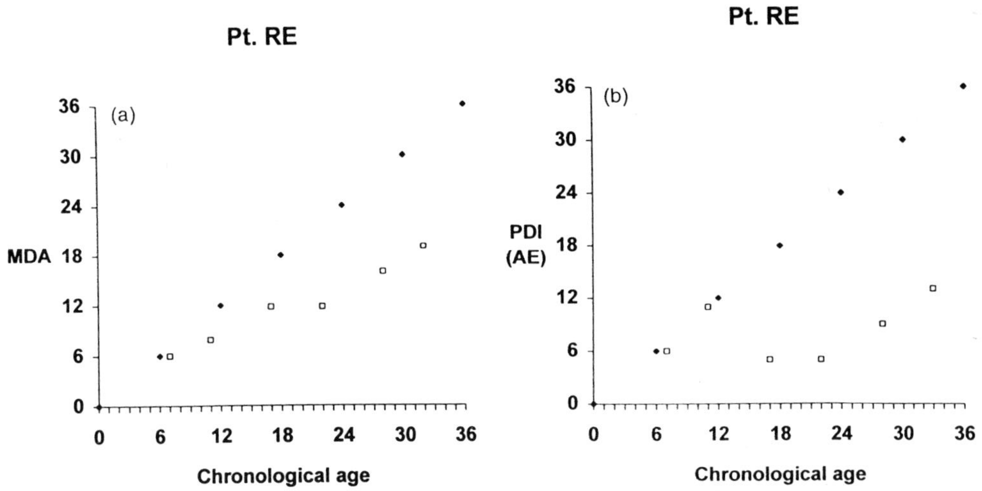

Figure 2 (a) Patient RE. Patient RE developed a "diparesis" syndrome in his second year of life. Note between ages 12–18 months he continued to acquire new "mental" skills; however, his rate of developmental progress slowed; between ages 18–24 months he gained few new skills; although mental development proceeds [between ages 24–36 months], his cognitive function deviates significantly from the norm. MDA = Mental developmental age (months); CA = chronological age (months); ◆ = MDA normative population; □ = MDA patient. (b) PDI (AE) scores for patient RE. Note the discrepancy between MDA and PDI (AE). PDI = Psychomotor Developmental Index of the BSID expressed as age equivalent (AE); ◆ = PDI (AE) normative population; □ = PDI (AE) patient.

they require orthotics to maintain independent ambulation. Severity in some children is more marked, and they become wheelchair bound within months. Some children will progress to quadriparesis (73,94).

Poor brain growth can usually be documented in younger patients by serial head circumference measurements. Serial neuorimaging studies may show atrophy and documented acquired microcephaly (64,73,74,93).

Cognitive impairment is frequent, although degree of impairment may range from "borderline" intelligence to mild or moderate ranges of retardation. Cognitive problems become evident as the rate of mental development deviates from the norm or declines. Over time, although the child may gain further cognitive, language, and socially adaptive skills, the rate of acquisition of these new skills deviates from the norm (Fig. 2) and, in some cases, from the child's previous rate of developmental progress (73). Serial psychometric evaluations show a decline in the composite cognitive score. The MDA, which reflects the "raw" scores, may gradually increase. There is an incremental rise over time, but the slope of the curve clearly deviates from the norm (see Fig. 2) (58). Less commonly, the MDA will remain the same for a period of months. Loss of milestones and previously acquired abilities is not observed.

A subset of these children who had a prolonged stable course will ultimately go on to further neurological deterioration—"plateau followed by further deterioration." The course then becomes similar to that of "subacute PE" (73). In contrast, other children with plateau show improvement. They steadily acquire additional developmental skills, and their rate of acquisition of new skills accelerates compared to their previous performance. This course then becomes similar to "stable/static" course (Fig. 3) (73).

It is noteworthy that we have now followed some children from birth in our prospective studies who had marked "delays" in motor and mental development (94,100,101). They continued to acquire milestones and skills although the rate and quality deviate from the norm. They manifested a "stable/static" course in infancy and early childhood. Many of these children did not have in utero exposure to drugs. This suggests that HIV-1 may compromise the normal developmental process.

School-Age Children. Cognitive decline, loss of interest in school performance, social withdrawal, increased emotional lability, worsening of attention deficit disorders (ADD), and psychomotor slowing are reported as signs of HIV-1–associated PE (73,95,102–104). With advancing disease, psychometric tests show a decline in composite IQ score (see Ref. 73). Motor involvement of varying severity is common. There is usually hyperreflexia, with or without increased extensor tone in the lower extremities. Clumsy and poor fine motor ability and coordination are often noted. Progressive long tract signs, movement disorders, cerebellar signs, and myelopathy may also develop. In the advanced stages of CNS disease, the child has cognitive impairment and at end stage is apathetic and abulic (105).

The term "static" encephalopathy was used by our group in the early years of the AIDS epidemic to describe a group of preschool and school-aged youngsters who had (1) varying degrees of cognitive and/or motor impairment, (2) histories of developmental abnormalities (delays in acquisition of language and motor milestones), and (3) *no history* of "loss of milestones" or progressive neurological deficits (73,74,105,106). Longitudinal follow-up documented a pattern of continued but impaired development. Developmental and intelligence quotients ranged from low average or borderline to retarded. These scores remained relatively stable during the study period (105–107). The children acquired new skills and abilities at a rate fairly consistent with their level of functioning at initial evaluation, although their rate was slower than expected for their age. Motor dysfunction was also common. The most frequent findings were hyperreflexia, increased tone in the lower extremities, and poor coordination and fine motor skills. Some children had a mildly spastic gait. This pattern was in direct contrast to the

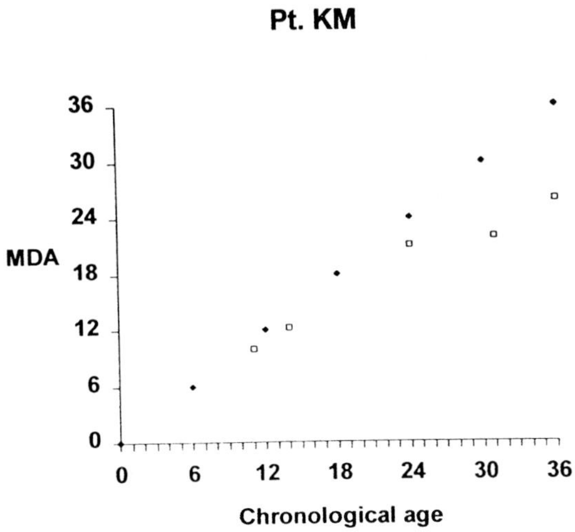

Figure 3 **MDA scores for a child whose neurological examination was considered abnormal in infancy. Although nonfocal, he had mild axial hypotonia and marked delays in motor development (sat unsupported at age 11 months, walked independently at age 23 months).**

deteriorating neurological pattern described above. It still remains unclear what role, if any, HIV-1 plays in this syndrome. It is possible that abnormalities are related to concurrent or previous effects of HIV-1 CNS disease. However, confounding uncontrolled factors (reviewed in Refs. 58 and 104) have made interpretation and analysis difficult. Continued follow-up of children who were enrolled as infants in controlled studies should help clarify this question.

Adolescents. It is as yet unknown whether HIV-1–associated CNS disease manifestations in adolescents differ in early signs and progression from that of adults or of children, although it is anticipated that manifestations will be similar to adults.

Neurobehavioral and Cognitive Profiles of HIV-1–Infected Children

The declining pattern of neuropsychological function as assessed by serial psychometric and neurodevelopmental measures in infants and children with HIV-1–associated CNS disease is described above. The question of early signs of HIV-1–related neuropsychological impairment and domains affected remains unanswered. Several domains of cognitive function have been reported to be affected in children with symptomatic HIV-1 infection who *did not* have overt clinical evidence of "PE" and who functioned in the borderline, low, or average range of cognitive ability (99,100,103,108–110). These include relative deficits in attention, perceptual motor function, and expressive language and memory. Mood and affective disorders were noted as well.

Attention. In adults, attentional problems are reported as an early manifestation of HIV-1–associated dementia. The *new* onset of difficulties with attention have also been described in some children who developed PE. Therefore, attentional problems may indeed be an early behavioral manifestation of HIV-1–associated CNS disease. However, the problem that confronts clinicians is that, although attention deficit hyperactivity disorders (ADHD) occur with significant frequency in children with HIV-1 infection, the prevalence of ADHD is relatively high in the general population, and particularly in children with in utero exposure to drugs, alcohol, those born prematurely, and those who have strong family histories of ADHD (confounding comorbid conditions) (104). Recent well-designed studies of HIV-1–infected children, HIV-1 seroreverters, and their controls have shown a high rate of ADHD and other disruptive behavior disorders in all three groups. The investigators suggested, as have others, that genetic and/or background factors common to this high-risk group of children may be important factors (109–113). Thus it is not yet certain if ADD/ADHD, as such, can be attributed to HIV-1 CNS disease unless it is of new onset.

Visual-Spatial and Organization Skills. Selective deficits in visual-spatial and organizational skills in HIV-1–infected children with "normal" composite IQ scores are reported from several different studies. Cohen et al. studied a cohort of asymptomatic and mildly symptomatic HIV-1–infected children who acquired infection via blood transfusions as neonates (114). Overall IQ test scores did not differ between the cohort and the HIV-1–seronegative control group. However, the investigators reported small but consistently significant differences in motor speed, visual scanning, and cognitive flexibility. This is in agreement with the earlier studies of Diamond and colleagues and, more recently, Tardieu et al. (108,109,115).

Language. Investigators have also noted language-related problems (58,98–100,103). As described above, infants with PE often stop vocalizing (58,95,98), and older children who previously spoke in full sentences may regress and only speak in single words or short phrases (103).

Many children who do not have overt clinical manifestations of HIV-1–associated disease and PE are also noted to have "delayed" language development and impairment of expressive language relative to receptive ability (99,100).

Havens et al. reported preliminary findings from a study of cognitive and language function in school aged HIV-1 infected children (110). The HIV-1–infected children were relatively well and were said to have no evidence of "encephalopathy." The HIV-1–infected cohort showed deficits in short-term memory relative to seroreverters and controls. There was no difference between the groups in general intelligence or language subsets.

However, Wolters et al. (99) recently studied language ability in a cohort of HIV-1–infected children and their controls (non–HIV-1-infected siblings of the case cohort). The HIV-1–infected children were stratified into two groups: "encephalopathic" and "nonencephalopathic." Expressive language impairment was noted in both groups but not their controls. Severity of language dysfunction was marked in the "encephalopathic" group and included impairment of both expressive and receptive ability, with expressive language more affected than receptive. Correlation neuroimaging evidence of atrophy was also noted in the "encephalopathic" group (99).

Mood and Affect. Signs and symptoms of neurobehavioral dysfunction associated with HIV-1 CNS disease were mentioned above. These include flattened affect, lack of social responsiveness, withdrawal, and declining interest in the environment. Manifestations may also include depression, mood swings, agitation, extreme impulsiveness, and new onset (or change) of attentional problems (116).

Coexisting Conditions

Antenatal and Perinatal Complications. The developing nervous system in HIV-1–infected infants, as in non–HIV-1-infected infants, may be adversely affected by maternal conditions and behaviors during gestation (58,95). "High-risk" maternal factors to the developing nervous system include maternal substance use, inadequate maternal nutrition, deficient prenatal care, and premature delivery. Maternal AIDS-associated illness or infections with pathogens other than HIV-1 also adversely affect the infant's developing nervous system.

The question of whether in utero exposure to HIV-1 has a deleterious effect on the neurological status of the uninfected infant was recently addressed in a prospective longitudinal study. Results suggest that maternal HIV-1 (per se) infection during gestation (per se) does not adversely affect the neurological outcome of the infant if the infant is not infected. The neurological and developmental status of "seroreverters" between ages 3 and 24 months was found to be no different from their controls (HIV-1–negative infants born to HIV-1–negative women) (101), although some of the infants were found to have neurological and neurodevelopmental abnormalities. These were present in both seroreverters and controls. Not surprisingly they were often associated with the "high-risk" maternal conditions discussed in this section.

The developing CNS in HIV-1–infected infants, as in non–HIV-1-infected infants, may be adversely affected by CNS complications in the perinatal period. Some of these are interlinked with the "high-risk" maternal factors described above.

Many drug-abusing women with HIV-1 infection are at high risk for premature delivery. The prematurely born HIV-1–infected infant, like any premature infant, is at high risk for developing perinatal CNS complications of the preterm infant. These conditions include hypoxic-ischemic encephalopathy, periventricular leukomalacia, intracranial hemorrhage (intraventricular, intraparenchymal), hydrocephalus, CNS infections caused by common and opportunistic pathogens, CNS "problems" related to systemic conditions, e.g., bronchopulmonary dysplasia, etc. (53).

Psychosocial Factors. Neurobehavioral and neurological function of infants and children with HIV-1 infection may also be affected by coexisting *psychosocial* stressors that occur with significant frequency in this population and that, at times, are both confounding and compounding. Some of these conditions are connected to HIV-1 infection (e.g., death of an HIV-1–infected parent or sibling), whereas others are not. During infancy and early childhood the HIV-1–infected child's development may be adversely affected by a myriad of complex psychosocial stressors, including unstable family units, poverty, maternal illness, death of parents and siblings, changing caretakers, impoverished environments, chronic illnesses, frequent hospitalizations, poor or no school attendance, and painful and unpleasant medical procedures and experiences.

Additional psychosocial stressors that may impact upon the older child and teenager (like children with other chronic illnesses) include, but are not limited to, poor self-esteem and body image, unresolved issues of sexuality, and struggles with issues related to death and dying. Moreover, the child with HIV-1 infection must contend with the societal stigma associated with HIV-1 infection and AIDS itself.

Transfusion-Acquired HIV-1 Infection: Disorders Related to Underlying Illness. Children with transfusion-acquired HIV-1 infection may also have nervous system disorders that predate HIV-1 infection and are related to the underlying disease or therapies for the disease that necessitated the transfusion of blood or blood products in the first place (e.g., hemophilia, other blood dyscrasias, cancer, sick neonates) (58,115,117). (Fortunately, since 1985, with the advent of blood and blood product testing, new cases of transfusion-acquired HIV-1 are virtually nonexistent in the United Sates.)

Cerebrospinal Fluid Findings

HIV-1 has been recovered from the CSF of children with HIV-1–associated CNS disease as well as neurologically normal children. Detectable levels of HIV-1 antigen, intrathecal production of anti–HIV-1 antibodies, oligoclonal bands, and cytokines may be found in some children with PE and static encephalopathy and in neurologically normal children (34,45,118–120). Markers of immune activation are reported to be elevated in children with PE (IL-6, IL-1B) (119). The prognostic significance of these findings is unclear, and to date data are still limited to a few cross-sectional studies of small numbers of patients.

Neuroimaging Findings

Computed Tomography. Computed tomography (CT) examinations of the brain in PE usually show variable degrees of cerebral atrophy and white matter (WM) abnormalities (Table 5) (64,73,74,83,104,121,122). There may be bilateral symmetrical calcification of the basal ganglia (BG) and, less frequently, of the frontal WM (Fig. 4). In general, calcification of the BG is more

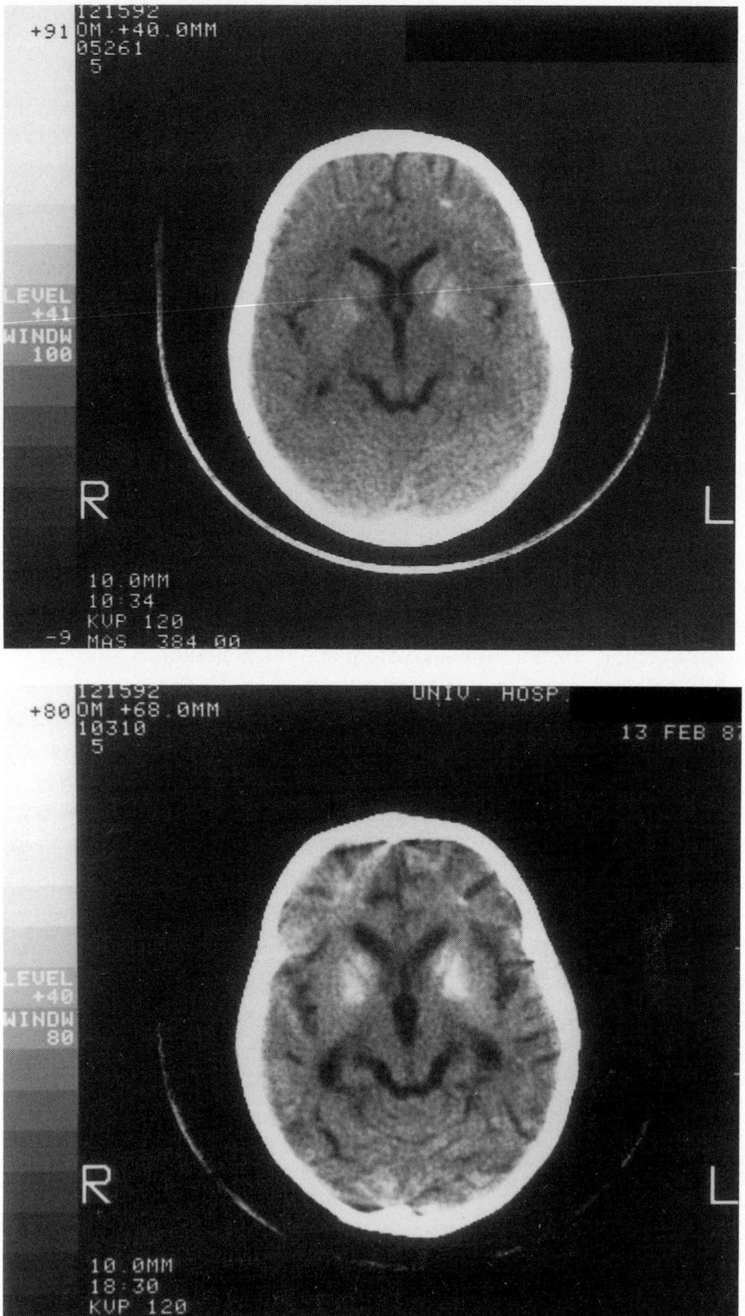

Figure 4 (A) CT scan shows mild cerebral atrophy and bilateral calcification in basal ganglia and frontal white matter. (B) CT 8 months later shows progressive atrophy and calcification.

frequently seen in younger children and those with clinical signs of HIV-1 CNS disease than in older children (121).

Serial studies often show progressive atrophy and WM changes (rarefaction) and, in some cases, progressive calcification of the BG. More recently, a direct correlation between the degree of cerebral atrophy and severity of "encephalopathy" has been reported (121), as has a correlation with behavior and mood (87), thus confirming earlier clinical observations described in early reports. However, it is noteworthy that in some children serial CT studies show no change, even though poor brain growth is demonstrated by serial head circumference and serial clinical examinations show "plateau" or marked delays in mental function (with or without progressive motor findings) (72). It is also noteworthy that some neurologically normal children may have mild to moderate atrophic findings.

Magnetic Resonance Imaging. Magnetic resonance imaging (MRI) may reveal atrophy on T1- and T2-weighted images. T2 images may show abnormal signal intensity in the WM and deep grey structures (58,95,104,123). Tardieu et al. found MRI abnormalities of WM in 40% of HIV-1–infected children (123). Because this finding was present in both neurologically normal and symptomatic children, the investigators suggested that it may serve as a marker for CNS HIV-1 infection. Leukomalacia and cerebral atrophy were found more frequently in patients with clinical evidence of HIV-1–associated PE than in the neurologically normal cohort.

MRI is more sensitive to image WM abnormalities, maturational changes in myelination, and structural abnormalities. CT is more preferable for detecting calcification. Cerebral atrophy is well demonstrated by both techniques.

PET. In a recent study of five neurologically normal children and three children with PE, diffuse hypometabolism and subcortical hypermetabolism were seen in the children with PE, whereas temporo-occipital cortical hypometabolism was seen in the neurologically normal children. Interestingly, Pizzo reported "normalization" of PET in one child after zidovudine (124).

Magnetic Resonance Spectroscopy. Magnetic resonance spectroscopic studies in a limited number of children suggest that there is a lower *n*-acetylaspartate/creatinine ratio in subcortical structures in children with encephalopathy (125).

Neurophysiological Studies

Electroencephalographic studies in children with HIV-1–associated PE may show diffuse mild to moderate slowing of background rhythm. Abnormal evoked potentials including increased central latencies (prolongation of the 1-V interwave latency) and abnormal responses to increased rate of stimulation have also been demonstrated (74,95,114,126–128).

Neuroepidemiology

The true incidence of pediatric HIV-1–associated CNS disease is not yet known. Information derived from the published literature is difficult to interpret because of lack of standardized definition (see terminology), differences in study populations, and difference in study design. A 23.8% prevalence is reported by Tovo et al. in their study of 433 HIV-1 perinatal infected P-2 classified children (129). Blanche and colleagues reported a 20% incidence of HIV-1 encephalopathy by age 3 years in their cohort of patients followed prospectively from birth (18,39). In contrast, studies of children with advanced symptomatic HIV-1 infection and AIDS estimate a frequency of 31–75% (73,75,130,131).

The frequency with which HIV-1–associated PE was reported as the initial AIDS-defining illness has ranged from 12 to 16% (4,86). This contrasts with the much lower figures reported for adults: 0.8–2.2% (132,133).

Extrapolating from the experiences of many investigators, it appears that in general HIV-1–associated CNS disease parallels progression and severity of immunodeficiency and systemic disease. However, it is also very clear that some patients will develop HIV-1–associated CNS disease as their first AIDS-defining illness (58,91,95,134–136).

DIFFERENTIAL DIAGNOSIS

The infant or child with congenital HIV-1 infection may present with several clinical manifestations. Differential diagnosis, therefore, is dependent on the presenting signs and symptoms and the age of the child.

Systemic Manifestations

In infancy, lymphadenopathy, hepatosplenomegaly, thrombocytopenia, anemia, or leukopenia may occur with other congenital or perinatal infections (toxoplasmosis, rubella, cytomegalovirus, herpes, syphilis, Epstein-Barr virus). Moreover, these infections are often associated with immunological abnormalities. However, each of these infections is usually associated with an increased concentration of specific immunoglobulin. Additionally, cytomegalovirus may be cultured in urine or blood, and syphilis can be determined by dark field exam, vRPR antibody titer, and immunoglobulin-FTA (38).

Later in infancy and in childhood if the presenting symptoms are chronic or recurrent infections or opportunistic infections, the most important and likely diagnosis is an immunodeficiency disorder. Primary congenital immunodeficiencies and secondary immunodeficiency disorders are included in the differential diagnosis.

Inherited forms of cellular congenital immunodeficiency diseases that may be considered include severe combined immunodeficiency or variants such as Nezelof syndrome, adenosine deaminase or nucleoside phosphorylase deficiency, Omenn's syndrome, Bare lymphocyte syndrome, severe combined immune deficiency with graft-versus-host disease, and DiGeorge syndrome. Other congenital immunodeficiencies include Wiskott-Aldrich syndrome, ataxia-telangiectasia, X-linked lymphoproliferative syndrome, mucocutaneous candidiasis, agammaglobulinemia, and dysgammaglobulinemia. An appropriate history, examination, and immunological analysis, including HIV-1 serological testing, can usually rule out these conditions.

Hematological disorders that should be considered in the differential diagnosis include neutrophil disorders, reticuloendotheliosis, lymphoma, and idiopathic thrombocytopenic purpura.

Secondary immunodeficiencies include malignancy, malnutrition, nephrotic syndrome, protein-losing enteropathy, and severe diarrhea (38).

Neurological Manifestations

The differential diagnosis in the infant or child who presents with progressive neurological dysfunction includes other neurodegenerative diseases (particularly the progressive genetic metabolic diseases and especially if the child has hepatosplenomegaly) and other CNS infections. A thorough history (including family history), physical and neurological examination, and laboratory studies including neuroimaging and anti–HIV-1-antibody testing (child $>$ 18 months) help to make the diagnosis (see below).

DIAGNOSIS

The goal of the diagnostic workup is to establish the presence or absence of HIV-1 infection and, if present, to determine the stage of the disease, extent of immune dysfunction, and presence or absence of neurological involvement (see Ref. 28).

HIV-1 Infection

Infants

Newborns and young infants (up to 18 months) present special diagnostic challenges. Although the detection of anti–HIV-1-specific IgG antibody in peripheral blood in older children and adults is taken as proof of HIV-1 infection, a positive antibody test in a well infant or young child is uninterpretable, as maternal IgG crosses the placenta and may persist for up to 18 months. Thus, a positive IgG antibody test only confirms the seropositivity of the mother. Other serological markers studied for the purpose of early diagnosis in neonates and infants include HIV-1-specific IgM and IgA. In the neonate, however, IgM studies do not provide consistent enough results for reliable early diagnosis. Studies of IgA (which does not cross the placenta and thus, if present, indicates a specific response of the infant to the virus) have been reported to have a 80% sensitivity in infants 2 months and older. Direct evidence for HIV-1 infection may be sought by HIV-1 culture, polymerase chain reaction (PCR), and assays of circulating p24 in the peripheral blood (137).

Virus Isolation

Viral isolation in infants provides definitive diagnosis of HIV-1 infection. This may be obtained by HIV-1 viral culture, detection of HIV-1 DNA by PCR, or detection of circulating p24 antigen in the peripheral blood (5,23,53,137–151). The diagnostic sensitivity is virtually 100% by age 6 months but less so in the newborn (as noted above).

Children

The initial laboratory evaluation of a child over age 18 months who is suspected of having HIV-1 infection should include HIV-1 serological testing (screening enzyme-linked immunosorbent assay and confirmatory Western blot), a complete blood count, and lymphocyte subsets [CD3, CD4, CD8 (and CD4:CD8 ratio)] enumeration. Other routine diagnostic tests, such as chest x-ray, urine analysis, appropriate cultures for pathogens, a chemistry panel, and IgA, IgM, and IgG levels, may also be warranted. Most children will have a normal blood count, a positive antibody test, elevated immunoglobulin levels, and variable T-cell abnormalities, dependent on the age of the patient and the stage of disease.

Currently, clinical prognostic and therapeutic decisions are based on virological markers of HIV-1 infection (p24 antigen or viral cultures of peripheral blood) and the degree of CD4 lymphopenia relative to normal values for age.

Evaluations of the competence of the immune system, such as lymphocyte proliferative responses to mitogens (phytohemagglutinin, pokeweed mitogen) and antigens (tetanus toxoid, *Candida*, etc.), delayed hypersensitivity skin tests, antibody titers to vaccine antigens (e.g., tetanus, diphtheria, rubeola, *Haemophilus*), and surrogate markers of immune activation, such as B_2-macroglobulin assays, may be used to determine immunological response to therapeutic protocols.

Neurological Involvement

The CNS in HIV-1–infected infants and children may be adversely affected by conditions directly associated with HIV-1 infection. It may also be affected by coexisting, and at times confounding and compounding, conditions that are not HIV-1 related but that occur with significant frequency in this population.

The CNS in HIV-1–infected children may be affected by (1) HIV-1 itself, (2) secondary CNS complications (infections, neoplasms, stroke), (3) metabolic and endocrinological derangements associated with systemic HIV-1 infection and AIDS-related disorders, and (4) toxic or metabolic complications of antiretroviral/antimicrobial therapy.

Therefore, the evaluation of the HIV-1–infected infant or child for neurological involvement requires the clinical skills and major diagnostic tools of the neurologist. The approach to the diagnosis of HIV-1–associated CNS disease, including differential diagnosis (secondary complications, confounding comorbid complications), involves a careful medical and developmental history, HIV-1 systemic disease history, current immunological status, neurological examination, psychological assessment, and neuroimaging studies (58,95).

HIV-Associated CNS Disease

The diagnosis of HIV-1–associated disease is relatively straightforward if the patient has been followed prospectively. Longitudinal assessments of the infant or child will reveal *progressive* dysfunction. The infant may stop vocalizing, lose head control, and develop axial hypotonia and upper motor neuron signs. The toddler or older child may have a change in gait, become hyperreflexic, refuse to walk and, over time, develop progressive CST signs or, less frequently, ataxia. Concomitant cognitive problems with a relative "plateau" or decline in psychometric test scores may also be documented.

The diagnosis is also fairly straightforward if the child, on initial examination, is found to have motor deficits (spasticity, ataxia, weakness, abnormalities of tone, change in gait, etc.), and, by a careful history, either the new onset or progression of motor impairment can be documented (again, when other causes for progressive motor dysfunction have been excluded). Confirmation of progression can at times be obtained by review of family photographs of the child.

However, diagnostic difficulties arise when an HIV-1–infected youngster who was not followed from birth or infancy by the examiner is found at the initial neurological evaluation to have neurological deficits or "delays." Because the frequency of neurological and developmental impairment in this population is high, it is often impossible for the clinician to ascribe these findings to HIV-1–associated CNS disease rather than to possible comorbid conditions. A careful history is paramount. If there are no other risk factors, the diagnosis is fairly certain. The child should have a formal psychological assessment and be reevaluated by the neurologist and psychologist in 2–6 months.

Neuroimaging studies are extremely helpful and in fact are critical. If calcification of basal ganglia is present, it is probable that the child has HIV-1–associated CNS disease. If cerebral atrophy is present in the absence of documented perinatal complications, steroid use, or other known causes of atrophy, the diagnosis becomes extremely likely. Follow-up neuroimaging studies should be requested in addition to the above-mentioned serial neurological and psychological evaluations.

Head circumference measurements are also very helpful. It has been our experience that a careful review of medical records will document at least one or two past head circumference measurements. This allows the examiner to plot serial measurements. The pattern of downward deviation and "crossing percentiles" makes the diagnosis of HIV-1–associated CNS disease likely. Thus, neuroimaging evidence of atrophy and clinical evidence of acquired microcephaly clearly strengthens the diagnosis.

TREATMENT

Antiretroviral agents clearly offer promising therapeutic interventions (see Refs. 35,124,134, 152-155). Improvement of cognition and mood, decrease of CT evidence of brain atrophy, improvement of auditory brain stem responses, and immunological parameters have been documented.

Clinical trials in progress are investigating various antiretroviral agents, different dosage regimens, combination therapies, and immunomodulating agents. New targets for therapy are under investigation, and new protocols are in development.

In parallel are rehabilitation programs, including "infant stimulation programs," therapeutic nursery schools, and special educational classes, physical and occupational therapy programs, and management of pain.

Antiretroviral Therapy

Drugs that treat HIV-1 infection attempt to interfere with the replication of HIV. Targeted points in the growth cycle of the virus include blockage of viral entry (soluble CD4+ preparations), prevention of transcription of RNA to DNA (reverse transcriptase inhibitors), interference with translation (drugs acting on regulatory genes or their proteins), inhibition of assembly (protease inhibitors), and release or virus (interferon) (reviewed in Ref. 47). In the United States, clinical trials with antiretroviral agents have been performed largely by the AIDS Clinical Trials Group of the National Institutes of Health and the National Cancer Institute. There are still relatively limited published data concerning antiretroviral therapy of children with HIV-1 infection.

In clinical trials, children treated with ZVD had improvement in weight gain and growth, stabilization of CD4 counts, a reduction in serum and CSF p24 antigen levels, decrease in immunoglobulin levels, and improvement or stabilization of cognitive function (39,134,152). At the time of this writing, the number of therapeutic agents available for the treatment of HIV-1 infection and its complications is limited. ZVD and DDI are the only antiretroviral agents approved by the FDA for treatment of HIV infection in children under age 13. The agents zalcitabine (ddC; Hivid), stavudine (d4T; Zerit), and lamivudine (3TC; Epivir) are approved for use in adult HIV disease and at the present time are available for investigational use in pediatric patients. In addition to the nucleoside analogue reverse transcriptase inhibitors mentioned above, two HIV protease inhibitors, saquinavir (Invirase) and ritonavir (Norvir), have recently been approved for adult use, and approval of a third protease inhibitor (indinavir; Crixivan) is expected. It is anticipated that these agents will be available for investigational use in pediatrics in the future.

The optimal time to initiate antiretroviral therapy in children is unknown. Currently antiretroviral therapy in recommended for children who either have evidence of significant immunodeficiency or who have defined HIV-associated symptoms (35). It is recommended that initial therapy should begin with DDL or DDI in combination with ZVD (with the caveat that combination therapy may carry a greater risk of toxicity). It should be noted that these recommendations are for HIV-1 infection and not specifically for HIV-1–associated CNS disease.

Several studies have shown improvements in neuropsychological function associated with HIV-1 disease after antiretroviral therapy (AZT, ddC, DDL). Improvements in cognitive and behavioral function were noted in many children who received AZT via continuous parenteral infusion. Intermittent orally administered antiretroviral agents have been efficacious in some children (although improvements were less dramatic than with continuous dosing) (134). With each of these agents, on an individual basis, some patients have shown improvement, some have remained stable, while some have continued to decline. Unfortunately, some children, after an initial favorable response to antiretroviral agents, "relapse" and develop progressive clinical and neuroimaging signs of HIV-1–associated CNS disease (87,156,157).

Infections

Intravenously administered immunoglobulins have been shown to be efficacious in reducing morbidity of infections (158,159).

Pneumocystis pneumonia is the most common serious opportunistic infection and is a major contributing cause of death for HIV-1–infected children with advanced disease. Pneumocystis pneumonia occurs most commonly between 3 and 8 months of age and can often be the presenting manifestation of HIV-1 infection in a previously apparently well infant. Prophylaxis with low doses of trimethoprim-sulfamethoxazole may prevent this infection. It is currently recommended that HIV-1–infected children who have CD4 counts that fall below age-adjusted normal values, or whose percentage of CD4 cells is less than or equal to 20%, or who experience an episode of pneumocystis pneumonia regardless of CD4 count receive prophylaxis.

Varicella-zoster virus, which in most children causes a one-time illness known as chickenpox, can cause significant morbidity in HIV-1–infected children. Primary varicella may be particularly severe, with multiple organ involvement, and may either persist or recur as severe herpes zoster infections. Varicella infections can potentially be prevented by administration of varicella immunoglobulin in exposed children, and complications in children with varicella can potentially be averted through use of acyclovir. The efficacy of varicella vaccine has not been investigated in HIV-1–infected children. HIV-1–infected children are at increased risk for tuberculosis from HIV-1–infected family members with tuberculosis. (HIV-1–uninfected children born to infected parents are also at increased risk for tuberculosis.)

Surveillance and early treatment of tuberculosis infections in family members should prevent tuberculosis in these children. Although BCG vaccine is given routinely to newborns in many countries, it is used infrequently in the United States. It is possible that it may prevent some tuberculosis disease for children of these infected families as well.

Measles can be particularly severe in HIV-1–infected children. Measles may have an atypical presentation in children with advanced HIV-1 disease, occurring without the characteristic rash, making diagnosis difficult and enhancing the opportunity for the child with measles to continue to spread the disease to contacts in the community or medical setting. It appears that measles vaccination is safe and relatively effective, particularly if given early in the HIV-1 disease course; immunoglobulin is also protective for exposed children.

NEUROLOGICAL COMPLICATIONS

Secondary CNS Complications

The common denominator of HIV-1 infection is the development of profound immunosuppression. The patient becomes susceptible to a variety of infections. Neoplasms (mainly lymphoma) may also develop. Stroke is another complication of pediatric HIV-1 infection and is related to infection or other AIDS-associated illnesses (73). Infants and children may have more than one complication and may also have coexisting HIV-1–associated CNS disease.

Secondary CNS complications must be considered in the differential diagnosis of the child with HIV-1 infection who presents with the new onset of neurological deficits, headache, seizures, or mental status changes.

CNS Infections

Infants and children with HIV-1 infection are at risk for CNS infections caused by the usual childhood pathogens as well as opportunistic organisms (reviewed in Refs. 37 and 47). Congenital CNS infections [toxoplasmosis, cytomegalovirus (CMV)] have also been reported in infants with vertically transmitted HIV-1 infection, although not frequently (160–162). Syphilis in women of childbearing age appears to be on the rise and as such must also be considered in infants. CMV encephalitis and *C. albicans* (meningitis and microabscesses) are the most frequent opportunistic infections reported (74,75,163,164). Measles encephalitis has also recently been described as an infrequent but devastating complication (165).

In adults most CNS opportunistic infections are due to reactivation of previously acquired infection (e.g., toxoplasmosis, CMV, HSV, and JC virus infection). Reactivation of latent organisms would not be expected in infants and young children, and indeed these CNS opportunistic infections are uncommon. However, due to more aggressive medical management as well as antiretroviral and immunomodulating therapy, children with HIV-1 infection and AIDS are living longer. Infections common in HIV-infected adults can now be anticipated to occur in older children and adolescents. In fact, PML, an extremely rare CNS disease in children, has now been reported in three HIV-1–infected children (166,167).

Neoplasms

Primary CNS lymphoma and systemic lymphoma metastatic to the CNS are well-documented complications of HIV-1 infection in children (73,75,168). Presenting signs of lymphoma include the new onset of focal neurological deficits, seizures, and/or a change in mental status. Neurological deterioration at times may be rapidly progressive and fulminant (73,169). CT characteristics of lymphoma include (1) hyperdense or isodense mass lesions with variable contrast enhancement, (2) diffusely infiltrating contrast enhancing lesions, and (3) periventricular contrasting lesions. Reduction in tumor size has been noted in some patients following radiation therapy, however, long-term survival rates have not been affected (170).

Strokes

Cerebrovascular accidents may also complicate the course of HIV-1 infection in children. Both hemorrhagic and nonhemorrhagic strokes have been described (73,168,170–172). Intracerebral hemorrhage usually occurs in the setting of immune-mediated thrombocytopenia. Clinical presentation is variable, reflecting the severity and location of the hemorrhage. Hemorrhage into tumor may also occur. Strokes may be catastrophic and fatal or clinically silent. Nonhemorrhagic infarctions are most often associated with pathological changes of cerebral blood vessels, meningeal infections, or cardiomyopathy.

The clinical presentation of stroke includes the new onset of focal neurological deficits, most commonly hemiparesis, with or without seizures.

Peripheral Nervous System Involvement

Although peripheral nervous system (PNS) involvement is well documented in adult patients with HIV-1 infection, there is little information concerning PNS complications in infants and children other than anecdotal reports (58,173). We and others have followed some infants and young nonverbal children who became markedly more irritable and distressed when their lower extremities were lightly touched, raising the possibility of painful dysesthesias of neuropathic origin. We have also followed a few children who developed a mononeuritis multiplex type syndrome reminiscent of HIV-1–associated neuropathy described in adults (M. Kaufman, unpublished information).

PNS toxicity associated with antiretroviral therapy has also been noted in children, as it has in adults.

PREVENTION

The most important and effective strategy for preventing maternal-infant HIV-1 transmission involves prevention of HIV-1 infection in the mother before pregnancy, and indeed in all women of childbearing age. Short of that, the second most important strategy is to identify HIV-1 infection in a pregnant woman in order to offer her medical treatment to prevent maternal–fetal transmission.

In a study conducted by the AIDS Clinical Trials Group (ACTG 076), it was shown that transmission of HIV-1 from mother to infant could be prevented by maternal antiretroviral therapy. This trial, begun in April 1991, was designed to evaluate the efficacy, safety, and tolerance of ZVD in preventing maternal transmission of HIV-1 to the fetus. Preliminary analyses in February 1994 indicated a substantial reduction in HIV-1 infection among infants born to women treated with ZVD. There was a 67% relative reduction in the risk of HIV infection for those infants whose mothers had taken ZVD. The rate of perinatal infection in the placebo group was 25.5%, consistent with the expected U.S. transmission rate, and only 8.3% in the treated group (28). Based on these findings, the U.S. Public Health Service provided guidelines and recommendations for treating pregnant HIV-1–infected women after the 14th week of gestation (see Ref. 28).

SUMMARY

Vertically transmitted HIV-1 infection occurs in an immature developing organism. The maturational stage of the nervous and immune system when exposed to the direct or indirect effects of the virus is likely to be of utmost importance. Innumerable dynamic interactions occur between these two systems during development, and these undoubtedly interact in complex ways with HIV-1 variables. In order to care for these children and to design rational approaches for treatment and prevention, it is now critical to develop a better understanding of how HIV-1 affects the developing nervous system (58).

Infants and children with HIV-1 infection are currently living longer. This is due in part to more reliable techniques for early diagnosis and thus identification of infants and children when they are still asymptomatic or mildly symptomatic. In part it is due to successful prophylactic therapy for life-threatening opportunistic infections as well as more aggressive and successful medical management of serious infections and other HIV-1–related conditions. It is also due to primary antiviral and immunomodulating therapies. Pediatric HIV-1 infection can now be considered a chronic multisystem disease as well as one with periods of progression and periods of relative stability.

REFERENCES

1. Rubenstein A. Acquired immunodeficiency syndrome in infants. Am J Dis Child 1983; 137:825–827.
2. Oleske J, Minnefor A, Cooper R, et al. Immune deficiency syndrome in children. JAMA 1983; 249:2345.
3. Ammann AJ, Cowan M, Wara DW, et al. Acquired immunodeficiency in an infant: possible transmission by means of blood products. Lancet 1983; 1:956–958.
4. Oxtoby MJ. Vertically acquired HIV infection in the United States. In: Pizzo PA, Wilfert CM, eds. Pediatric AIDS: The Challenge of HIV Infection in Infants, Children and Adolescents. 2nd ed. Baltimore: Williams & Wilkins, 1994:5–20.
5. Rogers MF, Ou CY, Rayfield M, et al. Use of polymerase chain reaction for early detection of the proviral sequences of human immunodeficiency virus in infants born to seropositive mothers. N Engl J Med 1989; 320:1649–1654.
6. European Collaborative Study. Risk factors for mother-to-child transmission of HIV-1. Lancet 1992; 339:1007–1012.
7. Mofenson LM, Wolinsky SM. Current insights regarding vertical transmission. In: Pizzo PA, Wilfert CM, eds. Pediatric AIDS: The Challenge of HIV Infection in Infants, Children and Adolescents. 2nd ed. Baltimore: Williams & Wilkins, 1994:179–203.
8. Lyman WD, Kressy Y, Kure K, et al. Detection of HIV in fetal central nervous system tissue. AIDS 1990; 4:917–920.

9. Jovaisas E, Koch MA, Schafer A, et al. LAV/HTLV-III in 20-week fetus (letter). Lancet 1985; 2:1129.
10. Krivine A, Firtion G, Gao L, Francoual C, et al. HIV replication during the first few weeks of life. Lancet 1992; 339:1187–1189.
11. Ehrnst A, Lindgren S, Dictor M, et al. HIV in pregnant women and their offspring: evidence for late transmission. Lancet 1991; 338:203–207.
12. Ehrnst A, Lingren S, Belfrage E, et al. Intrauterine and intrapartum transmission of HIV. Lancet 1992; 339:245–246.
13. Pizzo PA, Butler KM. In the vertical transmission of HIV, timing may be everything (editorial). N Engl J Med 1991; 325:652–654.
14. de Rossi A, Ometto L. Mammoano F, et al. Time course of antigenaemia and seroconversion in infants with vertically acquired HIV-1 infection. AIDS 1993; 7:1528–1529.
15. Delfraissy JF, Blanche S, Rouzioux C, Mayaux MJ. Perinatal HIV transmission facts and controversies. Immunodef Rev 1992; 3:305–327.
16. Rouzioux C, Burgard M, Blanche S, Costagliola D. HIV infection in newborns: French collaborative study. Estimate of the period of perinatal HIV-1 transmission (abst). J Cell Biochem 1993; 17E (suppl):100.
17. Bryson YJ, Luzariaga K, Sullivan JL, Wara DW. Proposed definitions for in utero versus intrapartum transmission of HIV-1. N Engl J Med 1992; 327:1246–1247.
18. Blanche S, Mayaux MJ, Rouzioux C, et al. Relation of the course of HIV infection in children to the severity of the disease in their mothers at delivery. N Engl J Med 1994; 330:308–312.
19. Boyer PJ, Dillon M, Navaie M, et al. Factors predictive of maternal-fetal transmission of HIV-1: preliminary analysis of zidovudine given during pregnancy and/or delivery. JAMA 1994; 271:1925–1930.
20. Goedert JJ, Duliege AM, Amos CI, Felton S, Biggar RJ. High risk of HIV-1 infection for first-born twins: the International Registry of HIV-exposed Twins. Lancet 1991; 338:1471–1475.
21. Report of a consensus workshop, Siena, Italy, January 17–18, 1992: Early diagnosis of HIV infection in infants. J AIDS 1992; 5:1169–1178.
22. Connor EM, Sperling RS, Gelber R, et al. Reduction of maternal-infant transmission of human immunodeficiency virus type 1 with zidovudine treatment. N Engl J Med 1994; 331:1173–1180.
23. Burgard M, Mayaux MJ, Blanche S, et al. The use of viral culture and p24 antigen testing to diagnose HIV infection in neonates. N Engl J Med 1992; 327:1192–1197.
24. St. Louis ME, Kalish M, Kamenga M, et al. The timing of perinatal HIV-1 transmission in an African setting (abstract). First National Conference on Human Retroviruses and Related Infections, Washington, DC, 1993.
25. Centers for Disease Control. Revision of the case definition of acquired immunodeficiency syndrome for national reporting—United States. MMWR 1985; 34:373–377.
26. Centers for Disease Control. Revision of the CDC surveillance case definition for acquired immunodeficiency syndrome. MMWR 1987; 36(suppl 1S):1S–13S.
27. Centers for Disease Control. Classification system for human immunodeficiency virus (HIV) infection in children under 13 years of age. MMWR 1987; 36:225–230, 235.
28. Centers for Disease Control. 1994 revised classification system for human immunodeficiency virus infection in children less than 13 years of age; official authorized addenda—human immunodeficiency virus infection codes and official guidelines for coding and reporting ICD-9-CM. MMWR 1994; 43(No. RR-12).
29. Chin J. Current and future dimensions of the HIV/AIDS pandemic in women and children. Lancet 1990; 336:221–224.
30. Chin J, Mann J. Global surveillance and forecasting of AIDS. Bull WHO 1989; 67:1–7.
31. Futterman D, Hein K. Medical management of adolescents. In: Pizzo PA, Wilfert CM, eds. Pediatric AIDS: The Challenge of HIV Infection in Infants, Children and Adolescents. 2nd ed. Baltimore: Williams & Wilkins, 1994:546–560.
32. D'Angelo LJ. HIV infection and AIDS in adolescents. In: Pizzo PA, Wilfert CM, eds. Pediatric AIDS: The Challenge of HIV Infection in Infants, Children and Adolescents. 2nd ed. Baltimore: Williams & Wilkins, 1994:71–78.

33. Burger H, Belman AL, Grimson R, et al. Long HIV-1 incubation periods and dynamics of transmission within a family. Lancet 1990; 336:134–136.
34. Johnson RT, McArthur JC, Narayan O. The neurobiology of human immunodeficiency virus infections. FASEB J 1988; 2:2970–2981.
35. Pizzo PA, Wilfert CM. Antiretroviral treatment for children with HIV infection. In: Pizzo PA, Wilfert CM, eds. Pediatric AIDS: The Challenge of HIV Infection in Infants, Children and Adolescents. 2nd ed. Baltimore: Williams & Wilkins, 1994:651–687.
36. Koot M, Keet I, Vos A, et al. Prognostic value of HIV-1 syncytium-inducing phenotype for rate of CD4+ cell depletion and progression to AIDS. Ann Intern Med 1993; 118:681–688.
37. Bernstein LJ, Ochs HD, Wedgewood RJ, Rubinstein A. Defective humoral immunity in pediatric acquired immunodeficiency syndrome. J Pediatr 1985; 107:352–357.
38. Koup RA, Wilson CB. Clinical immunology of HIV-infected children. In: Pizzo PA, Wilfert CM, eds. Pediatric AIDS: The Challenge of HIV Infection in Infants, Children and Adolescents. 2nd ed. Baltimore: Williams & Wilkins, 1994:129–157.
39. Blanche S, Tardieu M, Duliege AM, et al. Longitudinal study of 94 symptomatic infants with materno fetal HIV infection: evidence for a bimodal expression of clinical and biological symptoms. Am J Dis Child 1990; 144:1210–1215.
40. Papiernik M, Brossard Y, Mulliez N, et al. Thymic abnormalities in fetuses aborted from human immunodeficiency virus type 1 seropositive women. Pediatrics 1992; 89:297–301.
41. Rosenberg ZF, Fauci AS. Immunopathologic and pathogenesis of HIV infection. In: Pizzo PA, Wilfert CM, eds. Pediatric AIDS: The Challenge of HIV Infection in Infants, Children, and Adolescents. 2nd ed. Baltimore: Williams & Wilkins, 1993:82–94.
42. Connor RI, Ho DD. Transmission and pathogenesis of human immunodeficiency virus type 1 (review). AIDS Human Retrovir 1994; 10:321–323.
43. Levy JA, Shimabukuro J, Hollander H, et al. Isolation of AIDS associated retrovirus from cerebrospinal fluid and brain of patients with neurological symptoms. Lancet 1985; 2:586–588.
44. Ho DD, Rota TR, Schooley RT, et al. Isolation of HTLV-III from CSF and neural tissues of patients with AIDS related neurologic syndromes. N Engl J Med 1985; 313:1493–1497.
45. Epstein LG, Goudsmit J, Paul DA, et al. Expression of human immunodeficiency virus in cerebrospinal fluid of children with progressive encephalopathy. Ann Neurol 1987; 21:397–401.
46. Sprecher S, Soumenkoff G, Puissant F, DeGeldra M. Vertical transmission of HIV. Lancet 1985; 2:288–289.
47. Pizzo PA, Wilfert CM, eds. Pediatric AIDS: The Challenge of HIV Infection in Infants, Children and Adolescents. 2nd ed. Baltimore: Williams & Wilkins, 1994:651–687.
48. Dickson DW, Lee SC, Hatch W, Mattiace LA, Broshan C, Lyman WD. Macrophages and microglia in HIV-related CNS neuropathy. In: Price RW, Perry S, eds. HIV; AIDS and the Brain. New York: Raven Press, 1993:99–118.
49. Tornatore C, Meyers K, Atwood W, Conant K. Major E temporal patterns of human immunodeficiency virus type 1; transcripts in human fetal astrocytes. J Virol 1994; 68:93–102.
50. Epstein LG, Gendelman HE. Human immunodeficiency virus type 1 infection of the nervous system: pathogenetic mechanisms. Ann Neurol 1993; 33:429–436.
51. Pulliman L, Herndier BG, Tang N, et al. Human immunodeficiency virus-infected macrophages produce soluble factors that cause histological and neurochemical alterations in cultured human brains. J Clin Invest 1991; 87:503–512.
52. Benos DJ, Hahn BH, Bubien JK, et al. Envelope glycoprotein gp120 of human immunodeficiency virus type 1 alters ion transport in astrocytes: implication for AIDS dementia complex. Proc Natl Acad Sci 1994; 91:494.
53. Volpe J. Neurology of the Newborn. 2nd ed. Philadelphia: WB Saunders Co., 1994.
54. Barks JD, Nair MP, Schwartz SA, et al. Potentiation of N-methyl-p-aspartate–mediated brain injury by a human immunodeficiency virus-1-derived peptide in perinatal rodents. Pediatr Res 1993; 34: 192–198.
55. Toggas SM, Masliah E, Rochenstein EM, et al. Central nervous system damage produced by expression of the HIV-1 coat protein gp120 in transgenic mice. Nature 1994; 367:188–193.

56. Grulian D, Vaca K, Noonan CA. Secretion of neurotoxins by mononuclear phagocytes infected with HIV-1. Science 1990; 250:1593–1596.
57. Kure K, Weidenheim KM, Lyman WD, Dickson DW. Morphology and distribution of HIV-1 qp 41 positive microglia in subacute AIDS encephalitis. Acta Neurophathol (Ber 1) 1990; 80:393–400.
58. Belman AL. AIDS and pediatric neurology. Neurol Clin North Am 1990; 8:571–603.
59. Price RW, Perry S, ed. HIV; AIDS and the Brain. New York: Raven Press, 1993.
60. Wiley CA, Masliah E, Morey, et al. Neocortical damage during HIV infection. Ann Neurol 1991; 29:651–657.
61. Wiley CA, Masliah E, Achim CL. Measurement of CNS HIV burden and its association with neurologic damage. Adv Neuroimmunol 1994; 4:319–325.
62. Masliah E, Achim CL, Ge N, DeTeresa R, Terry RD, Wiley CA. Spectrum of human immunodeficiency virus-associated neocortical damage. Ann Neurol 1992; 32:321–329.
63. Ketzlen S, Weiss S, Haug H, Budka H. Loss of neurons in frontal cortex in AIDS brains. Acta Neuropathol (Berl) 1990; 80:92–94.
64. Epstein LG, Sharer LR, Joshi VV, et al. Progressive encephalopathy in children with acquired immune deficiency syndrome. Ann Neurol 1985; 17:488–496.
65. Gonda MA, Wong-Stall F, Gallo RC, et al. Sequence homology and morphologic similarity of HTLV-III and visna virus, a pathogenic lentivirus. Science 1985; 227:173–177.
66. Goudsmit J, Wolters EC, Bakker M, et al. Intrathecal synthesis of antibodies to HTLV-III in patients without AIDS or AIDS related complex. Br Med J 1986; 292:1231–1234.
67. Gabuzda DH, Ho DD, de la Monte, et al. Immunohistochemical identification of HTLV-III antigen in brain of patients with AIDS. Ann Neurol 1986; 20:289–295.
68. Koenig S, Gendelman HE, Orenstein JM, et al. Detection of AIDS virus in macrophage in brain tissue from AIDS patients with encephalopathy. Science 1986; 233:1089–1093.
69. Pumarola-Sune T, Navia BA, Cordon-Cardo D, et al. HIV antigen in the brains of patients with the AIDS dementia complex. Ann Neurol 1987; 21:490–496.
70. Shaw GM, Harper ME, Hahn BH, et al. HTLV-III infection in brains of children and adults with AIDS encephalopathy. Science 1985; 227:177–181.
71. Wiley CA, Schrier RD, Nelson AS, et al. Cellular localization of human immunodeficiency virus infection within the brains of acquired immune deficiency syndrome patients. Proc Natl Acad Sci 1986; 83:7089–7093.
72. Wiley CA, Belman AL, Dickson D, Rubinstein A, Nelson JA. Human immunodeficiency virus within the brains of children with AIDS. Clin Neuropathol 1990; 1:1–6.
73. Belman AL, Diamond G, Dickson D, et al. Pediatric AIDS: neurologic syndromes. Am J Dis Child 1988; 142:29–35.
74. Belman AL, Ultmann MH, Horoupian D, et al. Neurologic complications in infants and children with acquired immune deficiency syndrome. Ann Neurol 1985; 18:560–566.
75. Epstein LG, Sharer LR, Goudsmit J. Neurological and neuropathological features of HIV in children. Ann Neurol 1988; 23(suppl):S19–S23.
76. Dickson DW, Belman AL, Kim TS, Horoupian D, Rubinstein A. Spinal cord pathology in pediatric acquired immunodeficiency syndrome. Neurology 1989; 39:227–235.
77. Dickson DW, Belman AL, Park YD, et al. Central nervous system pathology in pediatric AIDS: an autopsy study. APMIS 1989; 8(suppl):40–57.
78. Kozlowski PB, Sher JH, Rao, et al. Central nervous system in pediatric AIDS registry. Ann NY Acad Sci 1993; 693:295–296.
79. Brustels O, Spiegel H, Leib SL, Finn T, Stein H, Kleihues P, Wiestler OD. Distribution of HIV in the CNS of children with severe HIV encephalopathy. Acad Neuropathol 1992; 84:24–31.
80. Budka H. Neuropathology of human immunodeficiency virus infection. Brain Pathol 1991; 1: 163–175.
81. Budka H, Wiley CA, Kleihues P, et al. HIV-1 associated disease of the nervous system: review of nomenclature and proposal for neuropathology-based terminology. Brain Pathol 1991; 1:143–152.
82. Sharer LR, Dowling PC, Michaels J, et al. Spinal cord disease in children with HIV-1 infection: a combined molecular and neuropathological study. Neuropathol Appl Neurobiol 1990; 16:317–331.

83. Sharer LR, Epstein LG, Cho ES, et al. Pathologic features of AIDS encephalopathy in children: evidence for LAV/HTLV-III infection of the brain. Hum Pathol 1986; 17:271–284.
84. Vazeux R, Lacroix-Ciaudo C, Blanche S, et al. Low levels of human immunodeficiency virus replication in the brain tissue of children with severe acquired immunodeficiency syndrome encephalopathy. Am J Pathol 1992; 140:137–144.
85. Auger I, Thomas P, De Gruttola V, et al. Incubation periods for paediatric AIDS patients. Nature 1988; 336:575–577.
86. Scott G. Survival in children with perinatally acquired human immunodeficiency virus type infection. N Engl J Med 1989; 3211:1791–1796.
87. Brouwers P, DeCarli C, Civitelli L, et al. Correlation between CT-brain scan abnormalities and neuropsychological function in children with symptomatic HIV disease. Arch Neurol 1995; 52:39–44.
88. Persaud D, Chadwani S, Rigaud M, et al. Delayed recognition of human immunodeficiency virus infection in preadolescent children. Pediatrics 1992; 90:688–691.
89. Rogers MF, Schochetman G, Hoff R. Advances in diagnosis of HIV infection. In: Pizzo PA, Wilfert CM, eds. Pediatric AIDS: The Challenge of HIV Infection in Infants, Children and Adolescents. 2nd ed. Baltimore: Williams & Wilkins, 1994:219–240.
90. Joshi VV. Pathology of pediatric AIDS: overview, update and future direction. Ann NY Acad Sci 1993; 693:71–92
91. Srugo I, Wittek AE, Israele V, Brunell PA. Meningoencephalitis in a neonate congenitally infected with human immunodeficiency virus type 1. J Pediatr 1992; 120:93–95.
92. American Academy of Neurology AIDS Task Force. Nomenclature and research case definitions for neurologic manifestations of human immunodeficiency virus type 1. Neurology 1991; 41:778–785.
93. Epstein LG, Sharer LR, Oleske JM, et al. Neurologic manifestations of human immunodeficiency virus infection in children. Pediatrics 1986; 78:678–687.
94. Belman AL, Taylor FL, Nachman S, Milazzo M. HIV-1 associated CNS disease syndromes in infants and children. Neurology 1994; 44(suppl 2):A168.
95. Belman AL. AIDS and the child's central nervous system. Pediatr Clin North Am 1992; 39:691–714.
96. Belman AL, Preston T, Milazzo M. HIV-1 associated CNS disease syndromes in infants and children: a proposal for "working" research case definitions according to age. J Neuro-AIDS 1996; 2:31.
97. Tovo PA, Gabiano C, Favro-Paris S, et al. Brain atrophy with intracranial calcification following congenital HIV infection. Acta Paediatr Scand 1988; 77:776–779.
98. Belman AL, Diamond G, Park Y, et al. Perinatal HIV infection: a prospective longitudinal study of the initial CNS signs. Neurology 1989; 39(suppl):278–279.
99. Wolters PL, Brouwers P, Moss HA, Pizzo PA. Differential receptive and expressive language functioning of children with symptomatic HIV disease: comparison with the language of sibling controls and CT scan brain abnormalities. Pediatrics 1995; 1:112–119.
100. Condini A, Axia G, Cattelan C, D'Urso MR, Lavera AM, Viero F, Zacchello F. Development of language in 18–30 month old HIV-1 infected but not ill children. AIDS 1991; 5:735–739.
101. Belman AL, Muenz L, Marcus J, Durako S, Willoughby A. Neurologic status of infants born to HIV-1 infected mothers and their controls: a prospective study from birth to 24 months of age (abstr). Pediatrics (in press).
102. Lifschitz M, Hanson C, Wilson G, Shearer WT. Behavioral changes in children with human immunodeficiency virus (HIV) infection. T.B.P.175. V International Conference on AIDS, Montreal, June 4–9, 1989.
103. Brouwers E, Belman AL, Epstein L. Central nervous system involvement: manifestations and evaluation. In: Pizzo PA, Wilfert CM, eds. Pediatric AIDS: The Challenge of HIV Infection in Infants, Children and Adolescents. 2nd ed. Baltimore: Williams & Wilkins, 1994:433–455.
104. Belman AL, Lantos G, Horoupian D, et al. AIDS: calcification of the basal ganglia in infants and children. Neurology 1986; 36:1192–1199.
105. Sharer LR, Epstein LG, Cho ES, et al. Pathologic features of AIDS encephalopathy in children: evidence for LAV/HTLV-III infection of the brain. Hum Pathol 1986; 17:271–284.
106. Ultmann MH, Diamond G, Ruff HA, Belman AL, et al. Developmental abnormalities in infants and

children with acquired immune deficiency syndrome (AIDS): a follow up study. Int J Neurosci 1987; 32:661–667.
107. Levenson RL, Mellins CA, Zawadzki R, Kairam R, Stein Z. Cognitive assessment of human immunodeficiency virus exposed children. AJDC 1992; 146:1479–1483.
108. Tardieu M, Mayaux M-J, Seibel N, Funck-Brentano I, Straub E, Teglas J-P, Blanche S. Cognitive assessment of school age children with maternally transmitted HIV-I infection. J Pediatr 1995; 126: 375–379.
109. Diamond GW, Kaufman J, Belman AL, et al. Characterization of cognitive functioning in a subgroup of children with congenital HIV infection. Arch Clin Neuropsychol 1987; 2:1–6.
110. Havens J, Whitaker AH, Feldman JF, Ehrhardt AA. Psychiatric morbidity in school-aged children with congenital human immunodeficiency virus infection: a pilot study. J Dev Behav Pediatr 1994; 15(suppl):S18–25.
111. Alyward EH, Butz AM, Hutton N, et al. Cognitive and motor development in infants at risk for human immunodeficiency virus. Am J Dis Child 1992; 146:218–222.
112. Nozyce M, Hittleman J, Muenz L, et al. Effect of perinatally acquired human immunodeficiency virus infection on neurodevelopment in children during the first two years of life. Pediatrics 1994; 94: 883–889.
113. Ultmann MH, Belman AL, Ruff HA, Novick BE, Cone-Wesson B, Cohen HJ, Rubinstein A. Developmental abnormalities in infants and children with acquired immune deficiency syndrome (AIDS) and AIDS-related complex. Dev Med Child Neurol 1985; 27:563–571.
114. Cohen SL, Mundy T, Kaarassik B, et al. Neuropsychological functioning in children with HIV-1 infection through neonatal blood transfusion. Pediatrics 1991; 88:58–68.
115. Whitt JK, Hooper SR, Tennison MB, et al. Neuropsychological functioning of human immunodeficiency virus-infected children with hemophilia. J Pediatr 1993; 122:52–59.
116. Moss H, Brouwers E, Wolters P, Weiner L, Hersh S, Pizzo PA. The development of a Q sort behavioral rating procedure for pediatric HIV patients. J Pediatr Psychol 1994; 19:27–46.
117. Bales JF, Constant CF, Garg B, Tilton A, Kaufman DM, Wasiewski W. Neurologic history and examination results and their relationship to human immunodeficiency virus type I serostatus in hemophilic subjects: result from the hemophilia growth and development study. Pediatrics 1993; 91:736–741.
118. Laverda AM, Gallo P, Tavolato B, et al. Cerebrospinal fluid findings in neurologically symptomatic and asymptomatic HIV-1 infected children. Neuroscience of HIV-1 Infection (abstr). Satellite Conference, VII Int'l Conf. on AIDS, Padova, Italy, 1991, p. 120.
119. Gallo P, Laverda AM, DeRossi A, et al. Immunological markers in the cerebrospinal fluid of HIV-1 infected children. ACTA Pediatr Scand 1991; 80:659–666.
120. Mintz M, Rappaport R, Oleske M, et al. Elevated serum levels of tumor necrosis factor are associated with progressive encephalopathy in children with acquired immunodeficiency syndrome. AJDC 1989; 143:771–774.
121. Di Carli C, Civitello AL, Brouwers P, Pizzo PA. The prevalence of computed tomographic abnormalities of the cerebrum in 100 consecutive children symptomatic with the human immune deficiency virus. Ann Neurol 1993; 34:198–205.
122. Chamberlin MC. Pediatric AIDS: a longitudinal comparative MRI and CT brain imaging study. J Child Neurol 1993; 8(2):175.
123. Tardieu M, Blanche S, Brunelle F. Cerebral magnetic resonance imaging studies in HIV-1 infected children born to seropositive mothers. Neuroscience of HIV-1 infection (abstr). Satellite Conference, VII Int'l Conf. on AIDS, Padova, Italy, 1991, p. 60.
124. Pizzo PA, Butler K, Balis F, et al. Dideoxycytidine alone and in an alternating schedule with zidovudine in children with symptomatic human immunodeficiency virus infection. J Pediatr 1990; 17:799–808.
125. Pavlakis SG, Lu PF, Frank Y, et al. MRS of the basal ganglia: diagnosis of childhood AIDS encephalopathy. Neurology 1994; suppl 2A:44.
126. Schmidt B, Seeger J, Jacobi G. EEG and evoked potentials in HIV-infected children. Clin Electroencephalogr 1992; 23(3):111–117.

127. Brivio L, Tornaghi R, Musetti L, Marchisio P, Principi N. Improvement of auditory brainstem responses after treatment with zidovudine in a child with AIDS. Pediatr Neurol 1991; 7(1):53–55.
128. Frank Y, Vishnubhakat SM, Pahwa S. Brainstem auditory evoked responses in infants and children with AIDS. Pediatr Neurol 1992; 8(4):262–266.
129. Tovo PA, Demartino M, Gabiano C, et al. Prognostic factors and survival in children with perinatal HIV-1 infection. Italian Register for HIV infection in Children. Lancet 1992; 339:1249–1253.
130. European Collaborative Study. Cogo P, Laverda AM, Ades AE, et al. Neurologic signs in young children with human immunodeficiency virus infection. Ped Inf Dis J 1990; 9:402–406.
131. Mintz M, Epstein LE. Neurological manifestations, clinical features and therapeutic approaches. Semin Neurol 1992; 12:51–56.
132. Berger JR, Moskowitz L, Fischl M, Kelley RE. Neurologic disease as the presenting manifestation of acquired immunodeficiency syndrome. South Med J 1987; 80:683–686.
133. Jannsen RS, Cornblath DR, Epstein LG, McArthur J, Price R. HIV infection and the nervous system: report from the American Academy of Neurology task force. Neurology 1989; 39:111–122.
134. Brouwers P, Moss H, Wolters P, et al. Effect of continuous-infusion zidovudine therapy on neuropsychologic functioning in children with symptomatic human immunodeficiency virus infection. J Pediatr 1990; 117:980–985.
135. Belman AL, Calvelli T, Nozyce M, et al. Neurologic and immunologic correlates in infants with vertically transmitted HIV infection. Neurology (Suppl) 1990; 40(1):409.
136. Davis SL, Halsted C, Levy N, Ellis W. Acquired immunodeficiency virus syndrome presenting as progressive infantile encephalopathy. J Pediatr 1987; 110:884–888.
137. Centers for Disease Control. HIV counseling, testing, and referral: standards & guidelines. Atlanta: U.S. Department of Health & Human Services, Public Health Service, CDC, 1994.
138. Newell ML, Peckham C. Risk factors for vertical transmission of HIV-1 and early markers of HIV-1 infection in children. AIDS 1993; 7:S91–S97.
139. Rogers MD, Ou C-Y, Kilbourne B, et al. Advances and problems in the diagnosis of human immunodeficiency virus infection in infants. Pediatr Infect Dis J 1991; 10:523–531.
140. Husson RN, Comeau AM, Hoff R. Diagnosis of human immunodeficiency virus infection in infants and children. Pediatrics 1990; 86:1–10.
141. Krivine A, Yakudima A, Le May M, et al. A comparative study of virus isolation, polymerase chain reaction, and antigen detection in children of mothers infected with HIV. J Pediatr 1990; 116:372–376.
142. Frenkel LD, Gaur S. Pediatric human immunodeficiency virus infection and disease. Curr Opin Pediatr 1991; 3:867–873.
143. Martin NL, Levy JA, Legg H, et al. Detection of infection with human immunodeficiency virus (HIV) type 1 in infants by an anti-HIV immunoglobulin A assay using recombinant proteins. J Pediatr 1991; 118:354–358.
144. Hutto C, Owens C, Dumond D, et al. Early detection of perinatal HIV-1 infection with polymerase chain reaction (PCR), virus culture and p24 antigen88. Pediatr Res 1992; 26:164A.
145. Gwinn M, Redus MA, Granad TC, et al. HIV-1 serologic test results for one million newborn dried-blood specimens-assay performance and implications for screening. J AIDS 1992; 5:505–512.
146. Fauvel M, Henrard D, Delage G, et al. Early detection of HIV in neonates. N Engl J Med 1993; 329: 60–61.
147. Comeau AM, Hsu HW, Schwerzler M, et al. Identifying human immunodeficiency virus infection at birth: application of polymerase chain reaction to Guthrie cards. J Pediatr 1993; 123:252–258.
148. Suarez MA, Bianco B, Brion LP, et al. A rapid test for the detection of HIV antibodies in cord blood. J Pediatr 1993; 123:259–261.
149. Getchell JP, Hausler WJ, Ramirez MT, et al. HIV screening of newborns. Biochem Med Metab Biol 1993; 49:143–148.
150. Miles SA, Balden E, Magpantay L, et al. Rapid serologic testing with immune-complex dissociated HIV p24 antigen for early detection of HIV infection in neonates. N Engl J Med 1993; 328:297–302.
151. Brandt CD, Rakusan TA, Sison AV, et al. Human immunodeficiency virus infection in infants during the first 2 months of life. Arch Pediatr Adolesc Med 1994; 148:250–254.

152. Pizzo PA, Eddy J, Balis FM, et al. Effect of continuous intravenous infusion of zidovudine (AZT) in children with symptomatic HIV infection. N Engl J Med 1988; 319:889–896.
153. DeCarli C, Fugate L, Falloon J, et al. Brain growth and cognitive improvement in children with HIV induced encephalopathy after 6 months of continuous infusion therapy. AIDS 1991; 4:585–592.
154. McKinney RE, Maha MA, Conners EM, et al. A multicenter trial of oral zidovudine in children with advanced HIV disease. N Engl J Med 1991; 324:1018–1025.
155. Butler KM, Husson RM, Balis J, et al. Dideoxginosine in children with symptomatic human immunodeficiency virus infection. N Engl J Med 1990; 324:137–144.
156. Nozyce M, Hoberman M, Arpade S, et al. The effects of oral AZT on neurodevelopmental, immunological and clinical outcomes in vertically HIV infected children (abstr). Ann NY Acad Sci 1993; 693:1992.
157. Mintz M, Conners EM, Oleski JM, et al. Neurologic deterioration in children in long-term zidovudine treatment (abstr). 9th ACTG, July 1990.
158. NICHD/IVIG. 9th ACTG, July 1990 (abstract).
159. Mofenson LM, Wolinsky SM. Current insights regarding vertical transmission. In: Pizzo PA, Wilfert CM, eds. Pediatric AIDS: The Challenge of HIV Infection in Infants, Children and Adolescents. 2nd ed. Baltimore: Williams & Wilkins. 1994:179–203.
160. Mitchell CD, Erlich SS, Mastrucci MT, et al. Congenital toxoplasmosis occurring in infants perinatally infected with HIV-1. Pediatr Infect Dis J 1990; 9:512–518.
161. Taccone A, Fondelli MP, Ferra G, Marzoli A. An unusual CT presentation of congenital cerebral toxoplasmosis in an 8 month-old boy with AIDS. Pediatr Radiol 1992; 22(1):68–69.
162. Shanks GD, Redfield RR, Fischer GW. Toxoplasma encephalitis in an infant with acquired immunodeficiency syndrome. Pediatr Infect Dis 1987; 6:70.
163. McAbee GN, Belman AL, Knapik M, Solitare G, Ciminera P, Dickson D. Rapid and fatal neurological deterioration due to CNS candida infection in an HIV-1 infected child. J Child Neurol 1995; 10: 405–407.
164. Biggemann B, Voit T, Neuen E, et al. Neurological manifestations in three German children with AIDS. Hippokrates 1987; 1:99–106.
165. Sharer LR, Fischer B, Blumberg BM, Epstein LG. CNS measles virus infection in AIDS. J Neuro-AIDS 1994. In press.
166. Van der Steenhoven JJ, Dbaibo G, Boyko OB, et al. Progressive multifocal leukoencephalopathy in pediatric acquired immunodeficiency syndrome (abstr). J Neuropathol Exp Neurol 1990; 50:326.
167. Berger J, Albrecht J, Belman AL, et al. Progressive multifocal leukoencephalopathy in children with HIV infection. AIDS 1992; 6:837–841.
168. Park Y, Belman AL, Dickson DW, et al. Stroke in pediatric acquired immunodeficiency syndrome. Ann Neurol 1988; 24:359.
169. Epstein LG, Dicarlo F, Joshi V, et al. Primary lymphoma of the central nervous system in children with acquired immunodeficiency syndrome. Pediatrics 1988; 82:355–363.
170. Goldstein J, Dickson DW, Rubinstein A, Woods W, Miner F, Belman AL, Davis L. Primary CNS lymphoma in a pediatric patient with acquired immunodeficiency syndrome treatment with radiation. Cancer 1990; 66:2503–2508.
171. Frank Y, Lim W, Kahn E, et al. Multiple ischemic infarcts in a child with AIDS, varicella zoster infection and cerebral vasculitis. Pediatr Neurol 1989; 5:64–67.
172. Kure K, Park YD, Kim TS, et al. Immunohistochemical localization of an HIV epitope in cerebral aneurysmal arteriopathy in pediatric AIDS. Pediatr Pathol 1989; 9:655–662.
173. Raphael SA, Price ML, Lischner HW, et al. Inflammatory demyelinating polyneuropathy in a child with symptomatic human immunodeficiency virus infection. J Pediatrics 1991; 118:242–245.

4

Neurological Complications of Immunization

Hema Patel and Bhuwan P. Garg
Indiana University Medical Center, James Whitcomb Riley Hospital for Children, Indianapolis, Indiana

INTRODUCTION

Routine large-scale immunization against common childhood infections such as poliomyelitis, pertussis, and measles has resulted in a significant decline in the incidence, morbidity, and mortality from these diseases. The current schedule recommended by the American Academy of Pediatrics Committee on Infectious Diseases for childhood immunization is outlined in Table 1.

Immunization is not without risk, and the most serious vaccine-related complications are neurological. The incidence of these complications has been a matter of debate. Case reports were for many years the only source of information of these complications; they are rarely useful in establishing a causal relationship between the two. Simultaneous administration of several vaccines, e.g., measles-mumps-rubella (MMR) vaccine, further confounds this causality. Analytical, population-based studies of adverse reactions have only recently been undertaken to ascertain the frequency of vaccine-related complications.

The Monitoring System for Adverse Events Following Immunization (MSAEFI) of the Centers for Disease Control and Prevention (CDC) and the most recent Vaccine Adverse Event Reporting System (VAERS) have been established for collecting data on illness that is temporally associated with immunization. These are passive surveillance systems. The reported information is accepted without verification, and long-term follow-up is not attempted.

MEASLES VACCINE

Measles (rubeola) is a viral infection caused by a member of the paramyxovirus group. The disease can be quite debilitating, and complications include otitis media, croup, diarrhea, hemorrhagic skin rash, pneumonia, encephalitis, and subacute sclerosing panencephalitis (SSPE) (1).

Table 1 Recommended Schedule for Immunization of Healthy Infants and Children

Recommended age	Immunization(s)
2 months	DTP, Hib, OPV
4 months	DTP, Hib, OPV
6 months	DTP, Hib
6–18 months	OPV
12–15 months	MMR, Hib
15–18 months	DTaP or DTP
4–6 years	DTaP or DTP, OPV
11–12 years	MMR
14–16 years	Td

See text for varicella vaccine.
Source: Ref. 122.

The fatality rate due to measles infection is estimated at 1 per 10,000 cases in industrialized countries (2) and may be as high as 1000 per 10,000 in developing countries (3).

Immune gammaglobulins had been used in the past for prevention of measles (4). A killed virus vaccine was subsequently developed in which a virus derived from the Edmondston strain, initially isolated in 1954, was inactivated by formalin and precipitated by alum (5). This vaccine provided short-lived immunity, and some patients later became infected with the wild-type measles virus (6). Therefore, after only 4 years of use, the killed virus vaccine was replaced by the newer live attenuated virus vaccine in 1967.

The currently licensed measles vaccines use the Edmondston B strain of the measles virus, which is attenuated by prolonged passage in chick embryo cell culture (7). Two vaccines, each from a different attenuated strain (Enders and Schwarz strain) of the Edmondston B virus, are available. The Enders strain is the product of 40 passages of the Edmondston B strain of the measles virus through a chick embryo cell culture (8). The Schwarz strain is the product of 85 passages of the virus through a chick embryo cell culture (9). This further attenuation resulted in reduction of side effects such as skin rash and fever following vaccination. Other strains have also been developed and have been used in various smaller population groups. A different strain, the Beckenham-31 strain has been used in the United Kingdom. It is not known if there are differences in the adverse effects between the vaccines derived from the Edmondston strain versus the Beckenham strain. Therefore, it is difficult to compare epidemiological studies in the United Kingdom with those from the United States.

Immunization against measles, mumps, and rubella has been administered in a combined vaccine in the United States since 1975. By 1982, 97% of all children entering school had been vaccinated against measles. The reported incidence of measles fell from 500 cases per 100,000 population in 1950 to 0.5 cases per 100,000 in 1982. The annual deaths from measles were reduced from 700 to 2, and the reported cases of measles encephalitis fell from 300 to 1 in the same time period (10).

Adverse Reactions: Systemic

Administration of the live attenuated virus vaccine is intended to cause an asymptomatic case of measles. Fever, rash, or mild measleslike symptoms may develop in the second week following immunization. Children with vaccine-induced measles can develop any of the known complications of natural measles infection.

Adverse Reactions: Neurological Complications

Encephalopathy and Encephalitis

Encephalopathy is an acute or chronic acquired impairment of brain function. Encephalitis refers to an encephalopathy associated with an inflammatory response in the brain. These terms have often been used interchangeably in the literature.

Encephalitis following natural measles virus infection usually occurs 3–5 days after the appearance of skin rash and is characterized by an alteration in consciousness or behavior, convulsions, headache, and focal neurological deficits. The encephalitis is usually severe, often leading to brain damage or even death. Pathologically, there is edema and demyelination in the brain.

Neurological disorders following immunization with the live attenuated measles virus were the subject of two surveillance reports by the CDC. The first covered the period from January 1965 to February 1967. During this time, 15 million doses of vaccine were distributed for use and 23 cases of vaccine-associated neurological disease were reported. The interval from vaccination to the onset of symptoms ranged from 3 to 24 days. Eighteen of the 23 cases were reported to have encephalitis. Of the remaining 5, 2 patients had aseptic meningitis, 2 had cerebellar ataxia, and 1 had paralysis of extraocular muscles. The estimated rate of encephalitis within a 4-week period after vaccination in this study was 1.5 cases per 1 million distributed doses of vaccine (11).

A second report covered the period from 1963 to 1971. During this time 51 million doses of vaccine had been distributed and 59 cases of encephalitis or encephalopathy including 13 cases of encephalomyelitis were identified. The incidence of encephalitis or encephalopathy was estimated to be 1.16 cases per million distributed doses in this report. The background rate of encephalitis from any cause (unrelated to vaccination or other known parainfectious causes) is 2.8 cases per 1 million children in any 4-week period (12). Therefore, the association of the symptoms of encephalitis with the vaccination in these patients could also be explained by chance alone.

The National Childhood Encephalopathy Study, a case-control study, reported a higher risk of either convulsions or encephalopathy within 7–14 days following measles vaccination. The estimated attributable risk was one case per 87,000 immunizations. This estimate was based on the occurrence of neurological symptoms in 14 patients. Five of these 14 patients had encephalitis or encephalopathy; 3 of them recovered completely. The remaining 9 had simple febrile convulsions with no sequelae. This study suggested that there is an increased risk of febrile convulsions in children receiving measles vaccination, with no evidence of residual neurological deficits (13).

There have been 17 additional case reports of encephalitis or encephalopathy following measles vaccination in the VAERS between November 1990 and July 1992. The children's ages ranged from 5 months to 11 years, with onset of symptoms 1–14 days after immunization.

It has not been possible to specifically implicate the measles component of the MMR vaccine as the cause of the encephalitis. However, the clustering of cases in the second week after immunization (which is the time of maximal viral replication) suggests that the measles virus is the etiological agent of the encephalitis. Even if we assume that all of the reported cases were caused by measles vaccination, the incidence of postvaccine encephalitis (1.5 cases per one million distributed doses of vaccine) remains lower than that of encephalitis following natural measles infection (1 per thousand cases) (14). It is also lower than the risk of encephalitis from any other cause, which is 2.8 cases per one million children in any 4-week period (11,12).

Subacute Sclerosing Panencephalitis

Subacute sclerosing panencephalitis (SSPE) is a progressive degenerative disease of the central nervous system following measles infection. It is characterized by an insidious onset of mental deterioration, motor dysfunction, and myoclonus, leading to coma and death. The incidence of SSPE following natural measles infection is estimated to be 8.5 cases per one million cases of natural infection. In comparison, only 0.7 cases of SSPE occur per one million distributed doses of measles vaccination (15).

Since the first report in 1968, 15 children have been reported with SSPE who had been vaccinated and had no history of measles (12,16,17). The latency between the measles vaccination and SSPE was reported to range from 3 weeks (12) to 5 years (17).

The national registry for SSPE was founded in 1969 and documented a dramatic decline in the number of measles cases in the United States from 1964 to 1968 with a resultant decline in the number of cases of SSPE starting in the early 1970s. From 1967 to 1975, 41.3 new cases of SSPE per year were reported, whereas on average only 4.2 new cases of SSPE per year were reported from 1982 to 1986 (18). Only two new cases of SSPE in U.S. citizens have been reported to the SSPE registry since 1989; neither patient had a history of natural measles infection. This decline in the incidence of SSPE was attributed to the widespread use of the measles vaccine.

The risk of SSPE following vaccination against measles appears to be far less than the risk after natural infection and is not a contraindication to routine immunization against measles (15).

Immunosuppressive Measles Encephalopathy

A specific type of measles encephalopathy, immunosuppressive measles encephalopathy (IME), has been reported in two immunosuppressed children following vaccination against measles. This condition is distinct from SSPE or acute measles encephalitis and has an incubation period of 5 weeks to 6 months. In a 7-year-old girl with acute lymphocytic leukemia, measles virus, believed to be the vaccine strain, was isolated from the CSF approximately 10 weeks after she received MMR vaccine (19). Another case of IME occurred in a leukemic child and involved the Schwarz strain of the attenuated measles virus (20). Caution is advised in the use of the measles immunization in immunosuppressed individuals.

Seizures

Seizures may occur following measles immunization. Studies in the United States (21,22) and the United Kingdom (23) have indicated that febrile and less frequently nonfebrile seizures may occur 7–14 days following measles immunization. No permanent neurological sequelae have been observed, although some children may later have simple febrile convulsions.

Other Neurological Complications

Other neurological complications associated with natural measles infection may also occur following immunization. These include transverse myelitis (24) and Guillain-Barré syndrome (GBS) (25). However, there have only been isolated case reports, and the number of cases identified does not appear to be above the background rates of these disorders, which is around 0.5–1.5 cases per 100,000 population per year (26,27).

Adverse Reactions: Ophthalmological Complications

There are several case reports of optic neuritis (28,29) following measles vaccination. Bilateral chorioretinitis (30) and transient third nerve palsy including ptosis and complete third nerve involvement (31,32) have also been reported. At present it is difficult to support a positive association between measles vaccine and these complications.

MUMPS VACCINE

Mumps is generally not as devastating a disease as measles, but complications including epididymoorchitis, aseptic meningitis, meningoencephalitis, and deafness have prompted the development of a vaccine.

Vaccines prepared from two strains of the mumps virus were introduced in 1967. The Jeryl Lynn strain is used in the United States and the Urabe strain in Japan. The live virus used in these vaccines has been attenuated by passage through the chick embryo cell culture (33). The vaccine produces a subclinical noncommunicable infection, and a neutralizing antibody response can be detected in recipients 2–6 weeks after administration. Mumps vaccine has been administered with measles and rubella vaccine in a combined vaccine as MMR in the United States since 1975. As a consequence, it is difficult to distinguish the adverse effects of the individual antigens. However, no neurological complications have been directly attributed to the mumps vaccine.

Until 1981, MMR was usually administered concurrently with diphtheria-tetanus-pertussis vaccine (DTP) and oral polio vaccine (OPV) at 15 months of age. Since 1981, it has been recommended that MMR be administered at 12–15 months of age and DTP and OPV at 18 months. Booster MMR has generally been given at school entry at the age of 4–6 years, though recently, a booster dose at 11–12 years of age has been recommended instead (Table 1).

Aseptic meningitis has been reported following the use of the Urabe strain (either monovalent or as MMR containing the Urabe strain) in Japan, Canada, and the United Kingdom. Data concerning the occurrence of aseptic meningitis with the Jeryl Lynn strain used in the United States are scarce. Eleven cases of meningitis following immunization with MMR (containing the Jeryl Lynn strain of the mumps vaccine) were reported in VAERS between November 1990 and July 1992. The latency of the symptoms following the vaccination ranged from 3 days to 2 weeks. However, in no case was the virus identified or the strain isolated. Although cases of sensorineural deafness following administration of mumps vaccine have been reported (34–36), a cause-and-effect relationship has not been established.

RUBELLA VACCINE

Rubella (German measles) is generally a mild exanthematous disease that may rarely be associated with encephalomyelitis and peripheral neuropathy. The rubella virus, however, produces marked neurological damage to the fetus of a mother infected during pregnancy. The maternal infection may be so mild as to be inapparent. Intrauterine rubella infection is associated with severe morbidity, including cataracts, deafness, congenital heart disease, and mental retardation. The frequency of congenital defects is highest when infection occurs in the first trimester of pregnancy.

Rubella vaccine was licensed for use in the United States in 1969. Initially three rubella vaccines using live attenuated virus cultured from duck embryo, dog kidney, and rabbit kidney cells were used. In January 1979, these were replaced by a vaccine (RA 27/30) prepared by culturing the virus in human diploid cells because of a high incidence of arthralgias associated with the older vaccines. The RA 27/30 vaccine produces an immune response that closely parallels the natural infection.

Adverse Reactions: Systemic

Forty percent of people, usually adults, receiving the present rubella vaccine (RA 27/30) may develop transient arthralgias and paresthesias that begin 7–21 days after immunization and last for 1–3 days. These symptoms are, however, mild, especially when compared with those caused by the older vaccines (37).

Adverse Reactions: Neurological Complications

Neuropathy

Two fairly well-defined syndromes—brachial radiculoneuritis (arm syndrome) and lumbosacral radiculoneuritis (leg syndrome)—have been reported following immunization with the older vaccines, but not with the RA 27/30 vaccine (38,39). The arm syndrome occurred 10–62 days following immunization and was characterized by sudden, episodic, nocturnal pain and paresthesias in the hands and wrists occurring nightly for 2–35 days. The leg syndrome was characterized by the appearance of bilateral intense pain in the popliteal fossa causing difficulty in weight bearing on the legs. The symptoms usually occurred 29–70 days following immunization, lasted for 2–14 days, and recurred periodically during 2–2½ years of follow-up (40).

The Institute of Medicine recently reviewed studies concerned with neurological illness following rubella vaccine and concluded that there is insufficient evidence to indicate a causal relationship between the RA 27⁄30 rubella vaccine and radiculoneuritis or other neuropathies (41).

Demyelinating Diseases

There are a few case reports of young women who developed transverse myelitis associated with optic neuritis 4 days to 2 weeks following rubella immunization (42,43). In at least some of these women, this neurological dysfunction may have been the first manifestation of a latent multiple sclerosis, possibly triggered by the immunization-induced fever (43). The fact that transverse myelitis following immunization has been reported in adults only, and not in children in whom multiple sclerosis is less common, may also favor this explanation.

Adverse Reactions: Congenital Rubella Syndrome

Rubella immunization plays an important role in reducing the incidence of congenital rubella syndrome. Older vaccines, but not the RA 27/30 vaccine, may cross the placenta and infect the fetus (44–46). The CDC surveillance of vaccination during gestation included 44 susceptible women who had been vaccinated with the RA 27/30 vaccine within 1 week before to 4 weeks after conception, which is the highest risk period for fetal defect. No infant had evidence of congenital rubella syndrome (47).

The risk of congenital rubella syndrome after vaccination appears to be minimal, but even the small risk should be avoided by not vaccinating women who are pregnant or attempting to conceive. Women should be vaccinated only if not pregnant and advised not to become pregnant for 2 months following vaccination (44). Physicians should determine the immunization status of all women of childbearing age in their care and vaccinate the inadequately immunized.

POLIO VACCINE

Poliomyelitis is an acute infectious disease caused by an enterovirus. It can result in nonparalytic disease (aseptic meningitis) and, less commonly, paralytic poliomyelitis involving motor neurons in the spinal cord and brain stem. There are three types of poliovirus: types 1, 2, and 3 with no cross immunity.

Jonas Salk developed an inactivated polio virus vaccine (IPV), which was licensed in 1959 and resulted in a great reduction of paralytic poliomyelitis. This vaccine was administered subcutaneously. In 1963, the Sabin vaccine containing live attenuated polio virus types 1, 2, and 3 was developed. This trivalent vaccine (OPV) is administered orally. OPV is easier to administer than the inactivated vaccine (IPV) and produces secretory immunity within the gastrointestinal tract in addition to the serum humoral immunity. The attenuated virus is shed in the feces and spreads to unvaccinated persons in the community leading to herd immunity (48). The American Academy of Pediatrics and the Advisory Committee on Immunization practices have recommended that OPV be administered at 2, 4, and 15 months and again at 4–6 years of age; however, administration of the third dose at 6 months instead of 15 months is now being recommended. IPV, if used, may be administered according to the same schedule as OPV (Table 1). The relative value of using the original Salk vaccine versus the oral Sabin vaccine is being reevaluated. The latter preparation is still recommended except for individuals who are immunosuppressed.

Neurological Complications: Acute Paralytic Poliomyelitis

There are two types of vaccine-related poliomyelitis: one that occurs in vaccine recipients and the other in contacts of the vaccinated persons, especially those with impaired immunity (49). Vaccine-related poliomyelitis develops following administration of OPV and does not occur with use of the inactivated polio virus vaccine, which only causes transient low-grade fever in approximately 5% of children.

Most cases of paralytic poliomyelitis in the United States are vaccine related, and the incidence is low. About a third of the cases have occurred in OPV recipients, half in contacts of OPV recipients, and the remainder in individuals with impaired immunity who themselves were recipients or contacts of vaccinees (50). The CDC data for the years 1975–1984 show an incidence of one case of vaccine-associated paralytic polio per 3.2 million distributed doses of OPV (51). The incidence is greater following the first dose of vaccine, and approximately 94% of recipient cases and 82% of contact cases occur after the first immunization (52). In healthy individuals, the onset of symptoms generally occurs one month after exposure to the virus. In immunosuppressed individuals the latent period may be longer and the course of illness protracted. Unimmunized siblings and playmates of recipients are potentially at risk for contracting polio and may constitute a special risk group. This may be significant, as with increasingly younger age of entry into day care, there is a growing group of nonimmunized infants who may be exposed to infants recently immunized with OPV (53,54). Administration of a single dose of IPV before beginning OPV immunization to prevent OPV paralytic disease has been suggested (52).

Neurological Complications: Guillain-Barré Syndrome

Between February and March of 1985, an increased incidence of Guillain-Barré syndrome (GBS) was noted during and shortly following a nationwide program of immunization of children and adults in Finland (55). Ten patients with GBS were reported, with onset of symptoms within 10 weeks of vaccination. This increase in the number of cases of GBS temporally associated with the OPV immunization program was thought to be significant. The Institute of Medicine in their 1994 report concluded that there is a causal relation between OPV and GBS (55a). If symptoms develop within 5 days to 6 weeks after vaccination, subsequent vaccinations with OPV may be associated with a greater risk of developing GBS again.

PERTUSSIS VACCINE

Pertussis was first described in 1579; encephalopathy following pertussis was recognized in 1877. The pathogenesis of pertussis encephalopathy is not well understood. It is characterized by an alteration of consciousness or behavior, seizures, headache, and focal neurological deficits and is associated with significant neurological sequelae (56,57). Two percent of children younger than one year of age had seizures, and 0.4% had encephalopathy following pertussis during 1982–1983 (58).

Pertussis vaccine, standardized in 1947, is a whole cell vaccine in which the organism is inactivated by either mild heat, storage in the cold with thimerosal, or formalin or a combination of all three methods.

A newly licensed acellular or component vaccine has been developed to replace the fourth and fifth dose of the whole cell vaccine (59) and will probably be used exclusively in the future. The major advantage of this vaccine is that it contains two or more denatured elements of *Bordetella pertussis* bacillus that are required for immunity but little or none of the endotoxin. Therefore, side effects related to the endotoxin such as local reaction and fever are reduced. The incidence of crying, hypotonic-hyporesponsive episodes, and seizures is also reduced 10-fold using this vaccine as compared to the whole cell vaccine (52).

Efficacy

The most impressive evidence of pertussis vaccine efficacy was the largest epidemic of pertussis in the United Kingdom in 1978–1979 following a decline in the rate of pertussis immunization to 31% (60). In all, 102,500 cases of pertussis were reported. Eighty-three of these patients had seizures, and 36 patients died (61). In contrast, in the United States a precipitous drop in the incidence of pertussis occurred after the introduction of the vaccine in the 1940s, with present attack rates being 0.5–1 per 100,000 (58).

The vaccine significantly decreases the severity of disease and the number of cases of pertussis in populations of all ages (57). It has protection rates of 90–95% in vaccinated populations (58,62,63). Immunization does not prevent infection but does prevent disease. Therefore, immunized children may carry organisms and infect other individuals (64).

Adverse Reactions

Local Reactions

Triple immunization with DTP produces a much higher frequency of local reactions than DT alone. These include local redness and swelling, pain, fever, vomiting, anorexia, and persistent crying (65).

Hypotonic-Hyporesponsive Episodes

The hypotonic-hyporesponsive episode generally occurs within 4 h of immunization and is characterized by pallor, hypotonia, and unresponsiveness lasting from 10 min to 36 h. The pathogenesis of hypotonic-hyporesponsive episodes is poorly understood. In a prospective study of 15,752 children who received DTP, 9 developed hypotonic-hyporesponsive episodes and another 9 experienced convulsions (65). On follow-up 6–7 years later, none of these 18 children had permanent sequelae (66). There was no association between local reactions and major neurological complications, supporting the idea that local reactions are probably caused by endotoxin whereas major neurological complications are caused by some other toxin.

Neurological Complications

Seizures. The incidence of seizures after pertussis vaccination has been estimated at 1 per 1850 to 1 per 10,000 injections (65,67). This could be a chance association, as the expected incidence of seizures in this age group is 2–5% (68). Febrile convulsions are the most common adverse neurological reaction to pertussis immunization (69,70) and are not associated with permanent neurological sequelae (66). More than half of the children who develop febrile convulsions have a personal or family history of febrile convulsions (70). Febrile convulsions occur most often within 48 h of the third immunization (23), which is also the age when simple febrile convulsions are commonly seen. Postimmunization nonfebrile convulsions, on the other hand, occur less frequently, and these children are likely to have a personal but not a family history of seizures (70). It is not possible to differentiate a simple febrile seizure from a reaction to the pertussis vaccine which may lead to more serious neurological problems with subsequent vaccination. Therefore, any seizure developing after pertussis vaccination should be considered a contraindication to further vaccinations.

Infantile Spasms. The age at which DTP is administered is also the peak age for the onset of infantile spasms. A cause-and-effect association has been suggested, and independent surveys from Denmark, Japan, and the United Kingdom have examined this hypothesis.

In Denmark, the national immunization program was changed in 1970. Before 1970, DTP immunization was administered at 5, 6, and 15 months of age. Thereafter, DTP was abandoned and only pertussis vaccine was given at 5 weeks, 9 weeks, and 10 months of age. However, the peak age of onset of infantile spasms remained constant at 5 months of age before and after 1970. It was concluded that there was no causal relationship between pertussis immunization and infantile spasms (71).

In the Japanese report, 200 consecutive patients with infantile spasms at a single hospital were studied to evaluate the significance of previous immunization as an etiological factor for the infantile spasms. Children with other known risk factors were excluded. Only one child remained in whom pertussis immunization was the only risk factor prior to the onset of spasms. This rate of occurrence of one case of infantile spasms temporally related to pertussis immunization per 200 cases of infantile spasms can be explained by chance (72).

The National Childhood Encephalopathy Study in the United Kingdom received reports on 269 patients with infantile spasms. In 34% of these children, other antecedent factors such as perinatal history or tuberous sclerosis were identified. An excess risk of developing infantile spasms during the 28 days following immunization could not be demonstrated. There was, however, an increased risk in the first 7 days following either DTP or DT immunization that was later compensated for by a decreased risk in the following 21 days (73).

This pattern suggests that vaccination may either trigger the onset of infantile spasms or bring them to attention more quickly (73). Subsequent neurological outcome is no different in children whose infantile spasms are triggered by immunization than in those whose spasms begin spontaneously.

Encephalopathy. The risk of encephalopathy following pertussis immunization was first suggested in the United Kingdom. In 1974, 50 children were evaluated for neurological illness that was thought to be related to DTP. Thirty-two of these 50 children experienced seizures and 22 children were subsequently retarded. It was concluded that "the clustering of complications in the first 24 h following inoculation suggested a causal rather than coincidental relation" (74). Another retrospective study identified 197 patients with reported brain damage after pertussis inoculation and concluded that the incidence of brain damage was not less than 2 per 100,000 immunized children (75). These reports were widely circulated and the vaccination rate for pertussis in the United Kingdom fell from 80% to 31%, resulting in a pertussis epidemic.

In response to this professional and public concern, the National Childhood Encephalopathy Study was undertaken in 1976 to analyze the risks of neurological complications of pertussis immunization. All children from 2 months to 3 years of age who were hospitalized during a 3-year period with an illness satisfying the study criteria were identified. These criteria included encephalitis or encephalopathy, unexplained coma, convulsions more than 30 min long or followed by persistent neurological complications, infantile spasms, and Reye's syndrome. In all, a total of 1182 children were registered, and 2 control children matched for sex, age, and area of residence were selected for each child with encephalopathy. The excess risk of encephalopathy following DTP inoculation over the risk in controls was estimated at one in 110,000, and was greatest in the first 72 h following immunization. Seizures with or without fever occurring within this time were the most common adverse effect attributable to the vaccine. Children with seizures made a complete recovery. The risk of brain damage following DTP in previously normal children was estimated at one case per 310,000 injections. However, this estimate did not exclude patients with possible alternative explanations. The rate of one case per 310,000 injections was based upon a total of 11 affected children and included 2 children with prolonged convulsions, 5 with encephalitis (one thought to be due to coxsackievirus and another to rhinovirus), three with infantile spasms, and one with Reye's syndrome (60). If the three patients with infantile spasms, the 1 patient with Reye's syndrome, and 2 patients with known viral etiology of the encephalitis are excluded, only 5 patients with unexplained encephalopathy remain for whom attributable risk may be assessed. The estimated risk remained at one per 310,000, but the 95% confidence limits became so broad that the figure became meaningless (13).

In England, a separate study conducted over 7 years (23) found no convincing evidence to support the belief that DTP caused major neurological damage.

Data from the CDC for 1978–1981 suggested a rate for severe reactions of one per 230,000 doses of immunization but provided no information on sequelae. By comparison, 5 of 1277 children with natural pertussis infection developed encephalopathy in that same time period, suggesting a higher risk of encephalopathy with natural infection than with pertussis vaccine (58).

Contraindications

Absolute contraindications to pertussis vaccination include (1) occurrence within 48 h of vaccination of fever of ⩾40.5°C, (2) collapse or shocklike state, with a previous vaccination, (3) persistent screaming lasting 3 hours or longer with a previous vaccination, (4) seizures or encephalopathy within 7 days of previous vaccination, (5) evolving neurological disorders, and (6) hypersensitivity to the pertussis vaccine (76,77). Another contraindication included in the package insert distributed with the vaccine is a personal or family history of central nervous system disorders.

There is good evidence that children who have experienced one neurological reaction to pertussis vaccination are at significant risk for more severe reactions with further vaccination (67,78). In 1949, 38 cases of seizures after pertussis immunization were reported on the basis of responses to questionnaires; several of these children had a positive personal or family history of seizures (79). In 1974, one third of 50 children with neurological reactions to pertussis had some preexisting neurological disease (74). The most compelling evidence can be found in a review of 262 reports from the MSAEFI in 1985. This study found that children who had an adverse neurological event within one month of DTP had a 7.2 times higher incidence of prior personal history of convulsions and a 4.5 times higher incidence of family history of convulsions than children with an adverse effect not involving the nervous system (70). There is no conclusive evidence to suggest that a personal or family history of neurological disease is an absolute contraindication to pertussis vaccination. However, based on the above studies, it has been recommended that pertussis vaccination be withheld until the presence or absence of an evolving neurological disorder can be ascertained in patients with seizures or a positive family history. Opinion to the contrary also exists (80).

It is important to remember that pertussis is a dangerous and deadly disease and that pertussis immunization is effective in protecting against the disease. Pertussis vaccination should be given to all children unless absolute contraindications exist.

The Child Neurology Society in 1991 published a consensus statement (81) with the following conclusions:

1. Administration of pertussis vaccine is associated with a short-term increased risk of seizures, mostly febrile seizures, and complete recovery is expected.

2. Case reports have raised the issue as to whether there is an association between pertussis vaccine and progressive or chronic neurological disorders, but controlled studies have failed to prove such an association.
3. At the present time, there is no means by which a diagnosis of pertussis vaccine encephalopathy can be established in an individual case.

To this may be added that there is a causal relationship between pertussis vaccine and an unusual shocklike state also referred to as a "hypotonic-hyporesponsive" episode as well as inconsolable crying, probably caused by pain at injection site.

TETANUS AND DIPHTHERIA VACCINES

Tetanus is caused by infection with *Clostridium tetani*, which produces two exotoxins: tetanolysin and tetanospasmin. Tetanus results from tetanospasmin, which acts presynaptically to prevent neurotransmitter release (82). Tetanus toxoid, a modified exotoxin, prevents germination of spores in wounds, prevents binding and production of the toxin in the central nervous system, and induces antibody formation against the toxins. The accepted protective level of this antibody in the plasma is 0.01 U/ml. These protective levels are achieved in most children and adults after two doses given 4 or more weeks apart. Children less than one year of age may require three doses of tetanus toxoid (83). These protective levels are short-lived in infants and older adults, and a reinforcing booster dose is given 6–12 months after the primary series. Long-term immunity, usually exceeding 10 years, develops after a booster dose of tetanus toxoid (84). Complications may arise when this level of protection is already present and repeated injections are given (85).

Diphtheria is caused by *Corynebacterium diphtheriae*, which also produces an exotoxin. Diphtheria and tetanus toxoid are generally administered together as tetanus and diphtheria toxoid (Td) in adults and diphtheria and tetanus toxoid (DT) or DTP (a combination that also includes vaccine against pertussis) in children. It is therefore difficult to analyze adverse reactions to diphtheria and tetanus toxoid separately. The diphtheria and tetanus vaccines are produced by inactivating the toxins elaborated by the two organisms and adsorbing this antigen on aluminum phosphate. DT and Td differ in the lower concentration of the diphtheria toxoid in Td, the preparation for use in adults. Monovalent diphtheria and tetanus toxoid are also available. In the United States, the American Academy of Pediatrics and Advisory Committee on Immunization Practices recommend that diphtheria, tetanus toxoid, and pertussis vaccine (DTP) be given at 2, 4, and 6 months, between 15 and 18 months, and between 4 and 6 years of age. DT should be used in children younger than age 7 years in whom pertussis is contraindicated. Td should be used in individuals older than 7 years. Recall immunization is suggested in both children and adults at 10-year intervals (Table 1).

Adverse Reactions of Diphtheria Toxoid

There are no known adverse reactions of diphtheria toxoid.

Adverse Reactions of Tetanus Toxoid

Local Reactions

Minor local reactions such as tenderness, edema, and erythema occur within 48 h of immunization (86). Severe reactions such as swelling of the arm and systemic manifestations of fever and malaise may correlate with high antibody levels prior to immunization (85).

Anaphylactoid Reaction

Anaphylactoid reaction usually occurs within a few hours following immunization with tetanus toxoid. The patient may have urticaria, pruritus, wheezing, angioedema, shortness of breath, and hypotension (86).

Neurological Complications

Demyelinating Diseases. There are case reports of acute demyelinating encephalomyelitis (ADEM) (87,88), acute transverse myelitis (89,90) (VAER 11/90–7/92), and rarely optic neuritis (91) following immunization with diphtheria and tetanus toxoid alone or in combination.

In a survey of the literature, 29 cases of GBS or polyradiculoneuritis were found in association with tetanus toxoid immunization (92–94). The majority of these patients had received tetanus toxoid alone or tetanus toxoid and antitoxin serum. These case reports do not, however, demonstrate a proved cause-and-effect relationship between tetanus toxoid and polyradiculoneuropathy, mononeuropathy, or myelopathy. The exception is a patient in whom a demyelinating neuropathy developed after each of three injections of tetanus toxoid over 14 years. The latencies for the episodes of GBS were 21, 14, and 10 days, respectively. There were minimal residual neurological signs following the second episode, and full functional recovery followed the third (92). Two episodes of GBS were also described in a child, each following tetanus toxoid administration (52). In these individual patients, the cause-and-effect relationship is established, even though it has never been proved epidemiologically.

The MSAEFI lists four cases of GBS following vaccination with DT between 1979 and 1990. The VAER lists two cases of GBS following Td vaccination between November 1990 and November 1992. It is noteworthy that both of these patients also simultaneously received MMR.

Neuropathy. Mononeuropathy (95) and brachial neuritis following administration of tetanus toxoid has been described numerous times in the literature (96,97) with latencies ranging from 4 to 21 days. Transient cranial mononeuropathies have rarely been reported, developing from 5 to 10 days following administration of tetanus toxoid. They were thought to be related to a "neuroallergic" phenomenon following tetanus toxoid. The mechanism of these nerve disorders following tetanus immunization is not well understood.

Encephalopathy. Diphtheria and tetanus toxoids are not known to be associated with an increased risk of encephalopathy or seizures.

Although rare, tetanus still occurs in the United States, primarily in neonates and in unimmunized or inadequately immunized adults. A careful history of prior immunization should be taken before administering routine booster injections because there may be a possible risk of neuropathy with repeated injections (52,92). Clean minor wounds require no booster in a person who has received a booster within 10 years and is fully immunized. Persons with contaminated wounds should receive a tetanus booster if more than 5 years have elapsed since the last dose. The only contraindication to use of the toxoids is a history of neurological or severe hypersensitivity reaction following a previous dose.

Haemophilus influenzae TYPE b VACCINE

Prior to the 1970s, *Haemophilus influenzae* type b (Hib) was the leading cause of bacterial meningitis among children in the United States. The cumulative incidence of invasive Hib disease in the first 5 years of life was estimated at approximately one case per 200 children, with a mortality rate of 3–6%. Permanent sequelae, including hearing loss, mental retardation, and seizures, occurred in 20% of survivors (98). The majority (75%) of cases occurred in children younger than 2 years of age. This susceptibility probably correlated with lack of antibody to Hib capsular polysaccharide polyribosylribitol phosphate (PRP) in this age group (99).

A plain polysaccharide vaccine composed of purified PRP was developed in the 1970s. It had several limitations. Responsiveness to PRP was highly age dependent. It did not provide immunity in children less than 18 months of age. In addition, there was a possible increased incidence of Hib disease in the immediate (< 7 days) postimmunization period (100,101).

A series of Hib conjugate vaccines were developed in the late 1980s. PRP was conjugated to other compounds such as the outer membrane protein complex of *Neisseria meningitides* (PRP-OMP), tetanus toxoid (PRP-T), oligosaccharide conjugate Hib (HibOC), or diphtheria toxoid (Hib-D) to increase its efficacy. These vaccines differ not only in the molecular size of the Hib polysaccharide, but also in the protein used as carrier and the methods used to link the polysaccharide to the protein. Variations in the type or frequency of adverse effects of these vaccines may occur because of differences in the polysaccharide or protein components. The conjugate vaccine produce larger amounts of anti-PRP antibody in vaccinees of all ages and in immunosuppressed individuals who do not have adequate antibody responses to natural infection with Hib or plain PRP vaccine, e.g., patients with splenectomy, sickle cell disease, and malignancy (102,103).

Routine immunization of infants with Hib conjugate vaccine is now recommended in the United States. It is given simultaneously with DTP and OPV vaccine for parental convenience and to provide protective immunity during the high-risk period of infancy. The American Academy of Pediatrics and the Advisory Committee on Immunization recommend that Hib conjugate vaccine be administered in two or three doses starting at 2 months with a booster at 12–15 months of age (Table 1). The expected efficacy of the Hib conjugate vaccine is between 90 and 100%. Since the widespread distribution of the Hib conjugate vaccine there has been a marked decrease in the incidence of Hib disease in the United States (104).

Adverse Reactions: Local

Pain, tenderness, swelling, and erythema may occur in approximately 5–20% of children 24–72 h following immunization. Local reactions are seen less frequently with plain PRP vaccine than with the conjugate vaccine.

Adverse Reactions: Systemic

Low-grade fever and irritability are short-lived and are not felt to be serious complications (105).

Adverse Reactions: Neurological Complications

GBS has been reported following immunization with Hib conjugate vaccine. Seven cases of GBS have been described following immunization with the three Hib conjugate vaccines currently licensed for use in the United States, including HbOC, PRP-D, and PRP-OMP (106,107). Since its introduction in the late 1980s, several million doses of Hib conjugate vaccine have been administered. Only five patients have been reported who fit the criteria for possible vaccine-related GBS with onset of symptoms 6–12 days after vaccination. Two of these five had possible predisposing factors for GBS other than Hib vaccination, including infection and OPV immunization. Hib conjugate vaccine administration was the only potential predisposing factor in three patients (106,107). Therefore, these data are insufficient to support a definite causal link between GBS and Hib vaccine.

Adverse Reactions: Early Susceptibility to Hib

Early-onset Hib disease following immunization is defined as a case of serious systemic infection that occurs within 7 days following immunization for Hib. There have been several studies that suggest immunization of children over 18 months of age with unconjugated PRP vaccine is

Associated with an increased risk of disease in the following 7-day interval, with an incidence of 1.62 cases per 100,000 vaccines (100,101). Since the PRP vaccine contains only purified capsular polysaccharide, these cases could not have been caused by the infectious material in the vaccine itself. Several mechanisms have been postulated. A small portion of unimmunized children may have anti-PRP antibody concentrations. This group may develop a transient depression of free antibody levels immediately (1–3 days) following immunization with Hib vaccine. In children without preexisting anti-PRP antibody concentrations, susceptibility to early Hib disease could be secondary to delayed acquisition of the protective antibody (108,109). Another less likely mechanism was thought to be a transient suppression of antibody synthesis (110). It was also postulated that the clustering of cases in the first week after immunization and not in the second and third weeks suggests that immunization may shorten the incubation period in children already destined to be ill (100).

Vaccination did not alter the frequency of the different clinical manifestations associated with subsequent Hib infection, except in children who developed disease within 72 h, in whom meningitis was less frequent and epiglottitis and cellulitis more frequent (111).

There is no evidence of an early susceptibility to Hib disease with the conjugated vaccines (112). Although these vaccines are capable of causing a transient decline in the levels of preexisting serum antibodies following immunization, they produce a rapid and more predictable rise in the protective antibody levels. Thus the interval of increased risk, if any, is very short. As the vaccine is usually administered to young infants, who generally have little preexisting antibody to be decreased, it is more likely to provide protection, rather than suppression, of antibody.

INFLUENZA VACCINE

Regular immunization against influenza is not recommended for healthy children in the United States. It is used mainly for the elderly and those with chronic disease. A new vaccine is used each year depending on the prevalent virus strains expected to appear in the upcoming winter.

Neurological complications following influenza vaccination were rarely reported before 1976. In that year, a national immunization program was established against the "swine flu" (A/New Jersey) strain of the influenza virus. A passive surveillance system was simultaneously organized to evaluate the adverse effects related to the immunization. These adverse effects were reported to the state health department by the vaccinee or the physician who administered the vaccine. Over the next 2 months, an increase in cases of GBS was documented. An active surveillance program was subsequently initiated, and these initial findings were confirmed. The risk of GBS attributable to influenza immunization was estimated at one per 100,000 immunizations, with onset usually 5–10 weeks following the immunization. This association has not been confirmed again since the original report (113).

Other neurological complications reported in the passive surveillance program included occasional case reports of encephalopathy (114–116), brachial plexus neuropathy or neuralgic amyotrophy (117), acute transverse myelitis (118), and isolated cranial neuropathies (119). However, these complications were too infrequent to establish a definite causal link.

VARICELLA VACCINE

Varicella is a highly communicable disease caused by the varicella-zoster virus. It is characterized by fever, malaise, and a generalized vesicular pruritic rash that lasts about 2 weeks. Rarely it is associated with serious complications, e.g., pneumonia, encephalitis, Reye's syndrome, and/or death. Herpes zoster (shingles) is a secondary infection caused by reactivation of latent varicella-zoster virus. Varicella is potentially severe in adults and in immunocompromised individuals.

About 3.9 million cases of varicella are estimated to occur annually in the United States. Eighty-seven percent of healthy susceptible individuals develop varicella following household exposure.

A live attenuated varicella vaccine was developed in Japan in the 1970s and is licensed for routine use in Japan and Korea. A similar vaccine prepared from a cell-free preparation of OKA strain was licensed for use in the United States on March 17, 1995 (121). The Committee on Infectious Diseases of the American Academy of Pediatrics recommends that varicella vaccine be administered subcutaneously as a single dose to children 12 months to 12 years of age who lack a history of varicella infection. In adolescents older than 12 years and adults who have not been immunized previously (by infection or vaccine) two doses are given 4–8 weeks apart.

Adverse reactions associated with varicella vaccine include fever and tenderness at the injection site. Varicellalike rash at the injection site or in a generalized distribution may be seen in 7–8% cases within 1 month of vaccine administration. Other unusual side effects seen only rarely include upper respiratory symptoms, headache, and fatigue.

Contraindications for the use of the varicella vaccine include (1) history of hypersensitivity to any component of the vaccine, or history of anaphylaxis to neomycin, (2) immunocompromised state, due to congenital or acquired immunodeficiency, immunosuppressive agents or steroid therapy, (3) leukemias, lymphomas, or other malignant neoplasms affecting the bone marrow or the lymphatics and untreated tuberculosis, (4) febrile illness, and (5) pregnancy. If the vaccine is administered, pregnancy should be avoided for 3 months.

Vaccination should be deferred for at least 5 months following blood transfusions or immunoglobulin administration. Use of salicylates is avoided for 6 weeks after vaccination as Reye's syndrome has been reported following the use of salicylates during natural varicella infection. Vaccine recipients should avoid close association with susceptible individuals (e.g., newborns, pregnant women, immunocompromised persons).

The duration of protection provided by the vaccine is unknown at present. Therefore, the need for booster doses is not yet defined (120,121).

REFERENCES

1. Robbins FC. Measles: Clinical features, pathogenesis, pathology and complications. Am J Dis Child 1962; 103:266–273.
2. Babbott FL Jr., Gordon JE. Modern measles. Am J Med Sci 1954; 228:334–361.
3. Morley DC. Measles in the developing world. Proc R Soc Med 1974; 67:1112–1115.
4. Stokes JJ, Maris EP, Gelles SS. Chemical, clinical and immunologic studies on the products of human plasma fractionation. XI. The use of concentrated normal human serum gammaglobulin (human immune serum globulin) in prevention and attenuation of measles. J Clin Invest 1944; 23:531–540.
5. Enders JF, Peebles TC. Propagation in tissue culture of cytopathic agents from patients with measles. Proc Soc Exp Biol Med 1954; 86:277–286.
6. Centers for Disease Control. Recommendations of the Public Health Service Advisory Committee on Immunization Practices: measles vaccines. MMWR 1967; 16:169–271.
7. Meyer HM Jr, Hopps HE, Parkman PD, Ennis FA. Control of measles and rubella through use of attenuated vaccines. Am J Clin Pathol 1978; 70:128–135.
8. Hilleman MR, Buynak EB, Weibel RE, Stokes J Jr, Whitman JE Jr, Leagus MB. Development and evaluation of the Moraten measles virus vaccine. JAMA 1968; 206:587–590.
9. Schwarz AJ. Immunization against measles: development and evaluation of a highly attenuated live measles vaccine. Ann Paediatr 1964; 202:241–252.
10. Bloch AB, Orenstein WA, Stetler HC, Wassilak SG, Amler RW, Bart KJ, Kirby CD, Hinman AR. Health impact of measles vaccination in the United States. Pediatrics 1985; 76:524–532.
11. Nader PR, Warren RJ. Reported neurologic disorders following live measles vaccine. Pediatrics 1968; 41:997–1001.

12. Landrigan PJ, Witte JJ. Neurologic disorders following live measles-virus vaccination. JAMA 1973; 223:1459–1462.
13. Fenichel GM. Neurologic complications of immunization. In: Swaiman KF, ed. Pediatric Neurology. Principles and Practice. St. Louis: The C.V. Mosby Company, 1989:925–930.
14. Miller DL. Frequency of complications of measles, 1963: Report on a National Inquiry by the Public Health Laboratory Service in collaboration with the Society of Medical Officers of Health. Br Med J 1964; 2:75–78.
15. Subacute sclerosing panencephalitis surveillance: United States. MMWR 1982; 31:585–588.
16. Schneck SA. Vaccination with measles and central nervous system disease. Neurology 1968; 18(Part II):79–82.
17. Cho CT, Lansky LJ, D'Souza BJ. Panencephalitis following measles vaccination (letter). JAMA 1973; 224:1299.
18. Dyken PR, Cunningham SC, Ward LC. Changing character of subacute sclerosing panencephalitis in the United States. Pediatr Neurol 1989; 5:339–341.
19. Valmari P, Lanning M, Tuokko H, Kouvalainen K. Measles virus in the cerebrospinal fluid in post-vaccination immunosuppressive measles encephalopathy. Pediatr Infect Dis J 1987; 6:59–63.
20. Mitus A, Holloway A, Evans AE, Enders JF. Attenuated measles vaccine in children with acute leukemia. Am J Dis Child 1962; 103:243–248.
21. Hirtz DG, Nelson KB, Ellenberg JH. Seizures following childhood immunizations. J Pediatr 1983; 102:14–18.
22. Griffin MR, Ray WA, Mortimer EA, Fenichel GM, Schaffner W. Risk of seizures after measles-mumps-rubella immunization. Pediatrics 1991; 88:881–885.
23. Pollock TM, Morris JA. A 7-year survey of disorders attributed to vaccination in northwest Thames region. Lancet 1983; 1:753–757.
24. Clark C, Hashim G, Rosenburg R. Transverse myelitis following rubeola vaccination. Neurology 1977; 27:360.
25. Grose C, Spigland I. Guillain-Barré syndrome following administration of live measles vaccine. Am J Med 1976; 60:441–443.
26. Beghi E, Kurland LT, Mulder DW. Incidence of acute transverse myelitis in Rochester, Minnesota, 1970–1980 and implications with respect to influenza vaccine. Neuroepidemiology 1982; 1:176–188.
27. Winner SJ, Evans GJ. Age-specific incidence of Guillain-Barré syndrome in Oxfordshire. Q J Med 1990; 77(New Series):1297–1304.
28. Kazarian EL, Gager WE. Optic neuritis complicating measles, mumps and rubella vaccination. Am J Ophthalmol 1978; 86:544–547.
29. Riikonen R. The role of infection and vaccination in the genesis of optic neuritis and multiple sclerosis in children. Acta Neurol Scand 1989; 80:425–431.
30. Marshall GS, Wright PF, Fenichel GM, Karzon DT. Diffuse retinopathy following measles, mumps and rubella vaccination. Pediatrics 1985; 76:989–991.
31. Pampiglione G, Griffith AH, Bramwell EC. Transient cerebral changes after vaccination against measles. Lancet 1971; 2:5–8.
32. Chan CC, Sogg RL, Steinman L. Isolated oculomotor palsy after measles immunization. Am J Ophthalmol 1980; 89:446–448.
33. Buynak ZB, Hilleman MR. Live attenuated mumps virus vaccine. I. Vaccine development. Proc Soc Exp Biol Med 1966; 123:768–775.
34. Nabe-Nielsen J, Walter B. Unilateral deafness as a complication of the mumps, measles and rubella vaccination. Br Med J 1988; 297:489.
35. Brodsky L, Stanievich J. Sensorineural hearing loss following live measles virus vaccination. Int J Pediatr Otorhinolaryngol 1985; 10:159–163.
36. Healy CE. Mumps vaccine and nerve deafness. Am J Dis Child 1972; 123:612.
37. Preblud SR. Some current issues relating to rubella vaccine. JAMA 1985; 254:253–256.
38. Kilroy AW, Schatter W, Fleet WF, Lefkowitz LB, Karzon DT, Fenichel GM. Two syndromes following rubella immunizations: clinical observations and epidemiological studies. JAMA 1970; 214:2287–2292.

39. Gilmartin RC, Jabbour JT, Duenas DA: Rubella vaccine myeloradiculoneuritis. J Pediatr 1972; 80: 406–412.
40. Schaffner W, Fleet WF, Kilroy AW, Lefkowitz LB, Herrmann KL, Thompson J, Karzon DT. Polyneuropathy following rubella immunization. A follow-up study and review of the problem. Am J Dis Child 1974; 127:684–688.
41. Institute of Medicine. Adverse Effects of Pertussis and Rubella Vaccines. Washington DC: National Academy Press, 1991.
42. Holt S, Hudgins D, Krishnan KR, Critchley EMR. Diffuse myelitis associated with rubella vaccination. Br Med J 1976; 2:1037–1038.
43. Kline LB, Margulies SL, Oh SJ. Optic neuritis and myelitis following rubella vaccination. Arch Neurol 1982; 39:443–444.
44. Modlin JF, Brandling-Bennet D, Witte JJ, Campbell CC, Meyers JD. A review of five years experience with rubella vaccine in the United States. Pediatrics 1975; 55:20–29.
45. Wyll SA, Herrmann KL. Inadvertent rubella vaccination of pregnant women. Fetal risk in 215 cases JAMA 1973; 225:1472–1476.
46. Vaheri A, Vesikari T, Oker-Blom N, Seppala M, Parkman PD, Veronelli J, Robbins FC. Isolation of attenuated rubella-vaccine virus from human products of conception and uterine cervix. N Engl J Med 1972; 286:1071–1074.
47. Rubella vaccination during pregnancy: United States 1971–1983. MMWR 1984; 33:365–373.
48. Nightingale EO. Recommendations for a national policy on poliomyelitis vaccination. N Engl J Med 1977; 297:249-253.
49. Henderson DA, Witte JJ, Morris L, Langmuir AD. Paralytic diseases associated with oral polio vaccine. JAMA 1964; 190:41–48.
50. Nkowane BM, Wassilak SG, Orenstein WA, Bart KJ, Schonberger LB, Hinman AR, Kew OM. Vaccine-associated paralytic poliomyelitis, United States: 1973 through 1984. JAMA 1987; 257: 1335–1340.
51. Centers for Disease Control. Poliomyelitis prevention. MMWR 1979; 28:510–520.
52. Fenichel GM. Neurological complications of Immunization. In: Swaiman KF, ed. Pediatric Neurology: Principles and Practice. St. Louis: The C.V. Mosby Company, 1993:1189–1193.
53. Bergeisen GH, Bauman RJ, Gilmore RL. Neonatal paralytic poliomyelitis: a case report. Arch Neurol 1986; 43:192–194.
54. Wilson J, Robinson R. Poliomyelitis after contact with recently vaccinated infant (letter). Br Med J 1974; 2:53.
55. Kinnunen E, Farkkila M, Hovi T, Juntunen J, Weckstrom P. Incidence of Guillain-Barré syndrome during a nationwide oral polio virus vaccine campaign. Neurology 1989; 39:1034–1036.
55a. Institute of Medicine. Polio vaccines. In: Stratton KR, Howe CJ, Johnston RB, eds. Adverse events associated with childhood vaccines: evidence bearing on causality. Institute of Medicine. Washington, DC: National Academy Press, 1994:187–210.
56. Miller CL, Fletcher WB. Severity of notified whopping cough. Br Med J 1976; 1:117–119.
57. Harris F, Bush G, Lewis M. Death of infants after triple vaccine (letter). Lancet 1979; 2:472–473.
58. Cherry JD. The epidemiology of pertussis and pertussis immunization in the United Kingdom and the United States: a comparative study. Curr Probl Pediatr 1984; 14:11,25,36,40,53.
59. Centers for Disease Control. Pertussis vaccination: acellular pertussis vaccine for reinforcing and booster use—supplementary ACIP statement: recommendations of the Immunizations Practice Advisory Committee (ACIP). MMWR 1992; 41(RR-1):1–10.
60. Miller DL, Ross EM, Alderslade R, Bellman MH, Rawson NSB. Pertussis immunization and serious acute neurological illness in children. Br Med J 1981; 282:1595–1599.
61. Fenichel GM. The pertussis vaccine controversy. Arch Neurol 1983; 40:193–194.
62. Church MA. Evidence of whooping-cough-vaccine efficacy from the 1978 whooping-cough epidemic in Hertfordshire. Lancet 1979; 2:188–190.
63. Preston NW. Protection by pertussis vaccine. Lancet 1976; 1:1065–1067.
64. Cherry JD, Brunell PA, Golden GS, Karzon DT. Report of the Task Force in Pertussis and Pertussis Immunization—1988. Pediatrics 1988; 81:939–984.

65. Cody CL, Baraff LJ, Cherry JD, Marcy SM, Manclark CR. Nature and rates of adverse reactions associated with DTP and DT immunizations in infants and children. Pediatrics 1981; 68:650–660.
66. Baraff LJ, Shields D, Beckwith L, Strome G, Marcy M, Cherry JD, Manclark CR. Infants and children with convulsions and hypotonic-hyporesponsive episodes following diphtheria-tetanus-pertussis immunization: follow-up evaluation. Pediatrics 1988; 81(6):789–794.
67. Ouvrier RA. Whooping cough immunizations: a neurologist's viewpoint. Med J Aust 1978; 2:300.
68. Harker P. Primary immunization in febrile convulsions in Oxford in 1972–1975. Br Med J 1977; 2:490–493.
69. Hirtz DG, Nelson KB, Ellenberg JH. Seizures following childhood immunizations. J Pediatr 1983; 102:14–18.
70. Stetler HC, Orenstein WA, Bart KJ, Brink EW, Brennan JP, Hinman AR. History of convulsions and use of pertussis vaccine. J Pediatr 1985; 107:175–179.
71. Melchior JC. Infantile spasms and early immunization against whooping cough. Arch Dis Child 1977; 52:134–137.
72. Matsumoto A, Watanabe K, Negoro T, Sugiura M, Iwase K, Hara K, Miyazaki S. Infantile spasms: etiological factors, clinical aspects and long term prognosis in 200 cases. Eur J Pediatr 1981; 135: 239–244.
73. Bellman MH, Ross EM, Miller DL. Infantile spasms and pertussis immunization. Lancet 1983; 1:1031–1034.
74. Kulenkampff M, Schwartzman JS, Wilson J. Neurological complications of pertussis inoculation. Arch Dis Child 1974; 49:46–49.
75. Stewart GT. Toxicity of pertussis vaccine: frequency and probability of reactions. J Epidemiol Commun Health 1979; 33:150–156.
76. American Academy of Pediatrics. Report of the Committee on Infectious Diseases: pertussis vaccine. Pediatrics 1984; 74:303–305.
77. Recommendations of the Immunization Practices Advisory Committee: supplementary statement of contraindications to receipt of pertussis vaccine. MMWR 1984; 33:169–171.
78. Berg JM. Neurologic complications of pertussis immunization. Br Med J 1958; 2:24–27.
79. Toomey JA. Reactions to pertussis vaccine. JAMA 1949; 139:448–450.
80. Melin KA. Pertussis immunization in children with convulsive disorders. J Pediatr 1953; 43:652–654.
81. Child Neurology Society Consensus Report. Pertussis immunization and the central nervous system. Ann Neurol 1991; 29:458–460.
82. Bergey GK, Bigalke H, Nelson PG. Differential effects of tetanus toxin on inhibitory and excitatory synaptic transmission in mammalian spinal cord neurons in culture: presynaptic locus of action for tetanus toxin. J Neurophysiol 1987; 57:121–131.
83. Barkin RM, Samuelson JS, Gotlin LP. DTP reactions and serologic response with a reduced dose schedule. J Pediatr 1984; 105:189–194.
84. Peebles TC, Levine L, Eldred ML, Edsall G. Tetanus toxoid emergency boosters: a reappraisal. N Engl J Med 1969; 280:575–581.
85. Collier LH, Polakoff S, Mortimer J. Reactions and antibody responses to reinforcing doses of adsorbed plain tetanus vaccines. Lancet 1979; 1:1364–1369.
86. Jacobs RL, Lowe RS, Lanier BQ. Adverse reactions to tetanus toxoid. JAMA 1982; 247:40–42.
87. Schlenska GK. Unusual neurological complications following tetanus toxoid administration. J Neurol 1977; 215:299–302.
88. Schwarz G, Lanzer G, List WF. Acute midbrain syndrome as an adverse reaction to tetanus immunization. Intensive Care Med 1988; 15:53–54.
89. Whittle F, Roberton NRC. Transverse myelitis after diphtheria, tetanus and polio immunization. Br Med J 1977; 1:1450.
90. Read SJ, Schapel GJ, Pender MP. Acute transverse myelitis after tetanus toxoid vaccination (letter). Lancet 1992; 339:1111–1112.
91. Topaloglu H, Berker M, Kansu T, Saaci U, Renda Y. Optic neuritis and myelitis after booster tetanus toxoid vaccination (letter). Lancet 1992; 339:178–179.

92. Pollard JD, Selby G. Relapsing neuropathy due to tetanus toxoid: report of a case. J Neurol Sci 1978; 37:113–125.
93. Reinstein L, Pargament JM, Goodman JS. Peripheral neuropathy after multiple tetanus toxoid injections. Arch Phys Med Rehab 1982; 63:332–34.
94. Holliday PL, Bauer RB. Polyradiculoneuritis secondary to immunization with tetanus and diphtheria toxoids. Arch Neurol 1983; 40:56–57.
95. Blumstein GI, Kreithin H. Peripheral neuropathy following tetanus toxoid administration. JAMA 1966; 198:1030–1031.
96. Baust W, Meyer D, Wachsmuth W. Peripheral neuropathy after administration of tetanus toxoid. J Neurol 1979; 222:131–133.
97. Kiwit JC. Neurologic amyotrophy after administration of tetanus toxoid. J Neurol Neurosurg Psychiatr 1984; 47:320.
98. Cochi SL, Broome CV, Hightower AW. Immunization of US children with Haemophilus influenzae type b polysaccharide vaccine: a cost effectiveness model of strategy assessment. JAMA 1985; 253:521–529.
99. Ward J, Cochi S. Hemophilus influenzae vaccines. In: Plotkin SA, Mortimer EA, eds. Vaccines. Philadelphia: W.B. Saunders, 1988.
100. Black SB, Shinefield HR, Hiatt RA, Fireman BH, Beekly M, Callas ER, and the Kaiser Permanente Pediatric vaccine study group. Efficacy of Hemophilus influenzae type b capsular polysaccharide vaccine. Pediatr Infect Dis J 1988; 7:149–156.
101. Shapiro ED, Murphy TV, Wald ER, Brady CA. The protective efficacy of Haemophilus b polysaccharide vaccine. JAMA 1988; 260:1419–1422.
102. Frank AL, Labotka RJ, Rao S, Frisone LR, McVerry PH, Samuelson JS, Maurer H, Yogev R. Haemophilus influenzae type b immunization of children with sickle cell diseases. Pediatrics 1988; 82:571–575.
103. Feldman S, Gigliotti F, Shenep JL, Roberson PK, Lott L. Risk of Haemophilus influenzae type b disease in children with cancer and response of immunocompromised leukemic children to a conjugate vaccine. J Infect Dis 1990; 161:926–931.
104. Adams WB, Deaver KA, Cochi SL, Plikaytis BD, Zell ER, Broome CV, Wenger JD. Decline of childhood Hemophilus influenza type b (Hib) disease in the Hib vaccine era. JAMA 1993; 269: 221–226.
105. Ahonkhai VI, Lukacs LJ, Jonas LC, Matthews H, Vella PP, Ellis RW et al. Hemophilus influenzae type b conjugate vaccine (meningococcal protein conjugate) (PedvaxHIB): clinical evaluation. Pediatrics 1990; 85(4 Pt 2):676–681.
106. D'Cruz OF, Shapiro ED, Spiegelman KN, Leicher CR, Breningstall JN, Khatri BO, Dobyns WB. Acute inflammatory demyelinating polyradiculoneuropathy (Guillain-Barré syndrome) after immunization with Haemophilus influenzae type b conjugate vaccine. J Pediatr 1989; 115:743–746.
107. Gervaix A, Caflisch M, Suter S, Haenggeli CA. Guillain-Barré syndrome following immunization with Haemophilus Influenzae type b conjugate vaccine. Eur J Pediatr 1993; 152:613–614.
108. Sood SK, Daum RS. Disease caused by Haemophilus influenzae type b in the immediate period after homologous immunization: immunologic investigation. Pediatrics 1990; 85(4 Part 2):698–704.
109. Marchant CD, Band E, Froeschle JE, McVerry PH. Depression of anticapsular antibody after immunization with Haemophilus influenzae type b polysaccharide-diphtheria conjugate vaccine. Pediatr Infect Dis J 1989; 8:508–511.
110. Murphy TV, White KE, Pastor P. Declining incidence of Haemophilus influenzae type b disease since introduction of vaccination. JAMA 1993; 269:246–248.
111. Hiner EE, Frasch CE. Spectrum of Disease Due to Haemophilus influenzae type b occurring in immunized children. J Infect Dis 1988; 158:343–348.
112. Santosham M, Wolff M, Reid R, Hohenboken M, Bateman M, Goepp J, Cortese M et al. The efficacy in Navajo infants of a conjugate vaccine consisting of Haemophilus influenzae type b polysaccharide and Neisseria meningitidis outer-membrane protein complex. N Engl J Med 1991; 324:1767–1772.
113. Schonberger LB, Bregman DJ, Sullivan-Bolyal JZ, Keenlyside RA, Ziegler DW, Retailliau HF, Eddens

DL, Buyan JA. Guillain-Barré syndrome following vaccination in the national influenza immunization program, United States 1976–1977. Am J Epidemiol 1979; 110:105–123.
114. Cherington M. Locked-in syndrome after "Swine-flu" inoculation (letter). Arch Neurol 1977; 34:258.
115. Gens RD, Beecham HJ. Meningoencephalitis after influenza inoculation (letter). N Engl J Med 1978; 299:721–722.
116. Yahr MD, Lobo-Antunes J. Relapsing encephalomyelitis following the use of influenza vaccine. Arch Neurol 1972; 27:182–183.
117. Weintraub MI, Chia DTS. Paralytic brachial neuritis after swine flu vaccination (letter). Arch Neurol 1977; 34:518.
118. Wells CEC. A neurological note on vaccination against influenza. Br Med J 1971; 3:755–756.
119. Felix JK, Schwartz RH, Myers GJ. Isolated hypoglossal paralysis following influenza vaccination. Am J Dis Child 1976; 130:82–83.
120. American Academy of Pediatrics, Committee on Infectious Diseases. Recommendations for the use of live attenuated varicella vaccine. Pediatrics 1995; 95:791–796.
121. Varivax package insert. Merck and Co., West Point, PA. Issued March 1995.
122. American Academy of Pediatrics. Active Immunization. In: Peter G, ed. 1994 Red Book: Report of the Committee on Infectious Diseases. 23rd ed. Elk Grove Village, IL: American Academy of Pediatrics, 1994:23.

5

Bacterial Meningitis

Karen L. Roos
Indiana University School of Medicine, Indianapolis, Indiana

HISTORY OF MENINGITIS

The first description of meningococcal meningitis, or as it was called in 1805 "cerebrospinal fever," came from Geneva describing a small outbreak that occurred in that city (1). The first epidemic of spotted fever to be documented in America occurred in Medfield, Massachusetts, in 1806 (2). The classic diagnostic sign of meningitis, meningismus, was initially described in 1910 by a medical student, Nathan Strong, in a dissertation required for his medical degree entitled "Inaugural Dissertation on the Disease Termed Petechial or Spotted Fever." Vladimir Mihailovich Kernig described his technique for detecting meningeal irritation in 1882, and Jozef Brudzinski described his techniques for detecting meningismus in 1909 (3). Heinrich Quincke performed a lumbar puncture on a patient with meningococcal meningitis and described the technique of lumbar puncture in 1891.

In the late 1800s, meningitis was treated by drainage of cerebrospinal fluid by repeated lumbar punctures. At the turn of the century, meningococcal meningitis was treated with intrathecal injections of "antimeningitis serum" (4). The antibacterial activity of sulfonamides was discovered in the early 1930s. Patients with meningococcal meningitis were treated with an intrathecal injection of sulfanilamide solution after the removal of a slightly larger volume of spinal fluid. The solution was also given subcutaneously. Sulfonamide therapy dramatically improved survival of meningococcal meningitis (5).

Flemming discovered penicillin in 1931. The first successful treatment of cases of meningococcal meningitis with penicillin was reported in 1944 (6). Initially, comparatively low doses of parenteral penicillin were used to treat meningitis, and this therapy was combined with intrathecal penicillin injections in order to improve survival. The first clinical trials using high doses of systemic penicillin were reported in 1950; thereafter, the intrathecal instillation of penicillin was no longer necessary for therapeutic success (7). The outcome of bacterial meningitis was significantly improved with penicillin therapy.

Despite the availability today of effective antimicrobial therapy, bacterial meningitis continues to be one of the most devastating neurological diseases. An improvement in the quality of survival is dependent on our ability to decrease the incidence and severity of the neurological complications of this disease with therapeutic modalities that alter the pathophysiology of bacterial meningitis.

PATHOPHYSIOLOGY

Streptococcus pneumoniae, *Neisseria meningitidis*, and *Haemophilus influenzae* are the bacteria that most commonly cause community-acquired meningitis. These organisms initially colonize the nasopharynx by attaching to the nasopharyngeal epithelial cells. The organism is able to attach to the epithelial cell via an interaction between bacterial surface structures, such as the fimbriae of *N. meningitidis*, and host cell surface receptors. The bacteria are then either carried across the cell in membrane-bound vacuoles to the intravascular space or invade the intravascular space by creating separations in the apical tight junctions of columnar epithelial cells (8). These are encapsulated bacteria, and once they have gained access to the bloodstream, they are able to avoid phagocytosis by neutrophils and classical complement-mediated bactericidal activity because of the presence of a polysaccharide capsule. Bacteria that are able to survive in the circulation then enter the cerebrospinal fluid (CSF) from the bloodstream through the choroid plexus of the lateral ventricles and in other areas of altered blood-brain barrier permeability.

The cerebrospinal fluid has been called an area of impaired host defense because of a lack of sufficient numbers of complement components and immunoglobulins for the opsonization of bacteria, an essential step for phagocytosis by neutrophils. In addition, the fluid medium of the cerebrospinal fluid impairs the phagocytosis of bacteria by neutrophils (9,10). Consequently, bacteria multiply rapidly in the subarachnoid space.

The formation and presence of a purulent exudate in the subarachnoid space (Fig. 1) is the basis for the neurological complications of bacterial meningitis. The lysis of bacteria with the release of bacterial cell wall components in the subarachnoid space is the initial step in the induction of the inflammatory process and the formation of a purulent exudate in the subarachnoid space (Fig. 2). The lipooligosaccharide (LOS) component of the *H. influenzae* type b (Hib) cell wall (endotoxin) and the teichoic acid and peptidoglycan components of the pneumococcal cell wall have been demonstrated in experimental models of meningitis to induce meningeal inflammation by stimulating the production of the inflammatory cytokines, interleukin-1 and tumor necrosis factor. Interleukin-1 (IL-1) and tumor necrosis factor (TNF) are produced by monocytes, macrophages, and CNS macrophage equivalent cells—brain astrocytes and microglial cells.

One of the biological activities of TNF that contributes to inflammation in the subarachnoid space is its role in neutrophil adherence to vascular endothelial cells. One of the major contributors to the purulent exudate in the subarachnoid space that develops in the course of meningitis is the increased number of neutrophils in the CSF. The exact mechanism by which neutrophils traverse the blood-brain barrier is not known; however, it appears that the adherence of neutrophils to capillary endothelial cells through specific adhesion molecules on capillary endothelial cells is a necessary prerequisite. TNF promotes neutrophil adherence to vascular endothelial cells by inducing the formation of endothelial leukocyte adhesion molecules. TNF also stimulates the synthesis and release of IL-1 from activated astrocytes and microglial cells. Interleukin-1 is a chemoattractant for neutrophils and stimulates neutrophils to degranulate and release toxic oxygen metabolites that then increase blood-brain barrier permeability (11).

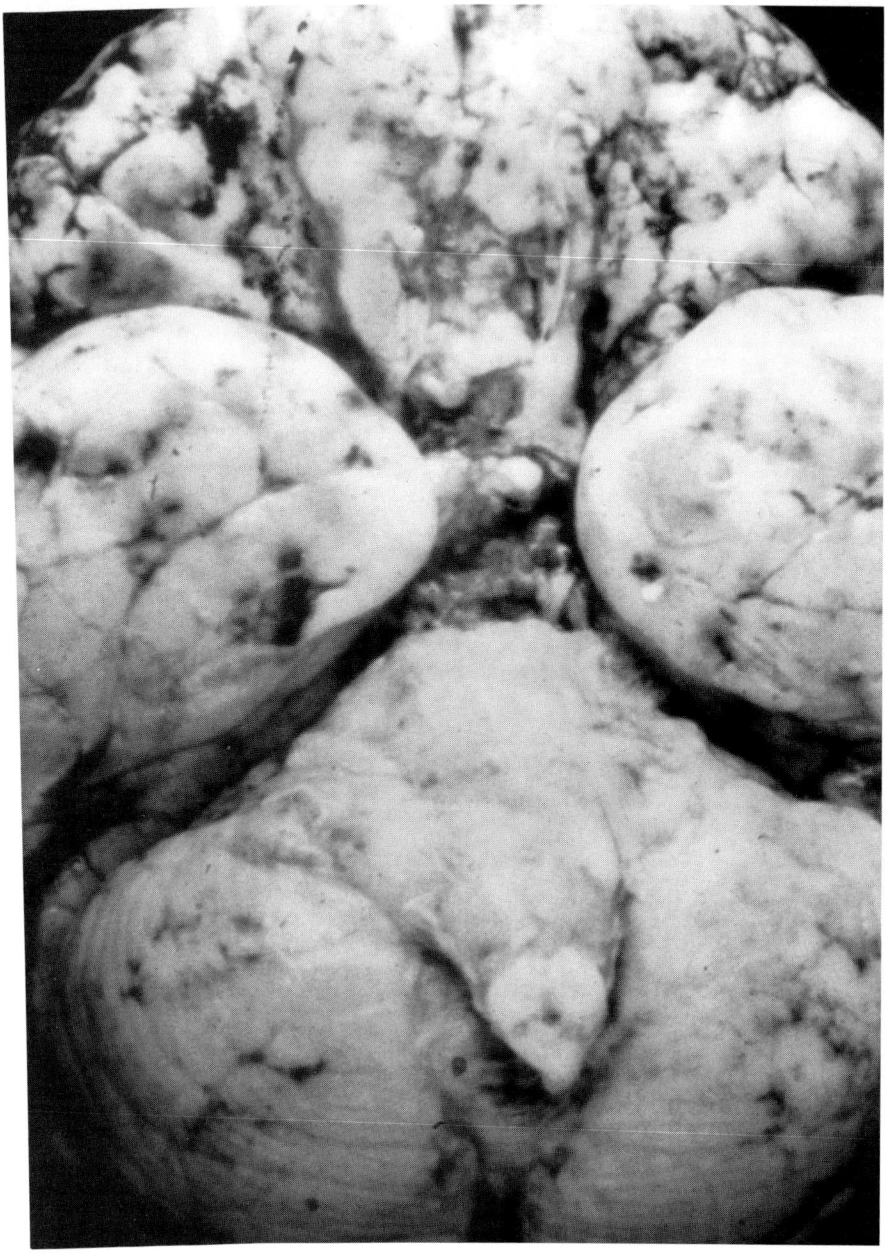

Figure 1 Purulent exudate surrounding the brainstem, cerebellum, temporal lobes, and optic chiasm. (From Ref. 89.)

The presence of TNF in CSF appears to be specific for bacterial meningitis. Elevated concentrations of TNF were detected in 42 (82%) of 51 patients with purulent bacterial meningitis and in only 5 of 78 individuals with nonbacterial meningitis. The individuals with nonbacterial meningitis and elevated concentrations of TNF in CSF had either herpes simplex type 2 or varicella-zoster virus meningitis (12). TNF activity was detected in the cerebrospinal fluid of 33

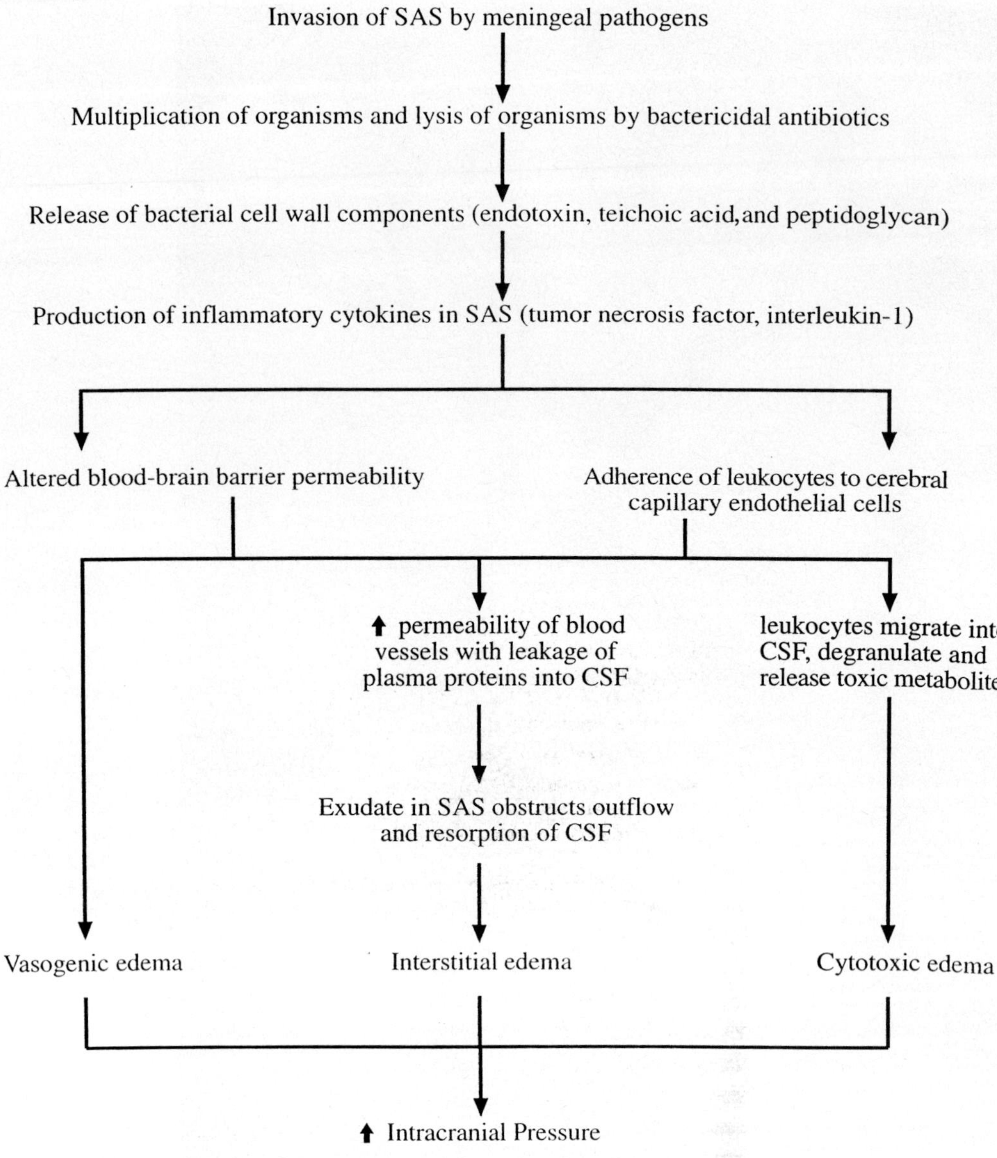

SAS = subarachnoid space

Figure 2 The inflammatory cascade is initiated by the multiplication and lysis of bacteria in the subarachnoid space.

of 38 children with bacterial meningitis but was undetectable in the CSF of 15 children with viral meningitis/encephalitis (13).

IL-1 may have a role in the altered level of consciousness and the production of fever in bacterial meningitis. It facilitates slow-wave sleep and produces fever by its affect on the hypothalamus (14,15). The initial CSF concentrations of IL-1 beta (IL-1β) may have predictive value for prognosis. In aliquots of CSF from 102 infants and children with bacterial meningitis there was a direct correlation between the initial CSF IL-1β concentrations and the CSF leukocyte count, lactate, protein, and TNF concentrations, and an inverse correlation with the CSF glucose concentration. Infants and children with initial CSF IL-1β concentrations of ⩾500 pg/ml were more likely to have neurological sequelae than infants and children with lower CSF IL-1β concentrations (16).

Other inflammatory cytokines have a role in the induction of meningeal inflammation. Interleukin-6 (IL-6) and interleukin-8 (IL-8) have been detected in serum from patients with septic shock and in CSF from patients with bacterial meningitis. IL-8 is a proinflammatory cytokine with chemoattractant effects on neutrophils. Other inflammatory mediators, such as platelet-activating factor (PAF), also appear to have a role in the pathophysiology of bacterial meningitis. Of the inflammatory mediators, TNF and IL-1 appear to be the principal cytokines in meningeal inflammation, and the roles of IL-6, IL-8, and PAF are not yet well defined.

Increased numbers of bacteria in CSF correlate with increased concentrations of TNF, and TNF concentrations in CSF correlate inversely with cerebral blood flow and cerebral oxygen uptake. There is an increased incidence of neurological sequelae among patients with large numbers of bacteria in CSF and high concentrations of TNF (17).

The inflammatory cytokines IL-1 and TNF act synergistically to alter the permeability of the blood-brain barrier. The alteration in blood-brain barrier permeability during bacterial meningitis results in vasogenic cerebral edema and increased intracranial pressure and allows for the exudation of serum proteins into the cerebrospinal fluid. The adherence of leukocytes to capillary endothelial cells also increases the permeability of blood vessels, allowing for the leakage of plasma proteins into the CSF and contributing to the inflammatory exudate in the subarachnoid space.

The cerebral edema that develops in the course of bacterial meningitis is due to a combination of vasogenic, interstitial, and cytotoxic edema (Fig. 2). Vasogenic edema is primarily a consequence of increased blood-brain barrier permeability. Interstitial edema is the result of diminished resorption of cerebrospinal fluid at the level of the arachnoid granulations due to the presence of a fibrinous exudate in the subarachnoid space. As resorption is obstructed, the flow of cerebrospinal fluid is altered and there is a transependymal movement of fluid from the ventricular system into the brain parenchyma (18). Cytotoxic edema develops secondary to swelling of the cellular elements of the brain as a result of toxic factors released from neutrophils and bacteria.

Increased intracranial pressure in bacterial meningitis is due to a combination of vasogenic, cytotoxic, and interstitial edema and, at least initially, an increase in cerebral blood volume. In experimental models of pneumococcal meningitis, cerebral blood flow is initially increased with a decline in blood flow later in the infection. Cerebral autoregulation is lost in bacterial meningitis so that an increase in systemic blood pressure initially leads to an increase in cerebral blood flow and a subsequent increase in intracranial pressure, and later in the infection a decrease in mean systemic arterial pressure results in a decrease in cerebral blood flow with resultant ischemia and infarction (17).

CLINICAL PRESENTATION

When the classic triad of headache, fever, and stiff neck are present, the diagnosis of bacterial meningitis is readily made. *Haemophilus influenzae* type b (Hib) meningitis is a disease of children between the ages of 6 months and 6 years, and of older adults. The symptoms of meningitis are often preceded by a history of an upper respiratory tract infection or an otitis media. The presentation of this illness is either that of a subacute infection that has been present for several days or that of an acute fulminant illness. Fever (⩾38.5°C), headache, photophobia, nausea and vomiting, lethargy, and/or irritability are the most common symptoms. Headache, vomiting, and neck stiffness are the most sensitive indicators of meningeal inflammation (19). The fulminant presentation is characterized by signs and symptoms of meningeal irritation and increased intracranial pressure.

A stiff neck is the pathognomonic sign of meningeal irritation from the presence of a purulent exudate or hemorrhage in the subarachnoid space. Nuchal rigidity or meningismus is present when the neck resists passive flexion. When neck stiffness is due to meningitis, the neck can usually be passively rotated from side to side. The neck may resist passive movement on examination due to cervical spondylosis, parkinsonism, or paratonic rigidity in the elderly. In these instances, passive movement of the neck in any direction meets with resistance.

Kernig's and Brudzinski's signs are also classic signs of meningeal irritation. Kernig's sign is best elicited with the patient in the seated position. Attempts to passively extend the knee are met with resistance in the presence of meningitis so that a "contracture of the extremities" is maintained (20). Brudzinski's "nape-of-the-neck sign" is elicited with the patient in the supine position and is positive when passive flexion of the neck results in spontaneous flexion of the hips and knees (Fig. 3) (19).

Seizures occur in 40% of patients with bacterial meningitis and typically occur during the first few days of the infection. In general, seizure activity is more frequent with pneumococcal meningitis and Hib meningitis than in meningococcal disease (21). The etiology of seizure activity in bacterial meningitis can be one or a combination of the following: (1) fever, (2) focal arterial ischemia or infarction, (3) cortical venous thrombosis with hemorrhage, (4) hyponatremia (due to the inappropriate secretion of antidiuretic hormone), (5) subdural effusion or subdural empyema producing a mass effect, or (6) antimicrobial toxicity. Seizure activity that has a focal onset is most likely a result of focal cerebrovascular disease due to one of the following: (1) narrowing of the major cerebral arteries at the base of the brain from encroachment on the vessel wall by the purulent exudate in the subarachnoid space, (2) vessel wall irregularities from vasculitis, or (3) thrombophlebitis of the cerebral cortical veins with hemorrhage. Focal seizure

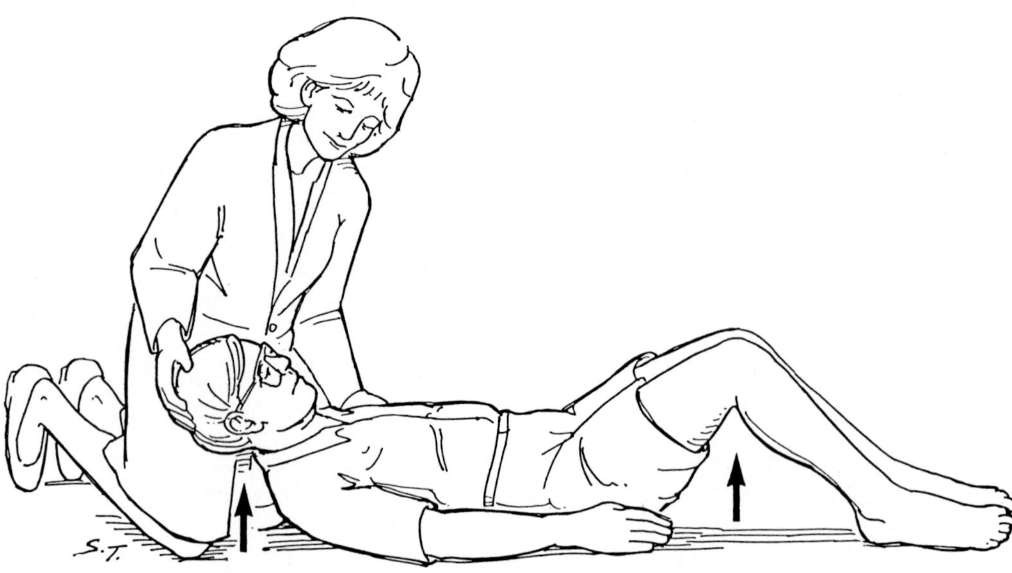

Figure 3 Brudzinski's sign of meningeal inflammation is elicited with the patient in the supine position, and is positive when passive flexion of the neck results in flexion of the hips and knees. (From Ref. 90.)

activity may also result from focal edema or mass effect from an expanding subdural effusion or empyema. Generalized seizure activity and status epilepticus may occur due to global hypoxia from decreased cerebral perfusion, hyponatremia, spread from a focal onset to a generalized tonic-clonic convulsion, or toxicity from antimicrobial agents.

The majority of patients with bacterial meningitis will have signs of raised intracranial pressure. The clinical signs of raised intracranial pressure are (1) an altered level of consciousness, (2) the Cushing reflex (bradycardia, hypertension, and irregular respirations), (3) unilateral or bilateral fixed and dilated pupils, (4) unilateral or bilateral cranial nerve six palsies, (5) papilledema, and (6) decerebrate posturing. The presence of raised intracranial pressure can be documented at the time of lumbar puncture by obtaining an opening pressure or measured with an ICP monitoring device. Raised intracranial pressure is the most likely etiology of an altered level of consciousness in the course of bacterial meningitis.

Meningococcal meningitis occurs in children and young adults. The typical symptoms of meningococcal meningitis are fever, vomiting, lethargy, neck stiffness, headache, and a petechial or purpuric rash on the trunk, the lower extremities, and in the mucous membranes, and conjunctiva. The petechial-purpuric rash of meningococcal septicemia is virtually diagnostic for this infection when present (Fig. 4). The rash of meningococcemia may vary from a few petechiae to extensive purpura with skin necrosis (21). A petechial rash is also seen in enteroviral meningitis, *Neisseria gonorrheae* sepsis, Hib and pneumococcal meningitis, and *S. aureus* endocarditis. The term Waterhouse-Friderichsen syndrome refers to a fulminating meningococcal septicemia characterized by the following: (1) sudden onset of a febrile illness, (2) large petechial hemorrhages in the skin and mucous membranes, (3) septic shock, and (4) disseminated intravascular coagulation. Fulminant meningococcal septicemia is reported in 10–20% of children with meningococcal infection (22,23).

The most common causative organism of community-acquired bacterial meningitis in the adult is *S. pneumoniae*. In a recent review of acute bacterial meningitis in adults 16 years of age or older, *S. pneumoniae* was responsible for 97 of 253 cases (38%) of community-acquired meningitis (24). An altered level of consciousness on presentation is common in community-acquired meningitis, and is particularly common in the older adult. In 279 episodes of community-acquired meningitis, 51% were confused or lethargic on presentation, 22% were responsive only to pain, and 6% were unresponsive to all stimuli (24). Similarly, in a review of 178 cases of community-acquired pneumococcal meningitis, 38% of patients were irritable or lethargic on admission, 29% were delirious or stuporous on admission, and 20% were comatose (25). Pneumonia and acute and chronic otitis media are common predisposing conditions for pneumococcal meningitis.

Cranial nerve palsies, and most notably sensorineural hearing loss, is a common complication of bacterial meningitis. Cranial nerve abnormalities develop as a result of the presence of an inflammatory exudate in the arachnoidal sheath surrounding the nerve (Fig. 5). Sensorineural hearing loss is a result of one of the following mechanisms: (1) cochlear dysfunction due to a direct invasion of bacteria into the cochlea via the cochlear aqueduct, (2) cochlear nerve inflammation secondary to the inflammatory exudate in the arachnoidal sheath of the nerve, (3) inflammation of the vascular supply to the nerve with subsequent ischemia, or (4) cochlear or nerve toxicity due to antimicrobial agents. Children with bacterial meningitis may also be ataxic as a result of labyrinthine dysfunction or vestibular neuronitis. The association of ataxia and sensorineural hearing loss suggests involvement of both the vestibular and cochlear divisions of the eighth nerve; alternatively, there is the simultaneous presence of cochlear and labyrinthine dysfunction due to inflammation.

Acute ischemic stroke may occur in the course of bacterial meningitis due to one of the following etiologies: (1) narrowing of the large arteries at the base of the brain due to encroachment on the vessel wall by the purulent exudate in the subarachnoid space or by infiltration of the

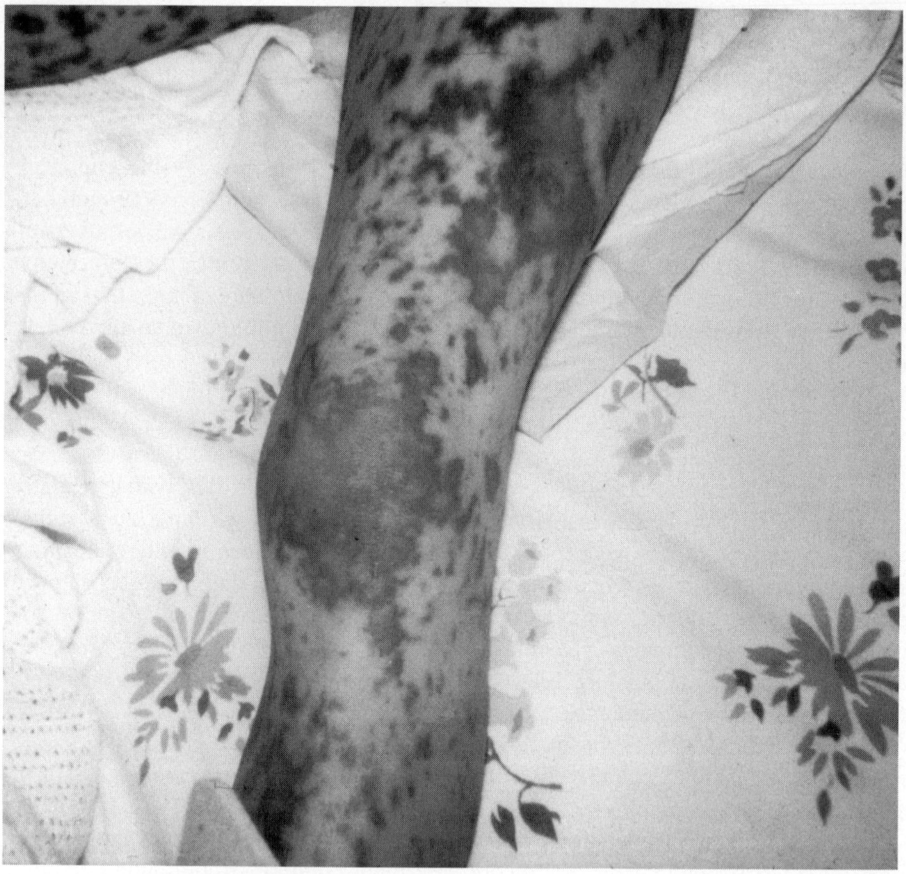

Figure 4 The petechial-purpuric rash of meningococcemia. (From Ref. 89.)

arterial wall by inflammatory cells (vasculitis) with thickening of the wall of the blood vessel and narrowing of the lumen, (2) vasospasm of the large or medium-sized arteries, (3) narrowing of medium-sized arteries and thrombotic or stenotic occlusion of branches of the middle cerebral artery, and (4) septic venous sinus thrombosis with thrombophlebitis of cortical veins. The clinical presentation of acute ischemic stroke in the course of bacterial meningitis is dependent on the territory of the vessels involved in the inflammatory process, but is most often a hemiparesis due to the frequent involvement of the supraclinoid portion of the internal carotid artery and the middle cerebral artery and its branches.

DIAGNOSIS

The gold standard for the diagnosis of bacterial meningitis is examination of the cerebrospinal fluid. A critical issue is the determination of the risk of cerebral herniation due to lumbar puncture in a patient with suspected bacterial meningitis and raised intracranial pressure. As neuroimaging procedures have become readily available, it has become standard practice to perform a computed tomographic (CT) or magnetic resonance (MR) scan prior to lumbar puncture. This procedure, however, often delays treatment, and a normal CT or MR scan does not rule out the presence of raised intracranial pressure. The risk of cerebral herniation following lumbar puncture has led to

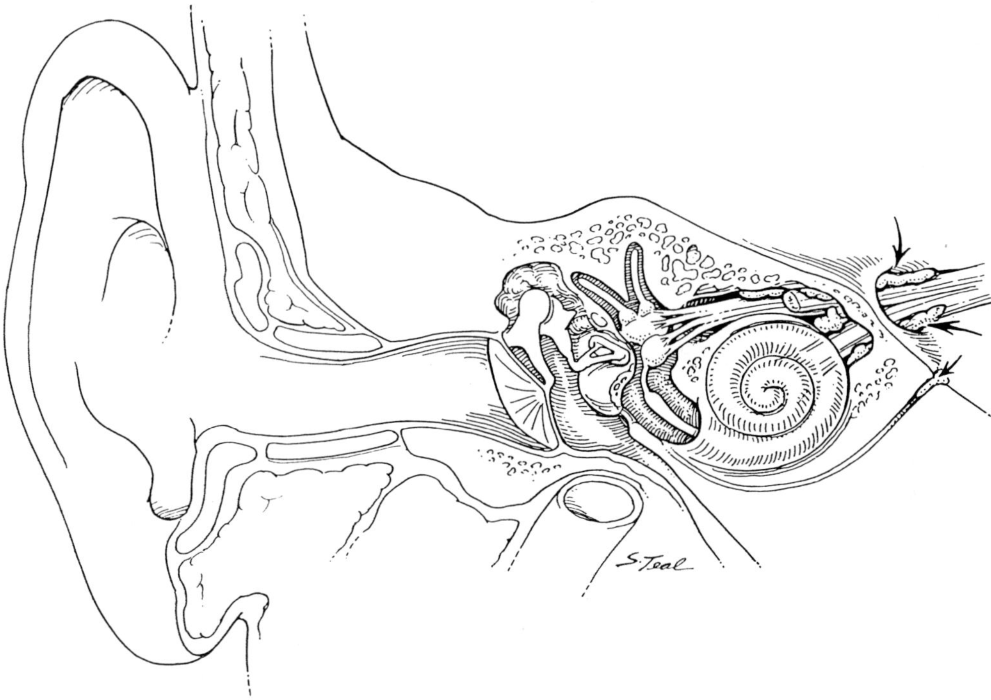

Figure 5 Sensorineural hearing loss in bacterial meningitis may develop due to the presence of an inflammatory exudate (black arrows) in the arachnoidal sheath of cranial nerve VIII. (From Ref. 90.)

the suggestion that lumbar puncture be avoided altogether when clinical signs of raised intracranial pressure are present and the patient be treated empirically. Unfortunately, the majority of patients with bacterial meningitis have a complicated course for at least the first 72 h after treatment is initiated. If cerebrospinal fluid has not been examined, the uncertainty of diagnosis increases the anxiety of the physician and affects the care of the patient. Cerebrospinal fluid should be obtained for examination in all patients with suspected bacterial meningitis unless there are clinical signs of impending cerebral herniation or CT or MR scan demonstrate a focal intracranial mass lesion. The clinical signs of impending cerebral herniation are (1) unilateral or bilateral dilated nonreactive pupils, (2) rapidly increasing deterioration in the level of consciousness, (3) the Cushing reflex (bradycardia, hypertension, and irregular respirations), and (4) decerebrate posturing. It is unreasonable to suggest that lumbar puncture be avoided in the presence of raised intracranial pressure as the majority of patients with bacterial meningitis have raised intracranial pressure. In order to perform a CSF examination in a patient with suspected raised intracranial pressure, a bolus dose of mannitol (1 g/kg of body weight) can be given intravenously, and lumbar puncture performed 30–60 min later. Lumbar puncture should be performed with a 22-gauge spinal needle, and only 3–5 cc of CSF need to be removed for analysis. Alternatively, the patient can be intubated and hyperventilated in addition to being treated with intravenous mannitol. If the decision is made to delay lumbar puncture until a neuroimaging study is obtained, broad-spectrum intravenous antimicrobial therapy should be initiated while awaiting the scan. An opening pressure should always be obtained at the time of lumbar puncture to determine if raised intracranial pressure is present. Opening pressure should be measured with the patient in the lateral recumbent position. The normal range of opening pressure for infants and children up to 6 years of age is 10–120 mmH_2O. The normal range of opening pressure for children older than age 6 and for adults is 10–180 mmH_2O. The upper limit of normal opening pressure in an obese adult is 250 mmH_2O. When obtaining cerebrospinal fluid for analysis, it is important to remember that infants and children have smaller amounts of CSF than adults. The volume of CSF in a neonate is 30–60 ml, in a child of 4–13 years of age is 65–140 ml, and in an adult is approximately 150 ml. While 10–12 ml of CSF is typically withdrawn from the adult for analysis, 3–5 ml is the appropriate amount to withdraw from a neonate or child (26,27).

The characteristic cerebrospinal fluid abnormalities in bacterial meningitis are (1) increased opening pressure, (2) polymorphonuclear pleocytosis, (3) decreased glucose concentration, and (4) elevated protein concentration. In uninfected CSF, the normal white blood cell (WBC) count ranges from 0 to 5 mononuclear cells/mm^3. In bacterial meningitis, the CSF WBC count is usually >100 cells/mm^3 and is typically >1000 WBC/mm^3 (27,28). There are reports of bacterial meningitis without an increased number of WBCs in which abnormalities of CSF glucose and protein concentrations were the only initial indicators of infection (29). A low initial CSF pleocytosis may occur in patients with bacterial meningitis who are immunosuppressed from alcoholism, extremes of age, organ transplantation, or cancer. In the case reports of bacterial meningitis with normal or low CSF WBC counts, bacteria have been detected in the CSF by Gram's stain or culture. Most cases of bacterial meningitis initially have a predominance of polymorphonuclear cells; however, a cerebrospinal fluid lymphocytosis has been reported in cases of bacterial meningitis when the cerebrospinal fluid WBC concentration was <1000 WBCs/mm^3 and in cases of bacterial meningitis due to *Listeria monocytogenes* (30,31). A high index of suspicion for bacterial meningitis should be maintained if the clinical presentation is suggestive of bacterial meningitis and the CSF glucose concentration is low, regardless of the presence of a CSF lymphocytic pleocytosis.

The CSF glucose concentration is normally lower than that of serum and is dependent upon not only the serum glucose concentration, but also the facilitated membrane carrier system that transfers glucose between blood and CSF and the rate of glucose metabolism by the various cellular elements close to and within the CSF. In bacterial meningitis, the decreased glucose concentration is due, in part, to increased glycolysis by polymorphonuclear leukocytes in the process of phagocytosis (32). The normal CSF glucose concentration is between 45 and 80 mg/dl, and concentrations below 40 mg/dl are abnormal. Hyperglycemia and/or hypoglycemia affect the CSF glucose concentration; therefore, it is recommended that the CSF glucose concentration be determined by the CSF:serum glucose ratio. The normal CSF:serum glucose ratio is 0.6. The differential diagnosis of a decreased CSF glucose concentration is listed in Table 1. A CSF:serum glucose ratio of ≤ 0.40 is highly predictive of bacterial meningitis (27,32). If the patient has

Table 1 Differential Diagnosis of Decreased CSF Glucose Concentration

Bacterial meningitis
Lymphocytic choriomeningitis
Mumps meningitis
Herpes simplex meningoencephalitis
Fungal meningitis
Tuberculous meningitis
Carcinomatous meningitis
Sarcoidosis
Hypoglycemia

received several 50-ml ampules of 50% glucose (D50) enroute to the emergency room, the CSF glucose concentration may be affected by this therapy. There is an estimated time range of 30 min to 4 h for the glucose concentration to reach an equilibrium between blood and CSF; therefore, an ampule of D50 will not influence the CSF glucose concentration until at least 30 min after it is given. The CSF glucose concentration may be spuriously low in the presence of hypoglycemia.

An increased CSF protein concentration is a nonspecific abnormality and is simply indicative of a process that is disrupting the permeability of the blood-brain barrier. An increased CSF protein concentration is typically seen in bacterial meningitis. The CSF protein concentration is increased if the value is >45 mg/dl in CSF obtained from the lumbar interspace and >30 mg/dl in CSF obtained from a cisternal puncture (33).

The best methods to determine the etiological organism of bacterial meningitis are Gram's stain and culture of CSF. A good rule of thumb is that the CSF culture should be sterile and the Gram's stain negative 24 h after the initiation of antimicrobial therapy if the organism is sensitive to the antibiotic. A common concern is how the analysis of the CSF will be affected by intravenous antibiotic therapy while awaiting a CT or MR scan and how the analysis of the CSF is affected by prior oral antimicrobial therapy. Children have often been treated with oral antimicrobial agents for 2–3 days or longer prior to presenting with signs and symptoms of meningitis. In general, antimicrobial therapy tends to decrease the likelihood of identifying the organism on Gram's stain or isolating the organism in culture but does not significantly alter the CSF white blood cell count or glucose concentration in the initial days of bacterial meningitis. In a series that examined CSF posttreatment in 161 patients cured of bacterial meningitis, the following was found (34):

1. In 36% of cases the posttreatment glucose concentration was <50 mg/dl; in 8% the posttreatment glucose concentration was <40 mg/dl.
2. In 38% of cases the posttreatment CSF protein concentration was >45 mg/dl; in 8% the protein concentration was >100 mg/dl.
3. Posttreatment CSF WBC counts were $<5/mm^3$ in only 28% of cases. The WBC count was $\geqslant 40/mm^3$ in 32% and $\geqslant 100/mm^3$ in 15%.

In the majority of patients, the CSF glucose concentration returns to normal within 3 days after therapy is initiated. The CSF WBC count often increases after the initiation of antimicrobial therapy. It appears unlikely, then, that delaying CSF examination for a few hours after initiating antibiotic therapy and while awaiting CT scan will significantly alter the CSF abnormalities. It is often the case, however, that in children pretreated with oral antimicrobial agents an organism cannot be detected on Gram's stain or grown in culture, but the CSF WBC count and glucose concentration will be suggestive of bacterial meningitis. In these cases, bacterial antigen tests on cerebrospinal fluid are very helpful in making the diagnosis of bacterial meningitis. Today most hospital laboratories use the latex particle agglutination test for the detection of bacterial antigens in the cerebrospinal fluid and the Limulus amebocyte lysate assay for detection of gram-negative endotoxin in CSF. The latex particle agglutination test has a sensitivity of 78–86% and a specificity of 100% for the detection of *H. influenzae* type b in CSF, a sensitivity of 69–100% and a specificity of 96% for the detection of *S. pneumoniae* in CSF, and a sensitivity of 33–70% and a specificity of 100% for the detection of *N. meningitidis*. The Limulus amebocyte lysate assay has a 77–99% sensitivity for the detection of gram-negative endotoxin in the CSF (35–39). One note of caution; a positive bacterial antigen test in a child who has recently been immunized against *H. influenzae* type b may be due to recent immunization and not due to bacterial meningitis. The positive Hib antigen test can be attributed to immunization if the CSF WBC count, protein, and glucose concentrations are normal and the clinical course is not typical of bacterial meningitis (40).

It is not necessary to repeat lumbar puncture at the end of treatment of bacterial meningitis in children and adults unless the clinical condition warrants this.

DIFFERENTIAL DIAGNOSIS

The differential diagnosis of bacterial meningitis includes the following: (1) viral meningitis, (2) viral meningoencephalitis, (3) subarachnoid hemorrhage, (4) fungal meningitis, (5) tuberculous meningitis, (6) Rocky Mountain spotted fever, (7) focal intracranial mass lesion, and (8) neuroleptic malignant syndrome.

In general, patients with viral meningitis appear less ill than those with bacterial meningitis. Patients with viral meningitis are typically able to give a history and complain of a "grippelike" headache, photophobia, nausea, and vomiting. Patients with viral meningitis may be lethargic but are not obtunded or comatose. Patients with viral meningitis may be febrile; however, the fever is lower in viral meningitis than in bacterial meningitis. Systemic viral illnesses and viral meningitis may be associated with a maculopapular, vesicular, or petechial rash, but not with a purpuric rash like that of meningococcemia. In viral meningitis, examination of the cerebrospinal fluid typically demonstrates a lymphocytic pleocytosis, a normal or mildly elevated protein concentration, and a normal glucose concentration. Meningitis due to mumps virus, vaccine strain mumps virus, and the lymphocytic choriomeningitis virus may have a decreased CSF glucose concentration with a lymphocytic pleocytosis.

The typical clinical presentation of herpes simplex virus (HSV) encephalitis includes (1) fever, (2) headache, (3) confusion or a change in behavior, (4) new onset seizure activity (from an epileptogenic area in the temporal lobe), and (5) a focal neurological deficit such as a hemiparesis or a visual field disorder. Behavioral abnormalities develop and get progressively worse, typically over a period of 7–12 days. The electroencephalogram (EEG) may demonstrate unilateral or bilateral periodic spike and slow wave activity localized to either the temporal lobe or the frontal and temporal lobes. Examination of the CSF demonstrates a lymphocytic pleocytosis, the presence of red blood cells, and an elevated protein concentration. Low CSF glucose concentrations are not unusual. The polymerase chain reaction (which allows for the detection of HSV DNA in CSF) is reported to have a sensitivity of $>95\%$ and a specificity that approaches 100% for the diagnosis of HSV encephalitis (41). The MR scan is also very useful in the diagnosis of this infection because it may demonstrate an area of increased signal intensity in the frontotemporal areas on T_2-weighted imaging.

The clinical presentation of a subarachnoid hemorrhage is the explosive onset of a severe headache with a transient loss of consciousness. Nuchal rigidity and vomiting may be present. The CT scan may demonstrate blood in the basilar cisterns; however, examination of the CSF is often required for diagnosis. Red blood cells are present in the cerebrospinal fluid within minutes of the rupture of an intracranial aneurysm. Xanthochromia can normally be detected in the CSF within 2–4 h of the rupture of an aneurysm. The appearance of blood-tinged CSF during the performance of a lumbar puncture necessitates distinguishing between a bloody tap and a subarachnoid hemorrhage. A red blood cell count should be determined on tube #1 and tube #4. In a traumatic puncture, the fluid typically clears between the first and the third or fourth tubes. In a subarachnoid hemorrhage, the fluid will remain blood-tinged in all tubes. A sample of the bloody CSF should be centrifuged. In a subarachnoid hemorrhage, the supernatant is yellow or xanthochromic. In a traumatic puncture, the supernatant is crystal clear (32).

The clinical presentation of fungal and tuberculous meningitis is more insidious than that of bacterial meningitis. Fungal meningitis typically presents with fever, headache, and photophobia and may be associated with an altered sensorium or cranial nerve palsies. In North America and Europe, tuberculous meningitis most often presents as a slowly progressive dementing illness with memory deficits and personality changes. In other areas of the world, however, the typical clinical presentation of tuberculous meningitis is coma, raised intracranial pressure, seizures, and focal neurological deficits.

Fungal, tuberculous, and bacterial meningitis are distinguished from each other by examination of the cerebrospinal fluid. Fungal meningitis is characterized by a lymphocytic pleocytosis and a decreased glucose concentration. The India ink stain is reported to be positive in cryptococcal meningitis in 50% of HIV-negative individuals but positive in 75–88% of HIV-infected individuals with cryptococcal meningitis (42,43). Latex agglutination test for the cryptococcal antigen is a highly sensitive and specific test.

The classic CSF abnormalities in tuberculous meningitis include a moderate lymphocytic pleocytosis, an elevated protein concentration and a decreased glucose concentration. Bacilli are typically difficult to detect on acid-fast smear. Cultures of CSF require 3–6 weeks for growth. The concentration of tuberculostearic acid in CSF has been reported to be a sensitive marker for tuberculous meningitis; however, this analysis is not routinely available and must be obtained through the Centers for Disease Control. The polymerase chain reaction technique for detection of tubercle bacilli DNA in CSF is under development.

Rocky Mountain spotted fever (RMSF) is included in the differential diagnosis because it is characterized by headache, fever, confusion or an altered level of consciousness, and a rash that may resemble the early rash of meningococcemia. The rash of RMSF consists of 1- to 5-mm pink macules, which are most often first detected on the wrist and ankles and then spread centrally to the chest, face, and abdomen. After a few days, the macules turn dark red or purple. Diagnosis can be made by biopsy of the skin lesions.

The symptoms of a focal infectious intracranial mass lesion, such as a brain abscess or a subdural empyema, are a hemicranial or generalized headache with focal neurological deficits and/or new-onset focal or generalized seizure activity and fever. A CT or MR scan is indicated prior to lumbar puncture if a focal infectious mass lesion is suspected.

Neuroleptic malignant syndrome (NMS) may look like bacterial meningitis because of the characteristic signs of generalized lead-pipe rigidity, fever, and fluctuating level of consciousness. NMS can be distinguished from bacterial meningitis by the finding of a marked elevation in the serum creatine kinase concentration, usually exceeding 10,000 IU/L, and a history of neuroleptic therapy when available.

TREATMENT

Antimicrobial therapy of bacterial meningitis is initially empiric (Table 2) based on the most likely etiological organism that can be predicted based on the age of the patient, whether the meningitis is community-acquired or nosocomial, and the presence of predisposing conditions, such as pneumonia, alcoholism, immunosuppression, splenectomy, or head trauma.

Children

The most common etiological organisms of bacterial meningitis in children are *H. influenzae* type b (Hib), *N. meningitidis*, and *S. pneumoniae*.

Haemophilus influenzae

H. influenzae meningitis is a disease of children between the ages of 6 months and 6 years and of older adults. Capsular type b strains account for >90% of cases of meningitis (44). The incidence of Hib meningitis has declined since licensure of the first conjugate Hib vaccine in December 1987 for routine use in children ≥18 months of age and in October 1990 for use in infants ≥2 months of age (45).

Table 2 Empiric Antimicrobial Therapy of Bacterial Meningitis

Children	Ceftriaxone 100 mg/kg/day IV in a once or twice daily dosing interval *or* Cefotaxime 225 mg/kg/day IV in divided doses every 8 h *plus* Vancomycin 40 mg/kg/day IV in divided doses every 6 h
Adults	
Community-acquired	Ceftriaxone 2 g IV every 12 h *or* Cefotaxime 8–12 g/day IV (in divided doses every 4 h) *plus* Vancomycin 2 g/day IV in divided doses every 6 h *plus* Ampicillin 12 g/day IV in divided doses every 4 h when indicated (see text)
Neurosurgical procedure	Ceftriaxone *or* cefotaxime *or* ceftazidime 6 g/day IV (for coverage of *P. aeruginosa*) in divided doses every 8 h *plus* Gentamicin or tobramycin 1.5 mg/kg every 8 h IV *plus* Oxacillin 12 g/day IV (in divided doses every 4 h) *or* Vancomycin 2 g/day IV (in divided doses every 6 h)
Alcoholism	Cefotaxime *or* ceftriaxone *plus* Vancomycin *plus* Ampicillin
Diabetes mellitus	Cefotaxime *or* ceftriaxone *plus* Vancomycin
Neutropenia	Ceftriaxone *or* cefotaxime *or* ceftazidime (for *P. aeruginosa*) *plus* Vancomycin
Organ transplant recipient and/or immunosuppressive therapy	Ampicillin *plus* ceftazidime
Cancer	Cefotaxime or ceftriaxone *plus* Ampicillin *plus* Vancomycin

A third-generation cephalosporin, either cefotaxime or ceftriaxone, is recommended for therapy of Hib meningitis (Table 3). A 7- to 10-day course of antimicrobial therapy is recommended.

Neisseria meningitidis

Penicillin G or ampicillin or a third-generation cephalosporin (ceftriaxone or cefotaxime) are recommended for antimicrobial therapy of meningococcal meningitis. A 7-day course of antimicrobial therapy is adequate for most cases of uncomplicated meningococcal meningitis. The doses of these antibiotics are listed in Table 3.

Streptococcus pneumoniae

The incidence of pneumococcal meningitis in children is expected to increase. The selection of an antibiotic for the treatment of pneumococcal meningitis in children must be based on antibiotic susceptibility testing of CSF isolates of *S. pneumoniae* because of the increased incidence of penicillin- and cephalosporin-resistant strains of pneumococci. A third-generation cephalosporin (i.e., cefotaxime or ceftriaxone) is recommended for relatively penicillin-resistant strains of pneumococci [penicillin minimal inhibitory concentrations (MICs) of 0.1–1.0 μg/ml]. Children with highly penicillin-resistant pneumococcal meningitis (MICs $\geqslant$ 2.0 μg/ml) are best treated with vancomycin and a third-generation cephalosporin. Children with intermediately penicillin-resistant pneumococcal meningitis (penicillin MICs of 0.1–1.0 μg/ml) who are treated with cefotaxime or ceftriaxone alone should be observed carefully for treatment failure (46). At least a 10-day course of antibiotics is recommended for pneumococcal meningitis (47).

The third-generation cephalosporin, cefuroxime, is not recommended for treatment of bacterial meningitis in children. In clinical trials, cefuroxime has been associated with delayed sterilization of CSF cultures and sensorineural hearing loss (48,49).

Gram-Negative Bacilliary Meningitis

Either a third-generation cephalosporin alone or a third-generation cephalosporin plus an aminoglycoside is recommended for the treatment of gram-negative enteric meningitis in children. The third-generation cephalosporins, with the exception of ceftazidime, are only minimally effective or not effective against *P. aeruginosa*. Ceftazidime is the recommended antibiotic for bacterial meningitis due to *Pseudomonas* species (50,51).

Listeria monocytogenes

The cephalosporins have limited or no activity against *L. monocytogenes*; therefore, meningitis due to this organism must be treated with ampicillin.

Fluid Management

The majority of children with bacterial meningitis are hyponatremic. Hyponatremia in bacterial meningitis is largely due to the syndrome of inappropriate antidiuretic hormone secretion (SIADH), which results in free water retention and a dilutional hyponatremia. The incidence of this complication in childhood bacterial meningitis in reported series ranges from 28 to 88% (52–54). The diagnostic criteria for SIADH are the following: (1) hyponatremia with hypo-osmolal serum, (2) inappropriately concentrated urine, (3) continued sodium excretion (urinary sodium of $>$25 mEq/liter), and (4) absence of renal or endocrine disease (55). For many years, the primary treatment of SIADH has been fluid restriction. Recently, however, this practice has received renewed attention because of the effect of fluid restriction on cerebral blood flow. Autoregulation of cerebral blood flow is lost in the course of bacterial meningitis. This means that a decrease in the mean systemic arterial pressure is associated with a decrease in cerebral blood flow. In experimental pneumococcal meningitis in rabbits, fluid-restricted rabbits had greater decreases in

Table 3 Antimicrobial Therapy for Bacterial Meningitis in Children and Adults

		Total daily dose (dosing interval)	
Organism	Antibiotic	Children	Adults
H. influenzae type b (Hib)	Cefotaxime *or*	225 mg/kg/day IV (every 6 h)	8–12 g/day IV (every 4 h)
	Ceftriaxone	100 mg/kg/day IV (in a once or twice daily dosing interval)	4 g/day IV (every 12 h)
N. meningitidis	Penicillin G *or*	250,000–400,000 U/kg/day (every 4 h)	20–24 million U/day IV (every 4 h)
	Ampicillin	200 mg/kg/day IV (every 4 h)	12 g/day IV (every 4 h)
S. pneumoniae	Cefotaxime *or* Ceftriaxone *plus*	Same doses as for Hib	Same doses as for Hib
	Vancomycin (see text)	40 mg/kg/day IV (every 6 h)	2 g/day IV (every 6 h)
Enteric gram-negative bacilli (except *P. aeruginosa*)	Cefotaxime *or* Ceftriaxone	Same doses as for Hib	Same doses as for Hib
P. aeruginosa	Ceftazidime	150 mg/kg/day IV (every 8 h)	6 g/day IV (every 8 h)
L. monocytogenes	Ampicillin	150–200 mg/kg/day IV (every 4 h)	12 g/day IV (every 4 h)
Staphylococcus aureus			
Methicillin-sensitive	Oxacillin	200–300 mg/kg/day IV (every 4 h)	12 g/day/IV (every 4 h)
Methicillin-resistant	Vancomycin	40 mg/kg/day IV (every 6 h)	2 g/day IV (every 6 h)
Enterobacteriaceae	Cefotaxime *or* Ceftriaxone	Same doses as for Hib	Same doses as for Hib

mean arterial pressures and cerebral blood flow after treatment with ceftriaxone than did euvolemic rabbits (56). The implication is that a rigid adherence to fluid restriction may adversely affect cerebral perfusion pressure. A revised set of recommendations for fluid management in children with bacterial meningitis and hyponatremia is not yet available. One reasonable approach to manage this problem would be to limit the initial rate of intravenous fluid administration to approximately three fourths of normal maintenance requirements (or 1000–1200 ml/m^2/24 h) rather than the well-established tradition of limiting the initial rate of intravenous fluid administration to one half of normal maintenance requirements. Body weight, serum sodium concentration, and urine specific gravity should be monitored every 6–12 h. In most cases, the rate of intravenous fluid administration will reach maintenance rates by 36–48 h after admission (1500–1700 ml/m^2/day) (18).

Seizure Activity

Seizure activity is an expected complication of bacterial meningitis. Seizure activity must be treated rapidly and aggressively because it can cause ischemic necrosis in the temporal lobes with loss of cortical neurons and anoxic ischemic changes in the cerebrum in general (18). Seizure activity may occur as a complication of the illness itself or as a result of hyponatremia, fever, cerebral edema, cerebral ischemia, cortical venous thrombosis with hemorrhage, or antimicrobial toxicity. The management of seizure activity is outlined in Table 4.

Subdural Effusion

Subdural effusions often develop in the course of bacterial meningitis and are usually self-limited. As the inflammatory process in the subarachnoid space subsides, fluid formation ceases and the fluid is resorbed. Some subdural fluid collections become infected and are then subdural empyemas. A subdural effusion can be distinguished from a subdural empyema on computed tomographic scan and on magnetic resonance scan. The indications for aspiration of a subdural fluid collection are the following: (1) clinical suspicion that the fluid is infected, (2) fever of unknown etiology, (3) rapidly enlarging head circumference in a child without hydrocephalus, (4) focal neurological findings, and/or (5) evidence of increased intracranial pressure (57).

Adults

In adults, the meningeal pathogen can be predicted and empiric antimicrobial therapy initiated based on the presence of predisposing or associated conditions (Table 2).

Table 4 Management of Seizure Activity

1. Administer oxygen by nasal cannula or mask.
2. Insert oral airway.
3. Maintain blood pressure at normal or high-normal values.
4. Measure ABG, serum electrolytes, and glucose.
5. Administer glucose by bolus injection:
   Adult: 50 ml of 50% glucose (intravenous thiamine, 100 mg, should precede glucose administration in adults)
   Child: 2 ml/kg of 25% glucose
6. Initiate anticonvulsant therapy with short-acting anticonvulsant:
   Diazepam
   - Adult: 5–10 mg intravenously
   - Child: 1 mg every 2–5 min up to a maximum of 10 mg

   Lorazepam
   - 0.1 mg/kg no faster than 2 mg/min
7. Administer intravenous phenytoin at a rate no faster than 50 mg/min in adults or 1 mg/kg/min in children. Monitor the electrocardiogram and blood pressure. The initial dose of phenytoin is as follows:
   - Adults: 18–20 mg/kg
   - Child: 20 mg/kg
8. If seizure activity continues, an additional 5 mg/kg of phenytoin can be given to a maximum dose of 30 mg/kg.
9. If seizure activity continues, endotracheal intubation and mechanical ventilation is necessary prior to or concomitant with the administration of phenobarbital in a dose of 20 mg/kg, at a rate of 100 mg/min.
10. If seizure activity continues, pentobarbital is given next in a loading dose of 5 mg/kg, followed by an infusion of 0.5–5.0 mg/kg/h to maintain a burst suppression pattern on EEG.

Community-Acquired

The most common causative organisms of community-acquired bacterial meningitis in adults are *S. pneumoniae* and *N. meningitidis*. A combination of a third-generation cephalosporin (cefotaxime or ceftriaxone) plus vancomycin is recommended for empiric therapy of community-acquired bacterial meningitis. Ampicillin is added if *L. monocytogenes* is a possible pathogen. An increasing number of *S. pneumoniae* strains are relatively or completely resistant to penicillin, precluding the use of penicillin for pneumococcal meningitis (21). Experimental studies have shown that the best clinical response is achieved with CSF antibiotic concentrations that exceed the minimal bactericidal concentration (MBC) of the meningeal pathogen by 10- to 20-fold. CSF cultures should be tested for antimicrobial susceptibilities. When the results of antibiotic susceptibility testing are known, vancomycin can be discontinued if the isolate is sensitive to ceftriaxone or cefotaxime. Pneumococcal meningitis is treated for 10–14 days. Meningococcal meningitis can be treated with either penicillin or ampicillin. Strains with relative resistance to penicillin have been reported, especially in Spain; however, conventional therapy with penicillin has been successful in treating most patients infected with these strains (58). Careful monitoring for penicillin resistance in the meningococci may become increasingly important. Meningococcal meningitis can be successfully treated in 7 days.

In the older adult ($\geq$50 years) the most common causative organisms of bacterial meningitis are *Streptococcus pneumoniae* and gram-negative bacilli. Gram-negative bacilli are likely to be the infecting organisms when meningitis is associated with chronic lung disease, sinusitis, a neurosurgical procedure, or a chronic urinary tract infection (59). The most common gram-negative bacilli causing meningitis in the older adult are *E. coli*, *K. pneumoniae*, *H. influenzae*, *Pseudomonas* organisms, *Enterobacter* species, and *Serratia* species (58,60). Empiric therapy of bacterial meningitis in the older adult should include a combination of a third-generation cephalosporin, either ceftriaxone or cefotaxime, with ampicillin. Vancomycin should be added if cephalosporin-resistant pneumococci could be the meningeal pathogens.

Neurosurgical Patient

The most common organisms causing meningitis in the neurosurgical patient are staphylococci and gram-negative bacilli such as *K. pneumoniae*, *E. coli*, *P. aeruginosa*, and *Acinetobacter* species. Empiric antimicrobial therapy of bacterial meningitis in the neurosurgical patient should include a combination of a third-generation cephalosporin, plus oxacillin or vancomycin, and an aminoglycoside. A third-generation cephalosporin is recommended for the treatment of gram-negative bacillary meningitis. Ceftazidime should be used because it is the only cephalosporin with sufficient activity against *P. aeruginosa* in the CNS. *P. aeruginosa* meningitis should be treated with ceftazidime plus an aminoglycoside for the first week of therapy.

Alcoholism

The most common causative organisms of bacterial meningitis in alcoholics are *S. pneumoniae*, *L. monocytogenes*, and *H. influenzae* (44). Empiric therapy of bacterial meningitis in the alcoholic should include a third-generation cephalosporin, either cefotaxime or ceftriaxone, plus vancomycin and ampicillin.

Diabetes Mellitus

The most common causative organisms of bacterial meningitis in the diabetic patient are *S. pneumoniae*, *Enterobacteriaceae*, and *S. aureus* (44). Empiric therapy of bacterial meningitis in these patients should include a combination of a third-generation cephalosporin, either cefotaxime or ceftriaxone, and either oxacillin or vancomycin.

Neutropenia

Meningitis in neutropenic patients is usually due to the gram-negative bacilli that reside in the gastrointestinal tract: *P. aeruginosa*, *E. coli*, *Klebsiella*, and *Enterobacter* species. Of these gram-negative bacilli, *P. aeruginosa* is the most common cause of bacterial meningitis in patients with neutropenia. These patients are also at risk for meningitis due to hematogenous dissemination of *S. aureus* and coagulase-negative staphylococci infections of hyperalimentation and other central intravenous lines (62,63). Empiric therapy in these patients should include a combination of ceftazidime plus vancomycin.

Organ Transplantation

Organ transplant recipients and patients receiving immunosuppressive agents are at risk for *L. monocytogenes* meningitis. The treatment of acute bacterial meningitis in these patients should include ampicillin.

Cancer

Patients with cancer and neutropenia are at risk for bacterial meningitis due to the organisms listed above that infect neutropenic patients in general. Patients with chronic lymphocytic leukemia, multiple myeloma, and Hodgkin's disease are at risk for meningitis due to the encapsulated bacteria, including *Streptococcus pneumoniae*, *H. influenzae* type b, and *N. meningitidis*. Patients with cancer are also at risk for meningitis due to *L. monocytogenes* and are at risk for meningitis due to staphylococci because of the tendency of staphylococci to infect indwelling intravenous catheters and Ommaya reservoirs. The empiric therapy of bacterial meningitis in patients with cancer should include a combination of cefotaxime or ceftriaxone plus ampicillin plus vancomycin.

Increased Intracranial Pressure

Raised intracranial pressure (ICP) is an expected complication of bacterial meningitis and can be determined either by obtaining an opening pressure at the time of initial lumbar puncture or by measuring the intracranial pressure by an ICP monitoring device. Patients that are awake and alert do not need ICP monitoring devices; however, patients that are stuporous or comatose should have an ICP monitoring device to manage elevations in intracranial pressure. Elevated intracranial pressure can cause death by brainstem compression and cardiopulmonary arrest and produces neurological morbidity by decreasing cerebral blood flow with resultant cerebral ischemia (64). The treatment of raised intracranial pressure is outlined in Table 5.

Seizure Activity

Seizure activity is managed as outlined in Table 4.

Stroke

The risk of an acute ischemic stroke is greatest during the first 5 days of bacterial meningitis (66). The etiology of cerebrovascular disease complicating bacterial meningitis may be one or more of the following: (1) narrowing of the large arteries at the base of the brain due to encroachment on the vessel wall by the purulent exudate in the subarachnoid space, (2) infiltration of the arterial wall by inflammatory cells (vasculitis) with thickening of the wall of the blood vessel, (3) vasospasm, (4) narrowing of medium-sized arteries and thrombotic or stenotic occlusion of branches of the middle cerebral artery, (5) focal hyperperfusion due to dilatation of arterioles and capillaries, and (6) septic venous sinus thrombosis and thrombophlebitis of cortical veins (66–70). Acute ischemic stroke in the course of bacterial meningitis is managed similarly to acute ischemic stroke of other etiologies. An emergency noncontrast cranial CT scan should be

Table 5 Management of Increased Intracranial Pressure

1. Elevate the head of the bed 30°
2. Hyperventilation to maintain $PaCO_2$ between 25–30 mmHg[a]
3. Hyperosmolar therapy—mannitol
   Loading dose: 1.0 g/kg bolus injection
   Maintenance dose: 0.25–0.5 g/kg every 3–5 h to achieve serum osmolarity of 295–320 mOsm/liter
4. Pentobarbital coma
   Loading dose: 5–10 mg/kg IV at a rate of 1 mg/kg/min
   Maintenance dose: 1–3 mg/kg/h. Titrate dose to achieve a therapeutic serum concentration of 25–40 μg/dl or a burst-suppression pattern on EEG

[a]Hyperventilation may compromise cerebral perfusion resulting in cerebral ischemia if $PaCO_2$ is lowered below 25 mmHg.
Source: Ref. 65.

obtained to rule out an intracranial hemorrhage. The head of the bed should be elevated and remain elevated at 30–45 degrees to prevent aspiration pneumonia. Oral feedings must be avoided until the patient is alert enough to swallow and the gag reflex has returned. For prophylaxis of deep vein thrombosis, low-dose heparin 5000 IUs should be given subcutaneously every 12 h in addition to the use of elastic compression stockings and intermittent pneumatic compression. Blood pressure should be controlled conservatively and is not treated unless the systolic or diastolic blood pressure is at or above 200 or 120, respectively (71). Arterial hypotension must be avoided. No firm recommendations can be made regarding the use of intravenous heparin at this time. Intermittent catheterization is preferable to an indwelling catheter to prevent urinary tract infections.

Dexamethasone Therapy

The American Academy of Pediatrics recommends the consideration of dexamethasone therapy for bacterial meningitis in infants and children 2 months of age and older. At the present time the recommended dose is 0.6 mg/kg/day in four divided doses (0.15 mg/kg/dose) given intravenously for the first 4 days of antibiotic treatment (72). For maximum benefit, the first dose of dexamethasone should be administered 20 min prior to the first dose of antibacterial therapy.

The results of the first prospective double-blind placebo-controlled trials to evaluate the efficacy of dexamethasone therapy in bacterial meningitis in infants and children was published in 1988 (73). The results of these clinical trials, involving 200 infants and children, demonstrated a significant reduction in the frequency of moderate, severe, or profound bilateral sensorineural hearing loss in children with *H. influenzae* meningitis treated with dexamethasone.

In a placebo-controlled, double-blind trial of dexamethasone therapy in 101 infants and children with bacterial meningitis in Costa Rica, dexamethasone therapy had a significant effect on meningeal inflammation. By 12 h of dexamethasone therapy, all indexes of inflammation in the cerebrospinal fluid (CSF lactate, leukocytes, glucose, and protein concentrations) had improved with dexamethasone therapy, whereas they had uniformly worsened in the patients given placebo. Neurological sequelae occurred significantly more often in the patients who were given placebo (74). In a clinical trial in Egypt, 210 patients with bacterial meningitis were treated with dexamethasone intramuscularly (8 mg to children younger than 12 years and 12 mg to adults every 12 h for 3 days), in addition to ampicillin and chloramphenicol therapy. Two hundred and nineteen patients received antibiotics alone. The case fatality rate was significantly lower in patients receiving dexamethasone; 20 of 210 patients treated with antibiotics and dexamethasone died, compared with 42 of 219 receiving antibiotics alone ($p < 0.01$). This reduction was significantly different for patients with pneumococcal meningitis; 7 of 52 (13.5%) of the patients treated with antibiotics and dexamethasone died compared with 22 of 54 (40.7%) of the patients treated with antibiotics alone ($p < 0.002$) (75).

In a retrospective review of 97 cases of pneumococcal meningitis in infants and children, 41 patients received corticosteroid therapy, 39 of whom were given dexamethasone 0.15 mg/kg/dose every 6 h for 4 days. Among the survivors, there were significantly fewer patients with an overall adverse neurological outcome, including hearing impairment, in those who received steroid therapy compared with those who did not (4 of 35 vs. 14 of 43). Twenty-seven of the 97 infants and children had evidence of fulminant meningeal infection. In this group, of the survivors, 1 of 8 steroid-treated patients compared with 7 of 13 non–steroid-treated patients had moderate or greater bilateral hearing loss. The one steroid-treated patient had severe neurological damage and brainstem auditory evoked response evidence of bilateral hearing loss before dexamethasone therapy was administered 31 h after the first parenteral dose of antibiotics (76).

In a prospective, placebo-controlled, double-blind trial of dexamethasone in 115 children with acute bacterial meningitis, dexamethasone (0.4 mg/kg) was started 10 min before the first dose of ceftriaxone and given every 12 h for 2 days. After 24 h of treatment, the cerebrospinal fluid glucose concentration had a significantly greater increase in the dexamethasone group than in the placebo group. This finding is significant in that there is a correlation between a low cerebrospinal fluid glucose concentration and sensorineural hearing loss. At follow-up examination 3, 9, and 15 months after hospital discharge, 3 of 60 (5%) dexamethasone-treated patients had one or more neurological or audiological sequelae compared to 9 of 55 (16%) placebo recipients ($p = 0.066$) (77).

In experimental models of meningitis, dexamethasone has been demonstrated to decrease the meningeal inflammatory response that is induced by the intracisternal injection of Hib LOS (endotoxin), to decrease cerebral edema and intracranial pressure, to decrease the leakage of serum proteins into the CSF, and to minimize the alteration in blood-brain barrier permeability (16,78). The rationale for giving dexamethasone 20 min prior to antibiotic therapy is that dexamethasone inhibits the production of TNF if administered to macrophages before they are activated by endotoxin, both by diminishing the quantity of TNF mRNA that is produced in response to endotoxin and by preventing its translation. Dexamethasone is unable to regulate TNF production once induction has occurred (16). The timing of the administration of dexamethasone to coincide with the lysis of bacterial organisms by antimicrobial therapy and the subsequent release of free endotoxin into the CSF allows dexamethasone to inhibit TNF production and limit the inflammatory cascade that follows (Fig. 6).

The efficacy of dexamethasone therapy in infants and children with Hib meningitis has been proven by clinical trials; however, the efficacy of dexamethasone in adults with bacterial meningitis and in infants and children with pneumococcal or meningococcal meningitis has not been clearly demonstrated by clinical trials to date. The decision to use dexamethasone as adjunctive therapy is left to the treating physician and should be based on the experimental and clinical data described above. When dexamethasone therapy is used, the recommended dose is 0.6 mg/kg/day in four divided doses given intravenously for the first 4 days of antibiotic treatment, just as is recommended for infants and children 2 months of age and older. The concomitant use of an H_2 antagonist is recommended with dexamethasone therapy to avoid gastrointestinal bleeding. Dexamethasone therapy does not appear to adversely affect the outcome in patients with viral meningitis when this is the eventual diagnosis. Waagner et al. found no adverse affects of dexamethasone therapy in patients with subsequently documented viral men-

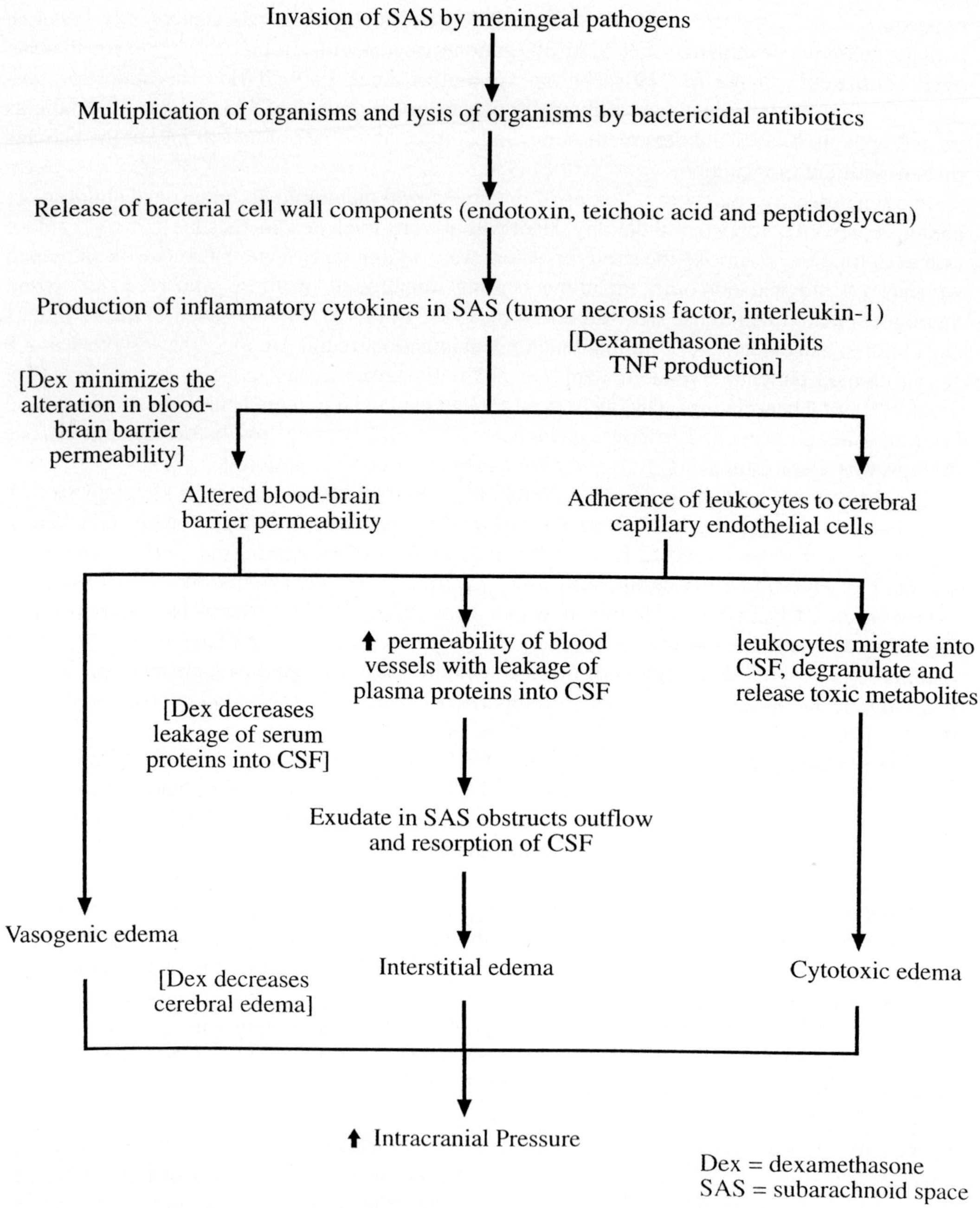

Figure 6 The effect of dexamethasone, as demonstrated in experimental models of meningitis, on the inflammatory cascade in bacterial meningitis.

ingitis (79). The main argument against using dexamethasone in bacterial meningitis is that dexamethasone will decrease meningeal inflammation, and a moderate degree of meningeal inflammation is required for the CSF penetration of many antimicrobial agents. In clinical practice, however, dexamethasone has not affected the early rate of sterilization of CSF cultures, with one exception (73). The addition of dexamethasone to vancomycin is not recommended in the therapy of highly penicillin-resistant pneumococcal meningitis, as vancomycin penetration into CSF is better in the presence of meningeal inflammation.

Dexamethasone therapy should be discontinued after 4 days because at this point in the treatment course, meningeal inflammation has been reduced substantially by dexamethasone therapy, and the penetration of antibiotics into CSF may be reduced. A 2-day course of dexamethasone therapy may also be efficacious.

PREVENTION

Immunization

The Committee on Infectious Diseases of the American Academy of Pediatrics recommends that all infants be immunized with an *H. influenzae* type b conjugate vaccine beginning at 2 months of age. Two *H. influenzae* type b conjugate vaccines are currently licensed in the United States for administration to infants beginning at 2 months of age. These are the HbOC vaccine and the PRP-OMP vaccine. If HbOC is used, infants 2–6 months of age should receive three doses given at least 2 months apart. An additional dose of HbOC should be given at 15 months of age at an interval not less than 2 months after the previous dose. If PRP-OMP is used, infants 2–6 months of age should receive two doses 2 months apart and a booster dose at 12 months of age. Vaccines should not be interchanged once a dose has been started, as the immunogenicities of HbOC and PRP-OMP are different. An additional dose of PRP-OMP should be given to all children at 15 months of age. Unvaccinated children 5 years of age or older with a chronic illness known to be associated with an increased risk of invasive Hib disease should be given a single dose of any licensed conjugate vaccine (80). Serious adverse reactions to the Hib conjugate vaccines are rare, the most common reaction being local reaction such as redness, swelling at the vaccination site, and low-grade fever (50). Three cases of an acute inflammatory demyelinating polyradiculoneuropathy (Guillain-Barré syndrome) have been reported in a child of 19 months, one of 20 months, and one of 33 months after immunization with an Hib PRP-D conjugate vaccine. The onset of the acute inflammatory demyelinating polyradiculoneuropathy occurred within one week after vaccination in all three patients (81). Invasive *H. influenzae* type b infections have been observed in the week after immunization with the PRP-D conjugate vaccine. A transient depression of antibody concentrations was documented in nine infants with preimmunization anticapsular antibody concentrations (>0.025 μg/ml) with recovery of antibody concentrations within 7 days of immunization (82). There may be an increased risk of disease in this 7-day interval. The reason for this depression of anticapsular antibody concentrations during the first week after immunization with the *H. influenzae* type b conjugate vaccine is not known.

Immunoprophylaxis of meningococcal disease currently uses a quadrivalent (serogroups A, C, Y, and W135) polysaccharide vaccine. The group A vaccine is efficacious in controlling local epidemics in third world countries where group A meningococcal disease is present in epidemics every few years. Vaccination is recommended for travelers to countries with endemic or epidemic disease, and immunity is not long-lasting. Serogroup C is responsible for meningococcal meningitis in outbreaks that occur in schools and military camps. Serogroup B is responsible for the majority of meningococcal disease in developed countries. The polysaccharide capsule of this organism is poorly immunogenic because anti-B polysaccharide antibodies are not bactericidal in the presence of human complement (83). In order to improve the immunogenicity of the serogroup B polysaccharide, the development of a polysaccharide-protein conjugate vaccine, similar to the *H. influenzae* type b conjugate vaccine, is expected to be effective (84).

The current pneumococcal vaccine consists of a group of capsular polysaccharides derived from up to 23 serotypes and is only 60–70% effective in adults (83,85). It is ineffective in children less than 2 years of age. The Immunization Practices Advisory Committee of the Public Health Service recommends the immunization of individuals 65 years of age and older and others at risk, including adults and children with chronic diseases, such as diabetes, congestive heart failure, pulmonary disease, hepatic or renal disease, and immunocompromised persons such as those infected with the human immunodeficiency virus, individuals with multiple myeloma or an asplenic state, and those with cancer (86).

Chemoprophylaxis

Rifampin is the currently recommended antibiotic for prophylaxis of meningococcal meningitis. The recommended dose is 600 mg every 12 h for 2 days in adults, 10 mg/kg every 12 h for 2 days in children older than 1 year, and 5 mg/kg every 12 h for 2 days in children younger than 1 year. Rifampin is used for the prevention of secondary cases once an index case has been identified. The risk of developing meningitis is highest immediately after contact with an index case, with the majority of secondary cases occuring within the first week after the index case (87). Close contacts of the index case should receive chemoprophylaxis as soon as a primary case is identified. Close contacts are defined as individuals who have had contact with the patient's nasopharyngeal secretions. Rifampin should not be used during pregnancy.

The risk of secondary disease from close contact with an individual with *H. influenzae* type b meningitis is age-dependent, being highest for children less than 2 years of age (87). The American Academy of Pediatrics recommends rifampin prophylaxis for all individuals in households with at least one child younger than 24 months of age or with a nonimmunized child 24–48 months of age. The recommended dose of rifampin is 20 mg/kg/day orally for 4 days, with a maximum dose of 600 mg/day (88). All members of the staff and school attendees of a daycare center should receive prophylaxis if children under 2 years of age attend for prolonged periods of more than 25 h/week (87).

REFERENCES

1. Vieusseux G. Memoire sur la maladie qui a regne a Geneve au printemps de 1805. J Med Chi Pharm 1806; 11:163–182.
2. Danielson L, Mann E. The history of a singular and very mortal disease which lately made its appearance in Medfield. In: Adams B, ed. The Medical and Agricultural Register. Boston: Manning and Loring, 1806:65–69.
3. Verghese A, Gallemore G. Kernig's and Brudzinski's signs revisited. Rev Infect Dis 1987; 9:1187–1192.
4. Flexner S. The results of the serum treatment in thirteen hundred cases of epidemic meningitis. J Exp Med 1913; 17:553–576.
5. McDermott W, Rogers DE. Social ramifications of control of microbial disease. Johns Hopkins Med J 1982; 151:302–312.
6. Rosenberg DH, Arling PA. Penicillin in the treatment of meningitis. JAMA 1944; 125:1011–1017.
7. Tauber MG, Sande MA. The impact of penicillin on the treatment of meningitis. JAMA 1984; 251:1877–1880.
8. Quagliarello V, Scheld WM. Bacterial meningitis: pathogenesis, pathophysiology, and progress. N Engl J Med 1992; 327:864–872.

9. Simberkoff MS, Moldover NH, Rahal J, Jr. Absence of detectable bactericidal and opsonic activities in normal and infected human cerebrospinal fluids: a regional host defense deficiency. J Lab Clin Med 1980; 95:362–372.
10. Zwahlen A, Nydegger UE, Vaudaux P, Lambert PH, Waldvogel FA. Complement-mediated opsonic activity in normal and infected human cerebrospinal fluid: early response during bacterial meningitis. J Infect Dis 1982; 145:635–646.
11. Dinarello CA. Interleukin-1. Rev Infect Dis 1984; 6:51–95.
12. Glimaker M, Kragsbjerg P, Forsgren M, Olcen P. Tumor necrosis factor-alpha (TNF-alpha) in cerebrospinal fluid from patients with meningitis of different etiologies: high levels of TNF-alpha indicate bacterial meningitis. J Infect Dis 1993; 167:882–889.
13. Arditi M, Manogue KR, Caplan M, Yogev R. Cerebrospinal fluid cachectin/tumor necrosis factor-alpha and platelet-activating factor concentrations and severity of bacterial meningitis in children. J Infect Dis 1990; 162:139–147.
14. Kruger J, Dinarello C, Chedid L. Promotion of slow wave sleep by a purified interleukin-1 preparation. Fed Proc 1983; 42:356.
15. Dinarello CA. An update on human interleukin-1: from molecular biology to clinical relevance. J Clin Immunol 1985; 5:287–296.
16. Mustafa MM, Ramilo O, Saez-Llorens X, Olsen KD, et al. Cerebrospinal fluid prostaglandins, interleukin-1 beta, and tumor necrosis factor in bacterial meningitis. Am J Dis Child 1990; 144:883–887.
17. Pfister HW, Fontana A, Tauber MG, Tomasz A, Scheld WM. Mechanisms of brain injury in bacterial meningitis: workshop summary. Clin Infect Dis 1994; 19:463–479.
18. Kaplan SL, Fishman MA. Supportive therapy for bacterial meningitis. Pediatr Infect Dis J 1987; 6: 670–677.
19. Feigin RD, McCracken GH, Klein JO. Diagnosis and management of meningitis. Pediatr Infect Dis J 1992; 11:785–814.
20. Kernig VM. Ueber ein Krankheitssymptom der acuten Meningitis. St. Petersburg Med Wochenschr 1882; 7:398.
21. Lambert HP. Meningitis. J Neurol Neurosurg Psych 1994; 57:405–415.
22. Fredericks JAM. Meningococcal meningitis. In: Vinken PJ, Bruyn GW, Klawans HL, Harris AA, eds. Handbook of Clinical Neurology. Amsterdam: Elsevier, 1988:21–40.
23. Ferguson JH, Chapman OD. Fulminating meningococcic infections and the so-called Waterhouse-Friderichsen syndrome. Am J Pathol 1948; 24:763–782.
24. Durand ML, Calderwood SB, Weber DJ, Miller SI, et al. Acute bacterial meningitis in adults: a review of 493 episodes. N Engl J Med 1993; 328:21–28.
25. Geiseler PJ, Nelson KE, Levin S, Reddy KT, Moses VK. Community acquired purulent meningitis: a review of 1316 cases during the antibiotic era, 1954–1976. Rev Infect Dis 1980; 2:725–745.
26. Dougherty JM, Roth RM. Cerebral spinal fluid. Emerg Med Clin North Am 1986; 4:281–297.
27. Bonadio WA. The cerebrospinal fluid: physiologic aspects and alterations associated with bacterial meningitis. Pediatr Infect Dis J 1992; 11:423–432.
28. Conly JM, Ronald AR. Cerebrospinal fluid as a diagnostic body fluid. Am J Med 1983; 102–106.
29. Fishbein DB, Palmer DL, Porter KM, Reed WP. Bacterial meningitis in the absence of CSF pleocytosis. Arch Intern Med 1981; 141:1369–1372.
30. Powers WJ. Cerebrospinal fluid lymphocytosis in acute bacterial meningitis. Am J Med 1985; 79: 216–220.
31. Cherubin CE, Marr JS, Sierra MF, Becker S. Listeria and gram-negative bacillary meningitis in New York City, 1972–1979. Am J Med 1981; 71:199–208.
32. Fishman RA. Composition of the cerebrospinal fluid. In: Fishman RA, ed. Cerebrospinal Fluid in Diseases of the Nervous System. Philadelphia: W.B. Saunders Company, 1992:183–252.
33. Greenlee JE. Approach to diagnosis of meningitis: cerebrospinal fluid evaluation. Infect Dis Clin North Am 1990; 4:583–598.
34. Durack DT, Spanos A. End-of-treatment spinal tap in bacterial meningitis. Is it worthwhile? JAMA 1982; 248:75–78.

35. Hoban DJ, Witwicki E, Hammond GW. Bacterial antigen detection in cerebrospinal fluid of patients with meningitis. Diagn Microbiol Infect Dis 1985; 3:373–379.
36. Maxson S, Lewno MJ, Schutze GE. Clinical usefulness of cerebrospinal fluid bacterial antigen studies. J Pediatr 1994; 125:235–238.
37. Burans JP, El Tayeb M, Abu-Elyazeed R, Woody JN. Comparison of latex agglutination with established bacteriological tests for diagnosis of cerebrospinal meningitis. Lancet 1989; 1:158–159.
38. Ingram DL, Pearson AW, Occhiuti AR. Detection of bacterial antigens in body fluids with the Wellcogen Haemophilus influenzae b, Streptococcus pneumoniae, and Neisseria meningitidis (ACYW 135) latex agglutination tests. J Clin Microbiol 1983; 18:1119–1121.
39. Dwelle TL, Dunkle LM, Blair L. Correlation of cerebrospinal fluid endotoxinlike activity with clinical and laboratory variables in gram-negative bacterial meningitis in children. J Clin Microbiol 1987; 25:856–858.
40. Darville T, Jacobs RF, Lucas RA, Caldwell B. Detection of Hemophilus influenzae type b antigen in cerebrospinal fluid after immunization. Pediatr Infect Dis J 1992; 11:243–244.
41. Whitley RJ, Lakeman F. Herpes simplex virus infections of the central nervous system: therapeutic and diagnostic considerations. Clin Infect Dis 1995; 20:414–420.
42. Treseler CB, Sugar AM. Fungal meningitis. Infect Dis Clin North Am 1990; 4:789–808.
43. Shaunak S, Cohen J. Clinical management of fungal infection in patients with AIDS. J Antimicrob Chemo 1991; 28 (Suppl A):67–81.
44. Tunkel AR, Scheld WM. Acute meningitis. In: Stein JH, et al., eds. Internal Medicine. 4th ed. St. Louis: Mosby, 1994:1886–1898.
45. Schoendorf KC, Adams WG, Kiely JL, Wenger JD. National trends in Haemophilus influenzae meningitis mortality and hospitalization among children, 1980 through 1991. Pediatrics 1994; 93: 663–668.
46. John CC. Treatment failure with use of a third-generation cephalosporin for penicillin-resistant pneumococcal meningitis: case report and review. Clin Infect Dis 1994; 18:188–193.
47. McCracken GH, Sande MA, Lentnek A, Whitley RJ, Scheld WM. Evaluation of new anti-infective drugs for the treatment of acute bacterial meningitis. Clin Infect Dis 1992; 15(suppl 1):S182–188.
48. Lebel MH, Hoyt MJ, McCracken GH Jr. Comparative efficacy of ceftriaxone and cefuroxime for treatment of bacterial meningitis. J Pediatr 1989; 114:1049–1054.
49. Schaad BV, Suter S, Borradori AG, Pfenninger J, Auckenthaler R, Bernath O, et al. A comparison of ceftriaxone and cefuroxime for the treatment of bacterial meningitis in children. N Engl J Med 1990; 322:141–147.
50. Kaplan SL. New aspects of prevention and therapy of meningitis. Infect Dis Clin North Am 1992; 6:197–214.
51. Jacobs RF. Cefotaxime treatment of gram-negative enteric meningitis in infants and children. Drugs 1988; 35 (suppl 2):185.
52. Laine J, Holmberg C, Anttila M, Peltola H, Perheentupa J. Types of fluid disorder in children with bacterial meningitis. Acta Pediatr Scand 1991; 80:1031–1036.
53. Kaplan SL, Feigin RD. The syndrome of inappropriate secretion of antidiuretic hormone in children with bacterial meningitis. J Pediatr 1978; 92:758–761.
54. Feigin RD, Dodge PR. Bacterial meningitis: newer concepts of pathophysiology and neurologic sequelae. Pediatr Clin North Am 1976; 23:541–556.
55. Diringer MN, Kirsch JR. Disturbances of sodium and osmolality. In: Johnson RT, Griffin JW, eds. Current Therapy in Neurologic Disease. 4th ed. St. Louis: B.C. Decker, 1993:347–352.
56. Tureen JH, Tauber MG, Sande MA. Effect of hydration status on cerebral blood flow and cerebrospinal fluid lactic acidosis in rabbits with experimental meningitis. J Clin Invest 1992; 89:947–953.
57. Klein JO, Feigin RD, McCracken GH. Report of the task force on diagnosis and managment of meningitis. Pediatrics 1987; 78:S959–S982.
58. Swartz M. Acute bacterial meningitis. In: Gorbach SL, Bartlett JG, Blacklow NR, eds. Infectious Diseases. Philadelphia: W.B. Saunders, 1992:1160–1177.
59. Rasmussen HH, Sorensen HT, Moller-Peterson J, Mortensen FV, Nielsen B. Bacterial meningitis in elderly patients: clinical picture and course. Age Ageing 1992; 21:216–220.

60. Gorse GJ, Thrupp LD, Nudleman KL, Wyle FA, Hawkins B, Cesario TC. Bacterial meningitis in the elderly. Arch Intern Med 1984; 144:1603–1607.
61. Fong IW, Tomkins KB. Review of Pseudomonas aeruginosa meningitis with special emphasis on treatment with ceftazidime. Rev Infect Dis 1985; 7:604–612.
62. Pruitt AA. Central nervous system infections in cancer patients. Neurol Clin 1991; 9:867–888.
63. Armstrong D. Central nervous system infections in the immunocompromised host. Infection 1984; 12:S58–S62.
64. Ropper AH, Rockoff MA. Physiology and clinical aspects of raised intracranial pressure. In: Ropper AH, ed. Neurological and Neurosurgical Intensive Care. New York: Raven Press, Ltd., 1993:11–27.
65. Ropper AH. Treatment of intracranial hypertension. In: Ropper AH, ed. Neurological and Neurosurgical Intensive Care. New York: Raven Press, Ltd., 1993:29–52.
66. Haring HP, Rotzer HK, Reindl H, et al. Time course of cerebral blood flow velocity in central nervous system infections: a transcranial Doppler sonography study. Arch Neurol 1993; 50:98–101.
67. Pfister HW, Borasio GD, Dirnagl U, Bauer M, Einhaupl KM. Cerebrovascular complications of bacterial meningitis in adults. Neurology 1992; 42:1497–1504.
68. Gado M, Axley J, Appleton B, Prensky AL. Angiography in the acute and posttreatment phases of Hemophilus influenzae meningitis. Radiology 1974; 110:439–444.
69. Igarashi M, Gilmartin RC, Gerald B, Wilburn F, Jabbour JT. Cerebral arteritis and bacterial meningitis. Arch Neurol 1984; 41:531–535.
70. Lyons EL, Leeds NE. The angiographic demonstration of arterial vascular disease in purulent meningitis. Radiology 1967; 88:935–938.
71. Adams RJ. Management issues for patients with ischemic stroke. Neurology 1995; 45(suppl 1): S15–S18.
72. Committee on Infectious Diseases. Dexamethasone therapy for bacterial meningitis in infants and children. Pediatrics 1990; 86:130–133.
73. Lebel MH, Freij BT, Syrogiannopoulos GA, Chrane DF, et al. Dexamethasone therapy for bacterial meningitis: results of two double-blind, placebo-controlled trials. N Engl J Med 1988; 319:964–971.
74. Odio CM, Faingezicht I, Paris M, Nassar M. The beneficial effects of early dexamethasone administration in infants and children with bacterial meningitis. N Engl J Med 1991; 324:1525–1531.
75. Girgis NI, Farid Z, Mikhail IA, Farrag I, et al. Dexamethasone treatment for bacterial meningitis in children and adults. Pediatr Infect Dis J 1989; 8:848–851.
76. Kennedy WA, Hoyt MJ, McCracken GH. The role of corticosteroid therapy in children with pneumococcal meningitis. Am J Dis Child 1991; 145:1374–1378.
77. Schaad UB, Lips U, Gnehm HE, Blumberg A, et al. Dexamethasone therapy for bacterial meningitis in children. Lancet 1993; 342:457–461.
78. Syrogiannopoulos GA, Olsen KD, Reisch JS, McCracken GH. Dexamethasone in the treatment of experimental Haemophilus influenzae type b meningitis. J Infect Dis 1987; 155:213–239.
79. Waagner DC, Kennedy WA, Hoyt MJ, McCracken GH Jr. Lack of adverse effects of dexamethasone therapy in aseptic meningitis. Pediatr Infect Dis J 1990; 10:922–923.
80. Committee on Infectious Diseases American Academy of Pediatrics. Haemophilus influenzae type b conjugate vaccines: recommendations for immunization of infants and children 2 months of age and older. Pediatrics 1991; 88:169–172.
81. D'Cruz OF, Shapiro ED, Spiegelman KN, et al. Acute inflammatory demyelinating polyradiculoneuropathy (Guillain-Barre syndrome) after immunization with Haemophilus influenzae type b conjugate vaccine. J Pediatr 1989; 115:743–746.
82. Marchant CD, Band E, Froeschle JE, McVerry PH. Depression of anticapsular antibody after immunization with Haemophilus influenzae type b polysaccharide-diphtheria conjugate vaccine. Pediatr Infect Dis J 1989; 8:508–511.
83. Jones DM. Current and future trends in immunization against meningitis. J Antimicrob Chemother 1993; 31 (suppl B):93–99.
84. Frasch CE, Zahradnick JM, Wang LY, Mocca LF, Tsai C-M. Antibody response of adults to an aluminum hydroxide-absorbed Neisseria meningitidis serotype 26 protein-group B polysaccharide vaccine. J Infect Dis 1988; 158:710–718.

85. Bolan G, Broome CV, Facklam RR, et al. Pneumococcal vaccine efficacy in selected populations in the United States. Ann Intern Med 1986; 104:1–6.
86. Recommendations of the Immunization Practices Advisory Committee: pneumococcal polysaccharide vaccine. MMWR 1989; 38:64–68, 73–76.
87. Cuevas LE, Hart CA. Chemoprophylaxis of bacterial meningitis. J Antimicrob Chemother 1993; 31 (suppl B):79–91.
88. Committee on Infectious Diseases. Revision of recommendation for use of rifampin prophylaxis of contacts of patients with Haemophilus influenzae infection. Pediatrics 1984; 74:301–302.
89. Roos KL, Bonnin JM. Acute bacterial meningitides. In: Mandell GL, ed. Atlas of Infectious Diseases. Vol. III. Central Nervous System and Eye Infections. Philadelphia: Churchill Livingstone, 1995:2–26.
90. Roos KL. Clinical presentation of bacterial meningitis. In: Roos KL. Meningitis: 100 Maxims. London: Arnold, 1996:20–35.

6

Viral Meningitis and Aseptic Meningitis

Karen L. Roos
Indiana University School of Medicine, Indianapolis, Indiana

INTRODUCTION

Aseptic meningitis, as defined by Wallgren in 1925, has the following characteristics: (1) acute onset, (2) signs and symptoms of meningitis, (3) a cerebrospinal fluid monocytic cell pleocytosis, (4) absence of bacteria on smear and by culture of cerebrospinal fluid, (5) no parameningeal focus of infection or systemic disease known to cause meningitis, and (6) a self-limited benign course (1,2). The classic cerebrospinal fluid abnormalities in aseptic meningitis are a mononuclear or lymphocytic pleocytosis with the absence of bacteria. The term *aseptic meningitis* is used today to describe any disease with signs and symptoms of meningitis, a cerebrospinal fluid lymphocytic pleocytosis, and negative smears and cultures for bacteria, fungi, and acid-fast bacilli (2). Since 1925 and until recently, the term aseptic meningitis has been synonymous with viral meningitis. With the increasing availability of laboratory diagnostic tests, such as the polymerase chain reaction, to make a timely and specific diagnosis of viral central nervous system infection, the term aseptic meningitis may become a term of historical interest only. This chapter will be divided into the viral and nonviral etiologies of aseptic meningitis.

VIRAL MENINGITIS

The most common viruses causing viral meningitis are the enteroviruses, the herpesviruses, and the human immunodeficiency virus.

Pathogenesis

Viruses initially enter the host by passively entering through the skin or through the mucosal surfaces of the respiratory, gastrointestinal, or genitourinary tract. Parainfluenza virus and respiratory syncytial virus are viruses that typically enter through the respiratory tract. Poliovirus enters through the gastrointestinal tract. The herpes simplex virus and human immunodeficiency virus are sexually transmitted viruses that enter the host through the mucosal surface of the genitourinary tract. Viruses may also be injected directly into the blood by a contaminated needle, via the transfusion of contaminated blood products, or by the bite of a mosquito. Viruses that produce neurological disease must spread from the initial site of entry to the central nervous system (CNS). There are two major pathways by which viruses may reach the CNS: the hematogenous route or the neuronal route. For virus that will reach the CNS via the hematogenous route, primary replication occurs at the site of entry and is followed by dissemination of the virus to the regional lymph nodes and eventually into the systemic circulation. Further replication of the virus in the reticuloendothelial system results in the continual release of virus into the systemic circulation. Virus may circulate as free virus in the plasma or in association with cellular elements. Enteroviruses circulate as free virus in plasma, lymphocytic choriomeningitis virus associates with platelets, Colorado tick fever virus with red cells, and HIV with CD4+ cells (3). Virus is carried through the systemic circulation to the cerebral circulation.

The second major mechanism for viral spread to the CNS is through neurons. Rabies virus, herpesviruses, and polio virus all enter the CNS via nerves innervating peripheral sites, mainly by retrograde intra-axonal transport (3). Herpes simplex virus type 1 (HSV-1) after an initial stomatitis becomes latent in the trigeminal ganglion. Herpes simplex virus type 2 (HSV-2) after an initial genital infection becomes latent in the sacral dorsal root ganglia. Varicella-zoster virus causes a generalized systemic infection and then becomes latent in dorsal root ganglia. During latency, virus replication ceases and clinical signs and symptoms are absent. Reactivation of the virus within the ganglion with renewed virus replication and subsequent spread of virus down the distal processes of infected neurons produces clinical disease (3).

Clinical Presentation

Viral meningitis is an acute illness characterized by a severe "grippelike" headache, photophobia, myalgias, fever (usually <40°C), and nausea and vomiting. There may be signs of meningeal irritation and the patient may be lethargic, but patients with viral meningitis are not obtunded or comatose. Focal neurological signs, new-onset seizure activity, and coma do not occur in a benign self-limited viral meningitis.

The enteroviruses are a family of viruses that include poliovirus, coxsackie viruses A and B, echoviruses, and human enteroviruses 68 to 72. They inhabit the alimentary tract and are spread from host to host by the fecal-hand-oral route of transmission. Enteroviral meningitis tends to occur in the summer and early fall and may be associated with the presence of a maculopapular, vesicular, or petechial exanthum or specifically recognizable enteroviral syndromes such as pleurodynia, herpangina, and hand-foot-and-mouth disease (2).

The diagnoses of HSV-2 aseptic meningitis may be suggested clinically by identification of genital vesicular lesions or complaints of urinary retention or radicular symptoms, in association with headache, fever, and mild photophobia. The meningitis usually occurs during a primary genital infection. A sacral radiculitis can also be seen in association with the meningitis and primary genital or rectal HSV-2 infection (4).

The human immunodeficiency virus (HIV-1) enters the CNS early in the infection. An acute meningitis may accompany primary infection with HIV-1 or present during the stage of clinical latency when the CD4+ T-lymphocyte count is between 200 and 500 cells/mm^3. When aseptic meningitis occurs early in HIV infection, serum antibodies for HIV-1 may be nonreactive as they do not typically become positive until 8–12 weeks after infection occurs (5).

Mumps virus and the vaccine strain mumps virus can cause meningitis. Meningitis may follow the onset of parotitis by several days to weeks or may precede the onset of parotitis or occur without associated parotitis. Meningitis may also follow the onset of the other manifestations of mumps, which are orchitis, oophoritis, and pancreatitis. Mumps virus and the vaccine strain mumps virus aseptic meningitis presents with fever, vomiting, irritability, lethargy, headache, and meningismus and is typically a benign self-limited illness (2).

The lymphocytic choriomeningitis (LCM) virus causes human disease due to contact with infected mice and hamsters. The disease tends to be more common in the winter months; however, infection with LCM virus may occur in any month. Meningeal symptoms are often preceded by a flulike illness with fever, arthralgias, myalgias, and occasionally pneumonitis, alopecia, parotitis, and orchitis. The clinical presentation of meningitis is typical of viral meningitis with fever, headache, stiff neck, nausea, and vomiting (4).

Symptomatic infections from arthropodborne viruses (arboviruses) typically present as an acute viral encephalitis, but may in their milder forms present as an aseptic meningitis. In the United States, the principal mosquitoborne viruses that may present as an aseptic meningitis are the St. Louis encephalitis virus and the California encephalitis virus. The St. Louis encephalitis virus is found throughout the United States and Canada with epidemics occurring typically in August through October. The LaCrosse variety of the California encephalitis virus is found in the midwestern and eastern United States, and infections typically occur between June and October. Their clinical presentations may be indistinguishable from enteroviral aseptic meningitis (2). The majority of infections due to the LaCrosse strain of the California encephalitis virus are either asymptomatic or present as an aseptic meningitis.

Diagnosis

The cerebrospinal fluid (CSF) findings suggestive of viral meningitis are (1) a lymphocytic pleocytosis, typically 200–2000 cells/mm^3, (2) a normal glucose concentration, (3) a normal or slightly elevated protein concentration, (4) negative bacterial antigen tests, (5) low concentrations of tumor necrosis factor, and (6) a CSF lactic acid concentration of <35 mg/dl (Table 1) (6–10). There may be a predominance of polymorphonuclear leukocytes in the CSF early in the course of viral meningitis. A repeat lumbar puncture within 24–48 h should demonstrate a shift to a lymphocytic predominance in the vast majority of cases of viral meningitis. The CSF lymphocyte count gradually decreases and usually returns to normal within a few days. In a minority of cases, the CSF pleocytosis may persist for 1–2 months. For this reason, repeating a lumbar puncture in a patient with viral meningitis who is clinically improving is not useful (4). Viral cultures will be positive in approximately 50% of CSF specimens. Cell culture is the "gold standard" for

Table 1 Cerebrospinal Fluid Abnormalities to Distinguish Viral from Bacterial Meningitis

Characteristic	Viral	Bacterial
Opening pressure	Normal or mildly elevated	> 250 mmH$_2$O
Cell count	200–2000 cells/mm^3	> 100 cells/mm^3
	Lymphocytic pleocytosis	Polymorphonuclear pleocytosis
Protein concentration	Normal or mildly elevated	> 45 mg/dl
Glucose concentration	⩾ 40 mg/dl	< 40 mg/dl
CSF: Serum glucose ratio	> 0.31	< 0.31
Gram's stain	Negative	Positive
Lactic acid concentration	< 35 mg/dl	⩾ 35 mg/dl

detecting viruses primarily because there are no false-positive results (10). An acute and convalescent serum sample should be obtained for antibody titers. The virus causing infection can be identified by detecting a fourfold or greater increase in antiviral IgG antibody between the serum samples or by the first-time appearance of virus-specific IgM antibodies (11).

In suspected enteroviral meningitis, cultures of CSF, stool, and oropharynx should be performed. The stool is the most likely source for virus isolation (4). If enterovirus is isolated from a non-CSF viral culture, a presumptive diagnosis of enteroviral meningitis can be made. A definitive diagnosis of enteroviral meningitis requires a positive CSF viral culture or a fourfold rise in serum virus antibody (12). A polymerase chain reaction–based assay for the diagnosis of enteroviral meningitis is currently under development. Earlier attempts at diagnosis with the use of DNA or RNA enteroviral probes were hampered by the low titers of virus in infected cerebrospinal fluid. The polymerase chain reaction, which allows for the amplification of short segments of DNA or RNA, should increase the sensitivity and specificity significantly and shorten the time required for the detection of viral infections of the CNS (10).

In HSV-2 aseptic meningitis examination of the CSF demonstrates a lymphocytic pleocytosis (median 300–400 cells/mm^3), a mildly elevated protein concentration, and a normal or decreased glucose concentration (13,14). A definitive diagnosis is made by either a positive CSF viral culture or by demonstrating a fourfold rise in HSV-2–specific IgG.

In HIV-1 meningitis, examination of the cerebrospinal fluid reveals a mononuclear pleocytosis (<200 cells/mm^3), an increased protein concentration (<100 mg/dl), and a normal or slightly decreased glucose concentration. HIV-1 may be isolated from the CSF (5). CSF abnormalities are very common on routine examination of the CSF in asymptomatic HIV-infected individuals without clinically detectable neurological disease (5). Cerebrospinal fluid examinations were performed on 459 asymptomatic, neurologically normal, HIV-positive individuals. At least one abnormality was detected in 60% of the CSF samples from these individuals. All of the individuals had T-helper cell counts of >400 cells/mm^3. CSF abnormalities included an elevated protein concentration in 6.4%, nucleated cell counts >10 cells/mm^3 in 15.6%, oligoclonal bands in 14%, an IgG synthesis rate of greater than 15 mg/dl (~4.5 times the upper limit of normal) in 10%, and an elevated CSF IgG concentration in 10%. There was a decline in the CSF glucose concentration and in the degree of CSF pleocytosis between a group of patients that were HIV-positive only with a T-helper cell count of >400 cells/mm^3 and a group of patients with HIV-positivity and decreased T-helper cells and/or opportunistic infections. Overall, there were greater CSF abnormalities for patients that were HIV-positive only compared to the group of patients that were HIV-positive and had decreased T-helper cells and/or opportunistic infections (15).

The typical cerebrospinal fluid abnormalities in mumps meningitis are (1) a mononuclear pleocytosis with a WBC count of 300–600 cells/mm^3, (2) a normal or slightly elevated protein concentration, and (3) a normal or decreased glucose concentration. The diagnosis is usually made from the presence of parotitis and isolation of the virus from the CSF, saliva, and urine (4).

Examination of the CSF in lymphocytic choriomeningitis virus meningitis demonstrates a lymphocytic pleocytosis typically more than 1000 cells/mm^3. LCM virus meningitis may have high CSF leukocyte counts up to several thousand and hypoglycorrhachia. The diagnosis of LCM can be established by culturing the virus from blood or spinal fluid early and later from urine. The diagnosis can also be made by demonstrating a fourfold antibody rise between acute and convalescent sera (2,4).

Treatment

Meningitis due to enteroviruses, HIV-1, mumps, and the LCM virus is self-limited, and treatment is supportive consisting of bedrest, fluids, antipyretics, and analgesics. Antiviral therapy is, however, recommended for HSV-2 meningitis that occurs in association with a primary genital herpes infection. Intravenous acyclovir therapy is slightly more effective than oral acyclovir therapy for a primary genital herpes infection; therefore, when aseptic meningitis develops during a severe primary genital herpes infection, acyclovir 5 mg/kg intravenous every 8 h for 5 days is recommended. Oral therapy (200 mg 5 times per day for 10 days) is nearly as effective as intravenous therapy and can be used in individuals with mild local disease without systemic complications (16). Valacyclovir recently became available for the treatment of recurrent genital herpes, but its role in the treatment of aseptic meningitis associated with recurrent genital herpes has not been defined.

Differential Diagnosis

The differential diagnosis of viral meningitis is the differential diagnosis of meningeal signs and symptoms with a cerebrospinal fluid lymphocytic pleocytosis. Table 2 lists the viral and nonviral infectious etiologies of an aseptic meningitis, as well as systemic diseases and medications that should be included in the differential diagnosis. The nonviral infectious etiologies of aseptic meningitis are discussed in length in other chapters in this volume.

NONVIRAL MENINGITIS

Partially Treated Bacterial Meningitis

Oral antimicrobial therapy prior to lumbar puncture may decrease the CSF protein concentration and decrease the likelihood of identifying the organism on Gram's stain or isolating the organism in culture, but will not significantly alter the CSF white blood cell count or glucose concentration (17–19). The presence of bacterial meningitis would be suspected from the detection of a polymorphonuclear pleocytosis and a low glucose concentration in cerebrospinal fluid, which should be seen despite prior oral antimicrobial therapy. The latex agglutination (LA) test for antigens to *Haemophilus influenzae* type b, *Streptococcus pneumoniae*, and *Neisseria meningitidis* is a useful technique in cases of suspected partially treated bacterial meningitis. In addition, the limulus amebocyte lysate (LAL) assay detects gram-negative endotoxin in CSF, and therefore is very sensitive in detecting gram-negative bacterial meningitis. Both the LA and LAL tests are very useful in the patient who has been pretreated with either parenteral or oral antibiotic therapy.

Tuberculous Meningitis

The clinical presentation of tuberculous meningitis is either that of an acute meningitis syndrome with headache, malaise, vomiting, meningismus, confusion, and cranial nerve deficits that progresses to coma or that of a slowly progressive dementing illness. The classic cerebrospinal fluid abnormalities in tuberculous meningitis are (1) elevated opening pressure, (2) elevated protein concentration in the range of 100–500 mg/dl, (3) white blood cell (WBC) count between 10 and 500 cells/mm^3 with a predominance of lymphocytes, and (4) a decreased glucose concentration. The gold standard for the diagnosis of tuberculous meningitis is the detection of acid-fast bacilli in smears of CSF or a positive culture result. Cultures of CSF require 3–6 weeks for growth to be detectable and are positive in approximately 75% of cases of tuberculous meningitis (20). The polymerase chain reaction (PCR) technique for detection of tubercle bacilli DNA in CSF is expected to be very sensitive and specific for the rapid detection of *Mycobacterium tuberculosis*. Radiographic evidence of pulmonary tuberculous, specifically hilar adenopathy, is found in 50–90% of cases of tuberculous meningitis in children (21,22). The

Table 2 Differential Diagnosis of Aseptic Meningitis

Viral infection	Drugs
Enteroviruses (poliovirus, Coxsackievirus types A and B, echovirus, human enterovirus 68 to 72)	Nonsteroidal anti-inflammatory agents
Mumps	OKT3
Herpes simplex virus types 1 and 2	Azathioprine (Imuran)
Varicella-zoster	Trimethoprim-sulfamethoxazole
HIV	Isoniazid
Adenoviruses	Intravenous immune globulin
Arboviruses	Spirochetes
Epstein-Barr virus	*Borrelia burgdorferi*
Lymphocytic choriomeningitis virus	*Treponema palllidum*
Influenza virus types A and B	Fungal infection
Colorado tick fever	*Cryptococcus neoformans*
Bacterial infection	*Histoplasma capsulatum*
Partially treated bacterial meningitis	*Coccidioides immitis*
Bacterial meningitis in cancer patient	*Blastomyces dermatitidis*
Parameningeal infection	Systemic disease
Listeria monocytogenes	Sarcoidosis
Mycoplasma pneumoniae	Leukemia, lymphoma
Mycobacterium tuberculosis	Adenocarcinoma, malignant melanoma, small-cell lung cancer
Human monocytic ehrlichiosis	Systemic lupus erythematosus
Human granulocytic ehrlichiosis	Behcet's disease
	Endocarditis
	Other
	Migraine
	Measles-mumps-rubella vaccine
	Vasculitis
	Parainfectious syndrome (acute disseminated encephalomyelitis)

association of pulmonary lesions and meningitis is not as high in adults, and the absence of pulmonary disease should not rule out a tuberculous etiology for the aseptic meningitis (22,23). The intradermal tuberculin skin test is helpful when positive, but a negative test does not rule out tuberculous meningitis. The clinical presentation of headache and cranial nerve palsies followed within days by an altered level of consciousness and the development of hydrocephalus on CT or MR scan and the presence of a CSF lymphocytic pleocytosis is highly suggestive of tuberculous meningoencephalitis.

Lyme Disease

Symptoms of Lyme meningitis typically begin several weeks after the appearance of the characteristic skin lesion, erythema migrans (EM), and can occur while EM is still present. The predominant symptom is headache. There may be evidence of mild neck stiffness, cranial neuropathies, specifically facial nerve palsy, and radicular symptoms. Examination of the cerebrospinal fluid demonstrates a mononuclear pleocytosis (generally <200 WBC/mm^3), with occasional plasma cells and atypical lymphocytes. The protein concentration may be elevated but is generally <100 mg/dl. A decreased CSF glucose concentration is unusual. The diagnosis is made by the detection of intrathecal Lyme antibody production (24).

The following characteristics of the meningitis of Lyme disease are thought to be helpful in distinguishing meningitis due to *B. burgdorferi* from meningitis due to *Mycobacterium tuberculosis*, fungal infections, or sarcoidosis:

1. Meningitis of Lyme disease is generally not associated with significant meningismus, raised intracranial pressure (tuberculous meningitis), or hypoglycorrhachia (tuberculous and fungal meningitis and sarcoidosis).
2. Facial nerve palsy, including bilateral facial nerve palsy, is common in Lyme disease and, if present, often helps separate Lyme disease from other entities.

Facial nerve palsy is also a common abnormality in sarcoidosis. A history of a tick bite and residence in or travel to an area endemic for Lyme disease greatly increases the likelihood of Lyme disease as the etiology of the aseptic meningitis.

The other tickborne infections—Colorado tick fever, human monocytic ehrlichiosis (HME), and human granulocytic ehrlichiosis (HGE)—may also present as an aseptic meningitis. Colorado tick fever is a viral infection, and HME and HGE are bacterial infections. All three diseases are characterized by leukopenia and thrombocytopenia during the acute illness, and serological studies using acute and convalescent sera are used to make the diagnosis.

Syphilitic Meningitis

The examination of the cerebrospinal fluid may be abnormal and suggestive of an aseptic meningitis in a syphilis patient without clinical signs or symptoms of neurological involvement; this is so-called asymptomatic neurosyphilis. The typical CSF abnormalities in asymptomatic neurosyphilis are an elevated CSF protein concentration, a mild mononuclear pleocytosis, and a reactive VDRL. Patients with asymptomatic neurosyphilis may also have primary or secondary syphilis (26,27). Acute, symptomatic syphilitic meningitis is characterized by headache, nausea and vomiting, signs of meningeal irritation, cranial nerve abnormalities, and papilledema. The classic cerebrospinal fluid abnormalities in cases of syphilitic meningitis are an increased opening pressure, a mononuclear pleocytosis, an elevated protein concentration, and a positive VDRL. The diagnosis is often made and treatment initiated in the presence of a mononuclear pleocytosis and a positive VDRL and in the presence of a positive VDRL only. A nonreactive CSF VDRL does not rule out neurosyphilis. A reactive CSF VDRL virtually confirms the diagnosis of neurosyphilis except when the CSF is blood-tinged (26,28). A nonreactive CSF microhemagglutination test for *T. pallidum* (MHA-TP) excludes a diagnosis of syphilitic meningitis. Unlike the CSF VDRL, a reactive CSF MHA-TP does not establish the diagnosis of neurosyphilis. The serum treponemal serological tests (FTA-ABS and MHA-TP) should be reactive in patients with syphilitic meningitis.

Fungal Meningitis

Headache and fever are the most common symptoms of fungal meningitis, and a fungal etiology for the aseptic meningitis should be suspected particularly in patients that are immunosuppressed due to one of the following: (1) the acquired immunodeficiency syndrome (AIDS), (2) organ transplantation, (3) immunosuppressive chemotherapy or chronic corticosteroid therapy, or (4) lymphoreticular malignancies. Cryptococcal meningitis may occur in immunocompetent individuals. The typical CSF abnormalities in fungal meningitis are (1) a normal or slightly elevated opening pressure, (2) a lymphocytic pleocytosis, (3) an elevated protein concentration, and (4) a decreased glucose concentration. The latex agglutination test for the cryptococcal antigen is a highly sensitive and specific test and should be performed on all CSF specimens. In areas endemic for *Coccidioides immitis*, specifically California, Arizona, New Mexico, and Texas, the complement fixation antibody test for *C. immitis* is performed on CSF (29). In areas endemic for *Histoplasma capsulatum*, specifically the midwestern United States, principally Indianapolis, Kansas City, Memphis, and Nashville Tennessee, the histoplasma polysaccharide antigen (HPA) should be measured in urine, blood, and CSF. This test has the same diagnostic significance as detection of the cryptococcal polysaccharide antigen in patients with cryptococcal meningitis (30). Large volumes (>10 ml) of CSF should be cultured on at least three occasions to increase the yield for isolation of fungi. When fungal meningitis is suspected and multiple cultures of lumbar fluid do not reveal the organism, CSF should be obtained by a cisternal puncture.

Sarcoidosis

Cranial neuropathy is the most frequent manifestation of sarcoidosis of the nervous system, and a facial nerve palsy is the single most common abnormality. Aseptic meningitis characterized by headache, meningismus, and a CSF lymphocytic pleocytosis may be a recurrent problem in patients with neurosarcoidosis (31). The CSF abnormalities in sarcoidosis are nonspecific, including an elevated protein concentration, a lymphocytic pleocytosis, and a decreased glucose concentration. A measurement of the CSF angiotensin-converting enzyme (ACE) may be helpful in making the diagnosis of neurosarcoidosis. ACE is produced in the epithelioid and giant cells of sarcoid granulomas, which are usually widespread throughout the meninges. ACE has a molecular weight of 150,000 and does not passively leak through the blood-brain barrier; therefore, its presence in CSF is due to synthesis in the CNS granulomas (32). Several investigators have demonstrated significant elevations of CSF ACE activity in patients with neurosarcoidosis (32–34). Normal CSF ACE values do not rule out neurosarcoidosis.

When a patient with systemic sarcoidosis develops an aseptic meningitis, the diagnosis of neurosarcoidosis is frequently considered. The more difficult clinical problem is ruling out neurosarcoidosis in the setting of an aseptic meningitis without established systemic sarcoidosis. In this situation, a chest x-ray, a gallium scan, a serum ACE, and biopsy of an enlarged lymph node, salivary gland, conjunctiva, or skin lesion may confirm the diagnosis of sarcoidosis.

Leptomeningeal Carcinomatosis

Patients with acute lymphoblastic leukemia, acute myelogenous leukemia, and non-Hodgkin's lymphoma may develop leptomeningeal metastases with the appearance of a CSF lymphocytic pleocytosis. Solid tumors, specifically adenocarcinoma, small-cell lung cancer, and malignant melanoma, may metastasize to the leptomeninges. The clinical presentation of leptomeningeal metastases depends on the extent of disease along the neuraxis. Headache is a frequent complaint, and there is often associated neck pain and stiffness. Cognitive abnormalities consisting of lethargy, confusion, or memory loss are common initial complaints. Cranial nerve abnormalities manifest as diplopia, hearing loss, facial numbness, and loss of visual acuity are often present (35,36). Signs of spinal nerve root involvement, particularly affecting the lower extremities, are common and are related in part to the gravitation of malignant cells in the CSF into the cul-de-sac of the thecal sac, the slow flow of CSF in this region, and the fact that the nerve roots comprising the cauda equina have an extensive course in the subarachnoid space (37).

The presence of leptomeningeal metastases is indicated by the clinical presentation, supported by evidence of meningeal enhancement postcontrast administration on CT or MR scan, and established by the identification of malignant cells in the cerebrospinal fluid. On examination of the CSF, the opening pressure is typically elevated, the protein concentration is moderately to markedly increased (2000–3000 mg/dl), and the glucose concentration is either normal or low. A lymphocytic, monocytic, or polymorphonuclear leukocytic pleocytosis may be present. Malignant cells will be identified in the CSF on initial lumbar puncture in approximately 50–70% of patients and in a second lumbar puncture in 80–90% of cases (35–37). To increase the yield of a positive CSF cytology, CSF should be obtained from a site along the neuraxis close to the area of symptomatic disease; therefore, in the presence of encephalopathy or cranial neuropathies, CSF should be obtained from a cisternal puncture. In the presence of a cauda equina syndrome, CSF should be obtained from a lumbar interspace. At least 10 cc of CSF should be sent for analysis. Malignant cells in the CSF produce biochemical markers. A CSF beta-glucuronidase concentration of >80 mU/liter is strongly suggestive of leptomeningeal metastases (35,38). An elevated CSF carcinoembryonic antigen (CEA) is also helpful in making the diagnosis of leptomeningeal metastases.

Behcet's Disease

This disease is characterized by recurrent aphthous ulcerations of the lips, gingiva, tongue, and buccal mucosa, skin lesions that have the appearance of erythema nodosum–like lesions and folliculitis or acnelike lesions, subcutaneous thrombophlebitis, iridocyclitis or chorioretinitis, and genital ulcers. The most common manifestations of CNS involvement are brainstem dysfunction characterized by cranial nerve abnormalities, dysarthria, dysphagia, and emotional incontinence or upper motor neuron disease characterized by hemiparesis or paraparesis. A meningomyelitic syndrome and an organic confusional syndrome have also been classified as neuro-Behcet's syndrome. The disease is characterized by exacerbations and remissions. The examination of the CSF shows a slight to moderate lymphocytic pleocytosis with a significant number of polymorphonuclear leukocytes. The etiology of this disease has been attributed to a persistent immune response to an infectious agent, presumably a virus (39).

Medication-Associated Meningitis

The medications that have been associated with the development of aseptic meningitis are listed in Table 2. The occurrence of meningitis is defined by the appearance of fever, headache, and photophobia and a cerebrospinal fluid pleocytosis, typically with a predominance of polymorphonuclear leukocytes, and negative results on CSF Gram's stain, CSF cultures for bacteria, fungi, and viruses, and a negative CSF cryptococcal antigen. The meningitis is typically self-limited, and there may be resolution of symptoms despite continuation of therapy (40–42).

Both of the contrast agents used for myelography—iophendylate (Pantopaque) and metrizamide (Amipaque)—have been associated with symptomatic meningeal irritation characterized by nuchal rigidity, a low-grade fever, and a mild CSF pleocytosis. Metrizamide is a water-soluble agent that has replaced iophendylate for myelography because of the additional occurrence of an adhesive arachnoiditis following iophendylate myelography and the necessity to remove iophendylate following myelography (43,44).

Measles-Mumps-Rubella Vaccine

The measles-mumps-rubella (MMR) vaccine has been associated with a vaccine-related mumps meningitis. A live attenuated virus is used in this vaccine. A Jeryl Lynn mumps virus strain has been used in the United States for many years, and the Urabe virus strain was used in the United Kingdom until a reported reduction in vaccine-associated aseptic meningitis in Canada following a change from Urabe to Jeryl Lynn–containing MMR vaccine in 1989 led to the decision to replace Urabe with Jeryl Lynn vaccine in the United Kingdom. The risk of aseptic meningitis following vaccination with the Jeryl Lynn strain appears to be extremely low (45–47).

Migraine

The presence of a CSF pleocytosis with a clinical presentation typical of migraine is most likely an aseptic meningitis with migrainelike symptomatology, rather than classic migraine, with cells in the CSF. In the syndrome of migrainous symptoms with a lymphocytic CSF pleocytosis, the onset of the illness begins with either a focal neurological deficit or a visual disturbance followed by headache. Some of the patients have fever early in the illness. CSF viral cultures are negative, and acute and convalescent serology for California virus, herpes simplex virus, mumps virus, St. Louis encephalitis virus, and Western equine encephalitis virus are negative. The syndrome is typically self-limited, although the neurological deficit and/or headache may recur in a series of attacks for a brief period of time (48). It is very likely that as our ability to identify viral agents in the CSF and to accurately make a diagnosis of a viral etiology of aseptic meningitis improves, the syndrome of migrainous symptoms with a lymphocytic CSF pleocytosis will be clarified. It is recommended that patients that present with a combination of migrainous symptoms and a CSF lymphocytic pleocytosis have viral cultures, polymerase chain reaction technique as available, and acute and convalescent viral serological studies.

Mollaret's Meningitis

In 1944, Mollaret described a syndrome of recurrent benign endothelioleukocytic meningitis (49). Mollaret's meningitis consists of recurrent brief episodes of meningitis alternating with symptom-free intervals. The attacks occur suddenly, and the symptoms reach maximum intensity within a few hours. Signs and symptoms include headache, neck pain, backache, muscle aches, and neck stiffness, which persist for 1–3 days. Transitory neurological abnormalities may occur.

Table 3 Laboratory Studies for Meningitis with a Lymphocytic Pleocytosis

1. CSF viral culture, virus-specific IgM antibodies, and acute and convalescent sera for virus-specific IgG antibodies to the following:
   - Enteroviruses
   - HSV-2
   - Arboviruses, adenoviruses
   - Influenza virus types A and B
   - Lymphocytic choriomeningitis virus
   - Epstein-Barr virus
2. Serology and CSF viral culture for HIV
3. CSF Gram's stain and bacterial culture; latex agglutination for *Haemophilus influenzae* type b, *Streptococcus pneumoniae*, and *Neisseria meningitidis*; limulus amebocyte lysate assay for gram-negative endotoxin
4. Acid-fast bacilli smear and culture; chest x-ray for pulmonary tuberculosis; intradermal tuberculin skin test; PCR for tubercle bacilli DNA in CSF
5. Lyme serology and CSF for detection of intrathecal Lyme antibody production
6. Serum treponemal tests (FTA-ABS and MHA-TP) and CSF-VDRL.
7. Latex agglutination test for cryptococcal antigen, urine-blood-CSF for Histoplasma polysaccharide antigen (HPA), CSF complement fixation antibody test for *C. immites*; fungal culture
8. Serum and CSF ACE
9. CSF cytology
10. Viral culture from CSF, saliva, and urine for mumps virus when indicated
11. Fourfold increase in *E. chaffeenis* antibody titer between acute and convalescent sera for human monocytic ehrlichiosis; a fourfold increase in *E. equi* antibody titer between acute and convalescent sera for human granulocytic ehrlichiosis

There may be prominent meningeal signs. Fever is present during the episodes, and nausea and vomiting may occur. All the symptoms and signs resolve as rapidly as they develop, and the patient is symptom-free and entirely well until the next episode. There are no residual neurological abnormalities. The abnormalities in the CSF are defined by "three stages of pleocytosis." During the first 12–24 h, the CSF demonstrates a polymorphonuclear neutrophilic pleocytosis up to several thousand cells per cubic millimeter, and a large type of cell is seen, which Mollaret called an "endothelial-leukocytic" cell. This is a mononuclear cell characterized by an irregular, vague outline of the nuclear and cytoplasmic membranes. These cells are difficult to identify because they rapidly disintegrate, and a number of these cells can be seen only as "ghosts" and are rarely detected after the first day of an attack. The polymorphonuclear neutrophilic pleocytosis disappears and is replaced by a predominantly lymphocytic pleocytosis in cerebrospinal fluid. The lymphocytic cells also rapidly disappear, and within a matter of days after an episode, the pleocytosis is almost completely resolved (50). Patients with Mollaret's meningitis have recurrent, separate episodes of meningitis over a period of 1 year or more, with symptom-free intervals lasting weeks, months, and sometimes years. The diagnosis of Mollaret's meningitis is rarely made today because "endothelial-leukocytic" cells are no longer identified in CSF.

A common clinical problem is identifying an etiological agent in patients with recurrent aseptic meningitis with a lymphocytic pleocytosis. With our increasing ability to identify specific viruses in CSF by laboratory techniques, the ambiguity that has surrounded the syndrome of recurrent aseptic meningitis with lymphocytic pleocytosis will more than likely be resolved. Table 3 provides an approach to the patient with meningitis with a lymphocytic pleocytosis that does not resolve over the course of several days.

REFERENCES

1. Wallgren A. Une nouvelle maladie infectieuse du systeme nerveux central (meningite aseptique aique). Acta Paediatr 1925; 4:158–182.
2. Connolly KJ, Hammer SM. The acute aseptic meningitis syndrome. Infect Dis Clin North Am 1990; 4:599–622.
3. Stroop WG. Viral pathogenesis. In: McKendall RR, Stroop WG, eds. Handbook of Neurovirology. New York: Marcel Dekker, 1994:27–54.
4. Rubeiz H, Roos RP. Viral meningitis and encephalitis. Semin Neurol 1992; 12:165–177.
5. Berger JR, Levy RM. The neurologic complications of human immunodeficiency virus infection. Med Clin North Am 1993; 77:1–23.
6. Leist TP, Frei K, Kam-Hansen S, Zinkernagel RM, Fontana A. Tumor necrosis factor alpha in cerebrospinal fluid during bacterial, but not viral, meningitis. J Exp Med 1988; 167:1743–1748.
7. Glimaker M, Kragsbjerg P, Forsgren M, Olcen P. Tumor necrosis factor-alpha (TNF alpha) in cerebrospinal fluid from patients with meningitis of different etiologies: high levels of TNF alpha indicate bacterial meningitis. J Infect Dis 1993; 167:882–889.
8. Bonadio WA. The cerebrospinal fluid: physiologic aspects and alterations associated with bacterial meningitis. Pediatr Infect Dis J 1992; 11:423–32.
9. Brooke I, Bricknell KS, Overturf GD, Finegold SM. Measurement of lactic acid in cerebrospinal fluid of patients with infections of the central nervous system. J Infect Dis 1978; 137:384–390.
10. Overall JC. Is it bacterial or viral; laboratory differentiation. Pediatr Rev 1993; 14:251–261.
11. Bale JF. Meningitis and encephalitis. In: McKendall RR, Stroop WG, eds. Handbook of Neurovirology. New York: Marcel Dekker, 1994:141–158.
12. Johnson GM, McAbee GA, Seaton ED, Lipson SM. Suspect value of non-CSF viral cultures in the diagnosis of enteroviral CNS infection in young adults. Dev Med Child Neurol 1992; 34:876–884.
13. Brenton DW. Hypoglycorrhachia in herpes simplex type 2 meningitis. Arch Neurol 1980; 37:317.
14. Corey L, Adams HG, Brown ZA, Holmes KK. Genital herpes simplex virus infections: clinical manifestations, course, and complications. Ann Intern Med 1983; 98:958–972.

15. Marshall DW, Brey RL, Cahill WT, et al. Spectrum of cerebrospinal fluid findings in various stages of human immunodeficiency virus infection. Arch Neurol 1988; 45:954–958.
16. Whitley RJ, Gnann JW. Acyclovir: a decade later. N Engl J Med 1992; 11:782–789.
17. Davis SD, Hill HR, Feigl P, Arnstein EJ. Partial antibiotic therapy in *Haemophilus influenzae* meningitis: its effect on cerebrospinal fluid abnormalities. Am J Dis Child 1975; 129:802–807.
18. Feldman WE. Effect of prior antibiotic therapy on concentrations of bacteria in CSF. Am J Dis Child 1978; 132:672–674.
19. Kaplan SL, Smith EO, Wills C, Feigin RD. Association between preadmission oral antibiotic therapy and cerebrospinal fluid findings and sequelae caused by *Haemophilus influenzae* type b meningitis. Pediatr Infect Dis 1986; 5:626–632.
20. Leonard JM, Des Prez RM. Tuberculous meningitis. Infect Dis Clin North Am 1990; 4:769–787.
21. Zarabi M, Sane S, Girdany BR. The chest roentgenogram in the early diagnosis of tuberculous meningitis in children. Am J Dis Child 1971; 121:389–392.
22. Lincoln EM, Sordillio VR, Davies PA. Tuberculous meningitis in children; a review of 167 untreated and 74 treated patients with special reference to early diagnosis. J Pediatr 1960; 57:803–823.
23. Molavi A, LeFrock JL. Tuberculous meningitis. Med Clin North Am 1985; 69:315–331.
24. Coyle PK. Neurologic Lyme disease. Semin Neurol 1992; 12:200–208.
25. Pachner AR, Steere AC. The triad of neurologic manifestations of Lyme disease: meningitis, cranial neuritis, and radiculoneuritis. Neurology 1985; 35:47–53.
26. Johnson RA, White M. Syphilis in the 1990s: cutaneous and neurologic manifestations. Semin Neurol 1992; 12:287–298.
27. Marra CM. Syphilis and human immunodeficiency virus infection. Semin Neurol 1992; 12:43–50.
28. Merritt HH, Moore M. Acute syphilitic meningitis. Med 1935; 14:119–183.
29. Treseler CB, Sugar AM. Fungal meningitis. Infect Dis Clin North Am 1990; 4:789–808.
30. Wheat JJ, Batteiger BE, Sathapatayavongs B. *Histoplasma capsulatum* infections of the central nervous system: a clinical review. Medicine 1990; 69:244–260.
31. Stern BJ, Krumholz A, Johns C, Scott P, Nissim J. Sarcoidosis and its neurological manifestations. Arch Neurol 1985; 42:909–917.
32. Oksanen V, Fyhrquist F, Somer H, Gronhagen-Riska C. Angiotensin converting enzyme in cerebrospinal fluid: a new assay. Neurology 1985; 35:1220–1223.
33. Schweisfurth H, Schioberg-Schiegnitz S, Kuhn W, Parusel B. Angiotensin-I-converting enzyme in cerebrospinal fluid of patients with neurological diseases. Klin Wochenschr 1987; 65:955–958.
34. Seem CPC, Norfolk G, Spokes EG. CSF angiotensin-converting enzyme in neurosarcoidosis. Lancet 1985; 1:456–457.
35. Wasserstrom WR, Glass JP, Posner JB. Diagnosis and treatment of leptomeningeal metastases from solid tumors: experience with 90 patients. Cancer 1982; 49:759–772.
36. Theodore WH, Gendelman S. Meningeal carcinomatosis. Arch Neurol 1981; 38:696–699.
37. Little JR, Dale AJD, Okazaki H. Meningeal carcinomatosis: clinical manifestations. Arch Neurol 1974; 30:138–143.
38. Schold SC, Wasserstrom WR, Fleisher M, Schwartz M, Posner JB. Cerebrospinal fluid biochemical markers of central nervous system metastases. Ann Neurol 1980; 8:597–604.
39. Inaba G. Behcet's disease. In: McKendall RR, ed. Handbook of Clinical Neurology: Viral Disease. 1989; 12(56):593–610.
40. Martin MA, Massanari M, Nghiem DD, Smith JL, Corry RJ. Nosocomial aseptic meningitis associated with administration of OKT3. JAMA 1988; 259:2002–2005.
41. Haas EJ. Trimethoprim-sulfamethoxazole: another cause of recurrent meningitis. JAMA 1984; 252: 252–346.
42. Garagusi VF, Neefe LI, Mann O. Acute meningoencephalitis associated with isoniazid administration. JAMA 1976; 235:1141–1142.
43. Junck L, Marshall WH. Neurotoxicity of radiological contrast agents. Ann Neurol 1983; 13:469–484.
44. Gelmers HJ. Adverse side effects of metrizamide in myelography. Neuroradiology 1979; 18:119–123.
45. Miller E, Goldacre M, Pugh S, Colville A, et al. Risk of aseptic meningitis after measles, mumps, and rubella vaccine in UK children. Lancet 1993; 341:979–982.

46. Anon. Mumps meningitis and MMR vaccination. Lancet 1989; ii:1015–1016.
47. Gray JA, Burns SM. Mumps vaccine meningitis. Lancet 1989; ii:927.
48. Bartleson JD, Swanson JW, Whisnant JP. A migrainous syndrome with cerebrospinal fluid pleocytosis. Neurology 1981; 31:1257–1262.
49. Mollaret P. La meningite endothelio-leucocytaire multirecurrente benigne: syndrome nouveau ou maladie nouvelle? (Document cliniques.) Rev Neurol 1944; 76:57.
50. Hermans PE, Goldstein NP, Wellman WE. Mollaret's meningitis and differential diagnosis of recurrent meningitis. Am J Med 1972; 52:128–139.

7

Viral Encephalitis

Karen L. Roos
Indiana University School of Medicine, Indianapolis, Indiana

Viral encephalitis is an acute infection of brain parenchyma characterized clinically by fever and an altered level of consciousness. The major etiological agents of viral encephalitis are herpes simplex virus type 1 (HSV-1), herpes simplex virus type 2 (HSV-2) in neonates, and the arthropod-borne viruses including LaCrosse virus, St. Louis encephalitis virus (SLE), eastern equine encephalitis (EEE) virus, western equine encephalitis (WEE) virus, Venezuelan equine encephalitis virus (VEE), and Japanese B virus encephalitis. Encephalitis is an unusual complication of enterovirus infections but can occur, particularly in patients with agammaglobulinemia. Varicella-zoster virus (VZV), Epstein-Barr virus, cytomegalovirus (CMV), and human herpesvirus-6 (HHV-6) are important etiological agents of viral encephalitis in the immunocompromised host (Table 1). Rabies virus encephalitis is discussed in detail in a separate chapter in this volume.

PATHOGENESIS

The pathogenesis of viral encephalitis is similar to that of viral meningitis in that viruses that cause encephalitis gain access to the central nervous system by either a neuronal or a hematogenous route. Neonatal HSV-2 infection is usually acquired either in utero or as a consequence of intrapartum contact of the fetus with maternal genital HSV-2 infection. There are two forms of neonatal HSV disease as it relates to encephalitis. Newborns may have either encephalitis alone or disseminated disease that is complicated by encephalitis. The pathogenesis of these two forms of neonatal HSV disease is different. In infants with encephalitis alone, CNS infection is thought to occur by intraneuronal routes and is often localized to one or both temporal lobes. In infants with disseminated disease, CNS infection is thought to occur by bloodborne spread of virus to the brain, and infection involves all areas of the brain (1).

The pathogenesis of herpes simplex virus encephalitis in older children and adults is most likely a reactivation of infection that initially occurred via retrograde transneuronal spread of

Table 1 Etiological Agents of Viral Encephalitis

Herpes simplex viruses	Tickborne viruses
Herpes simplex virus type 1	Powassan virus
Herpes simplex virus type 2 (neonates)	Colorado tick fever
Mosquitoborne viruses	Enteroviruses (neonates and agammaglobulinemia)
LaCrosse	Immunocompromised
St. Louis	Varicella-zoster
Japanese	Epstein-Barr
Eastern equine	Cytomegalovirus
Western equine	Human herpesvirus type 6
Venezuelan equine	

virus from a peripheral site of infection along a division of the trigeminal nerve. The virus then developed latency in the trigeminal ganglion. Reactivation of latent ganglionic infection with replication of virus leads to infection in the temporal cortex and limbic system structures. HSV-1 encephalitis may also be the result of primary infection via either intranasal inoculation of virus with direct invasion of the olfactory bulb and tract or spread of virus along a trigeminal nerve from a primary infection in the oral cavity. Whether infection is the result of reactivation or primary infection, inflammatory and necrotizing lesions are seen in the inferior and medial temporal lobes, the orbital-frontal cortex, and the limbic structures (2–4).

The arthropodborne viruses are inoculated into the host subcutaneously by a mosquito or tick bite and then undergo local replication at the skin site. A viremia follows, and if there is a large enough inoculum of virus, invasion and infection of the CNS occurs. Initial CNS infection by arboviruses appears to occur via cerebral capillary endothelial cells with subsequent infection of the neural parenchyma. Virus spreads from cell to cell, typically along dendritic or axonal processes. Arbovirus encephalitis is predominantly a disease of cortical gray matter and brainstem and thalamic nuclei. There may also be a meningeal exudate composed of lymphocytes, polymorphonuclear leukocytes, plasma cells, and macrophages (5).

CLINICAL PRESENTATION

Encephalitis is a febrile illness associated with headache and an altered level of consciousness. Focal or multifocal neurological signs and seizure activity may occur.

Herpes Simplex Virus

HSV-1 has a predilection to infect the temporal lobe; therefore, the clinical presentation is typically characterized by aphasia, focal neurological deficits, confusion, memory disturbance, behavioral abnormalities, and focal seizure activity. Patients with HSV-1 encephalitis may have had a headache for several days prior to the onset of an altered level of consciousness or a generalized confusional state. The most common etiological agent of focal encephalitis is HSV-1 (6). In a series of 113 biopsy-positive patients with herpes simplex encephalitis, 90% of patients had fever, 81% had headache, 97% had an alteration of consciousness that developed over a week to 12 days, 33% had hemiparesis, 67% had seizure activity, and 24% had memory loss (7).

Mosquitoborne Viruses

The clinical presentation of arthropodborne viral encephalitis is nonspecific, but the specific virus can be predicted based on the geographic location where the infection was acquired, the age of the patient, and some unique clinical features. The most common causes of arthropodborne encephalitis in the United States are LaCrosse virus and St. Louis encephalitis virus. The LaCrosse virus belongs to the California group of encephalitis viruses. It is responsible for nearly all infections due to California group viruses in the United States. The largest number of cases occur in wooded areas of the midwestern United States. Most cases occur in late summer to early fall. The vector, *Aedes triseriatus*, is a forest-dwelling mosquito. Clinically recognizable disease occurs primarily in children ages 4–11 years. A distinct prodromal phase characterized by fever, chills, headache, nausea, vomiting, and abdominal pain lasting 1–4 days commonly precedes the onset of symptoms of encephalitis (8). Encephalitis is characterized by fever, somnolence, and obtundation; seizures occur in about 50% of children. In adults, infection is either asymptomatic or causes a benign febrile illness or aseptic meningitis. Mortality is low, less than 1% (6), but personality changes or recurrent seizures occur in 15% of children following recovery (9).

St. Louis encephalitis virus causes large urban epidemics of encephalitis in the midwestern and southeastern United States. The ratio of asymptomatic to symptomatic infection is 100:1 or higher. St. Louis encephalitis may cause a mild febrile illness with headache, an aseptic meningitis, or an encephalitis. The majority of symptomatic infections are encephalitis. Adults older than 50 years are most commonly affected, and disease severity is greatest in this age group. Almost 90% of elderly patients develop encephalitis. The onset of encephalitis symptoms may be preceded by an influenzalike prodrome of malaise, myalgias, and fever. This is followed by symptoms of headache, nausea, vomiting, confusion, disorientation, irritability, stupor, tremors, and occasionally convulsions. St. Louis encephalitis has a mortality of 10–20%, and approximately 10% of survivors experience sequelae of memory loss, chronic fatigue, sleeplessness, headaches, and occasionally seizures or motor deficits (6,10). Cases of St. Louis encephalitis appear chiefly in late August and September and are greatest in years with heavy spring rains followed by a summer drought. The disease is transmitted by Culex mosquitoes that breed in stagnant water. A unique clinical feature of this form of encephalitis is the syndrome of inappropriate antidiuretic hormone secretion with hyponatremia, which can complicate this infection (9).

Japanese encephalitis virus is a member of the St. Louis complex of flaviviruses and is the most common cause of arthropodborne human encephalitis worldwide. Epidemic disease occurs in China (where more than 10,000 cases are reported annually), northern parts of Southeast Asia, and areas of India and Sri Lanka. The principal vector for Japanese encephalitis is the culicine mosquito, which breeds in the rice fields of Asia. The disease is primarily a disease of children, but nonimmune adults who enter an epidemic area are susceptible to severe encephalitis. The virus reaches the brain through hematogenous dissemination and tends to infect brainstem nuclei, leading to acute respiratory failure and death, and basal ganglia and thalamus, presenting as tremors during the acute disease and a parkinsonian masklike facies, rigidity and tremor, and dystonia in survivors. A factor predictive of outcome is the rapid appearance of antibodies in cerebrospinal fluid against Japanese B encephalitis, which apparently lessen the severity of the disease (5,6). Infection with Japanese encephalitis virus may be asymptomatic or appear as an influenzaelike syndrome of headache and low-grade fever that resolves over 4–5 days or a severe, fulminant encephalitis characterized by fever, vomiting, convulsions, and coma. Children most frequently have an encephalitis syndrome. Mortality rates during epidemics are in the range of 20–40%, with most deaths occurring within the first week of illness (10).

Eastern equine encephalitis virus causes the most severe arbovirus encephalitis, and in the United States most cases occur along the eastern coast from Massachusetts to Florida (10). The first human infection of eastern equine encephalomyelitis occurred in Massachusetts in the summer of 1938 (11). Eastern equine encephalitis virus can occur at all ages, but is more common in infants and children. The clinical manifestations of eastern equine encephalitis do not differ markedly from those of other arthropodborne encephalitis viruses except in the severity of the symptoms. There may be an influenzalike prodrome with fever, headache, vomiting, malaise, and lethargy, but more typically patients with eastern equine encephalitis have an abrupt onset of high fever, convulsions, and a rapid progression from stupor to coma. The fatality rate is 50–75%, and neurological sequelae are commonly characterized by mental retardation, seizures, spastic paralysis, and behavioral abnormalities (10,11). Disease in horses or pheasants precedes human disease by 2–3 weeks (9). Eastern equine encephalitis may present with focal signs or focal seizure activity, and thus mimic herpes simplex encephalitis.

Western equine encephalitis is a much milder encephalitis than eastern equine encephalitis; however, neurological sequelae are common in children who develop the disease when they are younger than 6 months of age (9). Western equine encephalitis virus infects horses and humans in western North America, with most cases occurring between April and September and peak activity in July and August. Inapparent infections with western equine encephalitis virus are more common than symptomatic cases, and attack rates are highest in young children. Like the other arthropodborne encephalitides, western equine encephalitis begins with an influenzalike syndrome of fever, malaise, myalgias, pharyngitis, and vomiting. As the disease progresses, lethargy, irritability, convulsions, or coma develop (10). The mortality rate is 3–4%, but morbidity is more common in children and typically consists of seizure disorders or developmental delay. Postencephalitic parkinsonism is reported occasionally in adults that survive western equine encephalitis (10,12).

Venezuelan equine encephalitis virus is endemic in South America and is a rare cause of encephalitis in Central America and the southwestern United States, particularly in Texas. Infection with Venezuelan encephalitis virus is typically mild, with encephalitis occurring only rarely. Children and the elderly are at greatest risk for encephalitis. Mortality is less than 1%, and neurological sequelae are rare.

Tickborne Viruses

Powassan virus and Colorado tick fever virus are transmitted to humans by ticks. Powassan virus is a flavivirus, more closely related to the tickborne flaviviruses of Europe (Central European encephalitis) and Asia (Russian spring-summer encephalitis) than to the mosquitoborne flaviviruses, such as SLE. Colorado tick fever virus is totally unrelated to Powassan virus, and is instead a member of the family Reoviridae. Both viruses are transmitted to humans by the *Dermacentor andersoni* tick. Isolates of Powassan virus have been obtained in the United States from hard ticks, principally ixodid ticks, and human cases of this disease have been documented in southern Canada, New York state, and Pennsylvania. Colorado tick fever virus has been isolated from humans and ticks in Colorado, Utah, Montana, California, Wyoming, Idaho, Oregon, South Dakota, Washington, New Mexico, Nevada, and southern Alberta and British Columbia, Canada. Physicians should be aware of the possibility of Colorado tick fever in patients who have vacationed in these areas during spring and early summer (13).

Powassan virus encephalitis may be preceded by prodromal symptoms of sore throat, lethargy, headache, and disorientation. These symptoms are then followed by the onset of fever to 40°C, vomiting, respiratory distress, lethargy, convulsions, and then coma. Neurological sequelae of hemiplegia and spasticity are common in survivors (13).

Colorado tick fever is a biphasic illness characterized by the abrupt onset of high fever, chills, myalgias and arthralgias, severe headache, conjunctival injection with ocular pain, and nausea. The patient may then defervesce to have fever recur in 2–3 days. Aseptic meningitis and encephalitis occur primarily in children and may be associated with a petechial or maculopapular rash or a more severe rash with purpura and petechiae. Disseminated intravascular coagulation and gastrointestinal bleeding may complicate the course of the illness (13).

Enteroviruses

Nonpolio enteroviruses are the most common etiological agents of aseptic meningitis, and aseptic meningitis is the most commonly identified CNS infection associated with enterovirus infections. Neonates and individuals with agammaglobulinemia are at increased risk for enterovirus meningoencephalitis. Unlike other viruses that are contained by cell-mediated immune mechanisms, the enteroviruses are cleared from the host by antibody-mediated immune mechanisms. For this reason, patients with agammaglobulinemia may have chronic meningitis or meningoencephalitis due to an enterovirus. Enterovirus infections are acquired by fecal-oral contamination. The viral inoculum is swallowed, and virus binds to specific receptors on enterocytes. The virus then traverses the intestinal lining cells, and a viremia ensues with dissemination of virus to the CNS. The clinical signs and symptoms of enterovirus meningoencephalitis is more often that of a generalized or multifocal encephalitis, but may have features of a focal encephalitis with a clinical presentation similar to that of herpes simplex virus encephalitis. The signs and symptoms of meningoencephalitis are often preceded by fever, headache, and nonspecific constitutional signs and symptoms of viral infection including vomiting, anorexia, rash, cough, diarrhea, and myalgias (14).

Varicella-Zoster Virus

Varicella-zoster virus encephalitis rarely develops in healthy individuals with shingles but may occur in patients with decreased cellular immunity due to cancer, chronic illness, the acquired immunodeficiency syndrome (AIDS), or immunosuppressive therapy including steroid therapy. Varicella-zoster virus encephalitis can complicate chickenpox (10). When encephalitis complicates chickenpox, neurological symptoms of headache, vomiting, and lethargy typically occur within 2 weeks of the onset of the vesicular exanthem. When encephalitis complicates zoster, neurological symptoms may begin days to weeks after the appearance of the vesicular rash or can occur without any history of a rash. The encephalitis that complicates chickenpox or shingles is characterized by fever, seizures, ataxia, and focal deficits (such as aphasia, hemiparesis, or cranial nerve palsies) (10,15). Neuroimaging may reveal ischemic and/or hemorrhagic infarctions and focal areas of demyelination (15).

Epstein-Barr Virus

Epstein-Barr virus encephalitis can affect children or adults and frequently occurs in association with other features of infectious mononucleosis such as headache, low-grade fever, and lethargy. The neurological manifestations of Epstein-Barr virus encephalitis consist of somnolence, disorientation, stupor, seizures, and occasionally focal deficits (10).

Cytomegalovirus

Cytomegalovirus (CMV) encephalitis occurs primarily in two groups of patients: organ-transplant recipients and HIV-infected individuals. In organ-transplant recipients, CMV encephalitis is a rapidly progressive fatal encephalopathic illness, whereas in HIV-infected individuals, CMV encephalitis is a subacute illness that is often difficult to distinguish from AIDS dementia. Both CMV encephalitis and HIV dementia develop late in HIV disease, but CMV infection typically does not occur until the CD4 count is <100; therefore, HIV dementia can develop somewhat earlier than CMV encephalitis in HIV-infected individuals. The clinical presentation of CMV encephalitis has a more acute onset and a more rapidly progressive cognitive decline than HIV dementia. In a retrospective review of 14 autopsy-confirmed cases of CMV encephalitis that were compared with a control group of patients with HIV dementia, confusion, disorientation, apathy, and withdrawal occurred significantly more frequently among patients with CMV encephalitis than with HIV dementia, and the patients with HIV dementia more often had complaints of depression and mental slowing. The clinical course of both diseases was characterized by a progressive dementia with episodic superimposed delirium, and the patients with CMV encephalitis had a shorter survival than the patients with HIV dementia (16).

A further distinction is made between CMV encephalitis and CMV ventriculoencephalitis. Cytomegalovirus ventriculoencephalitis has an acute onset of lethargy, disorientation, and a prominent clinical feature of ocular motor palsies and nystagmus. Cytomegalovirus retinitis is often diagnosed before the onset of encephalitis in these patients. Neuroimaging demonstrates progressive ventriculomegaly. The course from onset of disease to death is usually less than 5 weeks (17,18).

Human Herpesvirus-6

Human herpesvirus-6 (HHV-6) causes roseola infantum (exanthem subitum) in childhood and causes an acute illness in infants and young children characteized by high fever. Seizure activity may be associated with the fever or develop as a complication of roseola (19,20). Meningoencephalitis may complicate primary HHV-6 infection. It has been suggested that HHV-6 may persist in the CNS and be a cause of encephalitis in bone marrow transplant recipients (21).

DIAGNOSIS

Herpes Simplex Virus-Type 1

Neuroimaging, examination of the cerebrospinal fluid, and the electroencephalogram are the recommended diagnostic studies to make a diagnosis of HSV-1 encephalitis. Both computed tomography (CT) and magnetic resonance (MR) scans may be normal early in the infection. If the scan, however, is repeated in 2–4 days, evidence of focal edema in the inferiomedial temporal lobe may be appreciated. Lesions appear earlier on MR scan than on CT scan. A very characteristic abnormality on MR scan of HSV-1 encephalitis is a lesion in the medial and inferior temporal lobe extending up into the insula. Examination of the cerebrospinal fluid demonstrates the following: (1) an increased opening pressure, (2) a mild lymphocytic pleocytosis (500 cells/mm^3), (3) the presence of red blood cells and/or xanthochromia, (4) a modestly elevated protein concentration, and (5) a normal glucose concentration. The glucose concentration can be decreased, but if it is very low, suspect a diagnosis other than HSV-1 encephalitis. Cultures of CSF for HSV-1 are almost always negative in HSV encephalitis. Herpes simplex virus antibody can be detected in cerebrospinal fluid, but this is usually positive several days into the course of disease, 3–10 days after the onset of symptoms. The polymerase chain reaction (PCR) technique to detect HSV DNA in cerebrospinal fluid has emerged as a very specific and sensitive test for the diagnosis of HSV encephalitis. The polymerase chain reaction is often positive within the first 24–72 h of HSV encephalitis; however, if the PCR is negative initially, a repeat PCR analysis should be performed in 24–48 h. Herpes simplex virus DNA in CSF precedes the appearance of HSV antibody by several days. The PCR assay may be negative after 10 days to 2 weeks (22,23). The classic abnormalities on electroencephalography (EEG) in HSV-1 encephalitis are focal irregular polymorphic delta activity over one temporal region and/or periodic complexes localized to one temporal lobe (Chap. 31, Fig. 2). Although brain biopsy was historically used to make the diagnosis of HSV encephalitis, today it is primarily recommended for patients who do not respond to acyclovir therapy or patients who have unusual clinical or diagnostic features. It is anticipated that the widespread availability of PCR analysis for HSV DNA in CSF should certainly decrease the necessity of brain biopsy to establish a diagnosis of HSV-1 encephalitis.

Neonatal Herpes Simplex Virus

Neonatal herpes virus encephalitis is a diffuse rather than focal encephalitis, and therefore CT, MR, and EEG reveal diffuse or multifocal abnormalities. Cultures for HSV should be obtained from conjunctiva, throat, rectum, blood (circulating leukocytes), CSF, and skin lesions when present. Cerebrospinal fluid culture is positive for HSV in approximately 50% of cases of neonatal HSV encephalitis. (The diagnosis and therapy of neonatal HSV encephalitis is discussed in detail in Chap. 1.)

Mosquitoborne Viruses

When arthropodborne virus encephalitis is suspected, diagnosis depends on examination of the cerebrospinal fluid and viral serological studies. The cerebrospinal fluid abnormalities are as follows: (1) the opening pressure may be mildly elevated, (2) the glucose concentration is normal, (3) the protein concentration is normal or mildly elevated, and (4) there is initially a polymorphonuclear leukocytic pleocytosis early in infection with a shift to a lymphocytic or mononuclear pleocytosis later in the illness. LaCrosse virus has not been isolated from CSF. St. Louis encephalitis virus, eastern equine encephalitis virus, and western equine encephalitis are rarely isolated from CSF. In eastern equine encephalitis, there is typically a much more elevated leukocyte count in CSF than in the other arthropodborne encephalitides, with 200–2000 cells/mm^3, 60–90% of which are neutrophils. As has been discussed in the clinical presentation, St. Louis virus encephalitis may be associated with hyponatremia due to the inappropriate secretion of antidiuretic hormone (13). In cases of suspected arthropodborne encephalitis, an acute serum should be drawn at the onset of the illness and a convalescent serum obtained 4–6 weeks later. An etiological diagnosis is supported by detecting a fourfold or greater increase in virus-specific IgG in sequential serum samples. The etiological agent can also be identified on single specimens by detecting virus-specific IgM in serum or CSF (10).

Tickborne Viruses

The cerebrospinal fluid abnormalities in Powassan virus encephalitis are typical of the arthropodborne virus encephalitides, with a normal glucose concentration, a mild to moderately elevated protein concentration, and an initial polymorphonuclear pleocytosis shifting to a lymphocytic pleocytosis later in the disease course. Neutralizing antibody is usually detectable at the time of onset of illness, but brain biopsy may be necessary to make the diagnosis. Colorado tick fever is characterized by leukopenia and, in some instances, thrombocytopenia. Early in the disease, Colorado tick fever virus can be isolated from serum, but later on it is more easily isolated from blood clots and from erythrocytes. Antibody to Colorado tick fever virus is not detectable until 1–2 weeks after the onset of illness (13).

In both the mosquitoborne virus encephalitides and the tickborne virus encephalitides, the CSF demonstrates a mild polymorphonuclear pleocytosis with a shift to a lymphocytic pleocytosis, and the electroencephalogram has diffuse slowing of background activity. Focal abnormalities, either by neuroimaging or EEG, are uncommon but can occur. A general rule of thumb is that a markedly elevated CSF protein concentration should suggest a diagnosis other than mosquitoborne or tickborne encephalitis. A history of residence in or travel to an area endemic for arthropodborne virus encephalitis and a history of tick exposure or knowledge of a tick bite is critical to the diagnosis of these encephalitides.

Enteroviruses

The diagnosis of enterovirus encephalitis is made by isolating virus from CSF, or by PCR to detect enteroviral RNA in CSF, and is suggested by the occurrence of other enteroviral infections in family members. Cultures for enterovirus should be obtained from throat and stool, but only a positive CSF viral culture is definitive evidence of an enterovirus as the etiological agent of the encephalitis.

Varicella-Zoster Virus

In varicella-zoster encephalitis, neuroimaging may reveal multifocal enhancing lesions in the distribution of cerebrovascular territories consistent with infarction. In addition, varicella-zoster virus causes focal areas of demyelination, which appear as hyperintense lesions on T_2-weighted MR scan. These lesions of VSV encephalitis on MR scan resemble the lesions of progressive multifocal leukoencephalopathy. In immunocompromised patients, the presence of both multifocal lesions typical of cerebral infarction and demyelinative lesions should suggest the diagnosis of VSV encephalitis. The typical abnormalities on examination of the cerebrospinal fluid are a mild mononuclear pleocytosis, an elevated protein concentration, and a decreased glucose concentration. The detection of VSV DNA in CSF by PCR can confirm the diagnosis. Varicella-zoster antibody is often present in CSF, but viral culture is rarely positive (15).

Epstein-Barr Virus

The diagnosis of Epstein-Barr virus encephalitis is suggested by the association of encephalitis with other clinical features of infectious mononucleosis, a postive heterophil test, atypical lymphocytosis in a peripheral blood smear, and the presence of EBV nucleic acid in CSF.

Cytomegalovirus

The diagnosis of cytomegalovirus encephalitis is suggested by radiographic evidence of hydrocephalus and periventricular enhancement, a reflection of the predilection of the virus for subependymal areas. On magnetic resonance scan, the finding of a linear homogeneous increased signal on T_2-weighted scans around the ventricles is typical of CMV encephalitis. Meningeal or ventricular enhancement may be seen on MR scan. The typical abnormalities on examination of the CSF are a mild mononuclear pleocytosis with an elevated protein concentration. The specificity of the detection of CMV DNA by PCR in CSF for CMV encephalitis is presently unknown. CSF cultures for CMV are usually negative. Serum electrolyte abnormalities are common in patients with CMV encephalitis and are suggestive of adrenal insufficiency (16). Quantitative PCR techniques for detecting CMV in CSF may prove to be a useful technique in evaluating the extent of CNS disease, prognosis, and response to treatment (17).

Human Herpes Virus-6

HHV-6 DNA can be detected in the CSF of children during and after primary infection. It is not clear how long HHV-6 persists in the CNS, so that the finding of HHV-6 DNA in CSF in a child with meningoencephalitis suggests that HHV-6 may be the etiological agent but does not make a definitive diagnosis (20). In an adult bone marrow transplant recipient with encephalitis, the presence of HHV-6 DNA in CSF is suggestive that HHV-6 is the etiological organism (21).

Table 2 lists the recommended diagnostic studies for viral encephalitis.

Table 2 Diagnostic Studies for Viral Encephalitis

Virus	Diagnostic study
Herpes simplex virus type 1	EEG—periodic complexes localized to one or both temporal lobes
	MR—temporal lobe hyperintensity
	CSF HSV PCR (if negative, repeat in 48 h)
	CSF HSV antibody
Arthropodborne viruses	CSF viral-specific IgM
	Acute and convalescent sera
Enteroviruses	CSF viral culture
	Acute and convalescent sera
	Throat and stool culture
	CSF PCR for enteroviral RNA
Varicella-zoster virus	CSF VSV PCR
	Acute and convalescent sera
Epstein-Barr virus	CSF EBV PCR
Cytomegalovirus	CSF CMV PCR
	CSF CMV culture
	MR—linear, homogeneous periventricular hyperintensity on T_2-weighted MR
Human herpesvirus type 6	CSF HHV-6 PCR

CSF, Cerebrospinal fluid; PCR, polymerase chain reaction; EEG, electroencephalogram; MR, magnetic resonance scan.

TREATMENT

Herpes simplex virus encephalitis is currently treated with acyclovir (Zovirax) in a dose of 30 mg/kg/day (10 mg/kg intravenously every 8 h) for 14 days (1,10). A longer duration of therapy may occasionally be required. Patients with varicella-zoster virus encephalitis can also be treated with acyclovir in a dosing regimen similar to that for herpes simplex virus encephalitis. Patients with cytomegalovirus encephalitis, especially those with AIDS, should be treated with ganciclovir, although clinical trials have not yet been conducted to make firm recommendations. Ganciclovir has been successfully used in the treatment of CMV retinitis (16). Present practice is to use ganciclovir in a dose of 5 mg/kg intravenously every 12 h for a minimum of 2–3 weeks, followed by maintenance therapy. A combination of ganciclovir and foscarnet (60 mg/kg intravenously over 8 h) may also be efficacious. The treatment of arthropodborne virus encephalitis is aggressive supportive care. Many of these patients require intensive care unit monitoring for the management of raised intracranial pressure, electrolyte abnormalities, respiratory insufficiency, and seizure activity. Prophylaxis for deep venous thrombosis and gastrointestinal bleeding is recommended.

POSTINFECTIOUS ENCEPHALOMYELITIS

Postinfectious encephalomyelitis is an acute inflammatory, demyelinating disease of the brain, optic nerves, and spinal cord that occurs after upper respiratory infections, particularly influenza, measles virus and varicella virus infections, and immunizations, particularly the smallpox immunization with vaccinia virus. Postinfectious encephalomyelitis is also called acute disseminated encephalomyelitis, acute demyelinating encephalomyelitis, postviral encephalomyelitis, and allergic encephalomyelitis. Acute hemorrhagic leukoencephalitis or acute hemorrhagic necrotizing leukoencephalitis is a more severe form of postinfectious encephalomyelitis (24).

Postinfectious encephalomyelitis typically occurs a few days or weeks after a patient has had the systemic symptoms of viral infection. Prior to the discontinuation of vaccination against smallpox and prior to mandatory immunization with measles vaccine, the majority of cases of postinfectious encephalomyelitis were associated with viral exanthematous diseases such as measles, varicella, and rubella and following vaccination for smallpox. Today the majority of cases of postinfectious encephalomyelitis follow nonspecific upper respiratory tract infections and varicella (5). Postinfectious encephalomyelitis has been postulated to be an autoimmune disease because there is a period of time between viral infection and the onset of the neurological disease and because of the pathological similarities between postinfectious encephalomyelitis and the acute demyelinating disease that follows both the administration of rabies vaccine prepared in neural tissue and experimental allergic encephalomyelitis (5).

The clinical presentation of postinfectious encephalomyelitis is the abrupt onset of fever, obtundation, and multifocal neurological signs. The clinical differentiation of postinfectious encephalomyelitis from acute encephalitis is not often possible, but the former should be suspected when the encephalitis occurs a few days after a viral illness (24). The characteristic abnormalities on MR scan are multiple areas of hyperintensity on T_2-weighted images in the subcortical white matter consistent with a multifocal demyelinating disease. The abnormalities on MR scan closely resemble those of multiple sclerosis, and the radiographic differentiation of postinfectious encephalomyelitis and multiple sclerosis is sometimes difficult. Examination of the cerebrospinal fluid demonstrates a lymphocytic pleocytosis and an elevated protein concentration. The clinical presentation of an acute encephalitis occurring within 2–13 days of a viral exanthematous illness or upper respiratory tract infection, with magnetic resonance imaging evidence of multifocal demyelinating lesions, is suggestive of postinfectious encephalomyelitis. Current practice is to treat patients with this disorder with intravenous methylprednisolone, 1 g (250 mg every 6 h) for 5 days.

Acute hemorrhagic leukoencephalitis is a more aggressive form of acute disseminated encephalomyelitis presenting as a more fulminant illness with a more rapid progression to delirum and coma. The magnetic resonance scan demonstrates multifocal lesions involving white matter of the cerebral hemispheres, brainstem, spinal cord, and optic nerves similar to the MR abnormalities in acute disseminated encephalomyelitis. There is widespread demyelination and multiple hemorrhages. Gray matter may be involved as well. The cerebrospinal fluid is under increased pressure and typically has a predominantly neutrophilic pleocytosis, an increased protein concentration, and a normal glucose concentration. Hemorrhagic leukoencephalitis is also assumed to be an autoimmune disease like acute disseminated encephalomyelitis. T cells reactive to myelin basic protein have been cloned from the cerebrospinal fluid in a patient with postviral encephalomyelitis, but to date there are no reports of T cells reactive to myelin antigens in hemorrhagic leukoencephalitis. Nevertheless, current thinking suggests that a viral infection activates myelin-reactive T cells that migrate into the central nervous system and recruit other mediators of inflammation, including neutrophils, macrophages, and inflammatory cytokines that trigger demyelinating disease (25,26). The mortality rate is high, and current practice is to treat these patients with high-dose methylprednisolone and/or plasmapheresis, but no specific therapy has been proven to be effective by clinical trials to date.

REFERENCES

1. Whitley RJ, Lakeman F. Herpes simplex virus infections of the central nervous system: therapeutic and diagnostic considerations. Clin Infect Dis 1995; 20:414–420.

2. Johnson RT. The pathogenesis of herpes virus encephalitis. I. Virus pathways to the nervous system of suckling mice demonstrated by fluorescent antibody staining. J Exp Med 1964; 119:343–356.
3. Stroop WG, Schaefer DC. Production of encephalitis restricted to the temporal lobes by experimental reactivation of herpes simplex virus. J Infect Dis 1986; 153:721–731.
4. Barnett EM, Jacobsen G, Evans G, Cassell M, Perlman S. Herpes simplex encephalitis in the temporal cortex and limbic system after trigeminal nerve inoculation. J Infect Dis 1994; 169:782–786.
5. Johnson RT. The pathogenesis of acute viral encephalitis and postinfectious encephalomyelitis. J Infect Dis 1987; 155:359–364.
6. Whitley RJ. Viral encephalitis. N Engl J Med 1990; 323:242–250.
7. Whitley RJ, Soong SJ, Linneman C, Liu C, Pazin G, Alford CA. Herpes simplex encephalitis: clinical assessment. JAMA 1982; 247:317–320.
8. Johnson KP, Lepow ML, Johnson RT. California encephalitis: I. Clinical and epidemiological studies. Neurology 1968; 18:250–254.
9. Hanley DF, Ray G. Viral encephalitis: when it's likely. Patient Care 1992; (June 15):293–311.
10. Bale JF. Viral encephalitis. Med Clin North Am 1993; 77:25–42.
11. Feemster RF. Equine encephalitis in Massachusetts. N Engl J Med 1957; 257:701–704.
12. Schultz DR, Barthal JS, Garrett C. Western equine encephalitis with rapid onset of Parkinsonism. Neurology 1972; 27:1095.
13. Calisher CH. Medically important arboviruses of the United States and Canada. Clin Microbiol Rev 1994; 7:89–116.
14. Rotbart HA. Enteroviral infections of the central nervous system. Clin Infect Dis 1995; 20:971–981.
15. Amlie-Lefond C, Kleinschmidt-DeMasters BK, Mahalingam R, Davis LE, Gilden DH. The vasculopathy of varicella-zoster virus encephalitis. Ann Neurol 1995; 37:784–790.
16. Holland NR, Power C, Mathews VP, Glass JD, Forman M, McArthur JC. Cytomegalovirus encephalitis in acquired immunodeficiency syndrome (AIDS). Neurology 1994; 44:507–514.
17. McCutchan JA. Cytomegalovirus infections of the nervous system in patients with AIDS. Clin Infect Dis 1995; 20:747–754.
18. Kalayjian RC, Cohen ML, Bonomo RA, Flanigan TP. Cytomegalovirus ventriculoencephalitis in AIDS. Medicine 1993; 72:67–77.
19. Asano Y, Yoshikawa T, Kajita Y, Ogura R, et al. Fatal encephalitis/encephalopathy in primary human herpesvirus-6 infection. Arch Dis Child 1992; 67:1484–1485.
20. Caserta MT, Hall CB, Schnabel K, McIntyre K, et al. Neuroinvasion and persistence of human herpesvirus 6 in children. J Infect Dis 1994; 170:1586–1589.
21. Drobyski WR, Knox KK, Majewski D, Carrigan DR. Brief report: fatal encephalitis due to variant B human herpesvirus-6 infection in a bone-marrow transplant recipient. N Engl J Med 1994; 330:1356–1360.
22. Aurelius E, Johansson B, Skoldenberg B, Staland A, Forsgren M. Rapid diagnosis of herpes simplex encephalitis by nested polymerase chain reaction assay of cerebrospinal fluid. Lancet 1991; 337: 189–192.
23. Baringer JR, Pisani P. Herpes simplex virus genomes in human nervous system tissue analyzed by polymerase chain reaction. Ann Neurol 1994; 36:823–829.
24. Johnson RT, Griffin DE, Gendelman HE. Postinfectious encephalomyelitis. Semin Neurol 1985; 5: 180–190.
25. Case Records of the Massachusetts General Hospital (case 37-1995). N Engl J Med 1995; 333:1485–1493.
26. Hafler DA, Benjamin DS, Burks J, Weiner HL. Myelin basic protein and proteolipid protein reactivity of brain- and cerebrospinal fluid-derived T-cell clones in multiple sclerosis and postinfectious encephalomyelitis. J Immunol 1987; 139:68–72.

8

Tuberculous Meningitis

David A. Glander
Indianapolis, Indiana

HISTORY

Tuberculosis has plagued mankind through the centuries, and evidence of the disease has been found in the mummified remains of the ancient Egyptians dating back thousands of years. It remains the leading infectious cause of death in the world (1–3). One third to one half of the world's population is infected with *Mycobacterium tuberculosis*, and there are 8–10 million new cases reported per year in the world as estimated by the World Health Organization (2–4). Three million people die per year from tuberculosis (2,3). This "Captain of the Men of Death," as described by John Bunyan in 1700 when tuberculosis had a devastating effect in Europe, has claimed the lives of the poor and unknown as well as the famous such as Chopin, Keats, Thoreau, Paginini, Modigliani, and Elizabeth Browning (2,3). Once tuberculous drugs became available in this century, the prevalence of tuberculosis decreased (4). The United States began to monitor the incidence of tuberculosis infections in 1953. Eighty-four thousand cases were reported in that year. The number of cases then declined as noted in 1984 when only 22,000 cases were reported (4). From 1985 to 1992 the incidence rates of tuberculosis started to increase. In 1992, nearly 27,000 cases of tuberculosis were reported (5). The increase in incidence rates is felt to be due to many factors, such as the human immunodeficiency virus (HIV) epidemic and an increase in the numbers of homeless individuals, alcohol/substance abusers, correctional facility inmates, and immigrants from areas with a high prevalence of tuberculosis infection (3,4).

In 1836, P. H. Green coined the term "tubercular meningitis," and Robert Koch discovered the tubercle bacillus in 1882 (6). Tuberculous meningitis represents the most common form of central nervous system involvement in the patient infected with *M. tuberculosis*. Tuberculous meningitis has been reported to represent approximately 5–15% of the total number of extrapulmonary cases of tuberculosis reported in the United States each year (4,7). Tuberculous meningitis is a frequent complication in patients who are immunosuppressed, such as those infected with HIV (8). In

1988, it was estimated that HIV-associated extrapulmonary tuberculosis accounted for 21% of the total morbidity from extrapulmonary tuberculosis for that year (9).

PATHOPHYSIOLOGY

Mycobacteria are a genus of gram-positive bacilli. These are thin, rod-shaped organisms with a large proportion of lipids in their cell membranes. It is the abundance of lipids that makes the cell membranes difficult to Gram stain, however, once stained the bacilli resist decolorization with hydrochloric acid, and are thus termed "acid-fast" bacilli (3,10).

The transmission of *M. tuberculosis* is airborne via μm-sized droplets called "droplet nuclei," which are expelled from the host (humans) with active pulmonary infection while coughing, talking, or sneezing (3,11). The droplet nuclei may remain suspended in air for hours before finding a port of entry into the next host (2,11). The usual site of entrance is the lungs, but the gastrointestinal tract and skin are other possible sites. Once inhaled into the lungs, the droplet nuclei are small enough (<10 μm) to travel past the clearance defense mechanisms of the upper airways and eventually deposit in the alveoli and alveolar ducts to initiate infection (2,3,11). The bacilli then begin to multiply in the alveoli and are ingested (but not destroyed) by macrophages, which transport the bacilli to regional lymph nodes in the hilum or paratracheal regions of the lungs to form the primary complex (2,11).

Tuberculous infection is very common in humans, but tuberculous disease is not. The disease has been estimated to occur in only 5% of patients within the first year of infection (11). An individual's immunological response of cell-mediated immunity and delayed hypersensitivity reaction dictates how they will respond to the infection. The primary infection is defined as the response to infection in a person who has not been infected or sensitized to tuberculoproteins in the past (3).

During the primary infection and as the primary complex grows, subsequent spread of the tuberculous bacilli into the lymphatics and bloodstream occurs. This lymphohematogenous dissemination sends the bacilli to many parts of the body, such as the bones, liver, spleen, kidneys, brain, meninges, and spinal cord, and provides the groundwork for extrapulmonary reactivation in the future (2,11). Active miliary tuberculosis can occur in about 5% of hosts where the primary infection is not controlled (3). A devastating meningeal infection can also occur at this time in a young infant or an immunocompromised host (3). Two to 8 weeks after initial infection, hypersensitivity develops and the inflammatory response becomes more aggressive (2,3,11). This leads to caseation of the pulmonary lesions and the possibility of further dissemination. Since *M. tuberculosis* produces no toxins, the tissue destruction often seen with tuberculosis is thought to be due to the inflammatory response created by the cell-mediated immunity to *M. tuberculosis* and the delayed-type hypersensitivity to the tuberculoproteins (3,11).

Immunity to tuberculosis is affected by disorders that weaken the cell-mediated response such as HIV infection, malignancy, and use of immunosuppressive agents. The cell-mediated immune response and tissue hypersensitivity develop approximately 2–8 weeks after infection (2,3,11). Around this time, tubercles may develop. Tubercles are granulomas comprised of multinucleated giant cells (Langhans cells), epithelioid cells (macrophages), and lymphocytes around the periphery (2,3,11). The center of the tubercle may become soft or liquefy (caseating necrosis) and may eventually calcify. If this happens at the primary complex, it is referred to as the Ghon complex.

The primary lesions are usually self-limited, and after the development of the delayed-hypersensitivity reaction, the infection becomes asymptomatic in about 90% (3,11). Some bacilli, however, may remain viable in quiescent foci over many years to potentially reactivate the disease later if immunity weakens (3,11). Of those who recover from primary infection, approximately 10% will develop clinical disease later in their lifetime (3).

Tuberculous meningitis generally occurs months to years after recovery from primary infection. During the primary infection, lymphohematogenous seeding of tubercle bacilli may occur and form small foci in the brain, meninges, or spinal cord. These foci were determined to be the sites of origin of tuberculous meningitis by the pathologists Rich and McCordock in the 1930s (12). These "Rich foci," as they are called, are in a subpial or subependymal location (13). As these lesions enlarge and caseate, they may eventually extend to the surface of the brain or meninges and rupture into the subarachnoid space, releasing bacilli and tuberculous antigens to initiate the meningitic process (2–4, 13–15). It is well known that direct hematogenous spread of tubercle bacilli to the meninges rarely causes tuberculous meningitis during the primary infection (4). It is interesting to note that fate plays a role in determining if a patient will develop tuberculous meningitis due to the random distribution of bacilli during lymphohematogenous dissemination to form Rich foci close enough to the surface of the brain for potential rupture and subarachnoid invasion. Tuberculous meningitis occurs in approximately 0.7% of tuberculosis primary infections in the United States (4).

According to *Greenfield's Neuropathology* (15), the gross appearance of the brain at autopsy has five predominate characteristics: (1) the meninges have a slight gray-green appearance, (2) the exudate is thick and fills the basal cisterns, the pontine cisterns, and enters the Sylvian fissures and cisterna magna, (3) a focal exudate can be seen over a small area of the brain where there is an underlying tuberculoma, (4) communicating and obstructive hydrocephalus develops with white matter edema, and (5) cerebral infarctions are seen in the distribution of the middle cerebral arteries.

The primary pathological features of tuberculous meningitis are hydrocephalus, cerebral infarctions, cerebral edema, and cranial nerve palsies, which are, for the most part, complications due to the thick, gelatinous exudate that develops in tuberculous meningitis. The exudate forms in response to the hypersensitivity reaction that occurs in the subarachnoid space when tuberculoproteins are released by Rich foci (4,12). The predominant location of the exudate is at the basilar aspects of the brain, regardless of where the tuberculous bacilli were discharged into the subarachnoid space (4). The exudate tends to locate along the following areas: inferomedial frontal/parietal lobes, anteromedial temporal lobes, anterosuperior aspect of the cerebellar hemispheres, floor of the third ventricle, interpeduncular fossa, and the anterior portion of the pontomesencephalic junction (13). Spinal tuberculosis is typically due to spread of the exudate downward through the foramen magnum, but occasionally the meningitis may begin in the spinal subarachnoid space and spread upwards to cause intracranial tuberculosis (13). The exudate overlying brain parenchyma can create an inflammatory lesion of the brain tissue known as the border zone reaction. Edema, perivascular infiltration, and microglial cells characterize these lesions (16).

As the exudate develops along the basal aspect of the brain, the basal cisterns are filled and a resultant communicating type of hydrocephalus occurs. The hydrocephalus can progress rapidly and result in increased intracranial pressure (4,13). A communicating type of hydrocephalus may also be the result of disruption of cerebrospinal fluid resorption as exudate fills the arachnoid granulations (12). Obstructive hydrocephalus may develop due to (1) narrowing of the fourth ventricle or cerebral aqueduct as the exudate surrounds and mechanically compresses the brain stem or (2) prevention of the flow of cerebrospinal fluid (CSF) if exudate forms in the third ventricle (4,13,16).

Stroke has a major impact on the morbidity and mortality of patients who have tuberculous meningitis. The arteries that traverse the base of the brain are embedded in exudate that encroaches on the vessel and narrows the lumen. Inflammatory cells in the wall of the blood vessel (vasculitis) cause thickening of the arterial wall with subsequent narrowing of the lumen (4,14,16). In time, the intima of the blood vessel is affected, resulting in thrombosis of the blood vessel and ischemic infarction or hemorrhage of brain tissue. Most commonly, the branches of the middle cerebral artery and anterior cerebral artery are involved (16) to produce ischemic lesions in the basal ganglia and cerebral cortex. In a study by Hsieh et al. (17) 75% of cerebral infarctions in patients with tuberculous meningitis were located in the distribution of the medial striate and thalamoperforant arteries described as the "TB zone." The posterior circulation of the brain can also be involved as lesions of the pons and cerebellum are also seen (4).

The brainstem is the most common site of involvement from tuberculous meningitis in children, with injury to cranial nerves three, four, and seven (2). Cranial nerve abnormalities from tuberculous meningitis may be due to vasculitic infarction of the nerve or mechanical compression of the nerve by the thick, fibrous exudate (14).

As mentioned previously, tuberculous meningitis is frequently an infection associated with immunosuppression (8,15). Individuals with HIV and tuberculosis infection are at an increased risk for tuberculous meningitis (10%) as compared to patients with tuberculosis infection alone (2%) (8). As the incidence of HIV infection and acquired immunodeficiency syndrome (AIDS) increases, the number of cases of tuberculosis and extrapulmonary tuberculosis is expected to continue to increase (18). The primary pathophysiology of tuberculous meningitis in the HIV-infected patient does not differ from that in the absence of HIV infection in that the rupture of a subependymal or subpial caseating lesion (Rich foci) into the subarachnoid space is the initiating factor (18). However, tuberculosis infection may advance more rapidly, and latent infections may reactivate more frequently in patients with HIV (18).

CLINICAL PRESENTATION

Prior to the development of antituberculous agents, the diagnosis of tuberculous meningitis meant certain death after a progressive, stereotyped course of decline. Presently, patients with tuberculous meningitis have an improved chance for survival, but mortality remains high (approximately 20%) and the clinical course is quite variable (7,16). Classically, if tuberculous meningitis is untreated, clinical stages occur as defined by the British Medical Council in 1948 (16).

The disease begins with an indolent prodromal phase that includes fatigue, apathy, low-grade fevers, night sweats, occasional headaches, and, not uncommonly, personality changes (4,16). Children may have malaise, anorexia, irritability, nausea, vomiting, behavioral problems, and abdominal pain initially (1,2,16). Toward the end of this phase (2 or 3 weeks), signs of meningeal irritation, headache, vomiting, and stiff neck develop (4,16).

During the second phase, symptoms and signs of meningitis intensify and are associated with confusion, lethargy, and cranial nerve deficits. Nuchal rigidity and Brudzinski's and Kernig's signs can be elicited at this time. In the third phase, confusion and lethargy give way to obtundation or coma. If hydrocephalus develops, increasing intracranial pressure will manifest as papilledema in adults and a tense bulging fontanelle with increasing occipital-frontal circumference in children. Other signs of focal neurological deficits develop including seizures, hemiparesis, paraplegia, decerebrate or decorticate posturing, involuntary movements, pupillary and autonomic dysfunction. Death may occur within 5–8 weeks without treatment; however, cases lasting months are not uncommon (4).

The clinical presentation of tuberculous meningitis may not follow the three clinical stages described in 1948 and can be either an acute fulminant illness or an insidious subacute dementing process. The latter is more common and manifests as memory loss and personality changes similar to those seen in frontal lobe disease, with abulia and incontinence (12). Tuberculous meningitis may also present clinically as an acute pyogenic meningitis. The classic symptoms and signs of headache, vomiting, stiff neck, photophobia, decreased level of consciousness, and focal neurological deficits may appear acutely and progress rapidly (4,12).

A clinical syndrome of encephalopathy in patients with pulmonary tuberculosis was described in detail by Udani and Dastur in 1970. This "tuberculous encephalopathy" can occur with or without meningitis and is characterized by only mild inflammatory changes in the CSF. This syndrome is more common in children than adults, and may be manifest by seizure activity and altered level of consciousness or coma (16). Pathologically, there is diffuse cerebral edema and diffuse myelin loss in the white matter. The mechanism behind the injury is considered to be a cell-mediated immunity delayed type IV hypersensitivity reaction to tuberculoprotein (13).

HIV does not appear to change the clinical manifestations of tuberculous meningitis drastically. A study comparing two groups of patients with tuberculous meningitis (15 HIV-positive individuals and 16 HIV-negative individuals) revealed similar symptoms, signs, chest radiograph appearance, cerebrospinal fluid abnormalities, and mortality (9). The HIV-infected patients did have a higher incidence (60%) of intracerebral mass lesions. Berenguer et al. also found no difference in the clinical manifestations or outcome in tuberculous meningitis between patients with or without concurrent HIV infection (8).

DIAGNOSIS

The diagnosis of tuberculous meningitis is based on a comprehensive history and physical exam in conjunction with the appropriate ancillary investigations. However, the initiation of empiric antituberculous therapy should not await bacteriological proof of *M. tuberculosis* by smear or culture. A strong clinical suspicion should be maintained if the patient has had recent close contact with another person with tuberculosis. Such a history may be found in 20–30% of cases of tuberculous meningitis (16). A prevalence of tuberculosis in the area, family history of tuberculosis, history of alcohol and or drug abuse, immunodeficiency, malnourishment, and poor socioeconomic condition are risk factors for tuberculous meningitis. On general physical examination, the presence of retinal choroid tubercles, lymphadenopathy (scrofula), scrotal mass (due to epididymitis or orchitis), and bone lesions can raise the index of suspicion (4,16). Delay in diagnosis and initiation of antituberculous therapy may have a significant impact on the prognosis of patients with tuberculous meningitis. An overview of the diagnostic evaluation for tuberculous meningitis is given in Table 1.

Routine blood counts and chemistries often reveal nonspecific and nondiagnostic abnormalities. Common findings include a mild anemia, leukocytosis, mildly elevated erythrocyte sedimentation rate, and hyponatremia due to the inappropriate secretion of antidiuretic hormone. Kent et al. (19) reviewed 58 cases of tuberculous meningitis in an Australian institution and Davis et al. (20) reviewed 54 cases of tuberculous meningitis in a southwest American community. In these 112 cases, the white blood cell count was mildly elevated in 31–44% of cases. Serum

Table 1 Diagnosis and Therapy of Tuberculous Meningitis

1. Comprehensive history and physical examination
2. Electrolytes, complete blood count, erythrocyte sedimentation rate, and HIV
3. Chest radiograph
4. Tuberculin skin test
5. CT or MRI of head with contrast
6. Cerebrospinal fluid examination: elevated opening pressure, lymphocytic pleocytosis, hypoglycorrhachia, elevated protein concentration, AFB smear and culture (if available PCR, ELISA, or tuberculostearic acid)

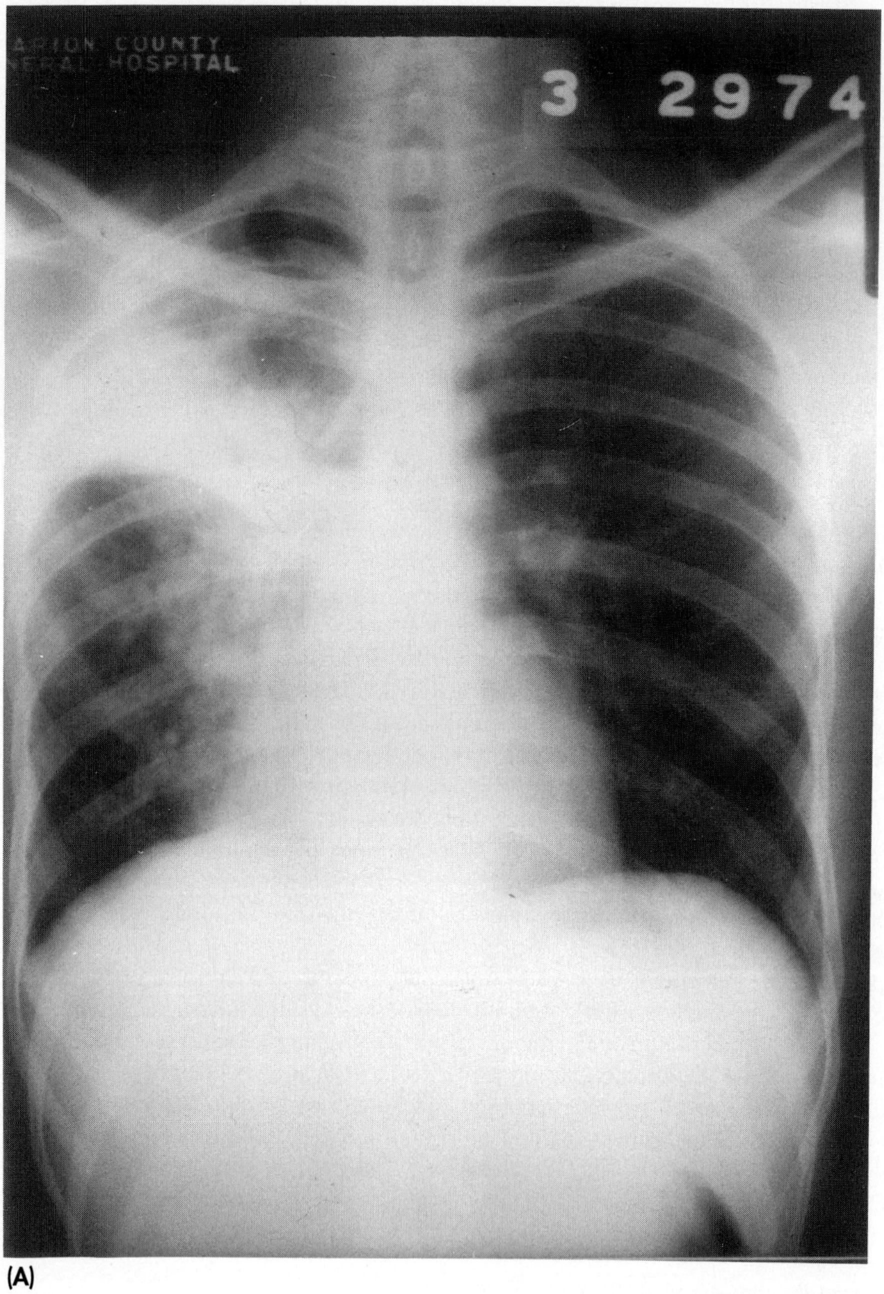

(A)

Figure 1 (A) Chest x-ray of pulmonary tuberculosis. (B) Chest x-ray posttreatment.

sodium was <135 mEq/liter in 50–79%, and erythrocyte sedimentation rate was >20 mm/h in only 28%.

The absence of radiographic evidence of pulmonary tuberculosis does not exclude the possibility of tuberculous meningitis. Findings associated with pulmonary tuberculosis found on chest x-ray include hilar adenopathy, Ghon complex, miliary pattern, infiltrates, cavitations, and

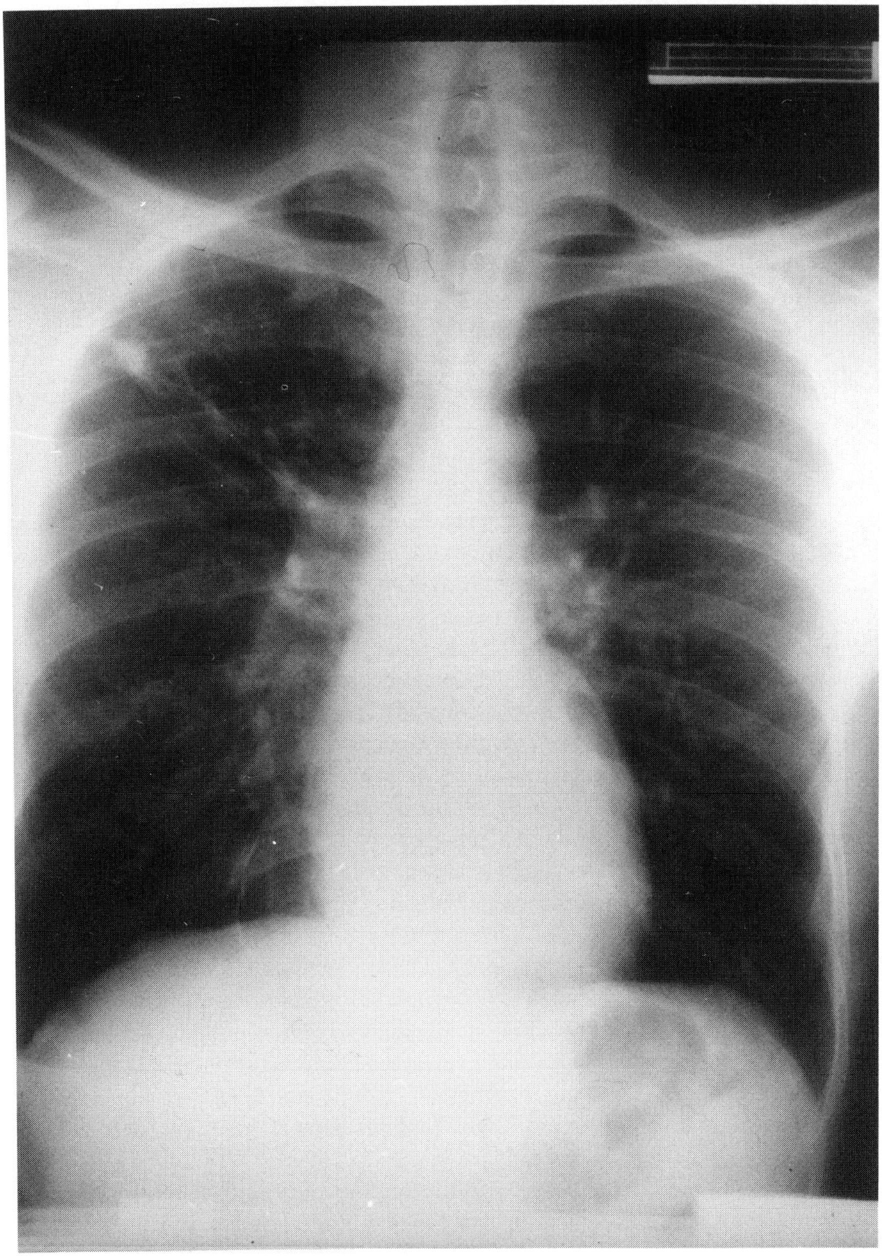

(B)

pleural effusions (Fig. 1) (2,16). Radiographic evidence of pulmonary tuberculosis is found in 50–90% of cases of tuberculous meningitis in children (16). The association of pulmonary lesions and meningitis is not as high in adults (16). Ogawa et al. reviewed 45 cases of tuberculous meningitis at a large urban medical center and found 14 patients with an abnormal chest x-ray on admission consistent with pulmonary tuberculosis (7). In the series by Kent and Davis, abnormal chest x-rays were noted in 41 and 53% of cases with tuberculous meningitis, respectively (19,20). The classic Ghon complex was seen in only 14% of those with abnormal chest x-rays in the latter study.

A positive tuberculin skin test can be helpful in establishing the diagnosis of tuberculous meningitis, but a negative test does not rule out tuberculous meningitis (12,16). Three recent series reported 50–75% of cases with tuberculous meningitis to have positive tuberculin skin tests (7,20,21). The test may be falsely negative in tuberculous meningitis and has been reported to be negative in 20–75% of cases, but often becomes positive during the course of treatment (1,4,16,21). An initial negative skin test may be secondary to immunosuppression, malnourishment, or severe infection. Previous vaccination with the bacillus of Calmette-Guérin (BCG) should not be considered in the interpretation of a tuberculin skin test (5,22,23). Fifty to 93% of individuals who are vaccinated with BCG do not convert to a positive tuberculin skin test (22).

Computed tomography (CT) and magnetic resonance imaging (MRI) are useful neuroimaging techniques in the evaluation of the patient with possible tuberculous meningitis. However, the findings are frequently nondiagnostic, and if the disease is in the early stages, the imaging studies without contrast may not reveal any abnormalities (18,24,25). The most common findings seen are enhancement of the basal cisterns, hydrocephalus, and infarctions. Hydrocephalus was reported in approximately 50% of cases of tuberculous meningitis in two recent series (7,20). Similar findings can be seen in other central nervous system diseases such as pyogenic meningitis, fungal meningitis, sarcoidosis, and carcinomatous meningitis. A noncontrasted CT often exhibits isoattenuated or hyperattenuated basal cisterns, whereas the image with contrast may reveal homogeneous enhancement of the basal cisterns and enhancement of the meninges over the convexities of the cerebral and cerebellar hemispheres (26). Disease of the cerebral cortex and underlying white matter may be seen on CT as hypodense areas (26). MRI with gadolinium is more sensitive than CT with contrast in demonstrating meningeal enhancement (18). MRI is also reported to be significantly more sensitive in detecting ischemic infarctions than CT (25). Enhancement of the choroid plexus or ependymal lining can be detected occasionally on MRI with gadolinium (25). Patients with AIDS may have an absence of meningeal enhancement on CT or MRI, possibly due to the lack of exudate associated with an impaired immune response (18).

CT can be a useful tool in the management of tuberculous meningitis enabling the clinician to follow the progression of hydrocephalus on serial exams (26). Likewise, MRI can be helpful in locating focal lesions associated with clinical deficits and in monitoring the response of antituberculous therapy since enhancement of meninges may resolve quickly after initiation of treatment (25). The basal aspects of the brain with thick exudate, however, continue to enhance on imaging even after initiation of therapy (25). MR angiography may be a beneficial and noninvasive technique to diagnose and follow vasculitis or mechanical compression of the vessels of the circle of Willis secondary to tuberculous meningitis (25).

Typical abnormalities on examination of the CSF in tuberculous meningitis include increased opening pressure on lumbar puncture, elevated protein concentration, lymphocytic pleocytosis, and hypoglycorrhachia. Not uncommonly, an opening pressure of >300 mm of water is measured (15).The fluid is usually clear to slightly milky and forms a thin film or weblike clot on the surface when allowed to stand (12,16). If the fluid is obtained in the early stages of infection, there may be only a mild increase of cells, which are predominantly polymorphonuclear leukocytes, the protein concentration may be elevated only slightly, and the glucose concentration may be normal (4,12). As repeat CSF examinations are performed, the protein concentration will progressively increase, the glucose concentration will decrease, and the cell count should shift to a mononuclear pleocytosis (12). The "therapeutic paradox" consists of a shift of cell type in the CSF from lymphocytic to polymorphonuclear leukocytes and deterioration of the patient clinically with initiation of antituberculous therapy (4,12).

The typical CSF white blood cell count in tuberculous meningitis is in the range of 10–500 cells/mm^3, and the median cell count in a recent series was 162 cells/mm^3 with a lymphocytic predominance in 68% of the cases (7). The CSF protein concentration is in the range of 100–500 mg/dl, but may be significantly higher in the presence of spinal block (4,16). CSF glucose concentration is ≤40 mg/dl in approximately 50% of cases (7). Other nonspecific CSF abnormalities in tuberculous meningitis include a decrease in the concentration of chloride and an increase in adenosine deaminase (16,27). The bromide partition ratio, which measures the ratio of serum to CSF bromide 24 h after the administration of oral or intravenous bromide, can be low in tuberculous meningitis. Again, this is a nonspecific abnormality that can occur with any process that increases the permeability of the blood-brain barrier (12,16).

The cornerstone to the diagnosis of tuberculous meningitis is in the identification of *M. tuberculosis* from the spinal fluid. This can be a difficult task as CSF cultures from patients with tuberculous meningitis have been reported to be positive in 45–90% of cases and require 3–8 weeks for growth (4,6,15,16). The detection of acid-fast bacilli (AFB) in smears of CSF also has a low yield, as positive smears are reported in 10–45% of cases (7,16,19). Recommended techniques to increase the yield of positive results on CSF smear or culture include (1) the examination of at least three serial samples of spinal fluid obtained from lumbar space or cisterna magna at daily intervals, (2) the examination of adequate amounts of spinal fluid (5–10 ml), and (3) careful microscopic examination of the smear for at least 30 min (2,4,12,16).

The initiation of empiric chemotherapy cannot await the results of CSF cultures or smears. Three to 8 weeks may be required to detect growth of *M. tuberculosis*, and, as noted above, AFB smears have a low yield. There is a need for methods of detection that are more sensitive, specific, and rapid. Several techniques have been described recently, but most are not currently available in commercial laboratories. One of these techniques detects a cell wall component (tuberculostearic acid) of *M. tuberculosis* that is almost uniquely associated with the organism. The concentration in the spinal fluid of tuberculostearic acid can be detected by gas chromatography and mass spectrometry with ion monitoring. This has been found to be a highly sensitive and fairly specific test, but it is currently available only through the Centers for Disease Control (CDC) and several research laboratories (2). Another technique, the enzyme-linked immunosorbent assay (ELISA), is used to detect *M. tuberculosis* antigens and antimycobacterial antibodies in CSF. This assay has been shown to produce reliable results in research settings and may be of value clinically in the future (4,12,16,28–31). Finally, the polymerase chain reaction (PCR) technique can be used to identify certain organisms in the spinal fluid by amplification of that organism's DNA. PCR can be used in the laboratory to detect the genome of *M. tuberculosis* within 24–72 h (32,33). Some researchers have found this technique to be highly specific and moderately sensitive (34). Studies have also shown that PCR can be a sensitive method to detect *M. tuberculosis* DNA up to 3 weeks after the initiation of therapy in patients with tuberculous meningitis (35). Larger studies using the PCR are needed to determine the true sensitivity and specificity of this technique before it can be recommended for routine use.

TREATMENT

It must be emphasized that the most important factor in the prognosis of tuberculous meningitis is the stage at which antituberculous therapy is begun. Early initiation of antimicrobial therapy when the clinical presentation and paraclinical studies suggest that the diagnosis is associated with an improved outcome (4,16). The potential benefits of beginning empiric therapy quickly in suspected tuberculous meningitis outweigh (in the short term) the possible toxic side effects of the currently recommended antituberculous agents. Additionally, empiric therapy will not endanger the diagnostic identification of the tubercle bacilli in subsequent CSF samples (16). Multiple

Table 2 Treatment of Tuberculous Meningitis

Child[a]	Immunocompetent adult[a]	Immunosuppressed individual[a]
1. Isoniazid 10–15 mg/kg/day 2. Rifampin 10–20 mg/kg/day 3. Pyrazinamide 20–40 mg/kg/day 4. Streptomycin 20–40 mg/kg/day 5. ± Corticosteroids[b] 6. ± VP shunt[c]	1. Isoniazid 5 mg/kg/day 2. Rifampin 10 mg/kg/day 3. Pyrazinamide 15–30 mg/kg/day 4. Pyridoxine 50 mg/day 5. ± Ethambutol or streptomycin 6. ± Corticosteroids[b] 7. ± VP shunt[c]	1. Isoniazid 10–15 mg/kg/day 2. Rifampin 10–15 mg/kg/day 3. Pyrazinamide or ethambutol 4. Streptomycin or rifabutin or clofazimine 5. Pyridoxine 50 mg/day 6. ± Corticosteroids[b] 7. ± VP shunt[c]

[a]See text for maximum daily dosages of all medications and duration of therapy.
[b]Recommended in the presence of altered mental status, focal neurological deficits, papilledema, visual impairment, hydrocephalus, or spinal block.
[c]Consider if hydrocephalus present secondary to increased intracranial pressure.
Source: Refs. 12, 37, 38.

agent regimens are the mainstay of treatment due to the presence of naturally occurring drug-resistant organisms (2). An overview of the therapy for tuberculous meningitis is given in Table 2. Even though mycobacterial populations in tuberculous meningitis are not as large as those in pulmonary disease, the potential severity of illness with meningitis necessitates the use of multi-drug regimens.

First-line agents against *M. tuberculosis* include isoniazid (INH), rifampin, pyrazinamide, and ethambutol. INH, streptomycin, and rifampin are bactericidal for *M. tuberculosis*; ethambutol is bacteriostatic at conventional doses; pyrazinamide has a role in destroying the bacilli but is not bactericidal in the lab (2). Drug-resistant strains are increasing in number in the United States as 10% of isolates are resistant to at least one drug (2). The two types of resistance are termed primary and secondary. Primary resistance occurs when initial infection occurs with a resistant strain. Secondary resistance occurs when a drug-resistant organism becomes the dominant organism during treatment. This can occur as a consequence of noncompliance to medications by the patient or by inadequate therapy (2). Penetration of the first-line agents into the CSF is variable. INH and pyrazinamide enter the CSF easily with or without meningeal inflammation, whereas rifampin, streptomycin, and ethambutol penetrate the CSF poorly without inflammation of the meninges (4,16).

If severe, the side effects of antituberculous medications can lead to alteration of the drug regimen. INH has been associated with an axonal sensorimotor polyneuropathy that occurs in about 10% of patients on conventional doses, usually occurring between 3 and 35 weeks after initiation of therapy (36). Symptoms begin with paresthesias in the lower extremities and sometimes in the hands. Mild weakness of distal extremities may occur. It is thought that INH may interfere with vitamin B_6-dependent coenzymes, which leads to a pyridoxine deficiency (36). Individuals who are slow acetylators of INH are susceptible to peripheral neuropathy. Conversely, fast acetylators are susceptible to hepatotoxicity. The combination of INH and rifampin is associated with hepatic injury (4) and liver function tests should be monitored during treatment.

Rifampin causes an orange discoloration to urine, tears, CSF, and saliva and can also cause a hypersensitivity reaction with neutropenia, thrombocytopenia, and hemolytic anemia (6). Pyrazinamide may be hepatotoxic at high doses, but is most commonly associated with arthralgias or gout during treatment (4,6). Streptomycin is ototoxic and can lead to hearing loss due to toxicity to the eighth cranial nerve; for this reason it is not to be used intrathecally (4,6). Ethambutol toxicity to the optic nerves occurs in 3% of individuals on standard doses. Visual exams should be done routinely; this may limit the use of the drug in patients who are not able to comply with this exam (such as young children or patients with altered mental status) (4).

The CDC recommends a combination of three drugs for the initial treatment of tuberculous meningitis in adults (12,37). Treatment should begin with

1. Isoniazid 5 mg/kg/day (max. daily dose 300 mg)
2. Rifampin 10 mg/kg/day (max. daily dose 600 mg)
3. Pyrazinamide 15–30 mg/kg/day (max. daily dose 2 g)

Pyridoxine 50 mg/day should be added to prevent the associated polyneuropathy. If drug resistant organisms are suspected, add either ethambutol (15–25 mg/kg/day; max. daily dose 2.5 g) or streptomycin (15 mg/kg/day IM; max. daily dose 1 g) to the initial regimen. If the patient improves clinically, pyrazinamide, ethambutol, and streptomycin can be discontinued after 8 weeks and isoniazid and rifampin continued alone. Total length of therapy should be at least 6 months, but 9–12 months is often recommended (4,6,12,16).

The American Academy of Pediatrics recommends a 12-month regimen of antimicrobial therapy for tuberculous meningitis in children. Initiation of the regimen uses the following:

1. Isoniazid 10–15 mg/kg day or 20–40 mg/kg/dose twice weekly (max. dose 300 mg daily or 900 mg twice weekly)
2. Rifampin 10–20 mg/kg/day or 10–20 mg/kg/dose twice weekly (max. daily dose 600 mg)
3. Pyrazinamide 20–40 mg/kg/day (max. daily dose 2 g)
4. Streptomycin 20–40 mg/kg/day (max. daily dose 1 g)

Streptomycin is used initially until the results of antibiotic susceptibility tests are known. Otherwise, this four-drug regimen is continued for 2 months, at which time pyrazinamide and streptomycin can be discontinued and isoniazid and rifampin can be given on a daily basis (or twice weekly if watched directly by medical personnel) (38). The Academy also recommends that (1) liver function tests be monitored during the first several months of treatment, (2) corticosteroids be considered in cases of tuberculous meningitis, (3) pyridoxine supplementation be given only if the patient is malnourished, lacks meat or milk in the diet, or is breast feeding, and (4) an expert in tuberculosis be consulted if drug-resistant organisms are suspected (38).

The recommended treatment of tuberculous meningitis in an immunosuppressed individual is the following:

1. Isoniazid 10–15 mg/kg/day (max. daily dose 300 mg)
2. Rifampin 10–15 mg/kg/day (max. daily dose 600 mg)
3. Pyrazinamide 20–30 mg/kg/day (max. daily dose 2 g) or ethambutol 25 mg/kg/day (max. daily dose 2.5 g)
4. Streptomycin 20–40 mg/kg/day (max. daily dose 1 g) or rifabutin 300 mg/day or clofazimine 300 mg/day

This regimen should be continued at least 6 months after cultures are negative and for a total length of at least 6–9 months of treatment (12,37).

The use of corticosteroids in the treatment of tuberculous meningitis is somewhat controversial. Steroids decrease the inflammation-induced increased permeability of the blood-brain barrier. This can theoretically decrease CSF concentrations of antituberculous agents that require meningeal inflammation for penetration. However, a clinical trial comparing the CSF concentrations of antituberculous agents in eight patients treated with isoniazid, rifampin, pyrazinamide, streptomycin, and dexamethasone to eight patients treated with the antituberculous agents alone found no difference in the CSF concentration of antituberculous agents in the two groups (39).

Although clinical trials demonstrating benefit from corticosteroid therapy in tuberculous meningitis are limited, most experts agree that steroids improve the clinical outcome in some patients with tuberculous meningitis (2,4,16,40,41). This may be the result of several mechanisms: (1) reduction in the inflammatory response to tuberculoproteins in the CSF, (2) treatment of cerebral arteritis, and (3) decrease in cerebral edema (2). By decreasing cerebral edema, corticosteroids decrease intracranial pressure. Also, as intracranial pressure decreases, cerebral perfusion increases allowing improved concentrations of antituberculous agents to the brain and meninges (2). The response to steroids may be quite dramatic, with improvement in mental status, normalization of CSF abnormalities, and improvement of focal neurological deficits (4,16). The use of steroids in tuberculous meningitis is recommended for patients with altered mental status, focal neurological deficits, papilledema, visual impairment, hydrocephalus, or spinal block (3,4,16).

Note should be made of the reports of paradoxical progression or enlargement of tuberculous lesions that can occur in some patients during therapy. The development of new tuberculomas or an increase in the size of preexisting tuberculomas can occur during the first 3 months of treatment leading to neurological decline. Steroids appear to be of benefit in such cases, and the lesions regress with continued antituberculous therapy (42,43).

Surgical treatment in tuberculous meningitis is often necessary in the setting of increased intracranial pressure secondary to hydrocephalus. If clinical deterioration occurs during the first few weeks of treatment, repeat imaging should be obtained. If hydrocephalus is found, ventriculoperitoneal or ventriculoatrial shunting should be considered. Other measures reported to be helpful in the treatment of increased intracranial pressure secondary to hydrocephalus include serial lumbar punctures, steroids, and acetazolamide (4,16).

DIFFERENTIAL DIAGNOSIS

The clinical presentation, cerebrospinal fluid abnormalities, and neuroimaging findings in tuberculous meningitis are often suggestive of a chronic meningitis. The disease process provoking a clinical picture of chronic meningitis could be infectious or noninfectious and the differential diagnosis moderately extensive. The list should include fungal meningitis, partially treated bacterial meningitis, viral meningitis, neurosyphilis, pyogenic brain abcess, CNS toxoplasmosis, parameningeal infections, carcinomatous meningitis, CNS sarcoidosis, and Behçet's disease (4,16).

PROGNOSIS AND PREVENTION

The prognostic factors that may adversely affect outcome in individuals with tuberculous meningitis include (1) age (the young and old being affected more severely), (2) malnutrition, (3) the presence of miliary disease, (4) alcoholism/substance abuse or other underlying debilitating disease, (5) hydrocephalus, (6) cerebrovascular complications, (7) hypoglycorrhacia, and (8) elevated CSF protein concentration (13). However, the most important determinant of morbidity and mortality in tuberculous meningitis is the stage of the disease at which therapy is initiated. Patients with little or no alteration in level of consciousness (stage 1) at the start of treatment generally survive with minor neurological sequelae, whereas patients who are comatose (stage 3) at the initiation of treatment have a mortality rate of greater than 50% (4,12,16).

Risk factors associated with contracting tuberculosis have been mentioned earlier. Third world countries with a high prevalence of HIV are reporting significantly more cases of tuberculosis (44). In the United States, the percentage of tuberculosis infection among the homeless may be five times that of the general population (45). Studies of BCG vaccination have been conflicting and of variable effect in protecting against pulmonary tuberculosis (46–48). However, BCG vaccination may be effective in limiting the dissemination of *M. tuberculosis* during primary infection and in turn preventing tuberculous meningitis at a later stage (47,48). Additional studies are needed to confirm this before recommendations regarding the use of BCG vaccination during primary infection can be made.

REFERENCES

1. Newton RW. Tuberculous meningitis. Arch Dis Child 1994; 70:364–366.
2. Starke JR. Tuberculosis. In: Jenson HB, Baltimore RS, eds. Pediatric Infectious Diseases. Principles and Practice. Norwalk, CT: Appleton & Lange, 1995:517–545.
3. Plorde JJ. Mycobacteria. In: Sherris, ed. Medical Microbiology. An Introduction to Infectious Diseases. 3d ed. Norwalk, CT: Appleton & Lange, 1994:401–415.
4. Leonard JM, Des Prez RM. Tuberculous meningitis. Infect Dis Clin North Am 1990; 4, No. 4:769–787.
5. Committee on Infectious Diseases. Screening for tuberculosis in infants and children. Pediatrics 1994; 93(1):131–134.
6. Bell WE. Bacterial meningitis in children. Selected aspects. Pediatr Neurology 1992; 39(4):651–668.
7. Ogawa SK, Smith MA, Brennessel DJ, Lowy FD. Tuberculous meningitis in an urban medical center. Medicine 1987; 66(4):317–325.
8. Berenguer J, Santiago M, Fernando L, Vicente T, Adrados M, Ortega A, Gonzalez-LaHoz J, Bouza E. Tuberculous meningitis in patients with the human immunodeficiency virus. N Engl J Med 1992; 326(10):668–672.
9. Dube MP, Holtom PD, Larsen RA. Tuberculous meningitis in patients with and without human immunodeficiency virus infection. Am J Med 1992; 93:520–524.
10. MacGregor RR. Tuberculosis: From history to current management. Sem Roentg 1993; 28(2):101–108.
11. Willet HP. Mycobacterium. In: Jolik WK, Willet HP, Amos DB, Wilfert CM, eds. Zinsser Microbiology. 19th ed. Norwalk, CT: Appleton and Lange, 1988:423–448.
12. Roos KL. Tuberculous meningitis. In: Meningitis 100 Maxims. London: Arnold, 1996, pp. 158–170.
13. Dastur DK, Manghani DK, Udani PM. Pathology and pathogenic mechanisms in neurotuberculosis. Radiol Clin North Am 1995; 33:733–752.
14. Cybulska E, Rucinski J. Tuberculous meningitis. Br J Hosp Med 1988; 39(1):63–66.
15. Reid H, Fallon RJ. Bacterial infections. In: Adams JH, Duchen LW, eds. Greenfield's Neuropathology. 5th ed. New York: Oxford University Press, 1992:302–321.
16. Molavi A, LeFrock JL. Tuberculous meningitis. Med Clin North Am 1985; 69(2):315–331.
17. Hsieh FY, Chia LG, Shen WC. Locations of cerebral infarctions in tuberculous meningitis. Neuroradiology 1992; 34(3):197–199.
18. Villoria MF, Fortea F, Moreno S, Munoz L, Manero M, Benito C. MR imaging and CT of central nervous system tuberculosis in patients with AIDS. Radiol Clin North Am 1995; 33(4):805–820.
19. Kent SJ, Crowe SM, Yung A, Lucas CR, Mijch AM. Tuberculous meningitis: a 30-year review. Clin Infect Dis 1993; 17:987–994.
20. Davis LE, Rastogi KR, Lambert LC, Skipper BJ. Tuberculous meningitis in the southwest United States: a community-based study. Neurology 1993; 43(9):1775–1778.
21. Janner D, Rutherford M, Azimi P. Tuberculous meningitis in children. Pediatr Emerg Care 1993; 9(5): 281–284.
22. Ciesielski SD. BCG vaccination and the PPD test: What the clinician needs to know. J Fam Pract 1995; 40(1):76–80.
23. Huebner RE, Schein MF, Bass JB. The tuberculin skin test. Clin Infect Dis 1993; 17:968–975.
24. Offenbacher H, Fazekas F, Schmidt R, Kleinert R, Payer F, Kleinert G, Lechner H. MRI in tuberculous meningoencephalitis: report of four cases and review of the neuroimaging literature. J Neurol 1991; 238:340–344.
25. Jinkins JR, Gupta R, Chang KH, Rodriguez-Carbajal J. MR imaging of central nervous system tuberculosis. Radiol Clin North Am 1995; 33(4):771–786.

26. De Castro et al. CT scans of cranial tuberculosis. Radiol Clin North Am 1995; 33(4):753–769.
27. Chawla RK, Seth RK, Raj B, Saini AS. Adenosine deaminase levels in cerebrospinal fluid in tuberculosis and bacterial meningitis. Tubercle 1991; 72(3):190–192.
28. Park SC, Lee BI, Cho SN, Kim WJ, Lee BC, Kim SM, Kim JD. Diagnosis of tuberculous meningitis by detection of immunoglobulin G antibodies to purified protein derivative and lipoarabinomannan antigen in cerebrospinal fluid. Tubercle Lung Dis 1993; 74(5):317–322.
29. Cocito CG. Properties of the mycobacterial antigen complex A60 and its applications to the diagnosis and prognosis of tuberculosis. Chest 1991; 100:1687–1693.
30. Curless R, Michell C. Central nervous system tuberculosis in children. Pediatr Neurol 1991; 7:270–274.
31. Srivastava L, Prasanna S, Srivastava VK. Diagnosis of tuberculous meningitis by ELISA test. Ind J Med Rsch 1994; 99:8–12.
32. Yuk-Fong Liu P, Shi Z, Lau Y, Hu B. Rapid diagnosis of tuberculous meningitis by a simplified nested amplification protocol. Neurology 1994; 44(6):1161–1164.
33. Folgueira L, Delgado R, Palenque E, Noriega AR. Polymerase chain reaction for rapid diagnosis of tuberculous meningitis in AIDS patients. Neurology 1994; 44(7):1336–1338.
34. Lin JJ, Harn HJ, Hsu YD, Tsao WL, Lee HS, Lee WH. Rapid diagnosis of tuberculous meningitis by polymerase chain reaction assay of cerebrospinal fluid. J Neurol 1995; 242(3)147–152.
35. Lin JJ, Harn HJ. Application of the polymerase chain reaction to monitor Mycobacterium tuberculosis DNA in the CSF of patients with tuberculous meningitis after antibiotic therapy. J Neurol Neurosurg Psychiatr 1995; 59(2):175–177.
36. Adams RD, Victor M. Diseases of the peripheral nerves. In: Principles of Neurology. New York: McGraw-Hill, 1993:1117–1169.
37. Holdiness MR. Management of tuberculosis meningitis. Drugs 1990; 39(2):224–233.
38. Committee on Infectious Diseases. Chemotherapy for tuberculosis in infants and children. Pediatrics 1992; 89:161–164.
39. Kaojarern S, Supmonchai K, Phuapradit P, Mokkhavesa C, Krittiyanunt S. Effect of steroids on cerebrospinal fluid penetration of antituberculous drugs in tuberculous meningitis. Clin Pharm Ther 1991; 49(1):6–12.
40. Girgis NI, Farid Z, Kilpatrick ME, Sultan Y, Mikhail IA. Dexamethasone adjunctive treatment for tuberculous meningitis. Pediatr Infect Dis J 1991; 10(3):179–183.
41. Alzeer AH, FitzGerald FM. Corticosteriods and tuberculosis: risk and use as adjunct therapy. Tubercle Lung Dis 1994; 74:6–11.
42. Afghani B, Lieberman JM. Paradoxical enlargement or development of intracranial tuberculomas during therapy: case report and review. Clin Infect Dis 1994; 19:1092–1099.
43. Rao GP, Nadh BR, Hemaratnan A, Srinivas TV, Reddy PK. Paradoxical progression of tuberculous lesions during chemotherapy of central nervous system tuberculosis. J Neurosurg 1995; 83:359–362.
44. Kochi A. The global tuberculosis situation and the new control strategy of the World Health Organization. Tubercle 1991; 72:1–6.
45. Barnes PF, El-Hajj H, Preston-Martin S, Cave MD, Jones BE, Otaya M, Pogoda J, Eisenach KD. Transmission of tuberculosis among the homeless. JAMA 1996; 275:305–307.
46. Wünsch-Filho V, Moncau JEC, Nakao N. Methodological considerations in case-control studies to evaluate vaccine effectiveness. Int J Epidemiol 1993; 22(1):149–155.
47. Rodrigues LC, Kiwan VK, Wheeler JG. Protective effect of BCG against tuberculous meningitis and miliary tuberculosis: a meta-analysis. Int J Epidemiol 1993; 22(6):1154–1158.
48. Clarke A, Rudd P. Neonatal BCG immunisation. Arch Dis Child 1992; 67:473–474.

9

Fungal Infections

Laurent Christin and Alan M. Sugar
Boston University Medical Center, Boston, Massachusetts

INTRODUCTION

Fungal infections of the central nervous system have been recognized for decades and characteristically occur with certain pathogenic fungi such as *Cryptococcus neoformans* or *Coccidioidomyces immitis*. Because of their increasing incidence, fungal infections have gained much attention over the last 20 years. The reasons for this observed trend are numerous, but pertain mainly to a growing population of immunologically deficient patients, be it from infection, malignancy, medications, or congenital conditions. In addition, increasingly invasive procedures and devices facilitate the entry of microorganisms beyond natural barriers like the skin or mucous membranes. The liberal use of potent broad-spectrum antibacterials results in the selection of intrinsically resistant microorganisms, including fungi. This chapter focuses on the predisposing conditions, clinical presentation, diagnosis, and management of the major central nervous system fungal infections.

CRYPTOCOCCOSIS

Epidemiology and Microbiology

Cryptococcus neoformans has been recognized for decades as a major fungal pathogen in humans (1). This encapsulated yeastlike fungus has a worldwide distribution, and a rising incidence of cryptococcosis had been documented well before the onset of the acquired immunodeficiency syndrome (AIDS) epidemic (2). Cryptococcosis is of special interest to neurologists since meningitis is the most common clinical manifestation of cryptococcosis in AIDS and non-AIDS patients (1,3,4). A rarity 15 years ago, this disease is now quite familiar to physicians who care for AIDS patients. Cryptococcal meningitis affects 6–10% of patients with AIDS, typically when the circulating CD4–T–lymphocyte count is less than 100 cells/mm^3 (5). These epidemiological trends and the improvements of outcome yielded by effective treatment call for a high awareness of a disease otherwise inevitably fatal when untreated.

The ecology and epidemiology of *C. neoformans* has recently been reviewed (6). Five serogroups have been defined—A,B,C,D, and AD—according to antigenic characteristics of the fungus's typical capsule. Serogroups A, D (*Cryptococcus neoformans* var. *neoformans*), and AD predominate in temperate climates like Europe, Japan, or the United States, except southern California, where serogroups B and C (*Cryptococcus neoformans* var. *gatti*) are frequent, as they tend to be in subtropical and tropical areas. This ubiquitous fungus is readily grown at 30°C on appropriate media and can be characterized through pigment production, urease activity, and genetic probes.

Exposure to bird droppings and thus to the fungus is presumably extensive among all human and animal populations, but immune-competent hosts have no trouble containing and eradicating the microorganism (6). Once in the alveoli, the fungus builds up a thick capsule, which impairs efficient host defenses (7). When the process extends beyond a localized pneumonitis, extrapulmonary dissemination occurs, preferentially localizing in the meninges, the skin, and the urinary tract, although it can affect virtually any organ (1,4). Dissemination occurs chiefly in immune-compromised patients with deficient cell-mediated immunity such as transplant recipients, AIDS patients, patients with hematological malignancies or collagen vascular diseases, or patients receiving high-dose steroids. It is extremely common, particularly for AIDS patients, to present with isolated meningitis without simultaneous or prior manifestations of respiratory tract involvement (5). Structural constituents of the human immunodeficiency virus (HIV) (gp 120) have been shown to impair the phagocytic efficiency of macrophages (8). Although cryptococcosis has been reported in patients without identifiable immune dysfunction (9,10), current experience suggests that these patients most likely have an underlying predisposition to the disease yet to be characterized.

Several hypotheses have attempted to explain why the disease preferentially localizes in the central nervous system. The cerebrospinal fluid (CSF) is a good culture media for cryptococci; it lacks complement and other possible anticryptococcal factors found in the serum (11). In addition, cryptococci trigger a weak meningeal inflammatory response possibly because of the local scarcity of mediators of inflammation and the influence of the polysaccharide capsule. This accounts for the usual subacute presentation of cryptococcal meningitis. Parenchymal brain lesions (cryptococcomas) are unusual (12); however, disseminated parenchymal involvement occurs as an invasive continuum from meningeal infection.

Clinical Presentation

Many patients present only with longstanding fever and sometimes headaches. Neck stiffness, photophobia, nausea, or vomiting occur in approximately one third of the patients. Encephalopathy with lethargy, personality changes, or memory dysfunction affects a minority of patients and forewarns of a worst outcome (13). Seizures and focal neurological deficits are unusual. The fundoscopic examination can reveal papilledema; acute blindness from optic neuritis or intracranial hypertension is a rare but typically irreversible complication (14). Computerized tomography of the brain can show meningeal enhancement or rarely a ring-enhancing lesion of a cryptococcoma (12). Routine blood chemistry and blood count are not helpful; abnormalities may reflect unrelated underlying processes.

Diagnosis

A definitive diagnosis requires culture of the microorganism; blood and urine culture obtained as part of a fever workup can reveal the fungemia, especially in AIDS patients. The recovery of

Cryptococcus neoformans from any body fluid or tissue specimen mandates central nervous system evaluation. A skin or a bone marrow biopsy sometimes shows the typical yeast. In the appropriate clinical situation, a presumptive diagnosis is made through visualization of encapsulated yeasts in tissue sections or detection of the cryptococcal antigen in body fluids (1,3). The sensitivity of this test is high (99%) (15); a serum titer of ≥1:8 is usually considered positive and suggestive of disseminated infection (1,4). The cryptococcin skin test is poorly standardized and has no diagnostic utility. The CSF parameters are frequently minimally abnormal and are similar to those encountered in other chronic meningitides (15,16). There is usually a CSF pleocytosis of <100 cells/mm^3, mainly lymphocytes, and the protein and glucose concentrations are frequently within the normal range. Presumptive identification of the yeast by India ink stain of the CSF is achieved in 74% of AIDS patients (15) and more than 50% of non-AIDS patients (1,16). An elevated opening pressure, a high protein concentration, a low glucose concentration, a leukocyte count of <20/mm^3, and a CSF cryptococcal antigen titer of >1:1024 at the onset are indicators of a worse prognosis (13,16).

Management, Treatment, and Outcome

Untreated cryptococcal meningitis is uniformly fatal, albeit there have been reports of extended survival of untreated patients (1). In addition to the use of an effective anticryptococcal agent, correction of the underlying immune deficiency should be attempted. Amphotericin B (AMB), 0.5–0.8 mg/kg/day, has been the antifungal agent of choice for the treatment of cryptococcal meningitis (3,17) (Table 1). 5-Fluorocytosine (flucytosine) is a valuable anticryptococcal agent, but it should never be used alone because resistance develops (18). Intrathecal AMB infused through a subcutaneous reservoir is rarely necessary (3).

The standard duration of treatment using both AMB and flucytosine in non-AIDS patients is 6 weeks, although a 4-week course has been successful in otherwise healthy patients (19). The main criterion for response to treatment is the patient's clinical course; ongoing treatment is classically indicated until four consecutive weekly CSF cultures return negative (3). Subsequent CSF analysis may not correlate closely with the clinical evolution. CSF India ink and cryptococcal antigen can remain positive while cultures become sterile (1). When comparing titers of cryptococcal antigen in any body fluid (including the CSF) in the same patient over time, it is recommended to use the same laboratory and to run all samples each time in parallel (1). This is frequently too cumbersome for clinical purposes, and therefore any change in cryptococcal antigen titer should be interpreted with respect to the patient's clinical course. By the end of the treatment course, the CSF glucose concentration should be normal or normalizing, if initially decreased (3). The protein concentration, on the other hand, is a poor indicator of response and can remain abnormal for months, bearing no predictive significance for outcome or risk of relapse (1,5). Patients in whom AMB cannot be used should be treated with fluconazole (400 mg/day PO or IV for 6–8 weeks followed by life-long suppressive therapy; see below) (13,20) or itraconazole (600 mg/day PO for 3 days then 400 mg/day PO for 6–8 weeks followed by life-long suppressive therapy; see Table 1) (21), bearing in mind that inferences from studies with AIDS patients may not apply to all patients. Chronic suppressive therapy with fluconazole should probably be offered for as long as the immune suppression is present, although no convincing data in non-AIDS individuals are available at this time. Monthly follow-up should occur for at least 1 year since relapses tend to occur most frequently during this period (1,3). The management of the relapse is similar to that of an initial episode; if a favorable outcome is achieved, prolonged secondary prophylaxis with an oral antifungal agent is advisable.

Whereas cure is the treatment intention in non-AIDS patients, clinical remission and prevention of relapse are currently the goals of cryptococcal meningitis management in AIDS patients

Table 1 Suggested Diagnostic Studies and Treatments of Disseminated Fungal Infections Involving the Central Nervous System

Fungus	Diagnostic studies	Treatment of choice	Alternative	Comments
Cryptococcus neoformans	Culture: (blood, CSF, urine, tissue) Antigen: (blood, CSF) Stains: GMS, India ink (sputum, BAL, biopsy)	Amphotericin B (0.5–0.8 mg/kg·d IV) ± Flucytosine (12.5–25 mg qid PO)	Fluconazole (400 mg/d PO/IV) ± Flucytosine (12.5–25 mg qid PO)	In meningitis, AMB usually given for the first 2 weeks, followed by fluconazole if clinical response is favorable. Patients who are at risk of relapse should be kept on secondary prophylaxis (fluconazole 200 mg/d PO; itraconazole 200 mg/d PO) (207). Steroids should be avoided.
Coccidioidomyces immitis	Culture: (blood, CSF, synovial, etc) Serology: IgM (TP) titer (blood) IgG (CF) titer (blood, CSF) Stains: GMS, (biopsy, BAL)	Amphotericin B (0.6–0.8 mg/kg·d IV) + Amphotericin B (0.5–1.5 mg/d IT or intraventricular)	Fluconazole[a] (800–1200 mg/d PO/IV) Itraconazole (200 mg bid PO) Ketoconazole (400–800 mg/d PO)	High-dose intrathecal (IT) AMB (with 25–50 mg hydrocortisone to decrease side effects) has had good results. Patients who are at risk of relapse should be kept on secondary prophylaxis (weekly AMB IV or fluconazole 200–400 mg/d PO). IV steroids are sometimes used when vasculitis is present.
Blastomyces dermatitidis	Culture: (biopsy, BAL, blood, CSF) Stains: GMS (BAL, biopsy)	Amphotericin B (0.5–0.8 mg/kg·d IV) for severe disease Itraconazole (200 mg bid PO)	Itraconazole (200 mg bid PO) Ketoconazole (400 mg bid PO)	There is no accepted alternative to AMB for severe disease and infections involving the central nervous system. Patients who are at risk of relapse should probably be kept on secondary prophylaxis (ketoconazole 400 mg/d PO).

Histoplasma capsulatum	Culture: (blood, CSF, tissue, etc) Stains: GMS (BM, lung, liver) Antigen: [HPA] titer? (CSF, blood) Serology: ? IgG (CF) titer (CSF)	Amphotericin B (0.6–0.8 mg/kg·d IV) for severe disease Itraconazole (200 mg bid PO)	Itraconazole (200 mg bid PO)	Intrathecal AMB not useful. Patients who are at risk of relapse should be kept on secondary prophylaxis (itraconazole 200 mg bid PO; fluconazole 200 mg/d PO).
Aspergillus sp.	Culture: (biopsy) Stains: GMS (BM, lung, liver) Serology: ? (IgG) Antigen: ?	Amphotericin B (0.8–1.0 mg/kg·d IV) ± Flucytosine (20–25 mg qid PO)	Itraconazole (200 mg bid PO)	Itraconazole not evaluated for CNS infection yet. Rifampin (600 mg/d) is controversial. Steroids are used for allergic bronchopulmonary aspergillosis. IgG serology has low specificity; antigen detection is experimental.
Candida sp.	Culture: (blood, CSF urine, biopsy, devices) Stains: GMS	Amphotericin B (0.5–0.7 mg/kg·d IV) ± Flucytosine (20–25 mg qid PO)	Fluconazole (200–400 mg/d PO/IV) or Itraconazole (200 mg bid PO)	Neither azole evaluated for CNS infection. Infected VP shunt must be removed.
Mucor sp.	Stains: GMS (biopsy) Culture: biopsy	Amphotericin B (1.0–1.5 mg/kg·d IV)	None	Treatment should start immediately once the fungus is suspected on biopsy specimen. Extensive surgical debridement of necrotic tissues is mandatory. Attempt to correct underlying predisposing conditions (ketoacidosis, neutropenia, etc).

AMB: Amphotericin B; BAL: bronchoalveolar lavage; BM: bone marrow; CF: complement fixation; CSF: cerebrospinal fluid; HPA: histoplasma polysaccharide antigen; GMS: Gomori methenamine silver stain; TP: tube precipitin.

[a]Fluconazole at this high dose is considered by some to be first-line therapy for coccidioidal meningitis.

(5). Although not routinely done because of a concern for bone marrow toxicity in already immunocompromised patients, flucytosine (75–100 mg/day PO in divided doses) can be successfully used with a reasonable range of safety in selected AIDS patients (22), in concert with AMB or an azole medication; close monitoring of serum flucytosine level is mandatory. Since the advent of oral triazole antifungal agents in the mid-1980s, several studies have compared their efficacy with that of AMB (13,22,23). Overall, AMB seems to offer some advantage over oral antifungal agents for initial treatment, mainly because of a more rapid CSF sterilization. A recent study, however, has shown that the association of fluconazole with flucytosine achieved CSF sterilization in 75% of patients after 10 weeks of treatment (24).

Hydrocephalus with elevation of the intracranial pressure is sometimes a major issue in the management of cryptococcal meningitis; ventricular shunting is required when vision or survival are at stake (5). Multiple, frequent large-volume lumbar punctures may be an alternative to shunting. The benefit and risk of using steroids in this situation are unknown, and they should be avoided. Acetazolamide has been used to decrease CSF production.

In non-AIDS patients, death from cryptococcal meningitis treated with AMB is in the range of 25–30%. Twenty-five percent of those initially cured eventually relapse; 40% have residual neurological deficits such as dementia, visual loss, and cranial nerve palsies; hydrocephalus can occur long after any evidence of active disease has vanished (1,3). In AIDS patients, the mortality rate of cryptococcal meningitis is 10–25% with most of the deaths occurring during the first 2 weeks of therapy. Response rates to AMB vary between 50 and 100%, but relapses occur in 50–60% of patients not taking suppressive therapy (5,25). Recurrence occurs as a consequence of reactivation rather than reinfection (22,26). Administration of oral fluconazole (200 mg/day) is now the standard management of these patients once clinical remission is achieved. The risk of relapse is markedly diminished with this suppressive regimen (27–29). Monitoring the serum cryptococcal antigen titer does not help predict impending relapse (29,30). There have been reports of *C. neoformans* resistant to fluconazole, and the chronic use of fairly low-dose antifungal prophylaxis may also have some impact on the sensitivity profile of other fungi such as *C. albicans* (5,30). Primary prophylaxis with oral triazoles for prevention of cryptococcosis in AIDS patients has shown some benefit (31) but needs additional evaluation.

COCCIDIOIDOMYCOSIS

Epidemiology and Microbiology

Coccidioides immitis is endemic to the southwestern United States and parts of Central and South America (32–34). In these arid areas, *C. immitis* grows as a mycelia, which releases airborne arthroconidia. These may be inhaled, and, once in the alveoli, they transform into spherules containing endospores. When the spherules rupture, they release numerous endospores, which resume a similar multiplication cycle, progressively invading the surrounding tissue.

In endemic areas of North America, *C. immitis* affects up to 100,000 persons per year (35). This incidence varies somewhat with each year's weather pattern, and recent outbreaks in California have been attributed to unusually high amounts of rainfall during spring following a protracted drought (36,37) or to high levels of airborne dust exposure (38).

Clinical Presentation

Serological surveys during outbreaks have demonstrated that most patients (>60%) remain asymptomatic despite seroconversion (34,36); few present with a limited pneumonitis with fever and some protracted cough; erythema nodosum and inflammatory arthritis sometimes follow the acute episode (39). Dissemination occurs in less than 1% of the patients, and among these, less than 5% will have CNS involvement—mainly chronic meningitis (40). Other sites of dissemination include skin, bone, and joints. The fungus has been isolated in numerous tissues (39). Patients of African-American, Hispanic, and Filipino descent have a higher risk of dissemination (33,39); the disease tends to be more severe in nonimmune pregnant patients, with the risk of dissemination increasing with the progression of the pregnancy (39,41). In AIDS patients, the disease is usually disseminated at the time of diagnosis and meningitis is a fairly common initial presentation in this population (42,43). Reactivation of dormant disease or de novo infection both occur in transplant recipients (44). Diabetes does not predispose to infection (39) or more severe disease.

Coccidioidal infection of the central nervous system (CNS) is a disastrous event and is invariably fatal if untreated. The delay between the initial infection and the symptoms of CNS involvement varies from weeks to years; meningitis can be the first manifestation of the disease in up to a third of patients (45). The spectrum of the clinical presentation is extremely variable (33,39,45,46). Patients can present with vague symptoms: headaches, low-grade fever, weight loss, and night sweats are common. Mental status changes, confusion, and lethargy are present in half of the patients. Nuchal rigidity and cranial nerve palsies are uncommon. Coccidioidal spinal arachnoiditis with lower extremity ataxia and spastic paraparesis has been described (47). Seizures and focal neurological deficits usually represent cerebral or spinal parenchymal involvement (48–51). Routine laboratory studies are nonspecific. Eosinophilia has been observed in some patients (52).

CNS computed tomography is abnormal in two thirds of the patients (53,54). Hydrocephalus, sometimes asymmetrical, and basilar enhancement are the most common findings. White matter lesions, usually subcortical, hypodense, and moderately enhancing (51), are encountered in up to 40% of the patients (54). Unless there is hemorrhage from a bleeding mycotic aneurysm, dense lesions are unusual (55).

The CSF opening pressure is sometimes elevated; analysis typically shows a lymphocytic pleocytosis, elevated protein, and moderately decreased glucose concentrations consistent with a chronic meningitis (40,45). Coccidioidal meningitis can present as an eosinophilic meningitis (>10% eosinophils) (56,57). The ventricular fluid tends to show less abnormal values than fluid obtained from lumbar or cisternal spaces (34). Visualization of spherules in the CSF is rare, but positive cultures can be obtained in up to a third of the patients, especially when large volumes of CSF are cultured (45).

Diagnosis

A definitive diagnosis is established by culture or visualization of typical *C. immitis* spherules in body fluids or biopsy specimens (39,45). The skin test is useful for epidemiological surveys but has no role in diagnostic evaluation since false-negative results are common and positive results only indicate prior exposure to the fungus. Positive blood cultures occur in 12–33%; fungemia is characteristic of severely immunocompromised patients, who rarely survive more than a month, and seems to correlate with the overall fungal load (58).

Serology is useful to diagnose coccidioidomycosis (39,59). The serum IgM or tube precipitin (TP) titer rises transiently in early infection. The serum IgG titer, or complement fixing (CF) antibody, rises later in the course of the disease; a serum CF titer of ≥1:16 is suggestive of extrathoracic infection (33) and a titer of ≥1:64 correlates with disseminated disease and a worse outcome (36). Unlike the TP titer, the CF antibody can be measured in CSF; the detection of specific IgG is virtually diagnostic of coccidioidal meningitis but can be negative early in the course of the disease. Despite their immune deficiency, most (90%) AIDS patients and transplant recipients have positive serologies (43,44). To some extent, the serum CF titer has a similar prognostic value in these patients. Their clinical presentation does not differ markedly from that of immunocompetent patients with the exception of a much higher frequency of positive CSF cultures (60% vs. <5%) (42,43). Disseminated (miliary) coccidioidomycosis with negative CF titer results occurs in AIDS patients (43), as it does in immune competent individuals, both early in the course and in far advanced disease.

The neuropathology of *C. immitis* infection is extremely diverse (49,60). In his report on 32 patients with premortem diagnosis of CNS coccidioidomycosis, Sobel et al. (60) identified meningitis in all of them; in six patients, the disease appeared limited to the CNS. Basilar meningitis is characteristic, with occasional obliteration of the subarachnoid space due to the inflammation. Microscopically, extensive fibrosis combines with lymphocytes, macrophages, and histiocytes and *C. immitis* spherules. Arteritis (endarteritis obliterans) affects small arteries and arterioles; endothelial proliferation, edema, and luminal obstruction are responsible for focal necrosis predominantly in the basal ganglia, thalamus, and white matter. Infarctions of the brain stem, spinal cord, and other areas are rare, as is miliary granulomatous dissemination involving the white matter. Fibrosing arachnoiditis with foci of necrosis sometimes affects the spinal cord. Brain abscess (51) and polyaneurysmal mycotic arteritis are unusual features (55).

Management, Treatment, and Outcome

The management of CNS coccidioidomycosis includes both antifungal therapy and treatment of complications. AMB given both intravenously (IV) (initial dose 0.6–0.8 mg/kg·day) and intrathecally (IT) (0.1–0.5 mg/day via reservoir), has been the standard treatment of CNS coccidioidomycosis (33,36,39) (Table 1); intraventricular infusion is used for ventriculitis (34). The need for IT AMB is supported by an excessive amount of treatment failure with systemic therapy alone. The duration of treatment is poorly defined but usually lasts for months, with progressive decrease in AMB infusion. This frequently requires the placement of an Ommaya reservoir (61), and the additional complications of arachnoiditis and bacterial superinfection (62). AMB has also been implicated in toxic vacuolar myelopathy with Brown-Séquard syndrome (63,64). The response to treatment should be evaluated clinically and by serial CSF analysis, cell count, cultures, and CF titers. Both the CSF glucose and protein concentrations can remain abnormal for years (33). The cell count is quite unreliable since it tends to decrease spontaneously in untreated CNS coccidioidomycosis (40) and may be affected by simultaneous arachnoiditis or IT AMB itself (65). Nevertheless, a sudden rise in cell count or CSF CF titer can herald a relapse and call for more intense antifungal therapy. Using a maintenance dose (up to 1.5 mg/dose every other day) of intrathecal AMB combined with 25–50 mg hydrocortisone (with simultaneous IV AMB administration), Labadie and Hamilton reported a survival rate of approximately 90% over a 75-month follow-up period (64). The use of steroids has been advocated when CNS coccidioidomycosis presents with vasculitic manifestations (stroke) (49). Overall, isolated meningitis has a better prognosis than CNS infection associated with other clinical indicators of disseminated disease (40).

Ketoconazole was the first oral antifungal agent used in the treatment of coccidioidomycosis (66–68). Control of CNS infection was obtained only with a high dose of ketoconazole and was associated with significant toxicity. Fluconazole as a single agent has had promising results (68,69) in non-HIV– as well as HIV-infected individuals, achieving a 79% response rate with minor side effects despite the use of a relatively low dose (400 mg/day PO). Patients with shunted hydrocephalus, in whom the administration of intrathecal AMB is frequently ineffective, had a similar good outcome (33,68). Itraconazole has been used with some success to treat relapse or meningitis refractory to AMB (IV and IT), miconazole, ketoconazole, or fluconazole (69,70). Consideration can now be given to the use of high-dose fluconazole (800–1200 mg/day PO) as initial therapy. Several years of treatment might be necessary since relapse tends to occur when treatment is stopped (69). Due to the low toxicity of these agents, it is customary to keep patients who relapse or who are at risk of relapse on suppressive therapy indefinitely, whether immune compromised or not (33,34).

BLASTOMYCOSIS

Epidemiology and Microbiology

Blastomyces dermatitidis is a dimorphic fungus growing as a mold at 25–30°C and a yeast at 37°C, the latter being the pathogenic form recovered from human infection. The thick-walled, broad-based single bud of this fungus makes it fairly easy to identify when found in clinical specimens. *B. dermatitidis* is found across Africa, in Central and North America (where it is endemic in the Southeast except Florida), along the Ohio and Mississippi River basins, and around the Great Lakes (71,72). Outbreaks of blastomycosis have been associated with outdoor activities like fishing, hunting, or construction work near waterways where decaying wood and animal dropping are found (73,74). Most commonly, the volatile conidia are inhaled; rare instances of percutaneous infections have been well documented (75,76). Although disseminated disease and serious complications are more frequently encountered in immunocompromised patients (77,78), the AIDS epidemic has not affected the epidemiology of blastomycosis to any extent comparable to its effect on the epidemiology of cryptococcosis (79).

Clinical Presentation

Blastomycosis is essentially a pulmonary disease (71). Dissemination most frequently affects the skin, bones, and prostate. Central nervous infection is rare and is almost exclusively a manifestation of disseminated disease (80). The alveolar macrophages are able to phagocytize the conidia and prevent its transformation into the pathogenic yeast (81,82). When these mechanisms are defective or overwhelmed, the disease becomes locally invasive and triggers a striking inflammatory reaction. Patients often complain of flulike illness with symptoms of community-acquired pneumonia (71,72,83). The chest radiograph often shows nonspecific infiltrates predominantly at the bases (83); extensive pneumonitis with adult respiratory distress syndrome is a feared manifestation of the infection (84). Many infections go unrecognized as demonstrated by serological surveys during outbreaks (74,85). Distant reactivation in the lung, the skin, the urinary tract, or the central nervous system occurs sometimes months to years after the initial infection (72).

CNS blastomycosis is diagnosed in 3–10% of all infected patients, although it is found at autopsy in as many as 30% of those dying of disseminated disease (80,86). CNS involvement is more frequent in non–HIV-immunocompromised patients (77) than in immunocompetent patients, and strikingly moreso in AIDS patients (77,87). The major role of macrophages and T-cell–mediated defense mechanisms has been stressed recently (82,88); like several other fungal infections, blastomycosis is typically a disseminated process in AIDS patients (89), owing to impaired T-cell–mediated immunity. A clinically identifiable focus of infection outside the nervous system is found in most patients. However, the manifestations of these various sites of infection can occur at different times, making the diagnosis quite challenging. Isolated CNS infections occur in less than 5% of patients (80,87); most are found to have a subclinical infection elsewhere at autopsy (80).

The symptoms of CNS blastomycosis can be subtle, and delayed diagnosis is common. Fever, fatigue, headaches, malaise, weight loss, and specific symptoms and signs from other affected organs are encountered with variable frequencies. The neurological manifestations of CNS blastomycosis are nonspecific and reflect the location of the infectious process. Lethargy, focal deficits, or seizures are suggestive of parenchymal brain infections (90,91). Headache with neck stiffness is present when meningeal inflammation is prominent. Chronic meningitis has a more smoldering course with subtle cranial nerve abnormalities or signs and symptoms of hydrocephalus (90–92). Parenchymal brain infections (cerebritis) or meningitis occur with somewhat similar frequencies (80,87,90). Out of 802 cases of disseminated blastomycosis reviewed by Roos, 8.9% had CNS involvement; of these, 40% had parenchymal brain infection (abscesses or granuloma), 37% had a suppurative meningitis, and 23% had a chronic meningitis (80).

Diagnosis

Some authors have suggested that the radiological features of CNS fungal infections have specific patterns depending upon the species of offending microorganism (93,94). *B. dermatitidis* presents sometimes with a single or multiple homogeneously enhancing lesions on computerized tomography, which correspond to granuloma or blastomycoma; little inflammation and edema surrounds these rather chronic forms of infection. Chronic blastomycotic meningitis predominantly involves the basilar meninges (90,93); computerized tomography has limitations for demonstrating meningeal disease but reliably detects hydrocephalus. The role of magnetic resonance imaging has yet to be defined in CNS blastomycosis (95).

Results of CSF analysis are extremely variable. A highly inflammatory meningitis is not unusual. Unlike other fungal meningitis, where a lymphocytic pleocytosis is usual, *B. dermatitidis* meningitis frequently presents with a polymorphonuclear neutrophil (PMN) CSF pleocytosis (96); a purulent CSF with cell count of $>5000/mm^3$ is not uncommon. A markedly decreased CSF glucose concentration (<30 mg/dl) is found in 64% of patients and protein concentrations average 199 mg/dl (96). These features are very similar to those of bacterial meningitis. Identification of *B. dermatitidis* on lumbar CSF examination is rare; cisternal or ventricular fluid may have better sensitivity. Also, the culture of cisternal or ventricular CSF has a better yield than that of lumber CSF (85% vs. 10%, respectively) (92). No reliable *B. dermatitidis* antigen detection test is currently available. *B. dermatitidis* has been isolated from blood cultures using lysis centrifugation (97). The diagnosis relies mainly on microscopic identification of the fungus in exudates or tissue samples from other organs such as the lung, skin, or prostate. Skin testing, serological diagnosis (complement fixation, immunodiffusion), and enzyme immunoassay are of limited use for diagnostic purposes (72,98).

Management, Treatment, and Outcome

The treatment of blastomycosis depends upon the extent of the disease and the patient's underlying condition (72,99). There have been case reports where ketoconazole cured a lung or skin infection while CNS involvement progressed on treatment (91,100); close follow-up is therefore essential. AMB remains the drug of choice for life-threatening disease and for CNS infections (Table 1). Initial AMB therapy (0.5–0.8 mg/kg·day) followed by lifelong suppressive therapy with itraconazole (200 mg/day PO) is recommended in AIDS patients (79); however, definitive recommendations cannot be provided for management of non-HIV–immunocompromised patients, it seems judicious to use similar suppressive measures until the immune dysfunction has been reversed (77,98). Fluconazole has been used with only moderate success at doses of 200–400 mg/day PO (101). Itraconazole has been used with good success and can be considered equivalent to ketoconazole for the treatment and suppressive therapy of blastomycosis not involving the CNS (102).

HISTOPLASMOSIS

Epidemiology and Microbiology

Histoplasma capsulatum is a dimorphic fungus with a worldwide distribution preferentially inhabiting areas with a warm and humid climate. It is heavily endemic to the Ohio and Mississippi river valleys of the Central United States and is also encountered in some areas of Central and South America, the Caribbean islands, and Asia (103,104). This fungus thrives as a mycelium on moist soils enriched with bird and bat excreta and decayed wood found in old buildings and caves. Microconidia can be inhaled when these sites are disturbed by excavation or sanitization of old buildings, for example. In hyperendemic areas, histoplasmosis occurs frequently in outbreaks (105). Following inhalation and conversion of the conidia into yeasts, the alveolar macrophages phagocytize the yeasts, which proliferate rapidly intracellularly in nonimmune individuals, leading to cell death. The fungus then continues to propagate into the surrounding tissues. The development of a competent cell-mediated immune response takes approximately 2 weeks and is essential in limiting the extent of the infection (104).

Clinical Presentation

Only 50% of affected individuals, mostly young children, develop symptoms of pneumonitis with fever and cough (103,104). Arthritis and erythema nodosum, pericarditis, and adult respiratory distress syndrome are sometimes encountered in immune competent individuals. Dissemination is rare (<10%) and is mainly encountered in patients with deficient cellular immunity: AIDS patients (104,106), patients with lymphoreticular malignancies, and transplant recipients (107), for example. Persistent fever, weight loss, and fatigue are associated with symptoms more specific to the various organs involved (108).

Prior to the HIV epidemic, disseminated disease and thus CNS involvement was fairly uncommon. However, autopsy series showed that 25% of patients with disseminated disease had CNS involvement (107–110); most of these patients (75%) had no neurological symptoms (110). AIDS was rapidly recognized as a significant predisposing condition to dissemination and therefore to CNS histoplasmosis (106,111).

CNS histoplasmosis consists of three main pathological entities: (1) a meningitis (≥60%), typically subacute or chronic, isolated (25%) or as part of a disseminated process, (2) a solitary abscess (histoplasmoma) (112) or multiple lesions, and (3) a combination of the above. The clinical picture can therefore consist of nonspecific symptoms like fever, sweats, weight loss, headaches (17–25%), lethargy (26%) and confusion (17%), cranial nerve palsy (17%), stroke (19%), seizure (10–28%), personality changes (10–17%) and coma; meningismus is rare (7%). Isolated spinal infection (<3%) is exceptional (112). Most patients (>90%) diagnosed with CNS histoplasmosis have abnormal brain computerized tomography showing hydrocephalus, basilar meningitis, solitary or disseminated contrast-enhancing lesions, or various combinations. The delay between a presumed or confirmed initial (pulmonary) infection and CNS manifestations varies from weeks to years (114); a trend toward earlier diagnosis has been attributed to the combined influences of AIDS and recent outbreaks of the disease in endemic areas, where health care providers are highly aware of the risk of fungal infection (111).

When meningitis is present, the CSF pleocytosis is typically moderate (≤100 cells/mm^3), essentially lymphocytic, though a predominance of PMN leukocytes occurs (111). As with other subacute or chronic meningitides, the CSF protein concentration is increased (⩾10%), whereas the glucose concentration is usually decreased (⩾80%). Identification of the fungus on CSF India ink stain is rare (115). In disseminated infections, and particularly so in AIDS patients, the CSF culture is frequently positive (25–50%) as are blood, bone marrow, or urine cultures (111,116); in most instances, one CSF culture out of several is positive, stressing the need for repetitive attempts (⩾3) to isolate the fungus using large volumes of centrifuged CSF (111); cisternal or ventricular sampling of CSF has better yield and should be considered when the diagnosis is uncertain. When the clinical presentation features predominantly parenchymal rather than meningeal symptoms, CSF abnormalities can be absent or minimal.

Diagnosis

The detection of anti-Histoplasma antibodies (CF) (IgG, complement fixing) in serum and CSF (117) is quite sensitive (69 and 75%, respectively) but does not allow for a definitive diagnosis since their presence can merely reflect long-standing immunity (118). In the CSF, a complement fixation titer (IgG) of >1:8 is nevertheless suggestive of meningitis. The histoplasma polysaccharide antigen (HPA) detection test has been developed recently (116,119); the presence of the antigen in the CSF is a reliable indicator of CNS involvement, but cross-reactions with *C. immitis*, *C. neoformans*, and *Candida* have been reported (106). Although useful in epidemiological surveys, the skin test has no role in the diagnosis of active histoplasmosis. Biopsy of a suitable parenchymal lesion can rapidly provide the diagnosis. Meningeal biopsy is rarely performed for diagnosis because of the propensity of the fungus to produce an inflammatory response predominately in the basilar cisterns and the morbidity associated with a biopsy of this area.

Histoplasma meningitis consists mainly of a basilar mononuclear infiltrate with granulomatous reaction and fibrosis, sometimes entrapping cranial nerves. The proliferative (112) and infiltrative (granulomatous, pseudotubercle) (120) vasculitis with occasional necrosis and thrombosis accounts for the ischemic manifestations. Parenchymal granulomata are sometimes encapsulated and can display central caseous necrosis. The yeast is occasionally identified at the interface of healthy tissue with vascular or parenchymal lesions (120). Isolated spinal arachnoiditis (113) or granuloma (121) are unusual. Endocarditis and adrenal infection are frequently associated with CNS histoplasmosis. Although routine evaluation for endocarditis is not warranted, the assessment of adrenal function should be performed since any abnormalities are readily correctable (111).

Management, Treatment, and Outcome

Intravenous AMB (initial dose 0.6–0.8 mg/kg·day) (Table 1) remains the mainstay of treatment of disseminated and CNS histoplasmosis (122), although reports of patients successfully treated with oral itraconazole (200 mg/day bid for 3 days, then 200 mg bid for several weeks) might eventually challenge this standard (102). Itraconazole has proven to be the best currently available oral agent against CNS histoplasmosis despite its poor penetration into the CSF. A favorable clinical response to treatment is expected within 7–10 days of initiating treatment. The cure rate of CNS histoplasmosis in non-AIDS patients is less than 50%; almost half relapse within 2 years of the diagnosis and ⩾20% die of the infection. This compares dismally with disseminated histoplasmosis not involving the CNS where the cure rate reaches 90% with AMB or itraconazole. The benefit of adding intrathecal to intravenous AMB administration to treat CNS histoplasmosis has not been thoroughly studied and appears to be limited (111). AIDS patients with histoplasmosis are unlikely to be cured by AMB or itraconazole (123). Chronic suppressive therapy with itraconazole or perhaps fluconazole is therefore recommended. As with all disseminated fungal infections, a close long-term follow up is essential.

ASPERGILLOSIS

Epidemiology and Microbiology

Aspergillus species belong to a group of filamentous fungi (124) and are ubiquitous. Of the numerous known species of *Aspergillus*, only a handful are opportunistic pathogens to humans, with *A. fumigatus* being the most frequently identified. This saprophytic mold thrives on decaying organic substrates and releases conidia, which are inhaled by the host. The mold is responsible for three main noninvasive manifestations, namely, extrinsic allergic alveolitis (sometimes known as "malt worker's lung"), allergic bronchopulmonary aspergillosis (which presents like asthma and has fairly strict diagnostic criteria), and aspergilloma such as found "colonizing" pulmonary cavities formed by a healed necrotizing process (125).

Clinical Presentation

In immune-competent hosts, inhaled conidia are normally readily killed by the combined effort of alveolar macrophages and polymorphonuclear neutrophils (126). Conditions that will either alter the function or decrease the number of these potent effector cells are well known and include chronic granulomatous disease, prolonged neutropenia, high-dose steroid therapy, and other immunosuppressive medications for cancer treatment or organ transplantation (127–129).

Aspergillosis of the brain and adjacent structures is usually a result of a disseminated infection (130,131). Isolated aspergilloma are unusual (132), except for intravenous drug users, who are at particular risk for fungal brain abscesses (133,134). In bone marrow transplant recipients, fungi are the most common cause of brain abscesses (57%) and *Aspergillus* accounts for most (33%) of these (135). Invasive aspergillosis remains a fairly unusual occurrence in AIDS patients, suggesting a limited role of T-lymphocyte–mediated immunity in controlling this infection (136,137).

CNS aspergillosis is frequently an autopsy finding owing to difficulty in premortem diagnosis (138). *Aspergillus* has a characteristic affinity for vascular invasion leading to hemorrhage, hence the high occurrence of hemoptysis characteristic of pulmonary parenchymal vascular involvement. Once present in various tissues, multiplication occurs locally, allowing for further angioinvasive propagation, vascular necrosis, and thrombosis. Therefore, CNS aspergillosis typically occurs preferentially along major vascular territories, particularly the posterior circulation (139) and presents frequently as isolated or multiple ischemic infarctions or subarachnoid hemorrhage from a ruptured mycotic aneurysm. Extension into the subarachnoid space causes meningitis, a very unusual entity (138,140). In the appropriate setting, an acute focal neurological event should prompt the physician to include aspergillosis in the differential diagnosis. Hemiparesis, unilateral ataxia, dysarthria, focal or generalized seizures, confusion progressing rapidly to coma and death are common (138).

Parenchymal infarctions, hemorrhages, or abscesses are easily identified by computerized tomography (93); neutropenic patients, however, may only have focal CNS edema on computerized tomography. Isolated thoracic spinal cord involvement presenting with symptoms of compression has been reported (141).

Since meningitis is most unusual, CSF analysis is usually not helpful. When there is a parameningeal reaction to the infection, the CSF may have a nonspecific polymorphonuclear pleocytosis and elevation of the protein concentration, while the glucose concentration and opening pressure remain normal (138,140). Because of the fungus's vascular tropism, meningeal involvement can present with a hemorrhagic CSF (138). Aspergillosis is relatively rare in AIDS patients, but is almost always disseminated (141,142); 10–55% of the patients have CNS involvement (136,137); in these patients as well, meningitis is rare.

Diagnosis

A definitive diagnosis of invasive aspergillosis is infrequently made during the patient's lifetime (131,138) except in AIDS patients, possibly because of a greater vigilance by physicians for unusual opportunistic infections (143). In immunocompromised patients, isolation of *Aspergillus* in sputum culture is quite frequent. Although this may represent a risk factor for subsequent invasive aspergillosis (144), the presence of this mold in bronchial secretions is nonspecific. Identification of *Aspergillus* fungemia is exceptional (145), as is a positive CSF culture. Serological diagnosis has limited usefulness since healthy people can harbor antibodies to *Aspergillus* (146). Detection of circulating *Aspergillus* antigens is still experimental and tends to coincide with the extent of the disease (146,147). A presumptive diagnosis can be made from tissue biopsies showing the characteristic invasive septate hyphae; definitive distinction from other fungi, such as *Fusarium* spp., requires culture or the use of specific fluorescent antibodies (147). Access to brain tissue for diagnostic purpose is usually limited (148), but allows sometimes for simultaneous decompression and diagnosis (141,149,150).

Management, Treatment, and Outcome

CNS aspergillosis has a dismal prognosis with a mortality rate exceeding 95% (151), even when patients are receiving appropriate treatment empirically (152). The rare survivors may be left with irreversible sequelae. In addition to providing tissue for pathology and culture, excision of well-demarcated lesions may be of some benefit (135,151). The treatment of CNS aspergillosis relies mainly upon intravenous administration of high-dose AMB (0.8–1.0 mg/kg·day) with flucytosine (75–100 mg/day in four divided doses with close monitoring of serum levels and blood cell counts) (153); AMB should be given for an extended period of time. The benefit of intrathecal AMB in the treatment of CNS aspergillosis has not been ascertained (151). Itraconazole (200 mg tid PO for 3 days, followed by 200 mg bid PO for several weeks) has shown remarkable efficacy in the treatment of invasive pulmonary and bone and joint aspergillosis; its efficacy for treatment of CNS aspergillosis awaits thorough evaluation. The blood level of itraconazole should be measured after 4–7 days to assess its absorption and metabolism (151).

CANDIDIASIS

Epidemiology and Microbiology

Although CNS infections due to *Candida* are unusual, the prevalence of serious infection with this microorganism has increased dramatically recently. *Candida* now accounts for almost 8% of all acute bloodborne sepsis in large medical centers nationwide. This represents an up to 200% increase in candidemia in some major teaching hospitals, such as those managing transplant recipients and cancer patients. In addition to this exploding incidence, the microbiology of *Candida* infection is changing rapidly with increasing isolation of strains less sensitive to currently available antifungal medications.

The main reasons for this dramatic increase in *Candida* and other disseminated fungal infections have been mentioned earlier and include the increasing number of immunocompromised patients, the frequent use of invasive monitoring devices, and broad-spectrum antibiotics. Severe burns, gastrointestinal trauma, or surgery are additional characteristic risk factors associated with severe *Candida* infection. *Candida* adheres to artificial surfaces such as plastics; this is quite relevant to CNS infections since this microorganism can infect ventricular shunts.

Clinical Presentation

CNS infections due to *Candida* consist mainly of meningitis and cerebritis. Both can occur simultaneously, the latter being characterized by parenchymal abscesses of various size and number; granuloma and mycetoma are unusual (154,155). Acute *Candida* meningitis is extremely rare in adults but quite frequent in premature neonates (156,157). In 1978, Parker (158) identified a fungal CNS infection in 0.4% of all patients who were autopsied at the Jackson Memorial Hospital Medical Center over a 10-year period; of the 39 brain tissue specimens with positive histopathology for fungal infections, 49% (19) were determined to be infected by *Candida albicans* through review of available clinical data. Disseminated microabscesses, rarely non-caseating granuloma, were preferentially distributed in the middle cerebral artery territory; thrombotic vasculitis was found in two patients and mycotic aneurysms were demonstrated by angiography; no meningitis was found. This study also established the strong relationship between intravenous cannulation, particularly when used for hyperalimentation, and the onset of disseminated candidiases and subsequent CNS involvement.

The clinical presentation of CNS candidiases exhibits no special features and is rarely suspected while the patient is alive. Specific symptoms such as stiff neck, lethargy, stroke, or even seizures can be blunted by the sedation necessary for mechanical ventilation, for example. A persistent or recurrent fever despite several days of antibiotic treatment may be the only sign of the onset of disseminated candidiasis. Blood cultures have notably poor sensitivity (<50%) for identifying disseminated candidiases. Skin lesions suggestive of disseminated candidiasis should be biopsied and submitted for fungal culture and histopathology (159,160). In this context, a careful fundoscopic examination showing endophthalmitis warrants the initiation of antifungal therapy. Signs or symptoms suggestive of CNS involvement should prompt evaluation through imaging studies and/or CSF analysis. Computerized tomography typically reveals scattered irregular ring-enhancing lesions surrounded by edema (161), but enhancement can be minimal in severely neutropenic patients.

Acute *Candida* meningitis in the absence of systemic dissemination is very unusual and typically follows either an otolaryngological procedure (162,163) or introduction of the fungus into the ventricles or the subarachnoid space through ventricular shunt manipulation (164) or lumbar puncture (165). *Candida* meningitis has been reported long after an episode of disseminated candidemia (166). The manifestations of acute meningitis include fever, headache, and neck pain due to meningeal inflammation (164–167). Chronic or subacute *Candida* meningitis has similar but blunted manifestations (168). Spontaneous isolated meningitis has been reported in AIDS patients (169). The clinical manifestations tend to be similar to those found in non-AIDS patients except that the pleocytosis might be minimal due to the deficient inflammatory response characteristic of severe immune dysfunction.

Candida rarely infects VP shunts (170,171). Although spontaneous infections have been reported, they are frequently associated with shunt manipulation; simultaneous infection with one or more bacteria has been described (172,173). In severely ill patients, an underlying gastrointestinal condition such as a gastrostomy, peptic ulcer disease, or bowel perforation has also been associated with subsequent VP shunt infection by *Candida* (173).

Diagnosis

A definitive diagnosis is made through isolation of the yeast from the CSF or tissue biopsy and culture. The CSF usually shows a pleocytosis (average 600 cells/mm^3), hypoglycorrhachia and increased protein concentration (164). Identification of yeast forms on the CSF smear occurs in 17% of all patients (168), more frequently (43%) in patients with a positive CSF culture (164).

In their recent review of 24 cases of *Candida* VP shunt infections, Sanchez et al. (172) reported that the CSF pleocytosis is usually lymphocytic and moderate (average 78 cells/mm^3); the CSF glucose concentration is rarely less than 30 mg/dl, and the protein concentration is moderately increased (average 107 mg/dl).

Management, Treatment, and Outcome

Although fluconazole has recently been found to be equivalent to AMB for disseminated candidiasis in nonneutropenic patients (174), the standard treatment for CNS infection has been AMB (initial dose 0.6 mg/kg·day IV) with or without flucytosine (70–100 mg/kg·day PO in four divided doses; Table 1) (163,175). Flucytosine should never be used as a single agent since this has been associated with high rates of failure due to the emergence of resistant organisms. Flucytosine is associated with significant bone marrow toxicity. This is a significant concern when treating immunocompromised patients with borderline cell counts. The use of a lower dose (50 mg/kg divided in four daily doses) in adult patients (with normal renal function) with peak and trough serum levels of ≈50 μg/ml and ≤10 μg/ml, respectively, should help decrease toxic complications (175). Selected patients may be considered for therapy with fluconazole or itraconazole, but this decision needs to be made on an individual basis.

Management of *Candida* VP shunt infection includes mandatory shunt removal combined with systemic antifungal therapy (172). CSF sterility should be demonstrated regularly during treatment. If the need for permanent drainage persists, another VP shunt can be inserted at a different site. There are no definite guidelines to assess total treatment duration or when shunt replacement can safely be performed; similarly, the need for subsequent oral antifungal therapy is uncertain.

Overall, the outcome of *Candida* CNS infections is poor; most patients succumb to the complications of the underlying diseases. The direct contribution of CNS *Candida* infection to mortality is therefore difficult to ascertain.

When properly managed, *Candida* VP shunt infection is rarely fatal. As is true for infants, adults who die of *Candida* VP shunt infection frequently have concurrent bacterial meningitis or another underlying lethal condition (172,173).

MUCORMYCOSIS

Epidemiology and Microbiology

The fungi responsible for mucormycosis belong to the order Mucorales, a member of the class Zygomycetes, which also contains the order Entomophthorales (123). Within the order Mucorales, *Absidia*, *Rhizopus*, *Rhizomucor*, and *Mucor* are the most common species recovered from infected patients (176,177). These fungi are ubiquitous, growing on decaying organic materials. When favorable conditions are present, the inhalation of spores is followed by their germination and subsequent growth into blood vessels leading to hemorrhage, thrombosis, and necrosis.

Clinical Presentation

In addition to the rhinocerebral form, the most common manifestation of mucormycosis, the infection has been reported in almost every organ. Primary skin infections have followed trauma, surgery, spider bite, and intravenous catheterization (178). Gastrointestinal mucormycosis was recently reported following liver transplantation (179) and is typically encountered in severely immunocompromised patients. Other conditions predisposing to mucormycosis include diabetic ketoacidosis, malnutrition, and treatment with deferoxamine (175,180). Diffuse pulmonary and disseminated infection occur during prolonged neutropenia. Because of the absence of inflammatory cells, the clinical presentation and results of ancillary studies can be deceptive. Rhinocerebral mucormycosis has also been reported in patients without identifiable predisposing conditions (181,182).

Mucormycosis of the CNS occurs predominantly as a direct extension from the nasal cavity and adjacent sinuses. Isolated mucormycotic brain abscesses are rare but have been reported in intravenous drug abusers (134,183); immunocompromised patients with disseminated infection can present with manifestations of multiple brain infarctions. Alert patients with nasal mucormycosis may complain of fever, facial swelling and pain, headaches, and sometimes epistaxis. Periorbital cellulitis occurs with ophthalmoplegia and blindness, suggesting extension into the orbit (184); invasion of the cavernous sinus and internal carotid artery can present with cranial nerve palsies (185), altered sensorium, and hemiparesis. Extension into the frontal or temporal lobes or the posterior fossa are devastating complications (181,186). Early on, the physical examination should focus on identifying ischemic skin or mucosal areas, while necrotic and hemorrhagic nasal or oral ulcerations are signs of more advanced infection. Invasive disease can present with disseminated ecchymotic skin lesions (187).

Meningitis is not a primary manifestation of CNS infection with Mucorales. Unless the subarachnoid space is involved, the CSF is unremarkable (188) or shows minimal changes (189).

Computerized tomography is extremely helpful as it will distinctively show soft tissue involvement, sinusitis, intraorbital edema, bone destruction, venous thrombosis, brain edema, hemorrhagic infarctions, or space-occupying lesions. Magnetic resonance (MR) scan offers some advantages for assessing the extent of soft tissue involvement and for imaging the posterior fossa (190,191); rarely, the fungal mass has a very low signal and is poorly visualized by MR scan (192). Intravenous drug abusers tend to present with bilateral lesions in the basal ganglia (134).

Diagnosis

The diagnosis of rhinocerebral mucormycosis is usually suspected from a comprehensive clinical evaluation, which should prompt a biopsy of suspicious lesions. The characteristic nonseptate hyphae are easily recognized and mandate immediate treatment; definitive identification of the fungus is achieved through culture.

Management, Treatment, and Outcome

The treatment of disseminated and rhinocerebral mucormycosis includes debridement of all devitalized tissues, high-dose intravenous AMB (0.8–1.0 mg/kg·day), and reversal of identifiable predisposing conditions (176,193). Once the infection is under control, the dose of AMB can be decreased or changed to every-other-day therapy (176). The duration of treatment depends upon the patient's response. Liposomal AMB has been used with some success (194). Despite the currently available diagnostic and therapeutic modalities, rhinocerebral mucormycosis remains a highly lethal infection, with a mortality rate of 70% (134,195); diabetic patients have a better prognosis probably due to the possibility of rapidly correcting the ketoacidosis (196). Some preliminary data have suggested that hyperbaric oxygen might be of benefit in treating rhinocerebral mucormycosis (197,198). The more recent azole antifungal agents have not been thoroughly evaluated for rhinocerebral mucormycosis and should not be used to treat these severe infections.

Infection with HIV does not seem to predispose to mucormycosis (199). Mucormycosis is encountered in HIV-infected individuals as complications of intravenous drug injection, either as local cutaneous necrosis, brain abscesses, or sinusitis. Mucormycosis has been reported in HIV-infected patients who do not inject drug intravenously, at least one of whom was neutropenic (200). With treatment as outlined above, the outcome is expected to be the same as in non-AIDS patients. Long-term suppressive therapy with AMB should be considered.

MISCELLANEOUS AND RARE FUNGAL PATHOGENS

Other fungi, such as *Paracoccidioides brasiliensis* (201), can present with meningitis or parenchymal brain disease. This fungus is endemic in South America. Some additional fungi rarely encountered in CNS infections (202) include *Sporothrix schenkii* (203), the agent of sporotrichosis, which is essentially a cutaneous disease, *Pseudoallescheria* (204), *Dactylaria* (205), and *Fusarium*. More unusual opportunistic pathogens should be expected to cause significant diseases in humans as immunologically deficient patients live longer. For example, an alga (*Prototheca*) has caused meningitis in a patient with AIDS (206). Definitive diagnosis is usually obtained through culture or identification of the microorganism in tissue sections. Management and treatment of these unusual infections usually require some expertise owing to their rarity and unpredictability.

CONCLUSION

This chapter reviews the clinical presentations of fungal infections of the central nervous system. The intrinsic neurotropism of some pathogenic fungi like *Coccidioides* or *Cryptococcus* has been recognized for decades. Nevertheless, the epidemiology and clinical presentations of these classic diseases are changing. For example, the incidence of cryptococcal meningitis has increased enormously over the last 15 years, owing mainly to the increasing prevalence of AIDS. Immunocompromised patients tend to present with disseminated fungal infections and are therefore predisposed to CNS involvement. These trends also apply to fungi without significant neurotropism like *Histoplasma*. Fairly avirulent saprophytic molds and commensal yeasts may take advantage of immune dysfunctions to become invasive. Signs and symptoms of disseminated fungal infections are frequently nonspecific, and ancillary studies well validated for identifying other pathogens are commonly unreliable for fungal infections. A high awareness of these characteristics is essential when caring for immunocompromised patients. Although amphotericin B remains the drug of choice for most fungal infections involving the CNS, recently developed medications show promise, not only in preventing relapses or recurrences, but also in treating severe fungal infections.

REFERENCES

1. Perfect JR. Cryptococcosis. Infect Dis Clin North Am 1989; 3:77–102.
2. Fraser DW, Ward JI, Ajello L, et al. Aspergillosis and systemic mycoses. The growing problem. JAMA 1979; 242:1641–1645.
3. Diamond RD. Cryptococcus neoformans In: Mandell GL, Bennett JE, Dolin R, eds. Principles and Practice of Infectious Diseases. New York: Churchill Livingstone, 1995:2331–2340.
4. White MH, Armstrong D. Cryptococcosis. Infect Dis Clin North Am 1994; 8:383–398.
5. Powderly WG. Cryptococcal meningitis in AIDS. Clin Infect Dis 1993; 17:837–842.
6. Levitz SM. The ecology of Cryptococcus neoformans and the epidemiology of cryptococcosis. Rev Infect Dis 1991; 13:1164–1169.
7. Granger DL, Perfect JR, Durack DT. Virulence of cryptococcosis. Regulation of capsule synthesis by carbon dioxide. J Clin Invest 1985; 76:508–516.
8. Wagner RP, Lewitz SM, Tabuni A, Kornfeld H. HIV-1 envelope protein (gp 120) inhibits the activity of human bronchoalveolar macrophages against Cryptococcus neoformans. Am Rev Respir Dis 1992; 146:1434–1438.
9. Lewis JL, Rabinovich S. The wide spectrum of cryptococcal infections. Am J Med 1972; 53:315–322.
10. Walker BF, Gunthel CJ, Bryan JA, Watts NB, Clark RV. Disseminated cryptococcosis in apparently

normal host presenting as primary adrenal insufficiency: diagnosis by fine needle aspiration. Am J Med 1989; 86:715–717.
11. Igel AJ, Bolande RP. Humoral defense mechanism in cryptococcosis: substances in normal human serum, saliva and cerebrospinal fluid affecting the growth of Cryptococcus neoformans. J Infect Dis 1966; 116:75–83.
12. Tan CT, Kuan BB. Cryptococcus meningitis, clinical—CT scan considerations. Neuroradiology 1987; 29:43–46.
13. Saag MS, Powderly WG, Cloud GA, et al. Comparison of amphotericin B with fluconazole in the treatment of acute AIDS-associated cryptococcal meningitis. N Engl J Med 1992; 326:83–89.
14. Rex JH, Larsen RA, Dismukes WE, et al. Catastrophic visual loss due to cryptococcus neoformans meningitis. Medicine 1993; 72:207–224.
15. Chuck SL, Sande MA. Infections with Cryptococcus neoformans in the acquired immunodeficiency syndrome. N Engl J Med 1989; 321:794–749.
16. Diamond RD, Bennett JE. Prognostic factors in cryptococcal meningitis. A study of 111 cases. Ann Intern Med 1974; 80:176–181.
17. Sugar AM, Stern JJ, Dupont B. Overview: treatment of cryptococcal meningitis. Rev Infect Dis 1990; 12(suppl 3):S338–S348.
18. Utz JP. Flucytosine. N Engl J Med 1972; 286:777–778.
19. Dismukes WE, Cloud GA, Gallis HA, et al. Treatment of cryptococcal meningitis with combination amphotericin B and flucytosine for four as compared with six weeks. N Engl J Med 1987; 317: 334–341.
20. Stern JJ, Hartman BJ, Sharkey P, et al. Oral fluconazole therapy for patients with acquired immunodeficiency syndrome and cryptococcosis: experience with 22 patients. Am J Med 1988; 85:477–480.
21. Denning DW, Tucker RM, Hanson LH, et al. Itraconazole therapy for cryptococcal meningitis and cryptococcosis. Arch Intern Med 1989; 149:2301–2308.
22. Larsen RA, Leal MAE, Chan LS. Fluconazole compared with amphotericin B plus flucytosine for cryptococcal meningitis in AIDS. A randomized trial. Ann Intern Med 1990; 113:183–187.
23. de Gans J, Portegies P, Tiessens G, et al. Itraconazole compared with amphotericin B plus flucytosine in AIDS patients with cryptococcal meningitis. AIDS 1992; 6:185–190.
24. Larsen RA, Bozzette SA, Jones BE, et al. Fluconazole combined with flucytosine for treatment of cryptoccal meningitis in patients with AIDS. Clin Infect Dis 1994; 19:741–745.
25. Clark RA, Greer D, Atkinson W, Valainis GT, Hyslop. Spectrum of Cryptococcus neoformans infection in 68 patients infected with human immunodeficiency virus. Rev Infect Dis 1990; 12: 768–777.
26. Spitzer ED, Spitzer SG, Freundlich LF, Casadevall A. Persistence of initial infection in recurrent cryptococcus neoformans meningitis. Lancet 1993; 341:595–596.
27. Sugar AM, Saunders C. Oral fluconazole as suppressive therapy of disseminated cryptococcosis in patients with acquired immunodeficiency syndrome. Am J Med 1988; 85:481–489.
28. Bozette SA, Larsen RA, Chiu J, et al. A placebo-controlled trial of maintenance therapy with fluconazole after treatment of cryptococcal meningitis in the acquired immunodeficiency syndrome. N Engl J Med 1991; 324:580–584.
29. Powderly WG, Saag MS, Cloud GA, et al. A controlled trial of fluconazole or amphotericin B to prevent relapse of cryptococcal meningitis in patients with the acquired immunodeficiency syndrome. N Engl J Med 1992; 326:793–798.
30. Nelson MR, Fisher M, Cartledge J, Rogers T, Gazzard BG. The role of azoles in the treatment and prophylaxis of cryptococcal disease in HIV infection. AIDS 1994; 8:651–654.
31. Nightingale SD, Cal SX, Peterson DM, et al. Primary prophylaxis with fluconazole against systemic fungal infection in HIV-positive patients. AIDS 1992; 6:191–194.
32. Drutz DJ, Catanzaro A. Coccidioidomycosis—parts I and II. Am Rev Respir Dis 1978; 117:559–585, 727–771.
33. Galgiani JN. Coccidioidomycosis. West J Med 1993; 159:153–171.
34. Stevens DA. Coccidioidomycosis. N Engl J Med 1995; 332:1077–1082.

35. Galgiani JN. Coccidioidomycosis: changes in clinical expression, serological diagnosis and therapeutic options. Clin Infect Dis 1992; 14(suppl 1):S100–S105.
36. Einstein HE, Johnson RH. Coccidioidomycosis: new aspects of epidemiology and therapy. Clin Infect Dis 1993; 16:349–54.
37. Centers for Disease Control and Prevention. Update: coccidioidomycosis—California, 1991–1993. JAMA 1994; 272:585.
38. Centers for Disease Control and Prevention. Coccidioidomycosis following the Northridge earthquake—California, 1994. JAMA 1994; 271:1735.
39. Ampel NM, Wieden MA, Galgiani JN. Coccidioidomycosis: clinical update. Rev Infect Dis 1989; 11: 897–911.
40. Vincent T, Galgiani JN, Huppert M, Salkin D. The natural history of coccidioidal meningitis: VA-Armed Forces cooperative studies, 1955–1958. Clin Infect Dis 1993; 16:247–254.
41. Walker MP, Brody CZ, Resnik R. Reactivation of coccidioidomycosis in pregnancy. Obstet Gynecol 1992; 79:815–817.
42. Ampel NM, Dols CL, Galgiani JN. Coccidioidomycosis during human immunodeficiency infection: results of a prospective study in a coccidioidal endemic area. Am J Med 1993; 94:235–240.
43. Fish DG, Ampel NM, Galgiani JN, Dols CL, Kelly PC, et al. Coccidioidomycosis during human immunodeficiency virus infection. A review of 77 patients. Medicine 1990; 69:384–91.
44. Riley DK, Galgiani JN, O'Donnell MR, et al. Coccidioidomycosis in bone marrow transplant recipients. Transplantation 1993; 56:1531–1533.
45. Bouza E, Dreyer JS, Hewitt WL, Meyer RD. Coccidioidal meningitis: an analysis of thirty-one cases and review of the literature. Medicine (Baltimore) 1981; 60:139–172.
46. Kelly PC. Coccidioidal meningitis. In: Stevens DA, ed. Coccidioidomycosis: a text. Current topics in infectious diseases. New York: Plenum, 1980:164–193.
47. Winston DJ, Terrance OK, Fleischmann J, et al. Successful treatment of spinal arachnoiditis due to coccidioidomycosis—case report. J Neurosurg 1983; 59:328–331.
48. Wrobel CJ, Rothrock J. Coccidioidomycosis meningitis presenting as anterior spinal artery syndrome. Neurology 1992; 42:1840.
49. Williams PL, Johnson R, Pappagianis D, et al. Vasculitic and encephalitic complications associated with Coccidioides immitis infection of the central nervous system in humans: report of 10 cases and review. Clin Infect Dis 1992; 14:673–682.
50. Delaney P, Niemann B. Spinal compression by Coccidioides immitis abscess. Arch Neurol 1982; 39: 255–256.
51. Mendel E, Milefchik EN, Ahmadi J, Gruen P. Coccidioidomycotic brain abscess. Case report. J Neurosurg 1994; 80:140–142.
52. Harley WB, Blaser MJ. Disseminated coccidioidomycosis associated with extreme eosinophilia. Clin Infect Dis 1994; 18:627–629.
53. Shetter AG, Fischer DW, Flom RA. Computed tomography in cases of coccidioidal meningitis, with clinical correlation. West J Med 1985; 142:782–786.
54. Dublin AB, Phillips HE. Computed tomography of disseminated cerebral coccidioidomycosis. Radiology 1980; 135:361–368.
55. Hadley MN, Martin NA, Spetzler RF, Johnson PC. Multiple intracranial aneurysms due to Coccidioides immitis infection. Case report. J Neurosurgery 1987; 66:453–456.
56. Ismail Y, Arsura EL. Eosinophilic meningitis. West J Med 1993; 159:623.
57. Raglan AS, Arsura E, Ismail Y, Johnson R. Eosinophilic pleocytosis in coccidioidal meningitis: frequency and significance. Am J Med 1993; 95:254–257.
58. Ampel NM, Ryan KJ, Carry PJ, Wieden MA, Schifman RB. Fungemia due to Coccidioides immitis. An analysis of 16 episodes in 15 patients and a review of the literature. Medicine (Baltimore) 1986; 65:312–321.
59. Pappagianis D, Zimmer BL. Serology of coccidioidomycosis. Clin Microbiol Rev 1990; 3:247–268.
60. Sobel RA, Ellis WG, Nielsen SL, Davis RL. Central nervous system coccidioidomycosis: a clinicopathologic study of treatment with or without amphotericin B. Hum Pathol 1984; 15:980–995.

61. Diamond RD, Bennett JE. A subcutaneous reservoir for intrathecal therapy of fungal meningitis. N Engl J Med 1973; 288:186–188.
62. Graybill JR, Ellenbogen C. Complications with the Ommaya reservoir in patients with granulomatous meningitis. J Neurosurg 1973; 38:477–480.
63. Carnevale NT, Galgiani JN, Stevens DA, Herrick MK, Langston JW. Amphotericin induced myelopathy. Arch Intern Med 1980; 140:1189–1192.
64. Labadie EL, Hamilton RH. Survival improvement in coccidioidal meningitis by high-dose intrathecal amphotericin B. Arch Intern Med 1986; 146:2013–2018.
65. Winn WA. The treatment of coccidioidal meningitis. Calif Med 1964; 101:78–89.
66. Sugar AM, Alsip SG, Galgiani JN, et al. Pharmacology and toxicity of high dose ketoconazole. Antimicrob Agents Chemother 1987; 31:1874–1878.
67. Galgiani JN, Stevens DA, Graybill JR, Dismukes WE, Cloud GA. Ketoconazole therapy of progressive coccidioidomycosis—comparison of 400- and 800-mg doses and observations at higher doses. Am J Med 1988; 84:603–610.
68. Tucker RM, Galgiani JN, Denning DW, et al. Treatment of coccidioidal meningitis with fluconazole. Rev Infect Dis 1990; 12(suppl 3):S380–S389.
69. Galgiani JN, Catanzaro A, Cloud GA, et al. Fluconazole therapy for coccidioidal meningitis. The NIAID-Mycoses Study Group. Ann Intern Med 1993; 119:28–35.
70. Graybill JR, Stevens DA, Galgiani JN, Dismukes WE, Cloud GA. Itraconazole treatment of coccidioidomycosis. NAIAD Mycoses Study Group. Am J Med 1990; 89:282–290.
71. Sarosi GA, Davies SF. Blastomycosis. Am Rev Respir Dis 1979; 120:911–938.
72. Bradsher RW. Blastomycosis. Clin Infect Dis 1992; 14(suppl 1):S82–S90.
73. Klein BS, Vergeront JM, Davis JP. Epidemiologic aspects of blastomycosis, the enigmatic systemic mycosis. Semin Respir Infect 1986; 1:29–39.
74. Baumgardner DJ, Buggy BP, Mattson BJ, Burdick JS, Ludwig D. Epidemiology of blastomycosis in a region of high endemicity in north central Wisconsin. Clin Infect Dis 1992; 15:629–635.
75. Gnann JW Jr, Bressler GS, Bodet CA 3d, Avent CK. Human blastomycosis after a dog bite. Ann Intern Med 1983; 98:48–49.
76. Yen A, Knipe RC, Tyring SK. Primary cutaneous blastomycosis report of a case acquired by direct inoculation of a bullous pemphigoid lesion. J Am Acad Dermatol 1994; 31:277–278.
77. Pappas PG, Threlkeld MG, Bedsole GD, et al. Blastomycosis in immunocompromised patients. Medicine (Baltimore) 1993; 72:311–325.
78. Serody JS, Mill MR, Detterbeck FC, Harris DT, Cohen MS. Blastomycosis in transplant recipients report of a case and review. Clin Infect Dis 1993; 16:54–58.
79. Pappas PG, Pottage JC, Powderly WG, et al. Blastomycosis in patients with the acquired immunodeficiency syndrome. Ann Intern Med 1992; 116:847–853.
80. Roos KL, Bryan JP, Maggio WW, Jane JA, Scheld WM. Intracranial blastomycoma. Medicine (Baltimore) 1987; 66:224–235.
81. Sugar AM, Picard M. Macrophage- and oxidant-mediated inhibition of the ability of live Blastomyces dermatitidis conidia to transform to the pathogenic yeast phase implications for the pathogenesis of dimorphic fungal infections. J Infect Dis 1991; 164:371–375.
82. Sugar AM, Picard M, Wagner R, Kornfeld H. Interactions between human bronchoalveolar macrophages and Blastomyces dermatitidis conidia: demonstration of fungicidal and fungistatic effects. J Infect Dis 1995; 171:1559–1562.
83. Rabinowitz JG, Bush J, Buttram WR. Pulmonary manifestations of blastomycosis: radiological support of a new concept. Radiology 1976; 120:25–32.
84. Meyer KC, McManus EJ, Maki DG. Overwhelming pulmonary blastomycosis associated with the adult respiratory distress syndrome. N Engl J Med 1993; 329:1231–1236.
85. Vaaler AK, Bradsher RW, Davies SF. Evidence of subclinical blastomycosis in forestry workers in northern Minnesota and northern Wisconsin. Am J Med 1990; 89:470–476.
86. Gonyea EF. The spectrum of primary blastomycotic meningitis a review of central nervous system blastomycosis. Ann Neurol 1978; 3:26–39.

87. Harding CV. Blastomycosis and opportunistic infections in patients with acquired immunodeficiency syndrome. Arch Pathol Lab Med 1991; 115:1133–1136.
88. Jacobs RF, Marmer DJ, Balk RA, Bradsher RW. Lymphocytes subpopulations of blood and alveolar lavage in blastomycosis. Chest 1985; 88:579–585.
89. Tan G, Kaufman L, Peterson EM, de la Maza LM. Disseminated atypical blastomycosis in two patients with AIDS. Clin Infect Dis 1993; 16:107–111.
90. Buechner HA, Clawson CM. Blastomycosis of the central nervous system. II. A report of nine cases from the Veterans Administration Cooperative Study. Am Rev Respir Dis 1967; 95:820–826.
91. Pitrak DL. Cerebral blastomycoma after ketoconazole therapy for respiratory tract blastomycosis. Am J Med 1989; 86:713–714.
92. Kravitz GR, Davies SF, Eckman MR, Sarosi GA. Chronic blastomycotic meningitis. Am J Med 1981; 71:501–505.
93. Whelan MA, Stern J, deNapoli RA. The computed tomographic spectrum of intracranial mycosis: correlation with histopathology. Radiology 1981; 141:703–707.
94. Claveria LE, duBoulay GH, Moseley IF. Intracranial infections: investigations by computerized axial tomography. Neuroradiology 1976; 12:59–71.
95. Ostrow TD, Hudgin PA. Magnetic resonance imaging of intracranial fungal infections. Topics Mag Res Imag 1994; 6:22–23.
96. Harley WB, Lomis M, Haas DW. Marked polymorphonuclear pleocytosis due to blastomycotic meningitis: case report and review. Clin Infect Dis 1994; 18:816–818.
97. Musial CE, Wilson WR, Sinkeldam IR, Roberts GD. Recovery of Blastomyces dermatitidis from blood of a patient with disseminated blastomycosis. J Clin Microbiol 1987; 25:1421–1423.
98. Klein BS, Vergemont JM, Kaufman L, et al. Serological tests for blastomycosis: assessments during a large point-source outbreak in Wisconsin. J Infect Dis 1987; 155:262–268.
99. Sarosi GA, Davies SF, Klein BS, Dismukes W, Bradsher R. Recent developments in blastomycosis. Am Rev Respir Dis 1986; 134:817–818.
100. Yancey RW Jr, Perlino CA, Kaufman L. Asymptomatic blastomycosis of the central nervous system with progression in patients given ketoconazole therapy a report of two cases. J Infect Dis 1991; 164:807–810.
101. Pearson GJ, Chin TW, Fong IW. Case report: treatment of blastomycosis with fluconazole. Am J Med Sci 1992; 303:313–315.
102. Dismukes WE, Bradsher RW Jr, Cloud GC, et al. Itraconazole therapy for blastomycosis and histoplasmosis. NIAID Mycoses Study Group. Am J Med 1992; 93:489–497.
103. Goodwin RA, Des Prez RM. Histoplasmosis. Am Rev Respir Dis 1978; 117:929–956.
104. George RB, Penn RL. Histoplasmosis. In: Sarosi GA, Davies SF, eds. Fungal Diseases of the Lung. 2d ed. New York: Raven Press, 1993:39–50.
105. Wheat LJ, Slama TG, Eitzen HE, Kohler RB, French MLV, Bieseckler JL. A large outbreak of histoplasmosis: clinical features. Ann Intern Med 1981; 94:331–337.
106. Wheat LJ, French M, Batteiger B, Kohler R. Cerebrospinal fluid Histoplasma antibodies in central nervous system histoplasmosis. Arch Intern Med 1985; 145:1237–1240.
107. Karalakusingam R, Krishan KA, Adams G, et al. Meningoencephalitis caused by Histoplasma capsulatum. Occurrence in a renal transplant recipient and review of the literature. Arch Intern Med 1976; 136:217–220.
108. Smith JW, Utz JP. Progressive disseminated histoplasmosis. A prospective study of 26 patients. Ann Intern Med 1972; 76:557–565.
109. Schulz DM. Histoplasmosis of the central nervous system. JAMA 1953; 151:549–551.
110. Rubin H, Furcolow ML, Yates JL, Brasher CA. The course and prognosis of histoplasmosis. Am J Med 1959; 27:278–288.
111. Wheat LJ, Batteiger BE, Sathapatayavongs B. Histoplasma capsulatum infections of the central nervous system. A clinical review. Medicine (Baltimore) 1990; 69:244–260.
112. Cooper RA, Goldstein E. Histoplasmosis of the central nervous system—report of two cases and review of the literature. Am J Med 1963; 35:45–57.

113. Canlas MS, Dillon ML. Histoplasma capsulatum endocarditis: report of a case following heart surgery. Angiology 1977; 28:454–463.
114. Tan V, Wilkins P, Badve S, et al. Histoplasmosis of the central nervous system. J Neurol Neurosurg Psychiatry 1992; 55:619–622.
115. Nelson JD, Bates R, Pitchford A. Histoplasma meningitis: recovery following amphotericin B therapy. Am J Dis Child 1961; 102:96–101.
116. Wheat LJ, Kohler RB, Tewari RP, Garten M, French ML. Significance of Histoplasma antigen in the cerebrospinal fluid of patients with meningitis. Arch Intern Med 1989; 149:302–304.
117. Plouffe JF, Lambert RJ. Histoplasma meningitis: diagnostic value of cerebrospinal fluid serology. Ann Intern Med 1980; 92:189–191.
118. George RB, Lambert RS. Significance of serum antibodies to Histoplasma capsulatum in endemic areas. South Med J 1984; 77:161–163.
119. Wheat JL, Kohler RB, Tewari RP. Diagnosis of disseminated histoplasmosis by detection of Histoplasma capsulatum antigen in serum and urine specimen. N Engl J Med 1986; 314:83–88.
120. Shapiro JL, Lux JJ, Sprofkin BE. Histoplasmosis of the central nervous system. Am J Pathol 1955; 31:319–335.
121. Voelker JL, Muller J, Worth RM. Intramedullary spinal Histoplasma granuloma. J Neurosurg 1989; 70:959–961.
122. Saag SM, Dismukes WE. Treatment of histoplasmosis and blastomycosis. Chest 1988; 93:848–851.
123. Wheat J, Hafner R, Korzun AH, et al. Itraconazole treatment of disseminated histoplasmosis in patients with the acquired immunodeficiency syndrome. Am J Med 1995; 98:336–342.
124. Kwong-Chung KJ. Phylogenetic spectrum of fungi that are pathogenic to humans. Clin Infect Dis 1994; 19(suppl 1):S1–S7.
125. Levitz SM. Aspergillosis. Infect Dis Clin North Am 1989; 3:1–18.
126. Diamond RD. Invasive aspergillosis: host defenses. Recent Results Cancer Res 1993; 132:109–115.
127. Gerson SL, Talbot GH, Hurwitz S, et al. Prolonged granulocytopenia: the major risk factor for invasive pulmonary aspergillosis in patients with acute leukemia. Ann Intern Med 1984; 100:345–351.
128. Saral R. Candida and Aspergillus infections in immunocompromised patients: an overview. Rev Infect Dis 1991; 13:487–92.
129. Hibberd PL, Rubin RH. Clinical aspects of fungal infection in organ transplant recipients. Clin Infect Dis 1994; 19(suppl 1):S33–S40.
130. Young RC, Bennett JE, Vogel CL. Aspergillosis: the spectrum of the disease in 98 patients. Medicine 1970; 49:147–173.
131. Rinaldi MG. Invasive aspergillosis. Rev Infect Dis 1983; 5:1061–1077.
132. Bjorkholm B, Elgefors B. Cerebellar aspergilloma. Scand J Infect Dis 1986; 18:375–378.
133. Morrow R, Wong B, Finkelstein WE, Sternberg SS, Armstrong D. Aspergillosis of the cerebral ventricles in a heroin abuser. Case report and review of the literature. Arch Intern Med 1983; 143: 161–164.
134. Hopkins RJ, Rothman M, Fiore A, Goldblum SE. Cerebral mucormycosis associated with intravenous drug use: three case reports and review. Clin Infect Dis 1994; 19:1133–1137.
135. Hagensee ME, Bauwens JE, Kjos B, Bowden RA. Brain abscess following marrow transplantation: experience at the Fred Hutchinson Cancer Research Center, 1984–1992. Clin Infect Dis 1994; 19: 402–408.
136. Chandler FW. Pathology of the mycoses in patients with the acquired immunodeficiency syndrome (AIDS). Curr Top Med Mycol 1985; 1:1–23.
137. Singh N, Yu VL, Rihs JD. Invasive aspergillosis in AIDS. South Med J 1991; 84:822–827.
138. Walsh TJ, Hier DB, Caplan LR. Fungal infections of the central nervous system: comparative analysis of risk factors and clinical signs in 57 patients. Neurology 1985; 35:1654–1657.
139. Bardana EJ Jr. The clinical spectrum of aspergillosis. Part 2: classification and description of saprophytic, allergic, and invasive variants of human disease. Crit Rev Clin Lab Sci 1981; 13:85–159.
140. Treseler CB, Sugar AM. Fungal meningitis. Infect Dis Clin North Am 1990; 4:789–808.
141. Hendrix WC, Arruda LK, Platts-Mills TA, et al. Aspergillus epidural abscess and cord compression

in a patient with aspergilloma and empyema. Survival and response to high dose systemic amphotericin therapy. Am Rev Respir Dis 1992; 145:1483–1486.
142. Woods GL, Goldsmith JC. Aspergillus infection of the central nervous system in patients with acquired immunodeficiency syndrome. Arch Neurol 1990; 47:181–184.
143. Khoo SH, Denning DW. Invasive aspergillosis in patients with AIDS. Clin Infect Dis 1994; 19(suppl 1):S41–48.
144. Yu VL, Muder RR, Poorsattar A. Significance of isolation of Aspergillus from the respiratory tract in diagnosis of invasive pulmonary aspergillosis. Results from a three-year prospective study. Am J Med 1986; 81:249–254.
145. Duthie R, Denning DW. Aspergillus fungemia: report of two cases and review. Clin Infect Dis 1995; 20:598–605.
146. Andriole VT. Infections with Aspergillus species. Clin Infect Dis 1993; 17(suppl 2):S481–S486.
147. Rogers TR, Haynes KA, Barnes RA. Value of antigen detection in predicting invasive pulmonary aspergillosis. Lancet 1990; 336:1210–1213.
148. Carpenter JL. Brain stem abscesses: cure with medical therapy, case report, and review. Clin Infect Dis 1994; 18:219–226.
149. Mukoyama M, Gimple K, Poser CM. Aspergillosis of the central nervous system. Report of a brain abscess due to A. fumigatus and review of the literature. Neurology 1969; 19:967–974.
150. Goodman ML, Coffey RJ. Stereotactic drainage of Aspergillus brain abscess with long-term survival: case report and review. Neurosurgery 1989; 24:96–99.
151. Denning DW, Stevens DA. Antifungal and surgical treatment of invasive aspergillosis: review of 2,121 published cases. Rev Infect Dis 1990; 12:1147–1201.
152. Weiland D, Ferguson RM, Peterson PK, et al. Aspergillosis in 25 renal transplants patients. Epidemiology, clinical presentation, diagnosis, and management. Ann Surg 1983; 198:622–629.
153. Denning DW. Treatment of invásive aspergillosis. J Infect 1994; 28(suppl 1):S25–S33.
154. Lipton SA, Hickey WF, Morris JH, Loscalzo J. Candidal infection in the central nervous system. Am J Med 1984; 76:101–108.
155. Black JT. Cerebral candidiasis: case report of brain abscess secondary to candida albicans, and review of the literature. J Neurol Neurosurg Psychiatry 1970; 33:864–870.
156. Weese-Mayer DE, Fondriest DW, Brouillette RT, Shulman ST. Risk factors associated with candidemia in the neonatal intensive care unit: a case-control study. Pediatr Infect Dis J 1987; 6:190–196.
157. Buchs S. Candida meningitis: a growing threat to premature and fullterm infants. Pediatr Infect Dis 1985; 4:122–123.
158. Parker JC, McCloskey JJ, Lee RS. The emergence of candidiasis: the dominant postmortem cerebral mycosis. Am J Clin Pathol 1978; 70:31–36.
159. Kressel B, Szewczyk C, Tuazon CU. Early clinical recognition of disseminated candidiasis by muscle and skin biopsy. Arch Intern Med 1978; 138:429–433.
160. Silverman RA, Rhodes AR, Dennehy PH. Disseminated intravascular coagulation and purpura fulminans in a patient with Candida sepsis. Biopsy of purpura fulminans as an aid to diagnosis of systemic Candida infection. Am J Med 1986; 80:679–684.
161. Thron A, Wietholter H. Cerebral candidiases: CT studies in a case of brain abscess and granuloma due to Candida albicans. Neuroradiology 1982; 23:223–225.
162. Chadwick DW, Hartley E, Mackinnon DM. Meningitis caused by Candida tropicalis. Arch Neurol 1980; 37:175–176.
163. Smego RA Jr, Devoe PW, Sampson HA, et al. Candida meningitis in two children with severe combined immunodeficiency. J Pediatr 1984; 104:902–904.
164. Bayer AS, Edwards JE Jr, Seidel JS, Guze LB. Candida meningitis. Report of seven cases and review of the English literature. Medicine (Baltimore) 1976; 55:477–486.
165. Chmel H. Candida albicans meningitis following lumbar puncture. Am J Med Sci 1973; 266:465–467.
166. Sarmiento R, Holubka J, Khatib R. Case report: Candida meningitis with an intradural filling defect 1 year after candidemia. Am J Med Sci 1994; 307:115–118.
167. Sulkava R, Jaaskelainen J, Paetau A, Valtonen V, Iivanainen M. Fatal Candida meningitis in a previously healthy adult. Ann Clin Res 1984; 16:201–203.

168. Voice RA, Bradley SF, Sangeorzan JA, Kauffman CA. Chronic candida meningitis: an uncommon manifestation of candidiasis. Clin Infect Dis 1994; 19:60–66.
169. Ehni WF, Ellison RT 3d, Ellison RT. Spontaneous Candida albicans meningitis in a patient with the acquired immune deficiency syndrome. Am J Med 1987; 83:806–807.
170. Gower DJ, Crone K, Alexander E Jr, Kelly Dl Jr. Candida albicans shunt infection: report of two cases. Neurosurgery 1986; 19:111–113.
171. Sugarman B, Massanari RM. Candida meningitis in patients with CSF shunts. Arch Neurol 1980; 37:180–181.
172. Sanchez-Portocarrero J, Martinez-Rabadan P, Saldana JS, Perez-Cecilia E. Candida cerebrospinal fluid shunt infection. Report of two new cases and review of the literature. Diagn Microbiol Infect Dis 1994; 20:33–40.
173. Forward KR, Fewer HD, Stiver HG. Cerebrospinal fluid shunt infections. J Neurosurg 1983; 59: 389–394.
174. Rex JH, Bennett JE, Sugar AM, et al. A randomized trial comparing fluconazole with amphotericin B for the treatment of candidemia in patients without neutropenia. N Engl J Med 1994; 331:1325–1330.
175. Anaissie E. Opportunistic mycoses in the immunocompromised host: experience at a cancer center and review. Clin Infect Dis 1992; 14(suppl 1):S43–S53.
176. Sugar AM. Mucormycosis. Clin Infect Dis 1992; 14(suppl 1):S126–S129.
177. Rinaldi MG. Zygomycosis. Infect Dis Clin North Am 1989; 3:19–41.
178. Adam RD, Hunter G, DiTomasso J, Comerci G Jr. Mucormycosis: emergence of cutaneous infections. Clin Infect Dis 1994; 19:67–76.
179. Singh N, Gayowski T, Singh J, Yu VL. Invasive gastrointestinal zygomycosis in a liver transplant recipient: case report and review of zygomycosis in solid-organ transplant recipients. Clin Infect Dis 1995; 20:617–620.
180. Boelaert JR, Roost GFV, Vergauwe PL, et al. The role of desferrioxamine in dialysis-associated mucormycosis: report of three cases and review of the literature. Clin Nephrol 1988; 29:261–266.
181. Nussbaum ES, Hall WA. Rhinocerebral mucormycosis: changing patterns of disease. Surg Neurol 1994; 41:152–156.
182. Radner AB, Witt MD, Edwards Jr JE. Acute invasive rhinocerebral zygomycosis in an otherwise healthy patient: case report and review. Clin Infect Dis 1995; 20:164–166.
183. Gollard R, Rabb C, Larsen R, Chandrasoma P. Isolated cerebral mucormycosis: case report and therapeutic considerations. Neurosurgery 1994; 34:174–177.
184. Larkin JG, Butcher IG, Frier BM, Brebner H. Fatal rhinocerebral mucormycosis in newly diagnosed diabetics. Diabet Med 1986; 3:266–268.
185. Rogers WD Jr. Facial paralysis and epistaxis in a diabetic: a typical presentation for rhinocerebral mucormycosis. Ann Emerg Med 1984; 13:560–561.
186. Soloniuk DS, Moreland DB. Rhinocerebral mucormycosis with extension to the posterior fossa: case report. Neurosurgery 1988; 23:641–643.
187. Fingeroth JD, Roth RS, Talcott JA, Rinaldi MG. Zygomycosis due to Mucor circinelloides in a neutropenic patient receiving chemotherapy for acute myelogenous leukemia. Clin Infect Dis 1994; 19:135–137.
188. Lim KKT, Potts MJ, Warnock NBN, Brown EM, Burns-Cox CJ. Another case report of rhinocerebral mucormycosis treated with liposomal amphotericin B and surgery. Clin Infect Dis 1994; 18:653–654.
189. Micozzi MS, Welti CV. Intravenous amphetamine abuse, primary cerebral mucormycosis, and acquired immunodeficiency. J Forensic Sci 1985; 30:504–510.
190. Press GA, Weindling SM, Hesselink JR, Ochi JW, Harris JP. Rhinocerebral mucormycosis: MR manifestations. J Comput Assist Tomogr 1988; 12:744–749.
191. McDevitt GR Jr, Brantley MJ, Cawthon MA. Rhinocerebral mucormycosis: a case report with magnetic resonance imaging findings. Clin Imaging 1989; 13:317–320.
192. Terk MR, Underwod DJ, Zee CS, Colletti PM. MR imaging in rhinocerebral and intracranial mucormycosis with CT and pathologic correlation. Magn Reson Imaging 1992; 10:81–87.
193. Parfrey NA. Improved diagnosis and prognosis of mucormycosis: a clinico-pathologic study of 33 cases. Medicine (Baltimore) 1986; 65:113–123.

194. Ericsson M, Anniko M, Gustafsson H, et al. A case of chronic progressive rhinocerebral mucormycosis treated with liposomal amphotericin B and surgery. Clin Infect Dis 1993; 16:585–586.
195. Siddiqi SU, Freeman JD. Isolated central nervous mucormycosis. South Med J 1994; 87:997–1000.
196. Blitzer A, Lawson W, Meyers BR. Patient survival factors in paranasal sinus mucormycosis. Laryngoscope 1980; 90:635–648.
197. Ferguson BJ, Mitchell TG, Moon R, Camporesi EM, Farmer J. Adjunctive hyperbaric oxygen for treatment of rhinocerebral mucormycosis. Rev Infect Dis 1988; 10:551–559.
198. De La Paz MA, Patrinely JR, Marines HM, Appling WD. Adjunctive hyperbaric oxygen in treatment of bilateral cerebro-rhino-orbital mucormycosis. Am J Ophthalmol 1992; 114:208–211.
199. Sanchez MR, Ponge-Wilson I, Moy JA, Rosenthal S. Zygomycosis and HIV infection. J Am Acad Dermatol 1994; 30:904–908.
200. Chavanet P, Lefranc T, Bonnin A, et al. Unusual cause of pharyngeal ulceration in AIDS. Lancet 1990; 336:383–384.
201. Nóbrega JP, Spina-França A. Neuroparacoccidioidomycosis. In: Paracoccidioidomycosis. Franco M, Lacaz CF, Restrepo Moreno A, Del Negro P, eds. Boca Raton, FL: CRC Press, 1994:321–330.
202. Salaki JS, Louria DB, Chmel H. Fungal and yeast infections of the central nervous system. Medicine (Baltimore) 1984; 63:108–132.
203. Ewing GE, Bosl GJ, Peterson PK. Sporothrix schenckii meningitis in a farmer with Hodgkin's disease. Am J Med 1980; 68:455–457.
204. Fisher JF, Shadomy S, Teabeaut JR, et al. Near-drowning complicated by brain abscess due to Petriellidium boydii. Arch Neurol 1982; 39:511–513.
205. Vukmir RB, Kusne S, Linden WP, et al. Successful therapy for cerebral phaeohyphomycosis due to Dactylaria gallopava in a liver transplant recipient. Clin Infect Dis 1994; 19:714–719.
206. Kaminski ZC, Kapila R, Sharer LR, Kloser P, Kaufman L. Meningitis due to Prototheca wickermanii in a patient with AIDS. Clin Infect Dis 1992; 15:704–706.
207. Kaplan JE, Masur H, Holmes KH et al. USPHS/IDSA guidelines for the prevention of opportunistic infections in persons infected with human immunodeficiency virus: an overview. Clin Infect Dis 1995; 21(suppl 1):S12–S31.

10

Seasonal (Spring-Summer) Encephalitides

Rahman Pourmand and Karen L. Roos
Indiana University School of Medicine, Indianapolis, Indiana

INTRODUCTION

The etiological agents of warm-weather encephalitis may be viral, arthropodborne or "arbovirus" infections, or nonviral infectious agents, such as *Rickettsia*, *Ehrlichia*, spirochetes, or amebae (Table 1). These infections are acquired during outdoor activities in the warm seasons of the year and are, to a degree, preventable. A knowledge of the clinical presentation of these unique causative agents of spring and summer encephalitis is critical to the management of patients with encephalitis during the warm months of the year.

ARTHROPODBORNE ENCEPHALITIDES

Arthropodborne or "arboviruses" are RNA viruses that are among the most important causes of encephalitis in the United States and worldwide. Four "arboviruses" are recognized as important causes of encephalitis in the United States: St. Louis encephalitis (SLE), eastern equine encephalitis (EEE), western equine encephalitis (WEE), and California encephalitis (CE) (1,2). In 1989, 108 cases of arboviral encephalitis were reported to the Centers for Disease Control (CDC); 65 cases of CE (LaCrosse encephalitis), 34 cases of SLE, and 9 cases of EEE (1,3).

The clinical spectrum of arbovirus infection varies from asymptomatic infections to aseptic meningitis to encephalitis. Arboviruses account for 5–10% of all cases of encephalitis reported to the CDC per year.

Mosquitoes are the main vectors for arboviral encephalitis in the United States. After the mosquito bites an infected animal, typically a bird, the virus replicates in the midgut and spreads to the brain and salivary gland, where it multiplies for a period of 1–2 weeks. The mosquito can then transmit the virus to a new host. Arboviral infections are at their peak during the summer and early fall, when mosquitoes are prevalent and are biting (1). The viruses reach the CNS via the

Table 1 Seasonal Encephalitides (Spring-Summer)

Viral	Nonviral
Arthropodborne encephalitis	Rocky Mountain spotted fever
	Ehrlichioses
Colorado tick fever	Free-living amebic encephalitis
	Leptospirosis
	Lyme meningoencephalitis

bloodstream (4). The annual incidence of each of these infections is affected by weather and its effects on mosquito populations. Mosquitoes breed in stagnant water; therefore, epidemics occur in years with greater rainfall.

St. Louis Encephalitis

St. Louis encephalitis was the first arbovirus infection identified in North America, when in 1933 it was the causative agent of an epidemic in the St. Louis area (5). The etiological agent was isolated from the brain of a fatal case (4). Hammon et al. (7) were the first to identify the mosquito vector, *Culex tarsalis*, for SLE. *Culex pipiens*, *Culex quinquefasciatus*, and *Culex nigripalpus* are other mosquito vectors for transmission of SLE. The last major outbreak of SLE occurred in 1975, when more than 2800 cases were recorded with a fatality rate of 10% (8,9).

SLE is most common in the Midwest (Indiana, Illinois, Kentucky), Texas, Florida, Mississippi, and Alabama, but it has been reported throughout the United States. Since the 1950s, well over 50,000 cases have been reported to the CDC (10,11). Disease occurs in late summer and early fall. In the western states the principal vector is *C. tarsalis* and in the central United States, disease is generally transmitted by *C. pipiens* and *C. quinquefasciatus*. Encephalitis due to this virus is more common in the elderly, and the case fatality rate in the elderly is higher as well (12).

Infection with SLE virus may be asymptomatic or may present as a headache with fever, an aseptic meningitis, or an encephalitis (1). Encephalitis accounts for the majority (75%) of symptomatic presentations. The typical symptoms include fever, headache, nausea, vomiting, and altered mental status (1). The clinical presentation of SLE is indistinguishable from other arboviral infections of the CNS (11). Examination of the cerebrospinal fluid (CSF) reveals a lymphocytic pleocytosis (50–500 cells/mm^3) with a normal or slightly elevated protein concentration and a normal glucose concentration. The identification of viral specific IgM by enzyme-linked immunosorbent assay (ELISA) has been successful for diagnosis (13). The evaluation of acute and convalescent sera by hemagglutination (HI) or complement fixation (CF) assays may be useful in the diagnosis. The clinical diagnosis of SLE should be suspected in patients with acute-onset febrile illness and signs of encephalitis in the late summer and early fall with residence in or travel to an endemic area (11).

The treatment of SLE is essentially supportive. Public education in endemic areas is the major method for prevention. Avoiding outdoor activity at dusk and wearing mosquito repellent during periods of outdoor activity is recommended.

Mortality is highest in the elderly. Approximately 25% of survivers of SLE will have permanent neurological deficits such as memory loss, speech impairment, or motor disability (14).

Western Equine Encephalitis

Western equine encephalitis was first isolated from the brains of horses in the San Joaquin Valley of California in 1930 (15) and subsequently isolated from the brain of a child who died of encephalitis in 1938 (11,16). The principal vector of WEE in the western United States is the *C. tarsalis* mosquito, which breeds in irrigated rural areas (1,11). The peak of disease occurs in early to midsummer. The disease is more severe in infants and children.

The majority of infections with WEE are subclinical. The ratio of asymptomatic to symptomatic clinical infection is reported to be 58:8 in children and over 1150:1 in adults. The clinical presentation of WEE is characterized initially by fever, headache, nausea, and vomiting followed several days later by somnolence, confusion, and then coma (1). Examination of the CSF reveals a pleocytosis of 10–300 cells/mm^3, a normal glucose, and an increased protein concentration. Diagnosis is usually confirmed by serological evaluation of acute and convalescent sera using HI or CF assays (11).

Treatment is supportive. Prevention includes mosquito control and public education of protective measures. An inactivated virus vaccine is available. Sequelae of mental retardation, seizures, and paralysis are most common in infants (17). Overall, the mortality is about 5% (18).

Eastern Equine Encephalitis

Eastern equine encephalitis virus was first isolated in 1933 from the brain of a horse that died from encephalitis (19). In 1938, the virus was isolated from a human who died during an epidemic of encephalitis (11,20).

Cases of EEE have occurred primarily along the Atlantic and Gulf coasts of the United States, with a few case reports from Michigan and the Dakotas. In the northeastern United States, epidemics occur in the late summer and early fall. The primary vector is *C. melanura*, and wild birds (swamp-dwelling birds) are the principal reservoir. *C. melanura* mosquitoes do not feed on humans, but humans become infected when the virus becomes established in the *Aedes* species of mosquitoes. EEE can occur at any age, but it is more common in children. EEE is the most severe encephalitis caused by an arbovirus (1). It has an abrupt onset with headache, focal neurological deficits, confusion, seizures, and coma.

Examination of the CSF reveals a lymphocytic pleocytosis (100–1000 cells/mm^3), a normal or slightly elevated protein concentration, and a normal glucose concentration. IgM antibody detection in CSF or serum permits early diagnosis. Evaluation of acute and convalescent serum by CF, HI, or neutralization assays can be useful in making the diagnosis.

The therapy is supportive care. Avoidance of swampy areas where contact with mosquitoes occurs is the most effective method for prevention. The mortality rate is between 50 and 75%. Survivors have severe neurological disability (1).

California Encephalitis

California encephalitis virus was first isolated from mosquitoes in Kern County, California (21,22). Presently, the California serogroup includes 14 viruses transmitted by mosquitoes (11). The LaCrosse virus is the protype of the California serogroup viruses and was identified in the brain of a child who died of encephalitis in LaCrosse, Wisconsin (11,23). LaCrosse virus infection is the most prevalent arthropodborne infection in the United States (11,24).

The largest number of cases of CE have been reported from the midwestern states—Wisconsin, Illinois, and Ohio. The vector is *Aedes triseriatis*, a forest-dwelling (woodland) mosquito. Small mammals, such as chipmunks and squirrels, serve as the reservoir (1). The mosquitoes have a very short flight range, and humans are bitten only when they go into the woods. The vector is a daytime feeder, and risk of being bitten is greatest during work and play in the woods. Cases occur in warm months (July through September). The disease is largely one of children between the ages of 5 and 15 years. The average number of reported cases per year is about 75 (25).

The clinical presentation of CE is similar to other arboviral infections and varies from an asymptomatic infection to an aseptic meningitis to a more severe form of encephalitis characterized by altered consciousness, focal seizures, and focal neurological deficits. Seizures occur in up to 50% of cases and may be either focal or generalized (2).

A CSF mononuclear pleocytosis, up to 500 cells/mm^3, is common. The CSF protein concentration is mildly elevated, and glucose concentration is normal. Serological tests using IgM-specific immunofluorescent assays appear to be promising diagnostic tests (16,27). Serological confirmation utilizing either CF or HI antibody assays are also useful.

Treatment is symptomatic and supportive. Patients who have seizures at the onset of their illness are at risk for recurrent seizures and should be maintained on antiepileptic drug therapy to prevent recurrence (28,29). The disease is relatively benign, but 15% of survivors have neurological sequelae, such as recurrent seizures, personality problems, and poor school performance (29,31).

ROCKY MOUNTAIN SPOTTED FEVER

Rocky Mountain spotted fever (RMSF) is caused by the bacteria *Rickettsia rickettsii* and is the most common rickettsial disease in the United States. The disease was first identified in Idaho, Montana, and Utah (32,33). In Montana it was known as "spotted fever" and had been recognized as a distinct entity by physicians of the Bitterroot Valley, Montana, for at least 20 years prior to the first publication of a rickettsial infection, which appeared in 1904 by Louis Wilson and William M. Chowning from Minnesota (34). In the Bitterroot Valley the disease was called spotted fever, "black fever," or blue disease. In 1906, Howard T. Ricketts traveled to Missoula, Montana, to identify the cause of spotted fever, also called "black measles" (35,36). He was able to show that an infectious agent was transmitted by a tick bite. Unfortunately, he died 4 years later from typhus fever while studying rickettsial infections in Mexico City. In 1919 rickettsiae were identified within endothelial cells (37). These small bacteria are capable of growth only within cells.

Epidemiology

RMSF is transmitted by various species of ticks. *Amblyomma americanum*, the Lone Star tick, is the vector in Texas. *Dermacentor andersoni*, the wood tick, is the vector in the Pacific coast states and mountains. *Dermacentor variabilis*, the dog tick, is the vector in the southern and eastern states. The latter is the most dangerous. The disease is found in all states as well as in Canada, Mexico, and South America. In the United States, the greatest number of cases have been reported in the southern states, the Piedmont area, and Oklahoma (38–40).

Virgina, North Carolina, and Tennessee are considered "hot spots" for this disease (40,41). The tick can survive over the winter and then becomes active in the spring, with the peak incidence of illness in early summer. Farmers, ranchers, miners, and bridge and construction workers are at increased risk for acquiring the disease because of their outdoor occupations. About 80% of patients have a history of a tick bite. In 1990, 649 cases of RMSF were reported to the CDC.

Pathology

After the rickettsiae invade the skin via a tick bite, they enter the vascular endothelial cells causing a vasculitis. The endothelial cell infection activates the intrinsic and extrinsic pathways of coagulation with the subsequent formation of thrombi. The vast majority of thrombi do not, however, occlude blood flow through the vessel. Injury to the endothelium results in an increase in vascular permeability, leading to hypovolemia, hypotension, hypalbuminemia, prerenal azotemia, and pulmonary edema. Vasculitis involves multiple organs, including eye, heart, kidney, liver, and gastrointestinal tract (42).

Clinical Features

After an incubation period of about 2–14 days, the disease begins with high fever, prostration, myalgias, headache, nausea, and vomiting, which lasts for 2–3 weeks. The rash is characteristic and usually appears 2–4 days after the onset of symptoms, but may be delayed for 2 weeks. The rash is initially a diffuse erythematous maculopapular rash that blanches with pressure. It progresses to a petechial rash, then to a purpuric rash and, if untreated, to skin necrosis or gangrene. The color of the lesions of the rash change from bright red to very dark red, then yellowish-green to black. The rash typically begins in the wrists and ankles and then spreads distally and proximally within a matter of a few hours, and involves the palms and soles (Fig. 1). Ten percent of patients do not have a rash (spotless RMSF) (43). The skin rash should be differentiated from other infections, such as meningococcemia, measles, and enterovirus infection, that are also associated with a maculopapular or purpuric rash (36). The classic triad of RMSF, which includes fever, rash, and a history of a tick bite, is present in only 3% of patients at the time of presentation but is seen in 45–60% of patients during the course of the illness according to 1990 CDC data (41).

Neurological manifestations of RMSF include severe bifrontal headache that is unresponsive to common analgesics, irritability, restlessness, photophobia, delirium, insomnia, confusion, seizures, and coma (44). Neurological findings such as hyperreflexia, spastic para or quadriparesis, pathological reflexes, hyperesthesia, facial diplegia, nystagmus, and ataxia are seen. Signs and symptoms of transverse myelitis, retinal vasculitis, and anterior uveitis have been reported (45). Signs of encephalitis—stupor and coma—occur in approximately 25% of cases and are associated with a poor prognosis with a mortality of 88% in the preantibiotic era (46,47). Without signs of encephalitis, the mortality rate is 20%. Neurological symptoms and signs sometimes occur prior to the appearance of the skin rash.

Renal failure is frequent in severe RMSF due to acute tubular necrosis or hypovolemia (42,48). Pulmonary manifestations of RMSF may be as mild as a cough to as severe as respiratory distress from pulmonary edema (42).

Diagnosis

In the summer months and in prevalent areas, RMSF should be considered in the differential diagnosis of any febrile illness associated with skin rash. The differential diagnosis includes viral illness such as rubella or measles, infectious mononucleosis, meningococcemia, and drug reactions. A rash that involves the palms and soles is characteristic of RMSF (Fig. 1). Ehrlichiosis has clinical similarities to RMSF and is also a tickborne infection, but a rash on the palms and soles is atypical of this infection (see below) (49).

Laboratory abnormalities in RMSF include thrombocytopenia, hyponatremia, and elevated liver enzyme concentrations. The white blood cell count is normal or low with a marked left shift. Cerebrospinal fluid abnormalities include a mild (rarely more than 100 cells/mm^3) lymphocytic pleocytosis and an elevated protein concentration. The CSF glucose concentration is usually normal but was reported to be decreased in 8% of patients in one study (48). The electroencephalogram is usually abnormal in cases of encephalitis, revealing diffuse slowing of background activity (50).

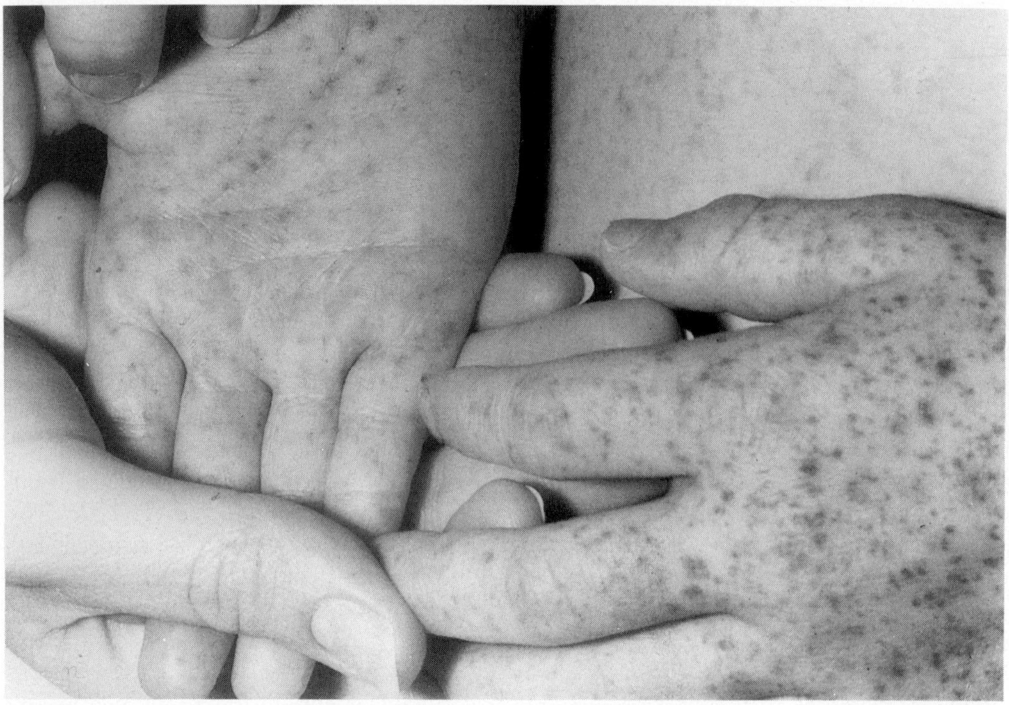

(a)

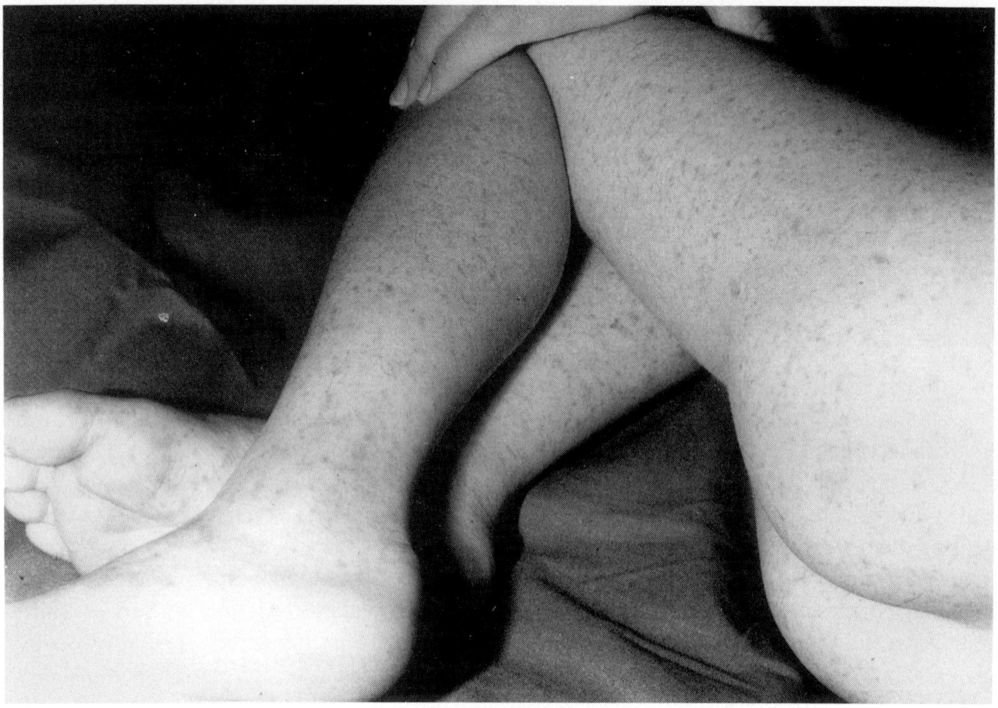

(b)

Figure 1 Petechial rash of RMSF. (Courtesy J. Q. Miller, MD.)

In the acute stage, diagnosis of RMSF can be made by skin biopsy and demonstration of rickettsiae in the endothelial cells of blood vessels by an immunofluorescence or immunoperoxidase technique. The rickettsiae are usually located at the center of the skin lesion (51–54).

Serological tests are useful for confirmation of the diagnosis. Currently, four serological tests are available; all use *R. rickettsii* antigen (55–57). These tests include indirect immunofluorescent antibody assay (IFA), indirect hemagglutination assay (IHA), latex agglutination (LA), and complement fixation (CF). According to the CDC, titers are diagnostic of 1:64 for IFA, 1:16 for CF, and a fourfold increase in titers between acute and convalescent sera for LA and IHA. Recently, polymerase chain reaction (PCR) has been utilized for the demonstration of DNA of *R. rickettsii* from blood samples of patients with severe disease (58,59).

The diagnosis and subsequent treatment of RMSF may be delayed because of the following (60):

1. Nonspecific symptoms at the onset resembling a viral illness
2. The occurrence of infection during the winter months in the southern states
3. Absence of typical rash (10% of cases)
4. Absence of a history of a tick bite
5. Presentation with symptoms other than fever, rash, and headache

Treatment

Treatment should be initiated as soon as the disease is suspected. Early treatment will drastically affect the outcome. Tetracycline, doxycycline, and chloramphenicol are the recommended antimicrobial agents for the treatment of this infection. The dose of these agents and duration of therapy is shown in Table 2. In patients with nausea, vomiting, or severe multisystem disease, antibiotics should be given intravenously.

Severely ill patients should be monitored in intensive care units. Anticoagulation is not recommended, as there is a risk of hemorrhage due to severe vasculitis from the infection.

The prognosis of RMSF has improved greatly since the introduction of antirickettsial therapy and intensive supportive measures. The case mortality rate is 3–7% in whites and 16% in blacks, possibly due to lack of recognition of skin lesions. The disease is more severe in patients with glucose-6-phosphate dehydrogenase deficiency (60–62). Elderly patients have a higher fatality

Table 2 Recommended Antimicrobial Therapy of Rocky Mountain Spotted Fever

Antibiotic	Dosage	Duration of therapy
Tetracycline		7–10 days
Child[a]	25–50 mg/kg/d (oral dose) in four divided doses	
Adult	500 mg (oral dose) qid	
Doxycycline		7–10 days
Adult	100 mg (oral dose) bid	
Chloramphenicol (recommended therapy for children under 8 years of age)		7–10 days
Child	50 mg/kg/d IV in four divided doses	

[a]Not recommended for children under the age of 8 years to avoid staining of the teeth.

rate. Neurological sequelae are common following RMSF and include headaches, learning disabilities, behavior abnormalities, and depression (63).

Prevention

The best means of prevention, particularly in endemic areas, is avoidance of contact with ticks by the use of repellents and protective clothing. Careful examination of the body twice a day for ticks in the scalp and axillary hair is suggested. Tweezers or forceps are recommended for removal of ticks. Following the removal, the area should be cleansed with soap and water. The tick should not be squeezed or crushed because tick tissues and fluids contain large quantities of *R. rickettsii* that may inoculate the individual removing the tick through a cutaneous lesion or the conjunctivae. Pets should be kept from roaming in tick-infested areas. Children living and playing in tick-infested areas, particularly in endemic areas, should be inspected daily for tick bites.

EHRLICHIOSES

Two human ehrlichioses occur in the United States: monocytic ehrlichiosis (HME), an infection of mononuclear phagocytes, and granulocytic ehrlichiosis (HGE), an infection of granulocytes. The *Ehrlichia* are bacteria, and infection is tickborne. Monocytic and granulocytic ehrlichiosis are separate diseases caused by different etiological agents. *Ehrlichia chaffeenis* is the etiological agent of HME. The etiological agent of HGE is not yet known. Most cases of HME occur in the southeastern and south central United States, but cases have been reported throughout the United States. Cases of HGE have been reported from Wisconsin, Minnesota, Connecticut, New York, California, and Florida. The tick vector of HME is most likely *A. americanum* and that of HGE the deer tick *Ixodes scapularis* and the dog tick *D. variabilis*.

The classic presentation of monocytic and granulocytic ehrlichioses is similar and includes fever, headache and myalgias, leukopenia, thrombocytopenia, anemia, and mild-to-moderate elevations in levels of aspartate and alanine aminotransferases, alkaline phosphatase, and lactate dehydrogenase. Liver enzyme abnormalities are present in approximately 80% of patients. Patients may present with pulmonary or gastrointestinal symptoms or signs and symptoms of meningitis. Over the course of several days, confusion, seizures, and coma may develop. Rash is present in only a minority of patients. Elderly patients are more prone to severe infection and to death. Secondary infections caused by nosocomial agents and opportunistic pathogens, including bacterial and fungal pneumonia, disseminated candidiasis, and necrotizing herpes esophagitis, often complicate the course of illness.

Diagnosis of ehrlichiosis in the acute stage of illness relies mostly on clinical suspicion. Serological confirmation requires acute and convalescent sera. Monocytic ehrlichiosis is diagnosed by use of the indirect fluorescent antibody assay (IFA) using an antigen to *E. chaffeenis*. A fourfold increase in *E. chaffeenis* antibody titer between acute and convalescent sera or a single high serum antibody titer ($\geqslant$128) is necessary for the serological diagnosis of HME. Although the etiological agent of HGE has not been determined, a serological reaction or fourfold increase in titer to *E. equi* antigen is presently recommended for seroconfirmation of HGE. A minimum titer of 80 is required.

Ehrlichia chaffeenis is susceptible only to doxycycline. The recommended therapy in adults or children for HME and HGE is doxycycline: 100 mg twice daily for adults and 3 mg/kg/day in two divided doses for children. A 7- to 10-day course of therapy is recommended. The total dose in children should be minimized to avoid staining of the teeth (49).

The important tickborne disease, Lyme disease, is discussed in the next chapter in this volume.

COLORADO TICK FEVER

Colorado tick fever is an acute viral illness acquired from a tick bite in the mountainous regions of the western United States, characterized by the abrupt onset of fever, headache, and myalgias. The illness may persist for 5–7 days, resolve, and recur, lasting for an additional 2–5 days. A petechial or macular rash may develop. During the acute illness, leukopenia or thrombocytopenia may develop. Neurological complications of encephalitis or aseptic meningitis are rare. Treatment is supportive care, and prognosis is excellent (63a).

FREE-LIVING AMEBIC MENINGOENCEPHALITIS

Amebae are single-cell organisms that infect humans world-wide. *Naegleria* and *Acanthamoeba* are free-living amebae (FLA) known to infect the central nervous system. *Naegleria* infections occur in healthy young individuals who acquire infection while swimming in freshwater lakes and, less often, swimming pools. *Acanthamoeba* infections occur in immunosuppressed and debilitated individuals and are usually not acquired by swimming. Both forms of amebic encephalitis are discussed in this section, although only *Naegleria* infections cause a spring and summer encephalitis.

In 1965, Malcolm Fowler and Rodney Carter reported four fatal cases of meningoencephalitis in young adults and children caused by amebae in South Australia along the Gulf of Spencer (64,65). The agent was thought to be *Acanthamoebae*; however, it was later shown to be *Naegleria fowleri*. In 1973, Robert and Rorke reported a case of granulomatous disease of the CNS produced by FLA in a 58-year-old male, who died (66). At autopsy, there was evidence of granuloma with giant cells and inflammatory infiltrates in the brain and brainstem area. In general, FLA infections manifest as two distinct clinical syndromes in humans: (1) an acute fulminant meningoencephalitis, referred to as primary amebic meningoencephalitis (PAM) due to *N. fowleri*, which occurs in healthy young adults and children after swimming in freshwater, and (2) subacute or chronic PAM or granulomatous amebic encephalitis (GAE) caused by *Acanthamoeba*.

Epidemiology

FLA are found worldwide (67). Since the first description in 1965, only 200 cases of PAM have been described worldwide (65). In endemic regions in Virginia, 16,174 autopsies were performed from 1920 to 1968, and 11 cases of PAM were attributed to FLA (68). Similarly, in a survey from an estimated one billion swimming episodes in Florida lakes, only seven fatal cases of CNS PAM have been seen (69).

Most United States cases of *N. fowleri* meningoencephalitis in humans are reported from the southeastern states. Characteristically, patients become ill after swimming and/or waterskiing in small, shallow freshwater lakes as a result of direct contamination through the nasal cavity. *N. fowleri* infection has been acquired from swimming in chlorinated pools. The organism may get into the pool through cracks in the pool (70). The contamination of swimming pools by these organisms has also been associated with failure of chlorination. Acute *Naegleria* meningoencephalitis usually affects children and young adults, particularly boys, and generally occurs during the hottest time of the year when people are most likely to swim (67). In Africa, cases have been reported during the dry and windy season by inhalation of the dust containing amebic cysts (71,72).

PAM due to *N. fowleri* generally occurs sporadically, although small outbreaks have been reported (67). Meningoencephalitis due to *Naegleria* is often a fatal disease.

Acanthamoeba infections are generally non–water-related and have been reported in individuals that are immunocompromised due to AIDS, chemotherapy, malnutrition, or chronic disease (73,74). *Acanthamoeba* has been isolated from the nasopharynx of asymptomatic individuals (75,76). *Acanthamoeba* usually causes a subacute or chronic form of meningoencephalitis (67). *Acanthamoeba* reaches the brain by way of the bloodstream from skin, eye, ear, or respiratory tract infections. Acanthamoeba keratitis has been reported in healthy contact lens wearers (77).

Pathogenesis and Pathology

Primary Amebic Meningoencephalitis

N. fowleri infects the CNS by invasion through the nasal cavity and then through the cribiform plate along the olfactory nerve (Fig. 2) (78,79). The pathogenesis of this infection has been observed experimentally in mice infected by instillation of a drop of *N. fowleri* into the nasal cavity. Ultrastructural studies show amebae invading the mucosa and ascending to the brain via the olfactory nerve (80). A purulent exudate develops around the olfactory bulbs.

Amebae can spread through the meninges to invade brain parenchyma directly or along blood vessels and induce extensive necrotizing inflammation in the cortex. The temporal and frontal lobes are most severely affected (78). The subcortical white matter is usually spared. Hemorrhagic and ischemic infarctions can occur (78–82).

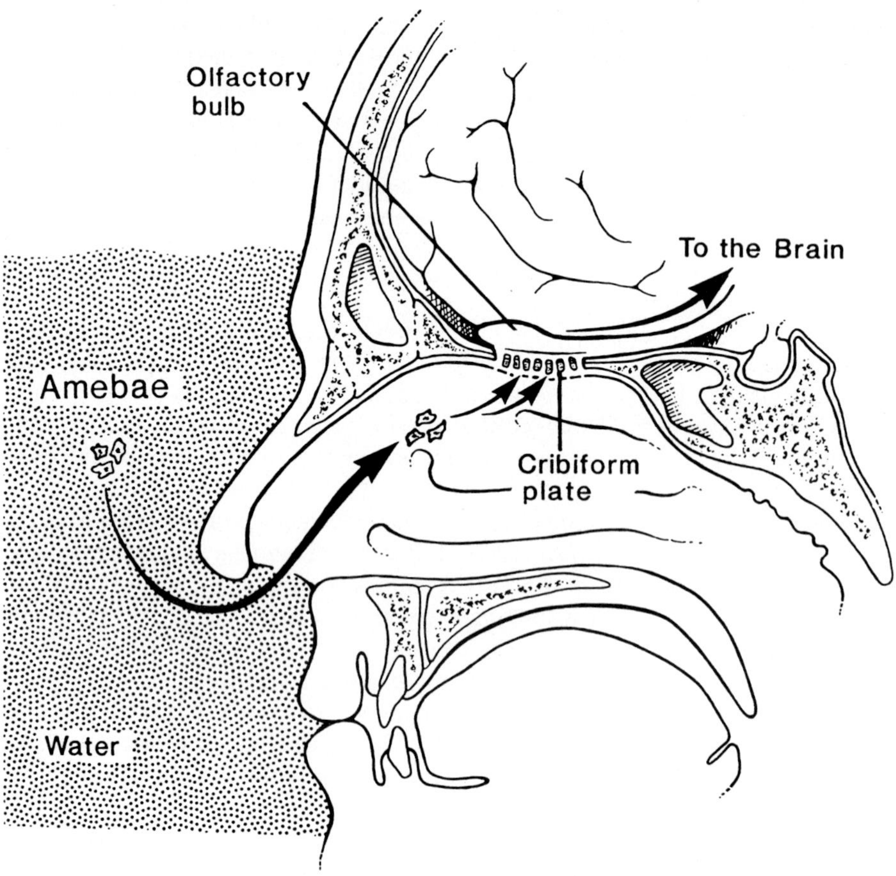

Figure 2 Invasion pathway of *Naegleria* into the CNS. (Adapted from Ref. 77a.)

Granulomatous Amebic Encephalitis

Acanthamoeba spp. reach the CNS through the bloodstream from a distant site of infection such as skin, cornea, or lung (83). *Acanthamoeba* spp. elaborate many enzymes, which may be directly or indirectly involved in the pathogenesis of tissue damage (78).

The neuropathology in GAE, as indicated previously, is a form of subacute or chronic PAM with focal inflammatory masses or abscesses in multiple areas of the brain, particularly white matter, and deep structures such as basal ganglia, brain stem, and cerebellum (66,84). Histology of the abscess shows granulomatous inflammation with histiocytes, mononuclear cells, and giant cells. A necrotizing vasculitis also occurs (78). In fixed tissue sections, amebae can be stained by H&E, but periodic acid Schiff (PAS) is required to identify cysts. In contrast to PAM, olfactory bulbs and tract are rarely affected. Ocular involvement manifested by uveitis may be the source of the CNS infection. Disseminated infection by *Acanthamoeba* has been reported in immunosuppressed patients (85).

Clinical Presentation

Primary Amebic Meningoencephalitis

The incubation period for infection by *N. fowleri* is usually 4–7 days. The initial presentation is often indistinguishable from bacterial meningitis. The patient presents with bifrontal severe headache, high fever, nausea and vomiting, anorexia, and neck stiffness. After 1 or 2 days, signs of encephalitis will appear, with focal neurological deficits, confusion, delirium, stupor, and finally coma. Death usually occurs within 2–4 days, although a few survivors have been reported (86). Because of involvement of the olfactory bulbs and tracts, early symptoms of abnormal smell (parosmia) or taste sensation (ageusia) have been reported (78,87).

The cerebrospinal fluid may have a cloudy appearance with a leukocytosis with a predominance of neutrophils, an increased protein concentration, a decreased glucose concentration, and red blood cells. The ameboid movements of the trophozoites can be seen on fresh or wet unstained specimens of CSF (78). Gram's stain is negative. Head computerized tomography (CT) scan may demonstrate hemorrhagic infarctions. Serological tests for *Naegleria* are basically of no value, because patients usually die before the results are available. After death, trophozoites can be demonstrated in the brain by light and/or electron microscopy. Death is commonly due to cerebral edema and increased intracranial pressure resulting in brainstem herniation (88).

Acute PAM clinically resembles acute bacterial meningitis. Examination of the CSF in bacterial meningitis reveals an increased opening pressure with a polymorphonuclear pleocytosis, an increased protein concentration, and a decreased glucose concentration. Gram's stain, bacterial culture, and latex agglutination tests on CSF are helpful in differentiating between these two infections. Other diseases in the differential diagnosis are brain abscess and herpes meningoencephalitis (89). These diseases can be diagnosed by neuroimaging, CSF examination, electroencephalogram, and brain biopsy.

Granulomatous Amebic Encephalitis

The incubation period of *Acanthamoeba* infections is longer than that of *Naegleria* infections, being weeks to months. The onset of encephalitis is insidious with symptoms and signs suggesting a focal cerebritis or abscess, i.e., seizures, hemiparesis, visual disturbances, and ataxia (90). A mild fever and headaches can occur. The patient may progressively deteriorate over several weeks. The disease is fatal, and only two cases of survival from GAE are reported (91,92). The cause of death is usually due to brainstem compression from cerebral edema and herniation.

Examination of the CSF shows a mild lymphocytic pleocytosis, normal to low glucose concentration, and a mild increase in protein concentration. Gram's stain and cultures of CSF are

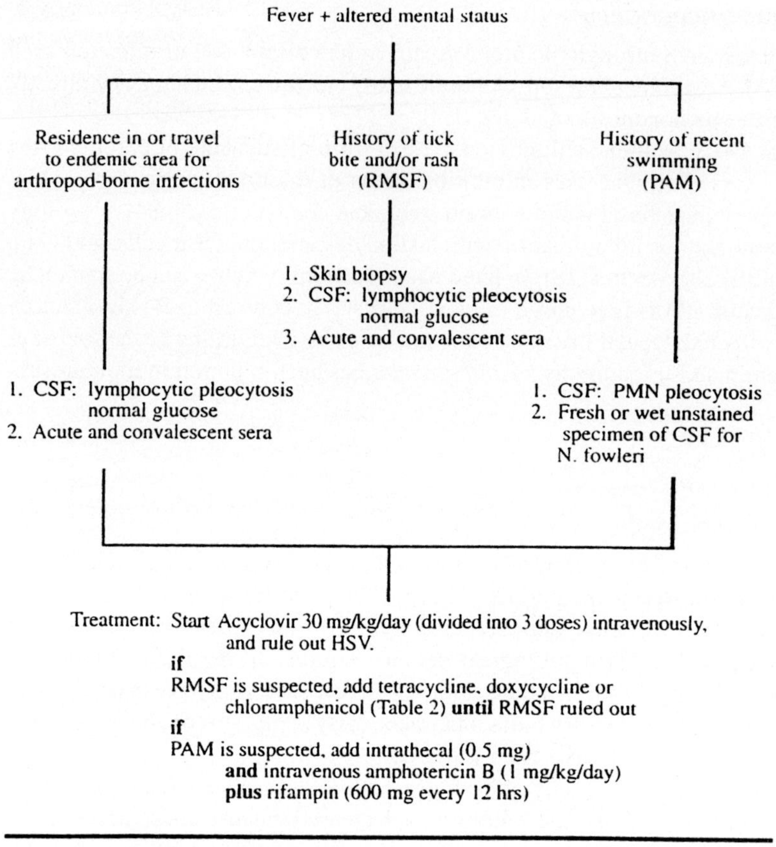

RMSF = Rocky Mountain spotted fever
HSV = Herpes simplex virus
PMN = polymorphonuclear
CSF = cerebrospinal fluid
PAM = Primary amebic meningoencephalitis

Figure 3 Diagnosis and management of spring and summer encephalitides.

negative. CT scan of the brain may show focal pathology that has the appearance of multiple brain abscesses or white matter demyelinating-type lesions (85,93). If the illness lasts more than 2–3 weeks, serological testing, complement fixation (CF), and indirect fluorescent antibody (IFA) tests are helpful in diagnosis.

The differential diagnosis of GAE is broader than that of acute PAM and includes viral meningoencephalitis, herpes encephalitis, tuberculous meningitis, cryptococcal meningitis, spirochetal infections, focal CNS lesions such as brain tumors, cysts of neurocysticerosis, and brain abscess. The diagnosis of GAE, therefore, is difficult on the basis of clinical and CSF examination. Brain biopsy can be diagnostic in these patients, but definite diagnosis is often established only at autopsy.

Prevention

PAM due to *Naegleria* is a fatal disease. Death usually occurs within 2–4 days. The most effective preventive measure for PAM is to prevent *Naegleria* from entering the nasal passages.

This can be done by avoiding swimming in freshwater lakes and/or stagnant water, particularly in high-temperature seasons. If one must enter these waters, nose clips should be worn. Chlorination is usually an effective measure to prevent FLA infection. Home-made saline solutions should not be used for cleaning or storing contact lenses, and lenses should not be worn when swimming in freshwater. As the epidemiology of *Acanthamoeba* is not known, no precautionary measures can be suggested. Since FLA infections are rare, routine use of vaccination is unnecessary.

Treatment

The drug of choice for acute *Naegleria* infection is amphotericin B, 1 mg/kg/day intravenously for 2–3 weeks (94). Rifampin, tetracycline, and/or minocycline have all been tried in combination with amphotericin B to treat PAM (95). The best documented survivor was treated with a combination of intravenous and intrathecal amphotericin B in combination with rifampin, sulfizoxole, and dexamethasone (78,96). Outcome may be improved by adding an intrathecal injection of amphotericin B (0.5 mg via a reservoir on alternate days) to the parenteral administration of this agent (97). There are four known survivors of PAM (96).

GAE should be treated with surgical excision of the focal granulomatous abscess followed by treatment with amphotericin B (78,98). A summary of the diagnosis and management of common seasonal encephalitides is shown in Figure 3.

LEPTOSPIROSIS

The term leptospirosis is derived from the Greek, meaning slender coil (*leptos* = slender; *spire* = coil), to describe the shape of the spirochete. Two forms of leptospirosis are recognized, a mild anicteric or benign form—the more common form of the disease—and a severe infection characterized by fever, jaundice, renal failure, hemorrhage, altered level of consciousness, and a high mortality rate

Rodents are the most important reservoir, but virtually all mammals can transmit the disease. In animals, leptospira produce a bacteremia and then localize to the tubules of the kidneys with persistent urinary excretion of the spirochetes into the environment (99).

Freshwater contaminated by rat urine is an important vehicle for transmission, particularly in North America (100). The peak season is late spring until late summer. Drinking water from a fountain also has been associated with infection (101). Sewer workers, miners, farmers (rice farmers), slaughterhouse workers, soldiers in jungle operations, and veterinarians have an occupational risk of infection (102).

Pathophysiology

The usual entry of spirochetes is through lacerations of the feet, skin, and mucosal membranes. Dissemination of organisms occurs through the bloodstream. Meningitis is characteristic of CNS infection. Meningeal reaction occurs only after the development of antibody, suggesting that meningitis is due to an antigen-antibody reaction (103,104).

Clinical Manifestations

The clinical spectrum of leptospirosis varies from mild to severe. The average incubation period is about 10 days. Leptospirosis generally is a biphasic illness. The first stage, or septicemic phase, is characterized by the sudden onset of severe headache, fever (100–105°F), chills, gastrointestinal complaints, myalgias (especially in the legs and lumbar area), and conjunctival injection. The onset of the disease is typically so sudden that it is said to have a "brutal beginning" based on the observation of farmers suddenly collapsing in the harvest fields with the illness (104). The headache is intense, unremitting, and intractable to analgesics. About 25% of patients have some disturbance in sensorium such as confusion or delirium (102,103). This stage usually lasts 5–7 days. During this stage, organisms can be isolated from the blood and cerebrospinal fluid. Improvement from this stage may occur; after 24–48 h the second stage, or immune phase, begins. This clinical stage correlates with the appearance of circulating IgM antibodies. This stage lasts 4–30 days. Leptospiruria is common and may continue for weeks to month.

Neurological manifestations of leptospirosis primarily occur in the second stage and are characterized by a meningitis. The incidence of meningitis in leptospirosis, either asymptomatic or symptomatic, is reported to be 80–90% if CSF analysis is performed during the second week of illness (103,105). Meningitis may be asymptomatic or may be manifest by intense headache, vomiting, and nuchal rigidity. Examination of the CSF reveals a normal or elevated opening pressure, a lymphocytic pleocytosis, and an increased protein concentration and often provides a striking relief of headache. This is a self-limited disease (103). Meningeal symptoms usually resolve within 1–2 days, and the CSF abnormalities resolve in 1–3 weeks (103).

Cerebral and subarachnoid hemorrhage and cerebral infarction have been reported in icteric leptospirosis (Weil's disease) (106).

Laboratory Diagnosis

The diagnosis of leptospirosis relies on either culture or serological studies. Multiple cultures should be obtained because the concentration of spirochetes in blood is low (107). In the first stage, the organisms can be cultured from blood or CSF, and in the second or convalescent phase, urine culture is the main source. CSF and blood cultures may be positive during the first 5–10 days of symptoms. Two weeks into the course of the illness, only the urine culture is likely to be positive.

Serological tests are often necessary for confirmation of leptospirosis. Antibodies appear from the 6th to 12th day of illness, reaching their highest concentration 3–4 weeks after the onset of symptoms. Several serological tests are available, including counterimmunoelectrophoresis, microscopic agglutination (MA) test, and IgM-specific dot ELISA. The MA test and the IgM-specific dot (ELISA) are considered the serodiagnostic tests of choice for leptospirosis (108,109).

Therapy

In mild cases, the disease is self-limited. For severe cases, the recommended antimicrobial agent is parenteral penicillin G.

Prevention

The following preventive measures should be considered: (1) avoidance of direct exposure to infected animal urine or tissues, (2) use of protective clothing (waterproof shoes, eye protection), and (3) chemoprophylaxis with doxycycline (200 mg weekly orally), which has provided up to 75% protection in U.S. soldiers undergoing jungle training (110).

ACKNOWLEDGMENTS

The author is grateful to J. Q. Miller, M.D., for providing photos of RMSF and to Linda Hagan for technical assistance.

REFERENCES

1. Rubeiz H, Roos RP. Viral meningitis and encephalitis. Semin Neurol 1992; 12:165–177.
2. Ho DD, Hirsch MS. Acute viral encephalitis. Med Clin North Am 1985; 69:415–429.
3. Centers for Disease Control. Arboviral infections of the central nervous system in United States, 11989. MMWR 1990; 39:407–417.
4. Johnson RT. Arboviral encephalitis. In: Warren KS and Mahmoud AF, eds. Tropical and Geographical Medicine. 2d ed. New York: McGraw-Hill, 1990:691–700.
5. Centers for Disease Control. St. Louis encephalitis outbreak—Arkansas, 1991. MMWR 1991; 40:605–607.
6. Kinsella RA, Braun GO. Clinical factors of epidemic (St. Louis) encephalitis. JAMA 1934; 103: 462–464.
7. Hammon W MCD, Reeves WC, Broukman B, et al. Isolation of the viruses of Western and St. Louis encephalitis from Culex tarsalis mosquitoes. Science 1947; 94:328–330.
8. Creech WB. St. Louis encephalitis in the United States, 1975. J Infect Dis 1977; 135:1014–1016.
9. Powell KE, Blakley DL. St. Louis encephalitis. JAMA 1977; 237:2294–2298.
10. Update: St. Louis encephalitis—Florida and Texas. 1990. MMWR 1990; 39:756–759.
11. Whitley RJ. Arthropod-borne encephalitides. In: Scheld WM, Whitley RJ, Durack DT, eds. Infections of the Central Nervous System. New York: Raven Press, 1991:87–111.
12. Tsai TF, Canfield MA, Reed CM, et al. Epidemiological aspects of a St. Louis encephalitis in Harris County, Texas, 1986. J Infect Dis 1988; 119:913–930.
13. Monath TP, Nystrom RR, Bailey RE, et al. Immunoglobulin M antibody capture enzyme-linked immunosorbent assay for diagnosis of St. Louis encephalitis. J Clin Microbiol 1984; 20:784–790.
14. Finley K, Riggs N. Convalescence and sequelae. In: Monath TP, ed. St. Louis Encephalitis. Washington, DC: APHA, 1980:535–550.
15. Meyer KF, Haring CM, Howitt B. The etiology of encephalomyelitis in horses in the San Joaguin Valley, 1930. Science 1931; 74:227–228.
16. Howitt BF. Recovery of the virus of equine encephalomyelitis from the brain of a child. Science 1938; 88:455–456.
17. Earnest MP, Goolishia HA, Calverley JR, Hayes RO, et al. Neurologic, intellectual and psychologic sequelae following Western encephalopathy. Neurology 1971; 21:969–974.
18. Centers for Disease Control. Arboviral infection of the central nervous system—United States, 1987. MMWR 1988; 37:506–515.
19. TenBroeck C, Merrill MH. A serological difference between eastern and western equine encephalomyelitis virus. Proc Soc Exp Biol Med 1933; 31:217–220.
20. Fothergill LD, Dingle JH, Faber S, et al. Human encephalitis caused by virus of the eastern variety of equine encephalomyelitis. N Engl J Med 1938; 219:411.
21. Reeves WC, Hammon WMcD. Epidemiology of the arthropod-borne viral encephalitides in Kern County, California, 1943–1952. Univ Calif Publ Health 1962; 4:257.
22. Hammon WMcD, Reeves WC. California encephalitis virus—a newly described agent. 1. Evidence of natural infection in man and other animals. Calif Med 1952; 77:303–309.
23. Thompson WH, Kalfoyan B, Anslow RO. Isolation of California encephalitis group virus from a fatal human illness. Am J Epidemiol 1965; 81:245–253.
24. LeDuc JW. Epidemiology and ecology of California serogroup viruses. Am J Trop Med Hyg 1987; 37:60S–68S.
25. Kappus KD, Monath TP, Kaminski RM, et al. Reported encephalitis associated with California serogroup virus infections in the United States, 1963–1981. In: Calisher CH, Thompson WH, eds. California Serogroup Viruses. New York: Alan R. Liss, 1983:31–41.
26. Calisher CH, Pretzman CT, Meth DJ, et al. Serodiagnosis of LaCrosse virus infection in humans by detection of immunoglobulin M class antibodies. J Clin Microbiol 1986; 23:667–671.
27. Calisher CH, Bailey RE. Serodiagnosis of LaCrosse virus infections in humans. J Clin Microbiol 1981; 13:344–350.

28. Baron RC, Hoffman RD, Powers JM, et al. Arboviral infections of the central nervous system in United States, 1987. MMWR 1988; 37:506–516.
29. Grabow JD, Mathews CG, Chun RWM, et al. The electroencephalographic and clinical sequelae of California arbovirus encephalitis. Neurology 1969; 19:394–404.
30. Balfour HH Jr, Siem RA, Bauer H, et al. California arbovirus (LaCrosse) infection. 1. Clinical and laboratory findings in 66 children with meningoencephalitis. Pediatrics 1973; 52:680–691.
31. Rie HE, Hilty MD, Cramblett HG. Intelligence and coordination following California encephalitis. Am J Dis Child 1973; 125:824–827.
32. Maxey EE. Some observations on the so-called spotted fever of Idaho. Portland Med Sent 1899; 7:433.
33. Hammarsten JF. The contributions of Idaho physicians to knowledge of Rocky Mountain spotted fever. Trans Am Cl Climatol Assoc 1982; 94:27–43.
34. Wilson LB, Chowning WM. Studies in pyroplasmosis brominis ("spotted fever" or "tick fever" of the Rocky Mountains). J Infect Dis 1904; 1:31–57.
35. Ricketts HT. The transmission of Rocky Mountain spotted fever by the bite of the wood tick (Dermacentor occidentalis). JAMA 1906; 47:358.
36. Weis E. History of rickettsiology. In: Walker DH, ed. Biology of Rickettsial Diseases. Vol 7. Boca Raton, FL: CRC Press 1988:15–32.
37. Wolbach SB. Studies on Rocky Mountain spotted fever. J Med Res 1919; 41:2–197.
38. Centers for Disease Control. Rocky Mountain spotted fever—United States, 1988. MMWR 1989; 38:513–515.
39. Kirk JL, Fine DP, Sexton DJ, Muchmore HG. Rocky Mountain spotted fever. A clinical review based on 48 confirmed cases, 1943–1986. Medicine 1990; 69:35–45.
40. Wilfert CM, McCormack JN, Kleeman K, et al. Epidemiology of Rocky Mountain spotted fever as determined by active surveillance. J Infect Dis 1984; 150:469–479.
41. Rocky Mountain spotted fever—United States, 1990. MMWR 1991; 40:451–9.
42. Marrie TJ, Raoult D. Rickettsial infections of the central nervous system. Semin Neurol 1992; 12: 213–224.
43. Helmick CG, Bernard KW, D'Angelo LJ. Rocky Mountain spotted fever: clinical, laboratory and epidemiological features of 262 cases. J Infect Dis 1984; 150:480–481.
44. Massey EW, Thomas T, Coffey CE, Gallis HA. Neurologic complications of Rocky Mountain spotted fever. South Med J 1985; 78:1288–1290.
45. Duffy RJ, Hammer ME. Ocular manifestations of RMSF. Ann Ophthalmol 1987; 19:301–306.
46. Horney LF, Walker DH. Meningoencephalitis as major manifestations of Rocky Mountain spotted fever. South Med J 1988; 81:915–918.
47. Katz DA, Dworzack DL, Horowitz ED, Bogard PJ. Encephalitis associated with Rocky Mountain spotted fever. Arch Pathol Lab Med 1985; 109:771–773.
48. Kaplowitz LG, Fisher JJ, Sparling FP. Rocky Mountain spotted fever: a clinical dilemma. In: Remington JB, Swartz HN, eds. Current Clinical Topics in Infectious Diseases. Vol. 2. New York: McGraw Hill, 1981:89–108.
49. Dumler JS, Bakken JS. Ehrlichial diseases of humans: emerging tick-borne infections. Clin Infect Dis 1995; 20:1102–1110.
50. Miller JQ, Price TR. The nervous system in Rocky Mountain spotted fever. Neurology 1972; 22: 561–566.
51. Woodward TE, Pederson CE, Oster CN, et al. Prompt confirmation of Rocky Mountain spotted fever: identification of rickettsiae in skin tissues. J Infect Dis 1976; 135:297–301.
52. Walker DH, Burdy JD, Fold MS. Laboratory diagnosis of Rocky Mountain spotted fever. South Med J 1980; 73:1443–1447.
53. Walker DH. Rocky Mountain spotted fever: a disease in need of microbiological concern. Clin Microbiol Rev 1989; 2:227–240.
54. Dumler JS, Gage WR, Peltis GL, et al. Rapid immunoperoxidase demonstration of Rickettsia rickettsii in fixed cutaneous specimens from patients with Rocky Mountain spotted fever. Am J Clin Path 1990; 93:410–414.

55. Kaplan JE, Schonbergar LB. The sensitivity of various serologic tests in the diagnosis of Rocky Mountain spotted fever. Am J Trop Med Hyg 1986; 35:840–844.
56. Hechemy KE, Michaelson EE, Amacker RL, et al. Evaluation of latex-Rickettsia rickettsii test for Rocky Mountain spotted fever in 11 laboratories. J Clin Microbiol 1983; 18:938–946.
57. Tzianabos T, Anderson BE, McDade JE. Detection of Rickettsia DNA in clinical specimens by using polymerase chain reaction technology. J Clin Microbiol 1989; 27:2866.
58. Carl M, Tibbs CW, Dobson ME, Paparello S, Dasch GA. Diagnosis of acute typhus infection using the polymerase chain reaction. J Inf Dis 1990; 161:791–793.
59. Fischer JJ. Rocky Mountain spotted fever: when and why to consider diagnosis. Postgrad Med 1990; 87:109.
60. Centers for Disease Control. Rocky Mountain spotted fever—United States, 1987. MMWR 1988; 37:388–390.
61. Fishbein DB, Kaplan JE, Bernard KW, Winkler WG. Surveillance of Rocky Mountain spotted fever in the United States, 1981–1983. J Infect Dis 1984; 150:609–611.
62. Walker DH, Kirkman HN. Rocky Mountain spotted fever and deficiency in glucose-6-phosphate dehydrogenase. J Infect Dis 1980; 142:771–777.
63. Gorman RJ, Saxon S, Snead OC. Neurological sequelae of Rocky Mountain spotted fever. Pediatrics 1981; 67:354–357.
63a. Spach DH, Liles WC, Campbell GL, Quick RE, Anderson DE, Fritsche TR. Tick-borne diseases in the United States. NEJM 1993; 329:936–947.
64. Carter RF. Primary amoebic meningoencephalitis: clinical, pathological and epidemiological features of six fatal cases. J Pathol Bacteriol 1968; 96:1–25.
65. Fowler M, Carter RF. Acute pyogenic meningitis probably due to acanthamoeba sp: A preliminary report. Br Med J 1965; 2:740–742.
66. Robert VB, Rorke LB. Primary amoebic encephalitis, probably from acanthamoeba. Ann Int Med 1973; 79:174–179.
67. Martinez AJ. Free-Living Amebas: Natural History, Prevention, Diagnosis, Pathology and Treatment of Disease. Boca Raton, FL: CRC Press, 1985.
68. Chang SL. Etiological, pathological, epdemiological and diagnostical consideration of primary amebic meningoencephalitis. Crit Rev Microbiol 1974; 3:135–159.
69. Wellings FM, Amuso PT, Chang SL, Lewis AL. Isolation and identification of pathogenic Naegleria from Florida lakes. Appl Environ Microbiol 1977; 34:661–667.
70. Cerva L. Studies of Limax amoebae in swimming pool. Hydrobiologic 1971; 38:141–161.
71. Lawande RV, John I, Dobbs RH, Engler LJ. A case of primary amebic meningoencephalitis in Zaria, Nigeria. Am J Clin Pathol 1979; 71:591–594.
72. Duma RJ, Helwig WB, Martinez AJ. Meningoencephalitis and brain abscess due to a free-living amoeba. Ann Intern Med 1978; 88:468–473.
73. Gonzalez MM, Gould E, Dickinson G, et al. Acquired immunodeficiency syndrome associated with Acanthamoeba and other opportunistic organisms. Arch Pathol Lab Med 1986; 110:869–879.
74. Martinez AJ. Acanthamoebiasis and immunosuppression. J Neuropathol Exp Neurol 1982; 41: 584–587.
75. Abraham SN, Lawande RV. Incidence of free-living amoebae in the nasal passages of local population in Zaria, Nigeria. J Trop Med Hug 1982; 85:217–222.
76. De Jonckheere JF, Michel R. Species identification and virulence of Acanthamoeba strains from human nasal mucosa. Parasitol Res 1988; 74:314–316.
77. Stehr-Green JK, Bailey TM, Brandt FH, et al. Acanthamoeba keratitis in contact wearers. A case-control study. JAMA 1987; 258:57–60.
77a. Niu MT, Duma RJ. Meningitis due to protozoa and helminths. Infect Dis Clin North Am 1990; 4: 809–839.
78. Cegielski JP, Durack DT. Protozoal infections of the central nervous system. In: Scheld WM, Whitley RJ, Durack DT, eds. Infections of the Central Nervous System. New York: Raven Press, 1991: 767–800.

79. Culbertson CG. Pathogenic Acanthamoeba (Hartmannelea). Am J Clin Pathol 1961; 35:195–202.
80. Martinez AJ, Duma RJ, Nelson EC, Moretta FL. Experimental Naegleria meningoencephalitis in mice. Penetration of the olfactory mucosal epithelium by Naegleria and pathologic changes produce: a light and electron microscopic study. Lab Invest 1973; 29:121–133.
81. Gutierrez Y. The free-living amebae. Naegleria and Acanthamoeba. In: Gutierrez Y, ed. Diagnostic Pathology of Parasitic Infection with Clinical Correlations. Philadelphia: Lea and Febiger, 1990: 80–93.
82. Butt CG. Primary amebic meningoencephalitis. N Engl J Med 1966; 274:1473–1476.
83. Jones DB, Visvesvara GS, Robinson NM. Acanthamoeba polyphagia keratitis and Acanthamoeba uveitis associated with fatal meningoencephalitis. Trans Ophthalmol Soc UK 1975; 95:221–232.
84. Callicott JH Jr, Jones MM, Nelson EC, et al. Meningoencephalitis due to free-living amoebae. JAMA 1968; 206:579–582.
85. Gullett J, Mills J, Hadley K, et al. Disseminated granulomatous Acanthamoeba infection presenting as an unusual skin lesion. Am J Med 1979; 67:891–896.
86. Duma RJ, Rosenblum M, McGehee RF, et al. Primary amebic meningoencephalitis caused by Naegleria. Two new cases and response to amphatericin B, and a review. Ann Intern Med 1971; 74: 923–931.
87. John DT. Primary amebic meningoencephalitis and the biology of Naegleria fowleri. Ann Rev Microbiol 1982; 36:101–123.
88. Duma RJ. Primary amebic meningoencephalitis. In: Warren KS, Mahmoud AF, eds. Tropical and Geographical Medicine. 2d ed. New York: McGraw-Hill 1990:321–326.
89. Jager BV, Stamm WP. Brain abscesses caused by free-living amoeba probably of the genus Hartmannella in patients with Hodgkin's disease. Lancet 1972; 2:1343–1345.
90. Martinez AJ. Is acanthamoeba encephalitis an opportunistic infection? Neurology 1988; 30:567–574.
91. Cleland PG, Lawande RV, Onyemelukwe G, Whittle HC. Chronic amebic meningoencephalitis. Arch Neurol 1982; 39:56–57.
92. Harwood CR, Rich GE, McAleer R, Cherian G. Isolation of Acanthamoeba from a cerebral abscess. Med J Aust 1988; 148:47–49.
93. Lalitha MK, Anadi V, Srivastava A, et al. Isolation of Acanthamoeba Culbertsoni from a patient with meningitis. J Clin Microbiol 1985; 21:666–667.
94. Stevens AR, Shulman ST, Lansen TA, Ciehon MJ, Willaert E. Primary amebic meningoencephalitis: a report of two cases and antibiotic and immunological studies. J Infect Dis 1981; 143:193–199.
95. Thong YH. Chemotherapy for primary amebic meningoencephalitis. N Engl J Med 1982; 306:1295–1296.
96. Seidel JS, Harmatz P, Visvesvara GS, Cohen A, Edwards J, Turner J. Successful treatment of primary amebic meningoencephalitis. N Engl J Med 1982; 306:346–348.
97. Anderson K, Jamieson A. Primary amoebic meningoencephalitis. Lancet 1972; i:902–903.
98. Kwame Ofori-Kwakye S, Sidebottom DG, Herbert J, Fischer EG, Visvesvara GS. Granulomatous brain tumor caused by *Acanthamoeba* (abstr). J Neurosurg 1986; 64:505–509.
99. Cohn AP, Howard AA. Common characteristics of leptospirosis: a report of 11 cases. Ann Intern Med 1961; 54:57–65.
100. Gillespie RW, Ryn I. Epidemiology of leptospirosis. Am J Public Health 1963; 53:950–955.
101. Cacciapuot B, Ciceroni L, Maffei C, et al. A waterborne outbreak of leptospirosis. Am J Epidemiol 1987; 126:535–545.
102. Heath CW Jr, Alexander AD, Galton MM. Leptospirosis in the United States. N Engl J Med 1965; 273:857–922.
103. Edwards GA, Domm BM. Human leptospirosis. Medicine 1960; 39:117–156.
104. Middleton JE. Canicola fever with neurological complications. Br Med J 1955; 2:25–26.
105. Cargill WH, Beeson PB. The value of spinal fluid examination as a diagnostic procedure in Weil's disease. Ann Intern Med 1947; 27:396.
106. Lessa I, Cortes E. Cerebrovascular accident as a complication of leptospirosis. Lancet 1981; 2:1113.
107. Sulzer CR, Jones WL. Leptospirosis: Methods in laboratory Diagnosis. Centers for Disease Control, U.S. Department of Health, Education and Welfare. Publication No. (CDC) 74-8275, 1974.

108. Myers DM. Serodiagnosis of human leptospirosis by counterimmunoelectrophoresis. J Clin Microbiol 1987; 25:897–899.
109. Watt G, Alquiza LM, Padre LP, et al. The rapid diagnosis of leptospirosis: a prospective comparison of the DOT enzyme-linked immunosorbent assay and the genus-specific microscopic agglutination test at different stages of illness. J Infect Dis 1988; 157:840–842.
110. Takafuji ET, Kirkpatrick J, Miller RN, et al. An efficacy trial of doxycline chemoprophylaxis against leptospirosis. N Engl J Med 1984; 310:497–500.

11

Lyme Disease

Patricia K. Coyle
State University of New York at Stony Brook, Stony Brook, New York

INTRODUCTION

Lyme disease (also called Lyme borreliosis) is a systemic bacterial infection produced by a tickborne spirochete, *Borrelia burgdorferi* (1). This infection targets specific body organs to cause disease of skin, joint, heart, eye, and central (CNS) and peripheral (PNS) nervous systems. Lyme disease is now recognized worldwide. There are endemic foci in North America, Europe, and northern Asia, with additional cases reported from Africa, Australia, and South America (2).

HISTORY

Lyme-related skin and neurological syndromes were first recognized in Europe (3). The earliest case report dates to 1883, when the German physician Buchwald described a patient with idiopathic skin atrophy. This lesion, which was subsequently named acrodermatitis chronica atrophicans (ACA) is now recognized as a late skin manifestation of Lyme disease. In 1909 the Swedish dermatologist Afzelius reported a patient with an expanding ringlike skin lesion following a tick bite. He called the lesion erythema migrans (EM). Thirteen years later the French neurologists Garin and Bujadoux described a patient with a similar red skin lesion and painful meningoradiculitis following tick bite. By 1930 the Swedish dermatologist Hellerstrom had associated EM with neurological involvement. The painful lymphocytic meningoradiculitis related to EM was subsequently named Bannwarth's syndrome. By 1951 it was recognized that EM responded to penicillin, but the causal infectious agent in Europe remained unknown.

The first reported case of EM in the United States was in 1969 and involved a Wisconsin physician who had been bitten by a tick while hunting (3). In 1975 a cluster of four EM cases was described in southeast Connecticut. By October 1975 Allen Steere had begun a study of children living near Old Lyme, Connecticut, who had developed a syndrome mimicking juvenile rheumatoid arthritis. In 1977 he reported this new clinical entity, Lyme arthritis, which was subsequently renamed Lyme disease. Willy Burgdorfer, working at the Rocky Mountain laboratories in 1981, isolated a novel spirochete from *Ixodid* ticks collected on Shelter Island. Identical spirochetes were soon shown to be present in European Ixodid ticks. In 1983 two separate groups cultured this spirochete, *B. burgdorferi*, from patients with Lyme disease (4,5).

PATHOPHYSIOLOGY

Organism

B. burgdorferi is technically a gram-negative bacteria that belongs to the spirochete family (6). Spirochetes encompass three genera (*Borrelia*, *Leptospira*, and *Treponema*) and cause four distinct neurological infections (Table 1) (6,7). Except for syphilis, all the infections are zoonotic or vectorborne.

B. burgdorferi is only visualized under phase contrast or darkfield microscopy. Organisms are difficult to culture, and require special growth (Barbour-Stoenner-Kelly, BSK) media. The organism divides by transverse fission every 8–12 h in vitro, with slower division in vivo. In addition to chromosomal DNA, *B. burgdorferi* contains extrachromosomal double-stranded DNA in the form of four to seven distinct supercoiled circular plasmids and linear plasmids. The chromosomal and extrachromosomal DNA code for many proteins. There are constant major proteins that are not unique to *B. burgdorferi*, such as the p41 flagellin (shared by other spirochetes), the p58-60 heat-shock protein, and additional p66 and 68 and p71 and 73 heat-shock proteins. These constant but nonspecific proteins cause serological cross-reactivity. There are also variable major proteins that are unique to *B. burgdorferi*. These include the plasmid-coded outer surface lipoproteins (Osp): the 31 kDa OspA, the 34 kDa OspB, and the 23 kDa OspC. Newly recognized Osp proteins include OspD, OspE, and OspF. Other important proteins are a unique p39 lipoprotein, and a unique p93 protein which appears to be a protoplasmic cylinder antigen. In addition to proteins, *B. burgdorferi* contains lipopolysaccharides with mitogenic and pyrogenic properties.

B. burgdorferi isolates show heterogeneity in their DNA, plasmids, and variable proteins (8,9).

Table 1 Spirochetal Infections

Definition
Flexible, helical bacteria with endoflagellum
Genera: *Treponema*
Leptospira
Borrelia
Neurological infections
Treponema pallidum (syphilis)
Leptospira interrogans (leptospirosis)
Borrelia recurrentis and other species (relapsing fever)
B. burgdorferi (Lyme disease)
Shared properties
Skin or mucous membrane entry sites
Early spirochetemia
Wide dissemination
Chronic infection with episodic clinical disease
Protean disease syndromes

The genospecies complex of *B. burgdorferi sensu lato* has been divided into more than three distinct species: *B. burgdorferi sensu stricto* (most of the North American isolates), *B. garinii*, *B. afzelii*, and one or more other species. Preliminary data suggest that different species cause different clinical disease patterns (10).

B. burgdorferi is believed to be a tissue-tropic but extracellular organism. Spirochetes can adhere to a number of different cell types, with attachment mediated by surface-exposed proteoglycans (11). Organisms adhere to and penetrate endothelial cells. This is an organism that is recognized to cause chronic infection. Although numbers are small, there are documented late isolations of *B. burgdorferi* from skin, cerebrospinal fluid (CSF), synovial tissue, flexor retinaculum, eye, myocardium, blood, and synovial fluid weeks to years after initial infection and despite the host immune response (12). In vitro, *B. burgdorferi* can invade fibroblasts to produce intracellular infection (12,13). In vivo, intracellular infection has not been shown. Whether viable spirochetes can persist inside a cell, protected from extracellular antibiotics, has therapeutic implications for treatment of chronic infection.

Vectors and Host

B. burgdorferi infects hard body *Ixodid* ticks (14). The infection geographically maps only to regions where these ticks are found. Except for a putative blood transfusion case and rare congenital cases, transmission of Lyme disease is confined to tick bite. There are exceptional examples of *B. burgdorferi* in other ticks (such as *Amblyomma americanum*) as well as in bloodsucking insects (fleas, mosquitoes, horseflies), but it is unproven whether these vectors can transmit infection (15,16). In North America the tick vectors are *Ixodes scapularis*, which has a northern (*I. dammini*) and southern form, and *I. pacificus*, the vector in the west. These vectors are established in 23 states and identified in 5 other states. The northern form of *I. scapularis* accounts for more than 80% of Lyme cases. Because the ticks prefer a moist environment, their preferred habitat is the ground, grass, bushes, and wooded undergrowth.

Hard body ticks have a 2-year life cycle, with larval, nymphal, and adult stages. There is only one blood meal per stage. Potential hosts include dozens of different mammals and bird species, which may help explain the geographic spread of the infection. Humans are accidental hosts and are most likely to be bitten by questing nymphs in the late spring and early summer. Nymphs are 1–2 mm, the size of a poppy seed, and easily missed. Tick saliva contains an anesthetic, so the tick bite is painless. The tick may also not bite at the site of initial skin contact, but may travel to intertriginous body parts (vaginal region, scrotum, axilla, retro-auricular region). *B. burgdorferi* is transmitted through the mouth parts of the tick by salivation and regurgitation. Transmission appears to occur only with prolonged attachment and feeding over 24 h, which activates spirochetes in the tick. A single tick may contain several different strains of spirochete.

Because transovarial transmission of *B. burgdorferi* is insignificant, reservoir hosts are critical to maintain the infection cycle. The white-footed mouse is the most important amplifying reservoir host in North America. Once infected, it maintains a spirochetemia for months without becoming ill. If an infected nymph feeds in the spring on such a mouse, any uninfected larvae that feed on that same mouse in the summer will be infected. In hyperendemic regions infection rates of *I. scapularis* approach 30–60%, compared to infection rates of only 1–6% for *I. pacificus*. These western ticks use lizards, which are incompetent reservoirs, as hosts.

Disease Pathogenesis

Infection with *B. burgdorferi* can result in a wide disease spectrum. Precisely how *B. burgdorferi* produces disease is not clear, and it is likely that several pathogenetic mechanisms are involved. Some syndromes, such as meningitis, reflect direct effects of tissue infection. Other syndromes may reflect indirect effects due to a secondary autoimmune response or due to bystander damage from a contiguous inflammatory or immune response. It is clear that *B. burgdorferi* can invade sequestered compartments, such as the CNS and joint, as part of the dissemination phase of infection. With regard to the CNS, *B. burgdorferi* binds in particular to galactocerebroside, has toxic effects on oligodendrocytes and astrocytes in vitro, and produces persistent infection of neural tissue (17–19). With regard to pathological changes associated with neurological disease, studies to date of brain, nerve, and muscle are striking for the lack of marked inflammatory changes and the paucity of organisms. CNS tissue has shown rare spirochetes, nonspecific microgliosis, and variable mononuclear infiltrates in parenchyma and meninges (20). Peripheral nerve has shown no spirochetes, no bound antibody or complement, limited axonal damage or loss, variable epineural, perineural, and perivascular mononuclear infiltrates, and angiopathy involving vasa nervorum suggestive of focal vasculitis (21,22). Muscle tissue has shown rare spirochetes, occasional focal myositis and interstitial inflammation, occasional focal necrosis, and a possible inclusion body myositis picture. The lack of striking neural tissue changes support the concept that certain neurological syndromes are due to indirect (immune or inflammatory) effects of the spirochete, rather than direct effects (23).

B. burgdorferi has many different effects on the immune system (24). Organisms are B-cell mitogenic (25), they activate T-cell subsets (26), and they induce cytokine production (including interleukins 1 and 6 and tumor necrosis factor α) (27–34). Within the nervous system, organisms effect specific B- and T-cell responses and formation of CSF immune complexes (35–37); they cause production of autoantibodies to axonal proteins, gangliosides, neurons, myelin components, and cardiolipin (38–41); they generate CSF T cells, which react to myelin, galactocerebroside, and cardiolipin (42); and they elevate CSF levels of interleukin 1, neopterin, and quinolinic acid (43,44). Myelin basic protein and the p41 flagellin share sequence homology (45), and certain monoclonal antibodies directed against *B. burgdorferi* epitopes will cross-react with CNS and PNS axons, Schwann cells, myelin, and other autoantigens (46,47). There is increasing data that chronic effects of Lyme disease are associated with a Thl response and induced proinflammatory cytokines (26,31–33).

CLINICAL PRESENTATION AND CLINICAL COURSE

Natural History

Infection with *B. burgdorferi* does not necessarily lead to disease, and up to 50% of infections are asymptomatic (48,49). This may reflect effects of inoculum dose, strain pathogenicity, or the host immune response. Similar to other human spirochetal infections, symptomatic illness may occur early or late in the infection. Clinical problems tend to be episodic, punctuated by asymptomatic periods (Table 2). There are discrete syndromes associated with early local (generally within one month of infection), early disseminated (within 3 months), and late disseminated infection. However, a patient may present with illness in one stage without manifesting features of other stages. Clinically, Lyme disease frequently causes very nonspecific manifestations at all stages, including prominent fatigue and malaise, headache, arthralgias, myalgias, meningismus, backache, and paresthesias.

Local Infection

Early local infection refers to the EM skin lesion, which is noted by 60–80% of Lyme patients (50). This is considered the sole pathognomonic clinical marker. EM is an expanding red lesion that occurs at the tick bite site an average of 8–9 (range 1–30) days after infection. The lesion is generally painless, although sometimes it itches or burns. The key feature of EM is expansion

Table 2 Clinical Stages of Lyme Disease

Early local infection
Erythema migrans (EM)
Mild viral-like illness
Early disseminated infection
Multifocal EM
Lymphocytoma (Europe)
Cardiac
Arthritis
Hepatitis
Conjunctivitis
Neurological
Late disseminated infection
Acrodermatitis chronica atrophicans (ACA) (Europe)
Cardiac
Arthritis
Keratitis, uveitis
Neurological

over time. The lesion begins as a macule, which evolves into a papule and then an annular erythematous plaque, which can enlarge to 42 cm. The center may be clear, vesicular, crusted, or edematous, and may form a bull's-eye lesion. There can be considerable variation in lesion configuration, size, color, center, and rate of expansion. Spirochetes can be detected in the EM lesion, particularly at the expanding edge, in as many as 60–86% of patients by culture, polymerase chain reaction (PCR) detection of Borrelial DNA, or immunohistochemical staining of a punch biopsy (50,51). This early skin lesion is the only high-yield biopsy or culture site in Lyme disease. Perhaps half of EM cases are associated with mild flulike symptoms (fever, headache, fatigue, myalgia, arthralgia). Untreated, EM typically resolves within weeks to months (average 4 weeks). Treated, EM typically resolves within days. Early infection with seroconversion has also been documented in children and adults with a flulike illness, without detectable concurrent EM.

Disseminated Infection

After a brief period of time, spirochetes disseminate to various body organs. Early dissemination may be associated with multifocal EM, joint, cardiac, or ocular problems. Elevated liver transaminases may be seen, consistent with mild hepatitis. Lymphocytoma, involving lymphocytic infiltration of earlobe or areola, is a skin lesion associated with dissemination, which occurs in 1% of European patients (50). Neurological syndromes of early dissemination are an "aseptic" meningitis or meningoencephalitis, cranial neuropathy, and radiculoneuritis (see below) (52–54,57).

Once spirochetes sequester within discrete body organs, they can cause late disease months to years after infection. ACA is a late atrophic skin lesion, an erythematous atrophic plaque, which occurs months to years after infection most typically on the leg. It is regularly seen as a feature of European Lyme disease, but only a handful of cases have been reported from North America (50). Very rare skin lesions associated with Lyme disease include lymphocytic skin infiltration, morphea, and other sclerodermatous lesions. Joint, cardiac, and ocular disease may be seen.

Neurological syndromes associated with late infection are encephalopathy, polyradiculoneuropathy, and encephalomyelitis (see below) (52,54–58).

Joint problems are very common in North American Lyme disease, and up to 60% of patients experience some rheumatological difficulties. The most characteristic joint problem of Lyme disease is an oligoarticular arthritis (defined as fewer than four joints involved) with intermittent painless swelling. The knee is most often involved, and there may be a Baker's cyst. Other joints involved in order of decreasing frequency are the shoulder, ankle, elbow, temporomandibular joint, wrist, hip, fingers, toes, and sternoclavicular joints. Lyme disease frequently causes migratory arthralgias, with large joints involved more commonly than small joints. This may begin shortly after the organism disseminates. There may also be migratory muscle, tendon, bone, or bursa pain. Typically, pain is present both at rest and with motion, tends to involve one or two regions at a time, and spontaneously clears over hours to days. Jaw pain, which occurs in up to 25% of patients, is an early suggestive feature. Arthritis in a minority of patients can even present as a septic joint or as a chronic process lasting over a year. Lyme disease may also produce a fibromyalgia syndrome with muscle tender points and chronic pain complaints. This is most commonly described as a posttreatment (post–Lyme syndrome) problem, which is felt to be antibiotic-unresponsive (59).

Cardiac involvement occurs in 8–20% of symptomatic Lyme infections and is three times more common in men than in women (60). The most characteristic cardiac manifestation is atrioventricular conduction block, which may be third degree (49%), second degree (16%), or first degree (12%). Other problems include sinus node problems, infra-His block, pericarditis, myocarditis, cardiomyopathy, congestive heart failure, and atrial or ventricular arrhythmias. Ocular manifestations include conjunctivitis, photophobia, periorbital edema, keratitis, and uveitis (61,62).

DIFFERENTIAL DIAGNOSIS

The clinical spectrum of Lyme disease is broad, and there is a wide differential diagnosis depending on the clinical syndrome and specific organ involvement. The major differential diagnosis for EM includes brown recluse spider bite, cellulitis, tinea, contact dermatitis, fixed drug reaction, reaction to an insect bite, and granuloma annulare. The differential diagnosis of flulike syndrome involves a variety of viral and other infections. The differential diagnoses of Lyme arthritis and Lyme carditis involve a variety of infectious and noninfectious causes of these syndromes. The differential diagnosis of neurological Lyme disease involves a wide variety of CNS and PNS disorders, which cause meningitis, cranial nerve palsy, radiculoneuritis, encephalopathy, encephalomyelitis, and polyradiculoneuropathy. Bilateral facial nerve palsy, for example, raises the possibility in particular of neurosarcoidosis, Guillain-Barré syndrome, acute viral infections (such as Epstein Barr or cytomegalovirus), or Melkersson's syndrome. Recently it has been appreciated that ticks can carry organisms other than *B. burgdorferi* that produce neurological problems. In particular, *Ehrlichia* and *Babesia* infections have been implicated as possible causes of symptoms in patients considered to have Lyme disease following tick bite (63,64). Both of these infections can be screened for serologically.

DIAGNOSIS

The diagnosis of Lyme disease is complicated by several factors. First, the clinical spectrum is not fully delineated, and this is particularly true for the neurological manifestations of infection. Second, no readily available active infection assay exists, and standard culture or stain techniques cannot be used to document infection. Antibody tests, which are the mainstay of the current laboratory diagnosis of Lyme disease, only document prior exposure to *B. burgdorferi*. Third, current antibody tests are not fully standardized. Screening ELISA tests in particular can give variable results. Fourth, there are seronegative Lyme cases. In well-studied populations at least 7% of infected patients are antibody negative (65,66). In high endemic areas, some practitioners have claimed that the seronegativity rate approaches 30–40%. Finally, many of the most common clinical complaints produced by Lyme disease are quite nonspecific and can result from many different disorders.

The CDC has created a case definition of Lyme disease for surveillance and study purposes (Table 3). However, for clinical purposes, this definition is too strict. The current diagnosis of Lyme disease is a clinical one, which should be supported by laboratory data. Of the suggested clinical criteria outlined in Table 4, EM is considered a pathognomonic marker. Only 60–80% of patients note an EM lesion, and other skin disorders can be misdiagnosed as EM. A truly definitive diagnosis of EM would require biopsy, culture, or PCR diagnosis (detection of Borrelial DNA within the skin lesion). The other clinical features are suggestive of the diagnosis. Exposure is more likely with recreational or occupational outdoor activity. With regard to tick bite, it is reported in less than 50% of neurological Lyme patients. Only the tiny *Ixodid* tick is a vector; the larger dog tick for all intents and purposes should not be considered a vector of Lyme disease. Disease is more likely when ticks are from recognized high endemic regions and when they have fed to engorgement. In experimental studies of *B. burgdorferi*–infected ticks, transmission is negligible if ticks feed for less than 24 h, increases to 50% if they feed 48 h, and is virtually 100% by 72 h (67). Since this is a systemic infection, antecedent flulike illness or suggestive extraneural involvement makes a diagnosis of Lyme disease more likely. Lyme disease is also more likely when the patient has one of the recognized characteristic neurological syndromes.

Unfortunately, there is nothing unique about the examination of the Lyme disease patient. Neurologically, a peripheral facial weakness (especially bilateral), radicular features, unexpected median nerve entrapment, and distal sensory loss support the diagnosis. Systemically a swollen joint, Baker's cyst, or cardiac/ophthalmological abnormalities would also be supportive in a neurological patient.

Unlike most bacterial infections, the laboratory diagnosis of Lyme disease does not depend on culture or stain of organism from various body fluids. Only the EM skin lesion has any reasonable yield in this regard, but in a recent study at a research facility, the success rate of lavage culture of

Table 3 CDC Surveillance Case Definition for Lyme Disease

EM (⩾5cm) diagnosed by a physician
or
Late manifestation
Recurrent brief swollen joints
Acute onset 2° or 3° atrioventricular conduction defect
Meningitis
Cranial neuropathy
Radiculoneuritis
Encephalomyelitis with intrathecal antibody production
and
Laboratory confirmation
Culture
Antibodies in serum or CSF
Acute and convalescent sera document rising titers

Table 4 Current Diagnosis of Lyme Disease

Clinical clues	Laboratory clues
EM	Blood studies
Exposure to endemic region	anti-*B. burgdorferi* antibodies
Antecedent tick bite	nonspecific tests
type (*Ixodes*)	tests to exclude other diagnoses
likelihood of infection (highest in Northeast)	CSF studies
duration of attachment	intrathecal anti-*B. burgdorferi* antibody production
engorgement	cell count
Antecedent constitutional syndrome	protein
Suggestive extraneural features	glucose
joint involvement	VDRL
jaw pain	other tests (oligoclonal bands, IgG index, myelin basic protein, etc.)
myalgias	experimental tests (antigen, PCR, culture, Borrelial immune complexes)
prominent fatigue	Ancillary studies
cardiac features (including palpitations)	neuroimaging (MRI preferred)
ocular features	neurophysiological (nerve conductions, evoked potentials, EMGs)
Characteristic neurological syndrome	neuropsychological testing
Examination clues	angiography or MR angiography
Facial nerve weakness	EKG
Radicular signs	synovial fluid studies
Median nerve entrapment	
Mild distal sensory loss	
Swollen joint	
Baker's cyst	
Cardiac or ophthalmological disease	

EM lesion was only 29% (68). Current laboratory diagnosis relies on documenting a specific host immune response.

Unfortunately, antibody assays have been fraught with problems, with poor inter- and intra-assay reliability (69–72). There may be false-positive and false-negative results, and early on serology will be negative (Table 5) (65,72–77). *B. burgdorferi* infection can also cause a false-positive FTA-Abs syphilis serology (78). Recently the CDC has moved to correct serological problems by standardizing Lyme disease Western blot tests (79). They now recommend that all borderline or positive ELISA assays be confirmed by Western blot. IgM blots are recommended

Table 5 Causes of Inaccurate Lyme Serology (anti–*B. burgdorferi* Antibodies)

False positives
Other infections (spirochetal, bacterial, rickettsial, HIV-1, EBV)
Hypergammaglobulinemia (polyconal B-cell activation)
Diseases with high autoantibody levels
Unreliable assay
False negatives
Early infection
Early antibiotics with blunted humoral response
Unreliable assay

only for patients within one month of onset of symptoms. Positive IgM Western blot must exhibit reactivity against at least two of the following protein bands: 23 (OspC), 39, and 41 (flagellin) kDa. IgG Western blots are used when patients have been ill for any length of time, but particularly past 1 month. A positive IgG blot must exhibit reactivity against at least five of the following protein bands: 18, 23, 28, 30, 39, 41, 45, 58, 66, and 93 kDa.

Once a patient is antibody positive, they may remain so for years after treatment or they may ultimately become seronegative. Serial serologies have not been useful to predict disease course or response to therapy (80). One peculiarity noted in some patients is the persistence of IgM, with an expanded antigenic profile over time (81). The significance of this finding is unknown, although it clearly suggests organism persistence.

It is hoped that standardized Western blot testing will correct the problem of false-positive ELISA assays. However, it will not address the issue of the seronegative patient. The most common feature in infected patients who remain seronegative is early antibiotic treatment, which aborts the mature humoral response. For example, 20% of treated EM patients never seroconvert. Ultimately, decisions on diagnosis must be dictated by reasonable clinical judgment rather than a single laboratory test.

In addition to documenting seropositivity, blood tests are useful to exclude other conditions (such as syphilis, vitamin B_{12} deficiency, thyroid disease, and collagen vascular disease) and other tickborne infections (such as babesiosis and ehrlichiosis). Lyme patients may show certain abnormal blood studies (elevated ESR, liver enzymes, circulating immune complexes, cryoglobulins, quantitative IgM, or IgM anticardiolipin antibodies) (82), but they are nonspecific.

For neurological Lyme disease, the most useful laboratory test is CSF examination. CSF studies allow one to examine a sequestered compartment, which *B. burgdorferi* is known to seed, they can provide objective evidence of CNS involvement, they provide a pretreatment baseline, and they can help guide therapy. However, North American patients tend not to show the marked inflammatory changes reported in European Lyme cases. In fact normal CSF does not exclude neurological infection by *B. burgdorferi*, and the organism has been cultured from normal CSF (83). The likelihood of abnormal CSF depends on the neurological syndrome. CSF is invariably abnormal in Lyme meningitis and radiculoneuritis cases, is often abnormal in cranial neuropathy and encephalomyelitis cases, can be normal in encephalopathy cases, and is generally normal in pure PNS syndromes. The most helpful CSF test is a paired Lyme antibody titer to look at intrathecal production of specific antibodies (84–86). With rare exceptions, this test documents CNS invasion. It is extremely unusual for CSF antibodies to be positive in the setting of peripheral seronegativity, but there have been a few early infection cases where the CSF titer was positive before serum. Other CSF abnormalities suggestive for Lyme disease are mononuclear pleocytosis, atypical plasma cells, and elevated protein. CSF glucose, VDRL, and myelin basic protein studies are generally normal or negative. In contrast to European patients, CSF oligoclonal bands or increased IgG index are found in a minority of North American Lyme patients.

More specific CSF tests to diagnose infection include detection of Borrelial DNA, antigens, immune complexes, and specific IgM antibodies (36,87,88). These tests are not yet widely available and have not been fully standardized, but in the future these tests will likely be used to document CNS invasion.

Ancillary laboratory studies can support the diagnosis of neurological Lyme disease. Neuroimaging (MRI is superior to CT) is abnormal in only 25% of patients, but there is no unique pattern (89). The most common finding is scattered small white matter lesions suggestive of vasculitis. Larger lesions in the basal ganglia or white matter, or even a single large granulomatous lesion, can also be seen on MRI, as well as enhancement of cranial or spinal nerves (90,91). Preliminary reports suggest that functional brain neuroimaging (using SPECT) may show abnormal cerebral blood flow patterns in some late CNS infections. Nerve conduction tests may document a multifocal axonal radiculoneuropathy, or silent median nerve entrapment. Cortical and brainstem auditory evoked potential tests have recently been reported as abnormal in some late infection cases. When there is a question of encephalopathy, formal cognitive function tests can document suggestive CNS abnormalities and can provide a pretreatment baseline. Angiography or MR angiography is reasonable in cerebrovascular cases. If muscle biopsy is indicated, it should be handled by a laboratory experienced in testing for *B. burgdorferi*. Other laboratory tests for diagnosis may include synovial fluid studies, synovial biopsy, cardiac studies, and cardiac biopsy.

TREATMENT

Lyme disease is a bacterial infection and typically responds well to appropriate antibiotic therapy, particularly when given in the early infection stage. However, there are several current treatment issues.

All of the drug regimens in current use have had treatment failures or relapses, although this is less likely with early aggressive treatment (92,93). Infections have persisted even when patients became seronegative after treatment. For the various stages and syndromes of Lyme disease, the optimal antibiotic, route of delivery, and duration of therapy have not been established. Very few controlled trials have compared different antibiotic regimens for Lyme disease. There are no reliable criteria to document antimicrobial cure. In vitro and in vivo antibiotic susceptibility studies have been inconsistent (94,95). Finally, it is a peculiarity of this infection that certain symptoms (fatigue, muscle and joint pain, headache, paresthesias, cognitive difficulties) may improve gradually weeks to months after treatment. The earlier in the infection the patient receives adequate antibiotics, the less likely they are to have prolonged symptoms or to develop a post-Lyme syndrome (defined as persistent complaints that are not improving more than 6 months after treatment).

Local infection is generally treated with several weeks of an oral antibiotic—either amoxicillin or doxycycline (Table 6) (96). There have been no convincing data that other alternatives (azithromycin, cefuroxime axetil) are superior (97–99), and clearly oral penicillin, erythromycin, or tetracycline, which do not give good levels or tissue penetration, are no longer recommended. Although probenecid has been added to amoxicillin to prolong blood levels, it increases the risk of allergic reactions. An alternative choice is the use of a higher dose of oral amoxicillin.

Neurological infections are generally treated with parenteral (intravenous) antibiotics (100). Ceftriaxone is the current drug of choice in North America and is preferred over penicillin, which has been associated with failure rates as high as 50% in late North American infections (101). Cefotaxime is an alternative third-generation cephalosporin. Studies from Europe (but not North America) support its efficacy in Lyme disease (102,103). It is less expensive than ceftriaxone, but is given on a less convenient tid rather than qd schedule. For North American Lyme disease, there is a greater experience with ceftriaxone, and this remains the drug of choice for most neurological Lyme disease patients. Doxycycline can also be given intravenously for severe infections. It can be given at higher doses to boost CSF concentrations (104).

Certain syndromes are treated with extended oral antibiotics. This is particularly true for mild PNS syndromes where there is no evidence of CNS involvement. There is debate about whether Lyme facial neuropathy can be treated with oral antibiotics, in light of experimental studies indicating CNS seeding in a good proportion of such patients. A recent study from Europe reported that oral doxycycline (100 mg bid) for 2 weeks was as effective as intravenous penicillin in treating neurological patients (105). There have also been reports of late-infection patients treated with oral antibiotics (106). The difficulty with generalizing such studies to North American patients is the increasing evidence that infection on the two continents differs in significant

Table 6 Antibiotic Treatment for Lyme Disease

A. Oral agents used for mild peripheral syndromes with negative CSF; duration of therapy usually 30 days.

Agent	Adult dose	Pediatric dose	Comments
Preferred			
Amoxicillin (amoxil, polymox, wymox)	500–1000 mg TID	50 mg/kg QD	Hypersensitivity reactions GI problems
Doxycycline	100 mg BID-TID	100 mg BID	Not used under age 9 (teeth discoloration) Photosensitivity Not used in pregnancy GI problems (do not take on empty stomach) Simultaneous antacids, calcium, iron medications may inactive drug
Alternative			
Azithromycin (zithromax)	500 mg QD	250 mg QD	Unclear duration of therapy
Cefuroxime axetil (ceftin)	500 mg BID	250 mg BID	Do not give with meals, antacids GI problems Bitter taste

B. Parenteral agents used for most neurological syndromes; when CSF is abnormal duration of therapy at least 2 weeks.

Agent	Adult dose	Pediatric dose	Comments
Preferred			
Ceftriaxone (rocefin)	2 g QD	75–100 mg/kg QD	GI problems Cholelithiasis Hypersensitivity reactions
Alternative			
Cefotaxime (claforan)	2 g TID	120–150 mg/kg	GI problems Hypersensitivity reactions Inflammation at injection site
Doxycycline	200–400 mg QD	200 mg QD	Same as for oral
Penicillin G	3–4 mU Q4H	0.3–0.5 mU/kg QD	Hypersensitivity reaction

ways. Congenital infection appears to be a very rare problem. Both ceftriaxone and amoxicillin have been used in pregnant infected women.

The issue of duration of therapy is controversial. In some endemic areas, patients are being treated for months to years. Neurological syndromes warrant therapy for a minimum of 2–4 weeks. Patients who require retreatment should be treated for at least 4 weeks.

A Jarisch Herxheimer reaction occurs in 10–20% of treated patients. This reaction is seen in the first 24–48 h after the initiation of antibiotic therapy and involves fever, headache, and worsening of symptoms. Problems that begin weeks into the therapy should not be considered Herxheimer reaction. Patients are treated symptomatically with antipyretics and anti-inflammatory agents.

As a general rule, corticosteroids are avoided in neurological Lyme disease because they have been associated with increased risk for treatment failure and persistent infection (101,107).

Treatment of Lyme disease includes symptomatic therapies, such as pain medications; appropriate rehabilitation therapy; and the use of plasmapheresis or intravenous immunoglobulin, in addition to antibiotics, for Lyme-related Guillain-Barré syndrome.

NEUROLOGICAL COMPLICATIONS

Overview

Neurological involvement occurs in up to 40% of symptomatic infections and includes both CNS and PNS involvement. Six characteristic neurological syndromes, as well as a variety of less well-established neurological syndromes, have been associated with early and late North American Lyme disease (Table 7) (20,52–57,108–110).

Early Syndromes

Meningitis

During the early dissemination phase of infection, spirochetes can seed the CNS to produce an "aseptic" meningitis or meningoencephalitis. This can occur while EM is still present and typically occurs within 12 weeks of infection. The meningitis syndrome is acute or subacute and rarely relapsing or chronic. It is often subtle, with the most prominent feature a fluctuating (typically frontal) headache that ranges from mild to severe. Meningismus is uncommon (20–30%) and tends not to be striking. Suggestive associated features of Lyme meningitis are facial nerve and spinal nerve root involvement (such as severe pain between the scapulae); associated fatigue, myalgia, arthralgia, or heart block; and an atypical lymphocytic or plasma cell component to the CSF pleocytosis. The median CSF pleocytosis is 52–170 cells, over 90% mononuclear. There is only one case of Lyme meningitis in the literature, which mimicked a septic neutrophilic meningitis (111). Protein is elevated in more than half of the patients, but the median value is less than 80 mg%. In North America less than half of Lyme meningitis cases are CSF oligoclonal band positive or have an elevated IgG index. Intrathecal Lyme antibody production occurs in 50–90%.

Table 7 Neurological Syndromes in North American Lyme Disease

Early characteristic syndromes:	"Aseptic" meningitis, meningoencephalitis
	Cranial nerve palsy (esp. uni- or bilateral Bell's)
	Radiculoneuritis
Early unusual syndromes:	Headache and stiff neck with normal CSF
	Confusional state
	Transient ischemic attack–type episode
Late characteristic syndromes:	Encephalopathy
	Sensorimotor polyradiculoneuropathy
	Encephalomyelitis, meningoencephalomyelitis
Late unusual syndromes:	Intracranial hypertension syndome (children, adolescents)
	Vasculitis
	Psychiatric syndrome
	Myositis

Borrelial antigen can be detected in 60% of cases, but PCR has been said to be positive in only 30%. This likely reflects current problems with PCR applied to CSF specimens.

Cranial Nerve Palsy

Cranial nerve palsy is the most frequent neurological abnormality noted in Lyme patients (54,112). During early dissemination in the first weeks to months after infection (most commonly during summer), Lyme disease can cause isolated cranial neuropathy. Cranial neuropathy can be the initial manifestation of Lyme disease and in rare cases has preceded the occurrence of EM (113). The facial nerve accounts for 80–90% of cranial neuropathies (54). This is the most frequent neurological manifestation of Lyme disease, occurring in 11–14% of symptomatic infections (113). In endemic regions up to 25% of facial nerve palsies are due to Lyme disease (114). This is especially true during summer and for children. Twenty-three to 37% of patients have bilateral involvement, which strongly suggests Lyme disease. The facial neuropathy is often accompanied by other features, such as headache, fever, or marked fatigue. In Lyme disease, facial neuropathy may result from a central or peripheral lesion and may or may not be associated with a CSF pleocytosis and an occult meningitis. When Lyme cranial neuropathy occurs without meningitis, specific intrathecal antibody production is found in <10%. However, experimental studies have detected Borrelial antigen and DNA in otherwise normal CSF. Patients may show an elevated ESR, IgM, and cryoglobulins. Corticosteroids are best avoided in the acute therapy of Lyme facial nerve palsy. Other cranial nerves involved in Lyme disease include the optic nerve (to give optic neuritis, ischemic optic neuropathy, or disc edema) (115); ocular palsies (VI, III, and IV); facial sensory problems (V); hearing loss or tinnitus (VIII) (116); and rarely lesions involving cranial nerves IX through XII (54). Cranial nerve involvement can be unilateral, bilateral, or multiple.

Radiculoneuritis

Painful radiculoneuritis is an unusual early dissemination complication in North America. It is much more common in Europe, where it is referred to as Bannwarth's syndrome or lymphocytic meningoradiculitis. Patients show asymmetrical and focal dermatomal and myotomal deficits, shooting radicular pains, and inflammatory (mononuclear cell) CSF changes (54,117). There may be an associated facial nerve palsy. This syndrome is much more common in adults than in children, and pain tends to be more severe in older individuals. There is severe radicular, burning, deep, or superficial pain, which is worse at night. Pain often migrates, but is most typical in the upper or lower back and between the scapulae. There are often associated patchy areas of skin dysesthesia. Objective sensory findings tend to be subtle. Sensory symptoms may be associated with focal motor weakness, depressed reflexes, and rarely with evidence of associated myelitis. Patients generally show inflammatory CSF changes (mononuclear pleocytosis, increased protein, intrathecal specific antibody production). Electromyography (EMG) may show loss of motor units, fibrillations, and positive sharp waves, increased duration of motor unit potentials, and increased polyphasic potentials. Studies overall suggest a predominantly axonal process. Variations of this radiculoneuritis syndrome include plexopathy, mononeuritis multiplex, and a Guillain-Barré–type syndrome (54,118,119). Such patients can show loss of reflexes with predominant motor involvement (119,120). An important clue that this is not typical Guillain-Barré syndrome is the finding of CSF pleocytosis. A second clue is that careful neurophysiological studies are more consistent with a polyradiculopathy and distal axonal damage, rather than a primary demyelinating process. In addition to this mimicking syndrome, true Guillain-Barré syndrome may occur as a postinfectious complication following *B. burgdorferi* exposure. Such patients do show cytoalbuminological dissociation and a demyelinating pattern on neurophysiological testing. As is true for all the early dissemination syndromes, patients will spontaneously improve even without antibiotic treatment.

Unusual Early Syndromes

Besides the above three syndromes, there has been experimental evidence for CNS seeding by *B. burgdorferi* in newly infected patients who develop problems with headache and stiff neck, confusional state, or transient ischemic attack (TIA)–type episode.

Late Syndromes

Encephalopathy

The most common late neurological syndrome of Lyme disease is a chronic encephalopathy, characterized by difficulty in word retrieval, slowed reaction time, and memory and attention problems (55,58,121). Cognitive difficulties range from mild to severe, but generally are not severe enough to produce dementia and the patient is able to continue to work. These cognitive problems are usually accompanied by prominent fatigue and malaise. Objective laboratory deficits reported in these patients include abnormalities on cognitive function tests not explained by fatigue, depression, or pain; abnormal cerebral blood flow on brain SPECT (122); delayed p300 on cortical evoked potential; and abnormal brain-stem auditory evoked potentials with hearing loss. Routine CSF abnormalities are not striking. Pleocytosis is noted in only 5%, increased protein in 17–46%, oligoclonal bands or increased IgG index in <5%, and intrathecal Lyme antibody production in less than 50%. CSF Borrelial antigen has been detected in 40–80% of such patients. Coincident with clinical improvement, deficits tend to improve after antibiotic treatment.

Sensorimotor Polyradiculoneuropathy

Mild chronic neuropathy and radiculopathy syndromes have been described as complications of late Lyme disease, distinct from the painful radiculoneuritis that occurs within a few weeks to months after *B. burgdorferi* infection. These late PNS syndromes may occur in association with late skin involvement (ACA), in isolation, or in association with late encephalopathy.

ACA develops in about 10% of European Lyme cases. It is more common in the elderly, and occurs typically 6 months to 8 years after initial infection (50). Spirochetes have been identified within the chronic skin lesion by culture and staining, even in a lesion present over 10 years. Approximately 40–60% of ACA patients show clinical or laboratory evidence of mild, chronic PNS disease (123,124). This takes the form of a predominantly distal sensory neuropathy. Variations include subclinical neuropathy, sensory cutaneous neuropathy, and asymmetrical or symmetrical polyneuropathy. Subjective complaints involve pain or paresthesias, and much less commonly weakness, muscle cramps, or restless legs. Objective deficits (generally sensory loss) are most marked in the region affected with ACA, but can also be found elsewhere. Nerve biopsy shows perivascular mononuclear cell infiltration around small and medium-sized epineural blood vessels, with occasional involvement of the vessel wall. Nerve fiber damage corresponds with inflammation.

A similar rather mild late peripheral nerve involvement has been noted in up to 40% of North American Lyme patients (56,120,125). These patients do not have ACA, but may have an associated late CNS syndrome (encephalopathy). Typically patients have been infected months to years earlier. The neuropathy may be so subtle as to be subclinical, but most patients note nonpainful distal paresthesias or mild radicular pains. Paresthesias tend to be intermittent, may be symmetrical or asymmetrical, and involve legs more often than arms (and rarely face). Radicular pains are also intermittent and generally asymmetrical. Unlike the early radiculoneuritis syndrome, these patients have no associated meningitis or facial neuropathy. Objective abnormalities are also subtle and include distal light touch and vibration sensory loss (most commonly in the toes) or stocking/glove sensory loss. Weakness, depressed reflexes, or muscle tenderness are uncommon.

Neurophysiological testing generally shows abnormalities suggestive of a rather diffuse neuropathy, even in clinically uninvolved limb and trunk regions. Nerve conduction abnormalities are particularly common in patients with paresthesias, and include mildly prolonged distal motor or sensory latencies and mild slowing of distal motor conduction velocities. Abnormalities suggestive of marked demyelination are exceedingly rare. EMG changes indicate minor motor nerve fiber abnormalities, with mild to moderate denervation of distal muscles, paraspinal muscles, and proximal limb muscles. Both active denervation changes, and chronic denervation-reinnervation changes (with prolonged, polyphasic motor potentials) are seen. Based on electrophysiological criteria, this neuropathy has been divided into a chronic axonal polyradiculoneuropathy syndrome, with evidence of root and distal nerve involvement; a chronic axonal polyradiculopathy syndrome, with evidence of root involvement only; a distal sensory polyneuropathy; and a distal sensorimotor polyneuropathy. CSF changes are unusual unless there is an associated Lyme encephalopathy.

Entrapment neuropathy is reported to be increased in patients with late Lyme disease. In a prospective evaluation of 68 patients with late infection, neurophysiological evidence of median nerve entrapment was noted in 25% (126). Although patients presented for rheumatological or systemic complaints, most who had objective entrapment also complained of intermittent hand paresthesias, particularly at night or with use. Only one patient had an associated wrist tenosynovitis. Median nerve entrapment was more common in men. Although paresthesias were often noted in both hands, objective deficits were bilateral in only 35%. Neurophysiological abnormalities included slowed sensory conduction, prolonged motor terminal latency, and decreased sensory potential amplitude. Median nerve entrapment could occur in isolation, as well as in the setting of a more diffuse late Lyme neuropathy. Following antibiotic treatment, 60% noted improvement in paresthesias and 30% had objective improvement in neurophysiological parameters. Entrapment neuropathy appears to be limited to adults and is not common in pediatric Lyme disease (112).

Encephalomyelitis

Encephalomyelitis is the least frequent late neurological syndrome in North American Lyme disease. Patients present with a variety of parenchymal brain or spinal cord problems that can mimic brain tumor, demyelinating disease, hemiparesis, movement disorders, spinal cord syndromes, cerebellar disease, or other problems (90,127–137). Unlike European Lyme encephalomyelitis cases, North American cases have not shown striking CSF changes. There may be a mild pleocytosis (40%), intrathecal Lyme antibody production (40%), elevated protein (33%), and oligoclonal bands or increased IgG index (<33%).

Unusual Late Syndromes

There are a variety of less well-characterized late neurological syndromes. Children and adolescents have developed an intracranial hypertension syndrome, manifested by headache and papilledema (112,138,139). Obesity is not a factor, and CSF is generally abnormal (pleocytosis or elevated protein). This syndrome has been associated with specific intrathecal immune complex formation. Cerebrovascular disorders (vasculitis, stroke, TIA) have also been reported in seropositive patients who had inflammatory CSF consistent with CNS seeding by *B. burgdorferi* (140–142). Psychiatric syndromes (depression, mania, anxiety disorder, acute psychosis) probably reflect encephalomyelitis (143). Although primary muscle involvement is unusual in Lyme disease, there are at least a dozen well-studied cases of myositis associated with *B. burgdorferi* infection in the literature, including a recent patient who developed dermatomyositis in the setting of multifocal EM (144–148). Myositis may occasionally complicate early infection and may be acute or gradual in onset. Most patients have had preceding skin manifestations of Lyme disease. Symptoms include weakness, muscle pain, and muscle swelling or atrophy. Oropharyngeal and orbital muscles may be involved, to give dysphagia, dysphonia, proptosis, or diplopia. Multiple muscle groups may be affected.

Creatine kinase has been normal or mild to moderately elevated. EMG may show myopathic features, may be normal, or may show spontaneous activity (perhaps due to accompanying neuropathy). Muscle biopsy has shown focal nodular, interstitial, or a necrotizing myositis. In rare cases a few spirochetes have been visualized within affected muscle by silver and immunogold-silver staining (144,146). Mononuclear cells (predominantly B cells, CD4 cells, macrophages, and scattered plasma cells) infiltrate the perimysium and muscle bundles, around small blood vessels. Sometimes there is an associated panniculitis and fasciitis. The myositis is antibiotic-responsive, with improvement (partial or complete) noted within weeks to months following treatment.

NEUROLOGICAL SEQUELAE

Neurological Syndromes

Neurological syndromes associated with early dissemination spontaneously remit even without antibiotic treatment, although they clear more rapidly with antibiotics. Complete recovery occurs in 86% of cranial neuropathy patients within weeks to months. Radiculoneuritis improves or clears within 2–16 weeks. Antibiotics result in more rapid improvement of pain. Paresthesias may persist for months, however, and in a minority of patients there is permanent mild weakness. Neurological syndromes associated with late infection do not spontaneously remit and tend not to respond as well to treatment. In Lyme encephalopathy, deficits improve after antibiotic treatment but may not entirely clear. Following treatment, the clinical and neurophysiological deficits of chronic neuropathy slowly improve over weeks to months.

Chronic Lyme Disease

It is not unusual for symptoms to gradually improve over months after treatment for Lyme disease, particularly when dissemination has occurred. In endemic areas, however, significant numbers of patients are being diagnosed as having "chronic Lyme disease" (149). These patients are believed to have a chronic *B. burgdorferi* infection, which has persisted for months to years and which seems refractory to standard antibiotic therapy. Many such patients are receiving a potpourri of antibiotics for months to years at a time, often in combination, and often in cycles (150). The therapy is generally symptom driven, with patients reporting that they feel worse if they are taken off antibiotics. Symptoms include severe fatigue, headache, diffuse pain, cognitive problems, and a variety of other complaints.

These patients are poorly characterized and often are not systematically investigated. They appear to fall into three categories. First, there are patients with a post-Lyme syndrome. These patients had bona fide Lyme disease, received a course of standard antibiotic treatment, and have continued to experience problems months to years after treatment (151–153). Second, there are seropositive patients with nonspecific symptoms. These patients have nonspecific and chronic complaints which remain unexplained, except for their seropositivity to *B. burgdorferi*. Third, there are seronegative patients who reside in Lyme endemic areas and who have chronic, nonspecific complaints. They receive a diagnosis of seronegative chronic Lyme disease in the absence of an alternative diagnosis.

It is clear that patients are misdiagnosed as having chronic Lyme disease (59). It is also clear that there are certain patients who continue to have problems long after their Lyme disease has been treated (151–153). Some of these patients appear to have a chronic or relapsing antibiotic-responsive infection, while others appear to have an ongoing immune or inflammatory process triggered by their prior infection. Chronic Lyme disease is now a major clinical issue, and future studies will hopefully clarify pertinent diagnostic, etiological, and management issues.

PREVENTION

Lyme disease is preventable by avoiding infected tick bite. Environmental manipulations have included eradication of deer, aerial application of insecticides, burning of habitat, and distribution of permethrin-treated cotton balls as rodent nesting material. Personal protection measures have included limiting exposure; wearing long-sleeved, light-colored, and tucked clothes; regular body inspection; application of insecticide (DEET, permethrin) to clothing; and early tick removal (154). Prophylactic treatment of Ixodid tick bite is controversial. A recent study based on cost-effective analysis recommended empiric antibiotics when the probability of tick infection was at least 3.6% and possibly even for infection rates over 1% (155). However, controlled studies have not been able to document the benefit of empiric therapy (156,157).

Vaccination offers the potential for a definitive preventive strategy (158). A canine Lyme vaccine has been in use for several years. For humans, two recombinant OspA vaccines are now under study. In addition a multivalent vaccine, based on recombinant chimeric proteins containing peptides from a number of *B. burgdorferi* antigens, is also under development. Table 8

Table 8 Current Recommended Diagnostic and Therapeutic Approach to Neurological Lyme Disease

	DIAGNOSIS
Test	Rationale
1. Screening Lyme serology (ELISA)	1. Document *B. burgdorferi* exposure
2. If borderline or positive, confirm by Western blot	2. Exclude false–positive ELISA
3. Check Babesia and Ehrlichia serologies	3. Look for evidence of coinfection
4. Proceed to CSF evaluation	4. Look for nonspecific (↑ cells, ↑ protein, ↑ plasma cells, VDRL) and specific (intrathecal *Borrelial* antibodies, *Borrelial* antigen, *Borrelial* DNA, *Borrelial* immune complexes, anti-*Borrelial* IgM) abnormalities
5. Proceed to ancillary studies based on initial evaluation nerve conductions, EMG neuropsychological tests neuroimaging (MRI, SPECT) muscle biopsy	5. Look for abnormalities consistent with Lyme disease
	TREATMENT
Drug	Rationale
1. Intravenous ceftriaxone 2 g QD (in one dose) for 2–4 weeks	1. CNS Lyme disease; abnormal CSF
2. Oral doxycycline 200–400 mg QD (in 2–4 doses) for 4 weeks	2. PNS Lyme disease; normal CSF
3. Appropriate symptomatic therapies	3. To improve clinical problems associated with Lyme disease

summarizes the present diagnostic and therapeutic approach to neurologic Lyme disease absent such a vaccine.

REFERENCES

1. Steere AC. Lyme disease. N Engl J Med 1989; 321:586–596.
2. Dennis DT. Epidemology. In: Coyle PK, ed. Lyme Disease. St. Louis: Mosby Year Book 1993:27–37.
3. Burgdorfer W. Discovery of Borrelia burgdorferi. In: Coyle PK, ed. Lyme Disease. St. Louis: Mosby Year Book, 1993:3–7.
4. Benach JL, Bosler EM, Hanrahan JP, Coleman JL, Habicht GS, Bast TF, Cameron DJ, Ziegler JL, Barbour AG, Burgdorfer W, Edelman R, Kaslow RA. Spirochetes isolated from the blood of two patients with Lyme disease. N Engl J Med 1983; 308:740–742.
5. Steere AC, Grodzicki RL, Kornblatt AN, Craft JE, Barbour AG, Burgdorfer W, Schmid GP, Johnson E, Malawista SE. The spirochetal etiology of Lyme disease. N Engl J Med 1983; 308:733–740.
6. Schmid GP. Epidemiology and clinical similarities of human spirochetal diseases. Rev Infect Dis 1989; 11:S1460–1469.
7. Lukehart SA, Hook EW III, Baker-Zander SA, et al. Invasion of the CNS by Treponema pallidum: implications for diagnosis and therapy. Ann Intern Med 1988; 109:855–862.
8. Barbour AG. Molecular biology of antigenic variation in Lyme borreliosis and relapsing fever: a comparative analysis. Scand J Infect Dis 1991; S77:88–93.
9. Wilske B, Anderson JF, Barcanton G et al. Workshop summary: taxonomy of Borrelia spp. Scand J Infect Dis 1991; S77:108–129.
10. Anthonissen FM, DeKesel M, Hoet PP, Bigaignon GH. Evidence for involvement of different genospecies of *Borrelia* in the clinical outcome of Lyme disease in Belgium. Res Microbiol 1994; 145: 327–331.
11. Isaacs RD. Borrelia burgdorferi binds to epithelial cell proteoglycans. J Clin Invest 1994: 93:809–819.
12. Klempner MS, Noring R, Rogers RA. Invasion of human skin fibroblasts by the Lyme disease spirochete, Borrelia burgdorferi. J Infect Dis 1993; 167:1074–1081.
13. Georgilis K, Peacocke M, Klempner MS. Fibroblasts protect the Lyme disease spirochete, B. burgdorferi, from ceftriaxone in vitro. J Infect Dis 1992; 166:440–444.
14. Anderson FJ. Epizootiology of Lyme borreliosis. Scand J Infect Dis 1991; S77:23–24.
15. Magnarelli LA, Anderson JF. Ticks and biting insects infected with the etiologic agent of Lyme disease, B. burgdorferi. J Clin Microbiol 1988; 26:1482–1486.
16. Teltow GJ, Fournier PV, Rawlings JA. Isolation of B. burgdorferi from arthropods collected in Texas. Am J Trop Med Hyg 1991; 44:469–474.
17. Garcia-Monco JC, Fernandez-Villar B, Alen JC, et al. B. burgdorferi in the CNS: experimental and clinical evidence for early invasion. J Infect Dis 1990; 161:1187–1193.
18. Garcia-Monco JC, Fernandez-Villar B, Benach JL. Adherence of the Lyme disease spirochete to glial cells and cells of glial origin. J Infect Dis 1989; 160:497–506.
19. Garcia-Monco JC, Fernandez-Villar B, Rogers RC, et al. B. burgdorferi and other related spirochetes bind to galactocerebroside. Neurology 1992; 42:1341–1348.
20. Pachner AR, Duray P, Steere AC. CNS manifestations of Lyme disease. Arch Neurol 1989; 46: 790–795.
21. Meier C, Grahmann F, Engelhardt A, Dumas M. Peripheral nerve disorders in Lyme borreliosis: nerve biopsy studies from 8 cases. Acta Neuropathol 1989; 79:271–278.
22. Vallat JM, Hugon J, Lubeau M et al. Tick bite meningoradiculoneuritis: clinical, electrophysiologic, and histologic findings in 10 cases. Neurology 1987; 37:749–753.
23. Szczepanski A, Benach JL. Lyme borreliosis: host responses to B. burgdorferi. Microbiol Rev 1991; 55:21–34.
24. Schutzer SE, ed. Lyme Disease: Molecular and Immunologic Approaches. Cold Spring Harbor Laboratory Press, Plainview, 1992.

25. Schoenfeld R, Araneo B, Ma Y, et al. Demonstration of a B lymphocyte mitogen produced by the Lyme disease pathogen, B. burgdorferi. Inf Immun 1992; 60:455–464.
26. Yssel H, Shanafelt M-C, Soderberg C, et al. B. burgdorferi activates a T helper type 1-like T cell subset in Lyme arthritis. J Exp Med 1991; 174:593–601.
27. Beck G, Benach JL, Habicht GS. Isolation of IL-1 from joint fluids of patients with Lyme disease. J Rheumatol 1989; 16:800–806.
28. DeFosse DL, Johnson RC. In vitro and in vivo induction of TNF-α by B. burgdorferi. Infect Immun 1992; 60:1109–1113.
29. Habicht GS, Beck G, Benach JL, et al. Lyme disease spirochetes induce human and murine IL-1 production. J Immunol 1985; 134:3147–3154.
30. Habicht GS, Katona LI, Benach JL. Cytokines and the pathogenesis of neuroborreliosis: B. burgdorferi induces glioma cells to secrete IL-6. J Infect Dis 1991; 164:568–574.
31. Kenefick KB, Lim LCL, Alder JD, Schmitz JL, Czuprynski CJ, Schell RF. Induction of interleukin-1 release by high-and-low-passage isolates of Borrelia burgdorferi. J Infect Dis 1993; 167:1086–1092.
32. Miller LC, Isa S, Vannier E, Georgillis K, Steere AC, Dinarello CA. Live Borrelia burgdorferi preferentially activate interleukin 1β gene expression and protein synthesis over interleukin-1 receptor antagonist. J Clin Invest 1992; 90:906–912.
33. Miller LC, Lynch EA, Isa S, Logan JW, Dinarello CA, Steere AC. Balance of synovial fluid IL-1β and IL 1 receptor antagonist and receptors from Lyme arthritis. Lancet 1993; 341:146–148.
34. Radolf JD, Norgard MV, Brandt ME, et al. Lipoproteins of B. burgdorferi and Treponema pallidum activate cachectin/TNF synthesis. J Immunol 1991; 147:1968–1974.
35. Beuche W, Siever A, Felgenhauer K. Specific antigen binding by activated CSF B lymphocytes in acute neuroborreliosis. J Neurol 1992; 239:322–326.
36. Coyle PK, Schutzer SE, Belman AL, et al. CSF immune complexes in patients exposed to B. burgdorferi: detection of Borrelia specific and nonspecific complexes. Ann Neurol 1990; 28:739–744.
37. Pachner AR, Steere AC, Sigal LH, et al. Antigen-specific proliferation of CSF lymphocytes in Lyme disease. Neurology 1985; 35:1642–1644.
38. Baig S, Olsson T, Hojeberg B, et al. Cells secreting antibodies to myelin basic protein in CSF of patients with Lyme neuroborreliosis. Neurology 1991; 41:581–587.
39. Garcia-Monco JC, Coleman JL, Benach JL. Antibodies to myelin basic protein in Lyme disease. J Infect Dis 1988; 158:667–668.
40. Ryberg B, Hindfelt B, Nilsson B, et al. Antineural antibodies in Guillain-Barre syndrome and lymphocytic meningoradiculitis (Bannwarth's syndrome). Arch Neurol 1984; 41:1277–1281.
41. Sigal LH, Tatum AH. Lyme disease patients' serum contains IgM antibodies to B. burgdorferi that cross react with neuronal antigens. Neurology 1988; 38:1439–1442.
42. Martin R, Ortlauf J, Sticht-Groh V, Bogdahn U, Goldmann SF, Mertens HG. B. burgdorferi specific and autoreactive T cell lines from CSF in Lyme radiculomyelitis. Ann Neurol 1988; 24:509–516.
43. Hagberg L, Dotevall L, Fuchs D, et al. CSF and serum neopterin levels in patients with Lyme neuroborreliosis. IV International Conference on Lyme Borreliosis. Stockholm, 1990, p. 55.
44. Halperin JJ, Heyes MP. Neuroactive kynurenines in Lyme borreliosis. Neurology 1992; 42:43–50.
45. Weigelt W, Schneider T, Lange R. Sequence homology between spirochete flagellin and human myelin basic protein. Immunol Today 1992; 13:279–280.
46. Aberer E, Brunner C, Suchanek G, Klade H, Barbour A, Stanek G, Lassmann H. Molecular mimicry and Lyme borreliosis: shared antigenic determinants between B. burgdorferi and human tissue. Ann Neurol 1989; 26:732–737.
47. Sigal LH. Cross reactivity between Borrelia burgdorferi flagellin and a human axonal 64,000 molecular weight protein. J Infect Dis 1993; 167:1372–1378.
48. Hanrahan JP, Benach JL, Coleman JL, Bosler EM, Morse DL, Cameron DJ, Edelman R, Kaslow RA. Incidence and cumulative frequency of endemic Lyme disease in a community. J Infect Dis 1984; 150:489–496.
49. Steere AC, Taylor E, Wilson ML, Levine JL, Spielman A. Longitudinal assessment of the clinical and epidemiological features of Lyme disease in a defined population. J Infect Dis 1986; 154:295–300.

50. Malane MS, Grant-Kels JM, Feder HM Jr, Luger SW. Diagnosis of Lyme disease based on dermatologic manifestations. Ann Intern Med 1991; 114:490–498.
51. Berger BW, Johnson RC, Kodner C, Coleman L. Cultivation of B. burgdorferi from erythema migrans lesions and perilesional skin. J Clin Microbiol 1992; 30:359–361.
52. Coyle PK. Neurologic complications of Lyme disease. Rheum Dis Clin North Am 1993; 19:993–1009.
53. Pachner AR, Steere AC. The triad of neurologic manifestations of Lyme disease. Neurology 1985; 35:47–53.
54. Reik LR Jr. Lyme Disease and the Nervous System. Thieme, New York, 1991.
55. Krupp LB, Masur D, Schwartz J, Coyle PK, Langenbach LJ, Fernquist SK, Jandorf L, Halperin JJ. Cognitive functioning in late Lyme borreliosis. Arch Neurol 1991; 48:1125–1129.
56. Logigian EL, Steere AC. Clinical and electrophysiologic findings in chronic neuropathy of Lyme disease. Neurology 1992; 42:303–311.
57. Logigian EL, Kaplan RF, Steere AC. Chronic neurologic manifestations of Lyme disease. N Engl J Med 1990; 323:1438–1444.
58. Kaplan RF, Meadows M-E, Vincent LC et al. Memory impairment and depression in patients with Lyme encephalopathy. Neurology 1992; 42:1263–1267.
59. Steere AC, Taylor E, McHugh GL, Logigian EL. The overdiagnosis of Lyme disease. JAMA 1993; 269:1812–1816.
60. Vlay S. Cardiac manifestations. In: Coyle PK, ed. Lyme Disease. St. Louis: Mosby Year Book, 1993:86–92.
61. Breeveld J, Rothova A, Kuiper H. Intermediate uveitis and Lyme borreliosis. Br J Ophthalmol 1992; 76:181–182.
62. Kesser RL, Kornmehl EW, Pachner AR, etc. Neuro-ophthalmologic manifestations of Lyme disease. Ophthalmology 1990; 97:699–706.
63. Dumler J, Bakken JS. Ehrlichial diseases of humans: emerging tick-borne infections. Clin Infect Dis 1995; 20:1102–1110.
64. Meldrum SC, Birkhead GS, White DJ, Benach JL, Morse DC. Human babesiosis in New York State: an epidemiological description of 136 cases. Clin Infect Dis 1992; 15:1019–1023.
65. Berardi VP, Weeks KE, Steere AC. Serodiagnosis of early Lyme disease: analysis of IgM and IgG antibody responses by using an antibody-capture enzyme immunoassay. J Infect Dis 1988; 158: 754–760.
66. Dattwyler RJ, Volkman DJ, Luft BJ, et al. Seronegative Lyme disease. N Engl J Med 1988; 319:1441–1446.
67. Piesman J, Maupin GO, Campos EG, et al. Duration of adult female Ixodes dammini attachment and transmission of B. burgdorferi with description of a needle aspiration isolation method. J Infect Dis 1991; 163:895–897.
68. Wormser GP, Forseter G, Cooper D et al. Use of a novel technique of cutaneous lavage for diagnosis of Lyme disease associated with EM. JAMA 1992; 268:1311–1313.
69. Bruckbauer HR, Preac-Mursic V, Fuchs R, Wilske B. Cross-reactive proteins of B. burgdorferi. Eur J Clin Microbiol Infect Dis 1992; 11:224–232.
70. Corpuz M, Hilton E, Lardis MP et al. Problems in the use of serologic tests for the diagnosis of Lyme disease. Arch Intern Med 1991; 151:1837–1840.
71. Hedberg CW, Osterholm MT, MacDonald KL, et al. An interlaboratory study of antibody to B. burgdorferi. J Infect Dis 1987; 155:1325–1327.
72. Luger SW, Krauss E. Serologic tests for Lyme disease. Arch Intern Med 1990; 150:761–763.
73. Coleman JL, Benach JL. Characterization of antigenic determinants of B. burgdorferi shared by other bacteria. J Infect Dis 1992; 165:658–666.
74. Magnarelli LA, Anderson JF, Johnson RC. Cross-reactivity in serological tests for Lyme disease and other spirochetal infections. J Infect Dis 1987; 156:183–188.
75. Magnarelli LA, Miller JN, Anderson JF, Riviere GR. Cross-reactivity of nonspecific treponemal antibody in serologic tests for Lyme disease. J Clin Microbiol 1991; 28:1276–1279.
76. Schwartz BS, Goldstein MD, Ribeiro JMC, et al. Antibody testing in Lyme disease. JAMA 1989; 262:3431–3434.

77. Raoult D, Hechemy KE, Baranton G. Cross-reaction with B. burgdorferi antigen of sera from patients with HIV infection, syphilis, and leptospirosis. J Clin Microbiol 1989; 27:2152–2155.
78. Hunter EF, Russell H, Farshy CE, et al. Evaluation of sera from patients with Lyme disease in FTA-Abs test for syphilis. Sex Trans Dis 1986: 13:232–236.
79. CDC/DVBID. Standardization of Lyme disease serodiagnosis: Working group meets to chart progress 1994; 5:1–3.
80. Zoller L, Haude M, Hassler D et al. Spontaneous and post-treatment antibody kinetics in late Lyme borreliosis. Serodiagn Immunother Infect Dis 1989; 3:345–353.
81. Craft JE, Fischer DK, Shimamoto GT, Steere AC. Antigens of B. burgdorferi recognized during Lyme disease. J Clin Invest 1986: 78:934–939.
82. Mackworth-Young CG, Harris EN, Steere AC et al. Anticardiolipin antibodies in Lyme disease. Arthritis Rheum 1988; 31:1052–1056.
83. Preac-Mursic V, Weber K, Pfister HW et al. Survival of B. burgdorferi in antibiotically treated patients with Lyme borreliosis. Infection 1989; 17:355–359.
84. Hansen K, Lebech A-M. Lyme neuroborreliosis: a new sensitive diagnostic assay for intrathecal synthesis of B. burgdorferi- specific IgG, A, and M. Ann Neurol 1991; 30:197–205.
85. Steere AC, Berardi VP, Weeks KE, et al. Evaluation of the intrathecal antibody response to B. burgdorferi as a diagnostic test for Lyme neuroborreliosis. J Infect Dis 1990; 161:1203–1209.
86. Wilske B, Schierz G, Preac-Mursic V, et al. Intrathecal production of specific antibodies against B. burgdorferi in patients with lymphocytic meningoradiculitis (Bannwarth's syndrome). J Infect Dis 1986; 153:304–314.
87. Coyle PK, Deng Z, Schutzer SE, Belman AL, Krupp LB, Luft B. Detection of Borrelia burgdorferi antigens in cerebrospinal fluid. Neurology 1993; 43:1093–1097.
88. Luft BJ, Steinman CR, Neimark HC, et al. Invasion of the CNS by B. burgdorferi in acute disseminated infection. JAMA 1992; 267:1364–1367.
89. Belman AL, Coyle PK, Roque C, Cantos E. MRI findings in children infected with B. burgdorferi. Ped Neurol 1992; 8:428–431.
90. Mokry M, Flaschka G, Kleinert G, et al. Chronic Lyme disease with an expansive granulomatous lesion in the cerebellopontine angle. Neurosurgery 1990; 27:446–451.
91. Nelson JA, Wolf MD, Yah WTC, Peeples ME. Cranial nerve involvement with Lyme borreliosis demonstrated by MRI. Neurology 1992; 42:671–673.
92. Diringer MN, Halperin JJ, Dattwyler RJ. Lyme meningoencephalitis: report of a severe, penicillin-resistant case. Arthritis Rheum 1987; 30:705–708.
93. Kohler J, Schneider H, Vogt A. High dose IV penicillin G does not prevent further progression in early neurological manifestation of Lyme borreliosis. Infection 1989; 17:216–217.
94. Dever L, Jorgensen JH, Barbour AG. In vitro antimicrobial susceptibility testing of B. burgdorferi: a microdilution MIC method and time-kill studies. J Clin Microbiol 1992; 30:2692–2697.
95. Luft BJ, Gorevic PD, Halperin JJ, et al. A perspective on the treatment of Lyme borreliosis. Rev Infect Dis 1989; 11:S1518–1525.
96. Dattwyler RJ, Volkman DJ, Conaty SM, et al. Amoxicillin plus probenecid vs doxycycline for treatment of erythema migrans borreliosis. Lancet 1990; 336:1404–1406.
97. Massarotti EM, Luger SW, Rahn D, et al. Treatment of early Lyme disease. Am J Med 1992; 92: 396–403.
98. Nadelman RB, Luger SW, Frank E, et al. Comparison of cefuroxime axetil and doxycycline in the treatment of early Lyme disease. Ann Intern Med 1992; 117:273–280.
99. Strle F, Ruzic E, Cimperman J. Erythema migrans: comparison of treatment with azithromycin, doxycycline and phenoxymethylpenicillin. J Antimicrob Chemother 1992; 30:543–550.
100. Rahn DW, Malawista SE. Lyme disease: recommendations for diagnosis and treatment. Ann Intern Med 1991; 114:472–481.
101. Dattwyler RJ, Halperin JJ, Volkman DJ, et al. Treatment of late Lyme borreliosis—randomized comparison of ceftriaxone and penicillin. Lancet 1988; 2:1191–1194.
102. Hassler D, Riedel K, Zorn J, Preac-Mursic V. Pulsed high-dose cefotaxime therapy in refractory Lyme borreliosis. Lancet 1991; 338:193.

103. Pfister H-W, Preac-Mursic V, Wilske B, Schielke E, Sorgel F, Einhaur KM. Randomized comparison of ceftriaxone and cefotaxime in Lyme neuroborreliosis. J Infect Dis 1991; 163:311–318.
104. Dotevall L, Hagberg L. Penetration of doxycycline into CSF in patients treated for suspected Lyme neuroborreliosis. Antimicrob Agents Chemother 1989; 33:1078–1080.
105. Karlsson M, Hammers-Berggren S, Lindquist L, Stiernstedt G, Svenungsson B. Comparison of intravenous penicillin G and oral doxycycline for treatment of Lyme neuroborreliosis. Neurology 1994; 44:1203–1207.
106. Gasser R, Dusleag J. Oral treatment of late borreliosis with roxithromycin plus cotrimoxazole. Lancet 1990; 336:1189–1190.
107. Steere AC, Pachner AR, Malawista SE. Neurologic abnormalities of Lyme disease: successful treatment with high dose intravenous penicillin. Ann Intern Med 1983; 99:767–772.
108. Finkel MJ, Halperin JJ. Nervous system Lyme borreliosis—revisited. Arch Neurol 1992: 49:102–107.
109. Reik L, Steere AC, Bartenhagen NH, et al. Neurologic abnormalities of Lyme disease. Medicine 1979; 58:281–294.
110. Reik L, Burgdorfer W, Donaldson JO. Neurologic abnormalities in Lyme disease without erythema chronicum migrans. Am J Med 1986; 81:73–78.
111. Bourke SJ, Baird AG, Bone FG, et al. Lyme disease with acute purulent meningitis. Br Med J 1988; 297:460.
112. Belman AL, Iyer M, Coyle PK, Dattwyler R. Neurologic manifestations in children with North American Lyme disease. Neurology 1993; 43:2609–2616.
113. Clark JR, Carlson RD, Sasaki CT, et al. Facial paralysis in Lyme disease. Laryngoscope 1985; 95:1341–1345.
114. Halperin JJ, Golightly M, LINCSG. Lyme borreliosis in Bell's palsy. Neurology 1992; 42:1268–1270.
115. Jacobson DM, Marx JJ, Dlesk A. Frequency and clinical significance of Lyme seropositivity in patients with isolated optic neuritis. Neurology 1991; 41:706–711.
116. Hanner P, Rosenhall U, Edstrom S, Kaijser B. Hearing impairment in patients with antibody production against B. burgdorferi antigen. Lancet 1989; 1:13–15.
117. Daffner KR, Saver JL, Biber MP. Lyme polyradiculoneuropathy presenting as increasing abdominal girth. Neurology 1990; 40:373–375.
118. Garcia-Monco JC, Beldarrain MG, Estrade L. Painful lumbosacral plexitis with increased ESR and Borrelia burgdorferi infection. Neurology 1993; 43:1269.
119. Sterman AB, Nelson S, Barclay P. Demyelinating neuropathy accompanying Lyme disease. Neurology 1982; 32:1302–1305.
120. Halperin J, Luft BJ, Volkman DJ, Dattwyler RJ. Lyme neuroborreliosis. Brain 1990; 113:1207–1221.
121. Szer IS, Taylor E, Steere AC. The long-term course of Lyme arthritis in children. N Engl J Med 1991; 325:159–163.
122. Logigian EL, Johnson KA, Becker JA, Kijewski MF, Kaplan RF, Holman BL, Steere AC. Cerebral hypoperfusion in Lyme encephalopathy: a quantitative SPECT study. Neurology 1994; 44:A186.
123. Hopf HC. Peripheral neuropathy in acrodermatitis chronica atrophicans (Herxheimer). J Neurol Neurosurg Psych 1975; 38:452–458.
124. Kristoferitsch W, Sluga E, Graf M, Partsch H, Neumann R, Stanek G, Budka H. Neuropathy associated with acrodermatitis chronica atrophicans. Ann NY Acad Sci 1988; 539:35–45.
125. Halperin JJ, Little BW, Coyle PK, Dattwyler RJ. Lyme disease: cause of a treatable peripheral neuropathy. Neurology 1987; 37:1700–1706.
126. Halperin JJ, Volkman DJ, Luft BJ, Dattwyler RJ. Carpal tunnel syndrome in Lyme borreliosis. Muscle Nerve 1989; 12:397–400.
127. Bendig JWA, Ogilvie D. Severe encephalopathy associated with Lyme disease. Lancet 1987; 1:681–682.
128. Berlit P, Pohlmann-Eden B, Henningsen H. Brown-Sequard syndrome caused by B. burgdorferi. Eur Neurol 1991; 31:18–20.
129. Broderick JP, Sandok BA, Mertz LE. Focal encephalitis in a young woman 6 years after the onset of Lyme disease: tertiary Lyme disease? Mayo Clin Proc 1987; 62:313–316.

130. Feder HM, Zalneraitis EL, Reik L. Lyme disease: acute meningoencephalitis in a child. Pediatrics 1988; 82:931–934.
131. Kohlhepp W, Kuhn W, Kruger H. Extrapyramidal features in central Lyme borreliosis. Eur Neurol 1989; 29;150–155.
132. Martin R, Meinck HM, Schulte-Mattler W, et al. B. burgdorferi myelitis presenting as a partial stiff man syndrome. J Neurol 1990; 237:51–54.
133. Midgard R, Hofstad H. Unusual manifestations of nervous system B. burgdorferi infection. Arch Neurol 1987; 44:781–783.
134. Reik L, Smith L, Khan A, Nelson W. Demyelinating encephalopathy in Lyme disease. Neurology 1985; 35:267–269.
135. Rousseau JJ, Lust C, Zangerle PF. Acute transverse myelitis as presenting neurological feature of Lyme disease. Lancet 1986; 2:1222–1223.
136. Weder B, Wiedersheim P, Matter L, et al. Chronic progressive neurological involvement in B. burgdorferi infection. J Neurol 1987; 234:40–43.
137. Wokke JHJ, Van Gijn J, Elderson A, et al. Chronic forms of B. burgdorferi infection of the nervous system. Neurology 1987; 37:1031–1034.
138. Jacobson DM, Frens DB. Pseudotumor cerebri associated with Lyme disease. Am J Ophthalmol 1989; 107:81–82.
139. Rauscher HS, Kaufman DM, Goldfarb J, et al. Pseudotumor cerebri and Lyme disease: a new association. J Pediatrics 1985; 107:931–933.
140. Brogan GX, Homan CS, Viccellio P. The enlarging clinical spectrum of Lyme disease: Lyme cerebral vasculitis, a new disease entity. Ann Emerg Med 1990; 19:572–576.
141. Uldry P-A, Regli F, Bogousslavsky J. Cerebral angiopathy and recurrent strokes following B. burgdorferi infection. J Neurol Neurosurg Psych 1987; 50:1703–1704.
142. Veenendaal-Hilbers JA, Perquin WVM, Hoogland PH, et al. Basal meningovasculitis and occlusion of the basilar artery in two cases of B. burgdorferi infection. Neurology 1988; 38:1317–1319.
143. Roelcke U, Barnett W, Wilder-Smith E, et al. Untreated neuroborreliosis: Bannwarth's syndrome evolving into acute schizophrenia-like psychosis. J Neurol 1992; 239:129–131.
144. Atlas E, Novak SN, Duray PH, Steere AC. Lyme myositis: muscle invasion by B. burgdorferi. Ann Intern Med 1988; 109:245–246.
145. Horowitz HW, Sanghera K, Goldberg N, Pechman D, Kamer R, Duray P, Weinstein A. Dermatomyositis associated with Lyme disease: case report and review of Lyme myositis. Clin Infec Dis 1994; 18:166–171.
146. Reimers CD, Pongartz DE, Neubert U, et al. Myositis caused by B. burgdorferi: report of 4 cases. J Neurol Sci 1989; 91:215–226.
147. Schoenen J, Sianard-Gainko J, Carpenter M, Reznik M. Myositis during B. burgdorferi infection (Lyme disease). J Neurol Neurosurg Psych 1989; 52:1002–1005.
148. Wokke JHJ, DeKoning J, Stanek G, Jennekens FGI. Chronic muscle weakness caused by B. burgdorferi meningoradiculitis. Ann Neurol 1987; 22:389–392.
149. Liegner KB. Lyme disease:the sensible pursuit of answers. J Clin Microbiol 1993; 31:1961–1963.
150. Ettestad PJ, Campbell GL, Welberl SF, Genese CA, Spitalny KC, Marchetti CM, Dennis DT. Biliary complications in the treatment of unsubstantiated Lyme disease. J Infect Dis 1995; 171:356–361.
151. Asch ES, Bujak DI, Weiss M, Peterson MGE, Weinstein A. Lyme disease: an infectious and postinfectious syndrome. J Rheumatol 1994; 21:454–461.
152. Coyle PK, Krupp LB, Doscher C, Amin K. Borrelia burgdorferi reactivity in patients with severe persistent fatigue who are from a region in which Lyme disease is endemic. Clin Infect Dis 1994; 18:S24–S27.
153. Shadick NA, Phillips CB, Logigian EL, Steere AC, Kaplan RF, Berardi VP, Duray PH, Larson MG, Wright EA, Ginsburg KS, Katz JN, Liang MH. The long-term clinical outcomes of Lyme disease. Ann Intern Med 194; 121:560–567.
154. Couch P, Johnson CE. Prevention of Lyme disease. AJHP 1992; 49:1164–1173.

155. Magid D, Schwartz B, Craft J, Schwartz JS. Prevention of Lyme disease after tick bites. N Engl J Med 1992; 327:534–541.
156. Costello CM, Steere AC, Pinkerton RE, Feder HM Jr. A prospective study of tick bites in an endemic area for Lyme disease. J Infect Dis 1989; 159:136–139.
157. Shapiro ED, Gerber MA, Holabird NB, et al. A controlled trial of antimicrobial prophylaxis for Lyme disease after deer-tick bites. N Engl J Med 1992; 327:1769–1773.
158. Keller D, Koster FT, Marks DH, Hosbach P, Erdile LF, Mays JP. Safety and immunogenicity of a recombinant outer surface protein A Lyme vaccine. JAMA 1994; 271:1764–1768.

12

Neurosyphilis

Christina M. Marra
University of Washington, Seattle, Washington

HISTORY

Overview

While syphilis has been a topic of investigation since the late fifteenth century, our current understanding of neurosyphilis comes primarily from studies conducted in the twentieth century. Much of this work was performed before recognition of neurological conditions that might be confused with neurosyphilis, such as viral (aseptic) meningitis (1), cerebral arteritis, or carotid and vertebrobasilar insufficiency (2), and before the widespread availability of penicillin and other antibiotics. Thus, questions regarding diagnostic criteria for neurosyphilis, optimal therapy, and response to therapy remain unanswered. These issues are particularly important because neurosyphilis is now most commonly described in patients also infected with the human immunodeficiency virus type 1 (HIV). The role of the host immune response in determining the clinical manifestations of syphilis and of neurosyphilis and in determining the outcome of treatment is currently a topic of intense debate.

Central Nervous System Invasion

Studies conducted in the preantibiotic era delineated the natural history of central nervous system (CNS) infection with *Treponema pallidum*. Cerebrospinal fluid (CSF) examination was routinely performed in all syphilis patients 6 months after initiating (nonpenicillin) therapy (3). Several studies showed that 10–20% of patients with primary syphilis and 30–70% of patients with secondary syphilis had CSF abnormalities such as pleocytosis, elevated protein concentration, or reactive CSF-Wassermann test [the predecessor of the Venereal Disease Research Laboratory (VDRL) test] (4–6). CSF abnormalities were more common in seropositive primary syphilis than seronegative primary syphilis, and a reactive CSF Wassermann test was more common with a longer duration of infection. *T. pallidum* could be demonstrated in CSF by rabbit inoculation in 30% of these patients, many of whom had normal CSF cell counts and protein concentrations (7). These data show that invasion of the CNS by *T. pallidum* occurs early in the course of infection.

This conclusion was recently confirmed by Lukehart and coworkers (8), who showed that 40% of patients with untreated primary and secondary syphilis had CSF pleocytosis. CSF-VDRL was reactive in 24% of patients with secondary syphilis, but in no patients with primary syphilis. *T. pallidum* was recovered from 30% of CSF samples by rabbit inoculation; one third of these samples were otherwise normal (8). As an aside, the similarity of these results to those obtained in the preantibiotic era show that 6 months of nonpenicillin therapy had a negligible effect on CSF abnormalities.

Despite frequent CNS invasion by *T. pallidum*, most syphilis patients do not develop symptomatic neurosyphilis. Less than 20% of syphilis patients seen by Merritt and coworkers at the Boston City Hospital had symptomatic neurosyphilis (9). In another series, only 62 (6.5%) of 953 patients with untreated early syphilis developed symptomatic neurosyphilis (10). In keeping with these observations, studies of serial CSF evaluations showed that CSF abnormalities spontaneously resolved in as many as 70% of individuals by the end of the secondary stage of syphilis (5) and that normalization of CSF carried a good prognosis, predicting a low likelihood of developing symptomatic neurosyphilis (11,12). Conversely, persistence of CSF abnormalities carried a poor prognosis (13). A study by Hahn and coworkers demonstrated that progression to symptomatic neurosyphilis was five times more likely in those patients in whom CSF was unchanged or worse on repeat examination 6 months to 10 years later, compared to those in whom CSF normalized or improved (14). In practical terms, these data allow us to discard the possibility of current or future neurosyphilis in patients with normal CSF, provided that proper therapy for uncomplicated syphilis is administered. However, we cannot predict which patients with abnormal CSF (asymptomatic neurosyphilis) will spontaneously clear these abnormalities and which ones will not. Thus, all patients with asymptomatic neurosyphilis are treated to prevent progression to symptomatic disease (see below).

PATHOPHYSIOLOGY

Overview

Neurosyphilis has been traditionally categorized into specific syndromes: asymptomatic neurosyphilis, symptomatic meningitis, meningovasculitis, general paresis, and tabes dorsalis. Asymptomatic neurosyphilis, meningitis, and meningovasculitis occur early after acquisition of infection (weeks to a few years) and may be seen in patients who also have primary and secondary syphilis. General paresis and tabes dorsalis occur late after acquisition of infection (decades) and are rarely seen in patients with primary and secondary syphilis (Fig. 1). Chronic meningeal inflammation is a feature of all types of neurosyphilis, with concomitant parenchymal involvement in late disease.

Early Neurosyphilis

Syphilitic meningitis is characterized by perivascular infiltration of the meninges with lymphocytes, plasma cells, and occasional neutrophils (9). This inflammatory reaction may also affect the ependyma. These changes are less extensive in asymptomatic, compared to symptomatic, meningitis. The inflammatory reaction may cause fibrosis and hydrocephalus. Focal meningeal inflammation may lead to the formation of hypertrophic meningitis or gummata that may eventually exert pressure on adjacent structures. Inflammation of vessel walls may cause arteritis, vascular occlusion, ischemia, and infarction of brain or spinal cord (see below). A combination of

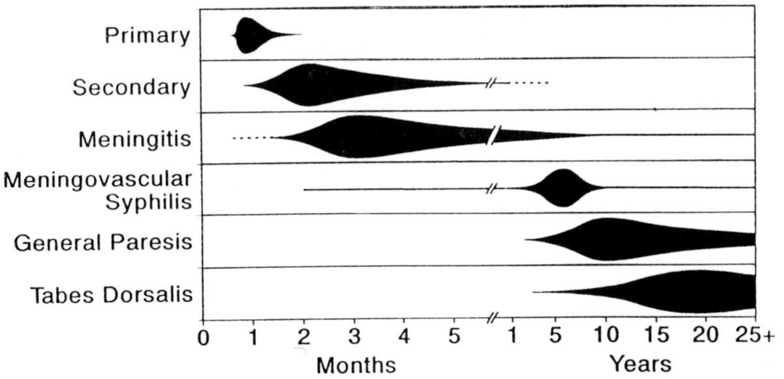

Figure 1 Approximate time course of the clinical manifestations of early syphilis and neurosyphilis. Neurosyphilis can occur at any time after primary infection. Meningeal and meningovascular disease occur early in the course of disease and may be seen in patients with primary or secondary syphilis. Paresis and tabes occur late in the course of infection. (Modified with permission from *The New England Journal of Medicine*, Hook EW III, Marra CM, 326, 1060–1069, 1992. Copyright (1992). Massachusetts Medical Society. All rights reserved.)

inflammation, fibrosis, and vascular occlusion may account for cranial neuropathy and spinal radiculopathy. Seizures may occur as a result of cortical irritation by meningitis, stroke, or gumma.

The pathological changes seen in meningovascular syphilis include meningeal inflammation, as described above, as well as more prominent vascular changes (9). Heubner's arteritis affects large or medium-sized vessels and is characterized by infiltration of the adventitia by lymphocytes and plasma cells. These cells may occasionally infiltrate the media and intima and may occlude the vasa vasorum. Fibroblasts proliferate and thicken the intima. In the late stages there is medial necrosis and replacement by connective tissue. Nissl-Alzheimer endarteritis affects small vessels and is characterized by noninflammatory endothelial and adventitial proliferation, which leads to obliteration of the vessel lumen.

Late Neurosyphilis

The pathological changes in general paresis are characteristic of a chronic spirochetal meningoencephalitis (9). The brain is atrophic and the meninges are thickened and cloudy. Meningeal and vascular changes are identical to those seen in meningeal neurosyphilis. Additionally, parenchymal involvement is characterized by neuronal degeneration and loss, gliosis, and deposition of iron pigment in vessel walls. Spirochetes have been identified within gray matter (9,15).

In early tabes dorsalis, the leptomeninges and preganglionic portion of the dorsal roots are infiltrated with lymphocytes and plasma cells, similar to the findings in meningeal neurosyphilis (9). These inflammatory changes disappear with time, and the posterior roots become thin and gray. Similar changes may be seen in the optic nerves. The posterior columns of the spinal cord become secondarily atrophic and gliotic, and the overlying arachnoid becomes opaque and thickened. Spirochetes are rarely demonstrated in dorsal roots or posterior columns.

CLINICAL PRESENTATION AND CLINICAL COURSE

Asymptomatic Neurosyphilis

Patients with asymptomatic neurosyphilis have no clinical signs or symptoms, but have CSF abnormalities including pleocytosis, elevated protein concentration, and reactive CSF-VDRL

Table 1 Cerebrospinal Fluid Abnormalities in Patients with Neurosyphilis in the Preantibiotic Era

	Cerebrospinal fluid measure		
Form of neurosyphilis	WBC (cells/μl)	Protein (mg/dl)	Wassermann test (% reactive)
Asymptomatic	0–100	<45–100	84%
Meningeal	200–400	100–200	91%
Meningovascular	11–100	100–200	81%
Paresis	25–75	50–100	100%
Tabes	10–50	45–75	72%

WBC, white blood cell count.
Source: Ref. 9.

(Table 1). As discussed above, these patients may also have primary or secondary syphilis. CSF abnormalities can be seen at any time after infection, but probably peak during the second year (3,16). Asymptomatic neurosyphilis is identified in about one quarter of all patients with syphilis. With increasing duration of infection, the proportion of patients with asymptomatic neurosyphilis declines relative to the total number of patients with neurosyphilis (Fig. 2), because previously asymptomatic patients become symptomatic and because many patients experience spontaneous normalization of the CSF (17).

Symptomatic Meningitis

Patients with acute, or symptomatic, syphilitic meningitis complain of headache, stiff neck, nausea, and vomiting. Signs of syphilitic meningitis include papilledema due to raised intracranial pressure from hydrocephalus, confusion, seizures, or focal abnormalities (9,18). Cranial

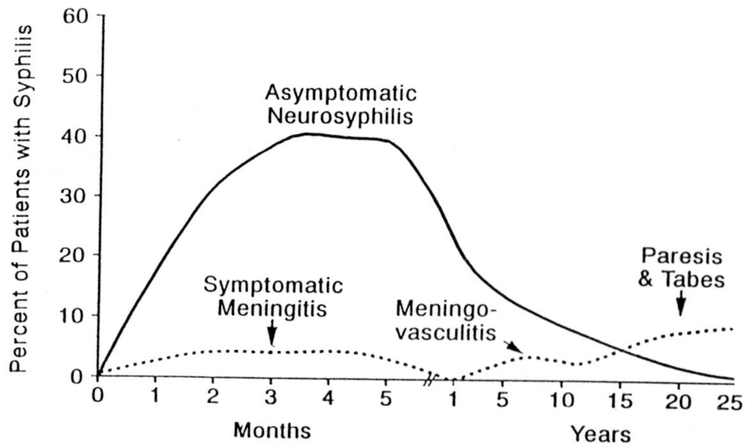

Figure 2 Time course for the development of neurosyphilis. Cerebrospinal fluid (CSF) abnormalities are common in early syphilis. Although the CSF becomes normal in most patients, about 25% have persistent asymptomatic neurosyphilis. A proportion of these patients subsequently develop symptomatic disease. Patients with asymptomatic neurosyphilis should be treated to prevent this progression. (From Marra CM, Syphilis and human immunodeficiency virus infection, *Seminars in Neurology*, 12, 43–50, 1995. Reproduced with permission.)

nerve (CN) abnormalities are relatively common, typically involving CN II, VII, and VIII (9,18). Syphilitic meningitis may cause hyperplastic pachymeningitis (19), and meningomyelitis (20–25) or radiculitis (26,27), which may be heralded by back pain, sensory loss, incontinence, leg weakness, or muscle atrophy. Rarely, one or more circumscribed masses of granulation tissue, or gummata, may develop as a result of localized meningitis involving the brain or spinal cord. Merritt defined a gumma as an area of caseous necrosis surrounded by varying degrees of chronic inflammation and fibrosis (9) that could occur in early or late neurosyphilis; modern authors do not always require pathological confirmation or demonstration of necrosis. Defined as such, gummata may be located in the basal cisterns (in proximity to the inflammatory infiltrate) (28–30), may arise from the leptomeninges (31–34), or may be located solely within the parenchyma (35). Gummata cause symptoms and signs by exerting pressure on adjacent structures. Neuroimaging studies of individuals with syphilitic meningitis may be normal or show meningeal enhancement (36); gummata enhance with contrast in a ring or homogeneous pattern and may have surrounding edema (28–35).

Merritt and Moore published detailed descriptions of 80 patients with syphilitic meningitis in 1935 (18). All patients had current or past syphilis, and, as expected, most patients complained of headache, nausea and vomiting, and stiff neck. All but one had CSF pleocytosis (the remaining patient had a reactive CSF Wassermann test); mean CSF white blood cell (WBC) count was 434 cells/μl. Cerebrospinal fluid protein was >45 mg/dl in 88%, and CSF glucose content was <50 mg/dl in 55%. Wassermann test on CSF was reactive in 91% at initial or follow-up examination, but Wassermann test on blood was reactive in only 64%, perhaps because most patients had been treated for uncomplicated syphilis before developing symptomatic meningitis. Overall, two thirds of cases occurred within a year of primary infection (range 2 months to 26 years), and 7.5% had concurrent secondary syphilis. In this publication and others, Merritt and coworkers observed that syphilitic meningitis was rare, occurring in less than 0.5% of individuals with syphilis (9,18,37). This form of neurosyphilis was most commonly seen in patients who had been inadequately or incompletely treated for early syphilis (3,6,38) and was often accompanied by syphilitic uveitis (39).

Meningovasculitis

Syphilitic arteritis can develop in any intracranial or intraspinal artery, leading to thrombosis, ischemia, and infarction. In the largest series of cerebral meningovascular syphilis, published by Merritt and coworkers in 1946, prodromal symptoms of headache, dizziness, and personality changes for days or weeks were common before symptoms of ischemia or stroke (9). These symptoms are likely due to underlying meningitis. The onset of vascular symptoms was abrupt in three fourths of patients. Hemiplegia, hemiparesis, or aphasia were most commonly described, consistent with the observation that the middle cerebral artery and its branches were more frequently affected than other vessels. Several recent reports describe brainstem infarctions as a consequence of meningovascular disease (40–42). Uncommonly, meningovascular syphilis affects spinal arteries, resulting in acute transverse myelitis with paraplegia, thoracic sensory level, and loss of sphincter control (22,43–46).

The neuroradiographic abnormalities of cerebral meningovascular syphilis augment Merritt and coworkers' clinical descriptions. Cerebral angiography may show beading or occlusion, or may demonstrate findings that resemble spasm associated with subarachnoid hemorrhage or other infectious or noninfectious vasculitides (47–49). Neuroimaging may show multiple areas of infarction, consistent with diffuse intracranial vasculitis (47,50,51).

In Merritt and coworkers' report (9), CSF WBC count was >10 cells/μl in 63% of patients. The CSF Wassermann was reactive in 81%, and the blood Wassermann was reactive in 95%.

Meningovascular syphilis developed an average of 7 years after infection, but some cases developed within months of primary disease (9,37). Like syphilitic meningitis, syphilitic meningovasculitis was uncommon, developing in 3% of patients with syphilis examined by Merritt and coworkers (9).

General Paresis

Early in the course of disease, patients with general paresis (also called paretic neurosyphilis, general paralysis of the insane, or dementia paralytica) may be forgetful and show personality changes (9). Psychiatric symptoms, such as mania, depression, or psychosis, develop in some patients. Progressive decline in memory and judgment leads to overt dementia, often with seizures. Neurological examination may show pupillary abnormalities; face and limb hypotonia; intention tremors of the face, tongue, and hands; and reflex abnormalities (9). However, if patients are examined early in the course, no abnormalities may be identified. Neuroimaging may show cerebral atrophy (52). Merritt and coworkers reported that CSF was always abnormal in untreated paresis (9): of 100 cases, 90% had mild CSF pleocytosis, 75% had mildly elevated protein concentration, and all had a reactive CSF Wassermann test. Serum Wassermann was reactive in at least 85% of patients. This high rate of reactive CSF and serum Wassermann tests has been corroborated by others (53). General paresis occurs 10–20 years after infection (range of 2 to >30 years) (9,53,54). Merritt and coworkers estimated that general paresis developed in 5% of all patients with syphilis (9).

Tabes Dorsalis

Patients with tabes dorsalis (also called locomotor ataxia) have sensory changes including loss of sensation, paresthesias, or hyperesthesia in radicular distributions (9). Impairment in position sense may be severe enough to produce sensory ataxia. Urinary retention with overflow incontinence and, more rarely, fecal incontinence may occur. Lancinating pains—sudden, brief stabs of pain in the legs, back, arms, or face that last for minutes to days—occur unpredictably and may be separated by prolonged remissions. Lancinating pains are frequently attributed in textbooks to tabes dorsalis (9), but some authors have suggested that they were not a consequence of syphilis infection, but were due to the heavy metal therapy used to treat neurosyphilis in the preantibiotic era (55).

Neurological examination of patients with tabes dorsalis shows impaired sensation to pain, touch, and vibration; loss of reflexes; optic atrophy with constriction of peripheral visual fields and central scotomata; and pupillary abnormalities, particularly Argyll Robertson pupils (9). When appearing as strictly defined—as small pupils that do not respond to light, contract normally to accommodation, dilate imperfectly to mydriatics, and do not dilate in response to painful stimuli—Argyll-Robertson pupils were present in almost half of Merritt and coworkers' patients with tabes dorsalis (9).

The CSF formula in early tabes dorsalis is similar to that seen in general paresis, but with time the meningeal process "burns out" and CSF becomes less abnormal. In fact, of Merritt and coworkers' 100 cases of tabes dorsalis, 50% had normal CSF WBC counts, 47% had normal protein concentration, and 28% had nonreactive CSF nontreponemal tests (Wassermann test or one of its predecessors) (9). However, 88% of their patients had reactive blood nontreponemal tests. Tabes has the longest latent period between primary infection and onset of symptoms, averaging about 20 years (range 3 to almost 50 years) (9). Tabes dorsalis was the most common form of neurosyphilis described in the preantibiotic era, occurring in 9% of patients with syphilis (9).

Clinical Manifestations of Neurosyphilis in Patients Also Infected with HIV

Syphilis is common in patients infected with HIV. In some urban health care settings, as many as 30% of HIV-infected patients have serological evidence of *T. pallidum* infection (56,57). Neurosyphilis is often reported in HIV-infected patients, most commonly as meningitis or meningovasculitis with stroke (40–42,58–63). Central nervous system gumma (31,34) and gummatous meningovascular neurosyphilis (64,65) have also been described. In order to determine the proportion of HIV-infected patients that ultimately develop neurosyphilis, several retrospective studies have described clinical or CSF abnormalities in HIV-infected patients with reactive syphilis blood tests. Asymptomatic neurosyphilis, defined strictly by reactive CSF-VDRL, has been identified in 2–54% of HIV-infected patients (66–68) and symptomatic neurosyphilis in 5.7–12.5% (69,70). Higher proportions are seen in patients who have not received prior treatment for syphilis (66) and in patients with higher-titer serum VDRL tests (66–68). When these estimates are compared to the proportion of syphilis patients that developed neurosyphilis in the preantibiotic era (see above), the proportion with asymptomatic neurosyphilis is similar, but the proportion with early symptomatic neurosyphilis is higher [5.7–12.5% in HIV-infected persons vs. 0.5–3% in Merritt and coworkers' experience (9)]. A recent retrospective study of neurosyphilis in HIV-infected and HIV-uninfected patients showed that syphilitic meningitis was more common in HIV-infected patients without AIDS than in HIV-uninfected patients [7 (64%) of 11 vs. 5 (23%) of 22, $p = 0.05$] (58). Although patients with HIV may be more likely to develop early neurosyphilis than their HIV-uninfected counterparts, the incubation period between primary infection and development of neurological disease is comparable. There is no evidence that neurosyphilis develops more rapidly in patients infected with HIV.

DIAGNOSIS

Serum

The diagnosis of symptomatic neurosyphilis is based on clinical findings, supported by results of serological tests on serum and CSF and the identification of CSF abnormalities. The diagnosis of asymptomatic neurosyphilis is based solely on identification of CSF abnormalities in an individual with reactive syphilis serological blood tests.

Merritt and coworkers reported a nonreactive serum nontreponemal test in 64–95% of their patients with neurosyphilis (9). These data have been criticized and attributed to diagnostic inaccuracy (1,2). However, even though today's nontreponemal tests [VDRL and Rapid Plasma Reagin (RPR)] are probably more sensitive than their predecessors, neurosyphilis continues to be reported in patients with nonreactive serum nontreponemal tests.

The likelihood of making a diagnosis of neurosyphilis in a patient with nonreactive serum VDRL or RPR tests clearly depends on the criteria chosen to define neurosyphilis. For example, Hooshmand and coworkers (71) diagnosed neurosyphilis in 241 (84%) of 289 hospitalized patients with reactive serum fluorescent treponemal antibody-absorbed (FTA-ABS) tests, a serological test that detects specific antibody to *Treponema pallidum*. Of the 241 patients diagnosed with neurosyphilis, 124 (51.5%) had a nonreactive serum nontreponemal serological test (71). In this series, diagnosis of neurosyphilis used unconventional criteria: (1) ophthalmological or neurological findings suggestive of neurosyphilis, or (2) reactive CSF FTA-ABS with CSF WBC $> 5/\mu l$ and no evidence of bacterial or viral meningitis, or (3) reactive CSF FTA-ABS in patients with progressive neurological symptoms in whom other etiologies had been excluded and who had either a temporary increase in CSF WBC count after treatment with penicillin or significant clinical improvement after treatment with penicillin (71). Almost half (43%) of the patients were admitted for evaluation of symptoms unrelated to syphilis and were incidentally found to have neurological examination findings that suggested this diagnosis. The most common examination abnormalities were reflex changes, including absent ankle jerks, pupillary changes, and sensory abnormalities.

In contrast to serum nontreponemal serological tests, serum treponemal serological tests [FTA-ABS or microhemagglutination test for *T. pallidum* (MHA-TP)] should be reactive in all patients with neurosyphilis. Without therapy, these tests remain reactive for life. Reversion to nonreaction has only been documented after therapy for a first episode of primary syphilis (72) and in HIV-infected persons with advanced immunosuppression who were previously treated for syphilis and have no current evidence of disease (73).

Cerebrospinal Fluid

A CSF profile characteristic of aseptic meningitis, with a mononuclear pleocytosis, and with a modestly elevated protein concentration is seen in patients with neurosyphilis (Table 1). Higher cell counts and protein concentrations are seen in early neurosyphilis compared to late neurosyphilis. Again, depending upon the criteria chosen to define neurosyphilis, the CSF-VDRL may be reactive in 0–100% of patients. In Merritt and coworkers' experience, CSF nontreponemal tests (the Wassermann test or its predecessors) were reactive in 72–100% of patients (9); in Hooshmand and coworkers' series, 56.7% of patients given a diagnosis of neurosyphilis had reactive CSF nontreponemal (VDRL) tests (71). While the specificity of the CSF-VDRL is high, the sensitivity has been estimated to be 22–69% (74); a reactive CSF-VDRL establishes the diagnosis of neurosyphilis, but a nonreactive test does not exclude it.

Several investigators have suggested that the CSF FTA-ABS and CSF MHA-TP may be more sensitive than the CSF-VDRL in the diagnosis of neurosyphilis (75,76). Thus, unlike the CSF-VDRL, lack of CSF FTA-ABS or CSF MHA-TP reactivity excludes a diagnosis of neurosyphilis with a high degree of certainty. However, the reverse does not hold true: reactivity of CSF treponemal tests does not establish the diagnosis of neurosyphilis. The specificity of these tests is not improved by calculating CSF indices that correct treponemal antibody titers in CSF for albumin or immunoglobulin concentrations. In a recent study of CSF findings in 39 individuals with primary and secondary syphilis, the CSF MHA-TP index [defined as (CSF MHA-TP titer/CSF IgG)/(serum MHA-TP titer/serum IgG)] was normal in two (28%) of seven patients with reactive CSF-VDRL (77). Similarly, in a study of 10 HIV-infected patients with suspected neurosyphilis, the TPHA index [defined as (CSF MHA-TP)/(1000 × CSF albumin/serum albumin)] was nonreactive in two (40%) of five patients with reactive CSF-VDRL (78). Identification of *T. pallidum* in CSF by rabbit inoculation, although quite specific and sensitive, is too cumbersome and expensive to be clinically useful (79). In addition, rabbit inoculation generally only identifies CSF organisms in early syphilis (8). The polymerase chain reaction (PCR) holds promise for sensitive detection of *T. pallidum* in CSF, but it remains a research tool at this time (34,80–82).

Diagnosis of Neurosyphilis in Patients Also Infected with HIV

Mild CSF pleocytosis and elevated CSF protein concentration are common in HIV-infected individuals, likely reflecting HIV infection of the CSF (83). Low sensitivity of the CSF-VDRL in the diagnosis of neurosyphilis may be especially problematic in these patients, because CSF abnormalities may be due to neurosyphilis, HIV, or both. Lack of CSF FTA-ABS or CSF MHA-

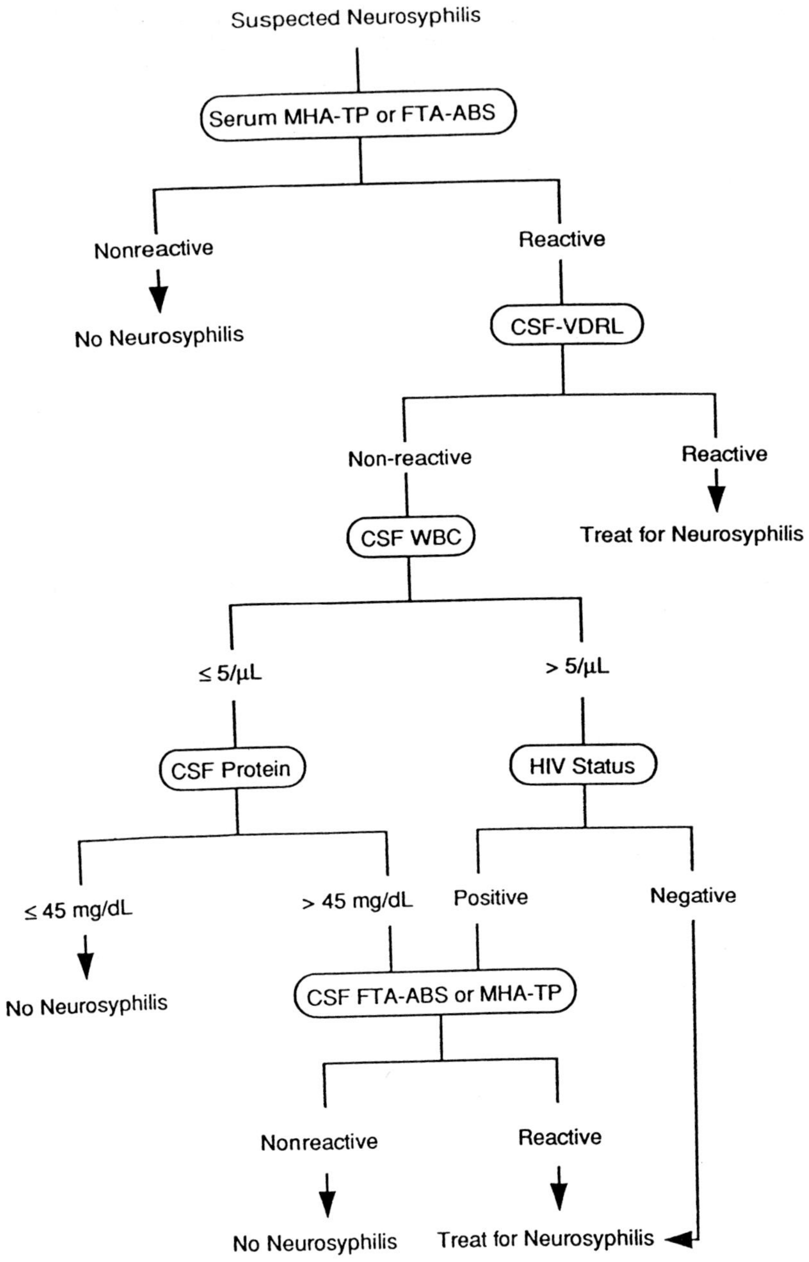

Figure 3 Algorithm for the laboratory diagnosis of neurosyphilis. MHA-TP, microhemagglutination test for *T. pallidum*; FTA-ABS, fluorescent treponemal antibody-absorbed test; CSF, cerebrospinal fluid; VDRL, Venereal Disease Research Laboratory test; WBC, white blood cell count; HIV, human immunodeficiency virus. (From Marra CM, Neurosyphilis: a guide for clinicians, *The Neurologist*, 1, 157–166, 1995. Reproduced with permission.

TP reactivity may be particularly useful in excluding the diagnosis of neurosyphilis in these equivocal cases (77). An algorithm for the laboratory diagnosis of neurosyphilis in HIV-infected and HIV-uninfected patients is shown in Figure 3.

TREATMENT

Antibiotics

Penicillin is the best-studied treatment for neurosyphilis, and the Centers for Disease Control and Prevention (CDC)–recommended regimens are outlined in Table 2 (84). Several alternative antibiotic regimens have been proposed. Most are based on their ability to produce treponemicidal antibiotic concentrations in CSF rather than on efficacy in clinical trials. The combination of (1) amoxicillin, 1.0 g orally six times per day during waking hours, plus probenecid, 500 mg orally four times per day (85), or (2) amoxicillin, 2.0 g orally three times per day, plus probenecid, 500 mg orally twice per day, achieves treponemicidal CSF concentrations (86). Similarly, doxycycline, 200 mg orally twice a day, achieves a CSF concentration that is 26% of the simultaneous serum concentration (87) and offers a promising approach that warrants further study.

Ceftriaxone is an appealing alternative to penicillin because it can be given intravenously or intramuscularly once a day and produces treponemicidal concentrations in CSF (88,89). Resolution of CSF abnormalities after treatment of asymptomatic neurosyphilis with ceftriaxone, 1.0 g intramuscularly daily for 14 days, has been reported (90). However, results from an animal model suggest that this dose of ceftriaxone may be associated with persistence of spirochetes in the CNS (91). A retrospective study of ceftriaxone for treatment of HIV-infected patients with neurosyphilis, latent syphilis, and presumed latent syphilis (many of whom were eventually found to have neurosyphilis) showed an unacceptably high (23%) failure rate using serological criteria (66).

Unless further study proves otherwise, alternative regimens to penicillin, including ceftriaxone, are not acceptable for treatment of neurosyphilis. Patients with a history of penicillin allergy should be skin tested, desensitized if necessary, and treated with penicillin.

Table 2 Diagnostic Tests and Treatment for Neurosyphilis

Diagnostic tests for neurosyphilis[a]	Therapy for neurosyphilis[b]
Serum VDRL or RPR FTA-ABS or MHA-TP Cerebrospinal fluid Cell count Protein concentration CSF-VDRL CSF FTA-ABS or CSF MHA-TP	Aqueous crystalline penicillin G, 2–4 million units IV every 4 h for 10–14 days or Procaine penicillin, 2.4 million units IM once daily, plus probenecid 500 mg orally four times a day, both for 10–14 days

[a]See Figure 3.
[b]From Ref. 84.
VDRL, Veneral Disease Research Laboratory test; RPR, rapid plasma reagin test; FTA-ABS, fluorescent treponemal antibody-absorbed test; MHA-TP, microhemagglutination test for *T. pallidum*; CSF, cerebrospinal fluid.

Adjunctive Treatment

Although dexamethasone is used in the treatment of some bacterial meningitides, it has not been commonly recommended for the treatment of neurosyphilis. The exception is treatment of CNS gummata, including gummatous meningeal disease, for which rapid and dramatic clinical and radiographic response to dexamethasone has been described (28,33).

Assessing Response to Treatment

Unlike many other bacterial infections of the CNS, the efficacy of neurosyphilis therapy cannot be proven by demonstration of CSF sterilization. The definition of response has therefore relied on improvement or stabilization of clinical abnormalities and resolution of serum and CSF abnormalities. Few guidelines are available concerning the rate or extent of resolution of these laboratory abnormalities. The CDC recommendations (based on consensus of a panel of experts) do not provide guidance concerning expected rate of decline of serum VDRL or RPR after treatment, but state that CSF should be examined every 6 months after neurosyphilis treatment until the cell count is normal (84). Retreatment is advised if the cell count has not decreased at 6 months or if the CSF is not entirely normal by 2 years after therapy (84).

Efficacy of Therapy in Patients Also Infected with HIV

Several reports describe failure of high-dose intravenous (IV) penicillin therapy for neurosyphilis in patients infected with HIV. Feraru et al. (27) described an HIV-infected patient who developed syphilitic polyradiculopathy 7 weeks after a 9-day course of 24 million units (MU)/day IV aqueous penicillin G for a reactive CSF-VDRL. Katz and coworkers described two HIV-infected patients who developed progressive neurological symptoms and worsening CSF parameters 4 and 6 months after treatment with high-dose IV aqueous penicillin G for neurosyphilis (58). A study of HIV-infected patients with symptomatic neurosyphilis treated with high-dose IV penicillin showed that three (43%) of seven patients examined 6 months after treatment failed therapy: two patients showed increases in serum RPR and worsening of all CSF parameters (including CSF-VDRL), and another patient failed clinically, with development of meningovascular neurosyphilis (82). Finally, a recent study documented serological relapse in three (60%) of five patients with asymptomatic neurosyphilis treated with high-dose IV penicillin G (92).

These reports suggest that the immune response may be even more important than antibiotic therapy in controlling neurosyphilis. In fact, some experts argue that neurosyphilis is not a curable disease in patients also infected with HIV (66,93).

Criteria for Defining Treatment Failure

Additional study of appropriate rates of decline in serum and CSF abnormalities after treatment of neurosyphilis is clearly warranted. Nonetheless, a reasonable approach to follow-up after therapy is to determine serum VDRL or RPR titers every 3 months and to examine CSF at 3 and 6 months and every 6 months thereafter. Serial serum examinations can be terminated when the serum VDRL or RPR becomes nonreactive or the titer drops by two dilutions (a fourfold reduction). Serial CSF examinations should continue until all CSF abnormalities resolve. Because of underlying CSF abnormalities in HIV-infected individuals (83), CSF pleocytosis and elevated protein concentration may persist, but CSF-VDRL should revert to nonreactive or the titer drop by two dilutions. Although it is easy to devise such criteria for "cure," there are insufficient data to determine whether failure to meet these criteria is equivalent to treatment failure. Until more information is available, retreatment after neurosyphilis therapy should be considered if the serum VDRL or RPR titer increases by two dilutions, if CSF pleocytosis persists at 6 months or later, if the CSF-VDRL titer increases, if all CSF parameters do not return to normal at 2 years after therapy, if existing neurological symptoms or signs worsen, or if new neurological symptoms or signs develop.

NEUROLOGICAL SEQUELAE

The best outcomes after treatment of neurosyphilis are seen in patients with meningitis. Because treatment will not reverse parenchymal damage, patients with meningovascular neurosyphilis, general paresis, and tabes dorsalis may be left with significant disability, although further disease progression may be prevented.

PREVENTION OF NEUROSYPHILIS

Ideally, neurosyphilis would be prevented by appropriate therapy for early syphilis. In fact, development of neurosyphilis after low-dose penicillin regimens for early syphilis (neurorelapse) is rare in immunocompetent individuals. In a study conducted by the U.S. Army (94), 5600 patients with primary and secondary syphilis underwent spinal fluid examinations 6–12 months after treatment with 2.4 MU IM penicillin given as 40,000 units IM every 3 h for 7.5 days). This penicillin regimen likely produces serum penicillin concentrations comparable to those produced by the depot regimen, 2.4 MU IM benzathine penicillin G (BPG), used for primary and secondary syphilis today (84). Only 24 (0.4%) CSF samples in this study were abnormal after therapy, suggesting that few patients were at risk for development of symptomatic neurosyphilis, and no patient developed clinical findings consistent with neurosyphilis (93).

In contrast, a striking feature of neurosyphilis in HIV-infected individuals is recent treatment with appropriate doses of BPG for early syphilis (neurorelapse). Of 42 HIV-infected patients with neurosyphilis reviewed by Musher (60), 16 (38%) had been previously treated with BPG for early syphilis, and 5 (31%) of these patients developed neurosyphilis within 6 months of treatment. Although reinfection cannot be excluded in all cases, the short time interval between treatment for early syphilis and development of neurosyphilis makes this explanation unlikely.

The high rate of neurorelapse in HIV-infected patients with syphilis indicates that these patients should undergo routine lumbar puncture to identify persistent CNS infection or asymptomatic neurosyphilis. Treatment with high-dose penicillin should prevent progression from asymptomatic to symptomatic neurosyphilis in this population, as it does in patients not infected with HIV. In addition, all patients with late latent syphilis, clinical or serological evidence of failure of therapy for early or latent syphilis, or early and latent syphilis who cannot be treated with penicillin should also undergo lumbar puncture to detect asymptomatic neurosyphilis, regardless of HIV status (84).

SUMMARY OF DIAGNOSIS AND TREATMENT

Neurosyphilis is associated with a spectrum of clinical manifestations including headache, cranial nerve abnormalities, stroke, dementia, and sensory ataxia. The clinical diagnosis is confirmed by reactivity of serological tests in blood and identification of CSF abnormalities. Appropriate diagnostic tests and recommended therapy are outlined in Table 2.

REFERENCES

1. Simon RP. Neurosyphilis. Arch Neurol 1985; 42:606–613.

2. Fishman RA. Cerebrospinal Fluid in Diseases of the Nervous System. 2d ed. Philadelphia: W. B. Saunders, 1992:297.
3. Moore JE. Studies in asymptomatic neurosyphilis II. The classification, treatment, and prognosis of early asymptomatic neurosyphilis. Bull Johns Hopkins Hosp 1922; 33:231–246.
4. Mills CH. Routine examination of the cerebrospinal fluid in syphilis: its value in regard to more accurate knowledge, prognosis and treatment. Br Med J 1927; 2:527–532.
5. Ravaut P. Le liquide céphalo-rachidien des syphiliques en période secondaire. Ann Dermatol Syphiligr 1903; 4:537–554.
6. Wile UJ, Stokes JH. A study of the spinal fluid with reference to involvement of the nervous system in secondary syphilis. J Cutan Dis 1914; 32:607–623.
7. Chesney AM, Kemp JE. Incidence of *Spirochaeta pallida* in cerebrospinal fluid during early stage of syphilis. JAMA 1924; 83:1725–1728.
8. Lukehart SA, Hook EW III, Baker-Zander SA, Collier AC, Critchlow CW, Handsfield HH. Invasion of the central nervous system by *Treponema pallidum*: implications for diagnosis and therapy. Ann Intern Med 1988; 109:855–862.
9. Merritt HH, Adams RD, Solomon HC. Neurosyphilis. New York: Oxford, 1946.
10. Clark EG, Danbolt N. The Oslo study of the natural course of untreated syphilis. An epidemiologic investigation based on a re-study of the Boeck-Bruusgaard material. Med Clin North Am 1964; 48: 613–623.
11. Moore JE, Kemp JE. The treatment of early syphilis II. Clinical results in 402 patients. Bull Johns Hopkins Hosp 1926; 39:16–35.
12. Hopkins HH. Prognostic import of a negative spinal fluid in early and in latent syphilis. Arch Derm Syphilol 1931; 24:404–408.
13. Moore JE, Hopkins HH. Asymptomatic neurosyphilis VI. The prognosis of early and late asymptomatic neurosyphilis. JAMA 1930; 95:1637–1641.
14. Hahn RD, Clark EG, Felsovanyi A, Keisselbach M, Koteen H, Potter R. Asymptomatic neurosyphilis: prognosis. Am J Syph Gonorrhea Vener Dis 1946; 30:513–548.
15. Noguchi H, Moore JW. A demonstration of *Treponema pallidum* in the brain in cases of general paralysis. J Exp Med 1913; 17:232–238.
16. Fordyce JA, Rosen I. Laboratory findings in early and late syphilis. Review of one thousand and sixty-four cases. JAMA 1921; 77:1696–1700.
17. O'Leary PA, Cole HN, Moore JE, Stokes JH, Wile UJ, Parran T, Vonderlehr RA, Usilton LJ. Cooperative clinical studies in the treatment of syphilis: asymptomatic neurosyphilis. Vener Dis Inf 1937; 18: 45–65.
18. Merritt HH, Moore M. Acute syphilitic meningitis. Medicine (Baltimore) 1935; 14:119–183.
19. Agdal N, Hagdrup HK, Wantzin GL. Pachymeningitis cervicalis hypertrophica syphilitica. Acta Dermatovenerol (Stockholm) 1980; 60:184–186.
20. Adams RD, Merritt HH. Meningeal and vascular syphilis of the spinal cord. Medicine (Baltimore) 1944; 23:181–214.
21. Fisher M, Poser CM. Syphilitic meningomyelitis. A case report. Arch Neurol 1977; 34:785.
22. Silber MH. Syphilitic myelopathy. Genitourin Med 1989; 65:338–341.
23. Strom T, Schneck SA. Syphilitic meningomyelitis. Neurology 1991; 41:325–326.
24. Berger JR. Spinal cord syphilis associated with human immunodeficiency virus infection: a treatable myelopathy. Am J Med 1992; 92:101–103.
25. Byrne TN, Bose A, Sze G, Waxman SG. Syphilitic meningitis causing paraparesis in an HIV-negative woman. J Neurol Sci 1991; 103:48–50.
26. Lanska MJ, Lanska DJ, Schmidley JW. Syphilitic polyradiculopathy in an HIV-positive man. Neurology 1988; 38:1297–1301.
27. Feraru ER, Aronow HA, Lipton RB. Neurosyphilis in AIDS patients: initial CSF VDRL may be negative. Neurology 1990; 40:541–543.
28. Case Records of the Massachusetts General Hospital (case 32-1991). N Engl J Med 1991; 325:414–422.
29. Standaert DG, Galetta SL, Atlas SW. Meningovascular syphilis with a gumma of the midbrain. J Clin Neurol Ophthalmol 1991; 11:139–143.

30. Vogl T, Dresel S, Lochmuller H, Bergman C, Reimers C, Lissner J. Third cranial nerve palsy caused by gummatous neurosyphilis: MR findings. Am J Neuroradiol 1993; 14:1329–1331.
31. Berger JR, Waskin H, Pall L, Hensley G, Ihmedian I, Post MJD. Syphilitic cerebral gumma with HIV infection. Neurology 1992; 42:1282–1287.
32. Tien RD, Gean-Marton AD, Mark AS. Neurosyphilis in HIV carriers: MR findings in six patients. Am J Roentgenol 1992; 158:1325–1328.
33. Herrold JM. A syphilitic cerebral gumma manifesting as a brain-stem mass lesion that responded to corticosteroid monotherapy. Mayo Clin Proc 1994; 69:960–961.
34. Horowitz HW, Valsamis MP, Wicher V, Abbruscato F, Larsen SA, Wormser GP, Wicher K. Brief report: cerebral syphilitic gumma confirmed by the polymerase chain reaction in a man with human immunodeficiency virus infection. N Engl J Med 1994; 331:1488–1491.
35. Punt J. Multiple cerebral gummata. Case report. J Neurosurg 1983; 58:959–961.
36. Brightbill TC, Ihmeidan IH, Donovan Post MJ, Berger JR, Katz DA. Neurosyphilis in HIV-positive and HIV-negative patients: neuroimaging findings. Am J Neuroradiol 1995; 16:703–711.
37. Merritt HH. The early clinical and laboratory manifestations of syphilis of the central nervous system. N Engl J Med 1940; 223:446–450.
38. Moore JE. The relation of neurorecurrences to late syphilis. A clinical study of eighty-one cases. Arch Neurol Psychiatry 1929; 21:117–136.
39. Moore JE, Gieske M. Syphilitic iritis. A study of 249 patients. Am J Ophthalmol 1931; 14:110–126.
40. Johns DR, Tierney M, Felsenstein D. Alteration in the natural history of neurosyphilis by concurrent infection with the human immunodeficiency virus. N Engl J Med 1987; 316:1569–1572.
41. Case SK, Levitz SM, Wolinsky JW, Sulis CA. Pontine pure motor hemiparesis due to meningovascular syphilis in human immunodeficiency virus-positive patients (letter). Arch Neurol 1988; 45:832.
42. Tyler KL, Sandberg E, Baum KF. Medial medullary syndrome and meningovascular syphilis: a case report in an HIV-infected man and a review of the literature. Neurology 1994; 44:2231–2235.
43. Harrigan EP, McLaughlin TJ, Feldman RG. Transverse myelitis due to meningovascular syphilis. Arch Neurol 1984; 41:337–338.
44. Lowenstein DH, Mills C, Simon RP. Acute syphilitic transverse myelitis: unusual presentation of meningovascular syphilis. Genitourin Med 1987; 63:333–338.
45. Tashiro K, Moriwaka F, Sudo K, Akino M, Abe H. Syphilitic myelitis with its magnetic resonance imaging (MRI) verification and successful treatment. Jpn J Psychiatr Neurol 1987; 41:269–272.
46. Terry PM, Glancy GR, Graham A. Meningovascular syphilis of the spinal cord presenting with incomplete Brown-Séquard syndrome: case report. Genitourin Med 1989; 65:189–191.
47. Vatz KA, Scheibel RL, Keiffer SA, Ansari KA. Neurosyphilis and diffuse cerebral angiopathy: a case report. Neurology 1974; 24:472–476.
48. Holmes MD, Brant-Zawadzki MM, Simon RP. Clinical features of meningovascular syphilis. Neurology 1984; 34:553–556.
49. Landi G, Villani F, Anzalone N. Variable angiographic findings in patients with stroke and neurosyphilis. Stroke 1990; 21:333–338.
50. Holland BA, Perrett LV, Mills CM. Meningovascular syphilis: CT and MR findings. Radiology 1986; 158:439–442.
51. Gabay EL, Hallinan J, Lovett MA. Computerized tomographic findings in meningovascular syphilis: a case report. Sex Transm Dis 1983; 10:39–40.
52. Kawai N, Baba A, Mizukami K, Sakai T, Shiraishi H, Koisumi J. CT, MR, and SPECT findings in a general paresis. Comput Med Imaging Graph 1994; 18:461–465.
53. Hahn RD, Webster B, Weickhardt G, Thomas E, Timberlake W, Solomon H, Stokes JH, Moore JE, Heyman A, Gammon G, Gleeson GA, Curtis AC, Cutler JC. Penicillin treatment of general paresis (dementia paralytica). Arch Neurol Psychiatry 1959; 81:557–590.
54. Dewhurst K. The neurosyphilitic psychoses today. A survey of 91 cases. Br J Psychiatry 1969; 115: 31–38.
55. Weismann K. Neurosyphilis, or chronic heavy metal poisoning: Karen Blixen's lifelong disease. Sex Transm Dis 1995; 22:137–144.

56. Ansell DA, Hu T-C, Straus M, Cohen M, Sherer R. HIV and syphilis seroprevalence among clients with sexually transmitted diseases attending a walk-in clinic at Cook County Hospital. Sex Transm Dis 1994; 21:93–96.
57. Schoenbaum EE, Webber MP, Vermund S, Gayle H. HIV antibody in persons screened for syphilis: prevalence in a New York City emergency room and primary care clinics. Sex Transm Dis 1990; 17: 190–193.
58. Katz DA, Berger JR, Duncan RC. Neurosyphilis. A comparative study of the effects of infection with human immunodeficiency virus. Arch Neurol 1993; 50:243–249.
59. Musher DM, Hamill RJ, Baughn RE. Effect of human immunodeficiency virus (HIV) infection on the course of syphilis and on the response to treatment. Ann Intern Med 1990; 113:872–881.
60. Musher DM. Syphilis, neurosyphilis, penicillin, and AIDS. J Infect Dis 1991; 163:1201–1206.
61. DiNubile MJ, Baxter JD, Mirsen TR. Acute syphilitic meningitis in a man with seropositivity for human immunodeficiency virus infection and normal numbers of CD4 lymphocytes. Arch Intern Med 1992; 152:1324–1326.
62. Savall R, Valls F, Cabré M. Syphilis and HIV infection (letter). Genitourin Med 1991; 67:353.
63. Gue J-W, Wang S-J, Lin Y-Y, Liao K-K, Wong W-W. Neurosyphilis presenting as tabes dorsalis in a HIV carrier. Chin Med J 1993; 51:389–391.
64. Morgello S, Laufer H. Quaternary neurosyphilis (letter). N Engl J Med 1988; 319:1549–1550.
65. Morgello S, Laufer H. Quaternary neurosyphilis in a Haitian man with human immunodeficiency virus infection. Hum Pathol 1989; 20:808–811.
66. Dowell ME, Ross PG, Musher DM, Cate TR, Baughn RE. Response of latent syphilis or neurosyphilis to ceftriaxone therapy in persons infected with human immunodeficiency virus. Am J Med 1992; 93: 481–488.
67. Holtom PD, Larsen RA, Leal ME, Leedom JM. Prevalence of neurosyphilis in human immunodeficiency virus-infected patients with latent syphilis. Am J Med 1992; 93:9–12.
68. Zisfein J, DiPietro D, Lugo-Torres O. CSF Venereal Disease Research Laboratory in neurologically asymptomatic HIV-infected patients with serological evidence for syphilis (abstract). Ann Neurol 1993; 34:283.
69. Berger JR. Neurosyphilis in human immunodeficiency virus type 1-seropositive individuals. A prospective study. Arch Neurol 1991; 48:700–702.
70. Brandon WR, Boulos LM, Morse A. Determining the prevalence of neurosyphilis in a cohort co-infected with HIV. Int J STD AIDS 1993; 4:99–101.
71. Hooshmand H, Escobar MR, Kopf SW. Neurosyphilis. A study of 241 patients. JAMA 1972; 219: 726–729.
72. Romanowski B, Sutherland R, Fick GH, Mooney D, Love EJ. Serologic response to treatment of infectious syphilis. Ann Intern Med 1991; 114:1005–1009.
73. Haas JS, Bolan G, Larsen SA, Clement MJ, Bacchetti P, Moss AR. Sensitivity of treponemal tests for detecting prior treated syphilis during human immunodeficiency virus infection. J Infect Dis 1990; 162:862–866.
74. Hart G. Syphilis tests in diagnostic and therapeutic decision making. Ann Intern Med 1986; 104: 368–376.
75. McGeeney T, Yount F, Hinthorn DR, Liu C. Utility of the FTA-ABs test of cerebrospinal fluid in the diagnosis of neurosyphilis. Sex Transm Dis 1979; 6:195–198.
76. Davis LE, Schmitt JW. Clinical significance of cerebrospinal fluid tests for neurosyphilis. Ann Neurol 1989; 25:50–55.
77. Marra CM, Critchlow CW, Hook EW III, Collier AC, Lukehart SA. Cerebrospinal fluid treponemal antibodies in untreated early syphilis. Arch Neurol 1995; 52:68–72.
78. Tomberlin MG, Holtom PD, Owens JL, Larsen RA. Evaluation of neurosyphilis in human immunodeficiency virus-infected individuals. Clin Infect Dis 1994; 18:288–294.
79. Turner TB, Hardy PH, Newman B. Infectivity tests in syphilis. Br J Vener Dis 1969; 45:183–196.
80. Burstain JM, Grimprel E, Lukehart SA, Norgard MV, Radolf JD. Sensitive detection of *Treponema pallidum* by using the polymerase chain reaction. J Clin Microbiol 1991; 29:62–69.

81. Noordhoek GT, Wolters EC, de Jonge MEJ, van Embden JDA. Detection by polymerase chain reaction of *Treponema pallidum* DNA in cerebrospinal fluid from neurosyphilis patients before and after antibiotic treatment. J Clin Microbiol 1991; 29:1976–1984.
82. Gordon SM, Eaton ME, George R, Larsen S, Lukehart SA, Kuypers J, Marra C, Thompson S. The response of symptomatic neurosyphilis to high-dose intravenous penicillin G in patients with human immunodeficiency virus infection. N Engl J Med 1994; 331:1469–1472.
83. Appleman ME, Marshall DW, Brey RL, et al. Cerebrospinal fluid abnormalities in patients without AIDS who are seropositive for the human immunodeficiency virus. J Infect Dis 1988; 158:193–199.
84. Centers for Disease Control and Prevention. 1993 Sexually transmitted diseases treatment guidelines. MMWR 1993; 42:27–46.
85. Faber WR, Bos JD, Rietra PJGM, Fass H, van Eijk RVW. Treponemicidal levels of amoxicillin in cerebrospinal fluid after oral administration. Sex Transm Dis 1983; 10:148–150.
86. Morrison RE, Harrison SM, Tramont EC. Oral amoxycillin, an alternative treatment for neurosyphilis. Genitourin Med 1985; 61:359–362.
87. Whiteside Yim C, Flynn NM, Fitzgerald FT. Penetration of oral doxycycline into the cerebrospinal fluid of patients with latent or neurosyphilis. Antimicrob Agents Chemother 1985; 28:347–348.
88. Cherubin CE, Eng HK; Norrby R, Modai J, Humbert G, Overturf G. Penetration of newer cephalosporins into cerebrospinal fluid. Rev Infect Dis 1989; 11:526–548.
89. Korting HC, Walther D, Riethmüller U, Meurer M. Comparative in vitro susceptibility of *Treponema pallidum* to ceftizoxime, ceftriaxone and penicillin G. Chemotherapy 1986; 32:352–355.
90. Hook EW III, Baker-Zander SA, Moskovitz BL, Lukehart SA, Handsfield HH. Ceftriaxone therapy for asymptomatic neurosyphilis. Case report and western blot analysis of serum and cerebrospinal fluid IgG response to therapy. Sex Transm Dis 1986; 13:185–188.
91. Marra CM, Slatter V, Tartaglione TA, Baker-Zander SA, Lukehart SA. Evaluation of aqueous penicillin G and ceftriaxone for experimental neurosyphilis (letter). J Infect Dis 1992; 165:396–397.
92. Malone JL, Wallace MR, Hendrick BB, LaRocco A Jr, Tonon E, Brodine SK, Bowler WA, Lavin BS. Syphilis and neurosyphilis in a human immunodeficiency virus type-1 seropositive population: evidence for frequent serologic relapse after therapy. Am J Med 1995; 99:55–63.
93. Hook EW III. Management of syphilis in human immunodeficiency virus-infected patients (editorial). Am J Med 1992; 93:477–479.
94. Altshuler L, Karpinos BD, Leifer W, Ozog JJ. Efficacy of penicillin treatment of early syphilis in the army. Am J Syph 1949; 33:126–138.
95. Marra CM. Syphilis and human immunodeficiency virus infection. Semin Neurol 1995; 12:43–50.

13

Neurological Complications of Human Immunodeficiency Virus Type 1 in Adults

Richard W. Price
University of California, San Francisco, and San Francisco General Hospital, San Francisco, California

Human immunodeficiency virus type one (HIV-1) is a retrovirus causing a chronic or "slow" infection, which in most, if not all, cases is eventually lethal although over a varying time course (1). This virus is classified among the lentiviruses because of its biological and genetic relationship to the visna-maedi virus, one of the prototypes included by Sigurdsson in his conceptualization of slow infections (2). The course of HIV-1 may be complicated by an array of neurological diseases. This chapter provides an overview of these neurological complications with an emphasis on the general principles of pathophysiology, diagnosis, and treatment and a lengthier discussion of the individual disorders not considered in detail in other chapters of this volume. Those complications discussed in other chapters are considered here principally in the context of differential diagnosis. The chapter is divided into three major sections, the first dealing with some general principles of diagnosis and treatment, the second with opportunistic diseases, and the third with the conditions that appear to be caused or triggered by HIV-1 itself, rather than another invading organism.

GENERAL PRINCIPLES OF NEUROLOGICAL DIAGNOSIS IN HIV-1 INFECTION

HIV-1 infection has a protracted time course that is determined by the biology of HIV-1 and its evolving interaction with the host, particularly with the immune system of the host. In approaching diagnosis, a conceptual framework based on certain pathophysiological variables is useful in providing a rationale for understanding the incidence and clinical profiles of the common disorders and for confronting new or less common neurological complications of this retroviral infection. Particularly important in this regard is the patient's phase in the evolving systemic HIV-1 infection and its resultant effects on immune reaction. Each phase confers a particular set of vulnerabilities and hence probabilities of differential diagnosis. The spectrum of neurological complications thus differs depending upon whether the patient has recently acquired HIV-1 infection, is in the phase of "clinical latency," or suffers from debilitating impairment of cell-mediated immune defenses. Additionally, like neurological diagnosis in most other settings, the neuroanatomical localization of the disease and its temporal profile are critical variables in diagnosis. The chronicity of HIV-1 infection and its progressive effect upon the host also determines certain aspects of therapy, particularly the need for protracted treatment of opportunistic infections.

Patient Background and Risk Profile

As with all neurological diagnoses, the HIV-1–infected patient's background has major implications for disease susceptibility and, hence, differential diagnosis. Two aspects of the patient's background assume particular importance. Foremost is the phase of systemic HIV-1 infection, but the risk for HIV-1 infection may also be associated with concomitant risks for other neurological complications.

Phase of Systemic HIV-1 Infection

HIV-1 infection exerts an increasing influence on neurological disease susceptibility as the course of systemic infection proceeds. This culminates in a strongly predominating influence late in the course of this infection when systemic host defenses against certain microorganisms are crippled, leading to opportunistic infections. While less potent, the earlier phases of infection also confer certain disease vulnerabilities as well, and these differ from those of late infection. For this reason it is critical to know the phase of the patient's systemic HIV-1 infection when formulating and evaluating differential diagnosis.

It goes largely without saying that HIV-1 infection should be documented in all individuals by standard serological testing. Following this, the phase of systemic infection can be defined either clinically on the basis of the history of other disease complications or by the results of laboratory studies. Thus, the HIV-1–seropositive patient who has suffered a major clinical AIDS-defining (3) infection has functionally demonstrated the phase of his or her systemic infection and immunosuppression, and hence his or her susceptibility to further opportunistic processes involving the nervous system. In those without known or defined evidence of such opportunistic infection, the blood CD4+ T-lymphocyte count is the most useful index of systemic disease status. This surrogate marker provides an index of the cumulative effect of systemic HIV-1 infection on its principal target, the helper-inducer subset of lymphocytes that express the CD4 surface marker. This marker is the principal cell receptor for HIV-1. Revision of the AIDS case definition to include individuals with CD4+ counts below 200 cells/mm^3 testifies to the prognostic utility of this measurement. Moreover, to a degree, the lower the level of this cell count, the higher the incidence of most of the major CNS complications (4). For patients presenting acutely without records of CD4+ counts, the total peripheral lymphocyte count can be used as a substitute, since this reflects the reduction of the CD4+ component.

Other Background Risks

The risk for HIV-1 infection may bear on other disease susceptibilities as well. Use of intravenous or other drugs—particularly ongoing use—may be accompanied by its own special nervous system complications, including, for example, pyogenic infection in the case of intravenous opiate injection or seizures and vascular disease with cocaine use. Low socioeconomic status may additionally predispose to infection by *Mycobacterium tuberculosis*, which is less common in more prosperous segments of the population. Some patients infected by homosexual or heterosexual transmission may harbor other sexually transmitted diseases, including syphilis. Hemophiliacs, of course, may be susceptible to hemorrhagic events. For this reason it is useful to know the patient's background risk for HIV-1 infection as well as other individual disease risks that may alter the spectrum or "weight" of other diagnoses.

Neuroanatomical Localization

As with other neurological diseases, a first step in considering diagnosis involves following the time-honored and empirically proven approach of the neurologist in segregating diagnostic possibilities on the basis of their neuroanatomical localization. This is founded upon the predilection of different pathological processes, including different infections, to select individual parts of the CNS or the PNS, whether meninges, brain, spinal cord, nerve roots, peripheral nerve or muscle, or a particular distribution within one or more of these neuroanatomical "compartments." For example, *Cryptococcus neoformans* infects primarily the subarachnoid space and only uncommonly invades the brain parenchyma, usually only after extending into the perivascular spaces. By contrast, *Toxoplasma gondii* causes focal parenchymal lesions in the gray matter and most commonly establishes infections in the diencephalon or cerebral cortex. Each invading microorganism has its particular propensity for localization, which is determined either by its route of invasion or by its predilection to replicate or grow within certain cells or spaces. These behaviors and resultant individual anatomical predilections provide the neuroanatomical basis for classification of the various disorders shown in Table 1.

Temporal Profile of Disease Evolution

Pathophysiology also determines the time frame within which individual diseases evolve, and the patient's history of the physician's direct observation of this temporal profile is often also helpful in assigning disease probabilities. Thus, abrupt membrane changes (as in a seizure) or substrate deprivation (as with an ischemic event) will cause acute symptoms, while inflammatory and neoplastic diseases evolve more slowly since they depend upon DNA replication (of the invading organism, the neoplastic cells or responding host defense cell populations) and often cell migrations. Unfortunately, most of the complications of late HIV-1 infection share this slower time course since they relate to opportunistic infections so that their temporal profiles are not distinctly different. However, there are some minor differences among the common conditions. For example, while the range of presentations among the three most common focal brain disorders overlaps, toxoplasmosis tends to evolve more quickly (over a few days) than primary CNS lymphoma (PCNSL; over 1–3 weeks), which in turn tends to be more rapid than progressive multifocal leukoencephalopathy (PML; over several weeks). These differences can be helpful, at least in the first approach, in diagnosis of both CNS and PNS diseases.

Principles of Treatment

By definition, the opportunistic infections that so often complicate the late stage of HIV-1 infection are caused by organisms that the normal, immunocompetent adult host can usually readily suppress with their repertoire of cell-mediated defenses involving particularly T lymphocytes and macrophages. Most of these organisms replicate within cells rather than freely in intracellular fluid spaces and also have the capacity to reside dormant within the host long after primary infection. For example, both *T. gondii* and JC virus (the virus that causes progressive multifocal leukoencephalopathy, PML) brain infections in AIDS patients are due to reactivation of endogenous organisms rather than reinfection. Other opportunistic pathogens are nearly ubiquitous in the environment, e.g., *C. neoformans*. Specific treatment with antimicrobials augments or substitutes for the weakened responses of the AIDS patient to these agents. However, usually such treatment does not fully eliminate the opportunistic pathogen from its intracellular

Table 1 A Classification of the Major Neurological Complications of Late HIV-1 Infection

- Brain
  - Predominantly nonfocal
    - *Common*
      - AIDS dementia complex
      - Cytomegalovirus (CMV) encephalitis (*clinical* impact uncertain)
      - Toxoplasmosis (encephalitic form)
      - Metabolic encephalopathies (alone or as exacerbating influence)
      - (See also Meninges, below)
    - *Rare*
      - Herpes simplex encephalitis
  - Predominantly focal
    - *Common*
      - Cerebral toxoplasmosis
      - Primary CNS lymphoma
      - Progressive multifocal leukoencephalopathy (PML)
    - *Uncommon/Rare*
      - Tuberculous brain abscess/Tuberculoma
      - Cryptococcoma
      - Varicella-zoster virus (VZV) encephalitis
      - Aspergillosis
- Spinal Cord
  - *Common*
    - Vacuolar myelopathy (part of AIDS dementia complex)
  - *Uncommon*
    - VZV myelitis (complicating herpes zoster)
    - Spinal epidural or intradural lymphoma
    - HTLV-I–associated myelopathy
- Meninges
  - *Common*
    - Cryptococcal meningitis
    - Aseptic meningitis (HIV-1?)
  - *Uncommon*
    - Lymphomatous meningitis (metastatic)
    - Tuberculous meningitis (*M. tuberculosis*)
    - Syphilitic meningitis
  - *Rare*
    - *Listeria monocytogenes* meningitis
- Peripheral nerve and root
  - *Very common*
    - Distal sensory polyneuropathy (? HIV-1–related)
  - *Common*
    - Autonomic neuropathy
    - Nucleoside toxic neuropathies (ddI, DDC)
    - Herpes zoster
  - *Uncommon*
    - Mononeuritis multiplex
      - Early limited form
      - Late malignant form
    - CMV polyradiculopathy

Table 1 Continued

Mononeuropathy associated with aseptic meningitis
Mononeuropathy secondary to lymphomatous meningitis
Muscle
Polymyositis
Noninflammatory myopathies
Zidovudine toxic myopathy

residence in the host or cannot prevent environmental reexposure and continuing vulnerability, so that these infections will recur when the antimicrobial therapy is stopped. For this reason, treatment of these infections must be lifelong rather than for the circumscribed period required for "ordinary" acute infections such as pyogenic meningitis.

OPPORTUNISTIC DISEASES

The hallmark of AIDS is the development of major opportunistic infections. The nervous system shares this susceptibility with other organ systems. This section individually considers the major central nervous system (CNS) opportunistic conditions of AIDS, selected on the basis of their frequency, and then more briefly discusses some of the less common CNS infections before considering the PNS opportunistic infections.

Cerebral Toxoplasmosis

Cerebral toxoplasmosis is the most frequent CNS opportunistic infection complicating AIDS and has been reported in 5–15% or more of patients, with the incidence depending on geographic origin (5–14). The varying incidence in different populations relates principally to the likelihood of earlier environmental exposure to this protozoan parasite. As noted above, cerebral toxoplasmosis almost invariably results from recrudescence of previously acquired infection and relates to the loss of immune defenses, which maintain *T. gondii* in an inactive encysted form. It has been estimated that about one quarter of HIV-1–infected patients with serum antibodies against this parasite will eventually develop cerebral toxoplasmosis (7). This incidence has declined where trimethaprim-sulfamethoxazole has been used as prophylaxis for *Pneumocystis carinii* pneumonia (PCP) since this regimen is also effective in reducing the development of cerebral toxoplasmosis (15,16).

As noted earlier, cerebral toxoplasmosis characteristically develops subacutely, evolving over several days from onset of symptoms to presentation with neurological deficit (5,11). While focal cerebral dysfunction usually predominates, this is often combined with nonfocal, "encephalitic" symptoms and signs, including fever, headache, lethargy, and confusion. In a minority of patients this diffuse brain dysfunction can predominate and cause a picture of subacute encephalitis without clear focal features. However, in most patients the focal manifestations are clear and usually relate to hemispheric lesions; these include hemiparesis, hemianesthesia, aphasia, apraxia, or focal seizures. Cerebellar ataxia and brain-stem abnormalities are less common but can also occur.

Pathologically, the disease is characterized by a variable number of cerebral abscesses (5,17). In the acute encephalitic form of the disease, the brain may exhibit numerous small lesions with variable cellular reaction (18). The more common, more slowly developing lesions are often larger and surrounded by mononuclear cells, edema, and sometimes vascular occlusion or microscopic hemorrhage. In untreated disease, free forms (tachyzoites) of *T. gondii* are seen pathologically, while after treatment these are usually no longer evident and only encysted forms persist.

The diagnosis of cerebral toxoplasmosis relies on a combination of clinical suspicion based on the clinical presentation, neuroimaging, blood serology, and therapeutic trial (5,11,19). In approaching AIDS patients with suspected toxoplasmosis or other focal disorders, MRI or, less optimally, CT scanning is critical both to confirm the presence of macroscopic focal disease and to determine the character of these abnormalities (20). Multiple lesions located in the cortex or diencephalic nuclei (thalamus, basal ganglia) surrounded by edema strongly favor cerebral toxoplasmosis. In most cases toxoplasma abscesses exhibit ringlike contrast enhancement on either MRI or CT, but either homogeneous contrast enhancement or nonenhancing hypodense lesions may be found occasionally. MRI is generally superior to CT in detecting toxoplasma abscesses and thus revealing the multiplicity of lesions. The most common diagnostic issue in these patients is the differentiation of cerebral toxoplasmosis form primary CNS lymphoma, since the appearance of these two conditions on CT or MRI may overlap (Table 2). The lesions of lymphoma commonly exhibit more diffuse or less clear-cut contrast enhancement (particularly on CT), tend to be radiologically less numerous, and are more often located in the white matter adjacent to the lateral ventricles with a tendency for subependymal extension. PML may also be considered clinically, but characteristically afflicts the white matter, often at the cortical junction, and does not cause mass effect. Recently, thallium SPECT imaging has been applied in the effort to distinguish cerebral toxoplasmosis from primary CNS lymphoma, with the former characterized by decreased uptake of the radionuclide and the latter with increased uptake (21). This is a promising methodology, but its utility and cost-effectiveness in otherwise ambiguous cases need to be evaluated further.

Toxoplasma serology is of ancillary help when appropriately interpreted. Since cerebral toxoplasmosis is almost invariably due to reactivation of earlier infection, patients rarely have negative serum IgG antibody titers (5,7). However, these titers may be low (occasionally an apparently negative titer will be positive when a more concentrated specimen, such as a 1:4 dilution, is tested) and characteristically do not rise during the course of the disease. A positive titer therefore indicates susceptibility, while a negative titer casts doubt on the diagnosis.

Table 2 Neuroimaging Features of Some Common CNS Complications of Late HIV-1 Infection

Disease	No. of lesions	Type of lesion	Location of lesion
Cerebral toxoplasmosis	Multiple	Mass effect; spherical ring enhancing	Basal ganglia, cortex
PCNSL	One or few	Mass effect; irregular; weakly enhancing	Often periventricular with subependymal spread, white matter
PML	Multiple	No mass effect; nonenhancing; white on T_2, black on T_1 MRI	White matter, often subcortical involving U-fibers
AIDS dementia complex	None, diffuse, or multiple	Cerebral atrophy; fluffy or diffuse T_2 signal, no mass effect or enhancement	Central white matter (sparing U-fibers), basal ganglia
CMV encephalitis	Few	Small, T_2 signal, enhancement	Ependymal, small cortical
Cryptococcal meningitis	Variable	Dilated perivascular spaces	Basal ganglia

Recently, the use of PCR to detect *T. gondii* nucleic acid in tissue samples, CSF, or serum has begun to be explored (22–25). While promising, further experience is needed before this technique finds its way to routine diagnosis. Practical diagnosis of cerebral toxoplasmosis now relies principally on the strategy of diagnostic therapeutic trial of antitoxoplasmosis treatment in those patients with the aforementioned clinical, neuroimaging, and serological features (5, 11,19,26). Brain biopsy is reserved for treatment failures or clinically atypical patients, such as those who are seronegative or have uncharacteristic MRI or CT studies. Fortunately, when treated promptly, toxoplasmosis responds with clear clinical and neuroimaging improvement, usually within a few days to a week. For this reason, treatment response has proved an effective and reliable diagnostic measure.

While the range of treatments for cerebral toxoplasmosis is growing and there is some uncertainty about optimal doses, the mainstay is a combined therapy with pyrimethamine and either sulfadiazine or clindamycin. These are usually administered at varying dosages, depending upon the phase of treatment. Thus, upon initial diagnosis (or considered diagnosis) pyrimethamine has been recommended at a loading dose of 200 mg, followed by 50–75 mg/day during the acute phase (27). This is accompanied by administration of folinic acid at 10–20 mg/day by oral, intravenous, or intramuscular routes. Additionally, sulfadiazine is given orally at 1–1.5 g every 6 h, or, in those allergic or intolerant, alternatively clindamycin is given usually at 600 mg every 6 h orally or intravenously and may be increased in some up to 1200 mg intravenously ever 6 hours. Once the patient has responded, maintenance therapy can be instituted at lower doses: for example, pyrimethamine at 25–50 mg with 10–20 mg folinic acid/day along with oral sulfadiazine at 1 g every 12 h or oral clindamycin at 300 mg every 6 h. Alternative regimens have included combining pyrimethamine/folinic acid with clarithromycin, azithromycin, atovoquone, or dapsone or trimethaprim/sulfamethoxazole alone.

An additional issue related to diagnosis and treatment of these patients involves the use of corticosteroids to reduce cerebral edema. In general, in treating cerebral toxoplasmosis, and indeed in all AIDS patients, *corticosteroids should be avoided when possible*. This is particularly important when considering a therapeutic trial to differentiate between toxoplasmosis and CNS lymphoma. Since the latter may respond symptomatically and radiologically to corticosteroids alone, clinical or neuroimaging improvement on combination antibiotic and steroid treatment can be difficult to interpret. More generally, corticosteroids exacerbate the impairment of immune defenses in AIDS patients, potentially worsening not only toxoplasmosis but other systemic opportunistic infections. Thus, corticosteroids should be used only if mass effect threatens brain herniation, and once there is sufficient improvement they should be rapidly tapered.

Primary CNS Lymphoma

Primary CNS lymphomas (PCNSL) develop in approximately 2–5% of AIDS patients (8,28–35). This incidence may be increasing related to the efficacy of prophylactic and therapeutic measures against various opportunistic infections and attendant extended longevity. Unlike the more varied timing of systemic lymphomas complicating HIV-1 infection in relation to the phase of disease, PCNSL is almost always a late complication and appears in the same context as the important AIDS-defining infections. They are B-cell lymphomas, and virtually all show evidence of Epstein-Barr virus (EBV) DNA, indicating a role for this herpesvirus in their development and perhaps a justification for classification with opportunistic infections (36). They usually present with progressive focal or multifocal neurological deficits similar to toxoplasmosis and PML, although the tempo of disease evolution is characteristically somewhere between these two other diseases, with patients presenting after several days to a few weeks of progressive symptoms. Symptoms and signs include change of personality or behavior, hemiparesis, dysphasia, or other indications of hemispheral dysfunction. Because of their frequent deep brain location and presumed slow growth, some patients may appear dull and apathetic with gait disturbance but only mild or subtle lateralizing signs. In these cases, the AIDS dementia complex may be a principal differential diagnosis. Headache is relatively common, while fever and constitutional symptoms are usually absent if there are no other simultaneous infections.

Neuroimaging is essential in evaluating these patients, and both MRI and CT usually detect symptomatic lesions, with MRI being more sensitive. Characteristically, PCNSL is microscopically multicentric, but often only one or two lesions show on MRI or CT scan (Table 2). Their location is characteristically deep in the brain adjacent to the lateral ventricles and involves the white rather than gray matter; MRI often shows characteristic subependymal extension. On CT scan they may enhance after contrast administration, but often this is either weak, assuming a diffuse rather than ringlike pattern, or absent. There is mass effect and variable surrounding edema. (Differentiation from toxoplasmosis was discussed above.) CSF cytology is unfortunately usually negative or equivocal, and definitive diagnosis therefore almost always relies on brain biopsy.

While brain biopsy is most often undertaken after failure of a trial of antitoxoplasma therapy to induce clinical improvement, early biopsy should be considered when neuroimaging of the lesion(s) is typical (for example, have the characteristic periventricular distribution with diffuse enhancement) and when blood toxoplasmosis serology is negative. Clinicians familiar with AIDS and PCNSL can often predict the correct diagnosis and accelerate the decision to proceed with biopsy. This is important because early diagnosis and therapy influences outcome. Thallium SPECT may also prove useful in supporting the diagnosis of lymphoma and early biopsy (21). The use of stereotaxic biopsy techniques has increased the access to these tumors and reduced the morbidity of biopsy.

The current standard therapy for lymphoma in AIDS patients consists of whole-brain radiation and corticosteroids (31,32). At present there is no defined role for systemic chemotherapy. Because aggressive chemotherapy has become the treatment of choice for PCNSL in non-AIDS patients (35) and for systemic lymphomas in HIV-1 infection, it might be conjectured that the same will eventually prove true for brain tumors in AIDS patients. However, because PCNSL characteristically occurs late in the course of HIV-1 infection at a time when these patients are more vulnerable both to the toxic effects of cytoreductive drugs and development of other systemic complications, patients cannot easily tolerate such aggressive treatment. In fact, these patients most often die of other HIV-1–related complications rather than lymphoma within a time frame before the recurrence that characterizes lymphoma in non-AIDS patients (28,31). Fortunately, primary CNS lymphomas in AIDS patients respond relatively well to radiation therapy, and some patients can remain "cured" for the remainder of their lives. Since early treatment will decrease morbidity and mortality, diagnosis should usually be pursued rapidly and thoroughly because of its palliative value. On the other hand, these patients are usually in a poor prognostic group vis-à-vis systemic disease, and their overall survival is limited.

Progressive Multifocal Leukoencephalopathy

PML is an opportunistic infection caused by the human papovavirus, JC virus, which induces little or no clinical disease in the normal host but causes demyelinating lesions of the CNS in certain immunosuppressed individuals, including AIDS (37–41). While previously noted as a rare complication of a variety of immunosuppressing conditions, the AIDS epidemic has markedly increased its incidence. It now complicates AIDS in 2–4% of patients. The disease is characterized by selective demyelination with pathological lesions beginning as small foci, most often in the white matter adjacent to the cortex, which then coalesce to form larger lesions, which eventually cavitate centrally as they also spread outward. In some cases a single lesion will spread centrifugally like a neoplasm—even follow white matter pathways—but without mass effect. Lesions of the hemispheres are most common, but the cerebellum and brain stem may also be affected. Microscopic appearance includes pathognomonic inclusion-bearing swollen oligodendrocyte nuclei and bizarre pleomorphic, hyperchromatic astrocytes. The oligodendrocyte inclusions are filled with JC virus nucleocapsids, which can be identified by electron microscopy, and the demyelinating lesions are caused by the death of these cells with secondary degeneration of their myelin-forming processes. Inflammation is inconspicuous in the majority of cases.

PML presents with focal neurological deficit and is the third most common cause of this type of presentation after toxoplasmosis and PCNSL. However, its clinical evolution is more protracted than these other two conditions, and altered consciousness or other "encephalitic" signs are usually not present. The picture is rather one of worsening focal deficits, including hemiparesis, hemianopia, aphasia, hemisensory deficit, ataxia, and the like. The hemispheres are more commonly involved than the posterior fossa structures. Based on this presentation, the diagnosis is often accurately suspected clinically, but neuroimaging is essential to support the diagnosis and rule out confounding diseases (42,43). MRI is again superior to CT and shows the characteristic white matter lesions that often begin adjacent to the cortex. They are usually most evident on T_2-weighted images with increased attenuation, i.e., appearing white, and on T_1-weighted sequences they may show low attenuation (appear black) (Table 2). They characteristically do not enhance with contrast, and there is no mass effect. These focal abnormalities correlate well with clinical deficits, and one should not confuse the white matter changes associated with the AIDS dementia complex with those of PML, since in the former there are no focal deficits. Neither serum nor CSF serologies are useful in diagnosis since positive serum titers against JC virus are found in the majority of the normal population and CSF titers are negative. Definitive diagnosis is made by brain biopsy or at autopsy. Light microscopy is usually adequate to establish the diagnosis, but occasionally either immunocytochemistry or in situ hybridization may be useful to detect JC antigens or nucleic acid. More recently, PCR amplification of nucleic acid in spinal fluid has been introduced and shows considerable promise, but both false-positive and false-negative results have been reported (44,45).

There is no proven effective therapy for the disease. Uncontrolled studies have suggested that zidovudine, gamma interferon, or cytosine arabinoside (administered either intrathecally or intravenously) may be helpful, and the latter is now being studied in a controlled trial (46,47). Surprisingly, spontaneous sustained remission of PML in AIDS can occur; this provides hope for developing new interventional strategies (48). At this time, patients should be placed on optimal antiretroviral treatment in the hope that this might reverse the host's loss of anti-JC virus defenses.

Cryptococcal Meningitis

Cryptococcal meningitis is the most common CNS fungal infection in AIDS, eventually affecting between 5 and 10% of patients (49–54). While most frequently presenting as a subacute meningitis with headache, nausea, vomiting, confusion, and lethargy, like in non-AIDS patients, in some AIDS patients both symptoms and signs are remarkably mild and nonspecific. Likewise, the CSF formula may be bland, with few or no cells and little or no perturbation in glucose or protein concentrations. Accordingly, one should routinely obtain CSF cryptococcal antigen titers, fungal cultures, and India ink preparations in all AIDS patients at lumbar puncture. Serum cryptococcal antigen is also almost always positive (55) and may therefore serve as a "screen" in those patients where the diagnostic suspicion is low, where the patient refuses a spinal tap or where a spinal tap should be avoided, for example, in the presence of thrombocytopenia or other bleeding diathesis. Neuroimaging is frequently negative or only nonspecifically abnormal, but MRI may show meningitis or meningoencephalitis, dilated Virchow-Robin spaces in the region of the basal ganglia, cystlike structures (gelatinous pseudocysts), and granulomas (cryptococcomas) of the choroid plexus, suggesting the diagnosis (50).

Further aspects of cryptococcal meningitis, including therapy, are discussed elsewhere in this volume. At present, optimal treatment is still somewhat uncertain and being studied in ongoing multicenter trials. It has been shown that the overall efficacy of oral fluconazole is similar to that of amphotericin B, although the latter results in more rapid clearing of organisms from the CSF at the price of somewhat higher toxicity (53,56–58). Consequently, one recommendation is that amphotericin be used initially in more severely ill patients (e.g., patients who are obtunded or have a CSF antigen titer of >1:256) and that fluconazole can be used in the remainder or after the severely affected patients improve and stabilize. Fluconazole is administered at a dose of 200–400 mg/day after a loading dose of 800 mg, while that for amphotericin B is 0.4–0.8 mg/kg/day. The role of 5-flucytosine (5-FC) is now being evaluated but is not yet routinely administered. As discussed earlier, patients with cryptococcal meningitis require maintenance therapy to prevent an otherwise high relapse rate. Usually this consists of a lower dose of the agent used for induction; for example, amphotericin may be given at 1 mg/kg one to three times a week or fluconazole at doses of 200–400 mg/day (59).

Attention must also be paid to dealing with secondary complications of meningitis including hydrocephalus. In some patients headache related to obstruction of CSF pathways can be relieved by repeated lumbar punctures, but in others with more persistent symptoms or neurological dysfunction, ventriculo-peritoneal shunt may be required to relieve elevated intracranial pressure and its sequelae.

CMV Encephalitis

The role of CNS CMV infection in the neurological morbidity of AIDS remains incompletely defined, perhaps in large measure because antemortem diagnosis is difficult. While minor brain CMV infection evidenced by inclusion-bearing cells within scattered microglial nodules is detected at autopsy in as many as one third of AIDS patients, the contribution of this level of infection to neurological dysfunction is uncertain (60–62). Clinical-pathological analysis suggests that it is generally minor and most often overshadowed by brain HIV-1 infection and the AIDS dementia complex (60). However, it is also clear that CMV may cause clinically overt encephalitis. According to one retrospective study where the diagnosis of CMV encephalitis was made by pathological examination of the brain, patients most often presented with a subacutely evolving confusional state (63). Approximately 20% had the additional finding of cranial neuropathies and 14% had seizures. Periventricular inflammation was detected by brain MRI in most of these patients. Hyponatremia was also common. Routine CSF studies did not show a distinct profile like that of CMV polyradiculopathy, and pleocytosis was observed in only approximately 20%, and in those cases it was predominantly lymphocytic. While amplification of CMV DNA from the CSF by the PCR was positive in only one third of these patients, other studies have found a higher positive yield (64–67), and this technology promises to improve characterization and diagnosis of CMV brain infection.

In cases where CMV infection of the brain is highly suspected, specific antiviral therapy should be administered, although the effectiveness of treatment for CMV is largely based on anecdotal experience rather than comparative clinical trials. At present it is uncertain whether ganciclovir, foscarnet, or a combination of these two drugs should be recommended, nor are optimal doses defined. The latter may depend upon previous therapy since many of these patients will have experienced CMV retinopathy.

Less Common CNS Opportunistic Diseases

A number of other CNS infections can complicate the late phase of HIV-1 infection. Since they are less common and in some cases less well characterized, they may be overlooked or present greater diagnostic difficulty.

Mycobacterial Infections

Although not strictly an opportunistic pathogen, *Mycobacterium tuberculosis* infection is more common in HIV-1–infected individuals than in the normal population, with this incidence additionally influenced by socioeconomic factors. Clinical tuberculosis is found predominantly in intravenous drug abusers and those from lower socioeconomic groups rather than in patients with homosexuality or transfusion as their major AIDS risk factors (68–70). However, even in AIDS patients with systemic tuberculosis, CNS involvement appears to be uncommon. While some have suggested that these infections may be more aggressive than in non–HIV-1-infected individuals, the spectrum and types of clinical presentations are similar and include meningitis, acute abscess and indolent, chronic tuberculoma (71,72). Diagnosis in some cases may be difficult and require brain biopsy, although PCR detection of nucleic acid in blood, spinal fluid, or brain biopsy specimens may aid both accuracy and speed of diagnosis (73). Although systemic atypical mycobacterial infections commonly complicate AIDS, only very rarely do they cause overt clinical CNS disease. Thus, while these mycobacteria have been detected in CSF or even brain, they have not been shown to infiltrate the brain parenchyma or cause clinical symptoms and signs (74).

Varicella-Zoster Virus and Herpes Simplex Virus Infections

Although uncommon, varicella-zoster virus (VZV) and, to a lesser extent, herpes simplex virus (HSV) 1 and 2 can cause CNS disease in AIDS patients. VZV infections are of several types, including (1) multifocal brain infection affecting principally the white matter and partially resembling PML (75–77), (2) cerebral vasculitis, which may involve medium-sized vessels and typically occurs in the setting of ophthalmic herpes zoster and causes contralateral hemiplegia (78,79) but may involve other arteries distant from or even in the absence of contemporaneous rash and cause single or multifocal infarctions of brain or spinal cord, and (3) myelopathy complicating herpes zoster and involving principally the corresponding segmental level (80). Some cases will involve a combination of these pathologies (81). While both HSV-1 and HSV-2 have been identified in brains of some AIDS patients, their frequency and clinical correlates have not yet been clearly delineated (82,83).

Syphilis

The influence of HIV-1 infection on the course, diagnosis, and treatment of syphilis in HIV-1 infection is presently somewhat controversial (84–91). There is some evidence that syphilis may have a more aggressive course, with neurological complications occurring at an earlier time in the course of the infection. This topic, including issues related to both diagnosis and treatment, is considered at length in Chapter 12.

Other Infections

While rare, cerebral *Aspergillus*, *Nocardia*, *Candida*, and *Listeria* CNS infections have all been reported in AIDS patients (92–104). These usually develop late in the course of infection, and in fact, their relative low frequency in AIDS compared to some other settings of immunosuppression such as organ transplantation or cancer treated with chemotherapy provide evidence that host defenses other than those typically impaired by HIV-1 infection are involved in protecting the brain against these organisms. Because these infections are more common in these other settings, more detailed discussion of diagnosis and treatment is presented elsewhere in this volume. Since susceptibility to several of these organisms is increased by neutropenia, one might anticipate an increased incidence in the setting of therapies that depress the bone marrow (for example, as a result of ganciclovir treatment of CMV). Diagnosis is difficult and depends upon early suspicion followed usually by direct identification of the organism by brain biopsy, in CSF, or outside the brain (in blood or lung, for example) since several of these occur as complications of well-established infections elsewhere. *Strongyloides stercoralis* hyperinfection has also been reported as a complication of HIV-1 infection (105).

Opportunistic PNS Diseases

Peripheral neuropathies of several types can complicate the various stages of HIV-1 infection (for reviews, see Refs. 106–109). Those in the late phase of HIV-1 infection are divided in this chapter into the opportunistic infections, discussed here, and the neuromuscular conditions that relate in some more fundamental way to HIV-1, itself, discussed below. One of the important neuropathies that is common in the transitional phase of infection as the phase of clinical latency gives way to more severe immunosuppression is herpes zoster. Surprisingly, while certainly more common in HIV-1 infection than in an age-matched population, this reactivated varicella-zoster virus (VZV) infection is most often self-limited, although, as discussed earlier, CNS complications can develop uncommonly.

CMV causes a more severe infection of nerve roots. This is a fairly stereotyped syndrome of severe ascending polyradiculopathy that usually begins with painful lumbosacral root involvement and progresses rostrally to involve sensory, motor, and autonomic components (110–112). Diagnosis is aided by the finding of a polymorphonuclear pleocytosis in the CSF, which is otherwise rare in late HIV-1 infection. Thickened spinal roots revealed by myelography or MRI scanning also have been reported. Although CMV can be cultured from the spinal fluid of these patients, viral replication and the appearance of cytopathology in culture are too slow to rely on as guides for therapy; PCR accelerates identification of this herpes virus, but processing laboratory specimens for this assay may also take unduly long. Therefore, clinical diagnosis should lead to rapid institution of specific antiviral therapy with ganciclovir, foscarnet, or a combination of these therapies.

CMV also causes a second neuropathic syndrome, a severe mononeuritis multiplex (106,113–116). This is one of two mononeuritis multiplex syndromes complicating HIV-1 infection, the second of which is discussed later in this chapter. This form occurs later in the course of systemic HIV-1 infection when CD4+ counts are lower and can be quite aggressive, leading to progressive paralysis and death in some patients. Definite diagnosis of this infection is difficult and requires nerve biopsy that is fortunate enough to sample a zone of infection. For this reason, clinical diagnosis of this neuropathy should be followed by aggressive anti-CMV therapy unless another etiology is proven.

NEUROLOGICAL DISEASES RELATED TO HIV-1 INFECTION

While progressive immunosuppression renders the host susceptible to a number of opportunistic infections of the nervous system, HIV-1 itself also appears to induce neurological disease without involvement of other microorganisms. Before considering these, it is pertinent to briefly consider certain aspects of the AIDS retrovirus, the biology of its systemic infection, and its interaction with the host immune system.

HIV-1 and Its Interaction with the Host

HIV-1 is a retrovirus with a complex genome containing not only virion structural and enzyme-coding genes, but a set of regulatory genes that assist in maintaining its protracted course of persistent infection and infectivity. Systemic infection is often segregated into three evolutionary phases. The initial phase is that of primary infection in which there is a high-titered systemic viremia that is then curtailed by virus-specific host immune defenses. While the most important components of this host response are still uncertain, T-cell–mediated defenses, perhaps particularly involving cytotoxic CD8+ lymphocytes, seem to be critical. While this viremia is suppressed, HIV-1 is unfortunately not eliminated. The second phase is often referred to as that of "clinical latency" or "asymptomatic seropositivity" in which patients are characteristically clinically well and immune defenses against opportunistic infections remain protective. However, the infection is not truly latent during this time; in fact, studies over the last few years document very active ongoing viral replication, most notably in lymph nodes. This chronic infection also gradually alters immune function, causing immune dysregulation and eventual immunodeficiency. In the third phase of infection, the loss of immune defenses reaches a threshold that predisposes to a number of clinical diseases, particularly opportunistic infections. As discussed earlier, the more severe the immunosuppression (and, as a marker of this, the lower the CD4+ T-lymphocyte count), the more likely are superimposed infections.

This loss of defenses against opportunistic infections also applies to defenses important in suppressing HIV-1 infection itself, and in this late stage of infection, HIV-1 replication accelerates and results in the return of high-level viremia. An additional facet of the interaction of HIV-1 with the immune system is the change in the profile of cytokines that are induced over the course of infection (117). Late in disease, cytokines that enhance rather than suppress infection become dominant and are reflected either directly (levels of the cytokines themselves) or indirectly (levels of certain markers that are stimulated as a result of or along with these cytokines) in blood or other body fluids. Chronic production of some of these cytokines may also have immunopathological sequelae, including effects on the nervous system.

For practical purposes, certain laboratory studies can provide insight into these "background" processes. Thus, as noted earlier, the blood CD4+ lymphocyte count can be viewed as an index of the cumulative effect of this chronic infection. It provides a view of the history of the effect of HIV-1 on its principal target, although it is now recognized that this is a dynamic process that reflects an equilibrium of constant loss and replacement of this cell population (118,119). Certain soluble immune markers in the blood also likely reflect this same history and dynamics since they serve as indicators of cytokine profiles. Among these, serum β_2-microglobulin (β_2M) and neopterin are used most commonly as prognostic markers. More recently, quantitative assessment of viral RNA in plasma has emerged as a useful index of active infection (120). RNA levels reflect the magnitude of viral replication at the time of sampling and fall with effective antiviral therapy only to rise again as the virus becomes resistant.

Treatment of HIV-1 infection has been the target of intensive investigation, including drug development and clinical trials. A number of antiviral drugs representing several mechanisms of action are now approved for clinical use and additional agents are undergoing trial and accelerated use. A review of these therapies is outside of the scope of this chapter. A few points warrant brief mention, however. The most effective therapies are targeted against virus-coded enzymes. The first group of drugs to see clinical use were nucleoside analogs directed against the viral RNA-dependent DNA polymerase, or reverse transcriptase (RT). Zidovudine (earlier referred to as azidothymidine or AZT) was the first of these to be approved, but several others have now achieved widespread use. More recently, inhibitors of the viral protease have been approved; these have marked antiviral potency and can dramatically lower viral RNA in plasma. However, as a general principal, none of the drugs eliminate latent virus, and hence none represents a cure of infection. Even more critical, all have been shown to allow emergence of resistant mutants and thus appear to lose their virus-suppressing efficacy over time. For this reason, various combination therapies of two or three drugs are now being advocated and used in clinical practice.

Early CNS HIV-1 Infection and Neurological Disease

Infection of the CNS appears to be an intrinsic part of the ecology of HIV-1 infection. Studies of CSF in clinically well patients have shown (1) abnormalities of routine studies, including cell count, total protein, and immunoglobulin, (2) local, intrablood-brain barrier synthesis of anti-HIV-1 antibody, and (3) culture isolation of virus or detection of viral nucleic acid after PCR amplification (121–128). These abnormalities have been noted in fully functional, asymptomatic patients who have remained well during follow-up care for a year or more. They imply that entry of HIV-1 into the nervous system is commonplace and likely begins during initial viremia (129) and continues through the asymptomatic and symptomatic phases, although perhaps with different intensities. They also indicate that HIV-1 can be relatively nonpathogenic for the CNS, since this biological process of CNS exposure and infected-cell traffic is asymptomatic (130–132). On a practical basis, such incidental abnormal levels in cell count, protein, immunoglobulin, oligoclonal bands, and HIV-1 detection must be taken into account when interpreting CSF results obtained for other diagnostic purposes or in following therapy.

In contrast to this early HIV-1 exposure, serious neurological disease uncommonly complicates the acute phase of systemic infection. However, a number of different diseases affecting both the CNS and PNS have been reported during this phase (127,133–143). These may occur from several days to weeks after the seroconversion-related illness that resembles mononucleosis or may occur in the absence of systemic symptoms. These early neurological complications usually evolve subacutely and manifest as focal or diffuse encephalitis or leukoencephalopathy, meningitis, ataxia, or myelopathy, either alone or together with PNS abnormalities, which include cranial neuropathy, brachial plexopathy, or neuropathy. They are characteristically monophasic, and most patients appear to recover within a number of weeks and resemble postinfectious immune-mediated disorders that complicate other infections. The cerebrospinal fluid (CSF) usually shows a mild lymphocytic pleocytosis with a modest increase in protein concentration. Results of neuroimaging using computed tomography (CT) have been normal, but experience with magnetic resonance imaging (MRI) has been less extensive. Although these early syndromes apparently are uncommon, it is possible that their incidence is underappreciated.

Neurological Complications During the Phase of "Clinically Latent" Systemic HIV-1 Infection

While defenses against opportunistic infections remain effective during this intermediate phase, the immune system is not normal and may show laboratory and clinical evidence of dysregulation. This likely underlies the development of what appear to be autoimmune neurological diseases during this phase. These processes affect the PNS more often than the CNS.

Demyelinating and Other Peripheral Neuropathies

Most common among the neurological complications manifesting during this phase of HIV-1 infection are demyelinating neuropathies. These resemble the subacute Guillain-Barré syndrome or chronic inflammatory demyelinating polyneuropathy (CIDP) seen in other contexts, with the exception that the CSF often exhibits a mild pleocytosis (107,144). These likely have an autoimmune pathogenesis and in that regard parallel the demyelinating neuropathies in other settings. Patients with these neuropathies appear to respond favorably to corticosteroids, plasmapheresis, and intravenous immunoglobulin (IVIG), with the latter two treatments currently preferred. The prognosis of demyelinating neuropathies in this setting may not be as good as that in the non–HIV-1-infected patient (106,145).

A second type of peripheral neuropathy may occur during this time, but is less-well characterized. This is a type of mononeuritis multiplex that appears to have a benign course (in contrast to a more malignant mononeuritis multiplex that complicates later infection, as discussed earlier). It may be due to vascular occlusions caused by immune complexes (146).

CNS Demyelinating Disease

An autoimmune demyelinating disorder also appears to affect the CNS, but is much less common than its PNS counterpart. This multiple sclerosis–like illness has been reported in HIV-1–infected patients in the latent phase of infection in the setting of preserved CD4 + T-lymphocyte counts (147,148). The presentation may include remissions and exacerbations, along with corticosteroid responsiveness. Although these cases may represent the concurrence of two diseases, more likely, as with the demyelinating neuropathies, they relate to an autoimmune process triggered by HIV-1 infection.

Complications of Late HIV-1 Infection

Just as with opportunistic infections, in the late stages of HIV-1 infection, several disorders that appear to relate to HIV-1 itself can complicate infection. These include (1) aseptic meningitis and headache, (2) a more interesting, common, and severe syndrome, the AIDS dementia complex, and (3) an important peripheral neuropathy.

Meningitis and Headache

Among the complications of the transition from the stage of clinical latency to late HIV-1 infection is a syndrome of aseptic meningitis that presumably relates to direct HIV-1 infection of the meninges (149,150). Clinically the aseptic meningitis may segregate into two types: an acute and a chronic form. Both usually present in the transitional phase (CD4+ T lymphocyte count $<200–500/mm^3$) or, somewhat less frequently, in the phase of overt AIDS (CD4+ cell count $<200/mm^3$). Both are accompanied by meningeal symptoms (e.g., headache and photophobia), although meningeal signs (e.g., nuchal rigidity) are more characteristic of the acute form. Cranial nerve palsies can complicate the course, affecting cranial nerves V, VII, and VIII, with Bell's palsy sometimes recurring. The CSF shows a mild mononuclear pleocytosis, usually with a normal or mildly depressed glucose concentration and a slightly elevated protein concentration. The presumption that this condition is due to direct HIV-1 infection is based on isolation of the virus from CSF of some patients and the absence of an alternative cause. While the syndrome itself is benign, it may indicate a poor prognosis in relation to impending progression to AIDS in some patients. The effects of antiretroviral therapies on this disorder have not been tested.

Headache may also occur in AIDS patients without accompanying meningeal reaction. In some patients, this occurs as a complication of systemic illness and resolves when that illness is treated. In others, however, a precipitating infection is not identified, and the term *HIV headache* has been used to describe this condition, which may be severe and protracted (151). Although some of these patients seem to be helped by tricyclic antidepressants, others are not and may even require narcotic analgesics.

AIDS Dementia Complex

The most important of the disorders thought to relate directly to HIV-1 infection, and especially to HIV-1 *brain* infection, is the AIDS dementia complex. This is a clinical syndrome characterized by a triad of cognitive, motor, and behavioral dysfunction (4,60,131,152–155). It is perhaps the most common CNS complication of HIV-1 infection and, if its mild form is included, may eventually afflict the majority of AIDS patients. It is generally a late complication of HIV-1 infection and characteristically appears during the same phase as the major opportunistic infections and neoplasms that define systemic AIDS, although patients can present with this syndrome before these major systemic complications occur (156). Results of prospective studies indicate that this syndrome is uncommon in patients who are systemically well (4,8,157–160). Early in the epidemic, some observers suggested that the majority of late-phase patients exhibited frank mild to severe AIDS dementia complex, while an additional number suffered subclinically. This no longer appears to be the case; it is not entirely clear whether this reflects inaccuracy of early reports because they reflected a biased hospital-based experience or represents a real change related to widespread use of zidovudine, other antiretrovirals, and supportive therapies. However, at least one study supports the second explanation (161,162).

Terminology and Classification. The term *AIDS dementia complex* was introduced to describe a cohesive constellation of symptoms and signs noted to be common in adult AIDS patients (130,152–155,163). *AIDS* was included in this terminology because the morbidity and prognosis of the condition are comparable to those of other clinical AIDS-defining complications of HIV-1 infection, *dementia* because of the acquired and persistent cognitive decline, marked by prominent mental slowing and inattention, and *complex* was added because the syndrome also, importantly, includes impaired motor performance and, at times, characteristic behavioral changes. An associated myelopathy and organic psychosis are encompassed within this term, but not neuropathy or functional psychiatric disturbance.

This terminology is made more useful when combined with a staging system based on functional and motor status for adult patients (Table 3) (154,164). This staging provides a common descriptive vocabulary for both clinical and investigative purposes. Although the World

Table 3 AIDS Dementia Complex Staging

ADC Stage	Characteristics
Stage 0 (Normal)	Normal mental and motor function.
Stage 0.5 (Equivocal/ subclinical)	Either minimal or equivocal *symptoms* of cognitive or motor dysfunction characteristic of ADC, or mild signs (snout response, slowed extremity movements), but *without impairment of work or capacity to perform activities of daily living* (ADL). Gait and strength are normal.
Stage 1 (Mild)	Unequivocal evidence (symptoms, signs, neuropsychological test performance) of functional intellectual or motor impairment characteristic of ADC, but able to perform *all but the more demanding aspects of work or ADL.* Can walk without assistance.
Stage 2 (Moderate)	Cannot work or maintain the more demanding aspects of daily life, but able to perform *basic activities of self-care.* Ambulatory, but may require a single prop.
Stage 3 (Severe)	*Major intellectual incapacity* (cannot follow news or personal events, cannot sustain complex conversation, considerable slowing of all output), *or motor disability* (cannot walk unassisted, requiring walker or personal support, usually with slowing and clumsiness of arms as well).
Stage 4 (End stage)	*Nearly vegetative.* Intellectual and social comprehension and responses are at a rudimentary level. Nearly or absolutely mute. Paraparetic or paraplegic with double incontinence.

Source: Refs. 154, 164.

Health Organization (WHO) and the American Academy of Neurology (AAN) have introduced an alternative terminology with certain useful features, including segregation of predominating myelopathy and predominating dementia and requiring greater severity when using the term dementia (165,166), I have continued to use the AIDS dementia staging scheme in my own studies and clinical practice because of its simplicity and parsimony. Moreover, the AIDS dementia complex staging and the WHO/AAN classification can be "cross-translated" (167).

Clinical Presentation. The AIDS dementia complex is classified as a subcortical dementia and shares some features with other conditions similarly classified. Patients' earliest symptoms usually consist of difficulties with concentration and memory. They begin to lose track of their train of thought and to complain of "slowness" in thinking. Complex tasks take longer to complete, and difficulty with concentration leads to missed appointments and the need to keep lists of simple daily chores.

In those only mildly affected, the insensitive bedside mental status examination may be within normal limits, although responses are often slow. As the condition progresses, however, patients begin to perform poorly on tasks requiring concentration and attention, such as word and digit reversals and subtracting serial 7s. With further worsening, a larger array of mental status tests becomes abnormal, although the core difficulty of mental slowing and poor attention/concentration remains most prominent. Afflicted individuals also may appear apathetic, with poor insight and indifference to their illness.

Symptoms of motor dysfunction are usually less prominent than those of cognitive difficulty, but when present, complaints most often include poor balance or incoordination. Gait disturbance can result in more frequent tripping or falling or a perceived need to exercise new care in walking. However, even when such symptoms are lacking, motor abnormalities can almost always be detected on examination early in the course of the disease. These include slowing of rapid successive and alternating movements of the extremities (for example, attempts to rapidly oppose the index finger and thumb or tap the foot) and impaired ocular smooth pursuits and saccadic eye movements. Abnormal reflexes also may be present, with a generalized increase in deep tendon reflexes (including the jaw jerk) and emergence of release signs, such as snout, glabellar, and, less commonly, grasp responses. As the disease evolves, spastic ataxia and, subsequently, leg weakness may limit walking. At the end stage of the AIDS dementia complex, patients are nearly vegetative, lying in bed with a vacant stare, seemingly unaware of their surroundings but awake.

Psychological depression is surprisingly infrequent. Patients appear uninterested and lack initiative but are without dysphoria. In a minority, a more agitated organic psychosis may be the presenting or predominant aspect of the illness (168). Such patients are irritable and hyperactive and may be overtly manic; however, there is always an element of confusion, and when their hyperactive state comes under control, the underlying cognitive impairment is evident.

Neuropsychological Test Profile. Formal neuropsychological studies may sometimes be helpful in clinically difficult cases in confirming either the presence of abnormalities or the characteristic profile of cognitive and motor impairment. They are also useful in longitudinally following the course of disease or response to therapy, particularly in the investigative setting. In general, the neuropsychological tests most useful in evaluating the AIDS dementia complex assess the following functions: performance under time pressure, motor speed, and alternation between two performance rules or stimulus sets (157,159,164,169,170).

Neuroimaging. Neuroimaging is an essential component in the evaluation of AIDS patients with CNS dysfunction, including those with the AIDS dementia complex. In this setting, imaging is most often used to exclude other neurological conditions that can present with overlapping symptoms and signs (such as PCNSL or CMV encephalitis), but can also be helpful in demonstrating characteristic, although diagnostically nonspecific, abnormalities. The latter include the nearly universal finding of cerebral atrophy with widened cortical sulci and enlarged ventricles detected by both CT scanning and MRI (153,171–175). Basal ganglia are also reduced in volume (176). Additionally, MRI of some patients detects patchy or diffuse T_2-weighted abnormalities in the hemispheric white matter and, less commonly, the basal ganglia or thalamus (20,172,177–179).

Cerebrospinal Fluid. CSF in patients with AIDS dementia complex often reveals abnormalities in both routine and more specialized analyses. However, routine studies are confounded by the CSF abnormalities described earlier in patients with asymptomatic HIV-1 infection, including HIV-1 isolation or detection of amplified nucleic acid. The likelihood of detecting HIV-1 p24 core antigen in the CSF increases with AIDS dementia complex severity, although free antigen is still a relatively infrequent finding and thus of lower sensitivity diagnostically (180,181). Whether quantitative studies of the CSF "viral burden" using PCR amplification will prove useful in diagnosis and longitudinal evaluation of patients awaits assessment of this newer technology on this body fluid. Measurement in the CSF of the surrogate markers reflecting immune activation discussed earlier, including CSF β_2-microglobulin and neopterin, can sometimes be useful since their concentrations correlate to some degree with the presence and severity of the AIDS dementia complex (182–185). Although nonspecific in that they are elevated in other CNS opportunistic infections and primary CNS lymphoma, these markers may be useful in efforts to distinguish mild AIDS dementia complex from psychiatric disease as well as in following response to therapy.

Neuropathology. A number of histological abnormalities can be found in AIDS dementia complex patients, although with inexact clinical correlation. In general, they most prominently affect subcortical structures and include (1) gliosis and diffuse white matter pallor, (2) multinucleated-cell encephalitis, and (3) vacuolar myelopathy. Less common are diffuse or focal spongiform changes in the cerebral white matter (60,61,186–188). The most common of these abnormalities is the central astrocytosis and accompanying diffuse white matter pallor that, in isolation, correlate with milder AIDS dementia complex. Inflammation is characteristically scant, consisting of a few perivascular lymphocytes and brown-pigmented macrophages accompanying the astrocytosis. This is accompanied by disruption of the blood-brain barrier (179).

Multinucleated cells are most characteristic but not invariant in patients with more severe clinical disease (60,189). The multinucleated cells are infected by HIV-1 and derive from macrophages and microglia and are accompanied by neighboring macrophage and microglial reaction, along with local edema and white matter rarefaction. They are concentrated most often in the white matter and deep gray structures. It is in these severe cases that neuronal change have been detected, including both selected loss of cortical neurons and alterations in their dendritic structures (190,191).

Although inflammation with multinucleated cells also may occur in the spinal cord, vacuolar myelopathy is more commonly associated with clinical evidence of spinal cord dysfunction (192). This pathologically resembles subacute combined degeneration resulting from vitamin B_{12} deficiency, but levels of this vitamin generally are normal in serum. Although there is a general correlation between the incidence of vacuolar myelopathy and the other pathological abnormalities found in the brain, the myelopathy can occur in the absence of the multinucleated cells and indeed does not appear to correlate with local productive HIV-1 infection (193–196). Its pathogenesis therefore remains elusive.

Etiology and Pathogenesis. Evidence from a variety of observations supports a central role for HIV-1 in the AIDS dementia complex, particularly in the subset of patients with more severe brain dysfunction (130–132,163,189). Numerous studies have now documented HIV-1 brain infection, and most indicate that macrophages and related microglia, along with multinucleated cells derived from these two cell types, are the principal participants in *productive* infection (197–204). Recent observations using combined PCR amplification in concert with in situ localization and other techniques to detect expression of nonstructural viral gene products suggest that other cell types in the brain, including the native astrocytes and neurons, as well as vascular endothelial cells, may be infected, although perhaps without the capacity to produce progeny virus (205–207). This is consistent with cell culture studies that have demonstrated low-level infection of astrocytic and other neuroectodermal cells and cell lines, involving a non-CD4 virus-cell interaction.

While this etiological association between AIDS dementia complex and HIV-1 brain infection has been made, this association is not an invariant finding, and there is still some controversy regarding the correlation of this viral load with the stage of the AIDS dementia complex (189,208,209). Characteristically, it is in the more severely affected patients (stages 2 and greater) that multinucleated-cell encephalitis or productive HIV-1 infection is commonly found, but there are some cases of severe clinical disease without a high viral burden and other examples of seemingly abundant infection without severe antemortem clinical dysfunction. An additional important aspect of brain infection is the observation that the viral "strains" cultured or directly cloned from brains of these patients exhibit a macrophage-tropic phenotype and may even have genetic characteristics that favor replication in brain macrophages and microglia (210–213).

Because of the seeming discrepancy between the severity of clinical deficits, on the one hand, and these pathological and virological features, on the other, indirect pathogenetic processes relating infection and brain injury have been proposed (for reviews, see Refs. 130–132, 214–216). To deal with the question of how the neuroectodermally derived elements of the brain, including neurons and oligodendrocytes, might be injured when they remain largely uninfected, a number of investigators have hypothesized that macrophage and microglial infection drives immunopathological processes that eventuate in neurotoxicity. Multicell models have been presented outlining a neurotoxic pathway in which infected cells either elaborate neurotoxic molecules or provide signals that secondarily activate more complex cell circuits that eventuate in neurotoxicity. Viral gene products, most notably the external glycoprotein gp120, have been shown to exert neurotoxic effects in cell culture and in animal models; the products of the *tat* and *nef* regulatory genes may also be toxic. Immunological reactions to the virus, especially ineffective ones, may also activate this pathway. At least part of this virus- and immune-mediated toxicity is effected by chronic activation of cytokine pathways. This likely involves circuits that both transduce and amplify neurotoxicity. In the broad sense, these toxic cytokine pathways can be considered to be immunopathological reactions that link infection to neurotoxicity and involve mechanisms that may also be important in other neurodegenerative diseases, including activation of *N*-methyl-D-aspartate receptors and production of nitric oxide. These theories and the accumulating observations that support and provide mechanistic details have been reviewed recently (131,215,217,218).

Treatment. The pathogenetic scheme outlining two linked processes, metastatic viral infection and host defenses in the brain on the one hand and a neuropathogenic pathway on the other, is useful in considering therapeutic strategies. Targeting the first process involves antiviral measures as the principal avenues of secondary prevention and treatment. Additionally, it may be necessary that these therapies have ready access to the brain. With respect to the second process, the "downstream" toxic pathways may provide additional targets for "adjuvant" therapeutic strategies. Thus far only the first of these has been shown to be worthwhile, although treatments aimed at inhibiting neurotoxic processes are now being tested.

A number of studies have now suggested that zidovudine has both therapeutic and prophylactic value in AIDS dementia complex and HIV-1 brain infection. These have included controlled clinical trials as well as anecdotal case reports and population "experiences" using a variety of measurements (161,219–223). Despite these observations, a number of practical clinical issues remain unresolved. These include the optimal dosage of zidovudine in this setting. In the only prospective, controlled trial of symptomatic AIDS dementia complex in adults, two high doses (1000 and 2000 mg/day) were found to be superior to placebo (219), but the study did not assess conventional, less toxic doses (300–600 mg/day). Importantly, the efficacy of other antiviral drugs in preventing or reversing AIDS dementia complex has not yet been assessed. This includes nucleosides other than zidovudine, nonnucleoside reverse transcriptase inhibitors, protease inhibitors, and the other antiviral therapies now in use or under investigation for systemic infection. This leaves the clinician without clear guidance in patients intolerant of or resistant to zidovudine. In the absence of proper studies, we currently recommend that zidovudine be given at the highest dose possible if there is not already prolonged exposure and either documented or likely antiviral resistance. This drug should also probably be given in combination with one or more other antiviral drugs just as for systemic infection. If the patient is resistant or cannot take zidovudine, other combination antiretroviral therapy should be given and "adjuvant" drugs that might inhibit the neurotoxic processes considered.

Secondary or adjuvant strategies to attenuate the toxic pathways leading to brain dysfunction can be divided into three therapeutic subcategories related to their sites of action: *immunosuppressive*, acting on immunopathology, *neuroprotective*, acting on the primary target cell, and *compensatory*, acting on the neural networks (163). These strategies, some involving drugs shown to have the desired effects in cell culture, are now beginning to be assessed in clinical trials. For example, the calcium channel blocker nimodipine and the *N*-methyl-D-aspartate receptor inhibitor memantine, both of which appear to block the neurotoxicity of HIV-1 gp120 in cell culture, are now the focus of early-phase clinical trials (215,224,225).

Peripheral Neuropathies and Myopathies Complicating Late HIV-1 Infection

Some of the peripheral neuropathies complicating late HIV-1 infection were discussed above in the context of opportunistic infections. This section includes a second group of neuromuscular disorders in which the etiology is uncertain but is suspected to relate in a more fundamental way to HIV-1 infection.

Distal Sensory (Axonal) Polyneuropathies. The most common and important neuropathy complicating AIDS is a distal, predominantly sensory and axonal neuropathy (8,109,144, 214,226). Characteristically, in this disorder sensory symptoms exceed either sensory or motor loss. While its prevalence is uncertain, in mild form it is clearly a very common complication of late HIV-1 infection. Afflicted patients complain of numb or painful, burning feet. When severe, this discomfort may be intolerable, and patients may be unable to walk, not because of sensory ataxia or weakness but rather due to the discomfort of their feet contacting the ground. The pathogenesis of this neuropathy is uncertain. The suspicion that it may relate to direct HIV-1 infection of either nerve or dorsal root ganglion has not been substantiated, and anecdotal experience suggests that it does not generally respond to zidovudine or other antiretroviral therapy. Most recent speculation centers on an indirect pathogenesis related to cytokine dysregulation and consequent axonal toxicity (109,214). Treatment now relies on symptom management with tricyclics and various analgesics, including narcotics in severe cases.

A second type of axonal, predominantly sensory neuropathy has more recently emerged as an important issue in AIDS differential diagnosis. This is the toxic neuropathy caused by several of the nucleoside antiretroviral drugs, including particularly dideoxyinosine (ddI) and dideoxycytidine (ddC). Both of these drugs can cause axonal neuropathy in a dose-related fashion (227). Their clinical features are similar to the AIDS distal sensory polyneuropathy discussed above and usually begins with foot pain that is described as "aching," "burning," or "bruiselike." Although symptoms in many patients worsen for a few weeks after discontinuation of the offending drug, a phenomenon known as "coasting," these neuropathies are reversible if recognized early. Since they may be difficult to distinguish from the spontaneous neuropathy and electrodiagnostic studies may be of little help in this differentiation, cessation or switch to alternative therapy may be necessary to confirm this diagnosis.

Autonomic neuropathy of varying severity has also been reported in AIDS patients (106, 228,229) and may be related to this sensory neuropathy, although in some cases the severity of autonomic and sensory dysfunction diverges. The clinical features of the former range from mild positional hypotension to cardiovascular collapse during invasive procedures. In addition, autonomic neuropathy may contribute to chronic diarrhea in some HIV-1–infected individuals (230).

Myopathies. Myopathies are less common and less well-characterized than the neuropathies and can occur at several stages of HIV-1 infection; however, they are most common late in infection (231–240). A wide range of presentations, from asymptomatic creatine kinase elevation to progressive severe proximal weakness, has been recognized. A polymyositislike or dermatomyositislike illness has been described in AIDS patients, but as with the other myopathies, the pathogenesis is not clear although suspected in some to be autoimmune. Viral antigens have been found in the inflammatory cells but not in myocytes (236), and there is at least one report of multinucleated giant cells in the inflammatory infiltrate (235).

Zidovudine therapy can also cause a toxic myopathy (232,241–248). The clinical and laboratory features of this disorder have not been delineated fully, but proximal muscles are affected causing weakness that fortunately is usually not profound. It is thought that this myopathy results from a cumulative toxic effect of the nucleoside on muscle mitochondria through interaction with mitochondrial DNA polymerase, and in many of these patients abnormalities of mitochondria are detected in muscle biopsy specimens. Clinical and laboratory improvement can occur after stopping zidovudine therapy.

CONCLUSION

As with other nervous system infections, precise diagnosis of the neurological complications of HIV-1 infection is important, particularly since an increasing number of these disorders can be treated with gratifying relief of morbidity or prevention of early death. These patients should be approached just like those with other neurological diseases and infections in which accurate diagnosis is paramount in implementing proper treatment, whether for cure or palliation.

REFERENCES

1. Haynes BF, Pantaleo G, Fauci AS. Toward an understanding of the correlates of protective immunity to HIV infection. Science 1996; 271:324–327.
2. Sigurdsson B, Palsson P, Grimson H. Visna, a demyelinating transmissible disease of sheep. J Neuropathol Exp Neurol 1957; 16:389–403.
3. Revision of the CDC surveillance case definition for acquired immunodeficiency syndrome. MMWR 1987; 36:3S–14S.
4. Neaton J, Wentworth D, Rhame F, Hogan C, Abrams D, Deyton L. Methods of studying interventions. Considerations in choice of a clinical endpoint for AIDS clinical trials. Stat Med 1994; 13:2107–2125.
5. Navia B, Petito C, Gold J, et al. Cerebral toxoplasmosis complicating the acquired immune deficiency syndrome: clinical and neuropathological findings in 27 patients. Ann Neurol 1986; 19:224.
6. Haverkos H. Assessment of therapy for Toxoplasma encephalitis. Am J Med 1987; 82:907.
7. Grant I, Gold J, Rosemblum M, et al. Toxoplasma gondii serology in HIV-infected patients: the development of central nervous system toxoplasmosis in AIDS. AIDS 1990; 4:519.

8. Bacellar H, Munoz A, Miller EN, et al. Temporal trends in the incidence of HIV-1-related neurologic diseases: Multicenter AIDS Cohort Study, 1985–1992. Neurology 1994; 44:1892–1900.
9. Climent C, De Vinatea ML, Lasala G, et al. Geographical pathology profile of AIDS in Puerto Rico: the first decade. Mod Pathol 1994; 7:647–651.
10. Kennedy PG, Kennedy D, Love C, Dow MG, Bone I. Neurological features of HIV-related disease in Glasgow. Scott Med J 1989; 34:433–437.
11. Luft BJ, Hafner R, Korzun AH, et al. Toxoplasmic encephalitis in patients with the acquired immunodeficiency syndrome. Members of the ACTG 077p/ANRS 009 Study Team. N Engl J Med 1993; 329:995–1000.
12. New LC, Holliman RE. Toxoplasmosis and human immunodeficiency virus (HIV) disease (review). J Antimicrob Chemother 1994; 33:1079–1082.
13. Wang F, So Y, Vittinghoff E, et al. Incidence proportion of and risk factors for AIDS patients diagnosed with HIV dementia, central nervous system toxoplasmosis, and cryptococcal meningitis. AIDS 1995; 8:75–82.
14. Gray F, Geny C, Lionnet F, et al. Neuropathologic study of 135 adult cases of acquired immunodeficiency syndrome (AIDS). (In French) Ann Pathol 1991; 11:236–247.
15. Gallant JE, Moore RD, Chaisson RE. Prophylaxis for opportunistic infections in patients with HIV infection (review). Ann Intern Med 1994; 120:932–944.
16. Mallolas J, Zamora L, Gatell JM, et al. Primary prophylaxis for Pneumocystis carinii pneumonia: a randomized trial comparing cotrimoxazole, aerosolized pentamidine and dapsone plus pyrimethamine. AIDS 1993; 7:59–64.
17. Falangola MF, Reichler BS, Petito CK. Histopathology of cerebral toxoplasmosis in human immunodeficiency virus infection: a comparison between patients with early-onset and late-onset acquired immunodeficiency syndrome. Human Pathol 1994; 25:1091–1097.
18. Gray F, Gherardi R, Wingate E, et al. Diffuse "encephalitic" cerebral toxoplasmosis in AIDS: Report of four cases. J Neurol 1989; 236:273.
19. Simpson DM, Tagliati M. Neurologic manifestations of HIV infection (review). (Published erratum appears in Ann Intern Med 1995 Feb 15; 122(4):317). Ann Intern Med 1994; 121:769–785.
20. Jarvik J, Hesselink J, Kennedy C, et al. Acquired immunodeficiency syndrome: magnetic resonance patterns of brain involvement with pathologic correlation. Neurology 1988; 45:731.
21. Ruiz A, Ganz WI, Post MJ, et al. Use of thallium-201 brain SPECT to differentiate cerebral lymphoma from toxoplasma encephalitis in AIDS patients. Ajnr: Am J Neuroradiol 1994; 15:1885–1894.
22. Johnson JD, Butcher PD, Savva D, Holliman RE. Application of the polymerase chain reaction to the diagnosis of human toxoplasmosis. J Infect 1993; 26:147–158.
23. Dupouy-Camet J, de Souza SL, Maslo C, et al. Detection of Toxoplasma gondii in venous blood from AIDS patients by polymerase chain reaction. J Clin Microbiol 1993; 31:1866–1869.
24. Ostergaard L, Nielsen AK, Black FT. DNA amplification on cerebrospinal fluid for diagnosis of cerebral toxoplasmosis among HIV-positive patients with signs or symptoms of neurological disease. Scand J Infect Dis 1993; 25:227–237.
25. Schoondermark-van de Ven E, Galama J, Kraaijeveld C, van Druten J, Meuwissen J, Melchers W. Value of the polymerase chain reaction for the detection of Toxoplasma gondii in cerebrospinal fluid from patients with AIDS. Clin Infect Dis 1993; 16:661–666.
26. Cohm J, McMeeking A, Cohen W, et al. Evaluation of the policy of empiric treatment of suspected Toxoplasma encephalitis in patients with the acquired immunodeficiency syndrome. Am J Med 1989; 86:521.
27. Wong SY, Israelski DM, Remington JS. AIDS-associated toxoplasmosis. In: Sande MA, Volberding PA, eds. The Medical Management of AIDS. Philadelphia: W. B. Saunders Company, 1995: 460–493.
28. So Y, Beckstead J, Davis R. Primary central nervous system lymphoma in acquired immune deficiency syndrome: a clinical and pathological study. Ann Neurol 1986; 20:566.
29. Levine AM. Non-Hodgkin's lymphomas and other malignancies in the acquired immune deficiency syndrome (review). Semin Oncol 1987; 14:34–39.

30. Meeker TC, Shiramizu B, Kaplan L, et al. Evidence for molecular subtypes of HIV-associated lymphoma: division into peripheral monoclonal, polyclonal and central nervous system lymphoma. Aids 1991; 5:669–674.
31. Baumgartner JE, Rachlin JR, Beckstead JH, et al. Primary central nervous system lymphomas: natural history and response to radiation therapy in 55 patients with acquired immunodeficiency syndrome. J Neurosurg 1990; 73:206–211.
32. Formenti SC, Gill PS, Lean E, et al. Primary central nervous system lymphoma in AIDS. Results of radiation therapy. Cancer 1989; 63:1101–1107.
33. Remick S, Diamond C, Migliozzi J, et al. Primary central nervous system lymphoma in patients with and without the acquired immune deficiency syndrome: a retrospective analysis and review of the literature. Medicine 1990; 69:345.
34. DeAngelis L. Primary CNS lymphoma: a new clinical challenge. Neurology 1991; 41:619.
35. DeAngelis L, Yaholom J, Heineman M. Primary CNS lymphoma: combined treatment with chemotherapy and radiotherapy. Neurology 1990; 40:80.
36. MacMahon E, Glass J, Hayward S, et al. EBV in AIDS primary CNS lymphoma. Lancet 1991; 338:969–973.
37. Richardson E. Progressive multifocal leukoencephalopathy. In: Vinken P, Bruyn G, eds. Handbook of Clinical Neurology. Vol. 34. Amsterdam: Elsevier, 1978:307.
38. Padgett B, Walker D, Zu Rhein G, et al. JC papovavirus in progressive multifocal leukoencephalopathy. J Infect Dis 1976; 133:868.
39. Houff S, Major E, Katz D, et al. Involvement of JC virus-infected mononuclear cells from the bone marrow and spleen in the pathogenesis of progressive multifocal leukoencephalopathy. N Engl J Med 1988; 318:301.
40. Schmidbauer M, Budka H, Shah K. Progressive multifocal leukoencephalopathy (PML) in AIDS and in the pre-AIDS era. Acta Neuropathol 1990; 80:375.
41. Berger J, Kaszovitz B, Donovan Post M, Dickinson G, Progressive multifocal leukoencephalopathy in association with human deficiency virus infection: a review of the literature with a report of sixteen cases. Ann Intern Med 1987; 107:78.
42. Krupp L, Lipton R, Swerdlow M, et al. Progressive multifocal leukoencephalopathy: clinical and radiographic features. Ann Neurol 1985; 17:344.
43. Mark A, Atlas S. Progressive multifocal leukoencephalopathy in patients with AIDS: appearance on MR images. Radiology 1989; 173:517.
44. Weber T, Turner RW, Frye S, et al. Specific diagnosis of progressive multifocal leukoencephalopathy by polymerase chain reaction. J Infect Dis 1994; 169:1138–1141.
45. Weber T, Turner RW, Frye S, et al. Progressive multifocal leukoencephalopathy diagnosed by amplification of JC virus-specific DNA from cerebrospinal fluid. Aids 1994; 8:49–57.
46. Conway B, Halliday W, Brunham R. Human immunodeficiency virus-associated progressive multifocal leukoencephalopathy: apparent response to 3′-azido-3′deoxythymidine. Rev Infect Dis 1990; 12:479.
47. Portegies P, Algra P, Hollak C, et al. Response to cytarabine in progressive multifocal leukoencephalopathy in AIDS. Lancet 1991; 1:680.
48. Berger J, Mucke L. Prolonged survival and partial recovery in AIDS-associated progressive multifocal leukoencephalopathy. Neurology 1988; 38:1060.
49. Saag, M. Cryptococcosis and other fungal infections (Histoplasmosis coccidioidomycosis). In: Sande M, Volverding P, eds. The Medical Management of AIDS, 5th ed. Philadelphia: WB Saunders, 1997:327–342.
50. Andreula CF, Burdi N, Carella A. CNS cryptococcosis in AIDS: spectrum of MR findings. J Comput Assist Tomogr 1993; 17:438–441.
51. Dismukes WE. Management of cryptococcosis (review). Clin Infect Dis 1993; 17:S507–S512.
52. Powderly WG. Cryptococcal meningitis and AIDS (review). Clin Infect Dis 1993; 17:837–842.
53. Saag MS, Powderly WG, Cloud GA, et al. Comparison of amphotericin B with fluconazole in the treatment of acute AIDS-associated cryptococcal meningitis. The NIAID Mycoses Study Group and the AIDS Clinical Trials Group (see comments). N Engl J Med 1992; 326:83–89.

54. Sugar AM. Overview: cryptococcosis in the patient with AIDS (review). Mycopathologia 1991; 114:153–157.
55. Chuck S, Sande M. Infections with Cryptococcus neoformans in the acquired immunodeficiency syndrome. N Engl J Med 1989; 321:794.
56. Stern J, Hartman B, Sharkey P, et al. Oral fluconazole therapy for patients with acquired immunodeficiency syndrome and cryptococcis: experience with 22 patients. Am J Med 1988; 85:477.
57. Larsen R, Leal M, Chan L. Fluconazole compared with amphotericin B plus flucytosine for cryptococcal meningitis in AIDS: a randomized trial. Ann Intern Med 1988; 85:481.
58. Sugar A, Saunder C. Oral fluconazole as suppressive therapy of disseminated cryptococcal in patients with the acquired immunodeficiency syndrome. Am J Med 1988; 85:481.
59. Powderly WG, Saag MS, Cloud GA, et al. A controlled trial of fluconazole or amphotericin B to prevent relapse of cryptococcal meningitis in patients with the acquired immunodeficiency syndrome. The NIAID AIDS Clinical Trials Group and Mycoses Study Group (see comments). N Engl J Med 1992; 326:793–798.
60. Navia B, Cho E-W, Petito C, Price R. The AIDS dementia complex: II. Neuropathology. Ann Neurol 1986; 19:525–535.
61. Petito C, Cho E-S, Lemann W, Navia B, Price R. Neuropathology of acquired immunodeficiency syndrome (AIDS): an autopsy review. J Neuropathol Exp Neurol 1986; 45:635–646.
62. Vinters H, Kwok M, Ho H, et al. Cytomegalovirus in the nervous system of patients with the acquired immunodeficiency syndrome. Brain 1989; 112:245.
63. Holland NR, Power C, Mathews VP, Glass JD, Forman M, McArthur JC. Cytomegalovirus encephalitis in acquired immunodeficiency syndrome (AIDS). Neurology 1994; 44:507–514.
64. Cinque P, Vago L, Brytting M, et al. Cytomegalovirus infection of the central nervous system in patients with AIDS: diagnosis by DNA amplification from cerebrospinal fluid. J Infect Dis 1992; 166:1408–1411.
65. Gozlan J, Salord JM, Roullet E, et al. Rapid detection of cytomegalovirus DNA in cerebrospinal fluid of AIDS patients with neurologic disorders. (Published erratum appears in J Infect Dis 1993 Apr; 167(4):995.) J Infect Dis 1992; 166:1416–1421.
66. Wolf DG, Spector SA. Diagnosis of human cytomegalovirus central nervous system disease in AIDS patients by DNA amplification from cerebrospinal fluid. J Infect Dis 1992; 166:1412–1415.
67. Weber T, Beck R, Stark E, et al. Comparative analysis of intrathecal antibody synthesis and DNA amplification for the diagnosis of cytomegalovirus infection of the central nervous system in AIDS patients. J Neurol 1994; 241:407–414.
68. Sunderam G, McDonald R, Maniatias T, et al. Tuberculosis as a manifestation of the acquired immunodeficiency syndrome (AIDS). JAMA 1986; 256:362.
69. Guarner J, Del Rio C, Slade B. Tuberculosis as a manifestation of the acquired immunodeficiency syndrome. JAMA 1986; 256:3092.
70. Bishburg E, Sunderam G, Reichman L, Kapila R. Central nervous system tuberculosis with the acquired immunodeficiency syndrome and its related complex. Ann Intern Med 1986; 105:210.
71. Dube MP, Holtom PD, Larsen RA. Tuberculous meningitis in patients with and without human immunodeficiency virus infection. Am J Med 1992; 93:520–524.
72. Berenguer J, Moreno S, Laguna F, et al. Tuberculous meningitis in patients infected with the human immunodeficiency virus (see comments). N Engl J Med 1992; 326:668–672.
73. Folgueira L, Delgado R, Palenque E, Noriega AR. Polymerase chain reaction for rapid diagnosis of tuberculous meningitis in AIDS patients. Neurology 1994; 44:1336–1338.
74. Jacob CN, Henein SS, Heurich AE, Kamholz S. Nontuberculous mycobacterial infection of the central nervous system in patients with AIDS. South Med J 1993; 86:638–640.
75. Horten B, Price R, Jimenez D. Multifocal varicella-zoster virus leukoencephalitis temporally remote from herpes zoster. Ann Neurol 1981; 9:251.
76. Ryder JW, Croen K, Kleinschmidt-DeMasters BK, Ostrove JM, Straus SE, Cohn DL. Progressive encephalitis three months after resolution of cutaneous zoster in a patient with AIDS. Ann Neurol 1986; 19:182–188.

77. Morgello S, Block G, Price R, et al. Varicella-zoster virus leukoencephalitis and cerebral vasculopathy. Arch Pathol Lab Med 1988; 112:173.
78. Hilt D, Bucholz D, Krumholz A, et al. Herpes zoster ophthalmicus and delayed contralateral hemiparesis caused by cerebral angiitis: Diagnosis and management approaches. Ann Neurol 1983; 14:543.
79. Eidelberg D, Sotrel A, Horopian D, et al. Thrombotic cerebral vasculopathy associated with herpes zoster. Ann Neurol 1986; 19:7.
80. Devinsky O, Cho E, Petito C, Price R. Herpes zoster myelitis. Brain 1991; 114:1181.
81. Gray F, Belec L, Lescs MC, et al. Varicella-zoster virus infection of the central nervous system in the acquired immune deficiency syndrome (review). Brain 1994; 117:987–999.
82. Levy RM, Bredesen DE. Central nervous system dysfunction in acquired immunodeficiency syndrome (review). J AIDS 1988; 1:41–64.
83. Rhodes R. Histopathology of the central nervous system in the acquired immunodeficiency syndrome. Hum Pathol 1987; 18:636.
84. Berger J. Neurosyphilis in human immunodeficiency virus type 1-seropositive individuals. Arch Neurol 1991; 48:700.
85. Johns D, Tierney M, Felsenstein D. Alteration in the natural history of neurosyphilis by concurrent infection with the human immunodeficiency virus. N Engl J Med 1987; 316:1569.
86. Berry C, Hooton T, Collier A, Lukehart S. Neurologic relapse after benzathine penicillin therapy for secondary syphilis in a patient with HIV infection. N Engl J Med 1987; 316.
87. Katz D, Berger J. Neurosyphilis in acquired immunodeficiency syndrome. Arch Neurol 1989; 46:895.
88. Davis L. Neurosyphilis in the patient infected with human immunodeficiency virus. Ann Neurol 1990; 27:211.
89. Lukehart S, Hook E, Baker-Zander S. Invasion of the central nervous system by Treponema pallidum: Implications for the diagnosis and treatment. Ann Intern Med 1988; 109:855.
90. Gordon SE, Eaton ME, George R, et al. The response of symptomatic neurosyphilis to high-dose intravenous penicillin G in patients with human immunodeficiency virus infection. N Engl J Med 1994; 331:1469–1473.
91. Simon R. Neurosyphilis. Neurology 1994; 44:2228–2230.
92. Carrazana EJ, Rossitch E, Jr., Morris J. Isolated central nervous system aspergillosis in the acquired immunodeficiency syndrome. Clin Neurol Neurosurg 1991; 93:227–230.
93. Decker CF, Parenti DM. Invasive aspergillosis in patients with HIV infection: report of two patients and a review of the literature (review). J AIDS 1991; 4:603–606.
94. Khoo SH, Denning DW. Invasive aspergillosis in patients with AIDS (review). Clin Infect Dis 1994; 19(suppl 1):S41–S48.
95. Pursell KJ, Telzak EE, Armstrong D. Aspergillus species colonization and invasive disease in patients with AIDS (review). Clin Infect Dis 1992; 14:141–148.
96. Kim J, Minamoto GY, Grieco MH. Nocardial infection as a complication of AIDS: report of six cases and review (review). Rev Infect Dis 1991; 13:624–629.
97. LeBlang SD, Whiteman ML, Post MJ, Uttamchandani RB, Bell MD, Smirniotopolous JG. CNS Nocardia in AIDS patients: CT and MRI with pathologic correlation. J Comput Assist Tomogr 1995; 19:15–22.
98. Long PF. A retrospective study of Nocardia infections associated with the acquired immune deficiency syndrome (AIDS) (letter). Infection 1994; 22:362–364.
99. Miralles GD. Disseminated Nocardia farcinica infection in an AIDS patient. Eur J Clin Microbiol Infect Dis 1994; 13:497–500.
100. Bruinsma-Adams IK. AIDS presenting as Candida albicans meningitis: a case report (letter). (Published erratum appears in AIDS 1991 Dec; 5(12):following 1547.) Aids 1991; 5:1268–1269.
101. Manfredi R, Mazzoni A, Cavicchi O, Santini D, Chiodo F. Invasive mycotic and actinomycotic oropharyngeal and craniofacial infection in two patients with AIDS. Mycoses 1994; 37:209–215.
102. Berenguer J, Solera J, Diaz MD, Moreno S, Lopez-Herce JA, Bouza E. Listeriosis in patients infected with human immunodeficiency virus (review). Rev Infect Dis 1991; 13:115–119.
103. da Silva LJ, Resende MR, de Abreu WB, et al. Listeriosis and AIDS: case report and literature review (review). Rev Inst Med Trop Sao Paulo 1992; 34:475–478.

104. Decker CF, Simon GL, DiGioia RA, Tuazon CU. Listeria monocytogenes infections in patients with AIDS: report of five cases and review (review). Rev Infect Dis 1991; 13:413–417.
105. Harcourt-Webster JN, Scaravilli F, Darwish AH. Strongyloides stercoralis hyperinfection in an HIV positive patient. J Clin Pathol 1991; 44:346–348.
106. Simpson DM, Olney RK. Peripheral neuropathies associated with human immunodeficiency virus infection (review). Neurol Clin 1992; 10:685–711.
107. Cornblath D. Treatment of the neuromuscular complications of human immunodeficiency virus infection. Ann Neurol 1988; 23:S88.
108. Fuller GN, Jacobs JM, Guiloff RJ. Nature and incidence of peripheral nerve syndromes in HIV infection. J Neurol Neurosurg Psychiatry 1993; 56:372–381.
109. Griffin JW, Wesselingh SL, Griffin DE, Glass JD, McArthur JC. Peripheral nerve disorders in HIV infection. Similarities and contrasts with CNS disorders. Res Publ Assoc Res Nervous Mental Dis 1994; 72:159–182.
110. Miller R, Parry G, Lang W, et al. AIDS-related inflammatory polyradiculoneuropathy: Successful treatment with plasma exchange (abstr). Neurology 1986; 36:206.
111. Eidelberg D, Sotrel A, Vogel H, et al. Progressive polyradiculopathy in acquired immune deficiency syndrome. Neurology 1986; 36:912.
112. Fuller G, Gill S, Guilloff R, et al. Ganciclovir treatment of lumbosacral polyradiculopathy in AIDS Lancet 1990; 335:48.
113. So Y, Olney R. The natural history of mononeuropathy multiplex and simplex in patients with HIV infection (abstr). Neurology 1991; 41(suppl):374.
114. Said G, Lacroix C, Chemouilli P, et al. CMV neuropathy in AIDS: A clinical and pathological study. Ann Neurol 1991; 29:139.
115. Fuller GN. Cytomegalovirus and the peripheral nervous system in AIDS (review). J AIDS 1992; 5:S33–S36.
116. Roullet E, Assuerus V, Gozlan J, et al. Cytomegalovirus multifocal neuropathy in AIDS: analysis of 15 consecutive cases. Neurology 1994; 44:2174–2182.
117. Pantaleo G, Graziosi C, Demarest J, et al. Role of lymphoid organs in the pathogenesis of human immunodeficiency virus (HIV) infection. Immunol Rev 1994; 140:105–130.
118. Pantaleo G, Graziosi C, Demarest J, et al. HIV infection is active and progressive in lymphoid tissue during clinically latent stages of the disease. Nature 1993; 362:355–358.
119. Embretson J, Zupancic M, Ribas J, et al. Massive covert infection of helper T lymphocytes and macrophages by HIV during the incubation period of AIDS. Nature 1993; 362:359–362.
120. Volberding PA. HIV quantitation: clinical applications. Lancet 1996; 347:71–73.
121. Resnick L, diMarzo-Veronese F, Schupbach J, et al. Intra-blood-brain-barrier synthesis of HTLV-III-specific IgG in patients with neurologic symptoms associated with AIDS or AIDS-related complex. N Engl J Med 1985; 313:1498–1504.
122. Resnick L, Berger J, Shapshak P, Tourtellotte W. Early penetration of the blood-brain-barrier by HIV. Neurology 1988; 38:9–14.
123. Goudsmit J, Wolters E, Bakker M, et al. Intrathecal synthesis of antibodies to HTLV-III in patients without AIDS or AIDS related complex. Br Med J 1986; 292:1231.
124. Marshall D, Brey R, Cahill W, Houk R, Zajac R, Boswell R. Spectrum of cerebrospinal fluid findings in various stages of human immunodeficiency virus infection. Arch Neurol 1988; 45:954–958.
125. McArthur J, Cohen B, Farzadegan H, et al. Cerebrospinal fluid abnormalities in homosexual men with and without neuropsychiatric findings. Ann Neurol 1988; 23(suppl):S34–S37.
126. Elovaara I, Nykyri E, Poutiainen E, Hokkanen L, Raininko R, Suni J. CSF follow-up in HIV-1 infection: intrathecal production of HIV-specific and unspecific IGG, and beta-2-microglobulin increase with duration of HIV-1 infection. Acta Neurol Scand 1993; 87:388–396.
127. Ho D, Sarngadhara M, Resnick L, et al. Primary human T lymphotropic virus type III infection. Ann Intern Med 1985; 103:880.
128. Conrad DI, Schmid P, Syndulko K, et al. Quantifying HIV-1 RNA using the polymerase chain reaction on cerebrospinal fluid and serum of seropositive individuals with and without neurologic abnormalities. J AIDS 1995; 10:425–435.

129. Davis LE, Hjelle BL, Miller VE, et al. Early viral brain invasion in iatrogenic human immunodeficiency virus infection. Neurology 1992; 42:1736–1739.
130. Price R, Brew B, Sidtis J, Rosenblum M, Scheck A, Cleary P. The brain in AIDS: Central nervous system HIV-1 infection and AIDS dementia complex. Science 1988; 239:586–592.
131. Price RW. Understanding the AIDS dementia complex (ADC). The challenge of HIV and its effects on the central nervous system (review). Res Publ Assoc Res Nervous Mental Dis 1994; 72:1–45.
132. Price R. The cellular basis of central nervous system HIV-1 infection and the AIDS dementia complex: introduction. J Neuro-AIDS 1995; 1:1–28.
133. Tindall B, Cooper D. Primary HIV infection: host responses and intervention strategies. AIDS 1991; 5:1.
134. Brew B, Perdices M, Darveniza P, et al. The neurological features of early and 'latent' human immunodeficiency virus infection. Aust NZ J Med 1989; 19:700.
135. Denning D, Anderson J, Rudge P, et al. Acute myelopathy associated with primary infection with human immunodeficiency virus. Br Med J 1987; 294:143.
136. Piette A, Tusseau F, Vignon D, et al. Letter to the editor. Lancet 1986; 1:852.
137. Wiselka M, Nicholson K, Ward S, Flower A. Acute infection with human immunodeficiency virus associated with facial nerve palsy and neuralgia. J Infect 1987; 15:189.
138. Hagberg L, Malmval B, Svennerholm L, et al. Guillain-Barre syndrome as an early manifestation of HIV central nervous system infection. Scand J Infect Dis 1987; 18:591.
139. Carne C, Smith A, Elkington S, et al. Acute encephalopathy coincident with serocoversion for anti HTLV-III. Lancet 1985; 2:1206.
140. Calabrese L, Proffitt M, Levin K, et al. Acute infection with the human immunodeficiency virus (HIV) associated with acute brachial neuritis and exanthematous rash. Ann Intern Med 1987; 107:849.
141. Clark SJ, Saag MS, Decker WD, et al. High titers of cytopathic virus in plasma of patients with symptomatic primary HIV-1 infection. N Engl J Med 1991; 324:954–960.
142. Gaines H, von Sydow M, Pehrson PO, Lundbergh P. Clinical pricure of primary HIV-1 infection presenting as a glandular-fever-like illness. Lancet 1988; 297:1363–1368.
143. Rabeneck L, Popovic M, Gartner S, et al. Acute HIV-1 infection presenting with painful swallowing and esophageal ulcers. JAMA 1990; 263:2318–2322.
144. Cornblath D, McArthur J. Predominantly sensory neuropathy in patients with AIDS and AIDS-related complex. Neurology 1988; 38:794.
145. Cornblath D, Chaudhry V, Griffin J. Treatment of chronic inflammatory demyelinating polyneuropathy with intravenous immunoglobin. Ann Neurol 1991; 30:104.
146. Lipkin W, Parry G, Kiprov D, Abrams D. Inflammatory neuropathy in homosexual men with lymphadenopathy. Neurology 1985; 35:1479–1483.
147. Berger J, Sheremata W, Resnick L, et al. Multiple sclerosis-like leukoencephalopathy revealing human immunodeficiency virus infection. Neurology 1989; 39:324–329.
148. Gray F, Chimelli L, Mohr M, et al. Fulminating multiple sclerosis-like leukoencephalopathy revealing human immunodeficiency virus infection. Neurology 1991; 41:105–109.
149. Hollander H, Stringari S. Human immunodeficiency virus-associated meningitis: clinical course and correlations. Am J Med 1987; 83:813–816.
150. Hollander H, McGuire D, Burack JH. Diagnostic lumbar puncture in HIV-infected patients: analysis of 138 cases. Am J Med 1994; 96:223–228.
151. Brew BJ, Miller J. Human immunodeficiency virus-related headache. Neurology 1993; 43:1098–1100.
152. Price RW, Sidtis JJ, Brew BJ. AIDS dementia complex and HIV-1 infection: a view from the clinic (review). Brain Pathol 1991; 1:155–162.
153. Navia B, Jordan B, Price R. The AIDS dementia complex: I. Clinical features. Ann Neurol 1986; 19:517–524.
154. Price R, Brew B. The AIDS dementia complex. J Infect Dis 1988; 158:1079–1083.
155. Price R. Management of AIDS dementia complex and HIV-1 infection of the nervous system. AIDS 1995; 9(Suppl A):S221–S230.
156. Navia B, Price R. The acquired immunodeficiency syndrome dementia complex as the presenting or sole manifestation of human immunodeficiency virus infection. Arch Neurol 1987; 44:65–69.

157. Selnes O, Miller E, McArthur J, et al. No evidence of cognitive decline during the asymptomatic stages. Neurology 1990; 40:204.
158. Selnes OA, Galai N, Bacellar H, et al. Cognitive performance after progression to AIDS: a longitudinal study from the Multicenter AIDS Cohort Study. Neurology 1995; 45:267–275.
159. Miller E, Selnes O, McArthur J, et al. Neuropsychological performance in HIV-1-infected homosexual men: The Multicenter AIDS Cohort Study (MACS). Neurology 1990; 40:197–203.
160. McArthur JC, Hoover DR, Bacellar H, et al. Dementia in AIDS patients: incidence and risk factors. Multicenter AIDS Cohort Study. Neurology 1993; 43:2245–2252.
161. Portegies P, de Gans JîAL, JM, Derix M, et al. Declining incidence of AIDS dementia complex after introduction of zidovudine treatment. Br Med J 1989; 299:819–821.
162. Portegies P, Enting RH, de Gans J, et al. Presentation and course of AIDS dementia complex: 10 years of follow-up in Amsterdam, The Netherlands. AIDS 1993; 7:669–675.
163. Price R. AIDS dementia complex and HIV-1 brain infection: a pathogenetic framework for treatment and evaluation. Curr Top Microbiol Immunol 1995; 202:33–54.
164. Sidtis JJ, Price RW. Early HIV-1 infection and the AIDS dementia complex (comment). Neurology 1990; 40:323–326.
165. Anonymous. Nomenclature and research case definitions for neurologic manifestations of human immunodeficiency virus-type 1 (HIV-1) infection. Report of a Working Group of the American Academy of Neurology AIDS Task Force (see comments). Neurology 1991; 41:778–785.
166. World Health Organization consultation on the neuropsychiatric aspects of HIV-1 infection. AIDS 1990; 49:935–936.
167. Price R, Worley J. Management of neurologic complications of HIV-1 infection and AIDS. In: Sande M, Volberding P, eds. Medical Management of AIDS. Philadelphia: WB Saunders Company, 1995:261–288.
168. Harris MJ, Jeste DV, Gleghorn A, Sewell DD. New-onset psychosis in HIV-infected patients (see comments). J Clin Psychiatry 1991; 52:369–376.
169. Tross S, Price R, Navia B, et al. Neuropsychological characterization of the AIDS dementia complex: a preliminary report. AIDS 1988; 2:81–88.
170. Sidtis JJ. Evaluation of the AIDS dementia complex in adults (review). Res Pub Assoc Res Nervous Mental Dis 1994; 72:273–287.
171. Post MJ, Berger JR, Quencer RM. Asymptomatic and neurologically symptomatic HIV-seropositive individuals: prospective evaluation with cranial MR imaging (see comments). Radiology 1991; 178:131–139.
172. Post M, Tate L, Quencer R, et al. CT, MR, and pathology in HIV encephalitis and meningitis. AJR 1988; 151:373.
173. Petty RK. Recent advances in the neurology of HIV infection (review). Postgrad Med J 1994; 70: 393–403.
174. Dal Pan GJ, McArthur JH, Aylward E, et al. Patterns of cerebral atrophy in HIV-1-infected individuals: results of a quantitative MRI analysis. Neurology 1992; 42:2125–2130.
175. Gelman B, Guinto FJ. Morphometry, histopathology, and tomography of cerebral atrophy in the acquired immunodeficiency syndrome. Ann Neurol 1992; 31:32–40.
176. Aylward EH, Henderer JD, McArthur JC, et al. Reduced basal ganglia volume in HIV-1-associated dementia: results from quantitative neuroimaging. Neurology 1993; 43:2099–2104.
177. Jakobsen J, Gyldensted C, Brun B, et al. Cerebral ventricular enlargement relates to neuropsychological measures in unselected AIDS patients. Acta Neurol Scand 1989; 79:59.
178. Moeller AA, Backmund HC. Ventricle brain ratio in the clinical course of HIV infection. Acta Neurol Scand 1990; 81:512–515.
179. Power C, Kong PA, Crawford TO, et al. Cerebral white matter changes in acquired immunodeficiency syndrome dementia: alterations of the blood-brain barrier. Ann Neurol 1993; 34:339–350.
180. Brew BJ, Paul MO, Nakajima G, Khan A, Gallardo H, Price RW. Cerebrospinal fluid HIV-1 p24 antigen and culture: sensitivity and specificity for AIDS-dementia complex. J Neurol Neurosurg Psychiatry 1994; 57:784–789.

181. Portegies P, Epstein L, Hung S, et al. Human immunodeficiency virus type 1 antigen in crebrospinal fluid: correlation with clinical neurological status. Arch Neurol 1989; 46:261–264.
182. Brew B, Bhalla R, Paul M, et al. Cerebrospinal fluid neopterin in human immunodeficiency virus type 1 infection. Ann Neurol 1990; 28:556–560.
183. Brew B, Bhalla R, Fleisher M, et al. Cerebrospinal fluid B2 microglobulin in patients infected with human immunodeficiency virus. Neurology 1989; 39:830–834.
184. Brew BJ, Bhalla RB, Paul M, et al. Cerebrospinal fluid beta 2-microglobulin in patients with AIDS dementia complex: an expanded series including response to zidovudine treatment. AIDS 1992; 6:461–465.
185. Griffin DE, McArthur JC, Cornblath DR. Neopterin and interferon-gamma in serum and cerebrospinal fluid of patients with HIV-associated neurologic disease. Neurology 1991; 41:69–74.
186. Budka H. Neuropathology of human immunodeficiency virus infection (review). Brain Pathol 1991; 1:163–175.
187. Rosenblum M. Infection of the central nervous system by the human immunodeficiency virus type 1: morphology and relation to syndromes of progressive encephalopathy and myelopathy in patients with AIDS. Pathol Ann 1990; 25:117–169.
188. Gray F, Haug H, Chimelli L, et al. Prominent cortical atrophy with neuronal loss as correlate of human immunodeficiency virus encephalopathy. Acta Neuropathol 1991; 82:229–233.
189. Brew B, Rosenblum M, Cronin K, Price R. The AIDS dementia complex and HIV-1 brain infection: clinical-virological correlations. Ann Neurol 1995; 38:563–570.
190. Masliah E, Achim CL, Ge N, DeTeresa R, Wiley C. Patterns of neurodegeneration in HIV encephalitis. J Neuro-AIDS 1996; 1(1):161–173.
191. Masliah E, Ge N, Achim C, De Teresa R, Wiley CA. Cellular neuropathology in HIV encephalitis (review). Res Publ Assoc Res Nervous Mental Dis 1994; 72:119–131.
192. Petito C, Navia B, Cho E, et al. Vacuolar myelopathy pathologically resembling subacute combined degeneration in patients with acquired immunodeficiency syndrome (AIDS). N Engl J Med 1985; 312:874.
193. Dal Pan GJ, Glass JD, McArthur JC. Clinicopathologic correlations of HIV-1-associated vacuolar myelopathy: an autopsy-based case-control study. Neurology 1994; 44:2159–2164.
194. Petito CK, Vecchio D, Chen YT. HIV antigen and DNA in AIDS spinal cords correlate with macrophage infiltration but not with vacuolar myelopathy. J Neuropathol Exp Neurol 1994; 53:86–94.
195. Rosenblum M, Scheck A, Cronin K, et al. Dissociation of AIDS-related vacuolar myelopathy and productive human immunodeficiency virus type 1 (HIV-1) infection of the spinal cord. Neurology 1989; 39:892–896.
196. Tan SV, Guiloff RJ, Scaravilli F. AIDS-associated vacuolar myelopathy. A morphometric study. Brain 1995; 118:1247–1261.
197. Shaw G, Harper M, Hahn B, et al. HTLV-III infection in brains of children and adults with AIDS encephalopathy. Science 1985; 227:177–182.
198. Koenig S, Gendelman H, Orenstein J, et al. Detection of AIDS virus in macrophages in brain tissue from AIDS patients with encephalopathy. Science 1986; 233:1089–1093.
199. Stoler M, Eskin T, Benn S, Angerer R, Angerer L. Human T-cell lymphotropic virus type III infection of the central nervous system—preliminary in situ analysis. JAMA 1986; 256:2360–2364.
200. Wiley C, Schrier R, Nelson J, Lampert P, Oldstone M. Cellular localization of human immunodeficiency virus infection within the brains of acquired immune deficiency patients. Proc Natl Acad Sci USA 1986; 83:7089–7093.
201. Gabuzda D, Ho D, De La Monte S, et al. Immunohistochemical identification of HTLV-III antigen in brains of patients with AIDS. Ann Neurol 1986; 20:289.
202. Vazeux R, Brousse N, Jarry A, et al. AIDS subacute encephalitis: identification of HIV-infected cells. Am J Pathol 1987; 126:403–410.
203. Pumarole-Sune T, Navia B, Cordon-Cardo C, Cho E-S, Price R. HIV antigen in the brains of patients with the AIDS dementia complex. Ann Neurol 1987; 21:490–496.
204. Michaels J, Price R, Rosenblum M. Microglia in the human immunodeficiency virus encephalitis of

acquired immune deficiency syndrome: proliferation, infection and fusion. Acta Neuropathol 1988; 76:373–379.
205. Nuovo G, Gallery F, MacConnel P, Braun A. In situ detection of polymerase chain reaction-amplified HIV-1 nucleic acids and tumor necrosis factor-α RNA in the central nervous system. Am J Pathol 1994; 144:659–666.
206. Tornatore C, Chandra R, Berger JR, Major EO. HIV-1 infection of subcortical astrocytes in the pediatric central nervous system. Neurology 1994; 44:481–487.
207. Saito Y, Sharer L, Epstein L, et al. Overexpression of nef as a marker for restricted HIV-1 infection of astrocytes in postmortem pediatric central nervous system tissues. Neurology 1994; 44:474–481.
208. Glass JD, Fedor H, Wesselingh SL, McArthur JC. Immunocytochemical quantitation of human immunodeficiency virus in the brain: correlations with dementia. Ann Neurol 1995; 38:755–762.
209. Wiley CA, Achim CL. Human immunodeficiency virus encephalitis and dementia. Ann Neurol 1995; 38:559–560.
210. O'Brien W. Genetic and biologic basis of HIV-1 neurotropism. In: Price R, Perry S, eds. HIV, AIDS and the Brain. New York: Raven Press, Ltd., 1994:47–70.
211. Sharpless N, O'Brien W, Verdin E, Kufta C, Chen I, Dubois-Dalcq M. Human immunodeficiency virus type 1 tropism for brain microglial cells is determined by a region of the env glycoprotein that also controls macrophage tropism. J Virol 1992; 66:2588–2593.
212. Westervelt P, Trowbridge D, Epstein L, et al. Macrophage tropism determinants of HIV-1 in vivo. J Virol 1992; 66:2577–2582.
213. Power C, McArthur JC, Johnson RT, et al. Demented and nondemented patients with AIDS differ in brain-derived human immunodeficiency virus type 1 envelope sequences. J Virol 1994; 68:4643–4649.
214. Tyor W, Wesselingh S, Griffin J, McArthur J, Griffin D. Unifying hypothesis for the pathogenesis of HIV-associated dementia complex, vacuolar myelopathy, and sensory neuropathy. J AIDS Human Retrovirol 1995; 9:379–388.
215. Lipton SA, Gendelman HE. Seminars in medicine of the Beth Israel Hospital, Boston. Dementia associated with the acquired immunodeficiency syndrome (review). N Engl J Med 1995; 332: 934–940.
216. Epstein LG, Gendelman HE. Human immunodeficiency virus type 1 infection of the nervous system: pathogenetic mechanisms (see comments). Ann Neurol 1993; 33:429–436.
217. Wesselingh SL, Glass J, McArthur JC, Griffin JW, Griffin DE. Cytokine dysregulation in HIV-associated neurological disease (review). Adv Neuroimmunol 1994; 4:199–206.
218. Genis P, Jett M, Bernton EW, Boyle T, Gelbard HA, Dzenko K, Keane RW, Resnick L, Mizrachi Y, Volsky DJ, Epstein LG, Gendelman HE. Cytokines and arachidonic metabolites produced during human immunodeficiency virus (HIV)-infected macrophage-astroglia interactions: implications for the neuropathogenesis of HIV disease. J Exp Med 1992; 176:1703–1718.
219. Sidtis JJ, Gatsonis C, Price RW, et al. Zidovudine treatment of the AIDS dementia complex: results of a placebo-controlled trial. AIDS Clinical Trials Group. Ann Neurol 1993; 33:343–349.
220. Schmitt F, Bigleg J, McKinnis R, et al. Neuropsychological outcome of azidothymidine (AZT) in the treatment of AIDS and AIDS-related complex: A double blind, placebo-controlled trial. N Engl J Med 1988; 319:1573–1578.
221. Pizzo P, Eddy J, Fallon J, et al. Effect of continuous intravenous infusion of zidovudine (AZT) in children with symptomatic HIV infection. N Engl J Med 1988; 319:889–896.
222. Vago L, Castagna A, Lazzarin A, Trabattoni G, Cinque P, Costanzi G. Reduced frequency of HIV-induced brain lesions in AIDS patients treated with zidovudine. J AIDS 1993; 6:42–5.
223. Gray F, Belec L, Keohane C, et al. Zidovudine therapy and HIV encephalitis: a 10-year neuropathological survey. J AIDS 1994; 8:489–493.
224. Lipton SA, Stamler JS. Actions of redox-related congeners of nitric oxide at the nmda receptor. Neuropharmacology 1994; 33:1229–1233.
225. Lipton SA. Neuronal injury associated with HIV-1 and potential treatment with calcium-channel and nmda antagonists. Dev Neurosci 1994; 16:145–151.

226. Miller R, Parry G, Pfaeffl W, et al. The spectrum of peripheral neuropathy associated with ARC and AIDS. Muscle Nerve 1988; 11:857.
227. Simpson DM, Tagliati M. Nucleoside analogue-associated peripheral neuropathy in human immunodeficiency virus infection (review). J AIDS Human Retrovirol 1995; 9:153–161.
228. Craddock C, Pasvol G, Bull R, et al. Cardiorespiratory arrest and automatic neuropathy in AIDS. Lancet 1987; 2:16.
229. Welby SB, Rogerson SJ, Beeching NJ. Autonomic neuropathy is common in human immunodeficiency virus infection. J Infect 1991; 23:123–128.
230. Batman P, Miller A, Sedgewick P, Griffin G. Autonomic denervation in jejunal mucosa of homosexual men infected with HIV. AIDS 1991; 5:1247–1252.
231. Simpson DM, Bender AN. Human immunodeficiency virus-associated myopathy: analysis of 11 patients. Ann Neurol 1988; 24:79–84.
232. Simpson DM, Citak KA, Godfrey E, Godbold J, Wolfe D. Myopathies associated with human immunodeficiency virus and zidovudine: can their effects be distinguished? Neurology 1993; 43: 971–976.
233. Dalakas MC, Pezeshkpour GH. Neuromuscular diseases associated with human immunodeficiency virus infection (review). Ann Neurol 1988; 23:S38–S48.
234. Dalakas MC, Pezeshkpour GH, Gravell M, Sever JL. Polymyositis associated with AIDS retrovirus. JAMA 1986; 256:2381–2383.
235. Bailey RO, Turok DI, Jaufmann BP, Singh JK. Myositis and acquired immunodeficiency syndrome. Human Pathol 1987; 18:749–751.
236. Illa I, Nath A, Dalakas M. Immunocytochemical and virological characteristics of HIV-associated inflammatory myopathies: similarities with seronegative polymyositis. Ann Neurol 1991; 29:474.
237. Gherardi RK. Skeletal muscle involvement in HIV-infected patients (review). Neuropathol Appl Neurobiol 1994; 20:232–237.
238. Manji H, Harrison MJ, Round JM, et al. Muscle disease, HIV and zidovudine. J Neurol 1993; 240: 479–488.
239. Nordstrom DM, Petropolis AA, Giorno R, Gates RH, Reddy VB. Inflammatory myopathy and acquired immunodeficiency syndrome. Arthritis Rheumatism 1989; 32;475–479.
240. Wrzolek MA, Sher JH, Kozlowski PB, Rao C. Skeletal muscle pathology in AIDS: an autopsy study. Muscle Nerve 1990; 13:508–515.
241. Chalmers A, Greco C, Miller R. Prognosis in AZT myopathy. Neurology 1991; 41:1181.
242. Dalakas M, Illa I, Pezeshkpour G, et al. Mitochondrial myopathy caused by long term zidovudine therapy. N Engl J Med 1990; 322:1098.
243. Arnaudo E, Dalakas M, Shanske S, Moraes CT, DiMauro S, Schon EA. Depletion of muscle mitochondrial DNA in AIDS patients with zidovudine-induced myopathy. Lancet 1991; 337:508–510.
244. Dalakas MC, Leon-Monzon ME, Bernardini I, Gahl WA, Jay CA. Zidovudine-induced mitochondrial myopathy is associated with muscle carnitine deficiency and lipid storage. Ann Neurol 1994; 35: 482–487.
245. Damati G, Lewis W. Zidovudine causes early increases in mitochondrial ribonucleic acid abundance and induces ultrastructural changes in cultured mouse muscle cells. Lab Invest 1994; 71:879–884.
246. Mhiri C, Baudrimont M, Bonne G, et al. Zidovudine myopathy: a distinctive disorder associated with mitochondrial dysfunction. Ann Neurol 1991; 29:606.
247. Modica-Napolitano JS. AZT causes tissue-specific inhibition of mitochondrial bioenergetic function. Biochem Biophys Res Commun 1993; 194:170–177.
248. Peters BS, Winer J, Landon DN, Stotter A, Pinching AJ. Mitochondrial myopathy associated with chronic zidovudine therapy in AIDS. Q J Med 1993; 86:5–15.

14

Neurological Complications of HTLV-I Infection

Walter Royal III
Johns Hopkins University School of Medicine, Baltimore, Maryland

INTRODUCTION

Human T-lymphotropic virus type I (HTLV-I), the first identified human retrovirus, was isolated in 1980 from a patient in the United States with mycosis fungoides, a cutaneous T-cell lymphoma, and later from a patient in Japan with acute T-cell leukemia/lymphoma (ATL). Five years later, researchers in Martinique and Japan reported that antibodies against HTLV-I could be demonstrated in serum and cerebrospinal fluid from patients in those regions with chronic myelopathy. The disorder, HTLV-I myelopathy, in Martinique, was referred to as tropical spastic paraparesis (TSP), and in Japan it is called HTLV-I–associated myelopathy (HAM). Subsequent DNA-sequencing data demonstrated that the viruses associated with these conditions were identical. The two diseases are clinically indistinguishable; therefore, HTLV-I myelopathy is frequently referred to as HAM/TSP.

EARLY CASES

The earliest record of cases of myelopathy in the Caribbean were reported by Cruickshank in Jamaica, who noted the occurrence of a chronic spastic paraplegia in residents of the island (1–3). The disorder, endemic TSP, was initially referred to as Jamaican neuropathy and was later grouped by Roman et al. with diseases referred to by the term *tropical myeloneuropathies* (4). The majority of cases of tropical myeloneuropathy are now known to have resulted from a number of distinct causes, including compressive, nutritional, neurodegenerative, and inflammatory etiologies. Endemic TSP occurred primarily in individuals of African descent and included diseases characterized by pyramidal tract weakness, bladder dysfunction, constipation, abnormal proprioception, and, in some individuals, retrobulbar optic neuropathy and auditory nerve dysfunction.

Similar cases of myelopathy had been also recognized for a number of years in Japan (5). Such patients were diagnosed with variant syndromes of spinal spastic paraparesis (SSP), either familial spinal spastic paraplegia or a disorder with features of primary lateral sclerosis. In 1975 the incidence of the SSP-like illness was reported by Osame et al. to be frequent among the Kagoshima Prefecture (3.25 cases per 100,000). The cases tended to occur in clusters and were characterized by a slow, progressive clinical course, prominent pyramidal weakness and spasticity, and slight sphincter and sensory abnormalities. In 1985, Gessain et al. reported the presence of antibodies against HTLV-I in the CSF and blood from a large percentage of patients with TSP in the French West Indies (6). The following year, Osame et al. reported that ATL-like cells can be demonstrated in CSF from patients with SSP and that a large percentage of SSP patients were also infected with HTLV-I (7).

VIROLOGY

HTLV-I is a type C retrovirus belonging to the subfamily, Onconaviridae (8). The virus infects cells, and, after release of the RNA into the cytoplasm, the RNA is converted to double-stranded DNA through the activity of the Mg^{2+}-activated, RNA-dependent DNA polymerase (reverse transcriptase). The double-stranded DNA is then integrated into the host cell DNA as a result of functions involving structures at the 5′ and 3′ ends of the viral genome, the long terminal repeat

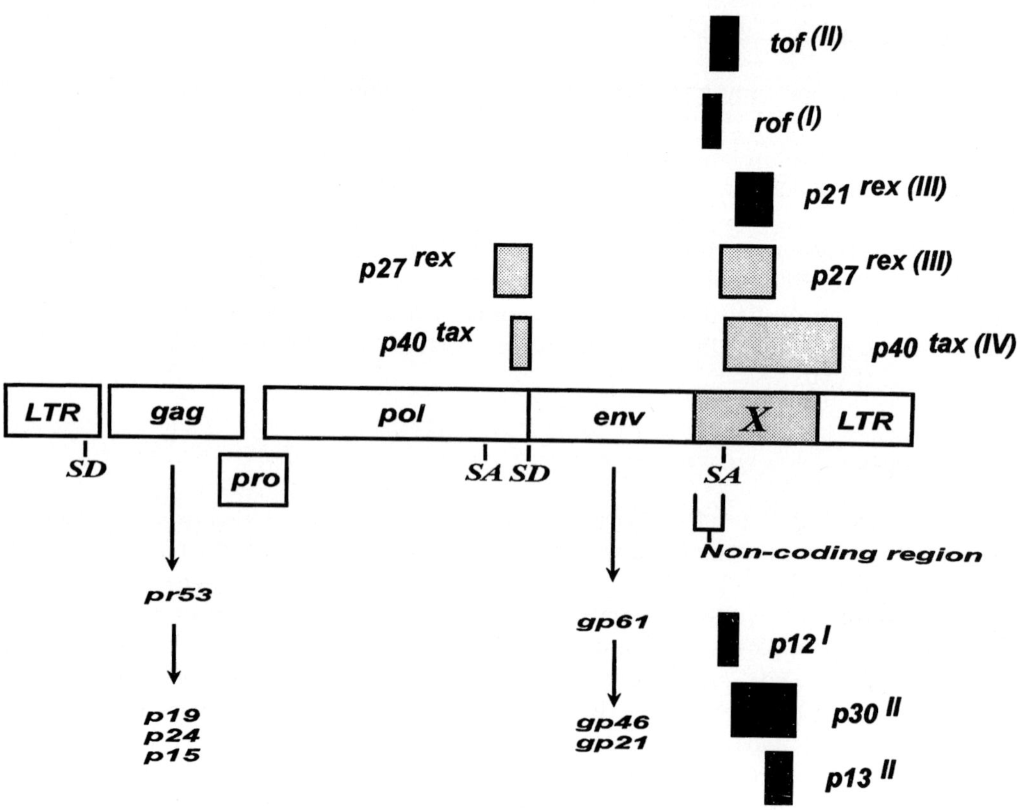

Figure 1 HTLV-I genomic organization and the respective gene products.

(LTR). The LTR also contain promoters for viral gene expression, which occurs through the action of several regulatory proteins and the reverse transcriptase.

The genomic organization of the virus is similar to that for other retroviruses with structural, or *gag* (group-specific antigen), *pol* (polymerase), and *env* (envelope) coding regions. The *gag* gene codes for a 53 kDa precursor protein (p53), which is cleaved into the p15, p19, and p24 core proteins (Fig. 1). The surface and transmembrane glycoproteins, gp46 and gp21, respectively, are produced by cleavage of the glycoprotein precursor, gp61, which is encoded by the *env* gene (9). The *pol* gene codes for the reverse transcriptase. Between the *env* region and the 3′ LTR is the *pX* region. The *pX* region contains four open reading frames, initially named x-I, x-II, x-III, and x-IV, which code for the major regulatory proteins, $p40^{tax}$(tax) and $p27^{rex}$ (rex), and minor proteins, $p21^{rex}$, tof, and rof and more recently identified proteins, $p12^{I}$, $p13^{II}$, and $p30^{III}$ (10–20).

Tax activates the transcription of specific viral and cellular genes resulting in efficient replication of virus and transformation of the infected cell. Increased levels of rex inhibit the expression of viral genes that code for HTLV-I regulatory proteins while increasing expression of viral structural proteins, resulting in production of progeny virus. $p12^{I}$ may be important in cell transformation by HTLV-I, as suggested by the fact that it enhances the transforming activity of the bovine papillomavirus E5 oncoprotein (14). The various functions of the other proteins encoded by the *pX* region are less clearly defined at this time.

The proviral LTR contains three cyclic AMP (cAMP) response elements (CRE), which bind complexes formed by tax and a family of proteins that include the cAMP response element binding protein (CREB), activation transcription factor (ATF), and CREB/ATF heterodimers (21). Gene transcription can be stimulated through the action of cyclic AMP and the phorbol ester, 12-O-tetradecanoylphorbol-13-acetate (TPA) on the viral LTR (22).

PATHOGENESIS

The induction of cellular gene activation by tax may be directly related to the occurrence of abnormalities associated with HTLV-I infection, including damage to nervous system tissue and neurological impairment. The products of these genes include the cytokines interleukin-2 (IL-2), IL-3, IL-4, and GM-CSF (granulocyte-monocyte colony-stimulating factor), IL-2R-α (the alpha chain of the interleukin-2 receptor), a factor responsible for the development of hypercalcemia, PTHrP (parathyroid hormone–related protein), TNF-α (tumor necrosis factor alpha), and TGF-β (transforming growth factor beta), the proto-oncogenes c-fos, c-jun, and c-egr, and MHC class 1 (23–25). Tax induction of NF κ-B and related proteins can also activate *cis*-acting elements in the human immunodeficiency virus LTR (26).

Immune cells infected by HTLV-I include CD4+ T-helper and CD8+ T-cytotoxic/suppressor cells and macrophages in the peripheral blood and microglia in the central nervous system. About 10–15% of peripheral blood lymphocytes from patients with HTLV-I myelopathy are infected with HTLV-I with polyclonal integration of virus (27). Lymphocytes from HTLV-I–infected patients with HTLV-I myelopathy also demonstrate greater spontaneous proliferation than subjects with asymptomatic infection or seronegative individuals due to, at least in part, increased expression of the IL-2 receptor (28,29). In these individuals, absolute numbers of CD4+ lymphocytes are elevated. Normal CD4+/CD8+ ratios are maintained due to proliferation of CD8+ lymphocytes, as well. However, these cells respond poorly to stimulation with phytohemagglutinin, pokeweed mitogen, and concanavalin A, suggesting that infection causes a functional immune impairment (29).

Cytotoxic lymphocytes can be demonstrated in blood and CSF from HTLV-I–infected subjects. These cells are HLA class I–restricted, CD8+, and specific for *pX* region gene products (30,31). A high frequency of these HTLV-I–specific cytotoxic lymphocytes is found in both cerebrospinal fluid and blood from patients with HTLV-I myelopathy and at greater numbers than for subjects with ATL or with asymptomatic infection (27,30,32,33). Using specific probes to detect tax in peripheral blood mononuclear cells from HTLV-I–infected subjects, it has been demonstrated that levels of tax proviral DNA expression is also higher for HTLV-I myelopathy patients than for patients with ATL and asymptomatic carriers (34). Among subjects with myelopathy and elevated lymphocyte tax proviral DNA levels, measurements were highest for those with earlier onset of symptoms as compared to those with later disease onset. In contrast, tax mRNA levels in infected lymphocytes are similar for myelopathy patients and asymptomatic carriers (35). Therefore, increased numbers of HTLV-I–specific cytotoxic blood and CSF lymphocytes and increased cellular integration of HTLV-I genome are found in patients with myelopathy as compared to subjects with ATL or infected individuals with no symptoms.

Human cerebellar and astroglial brain tumor cell explants, neuroblastoma and glioma cell lines, and microglial cell cultures have been demonstrated to be susceptible to infection by HTLV-I (36–39). Virus particles can be seen in spinal cord from patients with HTLV-I myelopathy using electron microscopy (40), and HTLV-I proviral DNA can be demonstrated in cerebrospinal fluid inflammatory cells (41,42). Using the polymerase chain reaction (PCR) assay, proviral DNA can be detected in DNA extracted from spinal cord obtained from patients with myelopathy and localized to tissue inflammatory cells using immunocytochemical stains for HTLV-I envelope glycoprotein and core protein (31,34,43,44). Inflammatory cells present in such infiltrates can be demonstrated to express restricted V-beta CD3 motifs that have been also identified in patients with multiple sclerosis and laboratory animals with experimental allergic encephalomyelitis (45). Virus can also be detected in astrocytes using in situ hybridization with pX region-specific probes (31,46).

It has been postulated that the occurrence of HTLV-I myelopathy in infected individuals may be related to *pX* region heterogeneity among virus strains, resulting in mutations in tax and, less frequently, rex (34,47,48). In patients from Tumaco, Columbia, tax-associated mutations were found in proviral DNA from all of 14 seropositive residents with myelopathy, in 5 of 14 patients in Japan, and in 8 of 11 in other regions of the world. In contrast, the tax-related mutations were found in proviral DNA from 2 of 21 patients without HTLV-I myelopathy from areas outside of Tumaco (48).

EPIDEMIOLOGY

Transmission of HTLV-I can occur as a result of sexual contact with an infected individual, due to sharing of contaminated needles and syringes by injection drug users, following transfusion of contaminated blood products, and by passage from mother to child. There are several known instances of transmission of HTLV-I infection among family members (49,50). Transfusion-related HTLV-I infection, first described in the early 1980s, most frequently occurs secondary to the transfusion of cellular products. Routine screening of donors in the United States was implemented in 1988, and the current risk of transfusion-associated HTLV-I infection in the United States is less than 1 in 50,000 (51).

The distribution of HTLV-I infection is worldwide, with cases concentrated along the tropical band that includes sub-Saharan Africa (52,53), South America (54,55), the Caribbean basin (56), and southern Japan (57) (Fig. 2). Cases have been also reported in diverse regions, such as in Western Europe and Canada among West Indian immigrants (58–60), in Australia and the Seychelles (61), and in the Middle East (62,63). In the United States, the greatest prevalence of HTLV-I infection is in the southeastern region (64). A lower prevalence of infection has been found in other regions of the United States, and the infection was recently reported among a small group of Alaskan Natives (65).

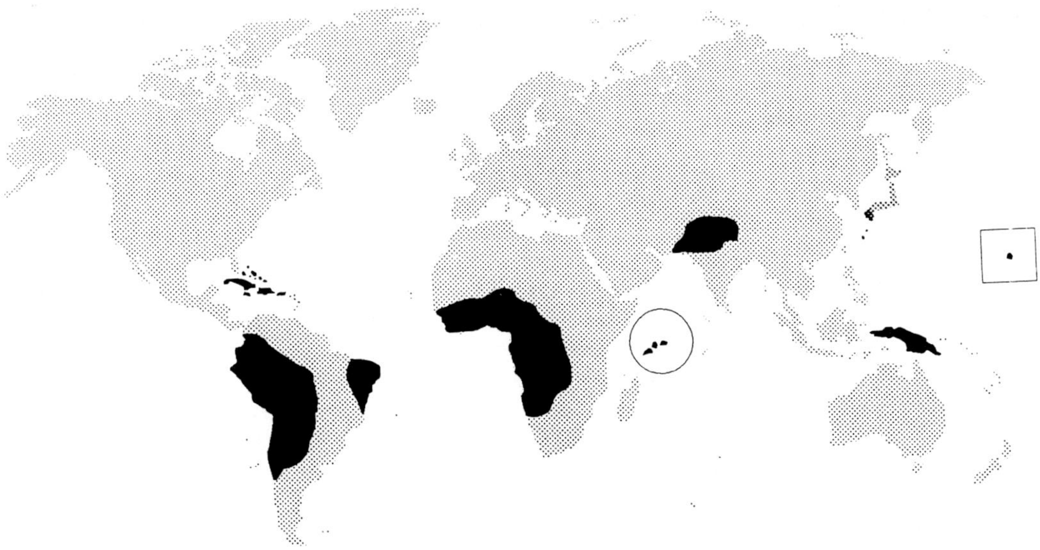

Figure 2 **Worldwide distribution of HTLV-I infection. Regions of high incidence of endemic infection are shaded. Circle: Seychelles; rectangle: Hawaii. (Adapted from Ref. 65a.)**

Between 1985 and 1986, 6.1% of 13,260 subjects tested in Jamaica were found to be seropositive for HTLV-I infection, predominantly older individuals and those of African descent (66). In Japan, surveys of blood donors between the ages of 40 and 64 years in 1984 demonstrated a seroprevalence for HTLV-I infection that ranged between 0.3 and 8.0% for prefectures on the mainland, with the highest incidence in the southwestern region of the country (67). Among the seven islands of the Yaeyama prefecture near southwestern Okinawa, the prevalence of infected donors ranged between 6.2 and 21.2%. With the introduction of mass screening of blood products at blood centers, the seroconversion rate among transfusion recipients showed a dramatic decrease (68–70).

Based on national surveys conducted in Japan between 1986 and 1988 performed by Kaplan et al. (71), the lifetime risk of developing HTLV-I myelopathy following infection at birth is approximately 0.25%, with a median age of onset of about 55 years and a range of 5–80 years of age. The lifetime risk of developing ATL has been estimated to be about 2–4% for residents of both Japan and Jamaica (72,73). The mortality data for HTLV-I–infected individuals without ATL are conflicting. Among 1997 community-based volunteers followed by Iwata et al. for 5.3 years with annual medical examinations, the mortality was about 1.9 times that for seronegative subjects (74). In contrast, the death rate for 3991 voluntary blood donors followed for 2.7 years was similar to that for an infected group (75).

CLINICAL MANIFESTATIONS

Clinical abnormalities secondary to HTLV-I infection may occur secondary to involvement of various areas of the nervous system (Table 1). However, less than 2% of HTLV-1–infected carriers will develop symptoms of any type from the infection. The occurrence of ATL secondary to adult infection has not been reported. A large percentage of patients with ATL develop neurological complications, which, in the majority of cases, are due to direct tumor cell invasion. These complications include altered consciousness, which may be related to hypercalcemia,

Table 1 Guidelines for the Diagnosis of HTLV-I Myelopathy

Clinical Criteria: The florid clinical picture of chronic spastic paraparesis is not always seen when the patient first presents. A single symptom or physical sign may be the only evidence of early HAM/TSP.

Age and sex incidence	Mostly sporadic and adult, but sometimes familial, occasionally seen in childhood; females predominant.
Onset	This is usually insidious but may be sudden.
Main neurological manifestations	Chronic spastic paraparesis, which usually progresses slowly, sometimes remains static after initial progression.
	Weakness of the lower limbs, more marked proximally.
	Sensory symptoms such as tingling, pins and needles, burning, etc. are more prominent than objective physical signs.
	Low lumbar pain with radiation to the legs is common.
	Vibration sense is frequently impaired, proprioception less often affected.
	Hyperreflexia of the lower limbs, and positive Hoffman's and Trömner's signs frequent; weakness may be absent.
	Exaggerated jaw jerk in some patients.
Other possible neurological manifestations	Muscular atrophy; fasciculation (rare); polymyositis; peripheral neuropathy; polyradiculopathy; cranial neuropathy; meningitis; encephalopathy.
Less frequent neurological findings	Cerebellar signs; optic atrophy; deafness, nystagmus; other cranial nerve deficits; hand tremor; absent or depressed ankle jerk.
	Convulsions, cognitive impairment, dementia, or impaired consciousness are rare.
Possible systemic nonneurological manifestations	Pulmonary alveolitis; uveitis; Sjögren's syndrome; arthropathy; vasculitis, ichthyoses; cryoglobulinemia; monoclonal gammopathy; adult T-cell leukemia/lymphoma.
Laboratory diagnosis	Presence of HTLV-I antibodies or antigens in blood and cerebrospinal fluid (CSF).
	CSF may show mild lymophocyte pleocytosis.
	Lobulated lymphocytes may be present in blood and/or CSF.
	Mild to moderate increase of protein may be present in CSF.
	Viral isolation when possible from blood and/or CSF.

Source: Ref. 65.

dementia, seizures, hemiparesis and pyramidal tract signs, cranial nerve deficits, meningeal irritation, and polyneuropathy.

In addition to HTLV-I myelopathy and ATL, HTLV-I infection has also been associated with a spectrum of systemic inflammatory disorders (Table 1). Patients may develop optic and eighth nerve involvement with impairment of vision and optic atrophy, tinnitus and decreased hearing, peripheral sensory and motor neuropathies, and polymyositis. Involvement of areas outside the nervous system may result in pneumonitis, iritis, hypothyroidism or hyperthyroidism, arthritis, and inflammation of the lacrimal and salivary glands, the latter resulting in symptoms similar to those seen in Sjögren's syndrome. Similar to what has been observed in patients with myelopathy, elevated levels of specific proviral DNA can be detected in infected peripheral blood lymphocytes from individuals with autoimmune complications (34).

Myelopathy

Among HTLV-I–seropositive individuals in Japan, the prevalence of HTLV-I myelopathy is less than 0.1%. HTLV-I has been observed to occur most frequently between the ages of 35 and 45 and to have a higher incidence in females than males by a ratio of about 2–3:1 (70,71). The disease latency for HTLV-I myelopathy following perinatal infection has been observed to be about 20–30 years. An earlier onset of disease has been noted in patients with transfusion-associated disease (76), perhaps due to the intravenous administration of a larger viral load. Rarely, HTLV-I myelopathy occurs in patients coincident with ATL (77–81). A possible explanation for the rare co-existence of the two diseases may be the existence of a genetic susceptibility for the development of either HTLV-I myelopathy or ATL (28).

The onset of symptoms is gradual in the majority of patients. Occasionally the clinical signs may be sudden and gradually progressive, rarely associated with acute relapses. Motor signs predominate in patients with HTLV-I myelopathy and are characterized by pyramidal tract weakness, spasticity, hyperreflexia, and bladder dysfunction (Table 1). Hyporeflexia in the ankles may suggest the presence of a nutritional distal neuropathy. Sensory abnormalities, including evidence of posterior column dysfunction, occur less frequently than motor impairment and primarily consist of numbness and paresthesias of the lower extremities. A thoracic sensory level tends to be poorly defined or not present. Cerebellar ataxia and upper extremity tremor may be seen in a small percentage of patients. The rate of progression of motor impairment tends to be variable. Among a group of patients who were followed for a mean duration of 6.5 years after onset of HTLV-I myelopathy, 40% maintained independent ambulation ability, 35% required unilateral support (e.g., use of a cane or single crutch), and 25% were dependent on bilateral support or a wheelchair (82).

Myelopathy has been documented in patients co-infected with HTLV-I and the human immunodeficiency virus type 1 (HIV-1) (83–86). In these cases, clinical disease was found to be due to HTLV-I based on serological studies, which demonstrated the presence of intrathecal synthesis of HTLV-I–specific antibody, and polymerase chain reaction assay results. Such patients may appear to be immunocompetent due to HTLV-I–induced lymphoproliferation. However, as stated previously, high CD4+ lymphocyte counts in these individuals do not function normally, as assessed by responses to mitogen stimulation (29). In addition, blood mononuclear cell fractions from such patients demonstrate impaired natural killer cell activity (87,88).

The lower thoracic cord generally shows the most severe involvement, containing the most advanced lesions. Lesions at an earlier stage tend to be located in the upper thoracic and cervical regions. Myelin staining of disease spinal cord from infected patients reveal pallor of the lateral funiculi due to inflammatory demyelination, especially in the lateral pyramidal tract (Fig. 3a). The posterior funiculi can also show severe involvement, but generally the neuropathological abnormalities in this area are mild. Abnormalities may be also seen in the anterior funiculi, primarily in the thoracic cord and with more irregular involvement (89). Tissue infiltrates are located primarily around venules (Fig. 3b,c) and consist of mainly T cells, macrophages, and microglial cells. B cells may be seen around larger vessels and in subarachnoid regions; the subarachnoid space may contain plasma cells and T cells (Fig. 3d). In early lesions, there is generally sparing of neuronal populations and intact axons. Chronic lesions reveal degeneration and loss of both myelin and axons with relatively little inflammation noted within the lesions, resulting in a spongiform appearance to the tissue. The vascular adventitia may also be thickened and hyaline changes noted within small vessels (89).

Myopathy

An inflammatory myopathy, or polymyositis, has also been reported with HTLV-I infection (90–92). Patients present with diffuse muscle tenderness and proximal muscle weakness. The weakness more severely involves the lower extremities and may be difficult to distinguish from myelopathic weakness. The serum creatine kinase is elevated in patients with HTLV-I–associated

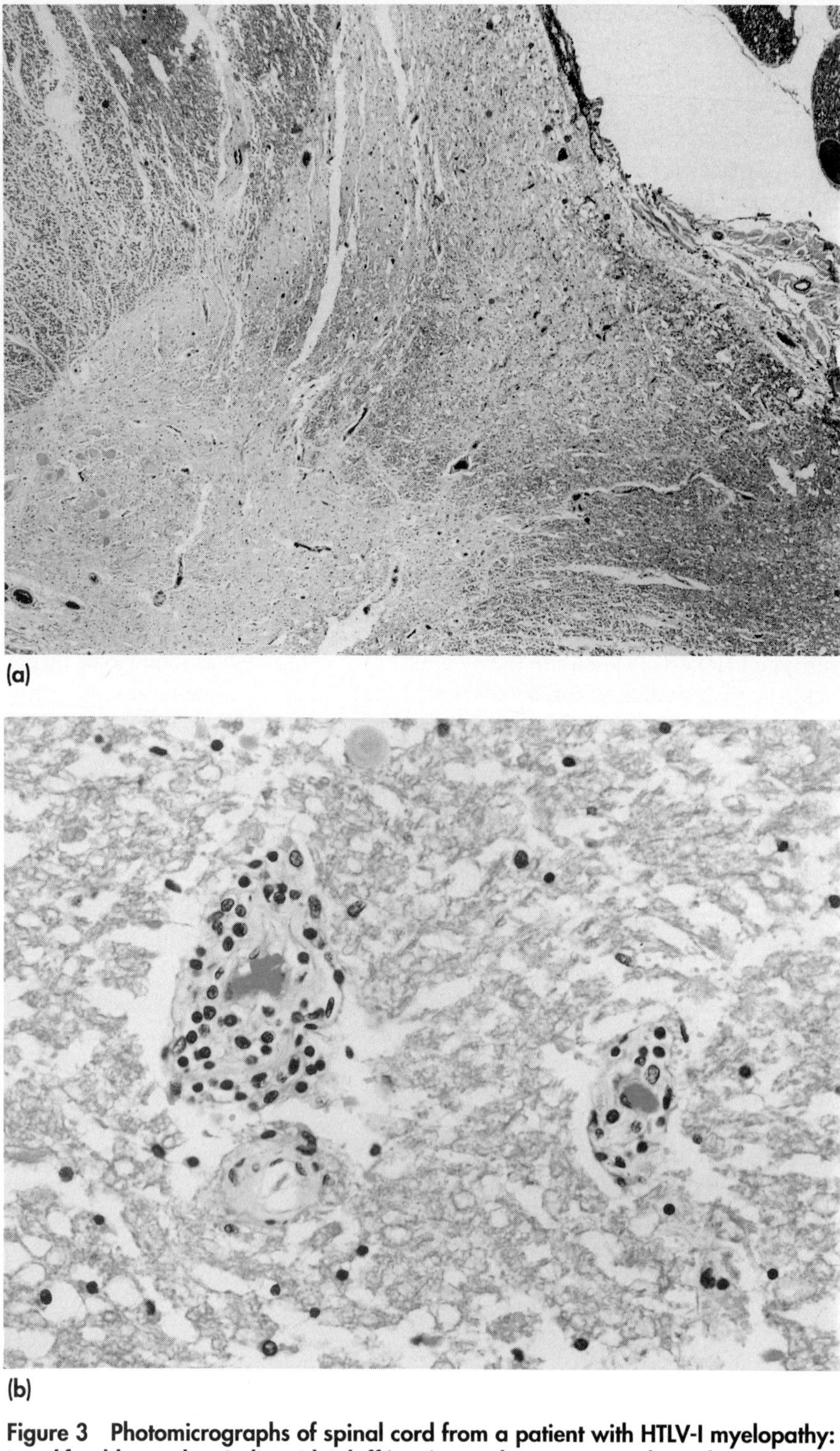

Figure 3 Photomicrographs of spinal cord from a patient with HTLV-I myelopathy: (a) stained with Luxol fast blue and periodic acid-Schiff (PAS) stain demonstrating demyelination of the lateral column;

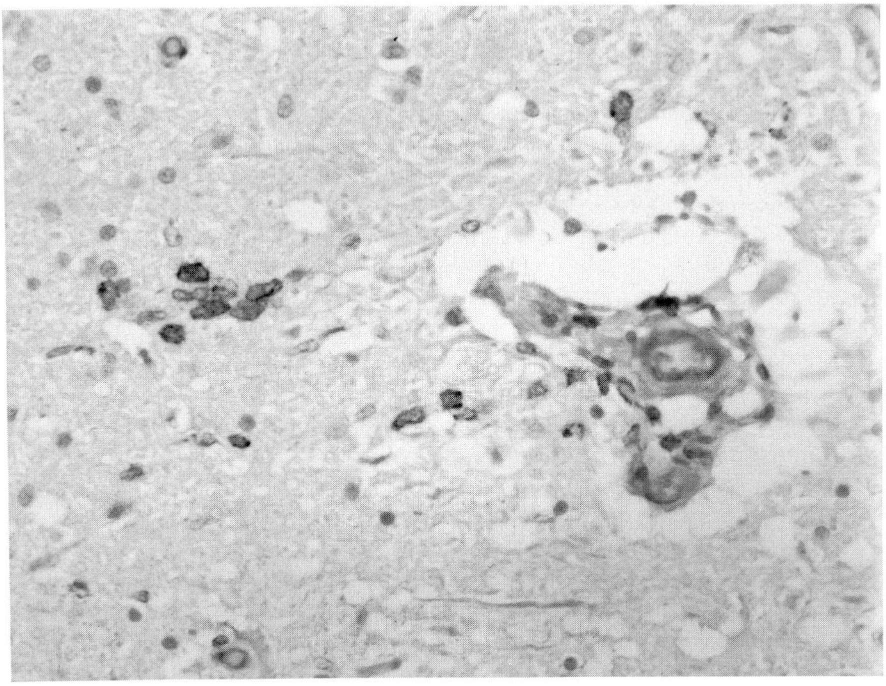

(c)

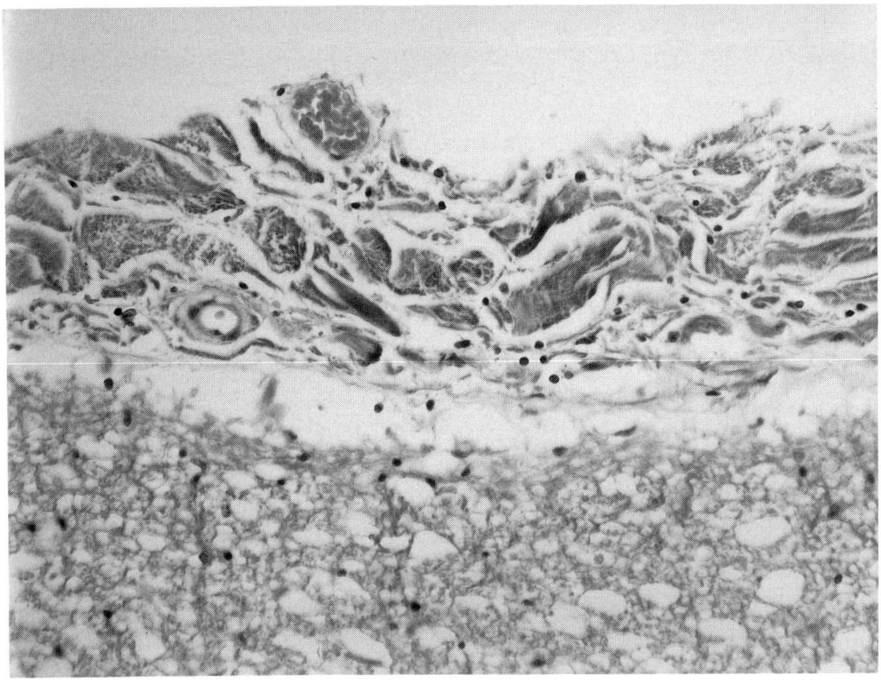

(d)

(b) mononuclear cell perivascular cuffs around spinal cord vessels; (c) positive staining of T cells in cuffs by immunoperoxidase with monoclonal anti-CD3 antibody; (d) thickened leptomeninges with scattered lymphocytes. (Courtesy of Dr. David Katz, National Institutes of Health.)

polymyositis, in some cases greater than 2000 U/liter. Electrophysiological studies demonstrate abnormalities consistent with muscle irritability with increased insertional activity, positive sharp waves, and fibrillation potentials. Patients typically show improvement in muscle strength and a decrease in serum creatine kinase levels in response to treatment with high-dose steroids (methyl-prednisone 1.0 g intravenously per day) followed by lower equivalent doses of oral prednisone. However, following the initiation of maintenance doses of corticosteroids, myopathic symptoms and muscle enzyme elevation often return.

Histologically the tissue may demonstrate type 2 fiber atrophy, a mixed mononuclear infiltrate (Fig. 4) comprised of primarily cytotoxic (CD8+) T lymphocytes in perivascular, interstitial, and endomysial regions with fascicular atrophy, muscle fiber necrosis, phagocytosis, and mixed fiber–type degeneration (93). Pathological specimens may also show noninflammatory myopathic changes (93). HTLV-I has been isolated from muscle of a patient with HTLV-I infection, and in a patient co-infected with human immunodeficiency virus type I (HIV-1) and HTLV-I, HTLV-I tax protein could be demonstrated histologically in muscle fibers, suggesting direct infection of muscle by HTLV-I in this case (92).

Motor Neuron Disease

Cases of an amyotrophic lateral sclerosis (ALS)–like syndrome have been reported both in the Caribbean and in Japan (94,95). These patients have wasting of the intrinsic hand muscles and proximal muscles of the upper extremities with no evidence of a primary sensory abnormality. Nerve conduction velocity studies show delayed motor and normal sensory nerve velocities.

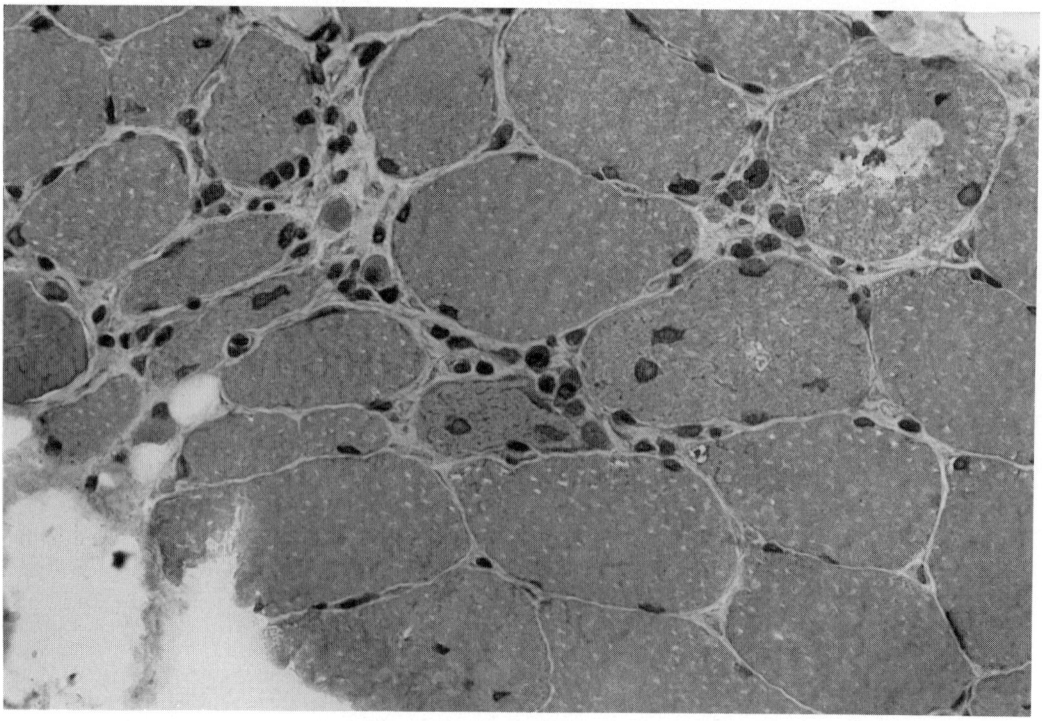

Figure 4 Muscle biopsy from a 64-year-old Jamaican woman with HTLV-I myelopathy and polymyositis. The specimen contains focal and diffuse mononuclear inflammatory infiltrates.

F-waves may be normal, though motor nerve conduction studies may suggest proximal motor nerve or anterior horn cell involvement (95,96). Denervation, fasciculation potentials, and giant motor unit potentials are seen on electromyography. On muscle biopsy, angular fibers and grouped atrophy may be seen.

LABORATORY STUDIES

Cerebrospinal Fluid and Serological Tests

Routine cerebrospinal fluid laboratory studies may reveal a pleocytosis comprised of mononuclear cells and an elevated protein concentration. Oligoclonal bands can be demonstrated in most patients. Infection with HTLV-I is made by serological tests, which include enzyme-linked immunosorbent assays, particle agglutination, and Western blot assays. High antibody titers to HTLV-I can be detected in blood and cerebrospinal fluid of patients with HTLV-I myelopathy using enzyme immunoassays and on Western blot (Fig. 5) with evidence of intrathecal synthesis of anti–HTLV-I antibodies (97,98). In about half of the patients studied, approximately 1% of

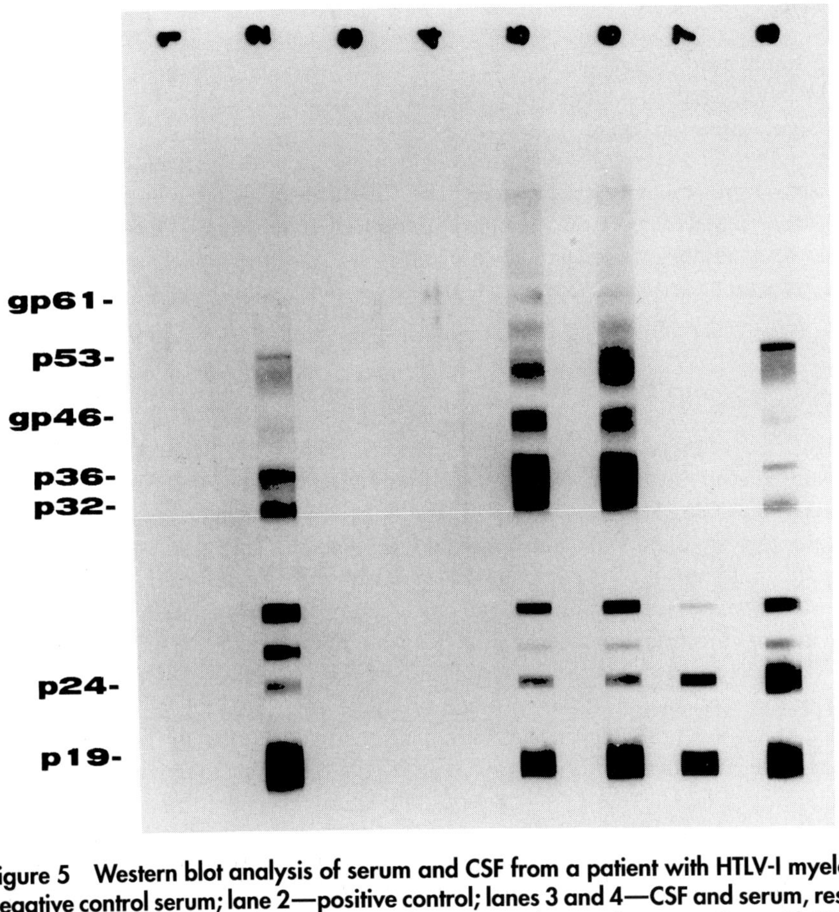

Figure 5 Western blot analysis of serum and CSF from a patient with HTLV-I myelopathy: lane 1—negative control serum; lane 2—positive control; lanes 3 and 4—CSF and serum, respectively, from a patient with multiple sclerosis; lanes 5 and 6—CSF and serum from a patient with HTLV-I myelopathy; lanes 7 and 8—CSF and serum samples from a patient co-infected with HTLV-I and HIV-1.

peripheral blood lymphocytes may have lobulated nuclei (ATL-like cells) (99), which can also be demonstrated in CSF (87).

Electrophysiology

Individuals with HTLV-I myelopathy may demonstrate abnormalities on electroencephalography (EEG), visual, auditory, and somatosensory evoked potential studies, and on nerve conduction and electromyographic testing. EEG abnormalities include diffuse background slowing and theta bursts with or without spikes. These findings have not been observed to correlate with the duration or severity of myelopathy or with cerebrospinal fluid antibody titers against HTLV-I. Somatosensory evoked potential (SSEP) studies show abnormalities more frequently than the visual and auditory studies (100). Latencies in the lower extremity SSEP tend to be prolonged more frequently than in the upper extremities (96,101). Imaging studies performed on individuals with abnormal auditory event-related potential abnormalities may demonstrate evidence of brain atrophy (102). Nerve conduction velocity studies may show delays in the F responses, and electromyography may reveal evidence of chronic denervation with high-amplitude motor unit potentials, which may be nonspecific or consistent with either a myeloradiculopathy or anterior horn cell disease.

Radiology

MR studies of the spinal cord of patients with HTLV-I myelopathy have been reported to show swelling or atrophy in up to half of patients (60). Magnetic resonance imaging (MRI) of the brain may reveal high-signal areas in white matter regions on T_2-weighted images (103,104). The lesions may be discrete or confluent and tend not to be contiguous with the lateral ventricles. In some cases, brainstem lesions may be seen as well. The abnormal areas in the brain may appear similar to plaques seen on MRI scans from patients with multiple sclerosis (105). However, when T_2-weighted MRI examinations on such patients are assessed using stringent criteria, the lesions in the majority of cases are found not to be consistent with the radiographic diagnosis of multiple sclerosis (103).

HUMAN T-LYMPHOTROPIC VIRUS TYPE II

HTLV-II was identified after being isolated from two patients with T-hairy-cell leukemia (106,107). It was subsequently determined that HTLV-II infection was not typical for the disease, and although the virus has been also recovered from patients with various leukemic syndromes, there is still no definite systemic disease entity linked with the virus infection (108,109). In the United States, endemic infection is found among Amerindian populations (110,111). Transmission of HTLV-II occurs as a result of transfusion of blood products and intimate sexual contact, and the infection is found among injection drug users and patients attending sexually transmitted disease clinics (112,113). The most frequent mode of transmission of HTLV-II infection is by exposure to infected blood or blood products. HTLV-II is found more frequently than HTLV-I in donated blood in the United States in all regions, except for in the South Atlantic and the Northeast (114).

The HTLV-II genome is about 60% homologous with HTLV-I (26), and the two viruses can be distinguished by type-specific enzyme immunoassays and using the polymerase chain reaction assay. There are known to be two molecular strains of HTLV-II, designated as strains A and B. Strain A viruses are found among North American non-Amerindian groups and strain B among Paleo-Amerindian groups, which include the Seminole in Florida, Guaymi in Panama, and the Toba, Chorote, and Chalupe in Argentina (115,116). Among these strains, a greater molecular diversity has been noted to exist for strain B than for strain A virus. The relationship between virus strain variations and the frequency and type of disease is unclear at this time.

The occurrence of a myelopathy that is indistinguishable from HTLV-I myelopathy has been described in several HTLV-II–infected patients who presented with lower extremity weakness, spasticity, urinary disturbance, and mild sensory complaints (117–119). HTLV-II infection was also found among two Amerindian sisters with an olivopontocerebellar atrophy variant and multisystem atrophy (120). Several cases of myelopathy have been reported in patients co-infected with HIV-1 (83). As stated previously, because of the presence of HTLV infection, these individuals may develop myelopathy in the setting of elevated CD4+ blood lymphocyte numbers. This is in contrast to the more common HIV-1–related spinal cord disorder, vacuolar degeneration (121), which typically occurs in the setting of significant immunosuppression characterized by decreased CD4+ lymphocyte numbers.

DIFFERENTIAL DIAGNOSIS

Since clinical abnormalities secondary to HTLV-I infection occur with very low frequency, patients should be evaluated for other potential diagnoses. The clinical and pathological abnormalities that occur in individuals with myelopathy are similar to those seen due to subacute combined degeneration, and, therefore, serum B_{12} levels should be measured. All patients should be tested for infection with HIV-1, both because the usual routes of transmission of infection by these viruses are identical and because co-infection may be associated with an increased risk for the development of spinal cord disease, peripheral neuropathy, and myopathy (64,122).

Patients should be evaluated with a cranial MRI for focal parenchymal abnormalities, such as mass lesions or ischemic areas, that may be responsible for the observed neurological symptoms. Imaging of the cervical, thoracic, and lumbar spine with MRI or myelography combined with computerized tomography may reveal spondylosis, which may also present with signs of spinal cord compression. Transmission of syphilis infection also typically occurs as a result of intimate sexual contact and may be associated with myelopathy, cranial neuropathies, and parenchymal brain lesions. Therefore, patients with known HTLV-I infection should be screened for syphilis infection with a rapid plasma reagin (RPR) test, and if the result is positive a fluorescent treponemal antibody (FTA) test in blood and a venereal disease research laboratory (VDRL) test in CSF should be obtained.

Other possible causes of myelopathy should be considered in patients with a history of injection drug use. These include vasculitis, presumably related to the injection of adulterants, and cervical trauma. Nitrous oxide use is a potential cause of myelopathy due to direct inactivation of vitamin B_{12} by the drug (123). Spinal cord damage may also result from the effects of the drug iodochlohrydroxquinoline (Chloroquinol) and from toxins such as the cresol phosphates. Parainfectious causes (enterovirus, mumps, and, in unvaccinated individuals, mumps, measles, and rubella) or idiopathic demyelination of the brain and spinal cord, mitochondrial encephalomyelopathy, and paraneoplastic syndromes due to bronchogenic carcinoma or lymphoma are other diagnostic possibilities.

TREATMENT

A number of immunosuppressive and immunomodulating therapies have been used to treat patients with ATL, and some of these approaches have been demonstrated to have short-term efficacy in the treatment of patients with HTLV-I myelopathy. Patients treated with plasmapheresis have been reported to show evidence of improved motor function associated with lower serum anti–HTLV-I antibody titers (124). In these patients, no change in specific antibody titers were seen in CSF. Similar improvement may occur following treatment with corticosteroids administered alone or in combination with other immunosuppressive agents (125,126). However, MRI abnormalities were noted to progress in a group of patients that demonstrated clinical improvement following treatment with high doses of oral corticosteroids (127). Administration of the anabolic steroid danazol has been associated with improvement in lower extremity weakness and bladder function (128,129). The drug zidovudine (3′-azidothymidine; AZT) has been used in the treatment of patients with HTLV-I myelopathy (130,131). However, no long-term benefit has been documented following initiation of treatment with this drug.

Lymphocytes infected with HTLV-I overexpress the IL-2-β (TAC) receptor, which has been associated with spontaneous proliferation of these cells. Studies are currently underway in which patients are administered monoclonal antibodies against the receptor. Such antibodies tagged with radioactive yttrium has been proven to be effective in eradicating malignant cells in patients with ATL (132). However, since activated immune cells normally express TAC expressing IL-2-β receptor, this therapy may potentially lead to the destruction of uninfected cell populations and result in significant impairment of specific immune responses (133).

REFERENCES

1. Cruikshank EK. A neuropathic syndrome of uncertain origin. West Indian Med J 1956; 5:147.
2. Montgomery RD, Cruikshank EK. Clinical and pathological observations on Jamaican neuropathy, a report on 206 cases. Brain 1964; 87:425.
3. Rogers PEB. The clinical features and etiology of the neuropathic syndrome in Jamaica. West Indian Med J 1965; 14:36.
4. Roman GC, Spencer PS, Schoenberg BS. Tropical myeloneuropathies: the hidden endemics. Neurology 1985; 35:1158–1170.
5. Osame M, Igata A. The history of discovery and clinico-epidemiology of HTLV-I-associated myelopathy (HAM). Jpn J Med 1989; 28:412–444.
6. Gessain A, Barin F, Vernant JC, Gout O, Maurs L, Calender A, de Thë G. Antibodies to human T-lymphotropic virus type-I in patients with tropical spastic paraparesis. Lancet 1985; 2:407–410.
7. Osame M, Usuku K, Izumo S, Ijichi N, Amitani H, Igata A, Matsumoto M, Tara M. HTLV-I associated myelopathy, a new clinical entity. Lancet 1986; 1:1031–1102.
8. Poiesz BJ, Ruscetti FW, Gazdar AF, Bunn PA, Minna JD, Gallo RC. Detection and isolation of type C retrovirus particles from fresh and cultured lymphocytes of a patient with cutaneous T-cell lymphoma. Proc Natl Acad Sci USA 1980; 77:7415–7419.
9. Seiki M, Hattori S, Yoshida M. Human adult T-cell leukemia virus: molecular cloning of the provirus DNA and the unique terminal structure. Proc Natl Acad Sci USA 1982; 79:6899–6902.
10. Sodroski J. The human T-cell leukemia virus (HTLV) transactivator (Tax) protein. Biochim Biophys Acta 1992; 1114:19–29.
11. Kiyokawa T, Seiki M, Iwashita S, Imagawa K, Shimizu F, Yoshida M. p27x-III and p21x-III, proteins encoded by the pX sequence of human T-cell leukemia virus type I. Proc Natl Acad Sci USA 1985; 82:8359–8363.
12. Hidaka M, Inoue J, Yoshida M, Seiki M. Post-transcriptional regulator (rex) of HTLV-1 initiates expression of virus structural proteins but suppresses expression of regulatory proteins. EMBO J 1988; 7:519–523.
13. Koralnik IJ, Fullen J, Franchini G. The p12I, p13II, and p30II proteins encoded by human T-cell leukemia/lymphoma virus type I open reading frames I and II are localized in three different cellular compartments. J Virol 1993; 67:2360–2366.
14. Franchini G, Mulloy JC, Koralnik EJ, Monico AL, Sparkowski JJ, Andresson T, Goldstein DJ, Schlegel R. The human T-cell leukemia/lymphoma virus type I p12I protein cooperates with the E5

oncoprotein of bovine papillomavirus in cell transformation and binds the 16-kilodalton subunit of the vacuolar H+ ATPase. J Virol 1993; 67:7701–7704.
15. Inoue J-I, Yoshida M, Seiki M. Transcriptional (p40x) and post-transcriptional (p27x-III) regulators are required for the expression and replication of human T-cell leukemia virus type I genes. Proc Natl Acad Sci USA 1987; 84:3653–3657.
16. Ciminale V, Pavlakis GN, Derse D, Funningham CP, Felber BK. Complex splicing in the human T-cell leukemia virus (HTLV) family of retroviruses: novel mRNAs and proteins produced by HTLV type I. J Virol 1992; 66:1737–1745.
17. Sodroski JG, Rosen CA, Haseltine WA. Transacting transcriptional activation of the long terminal repeat of human T lymphotropic viruses in infected cells. Science 1994; 226:177–179.
18. Fujisawa J, Seiki M, Kiyokawa T, Yoshida Y. Functional activation of long terminal repeat of human T-cell leukemia virus type I by trans-activator. Proc Natl Acad Sci USA 1985; 82:2277–2281.
19. Felber BK, Paskalis H, Kleinman-Ewing C, Wong-Staal R, Pavlakis GN. The pX protein of HTLV-I is a transcriptional activator of its long terminal repeats. Science 1985; 229:675–679.
20. Yoshida M. Host-HTLV Type I interaction at the molecular level. AIDS Res Hum Retroviruses 1994; 10:1193–1197.
21. Zhao LJ, Giam CZ. Human T-cell lymphotropic virus type I (HTLV-I) transcriptional activator, Tax, enhances CREB binding to HTLV-I 21-base-pair repeats by protein-protein interaction. Proc Natl Acad Sci USA 1992; 89:7070–7074.
22. Smith MR, Greene WC. Molecular biology of the type I human T-cell leukemia virus (HTLV-I) and adult T-cell leukemia. J Clin Invest 1991; 87:761–766.
23. Nicholas J, Nevins JR. Distinct DNA targets for trans-activation by HTLV-I tax and adenovirus EIA. Virology 1991; 182:156–167.
24. Ikeda K, Okazaki R, Inoue D, Ogata E, Matsumoto T. Transcription of the gene for parathyroid hormone-related peptide from the human is activated through a cAMP-dependent pathway by prostaglandin E1 in HTLV-I-infected T cells. J Biol Chem 1993; 268:1174–1179.
25. Sawada M, Suzumura A, Yoshida M, Marunouchi T. Human T-cell leukemia virus type I trans activator induces class I major histocompatibility complex antigen expression in glial cells. J Virol 1990; 64:4002–4406.
26. Sodroski JG, Rosen CA, Haseltine WA. Trans-acting transcriptional activation of the long terminal repair of human T lymphotropic viruses in infected cells. Science 1984; 225:381–385.
27. Jacobson S, Shida H, McFarlin DE, Fauci AS, Koenig S. Circulating CD8+ cytotoxic T lymphocytes specific for HTLV-I pX in patients with HTLV-I associated neurological disease. Nature 1990; 348: 245–258.
28. Usuku K, Sonoda S, Osame M, Yashiki S, Takahashi K, Matsumoto M, Sawada T, Tsuji K, Tara M, Igata A. HLA haplotype-linked high immune responsiveness against HTLV-I in HTLV-I-associated myelopathy: comparison with adult T-cell leukemia/lymphoma Ann Neurol 1988; 23(suppl):143–150.
29. Itoyama Y, Minato S, Goto I, Okochi K, Yamamoto N. Elevated serum antibody titers to Epstein-Barr virus in HTLV-I-associated myelopathy (HAM). Neurology 1988; 38:1650–1663.
30. Jacobson S, McFarlin DE, Robinson S, Voskuhl R, Martin R, Brewah A, Newell AJ, Koenig S. HTLV-I-specific cytotoxic T-lymphocytes in the cerebrospinal fluid of patients with HTLV-I-associated neurological disease. Ann Neurol 1992; 32:651–657.
31. Moore GRW, Traugott U, Scheinberg LC, Raine CS. Tropical spastic paraparesis: a model of virus-induced, cytotoxic T-cell-mediated demyelination? Ann Neurol 1989; 26:523–530.
32. Fujihara K, Itoyama Y, Yu F, Kubo C, Goto I. Cellular immune surveillance against HTLV-I infected T lymphocytes in HTLV-I associated myelopathy/tropical spastic paraparesis (HAM/TSP). J Neurol Sci 1991; 105:99–107.
33. Elovaara E, Koenig S, Brewah AY, Woods RM, Lehky T, Jacobson S. High human T cell lymphotropic virus type 1 (HTLV-1)-specific precursor cytotoxic T lymphocyte frequencies in patients with HTLV-I-associated neurological disease. J Exp Med 1993; 177:1567–1573.
34. Kira J, Koyanagi Y, Yamada T, Itoyama Y, Goto I, Yamamoto N, Sasaki H, Sakaki Y. Increased HTLV-I proviral DNA in HTLV-I-associated myelopathy: a quantitative polymerase chain reaction study. Ann Neurol 1991; 29:194–201.

35. Furukawa Y, Osame M, Kubota R, Tara M, Yoshida M. Human T-cell leukemia virus type-1 (HTLV-1) tax is expressed at the same level in infected cells of HTLV-1-associated myelopathy or tropical spastic paraparesis patients as in asymptomatic carriers but at a lower level in adult T-cell leukemia cells. Blood 1995; 85:1865–1870.
36. Macchi B, Caronti B, Pezzella M, Bonmassar E, Lauro G. Effect of human T lymphotropic retrovirus-I exposure on cultured human glioma cell lines. Acta Neuropathol 1991; 81:670–674.
37. Lehky TJ, Cowan EP, Lampson LA, Jacobson S. Induction of HLA class I and class II expression in human T-lymphotropic virus type-I-infected neuroblastoma cells. J Virol 1994; 68(3):1854–1863.
38. Hoffman PM, Dhib-Jalbut S, Mikovits JA, Robbins DS, Wolf AL, Bergey GK, Lohrey NC, Weislow OS, Ruscetti FW. Human T-cell leukemia virus type I infection of monocytes and microglial cells in primary human cultures. Proc Natl Acad Sci USA 1992; 89:11784–11788.
39. Akagi T, Hoshida Y, Yoshino T, Teramoto N, Kondo E, Hayashi K, Takahashi K. Infectivity of human T-lymphotropic virus type I to human nervous tissue cells in vitro. Acta Neuropathol 1992; 84: 147–152.
40. Liberski PP, Rodgers-Johnson P, Char G, Piccardo P, Gibbs CJ Jr., Gajdusek DC. HTLV-I-like viral particles in spinal cord cells in Jamaican tropical spastic paraparesis. Ann Neurol 1988; 23(suppl): S185–S187.
41. DeFreitas E, Wroblewska Z, Maul G, Sheremata W, Ferrante P, Lavi E, Harper M, di Marzo-Veronese F, Koprowski H. HTLV-I infection of cerebrospinal fluid T cells from patients with chronic neurologic disease. AIDS Res Hum Retroviruses 1987; 3:19–32.
42. Bhagavati S, Ehrlich G, Kula RW, Kwok S, Sninsky J, Udani V, Poiesz BJ. Detection of human T-cell lymphoma/leukemia virus type I DNA and antigen in spinal fluid and blood of patients with chronic progressive myelopathy. N Engl J Med 1988; 318:1141–1147.
43. Ionnone R, Sherman MP, Rodgers-Johnson PEB, Beilke MA, Mora CA, Amin RM, Tinsley SR, Papsidero LD, Poiesz BJ, Gibbs CF. HTLV-I DNA sequences in CNS tissue of a patient with tropical spastic paraparesis and HTLV-I-associated myelopathy. J AIDS 1992; 5:810–816.
44. Kira J, Itoyama Y, Koyanagi Y, Tateishi J, Kishikawa M, Akizuki S, Kobayashi, Toki N, Sueishi K, Sato H, Sakaki Y, Yamamoto N, Goto I. Presence of HTLV-I proviral DNA in central nervous system of patients with HTLV-I-associated myelopathy. Ann Neurol 1992; 31:39–45.
45. Hara H, Morita M, Iwaki T, Hatae T, Itoyama Y, Kitamoto T, Akizuki S, Goto I, Watanabe T. Detection of human T-lymphotrophic virus type I (HTLV-1) proviral DNA and analysis of T cell receptor V beta CDR3 sequences in spinal cord lesions of HTLV-I-associated myelopathy/tropical spastic paraparesis. J Exp Med 1994; 180:831–839.
46. Lehky TJ, Fox CH, Koenig S, Levin MC, Flerlage N, Izumo S, Sato E, Raine CS, Osame M, Jacobson S. Detection of human T-lymphotropic virus type I (HTLV-I) tax RNA in the central nervous system of HTLV-I-associated myelopathy/tropical spastic paraparesis patients by in situ hybridization. Ann Neurol 1995; 37:167–175.
47. Navarro-Roman L, Corin DO, Katz D, Callender DP, Prussia PR, Garriques S, Fraser HS, Jaffe ES, Roman GC. Human T-lymphotropic virus type I DNA in spinal cord of tropical spastic paraparesis with concomitant human T-lymphotropic virus type I-negative Hodgkin's disease. Hum Pathol 1994; 25:1101–1106.
48. Renjifo B, Borrero I, Essex M. Tax mutation associated with tropical spastic paraparesis/human T-cell leukemia virus type I-associated myelopathy. J Virol 1995; 69:2611–2616.
49. Liu H-F, Vandamme A-M, Kazadi K, Carton H, Desmyter J, Goubau P. Familial transmission and minimal sequence variability of human T-lymphotropic virus type I (HTLV-I) in Zaire. AIDS Res Hum Retroviruses 1994; 10:1135–1142.
50. McKhann G, Gibbs CJ, Jr., Mora CA, Rodgers-Johnson PE, Liberski PP, Gdula WJ, Zaninovic V. Isolation and characterization of HTLV-I from symptomatic family members with tropical spastic paraparesis (HTLV-I encephalomyeloneuropathy). J Infect Dis 1989; 160:371–379.
51. Dodd RY. The risk of transfusion-transmitted infection. N Engl J Med 1992; 327:419–421.
52. Saxinger W, Blattner WA, Levine PH, Clark J, Biggar R, Hoh M, Moghissi J, Jacobs P, Wilson L, Jacobson R, et al. Human T-cell leukemia virus (HTLV-1) antibodies in Africa. Science 1984; 225:1473–1476.

53. De The G, Giordano C, Gessain A, Howlett W, Sonan T, Akani F, Rosling H, Carton H, Mouanga Y, Caudie C, et al. Human retroviruses HTLV-I, HIV-1, and HIV-2 and neurological diseases in some equatorial areas of Africa. J AIDS 1989; 2:550–556.
54. Reeves WC, Saxinger C, Brenes MM, Quiroz E, Clark JW, Hoh MW, Blattner WA. Human T-cell lymphotropic virus type I (HTLV-I) seroepidemiology and risk factors in metropolitan Panama. Am J Epidemiol 1988; 127:532–539.
55. Maloney EM, Ramirez H, Levin A, Blattner WA. A survey of the human T-cell lymphotropic virus type I (HTLV-1) in south-western Columbia. Int J Cancer 1989; 44:419–423.
56. Blattner WA. Human T-lymphotrophic viruses and diseases of long latency. Ann Intern Med 1989; 111:4–6.
57. Hinuma Y, Komoda H, Chosa T, Dondo T, Kohakura M, Takenaka T, Kikuchi M, Ichimaru M, Yunoki K, Sato I, Matsuo R, Takuichi Y, Uchino H, Hanaoka M. Antibodies to adult T-cell leukemia-virus-associated antigen (ATLA) in sero from patients with ATL and controls in Japan: a nation-wide sero-epidemiologic study. Int J Cancer 1982; 29:631–635.
58. Donegan E, Lee H, Operskalski EA, Shaw GM, Kleinman SH, Busch MP, Stevens CE, Schiff ER, Mowicki MJ, Hollingsworth CG, Mosley JW. Transfusion transmission of retroviruses: human T-lymphotropic virus types I and II compared with human immunodeficiency virus type I. Transfusion 1994; 34:478–483.
59. Power C, Weinshenker BG, Dekaban GA, Ebers GC, Francis GS, Rice GP. HTLV-1 associated myelopathy in Canada. Can J Neurol Sci 1989; 16:330–335.
60. Cruickshank JK, Rudge P, Dalgleish AG, Newton M, McLean BN, Barnard RO, Kendall BE, Miller DH. Tropical spastic paraparesis and human T cell lymphotropic virus type 1 in the United Kingdom. Brain 1989; 112:1057–1190.
61. Bastian I, Gardner J, Webb D, Gardner I. Isolation of a human T-lymphotropic virus type I strain from Australian aboriginals. J Virol 1993; 67:843–851.
62. Achiron A, Pinhas-Hamiel O, Doll L, Djaldetti R, Chen A, Ziv I, Avni A, Frankel G, Melamed E, Shohat B. Spastic paraparesis associated with human T-lymphotropic virus type I: a clinical, serological, and genomic study in Iranian-born Mashhadi Jews. Ann Neurol 1993; 34:670–675.
63. Meytes D, Schochat B, Lee H, Nadel G, Sidi Y, Cerney M, Swanson P, Shaklai M, kilim Y, Elgat M, Chin E, Danon Y, Rosenblatt JD. Serological and molecular survey for HTLV-I infection in a high-risk Middle Eastern group. Lancet 1990; 336:1533–1535.
64. Levy RM, Bredesen DE, Rosenblum ML. Neurological manifestations of the acquired immunodeficiency syndrome (AIDS): experience at UCSF and review of the literature. J Neurosurg 1985; 62: 475–495.
65. Kaplan JE, Lal RB, Davidson M, Lanier AP, Lairmore MD. HTLV-I in Alaska natives. J AIDS 1993; 6:327–328.
65a. Roman GC, Osame M, Igata A. HTLV-I-associated myelopathy (HAM) and tropical spastic paraparesis. In: Roman GC, Vernant J-C, Osame M, eds. HTLV-I and the Nervous System. New York: Alan R. Liss, Inc., 1989:93–98.
66. Murphy EL, Figueroa JP, Gibbs WN, Holding-Cobham M, Cranston B, Malley K, Bodner AJ, Alexander SS, Blattner WA. Human T-lymphotropic virus type I (HTLV-I) seroprevalence in Jamaica. Am J Epi 1991; 133:1114–1124.
67. Kajiyama W, Kashiwagi S. Seroepidemiology of HTLV-I in Japan. In: Roman GC, Vernant J-C, Mitsuhiro O, eds. HTLV-I and the Nervous System. New York: Alan R. Liss, 1989:505–516.
68. Kamihira S, Nakasima S, Oyakawa Y, Moriuti Y, Ichimaru M, Okuda H, Kanamura M, Oota T. Transmission of human T-cell lymphotropic virus type I by blood transfusion before and after mass screening of sera from seropositive donors. Vox Sang 1987; 52:43–44.
69. Inaba S, Sato H, Okochi K, Fukada K, Takakura F, Tokunaga K, Kiyokawa H, Maeda Y. Prevention of transmission of human T-lymphotropic virus type I (HTLV-I) through transfusion, by donor screening with antibody to the virus. Transfusion 1989; 29:7–11.
70. Osame M, Janssen R, Kubota H, Nishitani H, Igata A, Nagataki S, Mori M, Goto I, Shimabukuro H, Khabbaz R. Nationwide survey of HTLV-I-associated myelopathy in Japan: association with blood transfusion. Ann Neurol 1990; 28:50–56.

71. Kaplan JE, Osame M, Kubota H, Igata A, Nishitani H, Maeda Y, Khabbaz RF, Janssen RS. The risk of development of HTLV-I-associated myelopathy/tropical spastic paraparesis among persons infected with HTLV-I. J AIDS 1990; 3:1096–1101.
72. Tokudome S, Tokunaga O, Shimamoto Y, Miyamoto Y, Sumida I, Kikuchi M, Takeshita M, Ikeda T, Fujiwara K, Yoshihara M. Incidence of adult T-cell leukemia/lymphoma among human T-lymphotropic virus type I carriers in Saga, Japan. Cancer Res 1989; 49:226–228.
73. Murphy EL, Hanchard B, Figueroa JP, Gibbs WM, Lofters WS, Campbell M, Goedert JJ, Blattner WA. Modelling the risk of adult T-cell leukemia/lymphoma in persons infected with human T-lymphotropic virus type I. Int J Cancer 1989; 43:250–253.
74. Iwata K, Ito S, Saito H, Ito M, Nagatomo M, Yamasaki T, Yoshida S, Suto H, Tajima K. Mortality among inhabitants of an HTLV-I endemic area in Japan. Jpn J Cancer Res 1994; 85:231–237.
75. Tokudome S, Maeda Y, Fukada K, Teshima D, Asakura T, Sueoka E, Motomura Y, Kusumoto Y, Imamura Y, Kiyokawa T, et al. Follow-up of asymptomatic HTLV-I carriers among blood donors in Kyushu, Japan. Cancer Causes Control 1991; 2:75–78.
76. Saxton EH, Lee H, Swanson P, Chen ISY, Ruland C, Chin E, Aboulafia D, Delamarter R, Rosenblatt JD. Detection of human T-cell leukemia/lymphoma virus type I in a transfusion recipient with chronic myelopathy. Neurology 1989; 39:841–844.
77. Morozov VA, Lagaye S, Saal F, Bazarbachi A, Gout O, Lyon-Caen O, Peries J. High level of HTLV-I specific protein expression in a patient with adult T-cell leukemia, chronic progressive myelopathy and Kaposi's sarcoma. Leukemia 1992; 6:746–750.
78. Sherman MP, Dube S, Spicer TP, Kane TD, Love JL, Saksena NK, Iannone R, Gibbs CJJr, Yanagihara R, Dube DK. Sequence analysis of an immunogenic and neutralizing domain of the human T-cell lymphoma.leukemia virus type I gp46 surface membrane protein among various primate T-cell lymphoma leukemia virus isolates including those from a patient with both HTLV-I-associated myelopathy and adult T-cell leukemia. Cancer Res 1993; 53:6067–6073.
79. Kawano F, Tsukamoto A, Satoh T, Sanada I, Shido T, Suzushima H, Asou M, Takatsuki K. HTLV-1 associated myelopathy/tropical spastic paraparesis with adult T-cell leukemia. Leukemia 1992; 6: 66–67.
80. Uozumi K, Iwahashi M, Ueda H, Otsuka M, Ishibashi K, Hanada S, Arima T. Adult T-cell leukaemia and HTLV-1-associated myelopathy in a family. Lancet 1991; 338:572.
81. Kawai H, Nishida Y, Takaaagi M, Nakamura K, Masuda K, Saito S, Shirakami A. HTLV-I-associated myelopathy with adult T-cell leukemia. Neurology 1989; 39:1129–1131.
82. Smadja D, Cabre P, Bellance R, Vernant JC. Paraplegia associated with HTLV1 in Martinique. Study of 271 cases. Bull Soc Path Ex 1993; 86:433–438.
83. Berger JR, Raffanti S, Svenningsson A, McCarthy M, Snodgrass S, Resnick L.The role of HTLV in HIV-1 neurologic disease. Neurology 1991; 41:197–202.
84. Berger JR, Svenningsson A, Raffanti S, Resnick L. Tropical spastic paraparesis-like illness occurring in a patient dually infected with HIV-1 and HTLV-II. Neurology 1991; 41:85–87.
85. Royal W, III, Griffin DE, McArthur JC, Johnson RT. Intrathecal synthesis of HTLV-I-specific IgG in a man with progressive myelopathy infected with HIV and HTLV-I (abstr). Neurology 1990; 40(suppl 1):454.
86. McArthur JC, Griffin JW, Cornblath DR, Griffin DE, Tesoriero T, Kuncl R, Gibbs CJ, Farzadegan H, Johnson RT. Steroid-responsive myeloneuropathy in a man dually infected with HIV-1 and HTLV-1. Neurology 1990; 40:938–944.
87. Johnson RT, Griffin DE, Arregui A, Mora C, Gibbs CJ,Jr., Cuba JM, Trelles L, Vaisberg A. Spastic paraparesis and HTLV-I infection in Peru. Ann Neurol 1988; 23(suppl):S151–S155.
88. Yu F, Itoyama Y, Fujihara K, Goto I. Natural killer (NK) cells in HTLV-I-associated myelopathy/ tropical spastic paraparesis-decrease in NK cell subset populations and activity in HTLV-I seropositive individuals. J Neuroimmunol 1991; 33:121–128.
89. Iwasaki Y. Pathology of chronic myelopathy associated with HTLV-I infection (HAM/TSP). J Neurol Sci 1990; 96:103–123.
90. Francis DA, Hughes RA. Polymyositis and HTLV-I antibodies. Ann Neurol 1989; 25:311.

91. Morgan OS, Rodgers-Johnson P, Mora C, Char G. HTLV-1 and polymyositis in Jamaica. Lancet 1989; 2:1184–1187.
92. Wiley CA, Nerenberg M, Cros D, Soto-Aguilar MC. HTLV-I polymyositis in a patient also infected with the human immunodeficiency virus. N Engl J Med 1989; 320:992–995.
93. Gabbai AA, Wiley CA, Oliveira AS, Smith R, Schmidt B, Nobrega JA, Bordin JO, Roman GC. Skeletal muscle involvement in tropic spastic paraparesis/HTLV-1-associated myelopathy. Muscle Nerve 1994; 17:923–930.
94. Vernant J-C, Buisson G, Bellance R, Francois MA, Madkaud O, Zavaro O. Pseudo-amyotrophic lateral sclerosis peripheral neuropathy and chronic polyradiculoneuritis in patients with HTLV-I-associated paraplegias. In: Roman GC, Vernant J-C, Mitsuhiro O, eds. HTLV-I and the Nervous System. New York: Alan R. Liss, 1989:361–365.
95. Arimura K, Nakashima H, Matsumoto W, Ohsako J, Hashiguchi K, Higuchi I, Osame M. HTLV-I-associated myelopathy (HAM) presenting with ALS-like features. In: Roman GC, Vernant J-C, Mitsuhiro O, eds. HTLV-I and the Nervous System. New York: Alan R. Liss, 1989:367–370.
96. Arimura K, Rosales R, Osame M, Igata A. Clinical electrophysiologic studies of HTLV-I-associated myelopathy. Arch Neurol 1987; 44:609–612.
97. Osame M, Matsumoto M, Usuku K, Izumo S, Ijichi N, Amitani H, Tara M, Igata A. Chronic progressive myelopathy associated with elevated antibodies to human T-lymphotropic virus type I and adult T-cell leukemialike cells. Ann Neurol 1987; 21:117–122.
98. Ceroni M, Piccardo P, Rodgers-Johnson P, Mora C, Asher DM, Gajdusek DC, Gibbs CJ, Jr. Intrathecal synthesis of IgG antibodies to HTLV-I supports an etiological role for HTLV-I in tropical spastic paraparesis. Ann Neurol 1988; 23(suppl):188–191.
99. Osame M, Igata A, Matsumoto M. HTLV-I-associated myelopathy (HAM) revisited. In: Roman GC, Vernant J-C, Mitsuhiro O, eds. HTLV-I and the Nervous System. New York: Alan R. Liss, 1989: 213–223.
100. Castillo JL, Cartier L, Araya F, Verdugo R, Mora C, Gibbs C. Evoked potential abnormalities in progressive spastic paraparesis associated to HTLV-1. Acta Neurol Scand 1991; 83:151–154.
101. Shibasaki H, Endo C, Kuroda Y, Kakigi R, Oda K, Komine S. Clinical picture of HTLV-I associated myelopathy. J Neurol Sci 1988; 87:15–24.
102. Fukushima T, Ikeda T, Uyama E, Uchino M, Okabe H, Ando M. Cognitive event-related potentials and brain magnetic resonance imaging in HTLV-I associated myelopathy (HAM). J Neurol Sci 1994; 126:30–39.
103. Kuroda Y, Matsui M, Yukitake M, Kurohara K, Takashima H, Takashima Y, Endo C, Kato A, Mihara F. Assessment of MRI criteria for MS in Japanese MS and HAM/TSP. Neurology 1995; 45:30–33.
104. Hara Y, Takahashi M, Ueno S, Yoshikawa H, Yorifuji S, Tarui S, MR imaging of the brain in myelopathy associated with human T-cell lymphotropic virus type I. J Comput Assist Tomogr 1988; 12:750–774.
105. Kreeger L, Gross M, Nieman E. Magnetic resonance imaging in an HTLV-I antibody positive patient with tropical spastic paraparesis (letter). J Neurol Neurosurg Psychiatry 1988; 51:999.
106. Kalyanaraman VS, Sarngadharan MG, Robert-Guroff M, Miyoshi I, Blayney D, Golde D, Gallo RC. A new subtype of human T-cell leukemia virus (HTLV-II) associated with a T-cell variant of hairy cell leukemia. Science 1982; 218:571–573.
107. Rosenblatt JD, Golde DW, Wachsman W, Giorgi JV, Jacobs A, Schmidt GM, Quan S, Gasson JC, Chen IS. A second isolate of HTLV-II associated with atypical hairy-cell leukemia. N Engl J Med 1986; 315:372–377.
108. Rosenblatt JD, Gasson JC, Glaspy J, Bhuta S, Aboud M, Chen ISY, Golde DW. Relationship between human T cell leukemia virus-II and atypical hairy cell leukemia: a serologic study of hairy cell leukemia patients. Leukemia 1987; 1:397–401.
109. Sohn CC, Blayney DW, Misset JL, Mathe G, Flandrin G, Moran EM, Jensen FC, Winberg CD, Rappaport H. Leukopenic chronic T cell leukemia mimicking hairy cell leukemia association with human retroviruses. Blood 1986; 67:949–956.
110. Ferrer JF, Del Pino N, Esteban E, Sherman MP, Dube S, Dube DK, Basombrio MA, Pimentel E,

Segovia A, Quirulas S, Poiesz BJ. High rate of infection with the human T-cell leukemia retrovirus type II in four Indian populations of Argentina. Virology 1993; 197:576–584.
111. Lairmore MD, Jacobson S, Gracia F, De BK, Castillo L, Larreategui M, Roberts BD, Levine PH, Blattner WA, Kaplan JE. Isolation of human T-cell lymphotropic virus type 2 from Guaymi Indians in Panama. Proc Natl Acad Sci USA 1990; 87:8840–8844.
112. Khabbaz RF, Darrow WW, Hartley TM, Witte J, Cohen JB, French J, Gill PS, Potterat J, Sikes RK, Reich R, et al. Seroprevalence and risk factors for HTLV-I/II infection among female prostitutes in the United States. JAMA 1990; 263:60–64.
113. Robert-Guroff M, Weiss SH, Giron JA, Jennings AM, Ginzburg HM, Margolis IB, Blattner WA, Gallo RC. Prevalence of antibodies to HTLV-I, II, and III in intravenous drug abusers from an AIDS endemic region. JAMA 1986; 255:3133–3137.
114. Sullivan MT, Williams AE, Fang CT, Notari EP. HTLV-I and HTLV-II infection in U.S. Blood donors: 1989–1993 (abstr). AIDS Res Hum Retroviruses 1994; 10:489.
115. Dube DK, Sherman MP, Saksena NK, Bryz-Gornia V, Mendelson J, Love J, Arnold CB, Spicer T, Dube S, Glaser JB, et al. Genetic heterogeneity in human T-cell leukemia/lymphoma virus type II. J Virol 1993; 67:1175–1184.
116. Hall WW, Takahasi H, Liu C, Kaplan MH, Sheewind O, Ijichi S, Nagashima K, Gallo RC. Multiple isolates and characteristics of human T-cell leukemia virus type II. J Virol 1992; 66:2456–2463.
117. Jacobson S, Lehky T, Nishimura M, Robinson S, McFarlin DE, Dhib-Jalbut S. Isolation of HTLV-II from a patient with chronic, progressive neurological disease clinically indistinguishable from HTLV-I-associated myelopathy/tropical spastic paraparesis. Ann Neurol 1993; 33:392–396.
118. Harrington WJJ, Sheremata W, Hjelle B, Dube DK, Bradshaw P, Foung SK, Snodgrass S, Toedter G, Cabral L, Poiesz B. Spastic ataxia associated with human T-cell lymphotropic virus type II infection. Ann Neurol 1993; 33:411–414.
119. Murphy EL, Engstrom JW, Miller K, Sacher RA, Busch MP, Hollingsworth CG. HTLV-II associated myelopathy in 43-year-old woman. REDS Investigators. Lancet 1993; 341:757–758.
120. Hjelle B, Appenzeller O, Mills R, Alexander S, Torrez-Martinez N, Jahnke R, Ross G. Chronic neurodegenerative disease associated with HTLV-II infection. Lancet 1992; 339:645–646.
121. Petito CK, Navia BA, Cho ES, Jordan BD, George DC, Price RW. Vacuolar myelopathy pathologically resembling subacute combined degeneration in patients with the acquired immunodeficiency syndrome. N Engl J Med 1985; 312:874–879.
122. McArthur JC. Neurologic manifestations of AIDS. Medicine (Baltimore) 1987; 66:407–437.
123. Green R, Kinsella LJ. Current concepts in the diagnosis of cobalamin deficiency. Neurology 1995; 45:1435–1440.
124. Matsuo H, Nakamura T, Shibayama K, Motomura M, Nagasato K, Takeo G, Tsujihata M, Nagataki S. Plasmapheresis to treat human T lymphotropic virus type I-associated myelopathy. Curr Stud Hematol Blood Transf 1990; 57:198–207.
125. Duncan J, Rudge P. Methylprednisolone therapy in tropical spastic paraparesis. J Neurol Neurosurg Psychiatry 1990; 53:173–174.
126. Levine PH, Blattner WA. The epidemiology of diseases associated with HTLV-I and HTLV-II. Infect Dis Clin North Am 1987; 1:501–510.
127. Kira J, Fujihara K, Itoyama Y, Goto I, Hasuo K. Leukoencephalopathy in HTLV-I-associated myelopathy/tropical spastic paraparesis: MRI analysis and a two year follow-up study after corticosteroid therapy. J Neurol Sci 1991; 106:41–49.
128. Harrington WJJ, Sheremata WA, Snodgrass SR, Emerson S, Phillips S, Berger JR. Tropical spastic paraparesis/HTLV-1-associated myelopathy (TSP/HAM): treatment with an anabolic steroid danazol. AIDS Res Human Retroviruses 1991; 7:1031–1034.
129. Harrington WJJ, Sheramata W, Cabral L. Danazol for urinary incontinence in tropical spastic paraparesis (letter). Lancet 1992; 339:368.
130. Gout O, Gessain A, Iba-Zizen M, Kouzan S, Bolgert F, De The G, Lyon-Caen O. The effect of zidovudine on chronic myelopathy associated with HTLV-1. J Neurol 1991; 238:108–109.

131. Sheramata WA, Benedict D, Aquilacote DC, Sazant A, DeFreitas E. High-dose zidovudine induction in HTLV-I-associated myelopathy: safety and possible efficacy. Neurology 1993; 43:2125–2129.
132. Tendler CL, Greenberg SJ, Blattner WA, Manns A, Murphy E, Fleisher T, Hanchard B, Morgan O, Burton JD, Nelson DL, Waldmann TA. Transactivation of interleukin 2 and its receptor induces immune activation in human T-cell lymphotropic virus type I-associated myelopathy: Pathogenic implications and a rationale for immunotherapy. Proc Natl Acad Sci USA 1990; 87:5218–5222.
133. Waldmann TA. The multichain interleukin 2 receptor. A target for immunotherapy in lymphoma, autoimmune disorders, and organ allografts. JAMA 1990; 263:272–274.

15

Subacute Spongiform Encephalopathies: Prion Infections of the Central Nervous System

Shigeru Sato and Raymond P. Roos
University of Chicago School of Medicine, Chicago, Illinois

INTRODUCTION

A short introduction is helpful reading for the neurologist trying to fathom the rapidly moving field pertaining to the subacute spongiform encephalopathies (SSEs). It is confusing because many of the diseases have more than one name; the term SSEs is interchanged with "prion diseases"; the abbreviation PrP stands for at least three other longer terms. The paragraph that follows has a few guiding statements.

The SSEs are a group of sporadic and inherited noninflammatory diseases of humans and animals with similar pathological features (Table 1) (for review see Refs. 2 and 3). These diseases are transmissible with a remarkably long incubation period. A scrapie form of the prion protein that is protease-resistant (PrP^{Sc}) is critical to the development of SSE by interacting with the normal cellular protease-sensitive form of the prion protein (PrP^{c}). PrP^{Sc} appears identical in sequence to PrP^{c} and is thought to only differ in structural conformation. Some forms of SSE are familial with an autosomal dominant inheritance and are associated with a mutation in PrP^{c}.

HISTORY

The history of the SSEs reads a bit like an Indiana Jones film. Perhaps this has to do with the colorful nature of the main characters—especially D. Carleton Gajdusek. There also seems to be a bit of Dickens in the story: diseases of sheep, mink, cows, New Guinea cannibalistic natives, and fatal insomniacs somehow get tied together with abstruse molecular biology.

This history is sometimes a bit difficult to be sure of, i.e., how much is an adventure film or Dickens novel, and how much is "true" historical account? This is best noted in a passage from Witold Gombrowicz provided by Gajdusek in his very lively foreword to Zigas's "Laughing Death: The Untold Story of Kuru" (4):

Table 1 Subacute Spongiform Encephalopathies[a]

Human Subacute Spongiform Encephalopathy (SSE)
- Nonfamilial SSE
  - Sporadic
    - Kuru
    - Creutzfeldt-Jakob disease (CJD)
  - Iatrogenic (associated with corneal transplants, dura mater grafts, contaminated electrode placement, growth hormone administration)
- Familial SSE (associated with mutation of PrP^{c})
  - Familial CJD
  - Gerstmann-Sträussler syndrome (GSS)
  - Fatal familial insomnia (FFI)

Animal SSE[b]
- Scrapie—sheep, goat, moufflon
- Transmissible mink encephalopathy—mink
- Bovine spongiform encephalopathy—domestic cattle
- Other—chronic wasting disease (mule, deer, elk), "bovid" spongiform encephalopathy (nyala, gemsbok, eland, greater kudu, Arabian oryx), feline spongiform encephalopathy (domestic cat, puma, cheetah)

[a]Transmissible diseases of long duration with neuropathological findings of neuronal loss, gliosis, and spongiform changes; affected brain tissue has a protease-resistant form (PrP^{Sc}) of the normal cellular form of a protein (PrP^{c}).
[b]From Ref. 1.

> Also the task is to evaluate and assess, and to decide whether the work is a novel, or a book of memoirs, or a parody, or a lampoon, or a variation on imaginative themes, or psychological study; and to establish its predominant characteristics; whether the whole thing is a joke, or whether it is just irony, sarcasm, ridicule…

We will try to keep to the "true" history in this brief account.

Gajdusek was trained as a pediatrician and virologist. In 1957, he was a visiting investigator under Dr. MacFarlane Burnet at the Eliza Hall Institute of Medical Research in Melbourne, Australia. Gajdusek was on his way home via Papua New Guinea because of his interest in child health and development among primitive peoples. He first heard of reports of kuru from Dr. Roy Scragg, the Director of Public Health in Port Moresby in Papua New Guinea. Gajdusek decided to investigate kuru further and, perhaps motivated by an inexhaustible *Wanderlust*, visit this remote region of the world.

In March of 1957 Gajdusek entered the kuru region with Dr. Vincent Zigas, who was then the medical officer at Kainantu in the Eastern Highlands District of the Territory of Papua and New Guinea. The best description of Gajdusek's experiences remain his correspondence—for example, the exciting letter of March 15, 1957, recounting the first confrontation with this new disease in this exotic area (5):

> I am in one of the most remote, recently opened regions of New Guinea (in the Eastern Highlands) in the center of tribal groups of cannibals, only contacted in the last ten years and controlled for five years—still spearing each other as of a few days ago, and cooking and feeding the children the body of a kuru case, the disease I am studying—only a few weeks ago. This is a sorcery-induced disease, according to the local populace, and that it has been the major disease problem of the region, as well as a social problem for the past five years, is certain. It is so astonishing an illness that clinical description can only be read with skepticism, and I was highly skeptical until two days ago, when I arrived and began to see the cases on every side. Classical advancing "Parkinsonism" involving every age, overwhelming in females although many boys and a few men also have had it, is a mighty strange syndrome. To see whole groups of well

> nourished healthy young adults dancing about, with athetoid tremors which look far more hysterical than organic, is a real sight. And to see them, however, regularly progress to neurological degeneration in three to six months, usually three, and to death is another matter and cannot be shrugged off. If psychological, we have the very best epidemic psychosis for study in the world, and the Institute of Mental Health should be most interested. If a heredo familial disease, we have the highest incidence concentrated "epidemic" ever seen, and the human geneticists should be "on the ball." If a post-encephalitic or toxic or allergic encephalitic epidemic of basal gangliar disease is here, then all of medicine should be interested.

Gajdusek quickly realized that this was a special disease that was new and potentially important (5).

> Should you be able to make a grant, based on little more than your assurance of my integrity and medical judgement—I tell you Joe [Smadel], this is no wild goose chase, but a really big thing. Everything in my medical training makes me confident—let me know, so that I can plan to extend my work here for at least several further months.... I stake my entire medical reputation on this matter.... This class of illness is not my specialty, but I can handle research on it as well as anyone. Thus, Joe, please let me know whether you can initiate or carry through even a temporary project-grant, on the promise of a paper which is already in draft form from the work. Do you not agree that such a situation is rare and not to be missed as a possible new clue in nervous system diseases, about which we know so little as yet?

Even then there were problems with funding. Fortunately, Smadel realized that Gajdusek was onto a "really big thing."

With remarkable energy, Gajdusek and Zigas were able to provide a comprehensive and accurate clinical description of this new disease in less than 6 months (6). At the same time an exhaustive search was made regarding possible etiologies. In another exciting twist to the story, a major clue to the unraveling of the transmissible nature of kuru came from studies of a little-known fatal disease of sheep, scrapie. These insights were supplied by Dr. William Hadlow, a veterinarian neuropathologist who was working in England at the time. In a letter to *Lancet* (7) Hadlow noted that scrapie bore a striking resemblance both clinically and pathologically to Kuru. Scrapie is manifest by a progressive gait disturbance; the term "tremblante" was used for scrapie because sick animals had localized or generalized muscular shivering—a feature certainly reminiscent of kuru (which means "trembling" as if from fear). He noted that scrapie was considered to be a slow virus infection, as first described by Sigurdsson (8); these diseases, although transmissible, have a long incubation period, long duration of disease, and narrow host range. With these characteristics in mind, Hadlow (7) suggested that kuru may also be a slow virus infection:

> While attempts to draw too close an analogy between diseases of man and lower animals are attended by numerous pitfalls, many valuable clues contributing to the understanding of the fundamental nature of a disease can be gained from a broad comparative viewpoint.... When viewed collectively, the general epizootiological, etiological, clinical and pathological features of scrapie closely parallel those that characterize kuru.... Thus, it might be profitable, in view of veterinary experience with scrapie, to examine the possibility of the experimental induction of kuru in a laboratory primate, for one might surmise that the pathogenetic mechanisms involved in scrapie—however unusual they may be—are unlikely to be unique in the province of animal pathology.

Gajdusek with his characteristic speed set off to attempt the transmission of kuru following inoculation into subhuman primates. In 1966, Gajdusek et al. reported the successful transmission of kuru from human brain to chimpanzee with an incubation period of almost 2 years (9). This was the first transmissible "slow virus infection" in humans.

We must return to the early years of kuru studies to understand how scientific interest became directed to Creutzfeldt-Jakob disease (CJD). Gajdusek and Zigas performed numerous autopsies in the field in order to characterize the neuropathology of the disease, kuru, that was killing the

Fore tribespeople. The tissues were dispatched to Dr. Igor Klatzo, a neuropathologist at the National Institutes of Health. In his letter of September 13, 1957, Klatzo (5) remarks that:

> I am afraid I am unable to give you any useful leads as far as the etiology of this disease is concerned. It seems to be definitely a new condition without anything similar described in the literature. The closest condition I can think of is that described by Jacob and Creutzfeldt. However, in cases reported the neuronal degeneration was most intense in the cerebral cortex, also no cases involving children or adolescents are mentioned. The etiology of Jacob–Creutzfeldt condition is entirely unknown (only about 20 cases have been reported). Since there are no known hereditary disorders resembling even remotely the kuru condition, I am inclined to suspect some toxic metabolism responsible for the process.

One is impressed by Klatzo's scholarship in both clarifying the pathology as well as identifying the resemblance of kuru to a rare disease that was little known at that time, Creutzfeldt–Jakob disease (CJD) (10). Following the transmission of kuru, Gajdusek was reminded of Klatzo's observations regarding the similarity of CJD and kuru. In 1968, Gibbs and colleagues (11) reported the development of SSE in a chimpanzee 13 months after inoculation with a filtered suspension of a brain homogenate from a CJD patient. The successful transmission of CJD led to the grouping of a number of human and animal diseases into the SSEs. The number of such entities has continued to grow, most recently with the addition of bovine spongiform encephalopathy (BSE) and fatal familial insomnia (FFI) to this list. The realization that diseases that fall into a group of noninflammatory degenerative processes can be transmissible has had an enormous impact on the field of neurology and medicine in general and won Gajdusek the Nobel Prize in 1976.

Along with these exciting aspects of the clinical, pathological, and transmissible features of the SSEs has been an equally fascinating story related to the nature of the transmissible agent. The transmissible agent possesses features that are remarkably different from conventional agents, e.g., extreme resistance to physical and chemical conditions that normally inactivate nucleic acid–containing agents. The unconventional properties of the agent led to varied hypotheses. This field opened up in 1982 as a result of a sentinel observation by Prusiner and colleagues (12), i.e., the presence of a protease-resistant protein called PrP^{Sc}, in SSE-affected tissue. Prusiner has relentlessly pursued the involvement of this protein in SSE with remarkable results. His studies have led to the concept that the SSEs are caused by "small proteinaceous infectious particles" or "prions." The importance of PrP in the development of the SSEs is now established as a result of experiments involving transgenic (13) and knock-out mice (14) (see next section).

The concept that a pathogenic modified host protein can interact with the normal host protein to produce increasing amounts of the pathogenic protein as well as disease is an extraordinarily important one. These original ideas provide a bit of healthy heresy with respect to Watson and Crick dogma; it is clear that the prion thesis will continue to provide insights that will have an enormous impact on neurology, medicine, and science.

PATHOPHYSIOLOGY

As noted above, the SSEs are transmissible following inoculation with filtered material, demonstrating the small size of the agent. The small size of the agent coupled with a long incubation period and long course led to the designation of these diseases as "slow virus infections," a term first used by Sigurdsson (8).

An impressive number of studies have been performed by Gibbs and colleagues clarifying details of the transmissibility of SSEs (reviewed in Refs. 2 and 15). Brain, cerebrospinal fluid (CSF), visceral tissue, and, at times, blood can transmit the disease experimentally. Transmission is most efficient following intracerebral inoculation. Although disease can result from inoculation by a peripheral route (e.g., subcutaneous and intravenous), transmission by this route generally requires larger amounts of virus and has a longer incubation period. For example, the incubation period of kuru among the Fore, which is thought to result from subcutaneous inoculation and possibly oral ingestion of contaminated brain during endocannibalistic rituals, can exceed three decades.

There appears to be a relative "species barrier" in transmission, a phenomenon originally noted by Sigurdsson regarding "slow virus infections" (8). In other words, SSE transmits most efficiently when inoculation of the affected tissue occurs in animals of the same species. For example, a variety of nonhuman primates are susceptible to experimental transmission of human SSEs; the average incubation period is 18 and 12 months following intracerebral inoculation into chimpanzees of kuru and CJD brain, respectively. Experimental transmission rates in nonhuman primates are 100% for iatrogenic cases of CJD, 95% for kuru, 90% for sporadic CJD, and 68% for familial SSE (15). Only *some* cases of human SSE, however, will transmit into rodents. Repeated (blind) passage into rodent brains may be necessary in order for the particular SSE "strain" to efficiently transmit to rodents and overcome this "species barrier." Recent data suggest the possibility that oral ingestion of BSE-infected tissues can produce human SSE (see below), thereby emphasizing that the "species barrier" is "relative."

The transmissible SSE agent is an unconventional one for a number of reasons. There is no evidence of any immune response and no evidence of virus particles by electron microscopy. Most remarkable is the extreme resistance of the agent to UV and x irradiation. In addition, the agent is resistant to heat and formalin. This chemical and physical resistance is very unusual for a nucleic acid–containing agent, prompting theories that the SSE agent is an unusual and unconventional one from a molecular point of view. In 1967, Gibbons and Hunter (16) proposed that the agent lacked nucleic acid, but was a "replicating membrane." Other investigators wondered whether the SSE agent could be a viroid—an infectious agent that causes a number of plant diseases and consists of naked, infectious nucleic acid (17). It remained for Prusiner and colleagues to add a critical direction to the field by identifying a protease-resistant form of a protein (that became known as PrP^{Sc}) in SSE tissue and proposing the prion concept (12).

Prusiner et al. were able to obtain sequence information from the protease-resistant protein and then clone it (18). It is now known that this protein is an isoform of a normal cellular protein (PrP^{c}). PrP^{c} is a highly conserved membrane-bound glycoprotein found in many *normal* cells and abundantly in neurons. It is anchored to the neuronal surface by glycosylphosphatidylinositol, suggesting a role in cell signaling or adhesion. PrP^{c} is encoded by a gene (*PRNP*) on the short arm of chromosome 20 (19). PrP^{Sc} differs from PrP^{c} (Table 2) primarily in its protease resistance (reviewed in Ref. 2). This resistance is not thought to result from a difference in sequence, but is believed to be a result of a conformational change or posttranslational modification. In addition, PrP^{Sc} accumulates during the disease duration. PrP^{Sc} is localized to amyloid filaments and plaques, however, these latter features may not be visible with standard light microscopy (20). This localization generated a concept that SSE is an "infectious amyloidosis" (21).

The initial observations concerning the presence of PrP^{Sc} were of interest to the scientific community; however, there was skepticism as to whether this protein merely served as a marker for disease (e.g., a pathological product) rather than the infectious particle itself. A variety of experimental observations (described below) now indicate that PrP^{Sc} should be considered a part or all of the infectious agent and critical for the development of the disease.

A key clue regarding the importance of what Prusiner calls "prions" in the SSEs was the discovery that patients with familial forms of the SSEs, such as Gerstmann-Sträussler-Scheinker disease (GSS), have mutations in the *PRNP* gene (22,23). These familial forms of disease

Table 2 Hypotheses for Pathogenesis of SSE

1. Experimental inoculation, iatrogenic disease, kuru	Presence of PrP^{Sc} converts PrP^{c} into more PrP^{Sc}
2. Familial	Mutant PrP change its conformation over time into PrP^{Sc}
3. Sporadic	PrP^{c} spontaneously changes its conformation into PrP^{Sc},or there is a somatic mutation of PrP^{sc} or spontaneous overexpression of PrP^{c}

generally transmit disease in experimental animals as readily as the sporadic form of SSE. All members that are affected from families with dominantly inherited forms of SSE carry the same particular mutation. A variety of different PrP^{c} mutations have been described in familial SSE (Fig. 1) (reviewed in Refs. 2,24,25). In some cases, a particular mutation appears associated with a particular clinical syndrome phenotype; e.g., GSS cases appear to be associated with mutations at varied locations including point mutations in *PRNP* codons 102, 117, 198, and 217. The most common mutation is in codon 200, which is associated with a cluster of familial CJD in Libyan Jews (26).

A number of studies suggest that other genetic factors have a major effect on disease. These genetic factors may be responsible for the variable disease and clinical onset in some pedigrees; in fact, modifying genes may allow some individuals that carry a mutation to remain unaffected. One critical factor is a polymorphism at *PRNP* codon 129: 62% of the general population have a methionine at this codon, while 38% have a valine (27). This polymorphism determines the disease phenotype of patients with a mutation at codon 178 and whether they have an FFI syndrome or a more typical (familial) CJD syndrome (27). The presence of homozygosity at codon 129 is also important in iatrogenic disease, significantly enhancing susceptibility (28). Clearly other genetic factors in addition to a particular PrP mutation affect clinical disease.

A critical experiment by Prusiner and colleagues in 1990 was the introduction of the mutant *PRNP* gene from GSS patients into mice as a transgene (13). Their landmark publication documented the development of SSE in a mouse that received this transgene. Of interest was the observation that the affected brain tissue of these transgenic mice inefficiently transmitted disease to nontransgenic mice (29). This finding indicated that interactions of the abnormal mutant PrP (and presumably proteinase-resistant PrP^{Sc} as well) with PrP^{c} are critical for the development of disease; it is presumed that the abnormal PrP leads to conversion of PrP^{c} into the protease-

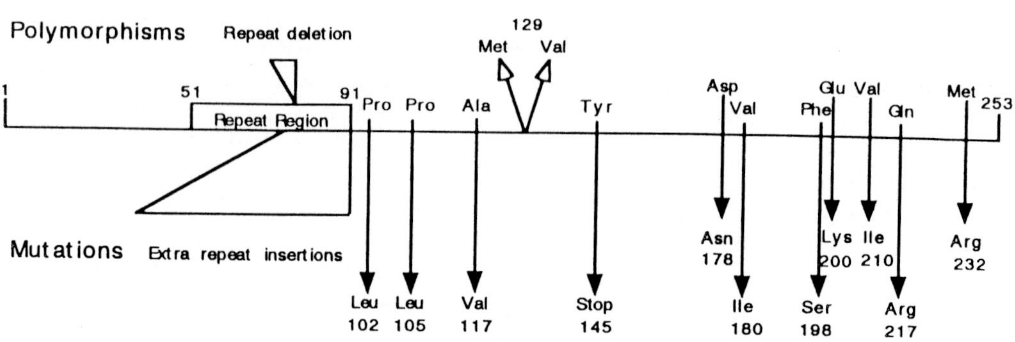

Figure 1 PRNP cDNA with some of the codons numbered. An arrow connects wild-type amino acids shown just above the line to mutant amino acids below the line. Polymorphisms are noted at a level above the line (and above these amino acids).

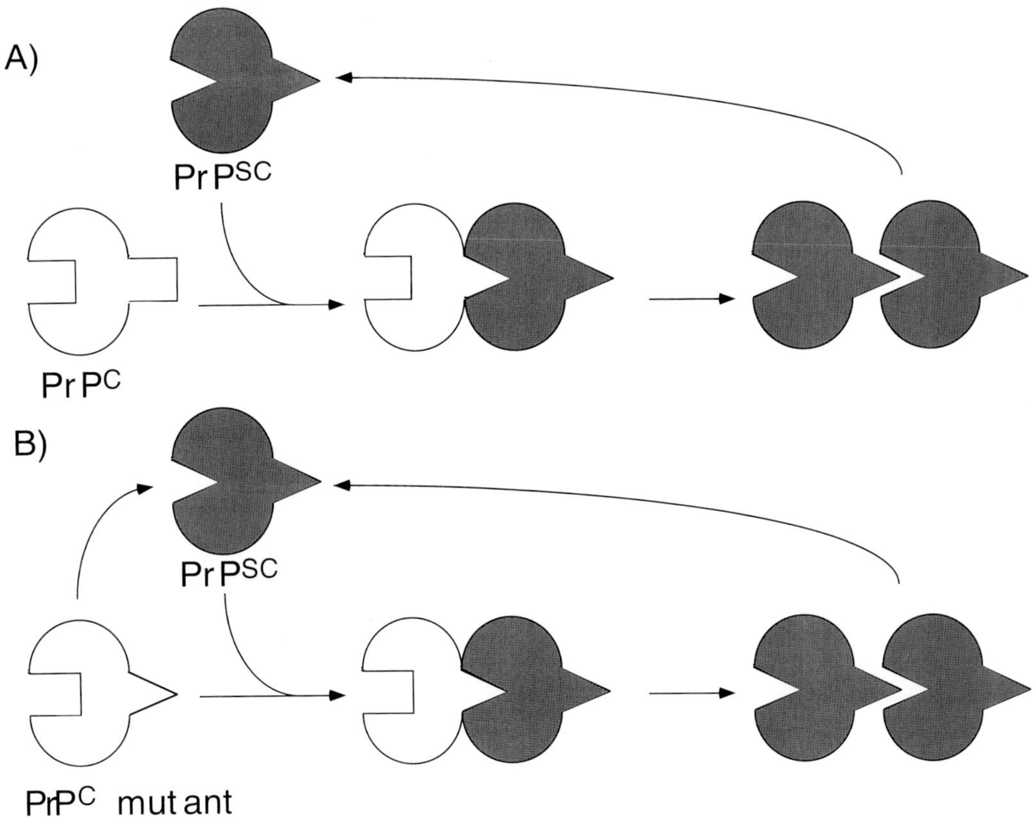

Figure 2 Schematic drawing showing hypothetical scheme in which (A) in iatrogenic and experimental SSE, PrP^{Sc} converts PrP^{c} into Prp^{Sc} and (B) in familial SSE, mutant PrP^{c} changes to PrP^{Sc}.

resistant form (Fig. 2). In vitro studies have demonstrated and confirmed the conversion of PrP^{c} into PrP^{Sc} (30). Interestingly, there appears to be a species-specificity in the interactions that lead to the conversion of PrP^{c} to PrP^{Sc} (31); this may be the molecular basis for the "species barrier." A protein that assumes alternative conformations and is apparently transmissible has been recently shown to underly a non-Mendelian element in yeast (32). Studies have demonstrated that the chaperone protein Hsp 104 may be required for the conformation of this protein in yeast (33). A chaperone protein interaction with PrP^{Sc} has also been proposed in the SSEs (34).

The importance of interactions between PrP^{Sc} and PrP^{c} in disease was further supported by PrP knock-out mice (14). These knock-out mice do not develop SSE following inoculation of (mouse-adapted) PrP^{Sc}; reintroduction of PrP^{c} as a transgene leads to a return in susceptibility of these mice. Recently, transgenic mice have been produced that have a chimeric human-mouse PrP^{c} (35); these mice have an enhanced susceptibility to human SSE, such as CJD, supporting the importance of interactions of PrP^{c} and PrP^{Sc}. Neural cell death may be at least partly related to the interactions of PrP^{c} with PrP^{Sc}, as suggested by transplant experiments (36).

Another issue related to the PrP knock-out mice is whether the mice demonstrate a specific abnormal phenotype and thereby provide clues to the function of PrP^{c}. Initial reports noted that the mice appeared completely normal (14), suggesting that another protein substitutes for the function of PrP in the knock-out mice, a situation that has been seen in other similar experiments.

Recent data demonstrate, however, that the PrP knock-out mice develop ataxia at about 70 weeks of age, and is associated with extensive loss of Purkinje cells (37); these results suggest that PrP plays a role in the long-term survival of Purkinje neurons. In addition electrophysiological abnormalities of the PrP knock-out mice have been described (38); this defect is rescued with a high copy number of a transgene encoding human PrP^c (39).

A recent surprising turn in the prion story is the discovery that transgenic mice that overproduce *normal* PrP^c also develop neurodegeneration, although very late (40). This result suggests that a protease-resistant form of PrP is not necessary for disease induction and that SSE may result from a protease-sensitive PrP^c that has an abnormal conformation or is present in an excessive amount. Transmission of these cases is much less efficient. Perhaps the difficulty in transmitting FFI despite the presence of mutations in PrP is also a reflection of the small amount of protease-resistant material in FFI-affected tissues (see later).

What do the above experiments tell us about the pathogenesis of SSE? Critical to our understanding is the concept that PrP^{Sc} promotes the conversion of PrP^c into more PrP^{Sc}. Perhaps it is useful to remember how cooled water changes (its conformation) into ice after the introduction of a crystal of ice. To follow up on this analogy, one should note that a variety of different structures (snowflakes) may be produced from the (frozen) water. Similarly, proteins can "nucleate" into different crystals, and different materials may trigger different patterns of crystal growth in the same protein (41). It can be postulated that the greater the difference in sequence (or conformation) between PrP^{Sc} with the host PrP^c, the less chance of successful transmission, thereby explaining the "species barrier." Biophysical studies of the structure of PrP^{Sc} (as well as mutant PrP) versus PrP^c are clearly necessary to put these theories on a more firm basis.

In the case of *experimental inoculation (or iatrogenic disease or kuru)* (Table 2), PrP^{Sc} is believed to enter the central nervous system and lead to the conversion of PrP^c into more PrP^{Sc} (Fig. 2). The accumulation of PrP^{Sc} interferes with neuronal function and causes SSE. It may be that the mutant PrP that is present in *familial SSEs* (Table 2) will change its conformation over time into PrP^{Sc} and lead to disease.

What is the means of spread of *sporadic CJD*? There is little evidence of horizontal transmission or of iatrogenic spread in the case of sporadic CJD. Epidemiological data do not support animal SSE-contaminated tissue (e.g., scrapie-contaminated meat) as a significant factor in the spread of CJD (42); this may be at least partly a result of the "species barrier." New data related to BSE, however, suggest that oral ingestion of animal tissue infected with some SSE strains may cause human disease (see later). The apparent clusters of CJD are infrequent and generally have been found to represent unrecognized familial CJD (26). For this reason, a number of investigators suspect that a spontaneous change in the conformation of PrP into PrP^{Sc} (or a somatic mutation of PrP^{Sc} or overexpression of PrP^c) may occur in the central nervous system and start the devastating cascade that leads to SSE. Unfortunately, this theory is a difficult one to test.

CLINICAL PRESENTATION AND CLINICAL COURSE

The SSEs are a group of animal and human diseases that have a similar pathology and are transmissible; affected tissues demonstrate an accumulation of PrP^{Sc}. The diseases tend to be gray matter processes characterized by neuronal loss with spongiform changes and gliosis (Fig. 3); there are cases, however, that have white matter pathology, especially among the Japanese (43). Plaques with the typical staining and ultrastructural appearance of amyloid occur in the SSEs to a variable degree and with a variable distribution. For example, plaques are seen in the cerebellum of kuru brains, in about 10% of cases of CJD, and in all cases of GSS rather diffusely. The plaques in kuru and CJD are compact, while those in GSS are multicentric (44–46). The plaques stain

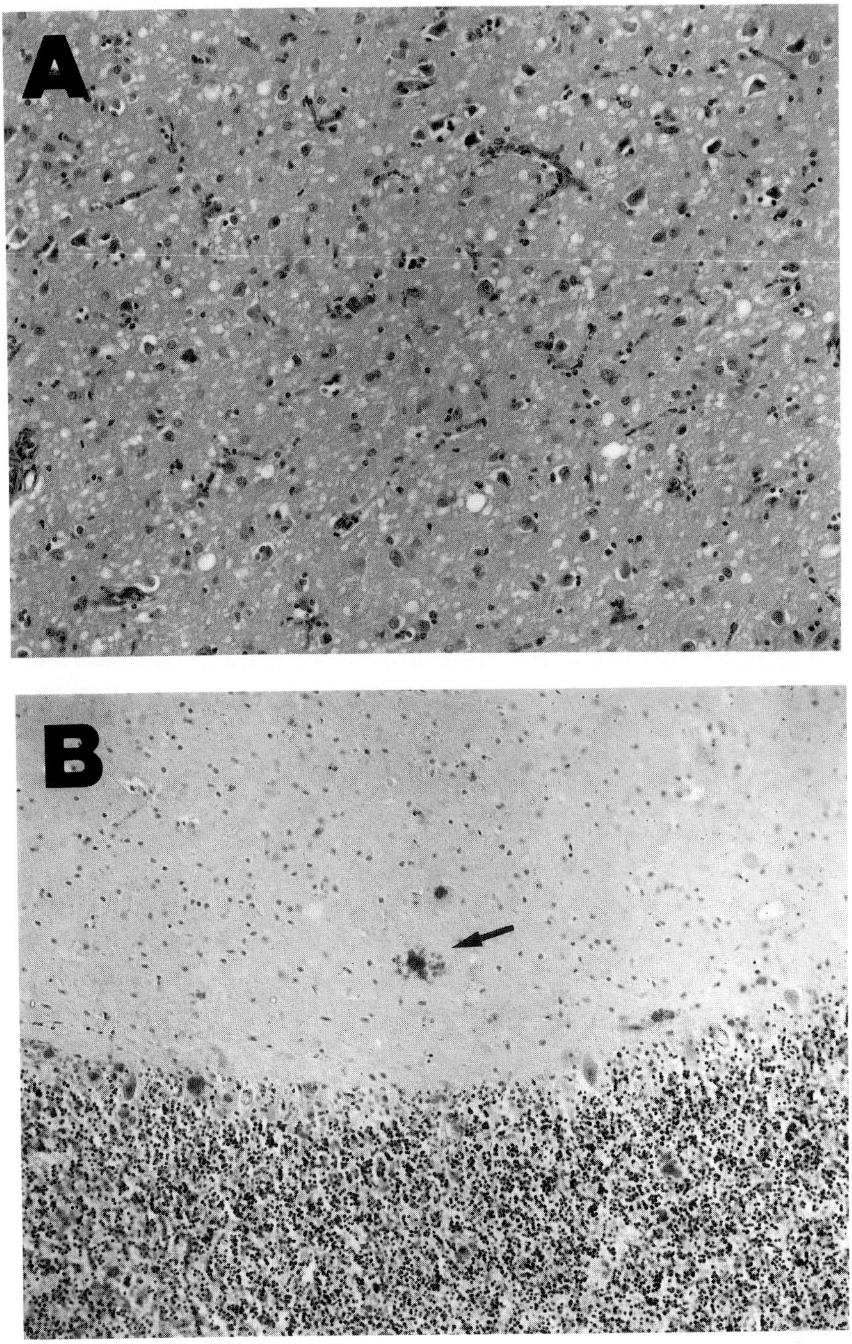

Figure 3 (A) Spongiform degeneration of cerebral cortex from CJD patient with loss of neurons and fibrillary astrocytosis. Hematoxylin and eosin stain (×450). (B) Amyloid plaques (one shown with arrow) in molecular layer of cerebellar cortex of CJD patient. Congo red stain (×225).

with anti-PrP antiserum, making immunohistochemical staining an important neuropathological diagnostic aid in differentiating SSE from Alzheimer's disease.

Kuru

Kuru is a subacute cerebellar disease that is confined to the Fore tribesmen, and adjoining tribes that they intermarry with, in the Eastern Highlands of New Guinea (reviewed in Refs. 2,46). The disease is a subacute cerebellar degeneration that generally affects adult females and children of both sexes. Patients complain of prodromal symptoms of headache and joint pain. Generally clinical signs appear within 6–12 weeks in the form of a gait disturbance; at first, this ominous sign is so subtle that it may only be apparent to the victim—probably because of the rigorous demands for agility in the wild terrain. Eventually patients require the use of a cane and become nonambulatory, usually after 6 months. Signs of cerebellar dysfunction invariably dominate the clinical picture. Patients at times develop a movement disorder, from which kuru derives its name. A lability of emotions, perhaps secondary to pseudobulbar disease, is the presumed reason that kuru has been called "the laughing death." "Frontal lobe" signs such as a snout, suck, etc., are seen, but patients do not develop the overt dementia of CJD. It is sobering to note that the disease generally progresses to death within a year, and all patients are dead within 2 years.

We now have some understanding of the epidemiology of kuru and its particular targeting of adult females and children. The Fore tribesmen were endocannibals who ate their dead relatives as a ritual form of mourning. The high-titered brain tissue was given to women and children, who ingested it and smeared it over their body. The importance of this route of transmission is confirmed by noting the disappearance of kuru since the cessation of cannibalism.

CJD

In contrast to kuru, CJD is a worldwide disease (reviewed in Refs. 2,3,46–49). There are occasional examples of clusters of cases of CJD, many of which represent foci of (vertically inherited) familial SSE (see below). CJD affects the sexes equally. The mean age of disease is approximately 60, although cases have been reported in teenagers as well as in individuals in their eighties. The approximate incidence has been remarkably uniform at about one per million individuals per year.

Most patients manifest a fairly uniform disease. More than a quarter of the patients have nonspecific symptoms that constitute a prodromal period. These symptoms include asthenia, anxiety, disturbances in sleeping patterns (with complaints of insomnia more frequently than drowsiness), changes in eating habits (usually with a decreased appetite), and weight loss. Disease is usually first manifest by sensory disturbances or confusion with inappropriate behavior; a cerebellar ataxia can also feature prominently in the initial signs. A constellation of neurological abnormalities is not infrequently seen, which includes: behavioral abnormalities, higher cortical dysfunction, visual disorder, signs of cerebellar, pyramidal and extrapyramidal disease, and lower motor neuron signs. Most patients develop myoclonic jerks during the course of the disease; the myoclonus, at times involving the whole body, can usually be precipitated by auditory or tactile stimulation. Patients generally have a characteristic electroencephalogram (EEG) at some time during the disease course with periodic or pseudoperiodic paroxysms of sharp waves or spikes against a slow background (Fig. 4). Over weeks or months, patients progress to a frank dementia and then a mute and akinetic state (except perhaps for persistent myoclonus). The average duration of the disease is approximately 4.5 months, with death usually occurring from respiratory complications.

The typical presentation and course of CJD described above is relatively stereotyped. A relentless subacute disease with a "clinical triad" of dementia, myoclonus, and a characteristic

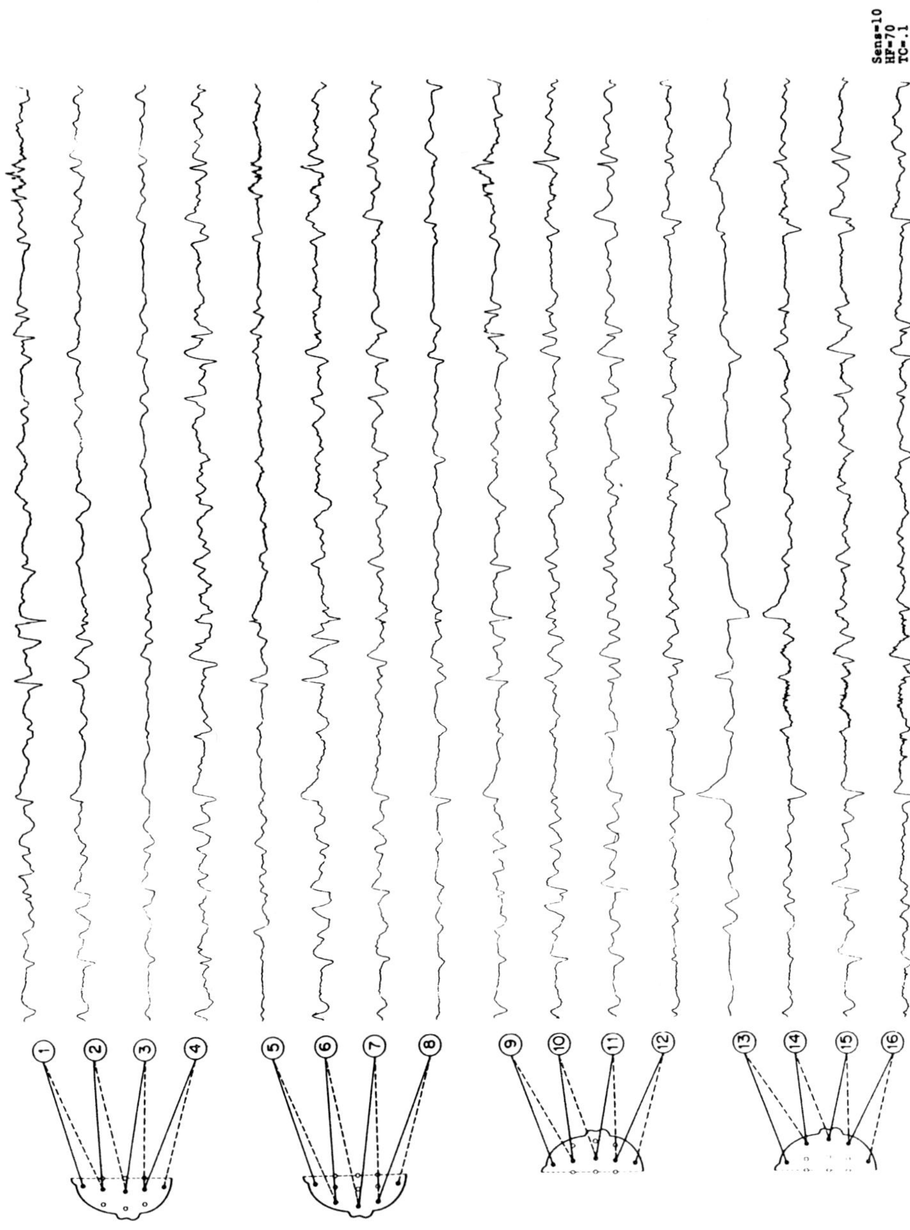

Figure 4 An EEG from a 58-year-old female with CJD shows pseudoperiodic triphasic complexes occurring symmetrically over both hemispheres at about one per second.

EEG makes the diagnosis fairly straightforward. In some cases, however, there may be significant variation in these symptoms and signs, causing diagnostic confusion. Insidious mental deterioration may occur initially in the absence of myoclonus or the characteristic EEG. Some patients may have a rather abrupt onset of confusion (or another neurological sign) without the prodrome, prompting consideration of other diagnoses. Some patients have psychiatric symptomatology; rare patients may even be admitted to psychiatric hospitals and administered electroconvulsive therapy. Some patients may manifest a surprisingly long disease duration. Some cases of CJD are familial (see next section).

A number of CJD variants reflect the variable focus of the pathology in the disease. The distinctive nature of these variants has resulted in the use of a multitude of names for CJD. Patients with the occipitoparietal or Heidenhain's syndrome have prominent disturbances in higher cortical function. The ataxic or Brownell-Oppenheimer variant can at times lead to diagnostic difficulties because of the early and prominent cerebellar dysfunction; this was apparently true in the celebrated case of George Balanchine. These latter cases may bear some similarity to those with kuru; in addition, some patients with CJD can manifest inappropriate laughter such as that seen with kuru. Interestingly, cases of CJD that have resulted from growth hormone treatment (see below) have had a characteristic cerebellar symptomatology (46,48). Patients with the amyotrophic variant or the classical form of Jakob's disease can also be diagnostically confusing; these patients have lower motor neuron signs early in disease with a late dementia and prolonged course, myoclonus, and an absence of the characteristic EEG findings.

Familial SSEs

The initial classification of the familial SSEs relied on clinical and pathological aspects of the disease. It then became clear that these syndromes were associated with *PRNP* mutations. In some cases, a particular familial SSE is associated with a distinctive *PRNP* mutation, such as the association of GSS with a codon 102 mutation. Confusion, however, has entered because particular mutations may be associated with varied clinical-pathological syndromes, and because diverse clinical pictures may even occur within the same pedigree. For example, there may be a pedigree with *PRNP* codon 102 mutations in which some cases have the typical clinical-pathological features of GSS, while others appear to have a clinical picture that more closely resembles sporadic CJD. In addition, new syndromes have been reported with unusual phenotypes, such as a PrP cerebral amyloid angiopathy associated with a PrP stop mutation at codon 145 of *PRNP* (50). Prusiner and Hsiao have recently suggested referring to familial cases as prion diseases followed by the mutation, thereby avoiding the necessity to subgroup them into a particular disease phenotype (3).

Familial CJD

About 10% of cases of CJD are familial, and autosomally dominantly inherited. As a group these cases tend to have a very similar clinical presentation and course compared to the sporadic form of CJD. Familial cases, however, tend to have a mean age of onset about 12 years earlier and a disease duration about 18 months longer than is true for sporadic CJD (46). As noted previously, the familial cases have mutations of the *PRNP* gene. At times there appears to be a fairly characteristic clinical syndrome associated with a particular mutation (reviewed in Ref. 46). For example, patients with codon 178 mutations (and an associated valine polymorphism at codon 129) have an insidious memory loss in the early stages of disease unaccompanied by cerebellar or visual signs or a periodic EEG activity (reviewed in Ref. 46). Patients with mutations of the octapeptide repeat have a lower incidence of cerebellar signs, myoclonus, and periodic EEG activity at the onset of disease. Patients with other mutations, such as codon 200, have a syndrome identical to that seen with sporadic CJD.

GSS

GSS is an autosomal dominantly inherited disease similar to CJD except that cerebellar and pseudobulbar symptoms are very frequent, myoclonus and periodic EEG activity are less frequent, and the disease duration is more prolonged with an average of $4\frac{1}{2}$ years (reviewed in Ref. 46). Cerebellar ataxia, dysarthria, ocular dysmetria, hyperreflexia, or areflexia in the lower extremities with extensor plantar responses, and mild wasting or weakness in the lower extremities may be found. Sensory disturbances, usually with an impairment of vibration and proprioception, may be present. Mental deterioration may occur, and dysphagia frequently develops later in the course. Although some cases of GSS manifest a typical clinical syndrome, the signs of GSS may be diverse, even among patients within the same pedigree. Molecular genetic studies coupled to neuropathological investigations have allowed a clarification of the spectrum of disease (46). The classical ataxic form of GSS is associated with a mutation of *PRNP* codon 102, while a "telencephalic" form is associated with codon 117 mutation. In the case of codon 198, ataxia is often accompanied by parkinsonism and dementia. In the codon 198 and 217 form of GSS, PrP amyloid plaques are found surrounded by numerous neurofibrillary tangles.

The potentially confusing nature of these diseases is made clear by noting a publication in 1966 (51) concerning a very large group with familial Alzheimer's disease. More than 30 years later (52), this group was realized to be one with GSS, not Alzheimer's disease. The diagnosis of GSS in this group was clarified by pathological studies of some of the affected individuals coupled with immunohistochemical staining studies of plaques with anti-PrP antiserum; further confirmation of the diagnosis was made by transmission of the disease. It is rather interesting to note the remarkable variation in clinical disease among individuals in this group.

FFI (Fatal Familial Insomnia)

In 1986, Lugaresi et al. (53) described a new autosomal dominantly inherited disease characterized by progressive intractable insomnia, dysautonomia, and motor signs; the pathology of this disease, designated FFI, showed selective atrophy of the anterior ventral and mediodorsal thalamic nuclei. Additional cases (54,55) have further delineated the clinical syndrome. The dysautonomia includes hyperhidrosis, hyperthermia, tachycardia, and hypertension. Ataxia, dysarthria, myoclonus, and pyramidal signs are seen. Memory loss and attention deficits are minimal initially, but progress over time.

The sleep disorder is characterized by a marked reduction or loss of slow-wave and rapid-eye movement phases; in advanced stages, patients have complex hallucinations, followed by stupor and coma. We recently treated a patient with FFI with gamma-hydroxybutyrate, which is used in the treatment of narcolepsy (54). This drug led to the induction of slow wave sleep.

There is an absence of hormonal circadian rhythm in FFI, presumably resulting from the abnormal sleep-wake cycle. Lugaresi (56) reported that both sleep-coupled (growth hormone and prolactin) and circadian-dependent (cortisone and melatonin) hormones have abnormal 24-h secretory profiles in FFI. In contrast, a patient we recently evaluated continued to manifest circadian variation in cortisol and melatonin (54).

FFI is a gray matter disease, as the other prion diseases tend to be. The pathology of the disease (53–55) is somewhat distinctive compared to these other diseases. There is selective targeting of neuronal loss and gliosis to the thalamus, especially particular regions of the thalamus. The rather focal area of involvement is reminiscent of kuru, although in the latter case the target is the cerebellum rather than the thalamus. There is minimal evidence of spongiform change in FFI; this is also the case in kuru.

In 1992, Medori et al. (57) reported that FFI can be classified as a prion disease because of the presence of a mutation at codon 178 of *PRNP*, changing aspartic acid to asparagine, in all affected individuals in all pedigrees. Interestingly, familial CJD cases have this same mutation.

In the case of FFI, the mutation is associated with a methionine at the polymorphic site at codon 129 on the same allele, while patients with the familial CJD syndrome and codon 178 mutation have an associated valine at codon 129 on the same allele (27).

Despite the classification of FFI as a prion disease, there are several unusual features that appear to differentiate it from the other human prion diseases. There is little evidence of protease-resistant PrP within the affected brain (54,58). This absence of PrP^{Sc} may also be responsible for the inefficient transmission of this disease (57,58). Perhaps the particular conformation of the PrP that is present in FFI and its biophysical properties are a bit different from PrP^{Sc}.

DIAGNOSIS

Overall, it should be stated that the diagnosis of the SSEs is not difficult because the typical CJD clinical presentation is usually so distinctive. As clearly articulated by Denny-Brown (59):

> Progressive dementia with no imminence of cause ... and the most fantastic degree of disintegration of the higher function of the brain occurring all in a few weeks, or a few months, with a galaxy of abnormal signs, is a startling syndrome.... The picture is so characteristic, once you have seen one or two cases, and are aware of the problem, that the diagnosis will seldom be missed.

Brain biopsy, which was frequently performed 20 years ago to aid in the diagnosis of this disorder, is rarely performed for these cases today for a number of reasons: the fairly stereotyped nature of typical CJD, the superb imaging studies now available (to rule out some diseases that might mimic CJD, such as subdural hematomas, strokes, gliomatosis cerebri, sarcoidosis, progressive multifocal leukoencephalopathy, metachromatic leukodystrophy, adrenoleukodystrophy, etc.), and the reluctance of neurosurgeons to perform this procedure because of concerns about exposure to the agent. In addition, most of the other diseases that may, in fact, lead to an erroneous diagnosis of CJD are nontreatable neurodegenerative ones, such as Alzheimer's disease (especially familial Alzheimer's disease), Pick's disease, and cerebellar degenerations. Nevertheless, brain biopsy can be valuable from a diagnostic point of view, since typical features of SSE are usually seen. Brain tissue can be immunostained with anti-PrP antiserum in cases where plaques are seen in order to differentiate SSE from Alzheimer's disease (which has plaques that are PrP-negative, but β-amyloid–positive). Brain tissue can be inoculated into experimental animals to determine its transmissibility; this may be the "gold standard" test, but it is a difficult, expensive, and slow one.

Despite the transmissibility of CJD, there is little laboratory evidence of an inflammatory disorder. Nevertheless, in order to rule out other inflammatory processes (e.g., vasculitis, sarcoid, acquired immunodeficiency syndrome, carcinomatous meningitis, lymphomatous meningitis, other CNS inflammatory diseases), the following studies should be performed: complete blood count, sedimentation rate, collagen vascular screen, complete CSF analysis, human immunodeficiency virus-1 antibody titers and angiotensin-converting enzyme level (Table 3). If a vasculitis is suspected, one should consider performing an arteriogram. A toxic screen with special attention to heavy metals is indicated to rule out conditions such as mercury poisoning, which may resemble CJD. Whipple's disease patients may have a primarily neurological disease picture with myoclonus, dementia, and eye-movement abnormalities with no evidence of a malabsorption; there may be a place for a small bowel biopsy in patients suspected of having this treatable disease. All patients should have imaging studies including magnetic resonance imaging with gadolinium infusion to rule out a structural lesion.

Although patients with SSE have no inflammation in the CSF, there is a not infrequent elevation of CSF protein; however, this finding probably results from degeneration of the central nervous system rather than an inflammatory process. Harrington et al. (60) described four

Table 3 Diagnosis and Treatment of SSE

1. Diagnostic studies
   - Recommended studies
     - Complete blood count
     - Sedimentation rate
     - Collagen vascular screen
     - HIV-1 antibody titers
     - Angiotensin-converting enzyme level
     - Complete CSF analysis
     - Imaging studies (MRI with gadolinium infusion)
     - EEG
   - Studies that may be helpful
     - Molecular genetic studies from blood leukocytes (especially for familial cases)
     - Arteriogram (if vasculitis is suspected)
     - Malabsorption test, small bowel biopsy (if Whipple's disease is suspected)
     - Brain biopsy (to examine tissue for typical spongiform pathology, etc., and to stain with anti-PrP antiserum)
     - Inoculation of brain tissue into experimental animals
     - Two-dimensional gel electrophoresis (needs confirmation)
     - Electroretinographic studies (needs conformation)
2. Treatment
   - There is no confirmed effective treatment

abnormal protein spots when the CSF was subjected to two-dimensional gel electrophoresis. Two of these spots were present in virtually every CJD patient studied but in no other neurological disease, except herpes simplex encephalitis (60,61). Recent information demonstrates that these spots correspond to 14-3-3 brain protein and that an immunoassay of CJD CSF can be used to detect these proteins with remarkable sensitivity and specificity (61a). This test will likely become commercially available.

The EEG is a widely used and valuable diagnostic aid. The great majority of CJD patients have abnormal EEG findings; in addition, the test is indicated to rule out disorders such as subclinical status epilepticus. The EEG is often normal early in the disease or shows only nonspecific slow-wave activity or a mildly disorganized background. With disease progression, the background becomes slow and irregular with a decreased amplitude. A variety of paroxysmal discharges (slow waves, sharp waves, spike-and-wave complexes) are frequently present, which are usually bilaterally synchronous but may be unilateral or focal. The EEG usually has an episodic burst-suppression high-voltage activity or, more typically, 1–2 cycles/s triphasic sharp waves against a diminished background activity. This typical periodic "burst-suppression" complex of high-voltage slow activity on EEG is usually seen at some time during the illness. If the characteristic EEG findings are not present, it is frequently advisable to perform serial EEGs at weekly intervals, since these abnormalities not infrequently appear as the clinical syndrome evolves. Visual, auditory, or somatosensory evoked response tracings generally add little to the information obtained by routine EEG studies.

Of interest is the fact that retinal pathology has been identified in both human and experimental SSEs (62,63). Electroretinographic studies have been reported as abnormal in three cases of (iatrogenic) CJD (64). This technique may have diagnostic value if the abnormality is found to be a consistent one.

Imaging studies are important in the diagnostic evaluation of a CJD patient, not to detect abnormalities specific to the latter disease, but to rule out other processes that might masquerade as CJD. Computed tomography and magnetic resonance imaging may show a variable degree of cortical atrophy and enlarged ventricles, especially late in the course of the disease.

Molecular genetic studies (namely, polymerase chain reaction) should be employed to detect PrP mutations if there is a history of familial neurological disease. This analysis is generally performed on DNA extracted from blood leukocytes. The DNA is amplified and examined by allele-specific hybridization or restriction enzyme analysis. Sequencing should be performed to confirm the mutation. These methods can be used for the diagnosis of an affected member of a familial SSE pedigree or for an at risk individual. There is therefore the possibility of making an in utero diagnosis (65) and then terminating the pregnancy if the genotype shows a mutation.

Sporadic CJD patients do not have PrP mutations unless there is a germline mutation in the patient (which is rare). One must, however, be aware of certain pitfalls that may cause sporadic and familial cases to be confused. There may be an unrecognized family history because of death of an affected parent from an unrelated disease prior to the onset of SSE or because of uncertain paternity. At times, family members will forget important features related to neurological disease of family members, or at times these will not be revealed. In addition, there are some examples of what appears to be incomplete penetrance in pedigrees that carry PrP mutations. For the above reasons, it may be valuable to perform *PRNP* genotyping on patients with no family history of SSE. This is especially true in patients that have distinctive syndromes normally associated with familial disease, such as FFI; in fact, a recent case with an FFI phenotype had the typical FFI mutation in PrP but no forthcoming family history of SSE (54).

TREATMENT

SSEs are fatal diseases without any effective treatment (Table 3). Remissions of CJD related to varied treatments have been claimed, but have not been confirmed when subsequently tested.

Patients are not infrequently treated symptomatically. For example, patients with many extrapyramidal signs may be treated with anti-Parkinsonian medication. Patients with potentially epileptiform activity on the EEG may be administered antiepileptic medication. Some patients receive a trial of high-dose steroids for a month or more as a desperate blind effort to treat an underlying occult inflammatory process, such as vasculitis. Unfortunately, these efforts rarely have any effect on the progressive disease. We were recently involved in the use of gamma-hydroxybutyrate, an experimental drug that is effective in narcolepsy, in order to enhance sleep in FFI patients (54). We questioned whether this treatment might also prolong life since sleep deprivation can produce death in experimental animals (66). Although the patient had the onset of slow-wave sleep and appeared to generally improve clinically with an increase in alertness, further cases must be treated before efficacy can be presumed.

Several substances—polyanions (HPA 23, carrageenan, and dextran sulfate) and amphotericin B—appear to be effective in interfering with the development of experimental scrapie (reviewed in Refs. 46,67). These treatments, however, do not reverse the disease once it is established; nevertheless, they may have a role in the treatment of asymptomatic individuals in a familial SSE group who are found to have a PrP mutation.

The recent identification of prions (PrP^{Sc}) as critical for the development of SSE has raised the possibility of a number of novel molecular approaches to treatment. If the process of protein replication requires a nucleation step in order to initiate autopatterned protein polymerization, as in the epitaxial growth of crystals, it may be possible to arrest its development by means analogous to "habit-modification poisoning" of in vitro crystal formation (46,67).

PREVENTION

Familial Cases

The association of particular mutations within the *PRNP* gene in the DNA of affected individuals signifies that in utero identification of these familial diseases can be accomplished (65). This provides the opportunity for elective therapeutic abortion of a fetus that carries the pathogenic mutation. Unfortunately, there is presently no method by which the disease can be prevented in individuals who carry the mutation but are not yet affected.

Issues Related to Horizontal Transmission and Iatrogenic Spread of CJD

Precautions Related to CJD and Decontamination of Tissues

A significant concern related to prion diseases pertains to high levels of infectious virus in affected tissues and the extraordinary resistance of the agent to decontamination. Brain tissue of CJD patients contains from a thousand to more than a million lethal doses of agent per gram of tissue when assayed in susceptible animals. The fact that scrapie-affected hamster tissue can have titers of over 10^{10} hamster lethal doses may indicate that levels of the agent could be even higher if there were no species barrier to contend with, i.e., if CJD tissue were inoculated inadvertently into humans (68,69). For these reasons, adherence to the current policy regarding universal precautions for handling CJD patient blood and body fluids—intended to prevent infection with hepatitis B and C viruses and HIV-1—should be followed to reduce the chance of accidental exposure. It is advisable to place patients on "stool and needle precautions."

All materials and surfaces that contact SSE-affected tissues must be treated with care (reviewed in Refs. 68,69). Whenever possible, contaminated instruments should be discarded by careful packaging and subsequent transport to sites of incineration. Although no method of sterilization can be relied upon to remove all infectivity from contaminated surfaces, several methods markedly reduce titers of infectivity: autoclaving (132°C for 60 min), 1.0 N sodium hydroxide (lye), and 2.5% sodium hypochlorite (bleach) for 60 min. Ethylene oxide gas, formaldehyde, and a variety of commercial liquid disinfectants are completely ineffective. The remarkable stability of the agent is realized when one notes that a section of tissue that has been formalin fixed and paraffin embedded is still infectious and successfully transmits disease; for this reason, Brown et al. (70) recommend formalin fixation with a 1-h immersion in formic acid.

Horizontal Spread of the SSEs and Iatrogenic Cases of CJD

A variety of occurrences emphasize the potential of SSEs for horizontal spread and epidemics. Perhaps the earliest example of such an event involved the spread of scrapie in sheep vaccinated with scrapie-contaminated louping-ill vaccine (prepared from formalin-inactivated louping-ill virus in sheep brain) (71).

> In September, 1937, two and a half years after vaccinating the sheep, two owners complained that scrapie, a disease which had not before been observed in the Blackface sheep was appearing in their stock of Blackface sheep and further that it was confined to animals vaccinated with louping-ill vaccine in 1935. At that stage it was difficult to conceive that the occurrence could be associated with the injection of the vaccine ... [however] the evidence indicated that: (1) the infective agent of scrapie was present in the brain, spinal cord and or spleen of infected sheep; (2) it could withstand a concentration of formalin of 0.35 per cent, which inactivated the virus of louping ill; (3) it could be transmitted by subcutaneous inoculation; (4) it had an incubative period of two years and longer.

Similarly, transmissible mink encephalopathy is believed to have spread by ingestion of scrapie-contaminated sheep or goat tissues (72). The most recent example of epidemic spread of disease because of contamination of infected tissue is BSE, which is discussed below.

BSE first appeared in England in the mid-1980s and has affected over 100,000 cattle (reviewed in Refs. 73,74). It has been called "mad cow disease" because of the "nervousness" and change in behavior of the affected animal. Cows also develop a progressive gait disturbance, with death usually occurring in less than 6 months. It is believed that this disease appeared because of the practice of feeding cattle ruminant-derived feed that was contaminated with scrapie-infected tissue, in other words, cross-species transmission. The material used for cattle feed has now been changed, and there appears to be some abatement in the epidemic.

There are serious concerns regarding this epidemic. One concern is that maternal transmission occurs from cow to cow which can prolong the epidemic. The other concern relates to the apparent transmission of BSE from cows to humans via ingestion of beef. This transmission had seemed unlikely because: the oral route is inefficient; there is a "species barrier" that must be overcome; there is little suggestion of spread to humans of the analogous disease, scrapie, which occurs worldwide and has clearly contaminated food in the past (42). Despite these issues, the possibility of transmission of BSE to humans was always a real one because: the present hypothesis regarding the origins of BSE into cows assumes an oral route of transmission and breach of the "species barrier," from sheep to cows; experimental studies have demonstrated that kuru, CJD, and scrapie can be orally transmitted to nonhuman primates (75); kuru is known to have been spread by ingestion and/or subcutaneous inoculation of kuru-contaminated brain tissue. A recent report notes 10 unusual cases of human SSE in Britain, suggesting the possibility of spread of BSE to humans (75a). The SSE resembles kuru and involves relatively young patients with cerebeller signs, an unremarkable EEG, and evidence of plaques in the central nervous system. Epidemiological studies will be important to clarify the impact of BSE on the incidence of human SSE.

There are a number of examples of iatrogenic transmission of CJD. The early cases occurred related to transplantation of a corneal transplant from a CJD patient and to implantation of stereotaxic EEG electrodes that had been used in a CJD case and then inadequately sterilized with paraformaldehyde vapor (reviewed in Refs. 46,48). Subsequent examples occurred related to dura mater or corneal homografts. The incubation period of CJD in the corneal transplant recipient was 18 months. More recent and dramatic examples of iatrogenic CJD were traced to human growth hormone administration. The incubation period in over 40 proven or highly suspect cases is approximately 11 years, with a range of over 30 years. The clinical picture of these cases has been somewhat atypical with a cerebellar presentation, no periodic EEG activity, and little or no dementia until comparatively late in the illness (46,48). Interestingly, some investigators have suggested that a preponderance of these patients have homozygosity at the *PRNP* polymorphic codon 129 (28,76), emphasizing the importance of host genetics in susceptibility to and development of SSE.

Just as the human growth hormone concern seemed to be ebbing—coincident with the availability of bioengineered hormone—a new problem arose related to potential contamination of human infected tissues, specifically related blood and blood products from CJD patients. It is known that the buffy coat of experimentally inoculated animals contains the SSE agent (77). Unfortunately, it is unknown how long peripheral blood white cells are infectious. The apparent absence of an increased incidence of CJD in a high-risk population such as hemophiliacs and the failure to find an increased incidence of a history of blood transfusion above control levels among CJD patients (78) is slightly reassuring. It is clearly necessary to have better quantification of the risk of disease from exposure to varied biological materials prepared from human and animal tissues. Unfortunately, experimental testing in subhuman primates may give a falsely low estimate of the actual risk in humans because of decreased susceptibility due to the "species barrier." Mice that carry the human *PRNP* as a transgene (35) may be a preferable system to use for transmission studies; however, the prolonged incubation following the oral route of transmission could exceed the life span of the mouse and cause a false sense of security. The real solution to problems related to the danger of contamination with PrP^{Sc} may have to await a reliable and quick detection of PrP^{Sc}.

SUMMARY

The SSEs have had an impressive impact on medicine and science and will undoubtedly continue to do so. The following are some of the lessons they have taught us:

1. Rare, unusual diseases from exotic areas may be important to investigate. Diseases such as kuru have given us a new understanding of human infectious disease and changed our thinking. For example, the long incubation periods and symptom-free durations of disease in the acquired immunodeficiency syndrome seem not as astonishing now as they would have prior to the recognition of SSEs and human "slow virus infections."
2. Noninflammatory diseases and inherited diseases may be transmissible. The finding that a transmissible disease in an immunocompetent host may trigger no antibody response, produce no inflammatory pathology, and be heritable is a startling one. This realization has brought a large number of other noninflammatory neurological diseases under scrutiny for evidence of transmissibility.
3. There may be transmissible agents not yet included in our present classification of infectious pathogens. There may be replicating agents that defy our present concepts of molecular biology.

The SSEs have also raised questions that remain unanswered:

1. What diseases will eventually be included in the group of "prion" diseases? A number of degenerative diseases of unknown cause have been under investigation for transmissibility over the years, including Alzheimer's disease, Parkinson's disease, progressive supranuclear palsy, etc. This seems an especially relevant issue with respect to Alzheimer's disease because of certain features analogous to those seen in the SSEs. The observation that 10% of Alzheimer's disease cases are autosomal dominantly inherited and that at least some of these familial cases have a mutation in an amyloidogenic protein resembles findings in familial SSE; however, in contrast to the SSEs, Alzheimer's disease tissue is apparently not transmissible. The fact that some prion diseases, such as FFI, are remarkably difficult to transmit (58) raises the possibility that Alzheimer's disease may also be difficult to experimentally transmit, but may have a similar pathogenesis to the prion-type diseases.
2. What is the nature of the transmissible agent? The concept of a pathogenic protein, PrP^{Sc}, that is key to the development and transmission of SSE is fairly well accepted now. Information regarding the differences between PrP^{Sc} and PrP^{c}, especially differences in their conformation, will clearly be important. In addition, other genetic and nongenetic factors that are necessary to or influence the disease will be critical to a more complete understanding of these processes and their treatment.
3. What is the cause of sporadic CJD? As discussed earlier, there are hypotheses related to the somatic mutation of PrP^{c} into PrP^{Sc}; supporting data are needed. It is unclear how much of sporadic CJD represents unrecognized iatrogenic disease or a result of oral ingestion of SSE-infected tissues. It is critical for public health reasons to obtain a firmer understanding

of these issues and of the risk of transmission secondary to certain medical procedures or dietary habits.

We look forward to answers to these questions with the excitement that has always surrounded the SSEs.

ACKNOWLEDGMENTS

We thank Ellie Orr for excellent secretarial assistance, Dr. R. Wollmann for supplying photographs, and Dr. J. P. Spire for providing the EEG tracing.

REFERENCES

1. Wells GAH. Pathology of nonhuman spongiform encephalopathies: variations and their implication for pathogenesis. In: Brown F, ed. Transmissible Spongiform Encephalopathies. Developments in Biological Standardization. Vol. 80. Basel: Karger, 1993:61–69.
2. Gajdusek DC. Subacute spongiform encephalopathies: transmissible cerebral amyloidoses caused by unconventional viruses. In: Fields BN, Knipe DM, Chanock RM, eds. New York: Raven Press Ltd., 1990:2289–2324.
3. Prusiner SB, Hsiao KK. Human prion diseases. Ann Neurol 1994; 35:385–395.
4. Gajdusek DC. Foreword. In: Zigas V. Laughing Death: the Untold Story of Kuru. Clifton, NJ: Humana Press, 1990:*v–vi*.
5. Gajdusek DC, ed. Correspondence on the discovery and original investigators of kuru. Smadel-Gajdusek Correspondence 1955–1958. Bethesda, MD: National Institutes of Health, 1975.
6. Gajdusek DC, Zigas V. Degenerative disease of the central nervous system in New Guinea: the endemic occurrence of "kuru" in the native population. N Engl J Med 1957; 257:974–978.
7. Hadlow WJ. Scrapie and kuru. Lancet 1959; 2:289–290.
8. Sigurdsson B. Rida, a chronic encephalitis of sheep: with general remarks on infections which develop slowly and some of their special characteristics. Br Vet J 1954; 110:341–354.
9. Gajdusek DC, Gibbs CJ Jr, Alpers M. Experimental transmission of a kuru-like syndrome in chimpanzees. Nature 1966; 209:794–796.
10. Klatzo I, Gajdusek DC, Zigas V. Pathology of kuru. Lab Invest 1959; 8:799–847.
11. Gibbs CJ Jr, Gajdusek DC, Asher DM, et al. Creutzfeldt-Jakob disease (spongiform encephalopathy): transmission to the chimpanzee. Science 1968; 161:388–389.
12. Bolton DC, McKinley MP, Prusiner SB. Identification of a protein that purifies with the scrapie prion. Science 1982; 218:1309–1311.
13. Hsiao KK, Scott M, Foster D, Groth DF, DeArmond SJ, Prusiner SB. Spontaneous neurodegeneration in transgenic mice with mutant prion protein. Science 1990; 250:1587–1590.
14. Büeler H, Aguzzi A, Sailer A, et al. Mice devoid of PrP are resistant to scrapie. Cell 1993; 73:1339–1347.
15. Brown P, Gibbs CJ Jr, Rodgers-Johnson P, et al. Human spongiform encephalopathy: the National Institutes of Health series of 300 cases of experimentally transmitted disease. Ann Neurol 1994; 35:513–529.
16. Gibbons RA, Hunter GD. Nature of the scrapie agent. Nature (Lond.) 1967; 215:1041–1043.
17. Diener TO, McKinley MP, Prusiner SB. Viroids and prions. Proc Natl Acad Sci USA 1982; 79:5220–5224.
18. Oesch B, Westaway D, Wälchli M, et al. A cellular gene encodes scrapie PrP 27-30 protein. Cell 1985; 40:735–746.
19. Sparkes RS, Simon M, Cohn VH, et al. Assignment of the human and mouse prion protein genes to homologous chromosomes. Proc Natl Acad Sci USA 1986; 83:7358–7362.
20. Bendheim PE, Barry RA, DeArmond SJ, Stites DP, Prusiner SB. Antibodies to a scrapie prion protein. Nature 1984; 310:418–421.

21. Gajdusek DC. Infectious and noninfectious amyloidoses of the brain: systemic amyloidoses as predictive models in transmissible and nontransmissible amyloidotic neurodegeneration of Creutzfeldt-Jakob disease and aging brain and Alzheimer's disease. In: Calne DB, ed. Neurodegenerative Diseases. Philadelphia: W.B. Saunders, 1994:301–317.
22. Goldgaber D, Goldfarb LG, Brown P, et al. Mutations in familial Creutzfeldt-Jakob disease and Gerstmann-Sträussler-Scheinker's syndrome. Exp Neurol 1989; 106:204–206.
23. Hsiao K, Baker HF, Crow T, et al. Linkage of a prion protein missense variant to Gerstmann-Sträussler syndrome. Nature (London) 1989; 338:342–345.
24. Prusiner SB. Inherited prion diseases. Proc Natl Acad Sci USA 1994; 91:4611–4614.
25. Goldfarb LG, Brown P, Gajdusek DC. The molecular genetics of human transmissible spongiform encephalopathy. In: Prusiner SB, Collinge J, Powell J, Anderton B, eds. Prion Diseases of Humans and Animals. New York: Ellis Horwood Limited, 1992:139–153.
26. Hsiao K, Meiner Z, Kahana E, et al. Mutation of the prion protein in Libyan Jews with Creutzfeldt-Jakob disease. N Engl J Med, 1991; 324:1091–1097.
27. Goldfarb LG, Petersen RB, Tabaton M, et al. Fatal familial insomnia and familial Creutzfeldt-Jakob disease: disease phenotype determined by a DNA polymorphism. Science, 1992; 258:806–808.
28. Brown P, Cervenáková L, Goldfarb LG, et al. Iatrogenic Creutzfeldt-Jakob disease: an example of the interplay between ancient genes and modern medicine. Neurology 1994; 44:291–293.
29. Hsiao K, Groth D, Scott L, et al. Serial transmission in rodents of neurodegeneration from transgenic mice expressing mutant prion protein. Proc Natl Acad Sci USA 1994; 91:9126–9130.
30. Kocisko DA, Come JH, Priola SA, et al. Cell-free formation of protease-resistant prion protein. Nature 1994; 370:471–474.
31. Kocisko DA, Priola SZ, Raymond GJ, et al. Species specificity in the cell-free conversion of prion protein to protease-resistant forms: a model for the scrapie species barrier. Proc Natl Acad Sci USA 1995; 92:3923–3927.
32. Wickner RB. [URE3] as an altered URE2 protein: evidence for a prion analogue in *Saccharomyces cerevisiae*. Science 1994; 264:566–569.
33. Chernoff YO, Lindquist SL, Ono B-I, et al. Role of the chaperone protein Hsp 104 in propagation of the yeast prion-like factor [psi+]. Science, 1995; 268:880–884.
34. Telling GC, Scott M, Mastrianni J, et al. Prion propagation in mice expressing human and chimeric PrP transgenes implicates the interaction of cellular PrP with another protein. Cell 1995; 83:79–90.
35. Telling GC, Scott M, Hsiao KK, et al. Transmission of Creutzfeldt-Jakob disease from humans to transgenic mice expressing chimeric human-mouse prion protein. Proc Natl Acad Sci USA 1994; 91:9936–9940.
36. Brandner S, Isenmann S, Raeber A, et al. Normal host prion protein necessary for scrapie-induced neurotoxicity. Nature 1996; 379:339–343.
37. Sakaguchi S, Katamine S, Nishida N, et al. Loss of cerebellar Purkinje cells in aged mice homozygous for a disrupted PrP gene. Nature 1996; 380:528–531.
38. Collinge J, Whittington MA, Sidle KCL, et al. Prion protein is necessary for normal synaptic function. Nature 1994; 370:295–297.
39. Whittington MA, Sidle KCL, Gowland I, et al. Rescue of neurophysiological phenotype seen in PrP null mice by transgene encoding human prion protein. Nature Genet 1995; 9:197–201.
40. Westaway D, DeArmond SJ, Cayetano-Canlas J, et al. Degeneration of skeletal muscle, peripheral nerves, and the central nervous system in transgenic mice overexpressing wild-type prion proteins. Cell 1994; 76:117–129.
41. Jarrett JT, Lansbury PT Jr. Seeding "one-dimensional crystallization" of amyloid: a pathogenic mechanism in Alzheimer's disease and scrapie? Cell 1993; 73:1055–1058.
42. Chatelain J, Cathala F, Brown P, Raharison S, Court L, Gajdusek DC. Epidemiologic comparisons between Creutzfeldt-Jakob disease and scrapie in France during the 12-year period 1968–1979. J Neurol Sci 1981; 51:329–337.
43. Mizutani T, Okumura A, Oda M, Shiraki H. Panencephalitic type of Creutzfeldt-Jakob disease: primary involvement of the cerebral white matter. J Neurol Neurosurg Psychiatry 1981; 44:103–115.
44. Masters CL, Gajdusek DC. The spectrum of Creutzfeldt-Jakob disease and the virus-induced subacute

spongiform encephalopathies. In: Smith WT, Cavanagh JB, eds. Recent Advances in Neuropathology. Vol. 2. Edinburgh: Churchill Livingstone, 1982:139–163.
45. Masters CL, Gajdusek DC, Gibbs CJ Jr. Creutzfeldt-Jakob disease virus isolations from the Gerstmann-Sträussler syndrome: with an analysis of the various forms of amyloid plaque deposition in the virus-induced spongiform encephalopathies. Brain 1981; 104:559–588.
46. Brown P. Transmissible human spongiform encephalopathy (infectious cerebral amyloidosis): Creutzfeldt-Jakob disease, Gerstmann-Sträussler-Scheinker Syndrome, and Kuru. In: Calne DB, ed. Neurodegenerative Disease. Philadelphia: W. B. Saunders, 1994:839–876.
47. Roos R, Gajdusek DC, Gibbs CJ Jr. The clinical characteristics of transmissible Creutzfeldt-Jakob disease. Brain 1973; 96:1–20.
48. Brown P. The clinical neurology and epidemiology of Creutzfeldt-Jakob disease, with special reference to iatrogenic cases. In: Bock G, Marsh, J. eds. Novel Infectious Agents and the Central Nervous System. Ciba Foundation Symposium 135. Chichester: John Wiley and Sons, 1988:3–23.
49. Brown P, Cathala F, Castaigne P, Gajdusek DC. Creutzfeldt-Jakob disease: clinical analysis of a consecutive series of 230 neuropathologically verified cases. Ann Neurol 1986; 20:597–602.
50. Ghetti B, Piccardo P, Spillantini MG, et al. Vascular variant of prion protein cerebral amyloidosis with τ-positive neurofibrillary tangles: the phenotype of the stop codon 145 mutation in PRNP. Proc Natl Acad Sci USA 1996; 93:744–748.
51. Heston LL, Lowther DLW, Leventhal CM. Alzheimer's disease. Arch Neurol 1966; 15:225–233.
52. Nochlin D, Sumi SM, Bird TD, et al. Familial dementia with PrP-positive plaques. Neurology 1989; 39:910–918.
53. Lugaresi E, Medori R, Montagna P, et al. Fatal familial insomnia and dysautonomia with selective degeneration of thalamic nuclei. N Engl J Med 1986; 315:997–1003.
54. Reder AT, Mednick AS, Brown P, et al. Clinical and genetic studies of fatal familial insomnia. Neurology. 1995; 45:1068–1075.
55. Manetto V, Medori R, Cortelli P, et al. Fatal familial insomnia: clinical and pathologic study of five new cases. Neurology 1992; 42:312–319.
56. Lugaresi E. The thalamus and insomnia. Neurology 1992; 42(Suppl 16):28–33.
57. Medori R, Tritschler H-J, LeBlanc A, et al. Fatal familial insomnia, a prion disease with a mutation at codon 178 of the prion protein gene. N Engl J Med 1992; 326:444–449.
58. Tateishi J, Brown P, Kitamoto T, et al. First experimental transmission of fatal familial insomnia. Nature 1995; 376:434–435.
59. Denny-Brown D. Discussion. Trans Am Neurol Assoc 1960; 85:149–150.
60. Harrington MG, Merril CR, Asher DM, Gajdusek DC. Abnormal proteins in the cerebrospinal fluid of patients with Creutzfeldt-Jakob disease. N Engl J Med 1986; 315:279–283.
61. Harrington MG, Merril CR. Cerebrospinal fluid protein analysis in diseases of the nervous system. J Chromatogr 1988; 429:345–358.
61a. Hsieh G, Kenney K, Gibbs CJ Jr, et al. The 14-3-3 brain protein in cerebrospinal fluid as a marker for transmissible spondiform encephalopathies. N Engl J Med 1996; 335:924–930.
62. Hogan RN, Kingsbury DT, Baringer JR, Prusiner SB. Retinal degeneration in experimental Creutzfeldt-Jakob disease. Lab Invest 1983; 49:708–715.
63. Croxson M, Brown P, Synek B, et al. A new case of Creutzfeldt-Jakob disease associated with human growth hormone therapy in New Zealand. Neurology 1988; 38:1128–1130.
64. Renault F, Richard P. Early electroretinogram alterations in Creutzfeldt-Jakob disease after growth hormone treatment. Lancet 1991; 338:191.
65. Collinge J, Poulter M, Davis MB, et al. Presymptomatic detection or exclusion of prion protein gene defects in families with inherited prion diseases. Am J Hum Genet 1991; 49:1351–1354.
66. Rechtschaffen A, Gilliland MA, Bergmann BM, Winter JB. Physiological correlates of prolonged sleep deprivation in rats. Science 1983; 221:183–184.
67. Brown P. A therapeutic panorama of the spongiform encephalopathies. Antivir Chem Chemother 1990; 1:75–83.
68. Gajdusek DC, Gibbs CJ Jr., Asher DM, et al. Precautions in medical care of, and in handling materials

from, patients with transmissible virus dementia (Creutzfeldt-Jakob disease). N Engl J Med 1977; 297:1253–1258.
69. Brown P. Guidelines for high risk autopsy cases: special precautions for Creutzfeldt-Jakob disease. In: Autopsy Performance and Reporting. Northfield, IL: College of American Pathologists, 1990:68–74.
70. Brown P, Wolff A, Gajdusek DC. A simple and effective method for inactivating virus infectivity in formalin-fixed tissue samples from patients with Creutzfeldt-Jakob disease. Neurology 1990; 40: 887–890.
71. Gordon WS. Advances in veterinary research: Louping-ill, tick-borne fever and scrapie. Vet Rec 1946; 47:516–520.
72. Marsh RF, Hanson RP. On the origin of transmissible mink encephalopathy. In: Prusiner SB, Hadley WJ, eds. Slow Transmissible Diseases of the Nervous System. Vol. 1. New York: Academic Press, 1979: 451–460.
73. Brown F, ed. International meeting on transmissible spongiform encephalopathies. Developments in Biological Standardization. Vol. 80. Basel: Karger, 1993.
74. Bovine spongiform encephalopathy in the United Kingdom: memorandum from a WHO meeting. Bull WHO 1993; 71:691–694.
75. Gibbs CJ Jr, Amyx HL, Bacote A, Masters CL, Gajdusek DC. Oral transmission of kuru, Creutzfeldt-Jakob disease, and scrapie to nonhuman primates. J Infect Dis 1980; 142:205–208.
75a. Will RG, Ironside JW, Zeidler M, et al. A new variant of Creutzfeldt–Jakob disease in the UK. Lancet 1996: 347:921–925.
76. Deslys JP, Marce D, Dormont D. Similar genetic susceptibility in iatrogenic and sporadic Creutzfeldt-Jakob disease. J Gen Virol 1994; 75:23–27.
77. Manuelidis EE, Gorgacs EJ, Manuelidis L. Viremia in experimental Creutzfeldt-Jakob disease. Science 1978; 200:1069–1071.
78. Esmonde TFG, Will RG, Slattery JM, et al. Creutzfeldt-Jakob disease and blood transfusion. Lancet 1993; 341:205–207.

16

Neurological Complications of Infective Endocarditis

Nina J. Solenski and E. Clarke Haley, Jr.
University of Virginia, Charlottesville, Virginia

INTRODUCTION

History

Infective endocarditis was described by Rudolf Virchow, a professor of pathological anatomy, nearly 150 years ago. He, along with other investigators, astutely observed the association between cardiac valvular vegetations and distal arterial emboli. By the end of the nineteenth century, further observations were made by Pajet, Goodhart, Kirkes, and Osler (1–3). In 1885, Sir William Osler, in his now famous Gulstonian Lectures, described to the Royal College of Physicians in London the classic triad of *fever*, *heart murmur*, and *hemiplegia* of "malignant endocarditis" (1). Though he was not the first to observe and emphasize the involvement of the central nervous system during endocarditis, he contributed greatly to the diagnosis of this potentially fatal disease. Since the nineteenth century, modern medical technological advancements have increased our understanding of the pathophysiology and clinical therapy of infective endocarditis (IE). The formation of operational clinically defined terms for infectious endocarditis by Pelletier and Petersdorf (4) and Von Reyn et al. (5) have further aided our study of this disease. However, despite these advances, neurological complications remain a major contributor to mortality during the course of infective endocarditis.

Incidence

Neurological complications occur in 20–40% of patients with infective endocarditis (6,7) and represent the heralding symptom in 12–23% (8,9). Usually complications are diagnosed when the patient becomes symptomatic, for example, with the development of hemiplegia from cerebral infarction or the onset of confusion from encephalopathy. However, the true frequency of neurological complications including asymptomatic neuropathology may be even higher.

Paradoxically, despite the widespread use of antibiotics over the past few decades, the incidence of infective endocarditis in some studies is rising (10,11). In particular staphylococcal IE is being reported with increasing frequency. The recent increasing incidence of IE may be due to the greater use of invasive techniques (intravascular monitoring, pacemakers, gastrointestinal or oropharyngeal procedures, and genitourinary examination techniques). The rising age of the patient population is another possible contributing factor. The mean age of incidence of IE is increasing, with current mean age between 52 and 60 years of age compared to the previous mean of between 34 and 43 years of age during the 1950s and 1960s.

It has been claimed that the overall incidence of neurological complications has not changed over the last several decades (6). However, no large patient series without intrinsic referral bias exists to determine this definitively. Mortality from neurological complications seems to be unchanged (12). Studies suggest that neurological complications during IE can double or triple the mortality rate of native valve endocarditis. The percent mortality in patients with IE and neurological complications is approximately 50%, with the range from 16 to 87% (12–15). Neurological complications are responsible for up to 36% of the deaths in patients with native valve IE and for 10–45% of those with prosthetic valve IE (4,7,16).

PATHOPHYSIOLOGY

Pathogenesis of Infective Endocarditis

During infective endocarditis, it is postulated that the antithrombotic nature of the endothelial surface of the heart is lost and the surface becomes prothrombotic (17,18). The actual mechanism of infection in humans is unknown; however, numerous animal models of IE reveal that even at low inocula, bacteria in the presence of damaged endothelium can adhere and colonize cardiac tissue. Minimal trauma leads to massive platelet-fibrin deposition and thrombus formation. Trauma of the endothelial surface can occur from cardiac conditions which favor a high velocity jet stream, especially if occurring across a narrow orifice, or from a high- to low-pressure chamber (19). For example, certain congenital or acquired cardiac lesions (see below) may produce a turbulent blood flow jet, damaging the endocardial lining. The highest concentration of bacteria is deposited immediately below the obstructed orifice (area of lowest pressure), making this area prone to vegetation formation (19).

During an acute infection with a virulent bacterial or fungal species, such as *S. aureus*, colonization of a preformed vegetation of platelet-fibrin and thrombin quickly occurs, resulting in significant endocardial surface damage. In this case the vegetation tends to be soft, friable, and larger, with a propensity for embolization. In subacute infections with "nonvirulent" organisms, the damaged endothelial surface may have adequate time to heal over, with reconstitution of the endothelial layer and varying degrees of fibrosis, or calcification.

Though the pathogenesis of IE clearly involves perturbation of the cardiac tissue, in at least one study there was no underlying cardiac disease noted prior to presentation in 40% of cases of IE (13). A decline in this number has been observed subsequently, which may be explained by better recognition of valvular heart disease and improved treatment of bacteremic infections (20).

Common Risk Factors for Neurological Complications

In one recent study, factors including *age*, *duration of prodrome*, *anticoagulation* at the onset of symptoms, and the presence of *atrial fibrillation* were found to have no predictive value for the development of neurological complications in patients with IE (13). An earlier smaller series also found no correlation between neurological complication frequency and age, sex, preexisting valvular disease, anticoagulant therapy, or cardiac dysrhythmias (21).

The following discusses the more common risk factors for the development of infective endocarditis with an emphasis on data describing their influence on the incidence of neurological complications. Table 1 summarizes the more common risk factors and their relationship to neurological complications.

Table 1 Risk Factors for the Development of Infective Endocarditis and Their Relationship to Neurological Complications

Risk factor	Additional factors contributing to neurological complications
I. Cardiac disease	
A. Valvular disease	Left-(versus right-)sided endocarditis more frequently associated
1. native	
rheumatic	
degenerative	
2. prosthetic valves	Risk of embolism higher than in native valve disease (some, but not all series)
mechanical	
bioprosthetic	
B. Primary disease (congenital)	
mitral valve prolapse	Greater risk if mitral regurgitant murmur is present
ventricular septal defect	
bicuspid aortic valve	
patent ductus arteriosus	
aortic stenosis	
coarctation of the aorta	
pulmonary stenosis/atresia	
tetralogy of Fallot	
Marfan's syndrome	
idiopathic hypertrophic subaortic stenosis	
II. Iatrogenic	
dental procedures	Any invasive procedure associated with transient bacteremia
indwelling cathethers	
GI/GU instrumentation	
surgical procedures	
chronic hemodialysis	
III. Domestic or personal habits	
IVDA	Infections with *S. aureus* associated with increased risk of ICH
dental hygiene	
IV. Underlying disease	
immunodeficiency state	Usually in association with IVDA
V. Other	
advancing age	
male gender	
prior endocarditis	Usually IVDA-related

GU, Genitourinary; ICH, intracerebral hemorrhage; GI, gastrointestinal; IVDA, intravenous drug abuse.

Valvular Disease—Native

Traditionally, rheumatic heart disease has been the most common valvular disease predisposing to infective endocarditis. With the advent of bioprosthetic and mechanical prosthetic valves and routine cardiothoracic surgery for valve replacement, the presence of a prosthetic valve has replaced rheumatic disease as the most frequent predisposing factor (see below).

Neurological complications are most frequently observed in left-sided infective endocarditis, most likely due to the direct access of the emboli through the aortic root into the carotid and more distal cerebral circulation. In right-sided endocarditis, vegetative emboli can rarely gain access to the distal cerebral circulation except in the setting of a patent foramen ovale (resulting in paradoxical emboli). Whether the mitral or aortic valve itself is more frequently affected is a matter of debate. A recent study revealed similar rates of infection in the aortic and the mitral valve (13).

Besides the well-established association between rheumatic mitral valve disease and IE, recent studies have implicated mitral valve prolapse (MVP) as a risk factor for IE. There exists an approximate five- to ninefold increased risk for infective endocarditis in patients with MVP (22,23). Despite the incidence of MVP in women being three times that of males, males with MVP have been found to be at higher risk for developing IE than females (22–24). In contrast, another study concluded that although mitral valve involvement was more common in women, neurological complications by valve involvement revealed no statistical difference between the two groups (13).

Other common valvular disorders, including bicuspid or unicuspid aortic valve, valvular stenosis/insufficiency, or atheromatous valvular changes (25,26), may also constitute predisposing factors for IE.

Valvular Disease—Prosthetic Valve Replacement

The incidence of prosthetic valve endocarditis is 2–4%, with an incidence of neurological complications from both early and late (>60 days following surgery) infection of 25–40% (13,27–29). In some series, neurological complications seem to occur with the same frequency in native and prosthetic valve endocarditis (13). In addition, those patients with prosthetic valves requiring anticoagulation and who are judiciously anticoagulated may have a similar risk of central nervous system (CNS) complications when compared to native valve IE. In a recent review by Jamieson (30) of randomized clinical trials, including the Veterans Administration Study on Valvular Heart Disease and the Edinburgh Heart Valve Trial (31,32), the prevalence rates of thromboembolism, thrombosis, and prosthetic valve endocarditis were the same for mechanical and biological prostheses.

Congenital Cardiac Disease

As discussed above, cardiac hemodynamic factors can predispose a patient to development of IE and subsequent vegetation formation. Cardiac defects characterized by an abnormal pressure gradient of blood flow, from high to low, or those possessing a high-pressure jet stream are particularly vulnerable for the development of IE. This type of hemodynamic dysfunction occurs in small interventricular septal defect, patent ductus arteriosus, and subaortic and valvular aortic stenosis (19,24). Other forms of cardiac disease associated with a higher risk of IE include coarctation of the aorta and hypertrophic cardiomyopathy. Since atrial septal defect of the secondum type involves no or minimal blood flow disruption, this cardiac defect does not carry a higher risk of IE.

Iatrogenic

Over the course of the last two decades, numerous invasive techniques have played a prominent role as etiologic factors in IE and ultimately contributed to the incidence of neurological complications. Dental procedures, including home oral irrigation devices, invasive surgical procedures including placement of arterial and intravenous lines and catheters, genitourinary instrumentation, and other invasive procedures create a transient bacteremia that can result in IE. Recognition of this source of infection has led to the development of prophylactic antibiotic treatment guidelines. The reader is referred to the more recent guidelines provided by the American Heart Association (Committee on Rheumatic Fever and Infective Endocarditis, 1990) (33).

Intravenous Drug Abuse

In contrast to nonaddicts with IE, patients with intravenous drug abuse (IVDA) and IE more commonly have right-sided cardiac disease. The subpopulation of patients using illicit intravenous drugs, who subsequently contract infective endocarditis, tend to be younger, with a mean age of 30 years. In addition, there is a male preponderance (3:1 male-to-female ratio) (34,35), and it is usually limited to chronic abusers. There is overwhelming evidence that the tricuspid valve is the most frequently infected valve, accounting for 40–60% of cases. Tricuspid valve involvement in IE may be underreported, due to the frequent lack of murmur and confusion with a pulmonary disease. Neurological complications are rare in isolated right-sided IE in IV drug abusers (35–37). In contrast, there is a high frequency of neurological complications in the intravenous drug abusers with left-sided IE ranging from 45 to 58% (9). One explanation for the higher incidence of neurological complications in intravenous drug abusers with left-sided IE as compared to the nonaddict population may be a higher rate of failure with compliance of a course of antimicrobial therapy (37).

Noncardiac Underlying Disease

Infective endocarditis can occur as a complication of immunosuppression from malignancy, diabetes, and human immunodeficiency virus (HIV) infection, especially when the latter is associated with IVDA. Systemic diseases, such as malignancies, that are also associated with hypercoagulable states have an additional increased risk of thromboembolic complications. Patients on chronic immunosuppressive drugs for lupus erythematosus, leukemia, etc., are also at risk for developing IE, particularly in the presence of cardiac murmur or known cardiac defect. These patients may be at risk for contraction of more virulent infective species including fungi, such as *Candida* or *Aspergillus* species.

Pathogenesis of Neurological Complications

Overview

Neurological complications of IE most commonly involve the central nervous system with the majority of pathology occurring from seeding of septic or nonseptic emboli within the cerebral vessels, the brain parenchyma, and/or the meningeal lining (Fig. 1). For example, the acute onset of a focal neurological deficit such as hemiplegia or aphasia is typical of embolic stroke, while global confusion with nuchal rigidity is typical of meningitis or meningoencephalitis.

Cerebral emboli are by far the most frequent neurological complication. In light of the pathophysiology of endocarditis (see below), this is not an unexpected observation. This complication is followed in decreasing frequency by meningitis, encephalopathy, headache, intracranial hemorrhage, seizure, abscess, and mycotic aneurysm (Fig. 2). Rarer neurological complications can occur in the spinal cord and bony spinal canal in the form of spinal artery emboli, space-occupying abscesses, or diskitis, in the retina (emboli), or involving the cranial or peripheral nerves. In addition there are case reports of various movement disorders, including dyskinesias, tremor, and myoclonus, implicating basal ganglia pathology. Psychiatric disorders including psychosis also have been reported (38,39).

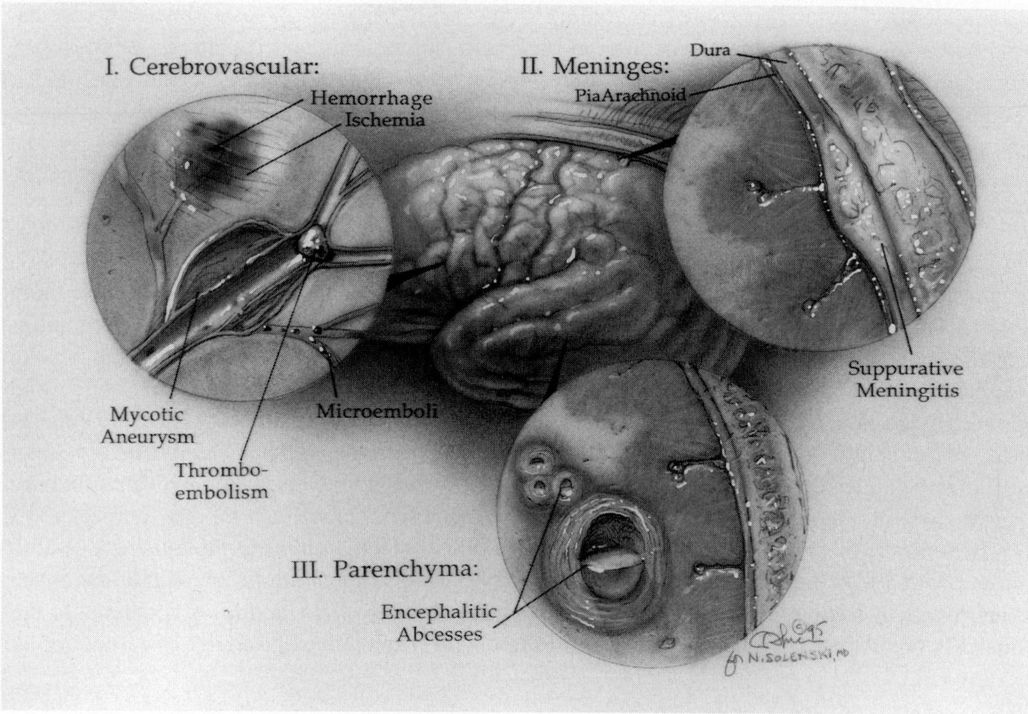

Figure 1 A variety of pathophysiological mechanisms lead to neurological complications of infective endocarditis. Involvement of brain parenchyma can result in meningoencephalitis or in abscess, while involvement of cerebral blood vessels can lead to arteritis, with thromboembolic infarction and/or the formation of a mycotic aneursym. Rupture of the vessel wall results in intraparenchymal and/or subarachnoid bleeding.

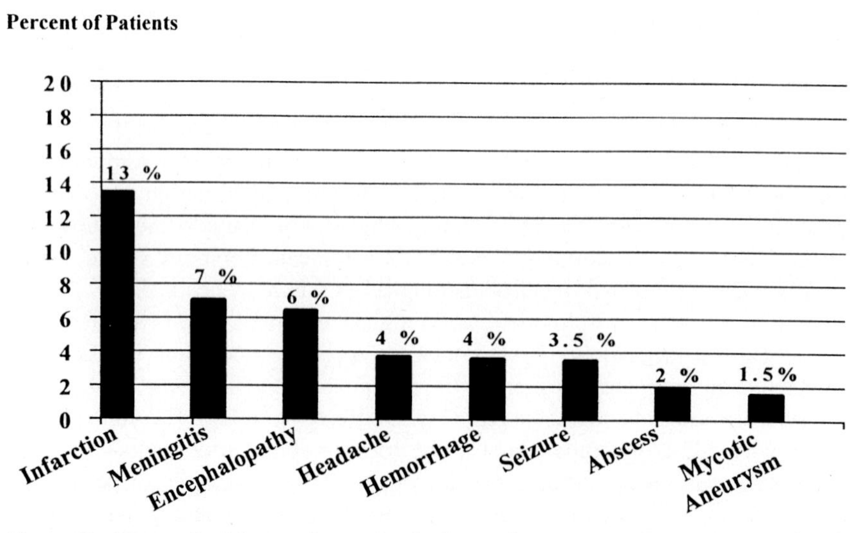

Figure 2 Percent incidence of neurological complications in 1014 patients with infective endocarditis. (From Ref. 9.)

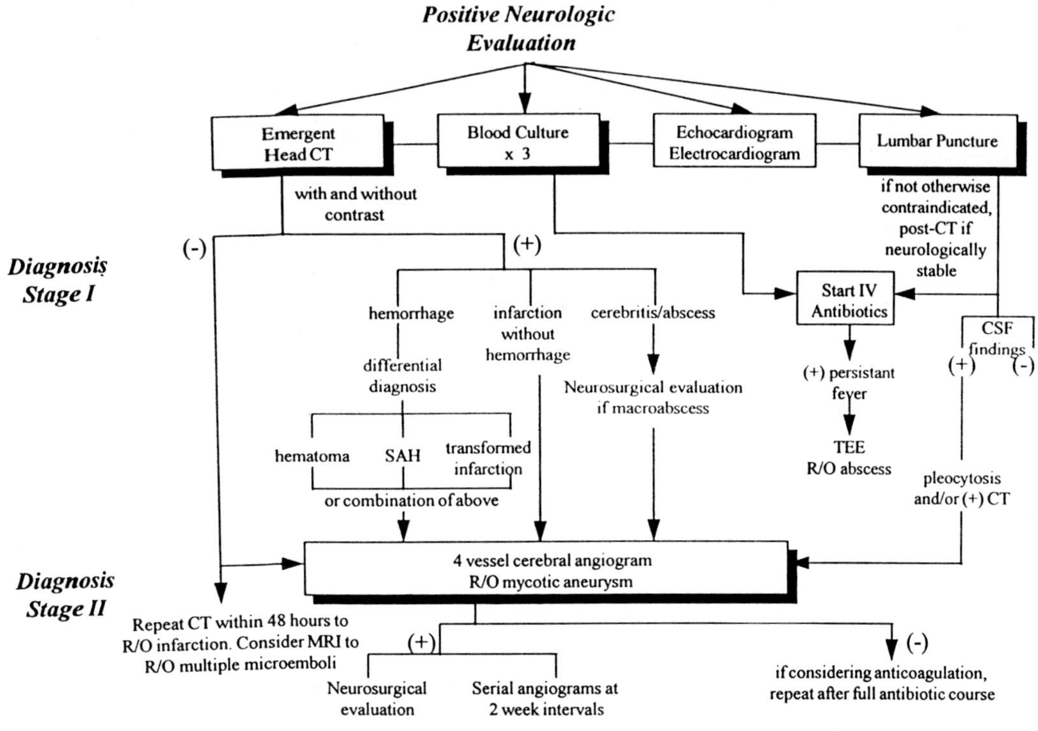

Figure 3 Management algorithm for the treatment of patients with known IE and a neurological complication and for the treatment of patients with the acute onset of a neurological deficit in the setting of suspected IE. CT—(cranial) Computerized tomography; IV—intravenous; CSF—cerebrospinal fluid; SAH—subarachnoid hemorrhage; TEE—transesophageal echocardiogram; R/O—rule out; MRI—magnetic resonance imaging; CNS—central nervous system.

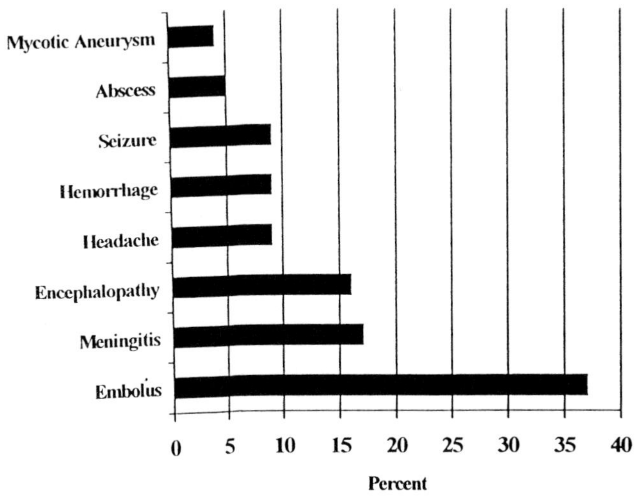

Figure 4 Proportion of individual neurological complications to total neurological complications during infective endocarditis. Data are based on a literature review of 1014 patients with infective endocarditis. (From Ref. 9.)

Table 3 Common Cerebral Embolic Infarction Syndromes

Occluded Cerebral Artery	CT Territory (coronal sections)	Neurologic Deficit	Management Issues
MCA proximal trunk	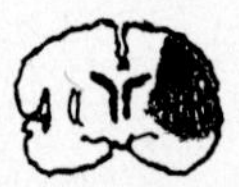	Contralateral hemiplegia hemianesthesia Head and eye deviation Homonymous hemianopia Global or mixed aphasia (dominant) Neglect (nondominant)	Large infarcted area-increased risk hemorrhage Possible mass effect with midline shift - requires intensive care monitoring for minimal 72 hours
superior division	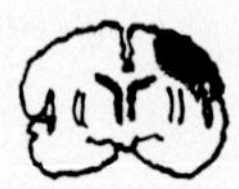	Contralateral hemiparesis hemianesthesia Expressive (motor) aphasia (dominant) Hemineglect	Oral motor dysfunction-poor clearing of oral secretions with increased risk of aspiration
inferior division	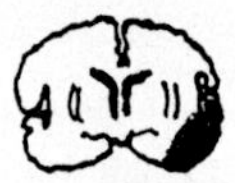	Contralateral hemianesthesia hemianopia Receptive (sensory) aphasia (dominant) or Conduction aphasia Apraxia	
ACA	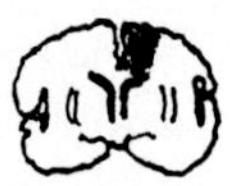	Hemiparesis leg>>arm mild leg sensory loss Dominant-transcortical motor aphasia Apathy, motor apraxia, incontinence	Behavioral changes result in significant morbidity

MCA - middle cerebral artery ACA - anterior cerebral artery CT - computerized tomography

of uncertain location. These same investigators noted that the majority of infarctions were small (58%) or of moderate size (33%). Though brain-stem syndromes are considered rare, nearly 10% of major cerebral embolic infarctions in the Massachusetts General Hospital series (4/38 episodes) were of this type (12). In this same series, there were three cases of cerebral infarction (in the "watershed" areas) due to hypotension.

In addition to the more easily recognized unifocal embolic cerebral infarction, which presents with a focal stroke syndrome, *multiple cerebral microemboli* can lead to significant neurological deficit as well. Microscopic infarctions have been associated with neurological complications including encephalopathy, focal or generalized seizures, and psychosis. Evidence of multiple microinfarctions (presumably from small vessel emboli) is common at autopsy, in as many as 50% of patients undergoing postmortem examination following IE.

Diagnosis

A neuroimaging study, usually a computerized tomography (CT) scan of the brain (with and without contrast), is mandatory for the initial evaluation of any patient with fever and evidence of a fixed or transient focal or multifocal neurological deficit. Serious life-threatening neurological complications, such as cerebral abscess and hemorrhage, must be ruled out emergently. In the setting of known infective endocarditis and cerebral infarction, the cranial CT may reveal signs of subacute cortical, subcortical, unifocal, or multifocal cerebral infarction (Fig. 5A). Hemorrhagic transformation of the infarcted site may be evident and, if present, must be distinguished from a primary parenchymal hemorrhage. In one series of 36 patients with MCA distribution strokes, early hypodensity within 4 h predicted hemorrhagic transformation in 72% of the patients

(48). In another recent study, hemorrhagic conversion following cerebral infarction was seen in nearly 43% of patients within 4 weeks (49). Clinically, the occurrence of a secondary hemorrhagic transformation may be suspected when the neurological deficit is large or there is a sudden neurological deterioration in the patient. Despite the emerging role of magnetic resonance imaging (MRI) for evaluation of the patient with IE with a neurological deficit, the CT scan remains the best choice as an initial imaging study because of its far greater sensitivity for detecting acute hemorrhagic pathology (Fig. 5B). The higher sensitivity of MRI for detecting small infarctions, notably in the posterior fossa (cerebellum and brain stem), make it a superior choice in patients with evidence of posterior circulation deficits (following an initial normal cranial CT). There are recent data suggesting a further role for MRI in diagnosing microabscesses or microemboli in the patient with IE particularly when the initial cranial CT findings are normal and the patient has neurological deterioration (50).

Therapy

Expeditious, organism-specific antibiotic therapy remains the single most important intervention for prevention of further embolic phenomena once cerebral infarction or ischemia has occurred during IE. In a 12-year retrospective follow-up study of neurological complications following IE, Salgado et al. found recurrent ischemic episodes were uncommon after initiation of antibiotic treatment. In this series of 175 patients, recurrent neurological events occurred acutely in only two patients; both patients had mechanical valves and had their episode prior to antibiotic therapy (13). The incidence of emboli is highest within the first 48 h chiefly during the acute uncontrolled infectious state. Following this period the risk of recurrent emboli falls significantly during adequate treatment.

In uncomplicated cases of IE, valve replacement, notably following a single initial cerebral embolic event, is rarely indicated. Two exceptions are the presence of fungal endocarditis or of cardiac hemodynamic failure due to valve incompetence.

Anticoagulation in Native Valve Endocarditis. In the patient with native valve endocarditis who survives the first episode of cerebral embolism, the recurrence rate is low following initiation of antibiotic therapy. The use of anticoagulation in this setting is difficult to justify. The potential benefit is exceeded by the potential risk for a hemorrhagic complication.

Anticoagulation in Prosthetic Valve Endocarditis. The overall rate of cerebral infarction in prosthetic valve endocarditis (PVE) is approximately 25%. Those patients with PVE not receiving anticoagulation therapy have a 20–71% rate of CNS complications including stroke (28,51). The current trend is to anticoagulate the patient with a newly infected prosthetic valve, mainly based on aggregate evidence suggesting that anticoagulation decreases the incidence of stroke in general. Some experts suggest the use of heparin sodium as soon as the diagnosis of late prosthetic valve endocarditis is suspected and its continuation during the course of antibiotic therapy (28,52). If a large cerebral infarction is detected on cranial CT, heparin should be discontinued and restarted greater than or at 48 to 72 h following the initial injury (52). In contrast, some investigators recommend discontinuance of anticoagulation at the time of the embolic event, with reinstitution following resolution of the infection.

Although some studies in the past have shown a high frequency of cerebral emboli with prosthetic valve endocarditis, more recent data indicate that the incidence of cerebral embolism may be similar between native and prosthetic valve IE (13). Recent studies have not found a dramatic decrease in cerebral embolic events by warfarin therapy for acute prosthetic valve IE (16). The potential for serious complications including cerebral hemorrhage and its associated mortality has led other authors to question and/or discourage the use of anticoagulation during PVE (47,53). These observations argue against the use of anticoagulation for the prophylaxis of cerebral embolic events in prosthetic valve IE.

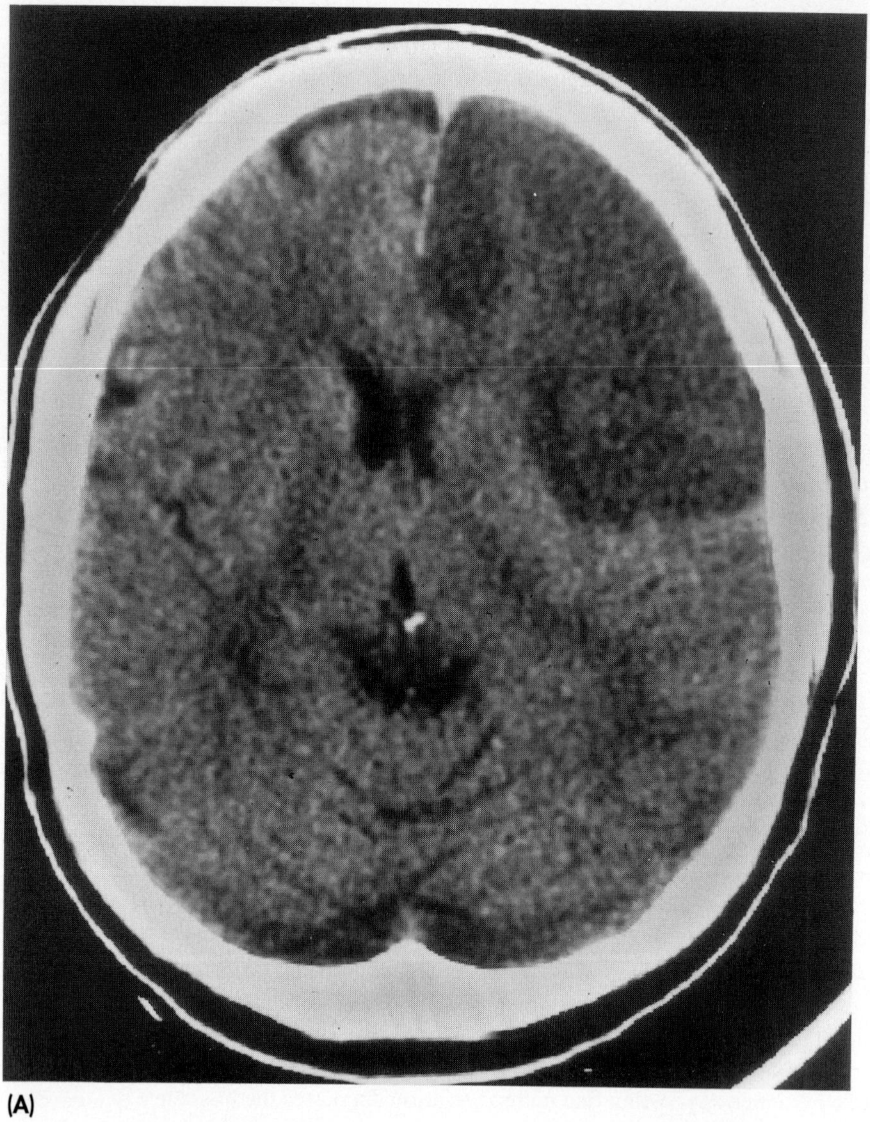

(A)

Figure 5 Cranial CT in the setting of IE can reveal single or multiple hypodensities. The noncontrasted CT (A) reveals a typical large left middle cerebral and anterior cerebral artery territory hypodensity consistent with a left hemispheric infarction. Cranial CT (B) in a 48-year-old with mental status changes revealed a large right frontoparietal parenchymal hemorrhage with associated intraventricular and subarachnoid extension. Follow-up cerebral angiography disclosed a mycotic aneurysm of one of the branches of the middle cerebral artery.

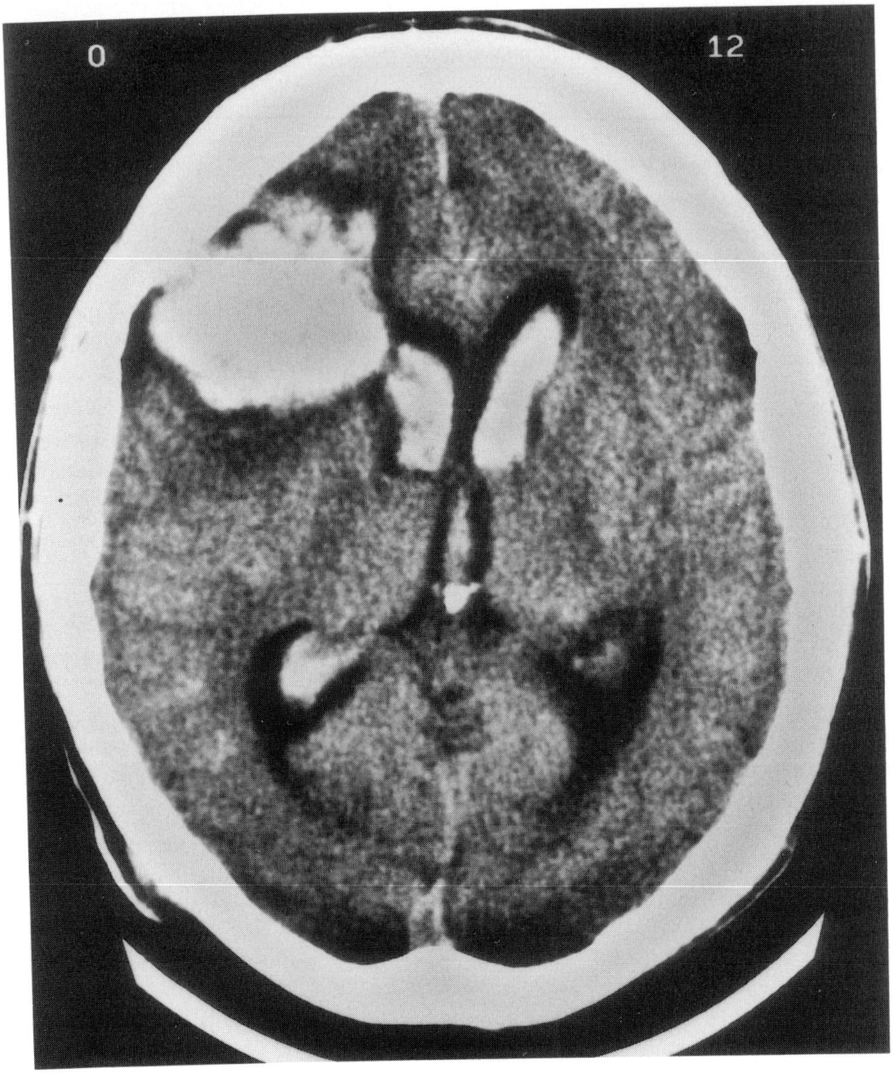

(B)

Direct comparison of individual studies is difficult due to inconsistent definitions of IE, type and degree of anticoagulation, type of PVE (early vs. late), type of valve (mechanical versus bioprosthetic), and length of patient follow-up. Until adequate prospective, randomized clinical trials are designed to assess the true risk-to-benefit ratio both as prophylaxis and as therapy for recurrent cerebral ischemia, a wide spectrum of use of anticoagulation in this patient subpopulation will be tolerated. Despite the controversy, there is agreement that if anticoagulation is deemed beneficial, careful and frequent monitoring of either the International Normalized Ratio (INR) or the Partial Prothrombin Time (PPT) is mandatory.

Aspirin and other antiplatelet drugs are currently being evaluated. In a recent study, the incidence of stroke on cranial CT was prospectively compared in a small series where patients with infective endocarditis were randomized to either low-dose aspirin (75 mg) or no aspirin for a mean period of 38 days. During the treatment period, one patient in the nontreated group developed a cerebral infarction. As the authors point out, a definite answer on the efficacy of aspirin prophylaxis for embolic infarction in the setting of IE will require a large, multicenter clinical trial (54).

Prognosis

In general the risk of recurrent stroke is extremely low in patients surviving the acute cerebral event and in those with controlled infection (12,13,47,55). In a large retrospective study, recurrent emboli were rare after the infection was controlled, leading the authors to conclude that anticoagulants and surgery are not warranted to prevent recurrent stroke in these patients (16). Higher rates of recurrent stroke have been reported. In a series from the Cleveland Clinic, of the patients discharged from the hospital with the diagnosis of IE and who were successfully followed for a median period of 2.2 years, 11% developed cerebrovascular complications, the majority of whom had prosthetic valves (13). In a retrospective review of the clinical literature, the Cerebral Embolism Task Force determined that the overall risk of a stroke with permanent adeficits is less than 2% per year and less than 1% per year for anticoagulated mechanical noninfected mitral and aortic prosthetic cardiac valves, respectively (55).

Encephalopathy

Incidence/Risk Factors

In numerous series, encephalopathy ranks second in frequency of neurological complications during IE (13). The term "encephalopathy" is nonspecific, and therefore a wide spectrum of CNS dysfunction is included within this diagnosis. Mild encephalopathy may be manifested by confusion and disorientation, while more severe encephalopathy may present as stupor or coma. Exacerbating factors for encephalopathy include age, iatrogenic causes (mainly from drug therapy), hypoxia, and metabolic changes. Pertinent metabolic complications include metabolic acidosis, hyponatremia (possibly a manifestation of inappropriate antidiuretic hormone syndrome), and elevated blood urea nitrogen level. Acute renal dysfunction in the form of focal glomerular nephritis can occur from multiple septic infarctions. The etiology of encephalopathy in most cases is multifactorial (56).

Pathogenesis

Nonmetabolic encephalopathy is attributed to microemboli, resulting in cerebral microinfarctions, with petechial hemorrhage and microabscess. These pathological features are not typically seen on routine cranial CT studies, but can be demonstrated by MR imaging (50). A total of 8 out of 218 patients (4%) in the Massachusetts General Hospital patient series had abscesses less than 1 cm^3 (microscopic) in size. Focal neurological findings were not present (12). Patients with microabscess frequently had a fulminate course of IE and were infected with *S. aureus*, *Enterococcus*, or *Serratia marcescans*.

Diagnosis

Some series define a type of encephalopathy known as "acute" or "toxic" encephalopathy in which psychiatric manifestations predominate, including personality change, hallucinations, or paranoid ideations. Disorientation and confusion may also be present (57). Similarly, cases of meningoencephalitis have also been described as "toxic encephalopathy." Additionally, encephalopathy in the elderly has been described as an "acute confusional syndrome." This encephalopathy occurs mainly in older adults and may be the predominant or presenting feature of endocarditis in 26% of this subgroup (58). The elderly patient with IE is particularly prone to misdiagnosis and delayed therapy (58). Misdiagnosis is due to frequent nonspecific complaints, in combination with an initial presentation of confusion, without fever or leukocytosis.

As suggested by previous authors, the multidefined terms "toxic encephalopathy" and "acute confusional syndrome" are best abandoned when possible (6). A clear description of the specific neurological cognitive deficit (delirium, comatose, etc.) and its etiology, if known, is far more useful for designing treatment protocols.

Therapy

Nearly any type of encephalopathy, regardless of cause, will be improved with aggressive antibiotic treatment of the primary infection. However, careful attention to drug allergies must be given since penicillin and other antibiotics may cause an encephalopathy. Other specific therapy includes correction of any metabolic abnormalities and careful administration of medications with possible CNS side effects. Common drugs, for example, histamine blockers (H_2), used in the intensive care setting are notable for their CNS effects in the elderly. In the stuporous or comatose patient, sedation should be avoided in order to adequately assess any change in neurological status.

Prognosis

Prognosis is highly dependent on etiology. Complicating conditions such as hyponatremia, renal azotemia, or drug reactions can usually be reversed. Elderly patients presenting with mental status changes may have a poorer prognosis. Errors in diagnosis often occur in the elderly patient, resulting in a delay in initiating appropriate therapy and thereby contributing to morbidity and death. In one series, an initial error in diagnosis was made in 11 of 16 elderly patients who ultimately died (58). Since the elderly are more prone to this neurological complication, it is difficult to determine if advanced age is an independent risk factor for a poor prognosis.

Intracranial Hemorrhage

Incidence/Risk Factors

The incidence of intracranial hemorrhage (ICH) in IE is 3–8% (8,59). Mechanisms leading to ICH include septic arteritis with vessel wall rupture, conversion of a bland cerebral infarction to a hemorrhagic one, rupture of a mycotic aneurysm, and primary parenchymal hemorrhage, especially in the setting of a bleeding diathesis (including anticoagulation). Although not always clinically recognized, antecedent embolism is most likely a prerequisite for ICH. Clinically recognized ipsilateral embolism precedes ICH in approximately 30–40% of cases (12,13,59,60). Hemorrhagic transformation of a cerebral infarction occurs in 6–24% of infarctions associated with native valve endocarditis and in 8–36% of infarctions with prosthetic valve endocarditis (61).

The role of anticoagulation as a risk factor for ICH is well recognized and has presented a serious therapeutic dilemma in the patient with IE and prosthetic valve replacement. In a large patient series, it was noted that 23% of the hemorrhagic events occurred in the 3% of the patients with IE who were on anticoagulation therapy (12). Anticoagulation potentially contributed to intracranial hemorrhage in 24% of patients in another analysis of patients with IE and ICH (59). In this series, approximately one-third of the patients who developed ICH in the setting of infective endocarditis were anticoagulated or had a bleeding diathesis at the time of the ICH. Another recent study to elucidate the pathological mechanisms of ICH noted 8/15 patients with IE and neurological symptoms were anticoagulated (prophylaxis for predisposing cardiovascular disorder), and an additional two patients were on hemodialysis prior to the discovery of the ICH (62).

The abrupt onset of severe neurological deficit and ICH is commonly associated with IE of *S. aureus* origin. These hemorrhages occur early in the clinical course (within 48 h of admission) and during uncontrolled infection (59).

Medical conditions predisposing to a bleeding diathesis include disseminated intravascular coagulation, thrombocytopenia, and vitamin K deficiency states. These conditions must be suspected in the alcoholic or otherwise debilitated patient and need to be treated expeditiously.

Clinical Presentation

There is a wide spectrum of neurological presentation with ICH in the setting of IE. The patient may present with encephalopathy including coma, meningismus, confusion, headache, generalized seizure, or with focal signs and symptoms, including hemiparesis or aphasia (59). Frequently, depending on the timing of presentation, there is a combination of both focal and generalized neurological deficits. For example, patients may present with confusion followed by the abrupt onset of hemiparesis. In addition, headache is a common complaint, and, in the febrile patient with known risk factors for IE, this symptom should alert the physician to the possibility of ICH.

As mentioned earlier, the occurrence of a TIA may precede intracerebral hemorrhage. In one series, 4 of 12 patients with TIA and subacute bacterial endocarditis subsequently developed a fatal intracerebral hemorrhage (63). In a review of 13 patients with ruptured mycotic aneurysm and IE, there was an average of 10 days between the onset of warning signs or symptoms and the subsequent catastrophic hemorrhage (64). There is a propensity for an expanding intracranial hematoma to result in rapid neurological deterioration with frequently fatal consequences if it is not recognized early on.

As with nonseptic emboli, hemorrhagic transformation of septic embolic infarction is usually asymptomatic but should be sought for whenever a large cerebral infarction occurs. Hemorrhagic conversion may be associated with acute neurological worsening in the anticoagulated patient.

Pathogenesis

Recognized mechanisms of intracranial hemorrhage in the patient with IE include the following:

1. Acute cerebral vessel rupture—this may occur due to septic necrosis of the arterial wall without aneurysm formation, or due to rupture of a mycotic aneurysm.
2. Hemorrhagic transformation of a bland infarction with or without additional hematoma formation.
3. Primary intracerebral hematoma formation.

The proportion of ICH attributable to each of the above mechanisms depends on the series. In one of the larger series of ICH from IE, 24% were from hemorrhagic infarction, 24% from necrotic arteritis, 12% from ruptured mycotic aneurysm, and the remaining 29% were unknown (59).

In the assessment of ICH there is normally a distinction between intraparenchymal hematoma and hemorrhagic infarction. In the IE patient with intracranial bleeding, this distinction may be difficult, especially if anticoagulated, since one pathology can quickly lead to the other. For example, a bland infarction that transforms into a hemorrhagic one can further worsen by forming a hematoma. The site of the hemorrhage varies, involving temporal, parietal, occipital, frontal lobes, or the entire hemisphere. Regardless of the initial cause of hemorrhage, the hemorrhage can remain confined within the parenchyma or extend into the subarachnoid or intraventricular space.

There is general agreement that most ICH is due to septic, necrotic arteritis from uncontrolled infection (47,55) rather than from mycotic aneurysm rupture (46). In a recent histopathological analysis of 16 patients with IE and ICH, 15 examined by autopsy, 13 of the patients had evidence of either septic emboli and/or pyogenic arteritis (62). In particular, *S. aureus* arteritis is associated with early hemorrhages (within 48 h) (59). ICH occurs in 17–32% of patients with *S. aureus* (21,55).

Diagnosis

The majority of current cases of ICH are diagnosed by cranial computerized tomography (CT). ICH is defined by a noncalcific hyperdensity on a noncontrasted CT. Depending on the mechanism of the hemorrhage, the cranial CT may reveal an expanding hematoma, or it may reveal a patchy distribution of hemorrhage within infarcted brain parenchyma. CT imaging of a *parenchymatous hematoma* reveals a homogenous, high-density, usually well-demarcated lesion, sometimes with prominent mass effect (Fig. 5B). This radiological finding is in contrast to a *hemorrhagic infarction*, which appears on CT as a more heterogeneous, patchy high-density lesion usually following the anatomy of the gyri. With the finding of ICH, the possibility of a mycotic aneurysm should be investigated with a four-vessel cerebral angiogram. A small area of focal cortical enhancement adjacent to the hyperdense clot on a contrasted CT is suspicious for an associated mycotic aneurysm (65).

While brain MRI is more sensitive for detecting subacute intraparenchymal hemorrhage, cranial CT remains the neuroimaging test of choice due to its greater sensitivity for diagnosing acute blood or any blood extending into the subarachnoid space. However, MRI can be useful to reveal abnormal vasculature, notably with the addition of MR angiography (MRA). MRA may be the only option for determining the cause of ICH for the patient that cannot tolerate conventional cerebral angiography. When the neuroimaging studies are nondiagnostic for the cause of the ICH, early cerebral angiography is indicated to rule out mycotic aneurysm.

Therapy

Patients with severe neurological deficits or signs of impending neurological deterioration should be immediately transferred to the intensive care setting where constant hemodynamic and neurological monitoring can be obtained. Parenteral antibiotic therapy should be started urgently upon suspicion of an infectious cause; this is particularly important if the organism could be *S. aureus*. Any potential source of bacteremia should be eliminated as well as potential contributors to a bleeding diathesis. Discontinuing antiplatelet therapy, correcting vitamin deficiencies, culturing, and removing any indwelling catheters may be necessary.

Craniotomy and evacuation of the hematoma in selected patients can be a life-saving procedure, although no strict guidelines exist for the determination of when craniotomy is best performed for ICH. A few generally agreed upon relative indications include (1) neurological deterioration, in the case that there is potentially salvageable brain tissue if surgery is performed acutely and (2) cerebellar hemorrhage, notably $>$ 3 cm in size and if there is minimal deficit. Cerebellar hemorrhage in the setting of IE is exceedingly rare, although there are case reports of mycotic aneurysms occurring in the vertebrobasilar system (66,67). Surgical treatment is less frequently advocated if there is a stable persistent neurological deficit or coma at the time of presentation.

Prognosis

Regardless of the initial mechanism of hemorrhage, the patient with symptomatic ICH in the setting of IE can have a high mortality of approximately 40–90% (21,52,59). In patients surviving the initial hemorrhage, there is evidence that recurrent hemorrhage is infrequent both during and following antibiotic therapy.

Cerebral Mycotic Aneurysm

Incidence and Risk Factors

The reported incidence of mycotic aneurysm in infective endocarditis is 1–10% (6,12,68,69). Mycotic aneurysms are clinically recognized in 2% of patients with diagnosed IE, and at autopsy in 5–10% of cases of IE (6). The true incidence remains unknown due to obliteration upon rupture and the fact that many patients may remain asymptomatic, especially if adequately treated with antibiotics. In addition, it has been suggested that mycotic aneurysm incidence may be falsely underestimated since many patients die from rupture prior to hospital admission (68). The overall incidence of mycotic aneurysm may be decreasing. In the early twentieth century, up to 30% of total intracranial aneurysms were mycotic aneurysms (70), compared to the current estimate of approximately 5%.

Clinical Presentation

The presentation of an unruptured mycotic aneurysm may mimic an embolic stroke by presenting with a focal neurological sign or may be associated with a severe localized headache suggesting subarachnoid hemorrhage (SAH) or other intracranial hemorrhagic event. Unfortunately, the initial presentation may be the abrupt onset of a neurological catastrophe (SAH or ICH) without a prior diagnosis of IE. In one large literature review of patients with the diagnosis of bacterial intracranial aneurysm in the setting of suspected or definite IE, the clinical presentation included hemorrhage (52%), infarction (20%), unknown (20%), infarction with hemorrhage (6%), and headache only (2%) (71).

Pathogenesis

Cerebral mycotic aneurysms are formed when septic emboli migrate and lodge within the cerebral vasculature. Once stagnant, the septic emboli may produce an inflammatory destruction of the arterial wall, starting on the luminal side and working through the adventitial layer (Fig. 6). Serial cerebral angiographic studies confirm that in some cases, an initial intraluminal septic clot may be the nidus for subsequent aneurysm formation (72). Alternatively, the embolus may become lodged within the vasa vasorum in the advential layer of the artery, leading to arterial dilatation (73). Mycotic aneurysms are typically located at bifurcation points within distal branches of the middle cerebral artery (MCA). Analysis of the location of the aneurysm in a total of 219 cases reveals involvement of the MCA in 39%, the anterior cerebral artery (ACA) in 5%, basilar artery in 5%, intradural internal carotid artery (ICA) in 4%, and posterior cerebral artery (PCA) in 4%, with location in remaining sites uncommon (70). This anatomical feature may help to distinguish mycotic aneurysms from congenital aneurysms, since the latter more commonly occur in the circle of Willis. Some investigators have suggested that drug abusers may be at increased risk for multiple mycotic aneurysm formation because of repeated episodes of bacteremia. Rarely, the mycotic aneurysm may be associated with an adjacent parenchymal abscess.

Diagnosis

Patients with evidence of cerebral emboli during the course of IE should undergo an urgent four-vessel angiogram unless otherwise contraindicated. If negative, serial angiograms should be done every 7–10 days and upon completion of antibiotic therapy if long-term anticoagulation is planned (53). Cerebral angiography should also be seriously considered in any patient with sterile meningitis and focal neurological symptoms or with unilateral headache (6). Cerebral angiographic findings in the patient with an unruptured aneurysm include nonfilling of major portions of the arterial branches, intra-arterial filling defects with embolic clot, and irregularly shaped fusiform or saccular arterial wall dilatation (72) (Fig. 7).

Therapy

The optimal therapeutic strategy for the unruptured aneurysm has not been defined. Appropriate bactericidal antibiotic therapy should be administered immediately upon diagnosis for a standard 4- to 6-week course. It is generally agreed that patients with ruptured aneurysm and with evidence

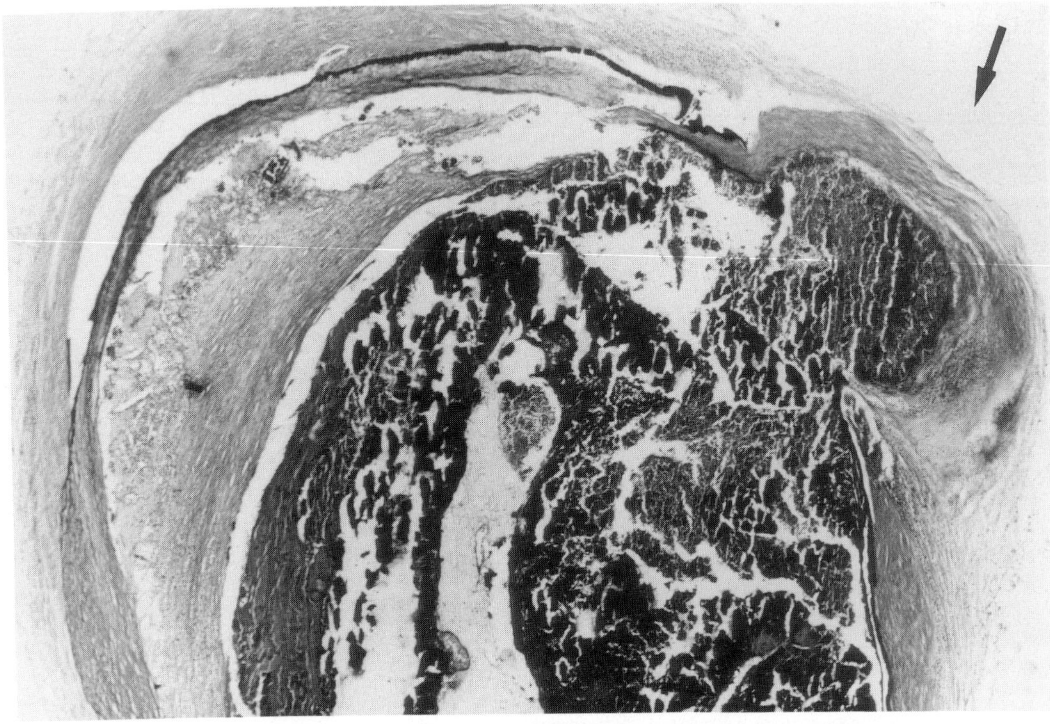

Figure 6 Autopsy histological slide of the left middle cerebral artery of a 71-year-old, who presented with a large left hemispheric stroke, while undergoing renal hemodialysis. The lumen is filled by a septic thrombus containing numerous gram-positive rods and neutrophils. Infiltrates of neutrophils are seen within the vessel media and adventitial layers. There is a small aneurysmal dilatation of the vessel wall (arrow). (10×)

of subarachnoid hemorrhage, intracranial hematoma, or evidence of a mass producing unruptured aneurysm should undergo neurosurgical treatment. Surgery may not be an option if the aneurysm is not easily accessible. In the case of the unruptured mycotic aneurysm, many experts advocate initial antibiotic therapy for 4–6 weeks, with serial angiography as often as every 2 weeks, until the aneurysm disappears. If at any point the aneurysm appears to enlarge (which may occur despite initial shrinking in size) or fails to reduce in size after 4–6 weeks of antibiotic therapy, neurosurgical intervention is indicated. In a review of the literature of 81 patients with intracranial mycotic aneurysm treated medically, follow-up cerebral angiography revealed that the aneurysm disappeared in 30%, enlarged in 22%, decreased in 19%, remained unchanged in 15%, and increased in number in 15% (71).

More difficult management decisions arise in the patient with multiple lesions or with an aneurysm in a proximal location. These factors are not necessarily a contraindication to neurosurgical therapy (64). In the patient with a known mycotic aneurysm who presents in cardiac failure requiring urgent valve replacement, some authors feel the patient may undergo valve replacement despite the heparinization required for cardiopulmonary bypass (74). In this clinical setting, replacement with a bioprosthetic rather than a mechanical valve may be preferable to avoid the need for chronic anticoagulation.

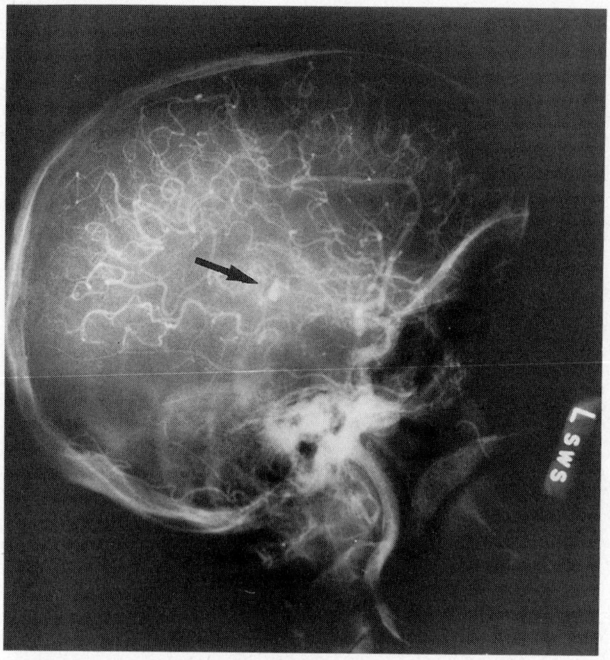

(A)

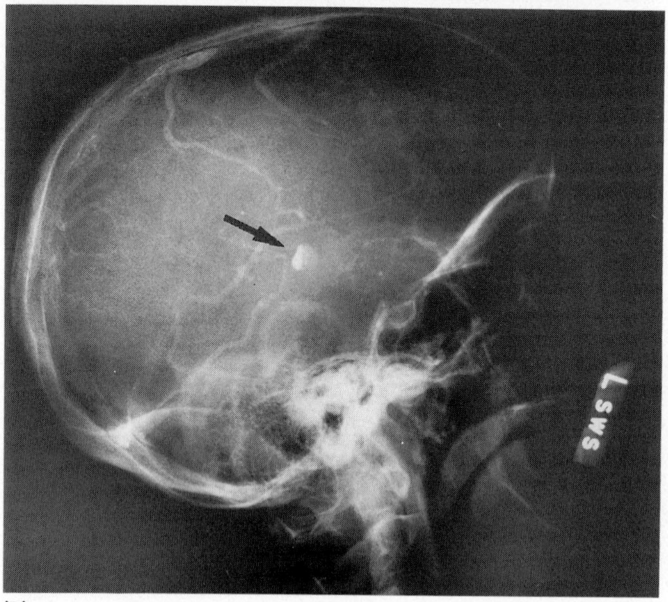

(B)

Figure 7 Cerebral angiogram (left sagittal views) of a 66-year-old female, who presented for evaluation of a subarachnoid hemorrhage. Both the arterial (A) and venous (B) phase contrast angiographic films demonstrate a large irregular mycotic aneurysm arising from the posteroparietal branch of the middle cerebral artery (arrow).

Prognosis

Rupture of a mycotic aneurysm is a catastrophic life-threatening event carrying a mortality rate of 60–90% (75), as compared to a rate of 30% if it remains unruptured (68). If the patient is fortunate to have a mycotic aneurysm diagnosed prior to its rupture, the risk of rupture following antibiotic therapy is lower. However, rupture has been reported as late as 6 months after successful treatment for IE, emphasizing the need for follow-up angiography (12).

Meningoencephalitis

Incidence and Risk Factors

Meningitis, once the most common neurological manifestation of infective endocarditis, has a decreasing incidence in the modern era of antibiotic therapy. The current incidence of meningitis with infective endocarditis has been reported in a large patient series as 1.4–3.5% (12,74). The incidence may be higher in certain areas of the world where antibiotics are less readily available (19%). In one series analyzing native valve endocarditis in 369 patients over a 14-year period, 17 patients had *Streptococcus pneumoniae* IE; 13 of the 17 also had purulent cerebrospinal fluid (CSF). Overall mortality was 59% mainly due to the purulent meningitis (74). In general, meningitis complicating IE due to virulent organisms such as *S. aureus*, enteric gram-negative rods, and *S. pneumoniae* has a purulent CSF (75), while meningitis complicating IE due to viridans streptococci has an aseptic or minimally abnormal or normal CSF (12). In the Massachusetts General Hospital patient series ($N = 218$), the results of cerebrospinal fluid analysis in 35 patients with meningeal signs or symptoms were as follows: purulent in 16 (46%), aseptic in 8 (23%), normal in 9 (26%), hemorrhagic in 2 (6%) (12).

Pathogenesis

Inflammation of the meninges during IE is commonly due to multiple septic emboli to meningeal vessels with direct vessel and CSF invasion. This microbial seeding may lead to parameningeal lesions including abscess. Cerebral inflammation can also be due to a secondary aseptic process, such as vasculitis, or hemorrhage from a leaking mycotic aneurysm. The incidence of left-sided endocarditis is far greater than right-sided infection, and it is more frequently associated with cerebral emboli. For this reason it has been suggested that septic emboli associated with bacteria may be more capable of disrupting the normal blood-brain barrier than simply bacteria alone (7).

Diagnosis

The clinical presentation of meningoencephalitis may be initially a change in mental status, ranging in severity from life-threatening coma to mild encephalopathy. In some instances, the latter may be interpreted as a change in personality, or the onset of mild confusion, especially in the elderly. These milder symptoms of disorientation can be inadvertently attributed to fever, or in the elderly to an iatrogenic drug effect, especially since fever in the elderly may not be a prominent sign. The symptoms of headache, disorientation, and fever may progress slowly and insidiously or depending on the organism, quickly progress to stupor, coma, and even death. A heightened awareness of the possibility of meningoencephalitis and a low threshold for obtaining CSF analysis is mandatory.

A cranial CT should be obtained prior to CSF examination in any patient with a focal deficit to rule out a space-occupying lesion, such as an abscess. The triad of a change in mental status with nuchal rigidity and fever are the classic features of meningoencephalitis. Meningeal symptoms or signs have been noted in approximately 6% of all patients with neurological complications during IE (15). The elderly may have meningitis without prominent meningeal signs; the diagnosis can also be confused with cervical degenerative disease, which is characterized by limitation in all planes of neck movement, rather than simply on flexion, which is typical of nuchal rigidity.

Therapy

The mainstay of treatment is timely administration of intravenous antibiotics that are specific for the suspected or isolated organism and which adequately cross the blood brain barrier. Antibiotic choice and therapy are described in detail below. Patients with meningoencephalitis may develop cerebral edema, which can be treated with a hyperosmolar agent, such as mannitol. The physician should be vigilant for possible seizure activity, and if of focal onset, rather than generalized, a cranial CT should be urgently obtained to rule out an abscess, hemorrhage, or embolic infarction.

Prognosis

Acute purulent meningoencephalitis from a virulent organism such as *S. aureus*, *S. pneumoniae*, or gram-negative bacilli carries a poor prognosis; in some patient series mortality in this setting was as high as 80%.

Headache

A diffuse, mild headache is a common complaint, occurring in 25–43% of patients with IE. Unrelenting severe or localized headache may indicate the presence of mycotic aneurysm, SAH, or meningoencephalitis. This type of headache should prompt cranial CT imaging and, if negative, a follow-up lumbar puncture to rule out an early warning leak of an aneurysm or infection in the subarachnoid space. Some experts suggest obtaining a cerebral angiogram in the setting of severe or localized headache in the course of IE to rule out mycotic aneurysm. In the elderly, severe headache and elevated erythrocyte sedimentation rate may be confused with temporal arteritis, obscuring the diagnosis of IE (especially if the patient is afebrile) (76).

Seizure

A seizure is rarely the presenting manifestation of IE, although in one series, 5 of 24 (21%) patients with a seizure complication had seizure as the initial symptom. In another series, approximately 10% of the IE cases had one or more seizures during the course of their illness (12). Focal seizures can occur from embolic cerebral infarction or can be a manifestation of microemboli. Generalized seizures may occur due to secondary metabolic derangements such as azotemia, hypoxia, or hyponatremia or due to drug effects including antibiotic therapy. Drugs such as high-dose penicillin, imipenem-cilastatin, haloperidol, and meperidine may lower the seizure threshold. Careful attention should be paid to the patient with renal dysfunction chiefly with the administration of renally excreted drugs, such as penicillin.

Abscess

Brain macroabscess (diameter $> 1\ cm^3$) rarely occurs during IE and accounts for less than 1% of all neurological complications of IE (56). Presenting symptoms include meningismus, focal neurological deficits, and seizures. Macroscopic abscesses have been documented 1–3 weeks following stroke; presumably the septic emboli provides the infectious nidus. Brain microabscess (diameter $< 1\ cm^3$) presenting clinically as encephalopathy occurs in 0.9–3.8% of cases of IE. A higher incidence is found in autopsy series and when MRI is performed. An abscess can also form as an extension of purulent meningoencephalitis or a mycotic aneurysm. The usual bacterial isolate from the abscess is *S. aureus* or streptococci.

Most abscesses are diagnosed by contrasted cranial CT or MRI. If CT is negative and MRI not possible, brain scan with Technetium-99 is a very sensitive supplementary test for detecting brain abscess or cerebritis (77).

Neuropathy

Mononeuropathy or multiple mononeuropathy (mononeuritis multiplex) occurs in 1% of cases of IE (78). Specific reported neuropathies include ulnar, median, peroneal, and sciatic nerves. Abnormalities of cranial nerves IV, VI, VII, IX, X, and XII have also been reported. Manifestations include paralysis of the face including bulbar palsy (bilateral), and weakness of the palate, tongue, larynx, and ocular muscles. On rare occasion, neuropathy is the initial manifestation IE, with viridans streptococci the causative organism in nearly all cases. Both septic embolic occlusion of the vasa vasorum and immune-mediated vasculitis are the proposed pathogenic mechanisms. Prognosis is usually good with little neurological deficit following antibiotic therapy.

Recently, a motor peripheral neuropathy has been recognized in severely critically ill patients. This polyneuropathy has been reported during sepsis, including during infective endocarditis, and may be associated with difficulty weaning from ventilatory support (79). Clinical signs include weakness chiefly in the lower limbs, amyotrophy, and symmetrically absent deep tendon reflexes. Electrophysiological studies are usually consistent with an axonal polyneuropathy, revealing fibrillations, reduced motor compound action amplitudes, normal or near normal motor nerve conduction, and normal distal latencies. No specific mechanism has been defined. Potential causes include septic microemboli effects on the microvasculature, a bacterial toxin effect, or an immuno-mediated vasculitis. Also common in the intensive care setting are drug-induced neuropathies, from antibiotics such as metronidazole, and pharmacologically induced weakness from muscular relaxant drugs, such as pancuronium bromide.

Ocular

Visual system involvement during IE has been reported in up to one fourth of the patients. The predominant mechanism is embolic occlusion of arteriolar flow producing either transient pathology, permanent infarction, or secondary infectious complications. Ophthalmic or central retinal artery occlusion is a rare consequence of emboli of endocarditis. Symptoms of sudden monocular blindness in the IE patient represent an ophthalmological emergency. Upon discovery, emergent neuro-ophthalmological or ophthalmological consultation should be obtained.

Immediate funduscopic examination occasionally reveals the embolus in place, interruption, or box-carring of retinal arteriolar flow, or venous dilatation. Within a period of hours, ischemic compromise of the inner retina, particularly the ganglion cells and nerve fiber bundle, leads to progressive retinal whitening, except at the fovea where absence of the ganglion cell and nerve fiber layer produces the classic "cherry red spot." Over the next several days, the retinal whitening resolves, eventually leading to optic disc atrophy over a period of 4–6 weeks. If recognized immediately, residual vision may be salvaged by encouraging the embolus to break up and move distally. This usually consists of a retrobulbar injection of anesthesia and digital massage to intermittently raise and then lower the intraocular pressure. Anterior chamber paracentesis may also be effective. More distal vascular infarction can result in retinal hemorrhages or soft exudate (representing localized edema of the nerve fiber layer). As the blood in retinal hemorrhages separates, the elevated white count in patients with endocarditis may cause a central collection or whitening resulting in so-called Roth spots. These are nonspecific and may be encountered in other causes of local retinal infarction when coupled with high white count (i.e., leukemia). Fundal findings have been documented in 35% of patients with neurological complications of infective endocarditis (15).

Small vessel disease may affect the adnexal structures as well as produce subconjunctival hemorrhage. Vascular involvement along the afferent visual pathways usually from mycotic aneurysms can produce various forms of visual field defect, commonly coupled with other neurological manifestations. Septic emboli may result in acute focal retinitis, followed by extension into the vitreous and endophthalmitis. IE represents one of the more common causes of the infrequently seen endogenous endophthalmitis. Extension of the infection to involve other orbital tissues can produce a panophthalmitis. Because of the frequency of ocular and visual involvement, a detailed ophthalmalogical evaluation, including funduscopic examination, should be part of the evaluation of every patient with suspected IE.

Other

Lumbar pain and diskitis occur in 3–10% of patients with infective endocarditis. An associated osteomyelitis and soft tissue abscess has been reported. Disc space infection with arachnoiditis can be reversed with antibiotic therapy. Myalgia can occur either diffusely or limited to one muscle location such as to the thigh or calf (80). Musculoskeletal complications typically resolve with appropriate antibiotic therapy. Rarer neurological manifestations exist, including spinal cord ischemia due to emboli or parameningeal abscesses compromising the vascular supply to the spinal cord. Movement disorders such as chorea and dyskinesia have also been reported. The etiology may be related to embolic infarction of the basal ganglia.

DIFFERENTIAL DIAGNOSIS

Noninfectious Etiology

In the febrile patient with neurological complications and repeatedly negative blood cultures (assuming they are drawn correctly), other considerations include atrial myxoma, primary cholesterol emboli, vasculitis, and nonbacterial thrombotic endocarditis (NBTE) (46). NBTE is associated with overt and occult carcinoma, uremia, connective tissue disease, and surrounding vascular incision sites. Similar to endocarditis, the erythrocyte sedimentation rate (ESR) and body temperature are frequently elevated in both carcinoma and connective tissue disease, complicating the diagnosis.

DIAGNOSTIC CONSIDERATIONS

Echocardiography

An echocardiographic study should be obtained acutely in any patient suspected of having IE. In the past decade the echocardiogram (ECHO) has been instrumental in understanding the pathological impact of vegetations on cardiac function. When performed by experienced personnel, two-dimensional echocardiography is a sensitive test for detecting cardiac vegetations. In the acute setting, the finding of a vegetation by ECHO prior to positive blood cultures can help in early diagnosis. A positive finding on ECHO is notably helpful in the setting of culture negative endocarditis or when the diagnosis is in question. *The lack of a vegetation, however, does not exclude the diagnosis of IE.* Serial ECHO examinations during an uncomplicated course of IE are not necessary. Vegetations can persist for months, and their persistence is not necessarily an indicator of therapeutic response (see below). In addition to imaging potential vegetations, ECHO is crucial for quickly determining the hemodynamic state of the heart, for elucidating the cause of hemodynamic failure if present, and for determining the extent of infection. Congestive heart failure due to left ventricular dysfunction has grave prognostic implications. Acute mortality rates are as high as 85% for patients with refractory congestive heart failure. The presence of valvular abscess (for example, aortic root abscess) may mandate surgical intervention.

Role of TTE versus TEE

Transthoracic echocardiography (TTE) detects vegetations in 40–80% of cases (81–83). The transesophageal echocardiogram (TEE) detects vegetations in up to 96% of cases, mainly due to its superior resolution. The sensitivity for vegetation identification is 33–63% for TTE and 90–100% for TEE. Frequently, TEE is performed following equivocal or poorly obtained TTE results or in cases with persistent fever despite antibiotic therapy in order to rule out possible perivalvular abscess.

Due to conflicting data, the role of ECHO in predicting risk of embolization in IE remains controversial. A recent study reviewing left-sided IE suggests that there is no statistically significant difference in the risk for embolus (systemic or to the central nervous system) among patients with detectable vegetations, compared to those patients without vegetations, when examined by two-dimensional ECHO. Furthermore, there was no increased risk for embolus with increasing size of the vegetation in patients with left-sided native valve IE (14). Another study, which included 77 patients with IE undergoing ECHO evaluation, concluded that patients with small vegetations were as likely to develop complications as those with larger vegetations (84). There was no relationship between change in lesion size or morphology during antimicrobial therapy and the incidence of embolization. In contrast, some investigators have found that in patients with acute IE, vegetations greater than 10 mm, as determined by transthoracic and/or transesophageal echocardiography, have a greater risk of embolization (85). In one study, this finding was only true in the subgroup of patients with native mitral valve endocarditis. Some series conclude that detection of a vegetation defines a high-risk subgroup of patients (83,86). Similarly, while some studies conclude that the presence of a vegetation on ECHO correlates with an increased risk of congestive heart failure, other studies find that severe heart failure and death were not significantly dependent on vegetation size.

Data to determine the prognostic value of ECHO for cerebral embolism are inconclusive. Available data from a few studies reveal no higher incidence of neurological complications from emboli based on the presence or absence of vegetative lesions (13,87). In a 12-year review of neurological complications of 175 patients with IE, vegetations were seen on echocardiography in approximately 37% of the patients with neurological complications (of all types) and in 28% of patients without neurological complications ($p = 0.26$, NS) (13).

Laboratory

In patients who have not had prior antibiotic therapy within 2 weeks of presentation, a total of three separate sets of venous blood cultures should be drawn over 24 h for both aerobic and anaerobic culture. Antibiotic therapy should not be delayed and can be initiated immediately after obtaining the first set of venous blood cultures. A minimal sample volume of 10–20 ml must be obtained to ensure adequate inoculum of organisms. Fungal cultures should be sent in patients who are known to be at risk for fungal infections. In patients with prior antibiotic therapy, blood should be collected in a beta-lactamase–supplemented tube. Three sets of cultures should be repeated at no less than hourly intervals. Blood cultures are negative in 2–31% of patients with infective endocarditis (20). Negative cultures can occur due to low blood sampling volume, prior empirical antibiotic therapy, or the presence of certain fastidious organisms, such as chlamydia, mycoplasma, brucella, and certain fungal species. Some gram-negative organisms grow poorly and may require long incubation periods, including *Haemophilus* sp., *Actinobacillus actinomycetemcomitans*, *Cardiobacterium hominis*, *Eikenella corrodens*, or *Kingella* species (also known as the HACEK group). Serum antibodies for Q fever should be obtained if cultures remain negative.

In the majority of patients with IE, blood cultures are positive, a direct result of the constant low-grade bacteremia that occurs. Blood cultures should be drawn prior to initiating antibiotic therapy. However, in partial antibiotic-treated patients, empirical therapy made be needed if there are signs of hemodynamic failure or severe neurological deterioration (e.g., meningitis with coma).

ESR and rheumatoid factor are frequently elevated, though this is a nonspecific finding and may depend on length of disease state and other unrelated factors, such as age. A normochromic normocytic anemia is often present. Leukocytosis occurs most often in acute IE and is present in 20–30% of cases. Immunological abnormalities including low circulating complement and/or hyperglobulinemia and elevated immune complexes can occur.

Neuroimaging

As discussed previously in the section on intracranial hemorrhage (ICH), the cranial CT is mandatory to distinguish hemorrhagic from nonhemorrhagic neurological complications in any patient presenting with a transient or fixed neurological deficit. CT may also suggest the presence of a mycotic aneurysm prompting angiographic confirmation or the presence of abscess or meningoencephalitis.

Magnetic resonance imaging is not the preferred test for early detection of hemorrhage in the initial evaluation of the patient with IE, since the signal intensity of acute subarachnoid hemorrhage is identical to CSF. However, MRI is more useful than CT for the diagnosis of microemboli, microabscess, aseptic meningitis, and vasculitis associated with meningeal involvement in IE. In addition, MR-angiography may be a useful alternative to cerebral angiography for the diagnosis and serial follow-up of mycotic aneurysms.

Cerebral Angiography

Four-vessel cerebral angiography is indicated in the patient suspected of IE with neurological complications to rule out life-threatening mycotic aneurysm(s). Cerebral angiography, if not otherwise contraindicated, is recommended in the following settings: (1) when cranial CT demonstrates hemorrhage (regardless of cause), (2) when cranial CT is normal but the history suggests an embolic phenomenon (e.g., TIA), and (3) when CSF examination reveals a pleocytosis and/or hemorrhage. The optimal timing of cerebral angiography is not well defined. Some experts suggest that angiography should be performed without delay, since in some patients mycotic aneurysm can rupture within 24 h of the onset of neurological symptoms.

Lumbar Puncture

Examination of the CSF most commonly reveals an "aseptic" CSF with a modest lymphocytic pleocytosis, moderately elevated protein concentration, normal glucose concentration, and a negative Gram stain. CSF can also be normal (up to 60%), grossly purulent, or hemorrhagic. Purulent CSF is typical of infection with more virulent organisms including *S. aureus*, enteric gram-negative bacilli, and *S. pneumoniae*, while aseptic or normal CSF tends to occur with less virulent organisms, such as viridans streptococci.

TREATMENT CONSIDERATIONS

Antimicrobial Therapy

The three key elements to antibiotic therapy are timely administration, appropriate specificity of the drug to achieve maximal bactericidal concentrations with adequate penetration of the blood-brain barrier, and sufficient length of treatment. It is clear that initiation of antibiotic therapy is associated with a sharp reduction in the number of embolic events, underscoring the need for prompt diagnosis and therapy. Prompt administration of antibiotics should be followed by vigilant monitoring of the patient's status for improvement of symptoms. Deterioration may warrant measurement of serum bactericidal titers and reevaluation of antibiotic choice. Follow-up blood cultures should be obtained at the end of a full course of therapy.

The chosen antibiotic must be bactericidal and is usually initially administered parentally for 2–6 weeks. Fungal infections may require both antifungal agents as well as surgery. If cultures are negative, broad-spectrum antimicrobial coverage is necessary.

In general, for the most common organism causing IE, penicillin-susceptible streptococci infections, aqueous crystalline penicillin G is recommended; for enterococci, amoxicillin in combination with gentamicin is recommended; oxacillin and gentamicin are recommended for *S. aureus* IE; a third generation cephalosporin and gentamicin for gram-negative bacilli; and for fungal infection, amphotericin B [in combination with 5-flucytosine for *Candida* species].

For a detailed description of antimicrobial therapy in the various forms of IE, the reader is referred to excellent recent reviews (7,88). Since the recommended antimicrobial therapy is continuously changing, the specific recommendations found in this chapter are based on current therapy at the time of this publication. The reader is advised to consult more recent publications, if applicable, including annually updated guides to antimicrobial therapy (89–91).

Anticoagulation

Based on evidence from both retrospective clinical studies and animal models of septic brain embolism, it is generally agreed that the routine use of anticoagulation is not recommended in patients with native valve IE because of the increased risk of hemorrhagic transformation. Exceptions to this rule include select cases of new-onset atrial fibrillation or in patients with evidence of pulmonary embolus or deep venous thrombosis.

In patients with prosthetic valve IE, anticoagulation is known to significantly decrease the risk of stroke (28,51). When anticoagulation is indicated, intravenous heparin sodium rather than warfarin is the drug of choice due to its easy reversibility. Excessive anticoagulation can convert a bland infarction into a hemorrhagic one; therefore, close monitoring of the PTT is necessary (60). The fact that the incidence of CNS thromboembolism in patients with prosthetic valve IE that are not receiving anticoagulation therapy is in the range of 46–71% (51,92), must be weighed against the fact that the incidence of hemorrhage in the same patient population while on anticoagulation therapy is as high as 36% (61).

Management of the patient with cerebral infarction and prosthetic valve IE can create a therapeutic dilemma. The increasing use of bioprosthetic valves that do not require long-term anticoagulation will make the decision to initiate anticoagulative therapy even more difficult. No large randomized trials exist to answer key questions concerning the risks and benefits of anticoagulation in this setting. Recent aggregate data on stroke morbidity in prosthetic valve endocarditis reveal a 42–70% incidence of CNS thromboembolic events and a 9–38% incidence of hemorrhage in nonanticoagulated patients versus a 9% incidence of stroke and an 11–43% incidence of hemorrhage in the anticoagulated patients (12,16,51). Aggregate data represent a

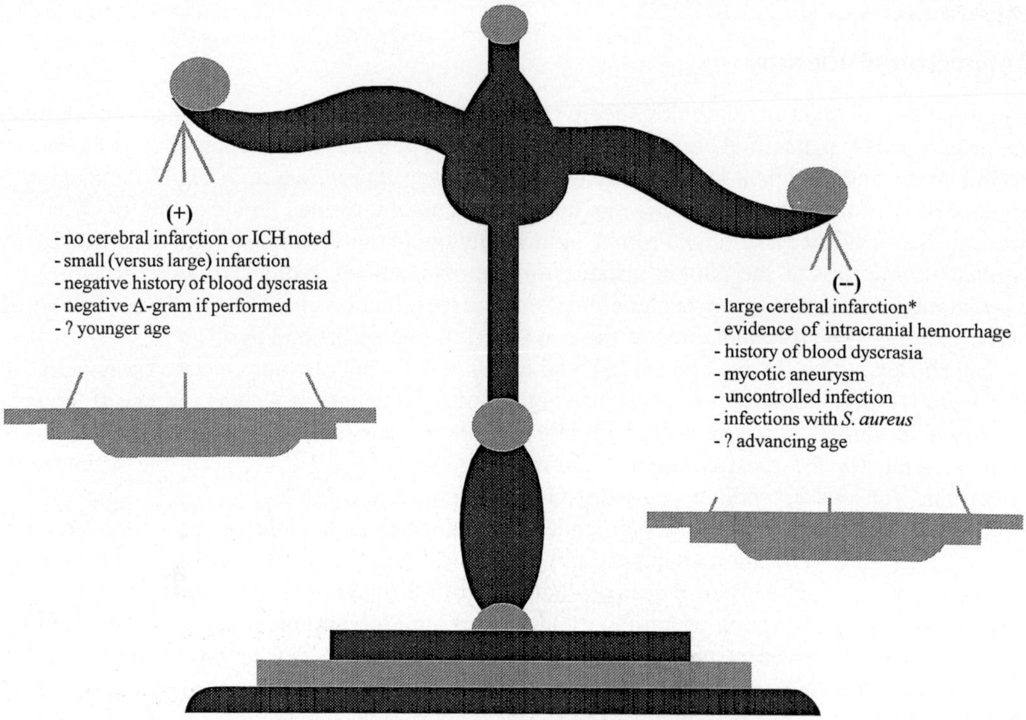

Figure 8 Factors either for (+) or against (−) the use of anticoagulation therapy in the patient with neurological complication and prosthetic valvular endocarditis. *As judged by neuroimaging study and/or presence of a severe neurological deficit. ICH—Intracerebral hemorrhage; A-gram—cerebral angiogram.

wide spectrum of therapeutic factors, including varying time of initiating antibiotic therapy, varying effectiveness of antibiotic therapy, type of anticoagulation chosen (warfarin versus heparin), and extent of anticoagulation [as assessed by INR and partial thromboplastin time (PTT) laboratory studies]. Figure 8 illustrates factors that, in addition to aggregate data studies, may be helpful in assessing the risk-to-benefit ratio of anticoagulation therapy, especially in the individual patient with prosthetic valve IE. Despite the potential benefit of anticoagulation in preventing thromboembolic events during IE, the single most important measure is timely, effective antibiotic therapy.

Role of Cardiac Surgery

Absolute indications for cardiac surgery include refractory heart failure, suppurative intracardiac disease (such as myocardial or perivalvular abscess), ineffective antibiotic therapy with repeated relapses of IE, the presence of an unstable prosthesis and a fungal endocarditis. When indicated, adjunctive surgical treatment for PVE with radical resection may provide a cure (92). Multiple embolic episodes and the presence of virulent organisms such as staphylococci and gram-negative bacilli are considered a relative indication (87). Cardiac valve replacement in patients who have had a single embolic event is controversial. Though often discussed, it is uncertain if the use of anticoagulation during cardiopulmonary bypass may confer an additional risk of an intracranial hemorrhagic event or lead to the transformation of a bland infarction into a hemorrhagic one.

It is unclear if patients with preoperative cardioembolic infarction are at increased risk of postoperative deterioration from either hemorrhagic conversion, increased cerebral edema, or new infarction site. For this reason, the optimal timing of cardiac surgery is controversial. The first 3–5 days following cerebral infarction represent the vulnerable time period for the development of cerebral edema, hence the recommendation that surgery be delayed, especially in those patients with a large stroke. One series consisting of 15 patients with IE revealed that open heart surgery (mainly valvular replacement) in patients with recent cardiogenic embolic stroke and CNS dysfunction could be safely performed (93). It should be noted that in this series the majority of patients were operated on more than 72 h following the diagnosis of cerebral infarction.

PROGNOSIS AND MORTALITY

The term "malignant," as found in Olser's lecture entitled "Malignant Endocarditis," accurately portrays the true nature of the neurological complications of IE. Mortality rates are higher in IE patients with neurological complications than in IE patients without neurological complications. Rupture of a mycotic aneurysm, intracerebral hemorrhage, and purulent meningoencephalitis are each associated with a mortality rate of nearly 80%. These high mortality rates emphasize the need for early recognition of predisposing factors and institution of appropriate preventive measures whenever possible. Equally important is early diagnosis. Early diagnosis demands constant vigilance to the many forms of presentation of IE. A high degree of suspicion is required in both the young and elderly patient.

SUMMARY

A substantial number of patients will experience a neurological complication during or following a course of IE. Despite recent innovations in antibiotic therapy, neurological complications continue to contribute significantly to the overall morbidity and mortality of this disease. Cerebral embolic infarction remains the most common neurological complication, followed by encephalopathy, intracranial hemorrhage, cerebral mycotic aneurysm, and meningoencephalitis. Other less common manifestations are headache, seizure, abscess, neuropathy, and ocular complications. Neurological complications can occur acutely but can also be delayed by months. The management of the patient with neurological complications frequently involves a multidisciplinary team approach involving the cardiologist, neurologist, infectious disease specialist, ophthalmologist, and neurosurgeon. The optimal treatment strategy is determined by the results of echocardiograms, neuroimaging studies, laboratory tests, and occasionally cerebral angiography. While some therapies, including the use of anticoagulants, are controversial, the expeditious initiation of specific antimicrobial therapy remains the undisputed single most important treatment.

ACKNOWLEDGMENTS

The authors thank M. Beatriz S. Lopes, M.D., Steven A. Newman, M.D., and John Dent, M.D., for their critical reviews. In addition, we also thank Ms. Sherri Alston for graphics and Ms. Sarah Hudson for editing of the manuscript.

REFERENCES

1. Osler W. Malignant endocarditis. (Gulstonian Lecture). Lancet 1885; 1:415–508.
2. Pajet J. On obstructions of the branches of the pulmonary artery. Med Chir Trans 1844; 27: 163–188.
3. Goodhart JD. A series of cases of ulcerative endocarditis. Transactions (Pathological Society of London) 1881; 33:52–61.
4. Pelletier LL, Petersdorf RG. Infective endocarditis: a review of 125 cases from the University of Washington Hospitals, 1963–72. Medicine 1977; 56:287–313.
5. Von Reyn CF, Levy BS, Arbeit RD, Freidland G, Crumpacker CS. Infective endocarditis: an analysis based on strict case definitions. Ann Intern Med 1981; 94:505–518.
6. Lerner PI. Neurologic complications of infective endocarditis. Med Clin North Am 1985; 69:385–398.
7. Francioli P. Central nervous system complications of infective endocarditis. In: Scheld WM, Whitley RJ, Durack DT, eds. Infections of the Central Nervous System. New York: Raven Press, 1991:515–559.
8. Salgado AV. Central nervous system complications of infective endocarditis. Stroke 1991; 22:1461–1463.
9. Tunkel AR, Kaye D. Neurologic complications of infective endocarditis. Neurol Clin 1993; 11: 419–440.
10. Kim EL, Ching DL, Pien FD. Bacterial endocarditis at a small community hospital. Am J Med Sci 1990; 299:87–93.
11. Grossman E, Holtzman T, Rosenthal T, Semesh E, Samra Y, Michaeli D. A comparative study of infective endocarditis. Isr J Med Sci 1984; 20:389–393.
12. Pruitt AA, Rubin R, Karchmer A. Neurologic complications of bacterial endocarditis. Medicine 1978; 57:329–343.
13. Salgado AV, Furlan AJ, Keys TF, Nichols TR, Beck GJ. Neurologic complications of endocarditis: a 12-year experience. Neurology 1989; 39:173–178.
14. Steckelberg JM, Murphy JG, Ballard D, Bailey K, Tajik AJ, Taliercio C, et al. Emboli in infective endocarditis: the prognostic value of echocardiography. Ann Intern Med 1991; 114:635–640.
15. Jones HR, Jr., Siekert RG, Geraci JE. Neurologic manifestations of bacterial endocarditis. Ann Intern Med 1969; 71:21–28.
16. Davenport J, Hart RG. Prosthetic valve endocarditis 1976–1987 antibiotics, anticoagulation and stroke. Stroke 1990; 21:993–999.
17. Ferguson DJP, McColm AA, Savage TJ, et al. A morphological study of experimental rabbit staphylococcal endocarditis and aortitis. I Formation and effect of infected and uninfected vegetations on the aorta. Br J Exp Pathol 1986; 67:667–678.
18. Weinstein L, Schlesinger JJ. Pathoanatomic, pathophysiologic and clinical correlations in endocarditis. N Eng J Med 1974; 291:832–837.
19. Rodbard S. Blood velocity and endocarditis. Circulation 1963; 27:18–28.
20. Von Reyn CF, Levy BS, Arbeit RD, Friedland G, Crumpacker CS. Infective endocarditis: an analysis based on strict case definitions. Ann Intern Med 1981; 94(Part 1):505–518.
21. Le Cam B, Guivarch G, Boles JM, Garre M, Carter F. Neurologic complications in a group of 86 bacterial endocarditis. Eur Heart J 1984; 5(suppl. C):97–100.
22. Clemens JD, Horwitz RI, Jaffe CC. A controlled evaluation of the risk of bacterial endocarditis in persons with mitral-valve prolapse. N Engl J Med 1982; 307:776–781.
23. Hickey AJ, MacMahon SW, Wilcken DEL. When is antibiotic prophylaxis necessary in mitral valve prolapse (abstract). Circulation 1984; 70:II–102.
24. Nagger CZ, Forgacs P. Infective endocarditis: a challenging disease. Med Clin North Am 1986; 70:1279–1294.
25. Lowes JS, Hamer J, Williams G. 10 years of infective endocarditis at St. Bartholomew's Hospital analysis of clinical features and treatment in relation to prognosis and mortality. Lancet 1980; 1: 133–136.
26. McKinsey DS, Ratts TE, Bisno AL. Underlying cardiac lesions in adults with infective endocarditis: the changing spectrum. Am J Med 1987; 82:681–688.

27. Keyser DL, Biller J, Coffman TT, Adams HPJ. Neurologic complications of late prosthetic valve endocarditis. Stroke 1990; 21:472–475.
28. Leport C, Vilde JL, Bricaire F, Cohen A, Pangon B, Valere PE, et al. Fifty cases of late prosthetic valve endocarditis: improvement in prognosis over a 15-year period. Br Heart J 1987; 58:66–71.
29. Madison J, Wang K, Gobel FL, Edwards JE. Prosthetic valve endocarditis. Circulation 1975; 51: 940–949.
30. Jamieson WRE. Modern cardiac valve devices—bioprostheses and mechanical prostheses: state of the art. J Card Surg 1993; 8:89–98.
31. Hammermeister KE, Sethi GK. Comparison of occurrence in bleeding systemic embolism, endocarditis valve thrombosis and re-operation between patients randomized between a mechanical prosthesis and a bioprosthesis. Results from a VA randomized trial. J Am College Cardiol 1991; 17:362A.
32. Bloomfield P, Wheatley DJ, Prescott RJ. Twelve year comparison of a Bjork-Shiley mechanical heart valve with porcine bioprostheses. N Engl J Med 1991; 324:573–579.
33. Dajani AS, Bisno AL, Chung KJ, Durack, DT, Freed, M. Gerber, MA, et al. Prevention of bacterial endocarditis. JAMA 1990; 250:2919–2922.
34. Levine DP, Crane LR, Zervos MJ. Bacteremia in narcotic addicts at the Detroit Medical Center. II. Infectious endocarditis: a prospective comparative study. Rev Infect Dis 1986; 8:374–396.
35. Chambers HF, Korzeniowski OM, Sande MA. Clinical manifestations in addicts and non-addicts. Medicine 1983; 62:170–177.
36. Ramsey RG, Gunnar RM, Tobin JR. Endocarditis in drug addicts. Am J Cardiol 1970; 25:608–618.
37. Openshaw H. Neurological complications of endocarditis in persons taking drugs intravenously. West J Med 1976; 124:276–281.
38. Antel JJ, Rome HP, Geraci JE, Sayre, GP. Toxic organic psychosis as a presenting feature in bacterial endocarditis in the elderly. Proc Mayo Clin 1955; 30:45–50.
39. Traut EF, Carter JB, Gumbiner SH, Hench RN. Bacterial endocarditis in the elderly. Geriatrics 1949; 4:205–210.
40. Sanabria TJ, Alpert JS, Goldberg R, Pape LA, Cheeseman SH. Increasing frequency of staphylococcal infective endocarditis. Arch Intern Med 1990; 150:1305–1309.
41. Thompson RL. Staphylococcal infective endocarditis. Mayo Clin Proc 1982; 57:106–114.
42. Gransden WR, Ekyn SJ, Leach RM. Neurological presentations of native valve endocarditis. Q J Med 1989; 73:1135–1139.
43. Parker SW, Apicella MA, Fuller CM. Hemophilus endocarditis. Two patients with complications. Arch Intern Med 1983; 143:48–51.
44. Felner JM, Dowell VR, Jr. Anaerobic bacterial endocarditis. N Engl J Med 1970; 283:1188–1192.
45. Bush M, Masferrer R, Teitel R, Pittman HW. Neurologic complications of infectious endocarditis. BNI Q 1985; 1:13–18.
46. Jones HR, Jr., Siekert RG. Neurological manifestations of infective endocarditis. Review of clinical and therapeutic challenges. Brain 1989; 112:1295–1315.
47. Hart RG, Foster JW, Luther MF, Kanter MC. Stroke in infective endocarditis. Stroke 1990; 21:695–700.
48. Bozzao L, Angeloni U, Bastianello S, Fantozzi LM, Pierallini A, Fieschi C. Early angiographic and CT findings in patients with hemorrhagic infarction in the distribution of the middle cerebral artery. Am J Neuroradiol 1991; 12:1115–1121.
49. Hornig CR, Dorndoff W, Agnoli AL. Hemorrhagic cerebral infarction—prospective study. Stroke 1986; 17:179–185.
50. Bertorini TE, Laster RE, Thompson BF, Gelfand M. Magnetic resonance imaging of the brain in bacterial endocarditis. Arch Intern Med 1989; 149:815–817.
51. Wilson WR, Geraci JE, Danielson GK, Thompson RL, Spittell JA, Washington JA, et al. Anticoagulant treatment and central nervous system complications in patients with prosthetic valve endocarditis. Circulation 1978; 57:1004–1007.
52. Delahaye JP, Malquarti PV, Beaune J, Gare JP, Mann JM. Cerebrovascular accidents in infective endocarditis: role of anticoagulation. Eur Heart J 1990; 11:1074–1078.

53. Salgado AV. Central nervous system complications of infective endocarditis. Curr Concepts Cerebrovasc Dis Stroke 1991; 26:19–22.
54. Taha TH, Durrant SS, Mazeika PK, Nihoyannopoulos P, Oakley CM. Aspirin to prevent growth of vegetations and cerebral emboli in infective endocarditis. J Intern Med 1992; 231:543–546.
55. Cerebral Embolism Task Force. Cardiogenic brain embolism—the second report of the cerebral embolism task force. Arch Neurol 1989; 46:727–743.
56. Kanter MC, Hart RG. Neurologic complications of infective endocarditis. Neurology 1991; 41:1015–1020.
57. Jones HR, Jr., Siekert RG, Geraci JE. Neurologic manifestations of bacterial endocarditis. Ann Intern Med 1969; 71:21–28.
58. Terpenning MS, Buggy BP, Kauffman CA. Infective endocarditis: clinical features in young and elderly patients. Am J Med 1987; 83:626–634.
59. Hart RG, Kagan-Hallet K, Joerns SE. Mechanisms of intracranial hemorrhage in infective endocarditis. Stroke 1987; 18:1048–1056.
60. Selky AK, Roos KL. Neurologic complications of infective endocarditis. Semin Neurol 1992; 12: 225–233.
61. Carpenter JL, McAllister C. Anticoagulation in prosthetic valve endocarditis. South Med J 1983; 76:1372–1375.
62. Masuda J, Yutani C, Waki R, Ogata J, Kuriyama Y, Yamaguchi T. Histopathological analysis of the mechanisms of intracranial hemorrhage complicating infective endocarditis. Stroke 1992; 23:843–850.
63. Siekert RG, Jones HR, Jr. Transient cerebral attacks associated with subacute bacterial endocarditis. Stroke 1970; 1:178–183.
64. Frazee JG, Cahan LD, Winter J. Bacterial intracranial aneurysms. J Neurosurg 1980; 53:633–641.
65. Simmons KC, Sage MR, Reilly PL. CT of intracerebral haemorrhage due to mycotic aneurysms: case report. Neuroradiology 1980; 19:215–217.
66. Calopa M, Rubio F, Aguilar M, Peres J. Giant basilar aneurysm in the course of subacute bacterial endocarditis. Stroke 1990; 21:1625–1627.
67. Davis KR. Case record 7—1988 of the Massachusetts General Hospital. N Engl J Med 1988; 318: 427–440.
68. Bohmfalk GL, Story JL, Wissinger JP. Bacterial intracranial aneurysm. J Neurosurg 1978; 48:369–382.
69. Ziment I. Nervous system complications in acute bacterial endocarditis. Am J Med 1969; 47:593–607.
70. Weir B. Special aneurysms (nonsaccular and saccular). In: Brown C, Eckhart C, eds. Aneurysms Affecting the Nervous System. Baltimore, MD: Williams & Wilkins, 1987:134–170.
71. Ojemann RG. Surgical management of bacterial intracranial aneurysms. In: Schmideck HH, Sweet WH, eds. Operative Neurosurgical Techniques, Indications, Methods, and Results. New York: Grune & Stratton, 1982:933–940.
72. Katz RI, Goldberg HI, Selzer ME. Mycotic aneurysm—case report with novel sequential angiographic findings. Arch Intern Med 1974; 134:939–942.
73. Molinari GF, Smith L, Goldstein MN, Satran R. Pathogenesis of cerebral mycotic aneurysms. Neurology 1973; 23:325–332.
74. Wolff M, Regnier B, Witchitz S, Gibert C, Amoudry C, Vachon F. Pneumoccocal endocarditis. Eur Heart J 1984; 5:C7780.
75. Greenlee JE, Mandell GL. Neurological manifestations of infective endocarditis: a review. Stroke 1973; 4:958–963.
76. Govindan S, Itani AL, Garcia JH. Inflammation of the temporal artery associated with subacute bacterial endocarditis and hepatitis B antigen. Arch Neurol 1980; 37:318.
77. Wispelwey B, Scheld WM. Brain abscess. Clin Neuropharmacol 1987; 10:483–510.
78. Jones HR, Jr., Siekert RG. Embolic mononeuropathy and bacterial endocarditis. Arch Neurol 1968; 19:535–537.
79. Coronel B, Mercatello A, Couturier J, Durand P, Holzapfell L, Blanc P, et al. Polyneuropathy: potential cause of difficult weaning. Crit Care Med 1990; 18:486–489.
80. Churchill MA, Jr., Geraci JE, Hunder GG. Musculoskeletal manifestations of bacterial endocarditis. Ann Intern Med 1977; 87:754–759.

81. Erbel R, Rohmann S, Dexler M. Improved diagnostic value of echocardiography in patients with infective endocarditis by transesophageal approach: a prospective study. Eur Heart J 1988; 1:43–53.
82. O'Brien JT, Geiser EA. Infective endocarditis and echocardiography. Am Heart J 1984; 108:386–394.
83. Buda AJ, Zotz RJ, LeMire MS, Bach DS. Prognostic significance of vegetations detected by two-dimensional echocardiography in infective endocarditis. Am Heart J 1986; 112:1291–1296.
84. Lutas EM, Roberts RB, Devereux RB, Prieto LM. Relation between the presence of echocardiographic vegetations and complication rate in infective endocarditis. Am Heart J 1986; 112:107–113.
85. Mugge A, Daniel WG, Frank G, Lichtlen PR. Echocardiography in infective endocardits: reassessment of prognostic implication of vegetation size determined by the transthoracic and the transesophageal approach. J Am College Cardiol 1989; 14:631–638.
86. Wann LS, Hallam CC, Dillon JC, Weyman AE, Feigenbaum H. Comparison of M-mode and cross-sectional echocardiography in infective endocarditis. Circulation 1979; 60:728–733.
87. Sanfilippo AJ, Picard MD, Newell JB, Rosas E, Davidoff R, Thomas JD, et al. Echocardiographic assessment of patients with infectious endocarditis: prediction of risk for complications. J Am Coll Cardiol 1991; 18:1191–1199.
88. Korzeniowski OM, Kaye D. Infective Endocarditis. In: Braunwald E, ed. Heart Disease—A Textbook of Cardiovascular Medicine. 4th ed. Philadelphia: W.B. Saunders Company, 1992:1078–1105.
89. Molavi A. Endocarditis: recognition, management, and prophylaxis. Cardiovasc Clin 1993; 23:139–174.
90. Mandell GL, Douglas RG, Bennett JE, Dolin R. Principles and Practice of Infectious Diseases—Antimicrobial Therapy. New York: Churchill Livingstone, 1993.
91. Sanford JP. Guide to Antimicrobial Therapy—1995. West Bethesda, MD: Antimicrobial Therapy, Inc., 1995.
92. Garvey CJ, Neu HC. Infectious endocarditis—an evolving disease. Medicine 1978; 57:105–127.
93. Maruyama M, Kuriyama Y, Sawada T, Yamaguchi T, Fujita T, Omae T. Brain damage after open heart surgery in patients with acute cardioembolic stroke. Stroke 1989; 20:1305–1310.

17

Central Nervous System Infections in Organ Transplant Recipients and Cancer Patients

Amy A. Pruitt
University of Pennsylvania Medical Center, Philadelphia, Pennsylvania

HISTORICAL PERSPECTIVE

Forty years ago Murray and colleagues performed the first successful renal transplantation between identical twins. During the next decade, organ transplantation was introduced for liver, cardiac, and bone marrow failure and has evolved into the treatment of choice for a wide variety of end-stage diseases. The procedures are performed in dozens of centers worldwide, more than three quarters taking place since 1985 (Table 1). Advances in tissue matching, immunosuppression, and perioperative management have increased the number of long-term survivors.

During roughly this same time period, a second medical success story developed. Improvements in diagnosis, radiation therapy, chemotherapy, and biological response modification greatly increased the long-term survival and cure rates of certain types of cancer. A corollary of these medical successes is the presentation to the neurological consultant of complicated patients whose associated diseases and their treatment may alter the presentation and course of familiar diseases and may even create some new diseases as well.

The incidence of neurological complications is high in both groups of patients. Between 30 and 60% of organ transplant recipients develop neurological complications (1). Approximately 5–10% of transplant recipients develop a central nervous system (CNS) infection at some point after transplant, 44–77% of which are fatal (2). CNS infections remain a major cause of morbidity and mortality among cancer patients as well. During the latter half of the decade 1980–1990, the rate of admissions for CNS infections increased by 30% at Massachusetts General Hospital. One of every six of these patients (17%) had an underlying malignancy (3). In an earlier series from the same institution, 60% of immunocompromised patients with CNS infection died as a result of their infection, many at a time when the underlying disease had an otherwise good prognosis (4). To improve these statistics, the neurological consultant must be aware of changing patterns in

Table 1 Frequency of Organ Transplantation

Organ type	First performed	No. performed (worldwide)	5-year survival (%)	Neurological complications (%)	CNS infections (%)
Kidney	1954	>10,000/year	>90[a]	30	4
Bone marrow[b]	1960	20,000	[c]	60–70	17
Heart	1967	15,000	70	60	0[d]–28[e]
Liver	1963	10,000	60	30	0–20[d] 23–43[e]
Pancreas	1966	5,000	NA	60	NA

[a]Nondiabetic patients.
[b]Allogeneic.
[c]Variable, dependent on underlying disease.
[d]Clinical study.
[e]Autopsy data.
NA—Not available, numbers too small.
Source: Refs. 1, 5–15.

bacterial, fungal, viral, and parasitic infections and must maintain a high index of suspicion in clinical situations with myriad diagnostic possibilities, both infectious and noninfectious.

APPROACH TO THE IMMUNOCOMPROMISED HOST WITH POTENTIAL CENTRAL NERVOUS SYSTEM INFECTION

Clinical Challenges

Several characteristics of CNS infections in the immunosuppressed host make their identification and treatment challenging.

1. The list of potential pathogens is large and includes many organisms of normally low pathogenicity in the intact host.
2. Infection with more than one agent or sequential infection is not uncommon. In one series, 40% of CNS infections had extraneural infections with an organism other than that infecting the CNS, and nearly 64% of CNS infections were associated with extraneural infections with the same pathogen (4).
3. The manifestations of CNS infections, such as headache, meningismus, and fever, may be mild or absent because of the host's diminished inflammatory response.
4. Coexisting conditions, such as metabolic encephalopathy, may complicate the picture, and the clinical syndrome due to infection may mimic a drug- or therapy-induced complication.
5. Meaningful survival without neurological deficit is dependent on rapid diagnosis and initiation of effective treatment. The appropriate duration of therapy for many CNS infections and the necessity for maintenance therapy is not yet resolved.
6. Drug therapy to the CNS is complicated by numerous factors, including the status of the blood-brain barrier and lipid solubility, molecular weight, protein binding, and removal of the drug from the cerebrospinal fluid (CSF). Neurotoxicity is a limiting factor for a number of anti-infectious agents.

Despite these problems, the vast majority of CNS infections in immunocompromised patients follow predictable patterns. Indeed, in the transplant population, despite the wide variety of potential pathogens, three organisms (*Listeria monocytogenes*, *Cryptococcus neoformans*, and *Aspergillus fumigatus*) cause more than 80% of CNS infections (2). Following a logical sequence of clinical and laboratory clues, the clinician should be able to narrow the spectrum of diseases quickly, apply specific diagnostic tests and institute empiric and then specific treatment in a timely fashion. This chapter will present a practical approach to the problem of infection in organ transplant recipients and patients with cancer. Pitfalls in diagnosis, including noninfectious causes specific to the underlying disease states, will be discussed along with specific therapeutic requirements and predictable setting-specific complications and sequelae.

Pathophysiology

Barrier Disruption

Several different levels of defenses protect the normal host from invasion by microorganisms. The skin and sebaceous glands represent the first such layer. Central lines and other monitoring devices break down this defense mechanism. Chemotherapeutic agents can break down mucous membranes. Neurosurgical procedures breach the skin barrier which may in turn be weakened by prior varicella-zoster infection, radiation therapy, or earlier surgery.

Colonization resistance refers to the protective mechanisms of the normal anaerobic gut flora preventing the overgrowth of unusual organisms such as fungi. This mechanism is impaired by the antibiotics used for prophylaxis or treatment of infections, though newer antibiotics such as the third-generation cephalosporins and carbapenems appear to preserve colonization resistance.

Neutrophil Dysfunction

Deficits in neutrophil function or number are usually associated with bacterial infections by organisms derived from the skin or gastrointestinal or respiratory tracts or introduced by the presence of indwelling catheters. Neutropenia represents the most common risk factor for the development of opportunistic infection in cancer patients and is the usual culprit in patients with leukemia, aplastic anemia, and pancytopenia due to marrow invasion or to intensive chemotherapy or radiation therapy. An increased risk of bacterial infections begins with an absolute neutrophil count of less than $1000/mm^3$ and increases as counts drop below $500/mm^3$. Neutropenia is also a risk factor for fungal infections such as *Aspergillus fumigatus* and *Candida* species.

B-Lymphocyte/Immunoglobulin Impairment

Deficiency of immunoglobulin synthesis is encountered in patients with chronic lymphocytic leukemia, multiple myeloma, or other blood dyscrasias. Encapsulated bacterial organisms such as *Hemophilus influenzae* and *Streptococcus pneumoniae* are the major pathogens in this setting. Splenectomy is a further risk factor for bacterial sepsis and CNS seeding in this setting.

Impaired T-Cell–Mediated Immunity

Disorders of cell-mediated immunity involving T lymphocytes and macrophages lead to a wider variety of CNS infection than do those involving deficient B-cell function. This type of host compromise occurs in patients with AIDS and in organ transplant recipients, but also in those with lymphoreticular malignancies and in patients receiving cytotoxic or chronic corticosteroid therapy. The typical pathogen spectrum varies somewhat depending on the underlying disease. For example, AIDS patients appear to be more prone to infection with *Mycobacterium tuberculosis* and *Toxoplasma gondii* than are those on chronic corticosteroid therapy (see Chaps. 3 and 13 for infections in pediatric and adult AIDS patients). All conditions involving impaired T-cell immunity, however, are associated with increased risk for infections by viruses, fungi, and intracellular pathogens such as *Listeria*.

The type of pathogen to be suspected in a CNS infection depends most importantly on the nature, intensity, and duration of the underlying immune deficiency. Table 2 summarizes pathogens associated with specific deficits in immunity.

Diagnosis

The response of the CNS to infection is limited to a relatively small, nonspecific repertoire of clinical signs and symptoms. Five sets of data help the clinician narrow the range of microorganism possibilities.

Table 2 Classification of Immunological Deficits and Common Pathogens

Immunological deficit	Granulocyte	B-lymphocyte/ immunoglobulin	T-lymophocyte/ macrophage	Barrier disruption
Associated diseases or risk factors	Infiltrating disorders of marrow (leukemia, lymphoma, solid tumors Chemotherapy Radiotherapy Bone marrow transplantation	Chronic lymphocytic leukemia Multiple myeloma Splenectomy	Lymphorecticular neoplasms Organ transplantation Chronic cortico-steroid or other immunosuppressive therapy AIDS	Indwelling ventricular reservoir Cranial surgery Hyperalimentation or other central IV lines Loss of cutaneous integrity[a]
CNS pathogens in rough relative order of importance	Bacteria *S. aureus* *S. epidermidis* *P. aeruginosa* *Enterobacter* *L. monocytogenes*	Bacteria *S. pneumonia* *H. influenzae* *Enterobacter* *P. aeruginosa*	Viruses HIV Cytomegalovirus Varicella-zoster Epstein-Barr virus[d] JC virus (PML) Measles Advenovirus	Bacteria *S. aureus* *S. epidermidis* *Enterobacter* *E. coli* *Klebsiella* Streptococci Diphtheroids
	Fungi *A. fumigatus* Mucoraceae *C. albicans* Viruses Cytomegalovirus[b] Herpes simplex Adenovirus[c]	Viruses Measles Enteroviruses (echo, polio)	Bacteria *L. monocytogenes* *N. asteroides* *M. tuberculosis* Fungi *C. neoformans* *A. fumigatus* *C. albicans* *Mucoraceae* *P. boydii* Parasites *T. gondii* *S. stercoralis*	Fungi *A. fumigatus* *C. albicans*

[a]Including prior varicella-zoster infection.
[b]After bone marrow transplantation.
[c]After blood transfusion.
[d]Posttransplant lymphoproliferative disorder.
Source: Adapted from Ref. 16.

Clinical Setting

Table 2 summarizes the major categories of immunocompromising diseases by the type of immune deficit. Patients with quite different diseases but similar immune deficits may resemble each other more than do patients with the same disease with different types of immune deficits. Thus, with respect to CNS infection risk, patients who have received chronic corticosteroids for more than 6 weeks for Hodgkin's or non-Hodgkin's lymphoma resemble patients chronically immunosuppressed for organ transplantation more than they do patients with other lymphoreticular disorders whose immune deficit at that point in time is neutropenia.

Pace of Illness

The time course of symptom progression may help raise suspicion of specific pathogens. In general, symptoms of less than 2 days' duration bespeak bacterial processes, often meningitis, from conventional gram-negative or gram-positive organisms, whereas a subacute presentation of fever and headache more often results from infection with *C. neoformans*, *M. tuberculosis*, *L. monocytogenes*, or herpesvirus infections. A chronically progressive focal neurological deficit or dementia is more likely to be due to progressive multifocal leukoencephalopathy (JC virus). However, because of the hosts' blunted immune response and the nonspecific nature of symptoms, the pace of illness is not always predictive of the responsible pathogen.

Extraneural Infection Sites

The finding of infection outside the nervous system should raise clinical suspicion of infection within the CNS. More than 20% of immunocompromised patients with cryptococcal meningitis have skin lesions that may have been present for months before examination of the CSF (2,4). The lungs are frequently infected by *A. fumigatus*, *N. asteroides*, and *C. neoformans* before dissemination to the CNS. Though varicella-zoster encephalitis can occur in the absence of skin lesions, their presence, along with a multifocal or diffuse encephalitic picture, should raise suspicion of this virus. Bacteria specifically associated with procedures performed for cancer or transplantation therapy also can help narrow the diagnostic spectrum. For example, *Listeria* is a likely pathogen when there has been gastrointestinal surgery, particularly in the setting of ongoing immunosuppression.

Neuroanatomic Distribution of Deficit

If the host's response is so blunted as to mask infection entirely or to indicate it only by mild headache and mental status changes, the clinical pattern of signs and symptoms may not be helpful. However, in some situations the presence of localizing findings with specific neuroanatomic distributions provides a diagnostic clue. Table 3 summarizes typical neuroanatomical deficits and their associated pathogens. The presence of a focal cerebral deficit should lead the clinician to consider infectious etiologies such as *Aspergillus*, *Toxoplasma*, *Listeria*, *Nocardia*, JC virus, or vasculitis related to remote or recent varicella-zoster infections.

The special clinical pattern of focal or multifocal disease with stepwise accumulation of deficits has a wide differential diagnosis. Depending on the clinical setting, this pattern could be due to the infections mentioned above or to stroke of several possible causes, including thrombocytopenia-related hemorrhage, nonbacterial thrombotic or infective endocarditis, superior sagittal sinus thrombosis, and vasculitis (24,28). In the appropriate setting, metastatic tumor or secondary malignancy may be a consideration.

Acute meningitis is most often caused by *Listeria* or conventional bacteria. The distinction between acute versus subacute presentation may be somewhat blurred in heavily immunosuppressed patients, but chronic meningitis in this population is most often due to either *Listeria* or *Cryptococcus*.

Table 3 Neuroanatomical Correlation of Infection Site and Possible Nervous System Infection

Typical pathogen	Focal cerebral deficit (localized mass)	Acute meningitis/ meningoencephalitis	Chronic meningitis	Myelopathy	Neuropathy or plexopathy	Myositis	Cranial nerve deficit
Bacteria	*S. aureus* *Anaerobes* *L. monocytogenes* *N. asteroides*	*L. monocytogenes* Gram-negatives *H. influenzae* *S. pneumoniae*	*L. monocytogenes*	Mycobacteria Epidural abscess due to organism causing sepsis	*L. interrogans* *T. pallidum*	*S. aureus* *S. pneumoniae* *E. coli*	*M. tuberculosis*
Fungi	*A. fumigatus* *C. neoformans* *Mucoraceae*	*C. neoformans*	*C. neoformans* *C. immitis*[a] *H. capsulatum*[a] *Candida* species				*Mucoraceae* *A. fumigatus*
Viruses	JC virus (PML) Varicella-zoster	Herpes simplex types 1 and 2 Cytomegalovirus Varicella-zoster		Cytomegalovirus Herpex simplex Varicella-zoster	Cytomegalovirus		Cytomegalovirus
Parisites	*T. gondii*	*T. gondii* *S. stercoralis*					

[a]Regional.
PML—Progressive multifocal leukoencephalopathy.
Source: Adapted from Ref. 16.

The picture of a progressive myelopathy should raise concern about epidural abscess due to the organism causing sepsis, mycobacteria, or several viral processes including cytomegalovirus (CMV), herpes simplex virus types 1 and 2, and varicella-zoster virus. Radicular, mononeuropathic, or plexus distribution of signs, when due to infection, raises the possibility of herpesvirus infections, CMV, or spirochetal disease. The presentation of progressive ascending polyradiculitis consistent with Guillain-Barré syndrome leads to the additional diagnostic consideration of leptospiral disease.

Cranial nerve palsies may occur with basilar meningitis of any etiology, but are most characteristic of meningitis due to tuberculosis and to fungi. The constellation of III, IV, V, and VI involvement unilaterally suggests cavernous sinus infection and should prompt an evaluation of the paranasal sinuses and ears. Infectious agents to considered in this situation are *Mucoraceae*, *Aspergillus*, and gram-negative bacteria, especially *Pseudomonas aeruginosa* (26,27).

Laboratory Data

A variety of readily available neuroradiological and laboratory procedures makes rapid diagnosis realistic. The clinician should use the previously discussed physical clues to guide his choice of appropriate tests.

Neuroimaging Studies (see also Chap. 30). Computed tomography (CT) without contrast enhancement excludes intraparenchymal hemorrhage and reveals ventricular size and mass effect. Addition of iodinated contrast material is contraindicated in patients with impaired renal function, and thus the utility of CT may be limited in many critically ill immunocompromised hosts. Magnetic resonance imaging (MRI) has some specific advantage over CT in the differentiation of CNS lesions, providing better definition of gray-white matter involvement, superior views of the posterior fossa and spine, and higher resolution of leptomeningeal disease. However, MRI cannot distinguish abscess from tumor reliably. Corticosteroids decrease contrast enhancement with both CT (iodinated contrast) and MRI (gadolinium diethylenetriamine pentaacetic acid) agents and retard ring formation. Lowered hematocrit may result in uncertainty about the presence or age of intracranial blood. Diffuse meningeal enhancement can be seen with breakdown of blood-brain barrier due to neoplastic, chemical, or infectious meningitis and is also seen on MRI after lumbar puncture. Therefore, this finding should be interpreted with caution when CSF evidence of meningeal infection is lacking.

Lumbar Puncture. The presence of fever and headache with or without meningismus mandates the performance of a lumbar puncture. Most clinicians would first perform contrast-enhanced CT or MRI if there is a suspicion of metastases or other mass lesion. In thrombocytopenic patients, a platelet count of less than 50,000 should prompt platelet transfusion before lumbar puncture.

Only rather general guidelines about CSF formulas are appropriate in the immunocompromised host. Predominantly polymorphonuclear leukocytes and CSF cell count of greater than 200 is suggestive of bacterial meningitis, and the finding of a CSF glucose level 50% or less than the concurrent blood glucose level supports this diagnosis. CSF pleocytosis with a lymphocytic predominance in the immunosuppressed patient could be consistent with *Cryptococcus*, *Listeria*, *Aspergillus*, *Nocardia*, or viral infection.

Two specific CSF formulas pose special diagnostic dilemmas. The first, aseptic meningitis, is summarized in Table 4. The differential diagnostic spectrum of aseptic meningitis in organ transplant recipients, and, in particular, in recipients of bone marrow transplants who may share both cancer and organ transplantation–related risk factors, is large. It should be remembered that at least two of the routinely used immunosuppressive drugs for organ transplantation, OKT 3 and antithymocyte or antilymphocyte globulin, can be associated with a prominent aseptic meningitis with meningeal and encephalopathic symptoms (27–29).

Table 4 Major Causes of Aseptic Meningitis Syndrome in Immunocompromised Hosts

Clinical setting	Infectious causes	Noninfectious causes
Cancer[a]	Viruses Varicella-zoster Conventional bacteria Partially treated bacterial meningitis Bacterial meningitis with profound neutropenia	Leptomeningeal carcinomatosis Chemical meningitis due to intrathecally administered drugs
Organ transplantation	Viruses Varicella-zoster *H. simplex* Types 1 and 2 Cytomegalovirus Adenoviruses Bacteria *M. tuberculosis* *Leptospira* Fungi *C. neoformans*	Drugs OKT 3 Antithymocyte globulin Trimethoprim-sulfamethoxazale Nonsteroidal anti-inflammatory drugs Azathioprine Isoniazid Neoplasia Posttransplant lymphoproliferative disorder Primary CNS lymphoma

[a]Recipients of bone marrow transplantation for malignancy span two clinical settings and may be at risk for infections listed in this table.
Source: Adapted from Refs. 27–29.

Table 5 lists the differential diagnostic considerations for a persistent neutrophilic meningitis in an immunocompromised host. This issue has been updated recently in a summary by Peacock (17). Serum and CSF antibody and antigenic studies are available to evaluate a number of the more common etiologies of this difficult clinical syndrome. Since many of the causes are treatable, including nocardiosis, several of the mycoses, brucellosis, tuberculosis, and herpes simplex viruses, every effort should be made to define a specific etiology before broad-spectrum antimicrobial treatment is undertaken.

Table 5 Etiologies of Persistent Neutrophilic Meningitis in Immunocompromised Hosts

	Infectious	Noninfectious
Common	Nocardiosis Candidiasis Aspergillosis Zygomycosis Herpes simplex virus (types 1 and 2)	Chemical meningitis OKT3 meningitis
Uncommon (but reported)	Brucellosis Tuberculosis Histoplasmosis Coccidioidomycosis Pseudoallescheriasis	

Source: Adapted from Ref. 17.

Indications for New CSF Diagnostic Tests. Increasingly, the clinician has access to and should understand the indications for a number of new organism-specific and nonspecific tests. These, along with the applicable organisms and potential problems in interpretation, are summarized in Table 6 and are discussed further in Chapter 29. Among the most widely available are *antigen detection* with commercial latex particle agglutination. Cryptococcal antigen and major bacterial pathogens (*H. influenza* type b, *N. meningitidis*, and *S. pneumoniae*) are the most common diagnostic applications of this test. RIA or ELISA antigen detection methods are more sensitive, though technically more difficult. Antigen detection is not synonymous with the presence of viable organisms.

Antibody detection serological tests generally measure organism-specific IgM, a marker of recent infection, and IgG. When the blood-brain barrier is intact, CSF antibody is 1% or less than that of blood. Since the blood-brain barrier is not intact in most CNS infections, antibody leakage, particularly IgG, must be taken into account. Organism-specific intrathecal antibody production is helpful in the diagnosis of Lyme disease as well as syphilis, cysticercosis, toxoplasmosis, and herpes simplex encephalitis. After treatment, the intrathecal humoral response may persist for prolonged periods. Antibody-capture ELISA obviates the problem of adjusting for blood-brain

Table 6 The Use of Newer Rapid Diagnostic Tests for Suspected CNS Infection

Test	Applicable pathogens	Problems
CSF antigen detection		
Latex particle agglutination	*H. influenzae* *N. meningitidis* *S. pneumoniae* *C. neoformans*	Does not indicate viable organism Prozone effect (false-negative due to antigen excess)
RIA or ELISA	*M. tuberculosis* *H. simplex* *Candida* *Aspergillus* *H. capsulatum* Cysticerci Retroviruses	Technically more difficult but more sensitive than latex agglutination
CSF antibody detection	*B. burgdorferi* *T. pallidum* Cysticerci *T. gondii* *H. simplex*	Positivity may persist well after successful treatment
Gas-liquid chromatography	*M. tuberculosis*	Not widely available
Polymerase chain reaction	*H. simplex* Varicella-zoster Epstein-Barr virus Retroviruses JC virus *M. tuberculosis* *B. burgdorferi* *N. meningitidis* *T. pallidum*	Detection of viral genome of latent viruses possible in absence of associated neurological disease

Source: Refs. 17–22.

barrier leakage and has been used to measure intrathecal antibody production in Lyme disease and herpes simplex encephalitis.

Gas liquid chromatography can be used for the rapid diagnosis of bacterial, fungal, and tuberculous infections based on the detection of metabolites or cell components such as tuberculostearic acid. It is not yet widely available.

Several nonspecific methods such as the limulate lysate test detect bacterial endotoxin in CSF. Sensitivity approaches 100%, but the results merely exclude or include gram-negative organisms. CSF adenosine deaminase is increased in tuberculous meningitis. Cytokines, including interleukin-1 beta, interleukin-6, and tumor necrosis factor alpha, are elevated during CSF infection but may be seen in inflammatory conditions as well.

Polymerase chain reaction (PCR) in the diagnosis of neurological disease has been the subject of several excellent reviews (20–22). PCR amplifies small quantities of DNA or RNA from a suspected pathogen. It can be applied to CSF or to CSF cells. PCR is rapid, extremely sensitive, and specific and does not require pathogen replication or a host immune response. Unfortunately, it is easy to contaminate the test sample or PCR apparatus, leading to false-positive results. PCR has been used successfully in the diagnosis of herpes simplex encephalitis, varicella-zoster infections, and retroviral diseases. One of its most promising uses is for the rapid diagnosis of tuberculous meningitis (30). JC virus, the etiological agent of progressive multifocal leukoencephalopathy, can be amplified in the CSF of 60–75% of PML patients, suggesting that the test is specific, but imperfectly sensitive for diagnostic purposes (31). A promising PCR-based CSF test for *T. gondii* along with PCR-based detection of Epstein-Barr virus genome in patients with primary CNS lymphoma makes it likely that the noninvasive diagnosis of common causes of mass lesions in AIDS patients soon will be feasible.

Arteriography. As MRI has become widely available, the use of arteriography has declined. However, there are several specific situations in which this procedure may be valuable in the diagnosis and management of CNS infections in the immunocompromised host. In a patient with known or suspected endocarditis, arteriography may be necessary to exclude mycotic aneurysm prior to anticoagulation. Arteriography may heighten suspicion of *A. fumigatus* infection, as this organism invades blood vessels with resultant subarachnoid hemorrhage. Subarachnoid hemorrhage may be delayed following successful treatment of infective endocarditis and may be related to ongoing vasculitis with the formation of immune complexes (32). Arteriography remains the procedure of choice for the diagnosis of vasculitis, which may be associated with some malignancies, particularly the lymphoproliferative disorders, and with many infections including varicella-zoster, mycobacteria, cryptococcosis, aspergillosis, mucormycosis, toxoplasmosis, CMV, and syphilis. Arteriography may help define an abnormal area to which brain or meningeal biopsy then can be directed (33,34).

Brain Biopsy. Despite the advent of several new noninvasive analyses for CSF, brain biopsy remains a useful adjunct to the diagnosis of CNS infections. Table 7 summarizes current indications for the procedure that should be undertaken to seek treatable infections and to offer prognostic information for those infections without definitive therapy. CT and MRI reveal nonspecific ring-enhancing lesions in a variety of situations. Depending on the clinical setting, empiric treatment can be initiated for *T. gondii*, for example, but failure of a lesion to respond rapidly should lead to consideration of definitive tissue diagnosis. Progressive abnormalities on MRI or CT should be considered for biopsy. Transcranial Doppler measurement of elevated velocity in intracranial vessels consistent with vasculitis or compatible arteriographic findings should prompt confirmatory biopsy of an involved area. Finally, meningeal biopsy may be the only remaining diagnostic tool for the undiagnosed case of persistent neutrophilic meningitis when all potential diagnoses and tests in Tables 5 and 6 have been exhausted.

Table 7 Indications for Brain/Meningeal Biopsy

1. Presence of a nonspecific ring-enhancing lesion or lesions whose bacterial, fungal, or neoplastic nature is unclear
2. Failure of a suspected toxoplasmosis lesion to respond to 2–3 weeks of appropriate therapy
3. A CT or MRI abnormality whose nature is unclear, but which seems to be progressive
4. Transcranial Doppler, arteriographic, or magnetic resonance angiographic data consistent with vasculitis
5. Persistent neutrophilic meningitis with negative results of all appropriate studies from Table 6

CNS INFECTIONS IN TRANSPLANT RECIPIENTS

Pathophysiology

More than 80% of allograft recipients have a significant infection in the first year after transplantation. CNS infection is common and often devastating, occurring in 5–10% of transplant recipients at some time after transplantation and resulting in the death of 40–77% of these patients (1,2). Many factors contribute to these high infection rates. Of these, by far the most important is the immunosuppression necessary to prevent rejection of the allograft. Regimens currently in use predominantly affect T cells and thus depress cellular immunity. However, many other factors also contribute to infection risk. After transplantation, patients may have indwelling catheters, which serve as a nidus or portal of entry for infection. Therefore these patients are at substantially increased risk of infections with common pathogens, often with atypical presentations, as well as opportunistic ones. The diseases necessitating transplantation and their metabolic complications (particularly hyperglycemia and uremia) further inhibit host defenses. Transplant patients are often acutely ill with more than one organ system affected by different pathological processes including rejection, organ failure, and potential drug toxicities. Finally, infection with certain agents increases the risk of other infections. Thus, patients with chronic hepatitis or CMV infection are particularly susceptible to infections by *L. monocytogenes* and *C. neoformans*.

Problems Common to All Transplant Recipients

As the consultant approaches the complicated clinical problem of a transplant recipient with potential CNS infection, he should consider both infectious and noninfectious etiologies. These can be grouped into four main types: (1) complications related to the underlying disease; (2) problems arising from the transplant procedure itself; (3) posttransplant disorders peculiar to the specific type of infection; and (4) side effects of immunosuppression. The first three types of problems differ according to the transplant procedure, but type 4 complications are common, to varying degrees, in all organ transplant recipients. Table 8 offers a differential diagnostic flow analysis to help with the often convoluted process of assessing the likelihood of infection and then arriving at a specific pathological diagnosis.

Neurotoxicity of Immunosuppressive Drugs

The major immunosuppressants in current use are cyclosporine (Sandimmune), azathioprine (Imuran), corticosteroids, polyclonal antilymphoblast and antithymocyte globulins, OKT3 (Muromonab-CD3), and FK506 (Tacrolimus). In addition to predisposing to CNS infection, direct neurotoxicity has been reported with all of these agents.

Cyclosporine. Introduced in 1978, cyclosporine is the most commonly used antirejection agent in use today. It is effective both for treatment of acute organ rejection and for chronic maintenance immunosuppression. It is not myelosuppressive, but inhibits lymphokine production and release and preferentially suppresses CD4+ T-cell function. It is not cleared by hemodialysis.

Table 8 Differential Diagnosis of CNS Infection in the Transplant Recipient

CONSIDER

↓

I. Underlying disease for which transplant performed A. ? metabolic abnormality B. ? drug complication C. ? stroke (? vasculitis) D. ? seizure E. ? tumor recurrence	→	II. Nature of transplant surgery A. ? hypoxia/hypotension B. ? stroke C. ? local nerve injury D. ? local infection		Immediate postoperative period
		↓		
IV. Organ-specific complications A. Kidney-uremic encephalopathy B. Liver-central pontine myelinolysis C. Cardiac-stroke D. Bone marrow-recurrent tumor, graft-vs.-host disease, nonbacterial thrombotic endocarditis	←	III. Acute rejection syndrome A. ? organ failure B. ? seizure C. ? raised intracranial pressure		At any time following transplantation
↓				
V. Toxicity of immunosuppressive drugs A. Aseptic meningitis: OKT3 B. Delirium, tremor: cyclosporine C. Psychosis: corticosteroids D. Delirium, tremor, seizures: FK506 E. Posttransplant lymphoproliferative disorder	→	VI. Possibility of CNS infection A. Intensity and duration of immunosuppression B. Pace of illness C. Extraneural sites of infection D. Anatomy of CNS involvement E. Laboratory data		

↓

Specific CNS Infection

Elimination involves the hepatic P450 enzyme system. There is considerable interindividual variability in pharmacokinetic properties, and cyclosporine has a narrow therapeutic index. Interactions with other drugs are important. Metabolism is enhanced by phenobarbital, phenytoin, carbamazepine, and rifampin leading to decreased levels and inhibited by ketoconazole, erythromycin, and beta-lactam antibiotics. Trough levels are more important than peak concentrations with a trough window being 150–400 ng/ml. Adverse effects correlate only approximately with blood levels in patients as a population.

The most important systemic complications of the drug are renal and hepatic toxicity and hypertension. It may also produce a vasculopathy with features of the hemolytic-uremic syndrome and thrombotic thrombocytopenic purpura (35).

Neurological complications occur in 15–40% of patients treated with cyclosporine. The risk of neurotoxicity from this agent is increased by drug-induced hypomagnesemia and hypocholesterolemia, the concomitant use of high-dose steroids or beta-lactam antibiotics, and by hypertension, uremia, previous intrathecal methotrexate, and previous CNS irradiation (36). Tremor is the most common manifestation of neurotoxicity. Motor syndromes include paraparesis, hemiparesis, or quadriparesis. Neuropathological studies reveal myelopathy in some patients and leukoencephalopathy in others. The clinical encephalopathy associated with cyclosporine has numerous manifestations including headache, confusion, depression, and prominent visual hallucinations or cortical blindness. Neuralgic symptoms including paresthesias and hyperesthesia of the limbs occurs frequently. Seizures occur in up to 6% of patients receiving cyclosporine. Fortunately, reduction or elimination of the drug is usually associated with reversal of even the most severe encephalopathic symptoms.

FK506. FK506 is a newer immunosuppressive agent, the use of which has been most extensively studied in liver transplant recipients. The mechanism of action is similar to that of cyclopsorine, and both the systemic and neurological symptoms also parallel those of cyclosporine (37). Most neurotoxic side effects of FK506 reverse completely after drug withdrawal.

Corticosteroids. Though the above immunosuppressive agents have helped reduce the doses of chronic corticosteroid therapy in the transplant population, most patients continue to receive corticosteroids in doses sufficient to affect both cellular and humoral immunity. The most common neurotoxic side effects are proximal myopathy, evident in patients on doses of steroids equivalent to 8 mg dexamethasone or greater for more than a few weeks and somewhat helped by change to a nonfluorinated drug (38). Steroid psychosis is common, and the range and duration of therapy necessary to produce psychotic symptoms varies considerably among individuals (39). The psychiatric reactions may be subacute, heralded by irritability, insomnia, or elation, or may be quite sudden. Reduction of dose may help, and small doses of haloperidol or other major tranquilizer can control the acute symptoms. Spinal cord or cauda equina compression from epidural lipomatosis caused by corticosteroids has been reported in transplant recipients. Surgical therapy may be necessary, though reduction or elimination of steroids has reversed symptoms in some patients (40).

OKT3. OKT3 (Muromonab CD3) is an anti–T-cell mouse monoclonal antibody administered intravenously to treat acute rejection. It also has been used prophylactically at the time of transplant. OKT3 causes T cells to release cytokines, including tumor necrosis factor alpha (TNF-alpha), gamma-interferon, and interleukin-2 (41). These are likely the mediators of both the systemic and neurotoxicty of this drug and other biological response modifiers (42). Most patients develop a transient flulike syndrome when the drug is first administered. The most common neurological toxicity is aseptic meningitis. Clinical symptoms include headache, photophobia, and meningismus, resolving in 1–5 days when the drug is stopped (43). Therefore, though infection must be excluded, patients usually may continue OKT3. Pretreatment with corticosteroids at doses of methylprednisolone (Solumedrol) 1 mg/kg IV 2–6 h before OKT3 administration may eliminate or reduce both the meningeal syndrome and the other major neurotoxicity, acute encephalopathy (44). Neutralizing anti–TNF-alpha antibodies have been effective experimentally in preventing adverse effects of anti-CD3 antibodies and eventually may prove clinically useful. Attention also should be directed to factors increasing the severity of OKT3-related adverse effects. These include volume overload and synergistic interaction with cyclosporine and nonsteroidal antiinflammatory drugs.

Lymphoproliferative Diseases

Following infection, the second most common complication of immunosuppression in the transplant patient population is neoplasia. Neoplasms occurring with increased frequency in this population often involve solely the skin (squamous cell, basal cell, and Kaposi's). The second most common proliferative disorders, not all of which are true neoplasia, are lymphoproliferative diseases. Posttransplant lymphoproliferative disorder (PTLD) is the term used to cover a wide spectrum of abnormal B-lymphocyte proliferations ranging from diffuse polyclonal lymphoid hyperplasia to malignant monoclonal lymphoma (45,46). Extranodal presentations are common in PTLD, occurring in up to 78% of patients in some series (47). The allograft is a frequent site of involvement, and organ failure due to PTLD must be distinguished from rejection. CNS involvement occurs in 15–25% of patients with PTLD and is the only site of detectable disease in about 85% of neurologically affected patients (46).

Several lines of evidence point to Epstein-Barr virus (EBV) infection as the mechanism of oncogenesis in PTLD. EBV is recoverable from 90% of transplant patients in the first year following surgery. EBV selectively infects B lymphocytes causing proliferation, which under normal circumstances is suppressed by cell-mediated immunity. The main risk factor for PTLD is the total extent of immunosuppression including the dose of agents such as cyclosporine and OKT3 and the duration of immunosuppression (48–50). PTLD is most common among heart and liver transplant recipients, followed by kidney and lastly BMT recipients.

The clinical presentation of PTLD involving the CNS may be quite nonspecific with altered mental status and systemic symptoms suggestive of a viral syndrome. Neuroradiographic studies usually reveal deep tumors in the periventricular white matter. There is leptomeningeal spread in 25% of cases. MRI findings also include single or multiple T_2 signal abnormalities in white matter with little mass effect and variable enhancement (51). Their appearance is difficult to distinguish from other entities occurring in transplant patients, and biopsy may be necessary for definitive diagnosis.

Therapy includes reduction of the level of immunosuppression. Radiation therapy may be necessary, but since many of these patients have other concurrent infections, organ failure, and metabolic abnormalities, the overall prognosis is poor (52).

Infection Patterns Common to All Transplant Recipients

Less Than One Month After Transplant

Three main periods of infection risk posttransplantation correlate well with the responsible microbial pathogens (1,2,4). The first period begins with the transplant procedure and lasts for approximately one month. At this time, although immunosuppressive drugs are used at their highest doses, duration of immunosuppression is as yet insufficient to place the patient at great risk for opportunistic infections. When infections occur they are often due to common pathogens found in the general population or to opportunistic organisms found in the transplant patient's environment (*Aspergillus* in the hospital ventilation system) or present before the surgery (*M. tuberculosis*, *S. stercoralis*).

One to Six Months After Transplant

The second risk period extends from roughly 1 to 6 months posttransplant. This is the period of highest immunosuppression and concomitantly the period of greatest risk for CNS infection. Viruses (EBV and CMV), which further depress the immune system and *Listeria*, *Aspergillus*, and *Nocardia* predominate.

More Than Six Months After Transplant

The third risk period begins 6 months following transplant. Earlier infections (i.e. cytomegalovirus retinitis) or their consequences (e.g., seizures) may persist, opportunistic infections may return, or more common pathogens may replace opportunistic ones as the degree of immunosuppression is reduced. Patients who continue to require high-dose immunosuppressive maintenance or have received additional antirejection therapy (usually with OKT3 or antilymphocyte globulin) continue to be at risk for *Cryptococcus*, *Listeria*, and *Nocardia*. Most cases of cryptococcal meningitis in transplant patients occur during this period, as do chronic disorders like PML.

CNS Complications and Infections Specific to Organ Transplant Type

Kidney Transplant

The most commonly performed transplant procedure, renal transplantation, is now the preferred therapy for patients with end-stage renal disease due to glomerulonephritis, diabetes, and hypertensive renal disease. Pretransplantation uremia may cause neurological impairment, and uremia may occur posttransplantation. Patients with diabetes or hypertension are predisposed to cerebrovascular complications perioperatively (53).

Altered metabolism of drugs due to uremia may complicate neurological assessment in the perioperative period (54). With decreased protein binding of drugs in uremia, high free levels of drugs like phenytoin or carbamazepine may cause neurological symptoms at "therapeutic levels" (of measured bound drug). Therefore, measurement of free drug levels may be necessary to assess the contribution of drugs to a new neurological syndrome. Neurotoxicity associated with antibiotics includes seizures due to beta-lactam antibiotics, cephalosporins, and imipenem, ototoxicity due to aminoglycosides, erythromycin, and vancomycin, peripheral nerve toxicity due to nitrofurantoin, and neuromuscular blockade with possible respiratory depression due to aminoglycosides and polymyxins. (See Chap. 33 for further discussion of neurotoxicity of commonly administered drugs.)

The syndrome of encephalopathy with acute rejection has been described only in renal transplant recipients (55). Systemic symptoms include fever and swelling and tenderness of the graft with renal failure. Neurological manifestations are a nonfocal encephalopathy with headache, altered mentation, and seizures. In the series described by Gross, this syndrome occurred between 6 and 652 days posttransplant. CSF examination showed increased opening pressure and protein. Patients were not receiving cyclosporine or OKT3, both of which can cause encephalopathy and seizures. There was a rapid rise in creatinine, and hypertension did not appear to be a factor. The pathogenesis is thought to be the release of soluble neuroactive cytokines. Recent information suggests that seizure control in the transplant population may be improved with the least risk of hepatic microenzyme induction and altered levels of immunosuppression with the new agent gabapentin (56).

Most of our understanding of the time course and type of infectious complications related to immunosuppression comes from renal transplant patients (2,57). In addition, renal transplant patients may have increased CD8 and decreased CD4 T-cell subsets, making them especially prone to CMV and EBV infections.

Heart Transplant

The underlying diseases for which cardiac transplantation currently is performed are primarily atherosclerotic disease and cardiomyopathies. Both conditions predispose to cerebrovascular events both pre- and posttransplant. Ischemic events during the procedure present clinically as either focal neurological deficits or as nonfocal encephalopathy with or without seizures. Compared to other transplant recipients, cardiac patients are most likely to have complications related to the transplant surgery itself. Patients may be on the pump for several hours and are sometimes subjected to hypotension and hypoxia. All newly transplanted hearts are prone to develop emboli (58,59).

Because the doses of immunosuppression required for heart and heart-lung transplantation are higher than those used for renal transplantation, the incidence of both drug-related neurological complications and CNS infections is slightly higher than with other organ transplantation. Aseptic meningitis is a particularly common complication occurring in 14 of 29 patients in one series who had lumbar puncture because of change in neurological function or fever of uncertain etiology (28). Four of these patients had an active infectious process including two cases of *Listeria*, one of aspergillosis and one of bacterial endocarditis. The CSF formulas did not help greatly in the differentiation among these cases and in the remaining 10 patients whose meningeal process was ascribed to OKT3. *Toxoplasma gondii* infection is more common among cardiac transplant recipients than among other organ transplant patients, and the source of the organism may be the transplanted heart itself (60). Other common infections in the largest adult series of 417 patients were *Aspergillus* and *Nocardia* among 13 patients with intracranial infections 2–143 weeks following transplantation (10). Cardiac transplant recipients have the highest incidence of posttransplantation lymphoproliferative disorders of any transplant group (78).

Liver Transplant

The 3-year survival rate among hepatic transplant recipients is now greater than 60% (61). The incidence of neurological complications varies greatly between clinical and autopsy series (see Table 1). In autopsy series, neuropathological lesions are present in more than 80% of liver transplant recipients and approximately 40% had evidence of intracranial infection. The underlying diseases for which transplantation is performed in the adult include alcoholic cirrhosis, viral hepatitis, primary biliary cirrhosis, hepatic neoplasms, and some congenital hepatic diseases. In children, the most common indication for liver transplantation is congenital biliary atresia. As a group, patients undergoing hepatic transplantation may be sicker than those receiving other organs. They may wait for a considerable time before their transplantation because of an organ shortage, and many have mild to moderate metabolic encephalopathy. These patients may also have some degree of coagulopathy prior to transplantation due to liver failure. Preoperative neurological assessment of these patients is important as the presence of an abnormal pretransplant neurological examination is associated with in-hospital CNS complications (62). The major short-term neurological complications of liver transplant include anoxic and septic encephalopathy and brain hemorrhage.

The liver transplantation procedure frequently necessitates large replacements of blood and electrolytes, and patients may have prolonged periods of hypotension. These may lead to diffuse hypoxic damage to the brain or to watershed infarctions. Though many liver transplant recipients have nonspecifically abnormal electroencephalograms postoperatively, epileptiform abnormalities were a specific, independent poor prognostic indicator in one series, indicating various serious structural changes such as infection and ischemic or hemorrhagic infarction (63).

At least one neurological syndrome appears much more commonly among hepatic organ recipients. This is central pontine myelinolysis (CPM), which has been found in up to 13% of liver transplant recipients at autopsy (64). MRI is the neurodiagnostic procedure of choice for documentation of this condition and is more sensitive than CT (65). Occasionally, the MRI manifestations of demyelination in the pons may be observed in patients who do not have clinical symptoms of CPM, and the incidence of neuropathological abnormalities consistent with CPM is higher than that seen during life (14). The clinical manifestations are altered mental status or coma, pseudobulbar palsy, and quadriplegia, often masked by other systemic problems. The rapid changes in serum sodium concentration with replacement of intraoperative blood loss may be the cause of this problem.

Liver transplant recipients are more sensitive to the toxic effects of immunosuppressive agents because of their hypocholesterolemia and frequent concurrent hypertension. For these reasons, tacrolimus (FK506), a newer immunosuppressive agent, has been studied largely in the liver transplant group. Tacrolimus is associated with a higher incidence of adverse effects in the form of nephrotoxicity and neurotoxicity than cyclosporine, with comparable results in terms of patient and graft survival (66).

Careful attention to perioperative management of blood pressure, electrolytes, and immunosuppressive drugs may lessen the frequency of neurological complications in liver transplant recipients. The Cleveland Clinic group reports a decrease in incidence of neurological complications from 47% to 19% in their most recent patients. Survival was comparable for patients with and without neurological complications. The authors attribute the improving statistics to immediate withdrawal of cyclosporine at the onset of mental status change and improvement in intraoperative and postoperative management (13).

The incidence of CNS infections among hepatic transplant recipients parallels that of cardiac transplant patients with whom they share a high level of immunosuppression. In addition, the presence of chronic active hepatitis predisposes liver patients to infections with *Listeria* and *Cryptococcus*.

Bone Marrow Transplant

Patients receiving bone marrow transplantation share features of those in the previous sections along with those in the next section on cancer. BMT has developed into an important method of treatment for aplastic anemia, inborn errors of metabolism, and a wide variety of hematological, lymphoreticular, and solid malignancies. The three types of BMTs are autologous, syngeneic, and allogeneic. Autologous marrow transplantation involves infusion of the patient's own marrow, which has been harvested and preserved while the patient receives high-dose chemotherapy. A syngeneic transplant involves transplantation between identical twins. These two types are associated with very few neurological infections, though early encephalopathy occurred in up to 39% of one representative series of patients transplanted for Hodgkin's disease. The main cause of encephalopathy was pulmonary (often infectious) or hepatic dysfunction. Sepsis with conventional bacteria was another common reason for CNS dysfunction (67).

Allogeneic BMT involves infusion of marrow from an unrelated donor. These recipients are often severely immunosuppressed and 60–70% of them experience neurological complications, which are the cause of death in 5–10% (68). Several features of allogeneic BMT recipients make them different from other organ transplant patients throughout the pre- and posttransplant periods. First, these patients may have been severely immunosuppressed for months because of their underlying disease. Therefore, infections which might occur later in the posttransplant period occur earlier in these patients. In addition, BMT patients are profoundly granulocytopenic for about 1 month before the new marrow begins to function. During this period, bacterial, viral, and fungal infections may become established. Even after granulocyte recovery, altered cell-mediated and humoral immunity persists for up to one year. CMV infections and *T. gondii* become common.

Second, the underlying disease for which allogeneic BMTs are performed may be the cause of neurological problems that are difficult to differentiate from CNS infections. Leukemias and lymphomas recur in the CNS (neoplastic meningitis), though the incidence of primary CNS lymphoma is lower in BMT recipients, possibly because of generally lower long-term levels of immunosuppression compared to other transplant patients. Prior radiation and chemotherapy may make BMT recipients more sensitive to the toxic effects of immunosuppression or appropriate antibiotic therapy for their diseases.

Third, several viral infections that appear unique to BMT patients have been described. These include a fatal adenovirus meningoencephalitis, possibly acquired from the infused marrow and a variant B herpesvirus-6 encephalitis that is untreatable (69,70).

Fourth, graft-versus-host disease (GVHD) produces several neurological syndromes including polymyositis, peripheral neuropathy, and myasthenia gravis. GVHD may affect the brain. However, in autopsy series a number of patients with lymphocytic infiltration of the brain also had evidence of possible CNS viral infectious (71).

Fifth, cerebrovascular complications are a relatively frequent problem in BMT patients. Infective endocarditis or nonbacterial thrombotic endocarditis (NBTE) may be the etiology. NBTE occurs in up to 9% of BMT patients, after both allogeneic and autologous BMTs (72,73). Associated with a hypercoagulable state, this condition may develop because of coagulation abnormalities in this group of patients, and chronic heparinization may be the only effective treatment (74). In the cancer patient population treated with BMT, focal or multifocal deficits must raise the consideration of metastatic disease or vasculitis in addition to the possibility of NBTE (25,75).

CNS INFECTIONS IN CANCER PATIENTS

During the past 20 years, as the lives of cancer patients with virtually all types of malignancies have been prolonged by surgery, radiation therapy, and chemotherapy, the growing problem of infection has been recognized, categorized, and, to a lesser extent, prevented (76–78). Between 1982 and 1990, 56 episodes of CNS infections were treated in 49 patients at Massachusetts General Hospital (MGH). Table 9 shows the distribution of cancers with associated neurological syndromes and organisms. As in previous reports, patients with leukemia and lymphoreticular malignancies represented a large percentage of the infected patients—in this series 13 of 49 (26%). Eight of the 49 patients (16%) had primary CNS tumors. Bacterial meningitis was the most common clinical syndrome. Two organisms accounted for nearly one-half of the meningitides: *S. pneumoniae* and *L. monocytogenes*. As in Lukas's series (23), neutropenia was the primary risk factor for bacterial meningitis in patients with leukemia or lymphoma, but seeding of the meninges from systemic sepsis was the likely mechanism in the nine patients with gram-negative meningitis. In the MGH series, only 16 of 30 cases (53%) of meningitis presented with a fulminant acute meningeal picture. Twelve patients with bacterial meningitis (36%) had between 2 and 10 days of mild headache and fever before the diagnosis was made, and two patients were symptomatic for more than 10 days before diagnosis. Five of nine gram-negative cases presented with a more indolent course of mental status deterioration over 2 or more days, as did three of the eight cases of *S. pneumoniae* meningitis. CSF formulas, as has been noted in Lukas's series (23), were not always predictive of bacterial organism in these patients, many of whom had been heavily pretreated with antibiotics. In the author's recent experience, half of the patients with bacterial meningitis had fewer than 5 white cells/mm^3 and only two had more than 100 inflammatory cells in the CSF. Four patients had completely normal CSF cell counts, glucose and protein concentrations, but culture was positive in 88% of the group as a whole, even though 55% were receiving antibiotics at the time (16). Hypoglycorrhacchia was both the single best indicator of bacterial meningitis and an independent poor prognostic sign in both series. Mortality in cancer patients with *S. pneumoniae* was 50%, compared with a 12% mortality rate among patients without malignancies with *S. pneumoniae* meningitis during this same time interval (23,79). In the latter half of the decade of the 1980s there appears to have been a slight decrease in *Pseudomonas* bacteremia and an increase in gram-positive bacteria as the cause of meningitis.

Bacterial brain abscess was the second most common type of neurological infection. Five of the 11 cases were due to *S. aureus* or *S. epidermidis*. Epidural abscess with *S. aureus* occurred in one patient following mastectomy.

Fungal diseases occurred in only nine patients. Forty-five cases of cryptococcal meningitis were seen at the Massachusetts General Hospital during this period, only four of which occurred in patients with cancer. These were successfully treated. All cases of *Candida* and *Aspergillus* infection, however, were fatal.

Two major risk factors emerged in the MGH cancer population. These were neutropenia and procedure-related infections. Procedure-related infections accounted for 19 of the 56 infectious

In the cancer patient population, multiple infections are frequent. An additional extraneural infection site was detected in 21 of the 56 CNS infectious episodes and provided a clue to the correct pathogen. Diagnostic errors were frequent, as clinical indicators of CNS infection were infrequent. Fever (45%) and headache (49%) were the most common clues. Consideration of epidemiological clues might have led to the suspicion of cysticercosis and Lyme disease in two patients.

Some specific trends can be identified. Gastrointestinal procedures preceded *Listeria* infections in three of five patients. Cephalosporin coverage for the procedure was not adequate, and *Listeria* coverage with a penicillin should be considered. The Hodgkin's disease population had fewer bacterial and fungal CNS infections compared with the previous decade at the MGH (3,4). Only one patient with Hodgkin's disease and CNS infection was seen in this most recent group, whereas 12 patients with cryptococcus and a variety of conventional bacteria were reported in the earlier Hooper series. Several factors may account for this: (1) there were fewer splenectomies as computed tomographic staging became standard; (2) neutropenia was less severe and persistent with recent chemotherapy regimens and with the use of hematopoietic growth factors; and (3) earlier prophylaxis was used to prevent *S. pneumoniae* infection.

A more disturbing trend was the tendency to ever broader antimicrobial coverage when bacterial infection was suspected. The reports from specialized cancer hospitals suggest that a wider spectrum of organisms needs to be considered in the differential diagnosis of sepsis (82). An additional concern is that bacteria resistant to all the major antimicrobials will become the predominant nosocomial pathogens. Jacoby and Archer provide a useful summary of current organism resistance and mechanisms (83).

CLINICAL MANIFESTATIONS AND MANAGEMENT OF SPECIFIC CNS INFECTIONS

Though most of the diseases discussed below have been covered in other chapters, this section will emphasize diagnostic and therapeutic issues common to immunocompromised hosts. Two types of bacterial pathogens, four groups of fungi, four viruses, and two parasites make an even dozen opportunistic infections with which the clinician should be familiar. He or she should also be aware of side effects of antimicrobial agents (discussed in Chap. 33).

Bacterial Diseases

Table 12 lists the appropriate antimicrobial regimens for various pathogens. Presumed bacterial meningitis with conventional organisms is usually covered with a third-generation cephalosporin, often with the addition of gentamicin until the identity of the organisms has been established.

Listeria monocytogenes

One of the most common agents causing bacterial meningitis in the immunocompromised host, *Listeria*, is not covered by third-generation cephalosporins. Therefore, initial broad-spectrum coverage for suspected meningitis in this population should include ampicillin. In studies of patients with impaired cell-mediated immunity, nearly 25% have harbored this organism in the gastrointestinal tract. *Listeria* produces bacteremia, meningitis, or cerebritis with focal dysfunction related to supratentorial or brain-stem invasion (Fig. 2). Evolution of symptoms ranges from fulminant progression over a few hours to a more indolent course up to 10 days. Approximately 75% of systemic *Listeria* infections result in CNS seeding in immunocompromised patients. In penicillin-allergic patients, trimethaprim sulfamethoxazole is an appropriate choice. The use of dexamethasone for bacterial meningitis in an immunocompromised host with bacterial meningitis has not been investigated prospectively.

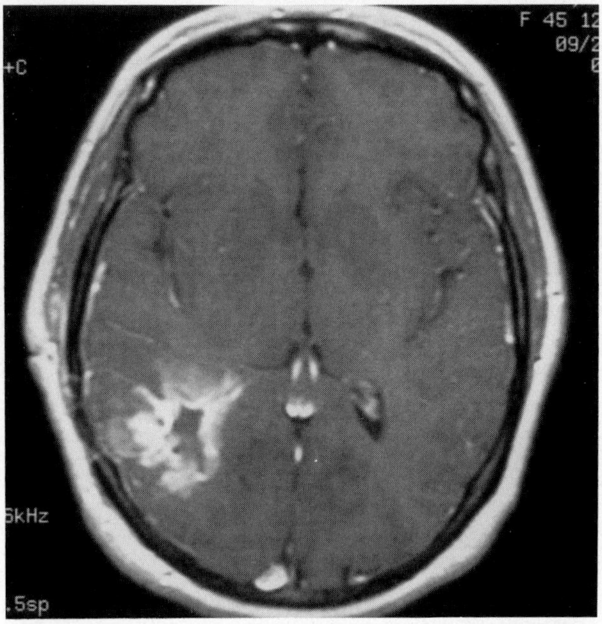

(A)

Figure 1 (A) MRI scan of patient with glioblastoma multiforme who had had three craniotomies and both conventional external and stereotactic radiosurgery for recurrent tumor and then developed rapid, marked worsening of symptoms with an enhancing mass in the tumor bed. The scan was felt to represent residual/recurrent tumor. (B) Axial view of the same patient 2 weeks later, when marked cerebritis and diffuse enhancement strengthened the suspicion of abscess. (C) Coronal view of the same patient from the same time as scan B shows the communication of enhancement with the extradural space. The patient had both recurrent tumor and *S. aureus* abscess. Treatment required removal of skull flap and 10 weeks of antibiotic therapy.

Nocardia asteroides

Chronic corticosteroid treatment is the most common predisposing factor for development of *Nocardia* infection. There is usually a pulmonary source of infection. CNS seeding typically results in a single or small number of brain abscesses (Fig. 3). Less commonly, meningitis is the clinical syndrome (84). If pulmonary infection cannot be documented, brain biopsy may be necessary. At least 6 weeks of therapy with trimethaprim sulfamethoxazole is recommended. Conservative medical therapy without surgical drainage has been associated with successful responses, decreasing the mortality rate in the immunocompromised host to the rate seen in the occasional immunocompetent patient with *Nocardia* (85).

Fungal Infections

Fungal infection is now as frequent a cause of death in patients with acute leukemia as bacterial infection. Some fungal infections take advantage of a neutrophilic deficit (candidiasis, aspergillosis, and mucormycosis), and others become established as a result of a disorder of T-lymphocyte–mediated immunity (cryptococcosis, histoplasmosis, and coccidioidomycosis). New fungal pathogens continue to be described in immunocompromised hosts, but two organ-

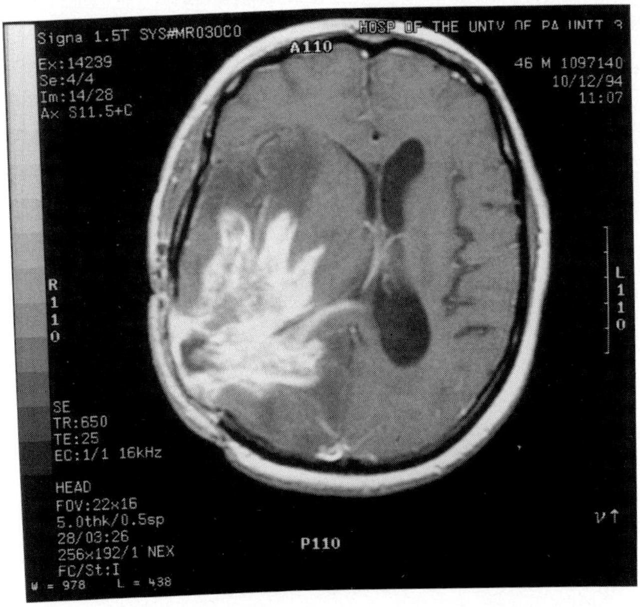

(B)

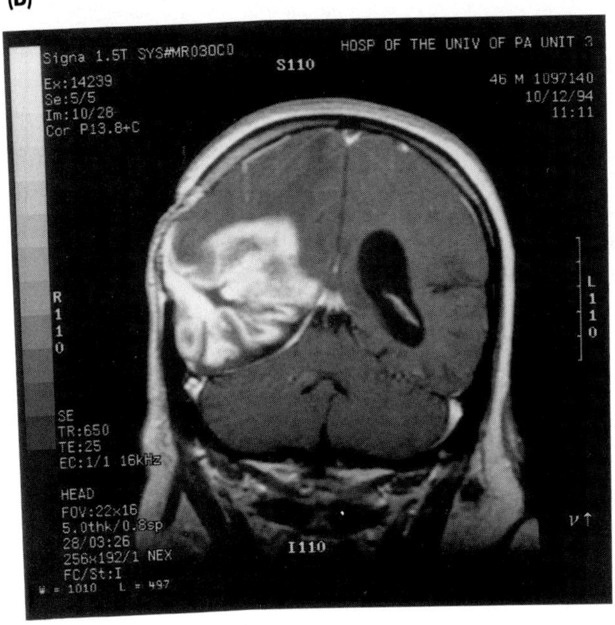

(C)

isms, *C. neoformans* and *A. fumigatus*, account for the vast majority of CNS infections in these patients.

Cryptococcus neoformans

Cryptococcus was the causative organism of one-third of CNS infections in one series of patients with defects in cell-mediated immunity, usually with immunosuppression of greater than 6 weeks duration (4). The organism usually enters through the respiratory tract or less commonly through

Table 12 Treatment of Specific Infections Associated with Immunodeficiency

Organism	Treatment[a]	Prophylaxis/Maintenance
Bacterial		
S. aureus	Nafcillin 2g q4h and Cefotaxime 2g q6h or Vancomycin 500 mg q6h	None
H. influenzae	Ceftriaxone 2g q12h or Ampicillin 3g q6h	None
S. pneumoniae	Penicillin 2mU q2h or Ceftriaxone 2g q12h	None
L. monocytogenes	Ampicillin 2–3g q4h plus Gentamicin 1–1.5mg/kg q8h (if blood cultures positive)	None
N. asteroides	Sulfadiazine 8–12g/day	None
Gram-negatives		
E. coli, Klebsiella, Proteus	Ceftriaxone 2g q12h plus Gemtamicin 1.5mg/kg q8h IM or IV	None
Pseudomonas	Ceftazidime 2g q8h plus Gentamicin 1.5mg/kg q8h IV or IM	None
Fungal		
C. neoformans	Amphotericin B 0.4–0.6mg/kg/d+ Flucytosine 150mg/kd/d	Fluconazole PO
Aspergillus species	Amphotericin B 0.6mg/kg/d	None
Candida species		
Viral		
CMV	Ganciclovir 5mg/kg q12h	Ganciclovir
Herpes simplex	Acyclovir 12mg/kg q8h × 10 days–14 days	IV Acyclovir in bone marrow recipients
Varicella-zoster	Acyclovir 12mg/kg q8h × 10 days	None
JC virus	Not established—see text	
Parasitic		
T. gondii	Pyrimethamine loading dose 50mg po than 25mg po qd and Sulfadiazine 1g po q6h	None
S. stercoralis	Thiobendazole 25mg/kg po bid	None

[a]All doses intravenous unless otherwise indicated.

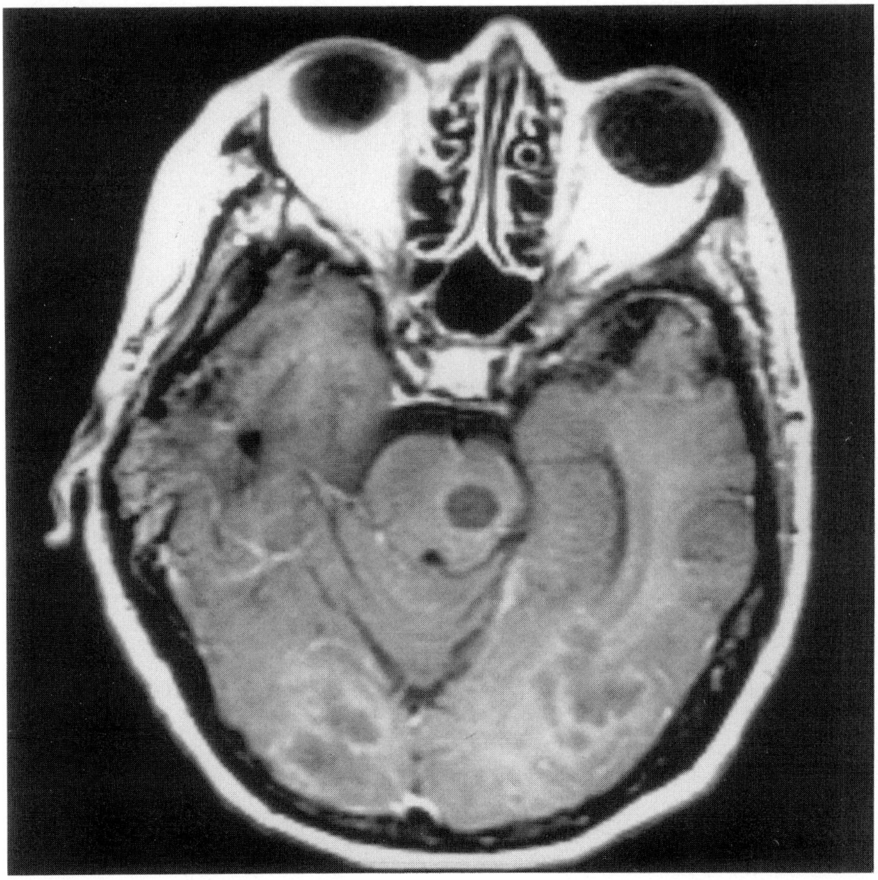

Figure 2 MRI of posterior fossa of patient one month post–liver transplant who was acutely ill with multiple metabolic abnormalities and fever despite antibiotic coverage with a third-generation cephalosporin and an aminoglycoside. These ring-enhancing lesions are unusually large for the *Listeria* demonstrated postmortem. Multiple abscesses, also large, were seen supratentorially as well (not shown).

the skin, where skin lesions are an important clue to the presence of infection. The most frequent neurological syndrome is meningitis, with mildly elevated CSF protein concentration and usually fewer than 300 WBCs/mm^3. Definitive diagnosis requires detection of cryptococcal antigen or culture of the organism. The initial antigen titer is a good prognostic indicator. Titers of less than 1:256 indicate a favorable prognosis. Six to 8 weeks of treatment with amphotericin B, preferably in combination with 5-flucytosine, has been reported to be curative in more than 60% of patients (86,87). Depending on the immune deficit present, lifelong prophylaxis with fluconozole may be beneficial (88,89).

Sequelae of cryptococcal meningitis include the development of hydrocephalus, compromised renal function due to amphotericin, and dose-limiting bone marrow suppression or hepatic dysfunction from 5-flucytosine. Unexpected deaths during the first week of treatment have been observed in some AIDS patients with cryptococcal meningitis, though this phenomenon is much less common in other immunocompromised populations. These patients had a dramatic increase in intracranial pressure, which did not appear to be a drug reaction, as a great variety of different

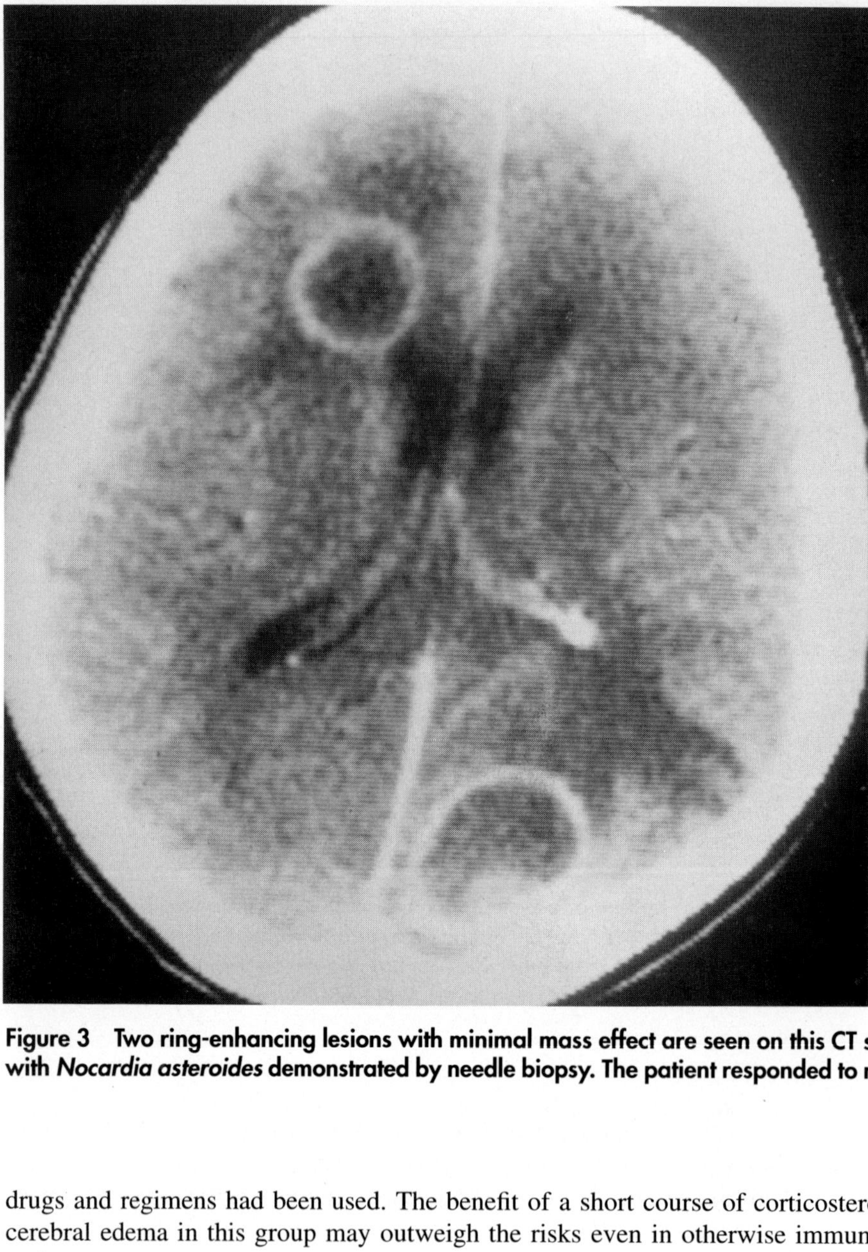

Figure 3 Two ring-enhancing lesions with minimal mass effect are seen on this CT scan of a patient with *Nocardia asteroides* demonstrated by needle biopsy. The patient responded to medical therapy.

drugs and regimens had been used. The benefit of a short course of corticosteroids to prevent cerebral edema in this group may outweigh the risks even in otherwise immunocompromised patients.

Aspergillus fumigatus

Aspergillus is a CNS pathogen in patients receiving high-dose corticosteroids or other chemotherapy and broad-spectrum antibiotics. Neutropenia and concurrent CMV infection are important risk factors for the development of this disease. CNS infection is almost invariably accompanied by invasive pulmonary disease (90). Affinity of the organism for blood vessels leads to the most characteristic neurological syndrome, multiple small hemorrhagic infarctions. Subarachnoid hemorrhage can occur when the vessels of the circle of Willis are invaded. A CSF pleocytosis, which can be either neutrophilic or lymphocytic, is seen. Abscess formation and granulomatous reactions are other intracranial manifestations of *Aspergillus* (91,92). While theoretically *Aspergillus* antigen can be detected in the CSF, proximity of lesions to the ventricular surface is a necessary requirement for this test, and failure to diagnose the organism antemortem is quite common (93). In the appropriate clinical setting and with one of the above syndromes, empiric therapy for *Aspergillus* can be instituted with amphotericin B and 5-flucytosine (Table 12).

Candida *Species*

Candida albicans causes most cases of invasive CNS candidiasis, although the incidence of other *Candida* species appears to be increasing as patients are given oral antimicrobial prophylaxis. *Candida* is also quite difficult to diagnose antemortem. The majority of patients with candidiasis have undergone operation, most commonly on the gastrointestinal tract, and virtually all have received several weeks of antibiotics. Bloodstream invasion and CNS dissemination also occur in the setting of intravenous catheter-related infection, particularly in association with hyperalimentation (91). Although the most common clinical manifestation of CNS candidiasis is meningitis, sometimes associated with base of the skull infiltration and cranial nerve palsies, endocarditis with cerebral embolism has been reported as well (94). In addition to amphotericin B and 5-flucytosine, treatment involves removal of all potential sources of infection including drains, shunt systems, and intravenous lines. Neutropenia and steroid use must be minimized. The likelihood of antemortem diagnosis may increase in light of recent reports of the detection of candida enolase by immunoassay in patients with invasive candidiasis (95).

Both *Aspergillus* and *Candida* are usually diagnosed only when the disease is advanced. Aggressive evaluation of pulmonary infiltrates in the neutropenic patient with persistent fever and timely use of CSF diagnostic techniques should improve diagnosis (96) (see Table 6). While lessening the period of neutropenia theoretically could improve host defenses against invasive mycoses, the use of hematopoietic growth factors such as granulocyte colony-stimulating factor (GCSF) and granulocyte/macrophage colony-stimulating factor (GMCSF) has not been studied systematically in the setting of CNS infection in the immunocompromised population (97).

Mucoraceae

The Mucorales or Zygomycetes organisms are a group of fungal species responsible for infections in neutropenic patients, particularly those with poorly controlled diabetes, hematological malignancies, or steroid therapy. They enter the CNS via adjacent structures such as the paranasal sinuses or orbit. Thus, there is concomitant facial-orbital pain and nasal discharge. Carotid artery thrombosis may occur. The palate and nasopharynx may contain necrotic areas that can be biopsied. The rhinocerebral type of infection is most often seen in organ transplant patients. Focal intracranial disease occasionally has been reported, mainly in intravenous drug abusers. Intracerebral mucormycosis must be considered in the differential diagnosis of a mass lesion in the appropriate clinical setting. Neurosurgical intervention usually is critical to obtain biopsy material. Early treatment with amphotericin B and subsequent maintenance amphotericin has been reported to control disease (25). Hyperglycemia should be treated promptly. There is no clear role for the use of anticoagulants to prevent carotid artery thrombosis.

Viral Infections

Four human herpesviruses account for the vast majority of clinically important CNS infections in the immunocompromised host. Epstein-Barr virus has been discussed in this chapter in the section on posttransplant lymphoproliferative disorder.

Varicella-Zoster Virus

Varicella-zoster virus (VZV) infection most frequently occurs in patients with lymphoma and leukemia, approximately 15% of whom develop symptomatic zoster infection. As many as 25% of these have symptomatic dissemination. Systemic complications of VZV include pneumonia, intestinal obstruction, and myocarditis. The risk of dissemination of VZV is significantly associated with the presence of active tumor at the time of infection and shows some correlation with dermatomal localization. Patients with gastrointestinal or genitourinary malignancies tend to have lower lumbar and sacral dermatomal involvement, whereas patient with breast or lung cancer have thoracic dermatomal sites of viral activation. Sixty-two percent of patients who had received radiation therapy before zoster infection developed their lesions in the previously irradiated site (98). The frequency of postherpetic neuralgia was two to three times that reported in zoster-infected patients without cancer. Seven to 9% of renal transplant patients, and a similar distribution of other organ transplant recipients, will have cutaneous zoster at some time following their surgery.

VZV is associated with numerous neurological syndromes. The major risk for development of CNS disease is dissemination of the virus. Patients with disseminated disease may have evidence of VZV encephalitis. This can take two forms, an acute, necrotizing encephalitis with marked inflammation and a multifocal, PML-like picture with little inflammation. These two syndromes probably represent part of a spectrum of host response. When the host is able to mount an inflammatory response, the first pattern develops. In cases with multifocal symptoms and signs resembling those of PML, microscopic examination of the brain revealed prominent necrosis and Cowdry type A eosinophilic intranuclear inclusions. Immunoperoxidase studies detected VZV temporally remote from cutaneous herpes zoster in these patients (99). The distinction from PML, by biopsy if necessary, is important, as VZV is a potentially treatable condition.

Other neurological syndromes associated with VZV include segmental motor weakness and myelopathy. The myelopathy may be exacerbating and remitting, acute or chronic. Detection of VZV DNA in the CSF months after the rash may be useful in diagnosis and in sorting out other causes of relapsing remitting myelopathy (100).

Several groups of patients with inflammatory neurological diseases and serological evidence of VZV activity without cutaneous vesicles have been described. These include cases of cranial polyneuropathy, aseptic meningitis, acute polyneuropathy, myelitis, and encephalitis. Chronic progressive VZV encephalitis in an AIDS patient without skin lesions has also been described (101,102). Fatal VZV meningoradiculitis is another variant that can occur without antecedent skin lesions (103). It seems likely that the advent of PCR diagnosis for VZV will expand our understanding of neurological syndromes associated with this virus. Acyclovir therapy for VZV infection is summarized in Table 12.

Patients with ophthalmic zoster should be referred urgently to an ophthalmologist for eye care. Acyclovir can reduce the severity and duration of the acute local pain but does not have any effect on the subsequent development of postherpetic neuralgia. The development of focal abnormalities referable to specific arterial territories suggests the presence of CNS arteritis, although other etiologies such as nonbacterial thrombotic endocarditis need to be considered (Fig. 4A,B). A multifocal granulomatous angiitis associated with isolation of HIV virus that appears quite similar to herpes zoster arteritis has been reported and consideration should be given to the possibility of HIV infection (104).

Herpes Simplex

Herpes simplex virus occurs in both immunocompetent and immunocompromised hosts. While herpes simplex virus is the most common cause of sporadic encephalitis in the immunocompetent population, the differential diagnosis of an acute encephalitis in the host with impaired immunity must include organisms more commonly causing encephalitis in this patient group, including *Listeria*, *Toxoplasma*, CMV, and VZV. Clinical and neuroimaging evidence of temporal lobe involvement with a hemorrhagic component to the CSF pleocytosis is strongly suggestive of herpes simplex virus encephalitis, but these findings are not specific. Many other diseases mimic herpes simplex virus, both in their clinical presentation and in their production of a modest CSF pleocytosis. These include embolic stroke, paraneoplastic processes, radiation and chemotherapy-related complications, and side effects of immunosuppressive drugs (105).

The advent of PCR technology for the detection of herpes simplex virus genome has greatly altered the diagnostic approach to patients with suspected encephalitis. Brain biopsy for suspected herpes simplex is now performed much less frequently.

Another clinical syndrome attributable to herpes simplex virus is myelitis with a rapidly progressive spinal cord syndrome. Neuropathology reveals extensive necrosis, and both clinically and pathologically the syndrome resembles what previously was thought to be a paraneoplastic process called subacute or acute necrotic myelopathy (106). Herpes simplex virus (usually type II in the myelitis syndrome) can be diagnosed by culturing the virus from CSF, and since it is a potentially treatable disorder, its recognition is important.

Cytomegalovirus

Cytomegalovirus (CMV), a DNA virus, is asymptomatic in the vast majority of immunocompetent hosts, though previously healthy individuals may develop extraneural manifestations such as esophagitis, pneumonitis, cholecystitis, cholangitis, and adrenalitis and occasional neurological manifestations such as Guillain-Barré syndrome. In the immunocompromised host, the most common manifestation is retinitis with or without an associated encephalitis. Autopsy studies in the two most prominently CMV-infected groups—HIV-infected persons and transplant recipients—have defined characteristic pathological abnormalities, which include microglial nodules, focal parenchymal necrosis, and a necrotizing ventriculoencephalitis with a predilection for the subependymal areas (107). CMV may cause a radiculomyelitis, sometimes involving the cranial nerves (108). Although the presence of PCR-detectable CMV genome in CSF does not necessarily prove that a neurological syndrome is due to CMV, it is worth considering this possibility if one of the above syndromes develops in an immunocompromised host. There are reports of neurological improvement following treatment with ganciclovir (109). Patients with CMV retinitis may develop resistance to ganciclovir. There is no information about amelioration of encephalitis or other neurological syndromes following treatment with foscarnet. In addition to its effects on the nervous system, CMV further directly depresses host immunity, predisposing the infected patient to bacterial and fungal infections. Extraneural clues to the presence of recent CMV infection are acute monoarticular arthritis, hepatitis, an infectious mononucleosis–like syndrome, myocarditis, and pneumonia.

Progressive Multifocal Leukoencephalopathy

Progressive multifocal leukoencephalopathy (PML) is a subacute progressive demyelinating disease caused by the JC virus of the papovavirus family and occurring most frequently in patients with defects in cell-mediated immunity. PML has been reported primarily in patients with carcinoma, transplant recipients, and AIDS patients (in whom the incidence of infection may approach 4%) (110). Clinical presentation is usually a progressive dementia or slowly progressive focal deficits mimicking a mass lesion. A visual deficit is the most common presenting sign, present in 35–45% of cases (111). The most frequent visual deficit is a homonymous hemianopsia, but up to 8% of patients may be cortically blind at the time of diagnosis, indicating bioccipital pathology. CSF is usually normal but PCR has been used to detect JC virus genome with excellent specificity but only a 75% sensitivity (20).

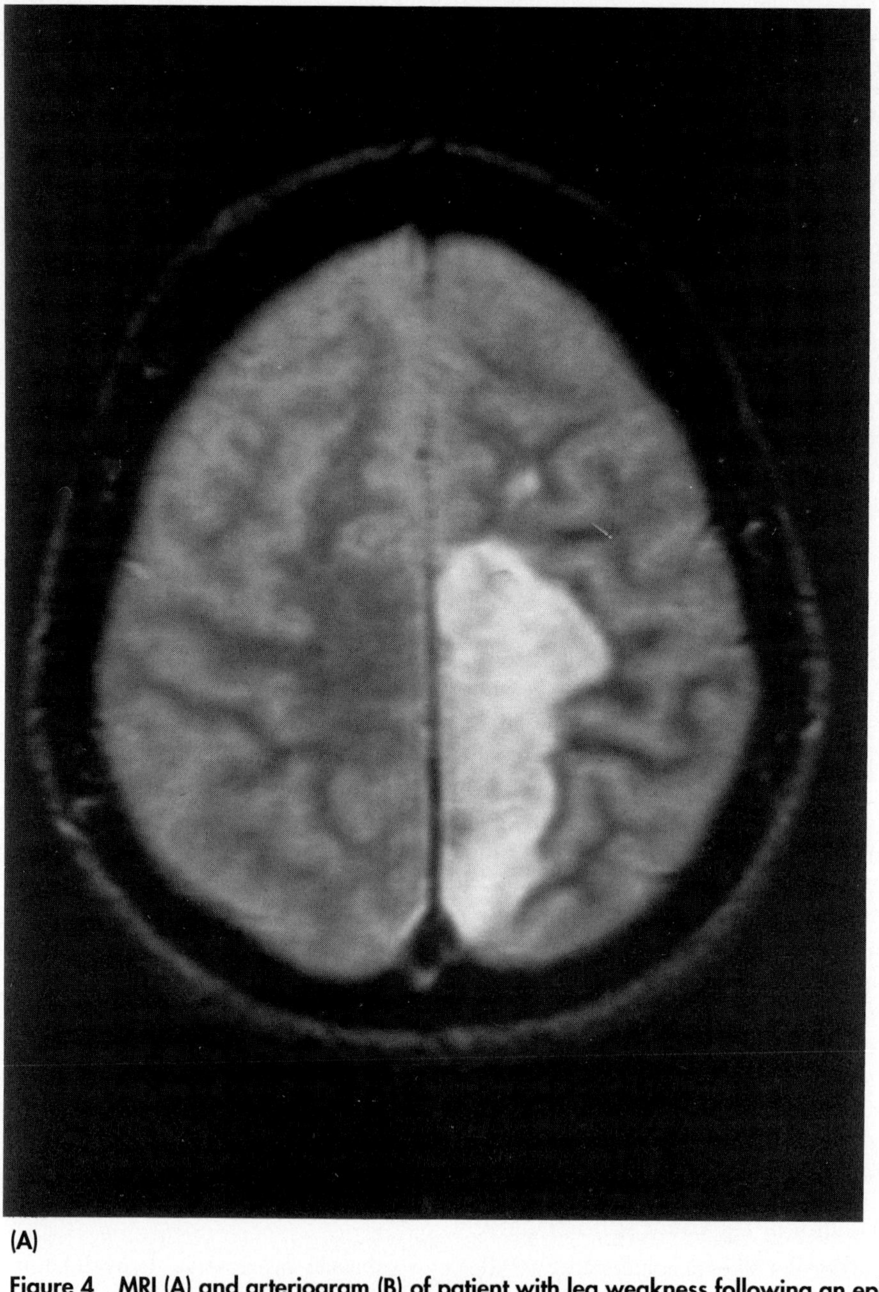

(A)

Figure 4 MRI (A) and arteriogram (B) of patient with leg weakness following an episode of herpes zoster ophthalmicus. The patient had been chronically immunosuppressed with steroids following renal transplantation. MRI shows an area of infarction in the anterior cerebral territory corresponding to the segmental narrowing seen on arteriography. (Photograph courtesy of Robert Hurst, M.D.)

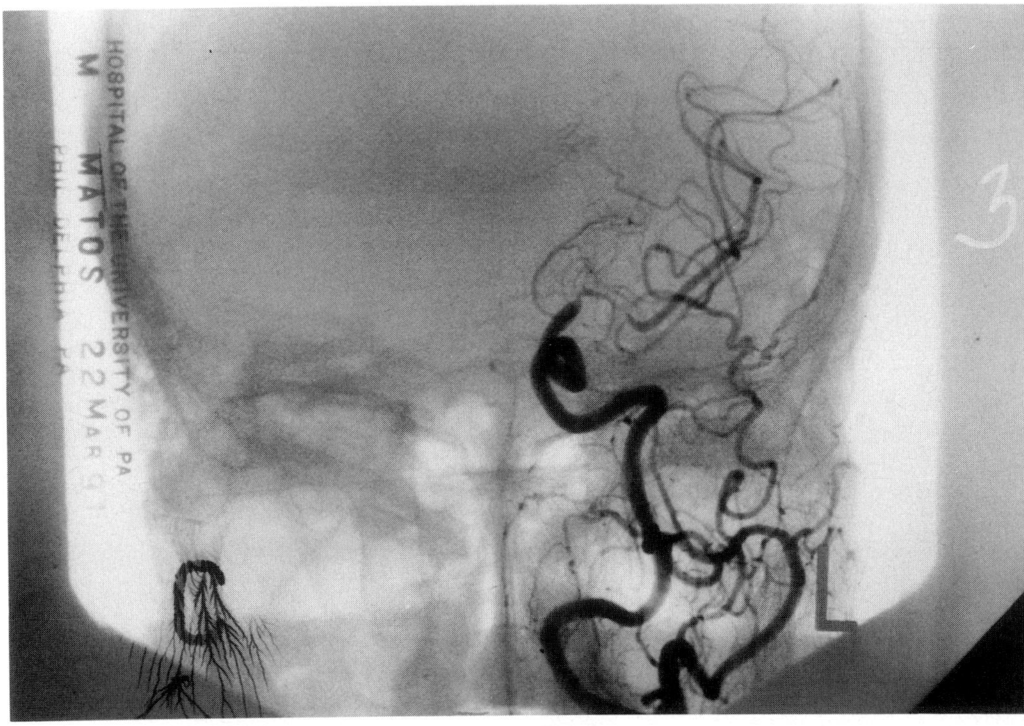

(B)

Neuroimaging is by far the most useful noninvasive study for the investigation of possible PML. CT scan shows areas of subcortical white matter hypodensity, which do not enhance. The ability of MRI to detect white matter abnormalities makes this technique even more useful than CT for suspected PML. However, the confluent areas of altered signal in the white matter on MRI are relatively nonspecific. Figure 5A shows a large area of T_2 signal abnormality in the right hemispheric white matter of a lung transplant recipient who presented with progressive mental status changes and left hemiparesis due to PML. Figure 5B shows very similar changes seen in a patient presenting with a similar clinical syndrome, but whose white matter abnormalities were due to prior radiation therapy. On MRI as well as on CT, enhancement of these areas is distinctly rare, but on MRI the lesions of PML occasionally may appear to involve the gray-white junction or the gray matter itself. Definitive diagnosis of PML still requires brain biopsy.

The natural course of PML is almost invariably one of relentless progression with a life expectancy of 3–18 months (110). Occasional partial recovery and prolonged survival in AIDS patients has been recognized. The course of the disease appears somewhat related to the intensity of underlying immunosuppression. Several therapies have been tried, all of which have been largely unsuccessful. The various proposed treatment regimens have been directed either at inhibition of the JC virus or at the enhancement of cellular immunity. No therapeutic regimens have been studied in a randomized fashion. Anecdotal reports exist on cytosine arabinoside, adenosine arabinoside (intrathecally or intravenously), AZT, alpha-interferon (subcutaneously), beta-interferon (intrathecally), heparin (subcutaneously), and oral or parenteral corticosteroids. One patient unresponsive to cytarabine and acyclovir had a dramatic improvement following the addition of interferon-alpha (112). It is recommended that an attempt be made to decrease the patient's immunosuppressive medication when PML is suspected or proven.

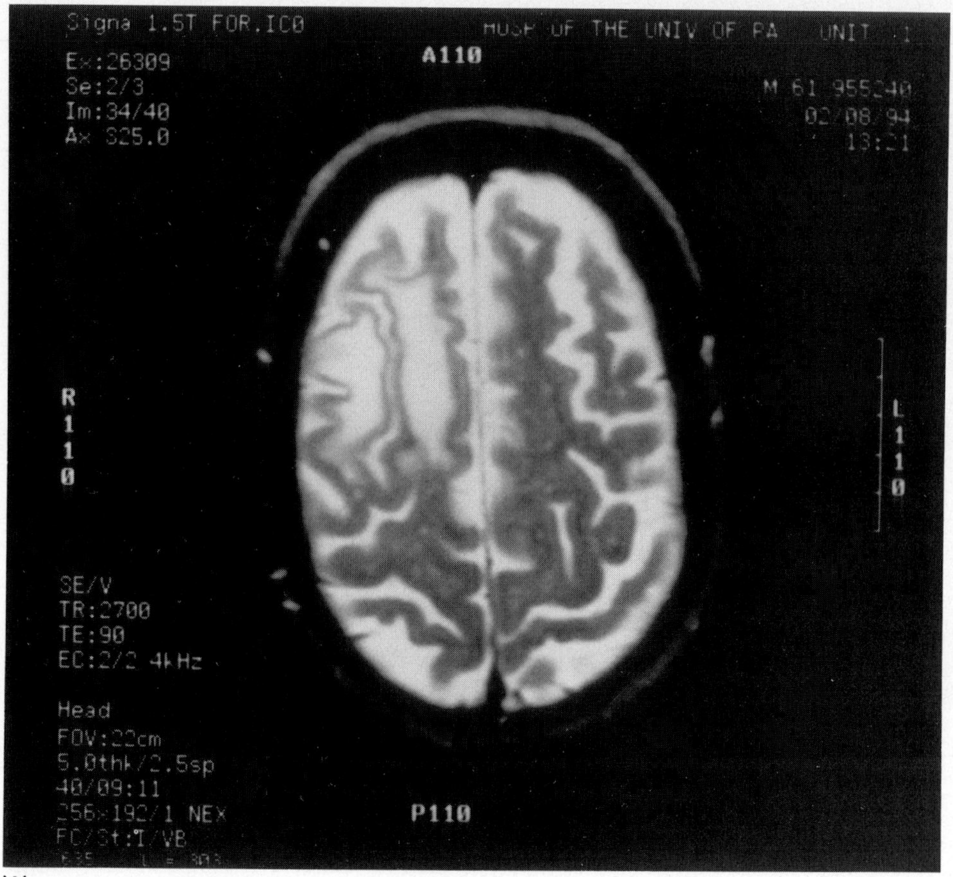

(A)

Figure 5 (A) This 57-year-old lung transplant recipient developed mental status changes and a left hemiparesis 3 months following transplantation. He died from progressive multifocal leukoencephalopathy, shown on this MRI as an area of right hemisphere white matter abnormality without mass effect. (B) A patient chronically on steroids following surgery and radiation for an anaplastic astrocytoma developed progressive hemiparesis and mental status changes. The MRI looks strikingly similar to that shown in (A), although the white matter abnormality, due in this case to radiation injury, extends to the opposite hemisphere.

Parasitic Diseases

Toxoplasma gondii

T. gondii is the most frequently occurring parasite of the CNS in the immunocompromised host. AIDS patients and patients with lymphoma represent the largest group at risk. The presentation is typically subacute, with a combination of focal neurological deficits due to intracranial mass lesions and a nonfocal encephalitis. The principal differential diagnostic consideration is primary CNS lymphoma. Recent reports suggest that PET scanning may be useful in differentiating enhancing lesions due to infection from those due to lymphoma in the appropriate population (113).

A therapeutic trial of pyrimethamine/sulfadiazine is the best approach in patients with suspected toxoplasmosis. Brain biopsy should be reserved for atypical cases or for those patients

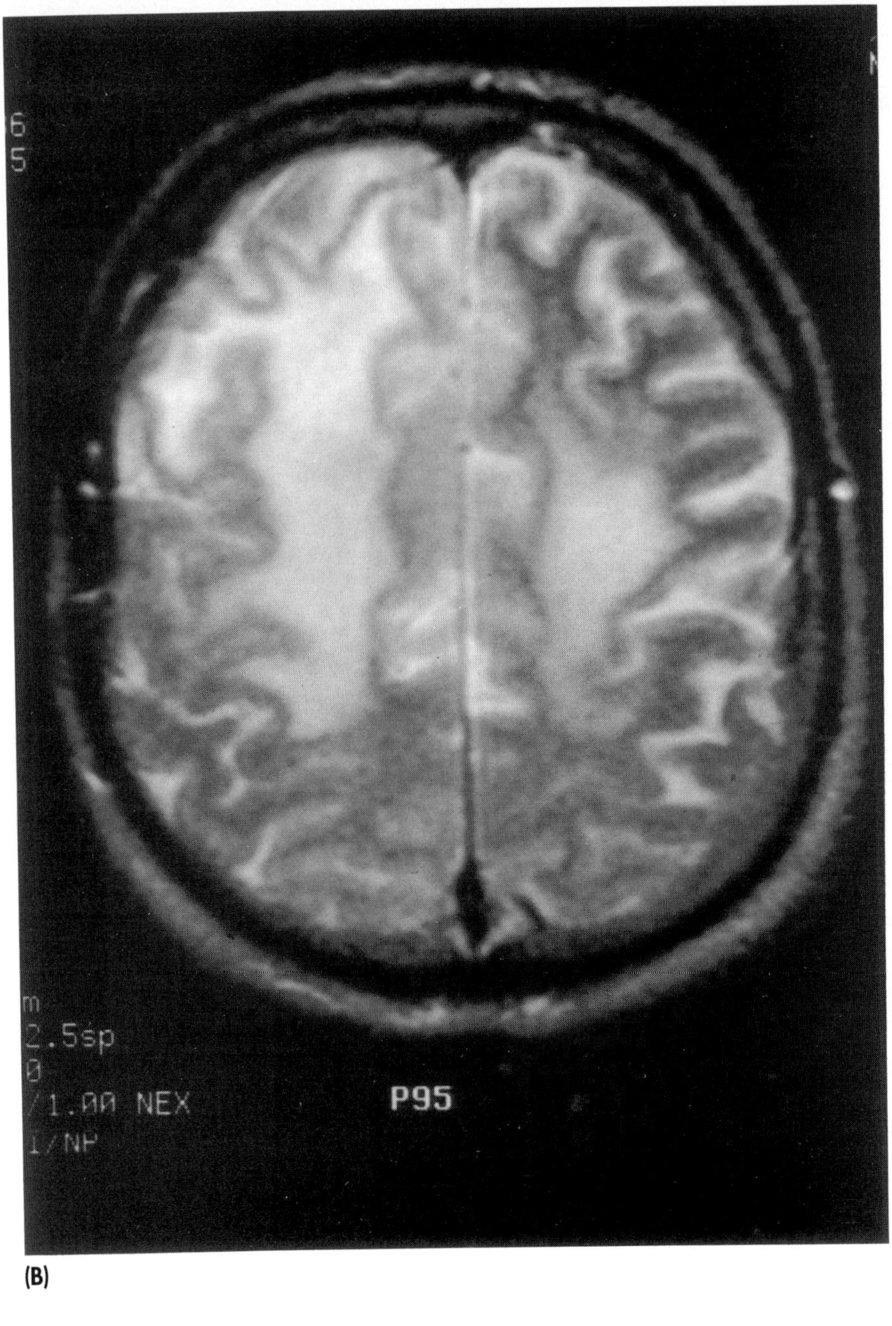

(B)

who have failed treatment. Patients should improve within 10–14 days. ELISA titers are unreliable in this population.

Strongyloides stercoralis

In patients with deficient cell-mediated immunity, *S. stercoralis* can cause overwhelming infection presenting as a pyogenic meningitis with diffuse microinfarctions or with brain abscess. The diagnosis should be suspected in an immunosuppressed patient with a history of travel to areas such as Asia, even when the travel occurred many years previously. Ova and parasites should be obtained on stool samples. The optimal therapy is oral thiobendazole. In addition, antibiotic therapy should be directed at the frequently coexisting gram-negative bacteremia and meningitis.

The above two parasites represent the major considerations in this class of organism in the immunocompromised host, but as this patient population increases, with longer survival and perhaps greater intensity of immunosuppression, other parasites are likely to surface. A recent report suggests that amebic meningoencephalitis can be diagnosed antemortem in patients with underlying immunosuppression (114).

PROPHYLAXIS OF CNS INFECTIONS

The high morbidity and mortality of CNS infections in immunocompromised patients, even when these patients are promptly diagnosed and appropriately treated, makes prophylaxis of infection of prime importance. Although the following discussion applies in a general way to all immunocompromised patients, it reflects the lessons learned from an aggressive approach to prophylaxis in bone marrow transplant recipients whose impaired host defenses span the spectrum of infection risk factors (Table 2).

Antibacterial prophylaxis has been achieved with hematopoietic growth factors, which reduce the period of neutropenia (97). Oral chemoprophylaxis has been greatly improved by the use of the fluoroquinolones, which, in contrast to nonabsorbable antibiotics, which cause gastrointestinal side effects and some myelosuppression and lack *Pseudomonas* coverage, are well tolerated and effective in reducing the incidence of gram-negative infections. Increased numbers of fungal superinfections or quinolone-resistant gram-negative bacteria have not been a problem thus far. Oral and intravenous immunoglobulin therapy for BMT patients also may lessen bacterial and fungal infections.

Empiric broad-spectrum antibiotic therapy for neutropenic fever remains the prime defense against bacterial infection. The frequency and severity of infections caused by gram-negative bacteria in the 1970s led to empiric antibiotic therapy regimens. During the 1980s, the frequency of infections caused by gram-positive bacteria increased in many cancer centers (82,115). Pizzo provides recommendations for the 1990s for the management of patients with neutropenia and fever (115). Table 13 outlines current recommendations for the management of neutropenic febrile patients, but the selection of any initial single or combination antibiotic regimen must be based on the microbial patterns at each institution, and additions or modifications to the initial regimen will be necessary as major isolates emerge or if the neutropenia continues.

Specific antifungal prophylaxis has been more problematic. There is no clearly effective oral antifungal agent for prophylaxis in granulocytopenic patients, although maintenance therapy with fluconazole reduces the recurrence rate of cryptococcal meningitis and is effective against *Candida*. Prophylactic measures against *Aspergillus* are particularly needed. Particulate air filters appear to be the best means of excluding this pathogen from the patient's environment. Itracanaxole has broad-spectrum activity that includes *Aspergillus*. Amphotericin B appears to be superior to placebo in preventing invasive candidiasis. Oral mycostatin troches have not prevented fungal dissemination (116). Ketoconazole is a difficult prophylactic agent in BMT, as it may interact

Table 13 Initial Management of Neutropenia and Fever

Clinical setting	Recommendation	Dosage regimen
Neutropenia[a] expected to last ≤5 days (and no evidence of infection)	Ceftazidime	2 g IV q8h
Neutropenia expected to last >5 days	Piperacillin + Gentamicin	4 g IV q6h; Dependent on creatinine clearance
↓		
Fever persists on above regimen without obvious source ≥72 h or evidence of clinical deterioration	Add aminoglycoside (if not already receiving) Add vancomycin if already on aminoglycoside and IV line present[b] Additional anaerobic coverage may be necessary for perirectal infection or oral abscess	
↓		
Fever persists >7 days on broad-spectrum antibiotics	Add amphotericin	0.6 mg/kg/d IV

[a]Absolute neutrophil count < 1000.
[b]Empiric use of vancomycin should be restricted to centers with high rates of methicillin-resistant *S. aureus*. Recently, strains of vancomycin-resistant enterocci have been reported.

with cyclosporine and requires an acid gastric environment for absorption. Prophylactic nasal sprays of amphotericin B are also being evaluated in neutropenic patients (117). Limiting the period of neutropenia and the early addition of antifungal therapy in patients with fever unresponsive to antimicrobial regimens remain the best measures for control of fungal infection. There is a great need for antifungal agents with less toxicity. Liposomal amphotericin B is being studied for chronic administration in CNS infection (118). Nephrotoxicity remains a limiting factor for conventional amphotericin B use, but neurotoxicity in the form of leukoencephalopathy, rarely reversible, has been reported, usually in the setting of BMT with multiple other therapies (119,120).

Antiviral prophylaxis of the four major human herpes viruses has been studied extensively. Acyclovir is now a regular part of the BMT prophylactic regimen and is effective for the treatment of established infection due to herpes simplex or varicella-zoster infection (121). Acyclovir is easily administered with only infrequent reports of neurotoxicity (hallucinations and tremor) (122). Patients receiving prophylactic acyclovir have significantly reduced CMV infections as well (121). CMV has otherwise been difficult to prevent. In BMT recipients seronegative for CMV, infection can be reduced by the use of blood products seronegative for CMV. Prophylactic ganciclovir has been effective in preventing the development of CMV interstitial pneumonia in BMT patients with asymptomatic infection (123).

A recent report of the use of intermittent courses of interleukin-2 in patients with human immunodeficiency virus infection represents an exciting possible new adjunctive method of CNS prophylaxis and treatment. This potent cytokine induces the proliferation and differentiation of peripheral-blood mononuclear cells. Infusion for 5 days every 8 weeks resulted in increased CD4 T-cell counts. Interleukin-2 merits further investigation as a treatment for patients with diseases characterized by decreased T-cell function, including infections with fungi or mycobacteria

(124). Neurotoxicities of interleukin have been reported and can be expected to increase as biological response modifiers are used more frequently (125).

Nonspecific measures to protect the CNS include attention to nutrition, as poor nutrition globally impairs both humoral and cell-mediated immunity, early broad-spectrum coverage of gastrointestinal and genitourinary sepsis, careful attention to intravenous lines, and aggressive evaluation of pulmonary infiltrates for bacterial, fungal, and parasitic infection. Splenectomized patients should report rigors or upper respiratory tract infections promptly. Minor fever or abdominal pain should be investigated promptly in patients on corticosteroids as this treatment may mask pulmonary infections and gastrointestinal as well as CNS infections. Indwelling Ommaya or Rickham reservoirs should always be entered cautiously and only after sterile preparation of the puncture site. The choice of broad-spectrum antibiotic coverage should reflect local trends in antibiotic resistance for nosocomial infections, and infectious disease consultation should always be obtained. It may be necessary to begin broad-spectrum antibiotic coverage for a CNS disease that is subsequently found to result from a viral illness or from a noninfectious cause. Undertreatment of those infections for which specific therapy can be offered should be avoided, and broad-spectrum treatment usually will not be regretted.

SUMMARY AND TRENDS

The continued improvement in survival statistics for patients with cancer of all types and for organ transplant recipients is a trend for which realistic hope can be offered. At the same time, the challenge to the neurological consultant becomes ever greater. The consultant must be familiar with new clinical syndromes including the neurological manifestations of microbial pathogens such as herpes simplex myelitis, varicella-zoster angiitis, and posttransfusion lymphoproliferative disorder. The consultant must be aware of the toxicities of new therapies such as FK506, interleukins, and OKT3 and be aware of new agents likely to cause infection such as *Pseudo-allesecheria boydii*, amoebae, and *Afipia felis* (126) as well as new microbial detection techniques and their indications. The consultant must advocate brain biopsy when diagnosis remains unclear. He or she must be aware of new diseases and new manifestations of them, such as smooth-muscle tumors developing in association with EBV after organ transplantation (127). He or she should remain vigilant for late sequelae or recurrence of infection with the same or a different opportunistic organism. Finally, for the patient's sake, the consultant must remain suspicious of minor findings and above all remain open-minded. After a thorough examination and appropriate neurodiagnositc studies, it is appropriate to consult with infectious disease colleagues to provide optimal care for this challenging group of patients.

REFERENCES

1. Patchell RA. Neurological complications of organ transplantation. Ann Neurol 1994; 36:688–703.
2. Conti DJ, Rubin RH. Infection of the central nervous system in organ transplant recipients. Neurol Clin 1988; 6:241–260.
3. Pruitt AA, unpublished data.
4. Hooper DC, Pruitt AA, Rubin RH. Central nervous system infection in the chronically immunosuppressed. Medicine 1982; 61:166–188.
5. Adams HP, Dawson G, Coffman TJ, et al. Stroke in renal transplant patients. Arch Neurol 1986; 43:113–115.
6. Patchell RA, White CL, Clark AW, et al. Neurologic complications of bone marrow transplantation. Neurology 1985; 35:300–306.

7. Mohrmann RL, Mah V, Vintgers HV. Neuropathologic findings after bone marrow transplantation: an autopsy study. Hum Pathol 1990; 21:630–639.
8. Armitage JO. Bone marrow transplantation. N Engl J Med 1994; 330:827–838.
9. Ang LC, Gillett JM, Kaufmann JCE. Neuropathology of heart transplantation. Can J Neurol Sci 1989; 16:291–298.
10. Hall WA, Martinez AJ, Dummer JS, et al. Central nervous system infections in heart and heart-lung transplant recipients. Arch Neurol 1989; 46:173–177.
11. Andrews BT, Hershon JJ, Calanchini P, et al. Neurologic complications of cardiac transplantation. West J Med 1990; 153:146–148.
12. Moreno E, Gomez SR, Gonzalez I, et al. Neurologic complications in liver transplantation. Acta Neurol Scand 1993; 87:25–31.
13. Stein DP, Lederman RJ, Vogt DP, et al. Neurological complications following liver transplantation. Ann Neurol 1992; 31:644–649.
14. Ferreiro JA, Robert MA, Townsend J, et al. Neuropathologic findings after liver transplantation. Acta Neuropathol 1992; 54:1–14.
15. Kiok MC. Neurologic complications of pancreas transplants. Neurol Clin 1988; 6:367–376.
16. Pruitt AA. Central nervous system infections in cancer patients. Neurol Clin 1991; 9:867–888.
17. Peacock JE. Persistent neutrophilic meningitis. Infect Dis Clin North Am 1990; 4:747–767.
18. French GL, Teoh R, Chan CY, et al. Diagnosis of tuberculous meningitis by detection of tuberculostearic acid in cerebrospinal fluid. Lancet 1987; 8551:117–119.
19. Daniel TM. Antibody and antigen detection for the immunodiagnosis of tuberculosis. Why not? What more is needed? Where do we stand today? J Infect Dis 1988; 158:678–680.
20. Tyler KL. Polymerase chain reaction and the diagnosis of viral central nervous system diseases. Ann Neurol 1994; 36:809–811.
21. Darnell RB. Polymerase chain reaction: application to nervous system disease. Ann Neurol 1993; 34:513–523.
22. Baringer JR, Pisani P. Herpes simplex virus genomes in human nervous system tissue analyzed by polymerase chain reaction. Ann Neurol 1994; 36:823–829.
23. Lukes SA, Posner JB, Nielsen S, et al. Bacterial infections of the CNS in neutropenic patients. Neurology 1984; 34:269–275.
24. Wen PJ, Scully RF, Mark EJ, et al. Case records of the Massachusetts General Hospital. Case 36-1991. N Engl J Med 1991; 325:714–726.
25. Skolnik PR, Scully RE, Mark EJ, et al. Case records of the Massachusetts General Hospital Case 52-1990. N Engl J Med 1990; 323:1823–1833.
26. Babiatzki A, Sade J. Malignant external otitis. J Laryngol Otol 1987; 101:205–210.
27. Coleman AE, Norman DJ. OKT3 encephalopathy. Ann Neurol 1990; 28:837–838.
28. Graus F, Rogers LR, Posner JB. Cerebrovascular complications in patients with cancer. Medicine 1985; 64:16–35.
29. Connolly KJ, Hammer SM. The acute aseptic meningitis syndrome. Infect Dis Clin North Am 1990; 4:599–622.
30. Kaneko K. Rapid diagnosis of TB meningitis by PCR. Neurology 1990; 40:1617–1618.
31. Gibson PE, Knowles WA, Hand JF, et al. Detection of JC virus DNA in the cerebrospinal fluid of patients with progressive multifocal leukoencephalopathy. J Med Virol 1993; 39:278–281.
32. Venger BH, Aldama A. Mycotic vasulitis with repeated intracranial aneurysmal hemorrhage. J Neurosurg 1988; 69:775–777.
33. Giang DW. Central nervous system vasculitis secondary to infections, toxins, and neoplasms. Sem Neurol 1994; 14:313–319.
34. Hurst RW, Grossman RI. Neuroradiology of central nervous system vasculitis. Sem Neurol 1994; 14:320–340.
35. Kahan BO, Cyclosporine. N Engl J Med 1989; 321:1725–1729.

36. deGroen PC, Aksamit AJ, Rakela J, et al. Central nervous system toxicity after liver transplantation. The role of cyclosporine and cholesterol. N Engl J Med 1987; 317:861–866.
37. Wijdicks EFM, Wiesner RH, Dahlke LJ, et al. FK506-induced neurotoxicity in liver transplantation. Ann Neurol 1994; 35:498–501.
38. Dropchow EJ, Soong S-J. Steroid-induced weakness in patients with primary brain tumors. Neurology 1991; 41:1235–1239.
39. Stiefel FC, Breitbart WS, Holland JC. Corticosteroids in cancer: neuropsychiatric complications. Cancer Invest 1989; 7:479–491.
40. Tobler WD, Weil S. Epidural lipomatosis and renal transplantation. Surg Neurol 1988; 29:141–144.
41. Agarwal RK, Ostaszewski ML, Feld LG, et al. Tumor necrosis factor and interleukin-6 in cerebrospinal fluid of a patient with recurrent adverse central nervous system events following OKT3. Transplant Proc 1993; 25:2143–2144.
42. Triozzi PL, Kinney P, Rinehart J. Central nervous system toxicity of biological response modifiers. Ann NY Acad Sci 1990; 594:347–354.
43. Adair JC, Woodley SL, O'Connell JB, et al. Aseptic meningitis following cardiac transplantation: clinical characteristics and relationship to immunosuppressive regimen. Neurology 1991; 41:249–252.
44. Shihab FS, Barry JM, Norman DJ. Encephalopathy following the use of OKT3 in renal allograft transplantation. Transplant Proc 1993; 25:31–34.
45. Swerdlow SH. Post-transplant lymphoproliferative disorders: a morphologic, phenotypic and genotypic spectrum of disease. Histopathology 1992; 20:373–385.
46. Cohen JI. Epstein-Barr virus lymphoproliferative disease associated with acquired immunodeficiency. Medicine 1991; 70:137–160.
47. List AF, Greco FA, Vogler LB. Lymphoproliferative diseases in immunocompromised hosts: the role of Epstein-Barr virus. J Clin Oncol 1987; 5:1673–1689.
48. Young L, Alfieri C, Hennessy, K, et al. Expression of Epstein-Barr virus transformation-associated genes in tissues of patients with EBV lymphoproliferative disease. N Engl J Med 1989; 321:1080–1085.
49. Purtilo DT, Strobach RS, Okano M, et al. Biology of disease: Epstein-Barr virus-associated lymphoproliferative disorders. Lab Invest 1992; 67:5–23.
50. Craig FE, Gulley ML, Banks PM. Posttransplantation lymphoproliferative disorders. Am J Clin Pathol 1993; 99:265–276.
51. Patchell RA. Primary central nervous system lymphoma in the transplant patient. Neurol Clin 1988; 6:297–303.
52. Benkerrou M, Durandy A, Fisher A. Therapy for transplant-related lymphoproliferative diseases. Hematol Oncol Clin North Am 1993; 7:467–475.
53. Bruno A, Adams HP. Neurologic problems in renal transplant recipients. Neurol Clin 1988; 6: 305–325.
54. Manian FA, Stone WJ, Alford RH. Adverse antibiotic effects associated with renal insufficiency. Rev Infect Dis 1990; 12:236–249.
55. Gross MLP, Sweny P, Pearson RM, et al. Rejection encephalopathy: an acute neurological syndrome complicating renal transplantation. J Neurol Sci 1982; 56:23–34.
56. Harden CL. New antiepileptic drugs. Neurology 1994; 44:787–795.
57. Kahan BD, Flechner SM, Lorber MI, et al. Complications of cyclosporine-prednisone immunosuppression in 402 renal allograft recipients exclusively followed by a single center for from one to five years. Transplantation 1987; 43:197–204.
58. Hotson JR, Enzmann DR. Neurologic complication of cardiac transplantation. Neurol Clin 1988; 6:349–365.
59. Adair JC, Call GK, O'Connell JB, et al. Cerebrovascular syndromes following cardiac transplantation. Neurology 1992; 42:819–823.
60. Michaels MG, Wald ER, Fricker J, et al. Toxoplasmosis in pediatric recipients of heart transplants. Clin Infect Dis 1992; 14:847–851.
61. Belle SH, Detre KM. Report from the Pitt-UNOS liver transplant registry. Transplant Proc 1993; 25:1137–1142.

62. Pujol A, Graus F, Rimola A, et al. Predictive factors of in-hospital CNS complications following liver transplantation. Neurology 1994; 44:1226–1230.
63. Wszolek ZK, Aksamit AJ, Ellingson RJ, et al. Epileptiform electroencephalographic abnormalities in liver transplant recipients. Ann Neurol 1991; 30:37–41.
64. Winnock S, Janvier G, Parmentier F, et al. Pontine myelinolysis following liver transplantation: a report of two cases. Transpl Int 1993; 6:26–28.
65. Brunner JE, Redmond JM, Haggar AM, et al. Central pontine myelinolysis after rapid correction of hyponatremia: a magnetic resonance imaging study. Ann Neurol 1988; 23:389–391.
66. The US Multicenter FK506 Liver Study Group. A comparison of tacrolimus (FK506) and cyclosporine for immunosuppresion in liver transplantation. N Engl J Med 1994; 331:1110–1115.
67. Patchell RA, White CL, Clark AW, et al. Neurologic complications of bone marrow transplantation. Neurology 1985; 35:300–306.
68. Davis DF, Patchell RA. Neurologic complications of bone marrow transplantation. Neurol Clin 1988; 6:377–387.
69. David D, Henslee PK, Markesbery WF. Fatal adenovirus meningoencephalitis in a bone marrow transplant patient. Ann Neurol 1988; 23:385–389.
70. Drobyski WR, Knox KK, Majewski D, et al. Brief report: fatal encephalitis due to variant B human herpesvirus-6 infection in a bone marrow-transplant recipient. N Engl J Med 1994; 330:1356–1360.
71. Iwasaki Y, Sako K, Ohara Y, et al. Subacute panencephalitis associated with chronic graft-versus-host disease. Bone Marrow Transplant 1990; 6:53–57.
72. Diez-Martin JL, Habermann TM, Gastineau DA, et al. Nonbacterial thrombotic endocarditis in autologous bone marrow transplantation. Am J Med 1988; 85:742–744.
73. Vukelja SJ, Baker WJ, Jeffreys P, et al. Nonbacterial thrombotic endocarditis clinically mimicking veno-occlusive disease of the liver complicating autologous bone marrow transplantation. Am J Clin Oncol 1992; 15:500–502.
74. Rogers LR, Cho ES, Kempin S, et al. Cerebral infarction from non-bacterial thrombotic endocarditis: clinical and pathological study including the effects of anticoagulation. Am J Med 1987; 83:746–756.
75. Amico L, Caplan aLR, Thomas C. Cerebrovascular complications of mucinous cancers. Neurology 1989; 39:745–749.
76. Chernik NL, Armstrong D, Posner JB. CNS infections in patients with cancer. Cancer 1977; 40: 268–278.
77. Bodey GP. Infections in cancer. Cancer Treat Rev 1975; 2:89–128.
78. Ketchel SJ, Rodriguez V. Acute infections in cancer patients. Sem Oncol 1978; 2:167–179.
79. Durand ML, Calderwood SB, Weber DJ, et al. Acute bacterial meningitis in adults—a review of 493 episodes. N Engl J Med 1993; 328:21–28.
80. Salzman C, Tauzon CU. Value of the ring enhancing sign in differentiating intracerebral hematoma and brain abscess. Arch Intern Med 1987; 147:951–952.
81. Phillips ME, Ryals TJ, Cambhu SA et al. Neoplastic vs. inflammatory meningeal enhancement with gd-DTPA. J Comput Assist Tomogr 1990; 14:536–541.
82. Elting LS, Bodey GP. Septicemia due to *Xanthomonas* species and non-aeruginosa *Pseudomonas* species: increasing incidence of catheter-related infection. Medicine 1990; 69:307–316.
83. Jacoby GJ, Archer GL. New mechanisms of bacterial resistance to antimicrobial agents. N Engl J Med 1991; 324:601–612.
84. Bross JE, Gordon G. Nocardial meningitis: case report and review. Rev Infect Dis 1991; 13:160–165.
85. Barnicoat MJ, Wierzbicki AS, Norman PM. Cerebral nocardiosis in immunosuppressed patients: five cases. QJ Med 1989; 72:689–698.
86. Dismukes WE, Cloud G, Gallis HA. Treatment of cryptococcosis meningitis with combination amphotericin B and flucytosine for four as compared to six weeks. N Engl J Med 1987; 317:334–339.
87. Perfect JR. Diagnosis and treatment of fungal meningitis. In: Scheld WM, Whitley RJ, Durack DT, eds. Infections of the Central Nervous System. New York: Raven Press, 1991:729–739.
88. Sugar AM, Saunders C. Oral fluconazole as suppressive therapy of disseminated cryptococcosis in patients with acquired immunodeficiency syndrome. Am J Med 1988; 85:481–489.

89. Yu YL, Lau YN, Woo E, et al. Cryptococcal infection of the nervous system. Q J Med 1988; 66: 87–96.
90. Walsh TJ, Hier DB, Caplan LR. Aspergillosis of the central nervous system: clinicopathological analysis of 17 patients. Ann Neurol 1985; 18:574–582.
91. Walsh TJ, Hier DB, Caplan LR. Fungal infections in the CNS: a comparative analysis of risk factors and clinical signs in 57 patients. Neurology 1985; 35:1654–1657.
92. Case Records of the Massachusetts General Hospital. Case 7—1988. N Engl J Med 1988; 318: 427–440.
93. Weiner MH. Antigen detection in the diagnosis of invasive aspergillosis. Ann Intern Med 1983; 99: 777–782.
94. Bodey GP. Fungal infections in cancer patients. Ann NY Acad Sci 1988; 544:431–441.
95. Walsh TJ, Hathorn JW, Sobel JD, et al. Detection of circulating candida enolase by immunoassay in patients with cancer and invasive candidiasis. N Engl J Med 1992; 324:1026–1031.
96. Armstrong D. Problems in management of opportunistic fungal diseases. Rev Infect Dis 1989; 11(suppl 7):S1591–S1599.
97. Lieschke GJ, Burgess AW. Granulocyte colony stimulating factor and granulocyte-macrophage colony stimulating factor. N Engl J Med 1992; 327:99–106.
98. Rusthoven JJ, Ahlgren P, Elhakim T. Varicella-zoster infection in adult cancer patients. Arch Intern Med 1988; 148:1561–1566.
99. Horten B, Price RW, Jimenez D. Multifocal varicella-zoster virus leukoencephalitis temporally remote from herpes zoster. Ann Neurol 1981; 9:251–266.
100. Gilden DH, Beinlich BR, Rubinstien MD. Varicella-zoster virus myelitis: an expanding spectrum. Neurology 1994; 44:1818–1823.
101. Mayo DR, Booss J. Varicella-zoster-associated neurologic disease without skin lesions. Arch Neurol 1989; 46:313–315.
102. Gilden DH, Murray RS, Wellish M. Chronic progressive varicella-zoster virus encephalitis in an AIDS patients. Neurology 1988; 38:1150–1153.
103. Devlin M, Dueland AN, Martin JR. Fatal varicella meningoradiculitis without skin involvement (abstr). Neurology 1991; 31(suppl 1);161.
104. Yankner BA, Skolnik BR, Shoukimas GH, et al. Cerebral granulomatous angiitis associated with isolation of human T-lymphotrophic virus type III from the central nervous system. Ann Neurol 1986; 20:362–364.
105. Whitley RJ, Cobbs CG, Alford CA et al. Diseases that mimic herpes simplex encephalitis: diagnoses, presentation and outcome. JAMA 1989; 262:234–239.
106. Folpe A, Lapham LW, Smith HC. Herpes simplex myelitis as a cause of acute necrotizing myelitis syndrome. Neurology 1994; 44:1955–1957.
107. Reyes MG. Cytomegalovirus encephalitis in acquired immunodeficiency syndrome. Ann Neurol 1988; 24:98.
108. Bale JF. Human cytomegalovirus infections and disorders of the nervous system. Arch Neurol 1984; 41:210–320.
109. Graveleau P, Perol R, Chapman A. Regression of cauda equina syndrome in AIDS patients being treated with ganciclovir. Lancet 1989; 2:511–512.
110. Berger JR, Kaszovitz B, Post JD, et al. Progressive multifocal leukoencephalopathy associated with human immunodeficiency virus infection. Ann Intern Med 1987; 107:78–87.
111. Major EO, Amemiya K, Tornatore CS, et al. Pathogenesis and molecular biology of progressive multifocal leukoencephalopathy, the JC virus-induced demyelinating disease of the human brain. Clin Microbiol Rev 1992; 5:49–73.
112. Steiger MJ, Tarnesby G, Gabe S, et al. Successful outcome of progressive multifocal leukoencephalopathy with cytarabine and interferon. Ann Neurol 1993; 33:407–411.
113. Ruiz A, et al. Use of thallium-201 brain SPECT to differentiate cerebral lymphoma from toxoplasma encephalitis in AIDS patients. Am J Neuroradiol 1994; 15:1885–1894.
114. Slater CA, Sickel JZ, Visvesvara GS, et al. Brief report: successful treatment of disseminated acanthamoeba infection in an immunocompromised patient. N Engl J Med 1994; 331:85–87.

115. Pizzo PA. Management of fever in patients with cancer and treatment-induced neutropenia. N Engl J Med 1993; 328:1323–1332.
116. Winston DJ, Ho WG, Champlin RE. Current approaches to management of infections in bone marrow transplants. Eur J Cancer Clin Oncol 1989; 25(suppl 2):S25–S35.
117. Klastersky J. Infections in compromised hosts: considerations on prevention. Eur J Cancer Clin Oncol 1989; 25(suppl 2):S53–S61.
118. Patterson TF, Andriole VT. The role of liposomal amphotericin B in the treatment of systemic fungal infections. Eur J Cancer Clin Oncol 1989; 25(suppl 2):S63–S68.
119. Walker RW, Rosenblum MK. Amphotericin B-associated leukoencephalopathy. Neurology 1992; 42:2005–2010.
120. Balmaceda CM, Walker RW, Castro-Malaspina H, et al. Reversal of amphotericin-B-related encephalopathy. Neurology 1994; 44:1183–1184.
121. Whitley RJ, Gnann JW. Acyclovir: a decade later. N Engl J Med 1992; 327:782–789.
122. Wade JC, Meyers JD. Neurologic symptoms associated with parenteral acyclovir treatment after marrow transplantation. Ann Intern Med 1983; 98:921–925.
123. Schmidt GM, Horak DA, Niland JC, et al. A randomized, controlled trial of prophylactic ganciclovir for cytomegalovirus pulmonary infection in recipients of allogeneic bone marrow transplants. N Engl J Med 1991; 324:1005–1011.
124. Kovacs JA, Baseler M, Dewar RJ, et al. Increases in CD4 T lymphocytes with intermittentt courses of interleukin-2 in patients with human inmmuodeficiency virus infection. N Engl J Med 1995; 332: 567–575.
125. Bernard ST, Ameriso S, Kempf RA. Transient focal neurologic deficits complicating interleukin-2 therapy. Neurology 1990; 40:154–155.
126. Meyers CA, Scheibel RS, Forman AD. Persistent neurotoxicity of systemically administered interferon-alpha. Neurology 1991; 41:672–676.
127. Berenguer J, Diaz-Mediavilla J, Urra D, et al. Central nervous system infection caused by *Pseudo-allescheria boydii*: case report and review. Rev Infect Dis 1989; 11:890–896.
128. Lee ES, Locker J, Nalesnik M, et al. The association of Epstein-Barr virus with smooth-muscle tumors occurring after organ transplantation. N Engl J Med 1995; 332:19–25.

18

Infectious Etiologies of Facial Palsy

Steven W. Huder
Burns Clinic Medical Center, Petoskey, Michigan

HISTORY

Acute Idiopathic Peripheral Facial Palsy

Lower motor neuron lesions affecting the seventh cranial (facial) nerve may be due to a number of possible etiologies, some of which are benign, self-limited, and have a good prognosis, others of which are associated with significant morbidity and mortality and are potentially treatable if detected early (see Table 1). It is, therefore, the goal of the clinician to distinguish between these two etiological groups of facial palsy. Sir Charles Bell (1774–1842), a Scottish surgeon and physiologist, classified and lent his name to an etiological subclass of facial palsy which has an acute onset, is an isolated lesion idiopathic in etiology, and from which a majority of patients recover spontaneously within 6 weeks, though some incompletely. Bell's palsy, or acute idiopathic peripheral facial palsy (AIPFP), is a diagnosis of exclusion of other causes of facial palsy; as such, it is not uncommonly seen as a misdiagnosis or misused term. But there is evidence that this so-called "idiopathic" disorder may actually be mediated by a viral inflammatory immune mechanism (1–3). Increases in antibody titers to herpes simplex virus, or to other viruses listed in Table 2, in presumed AIPFP patients lends support to the viral origin theory (3–5). Other etiologies of AIPFP include various infectious agents (see Table 2), vasospasm, vascular insufficiency, and secondary ischemia (see Table 1) (3).

Ramsay Hunt Syndrome (Herpes Zoster Oticus)

In June 1906, J. Ramsay Hunt, a neurologist, presented to the American Neurological Association a detailed description of herpetic inflammation involving the geniculate ganglion, its association with other cranial nerves and their ganglia, and its complications, a topic elaborated upon by Hunt in several manuscripts from 1907 to 1937 (6,7). Ramsay Hunt syndrome, also known as herpes

Table 1 Etiologies of Facial Palsy

Infection:	See Table 2 for details.
Birth:	Molding, forceps delivery, dystrophica myotonica, Möbius syndrome (congenital facial diplegia)
Trauma:	Basal skull fractures, facial injuries, middle ear injuries, altitudinal or scuba (barotrauma) injuries
Neurological:	Opercular syndrome (facial motor area lesion), Millard-Gubler syndrome (brainstem syndrome involving CNs VI, VII, and corticospinal tract)
Metabolic:	Diabetes mellitus, hypertension, hyperthyroidism, pregnancy, preeclampsia, acute porphyria, vitamin A deficiency
Neoplastic:	Parotid tumors, cholesteatoma, CN VII tumor, glomus jugulare tumor, leukemia, sarcoma, meningioma, hemangioblastoma, carcinoma (invasive or metastatic), vestibular schwannoma, anomalous sigmoid sinus, teratoma, tympanic hemangioma, hydradenoma of external canal, carotid artery aneurysm, fibrous dysplasia, Hand-Schüller-Christian disease (histiocytosis X)
Toxic:	Thalidomide (Miehlke syndrome), ethylene glycol, ethanol, tetanus, arsenic intoxication, diphtheria, carbon monoxide
Iatrogenic:	Mandibular anesthetic block, antitetanus serum, rabies vaccine, mastoid surgery, parotid surgery, postimmunization, posttonsillectomy
Idiopathic:	Bell's, familial, Melkersson-Rosenthal syndrome (recurrent facial palsy, facial edema, lingua plicata, cheilitis, and migraine), hereditary hypertrophic neuropathy (CMT or DS), autoimmune disease, amyloidosis, temporal arteritis, periarteritis nodosa, TTP, Guillain-Barré syndrome, MS, myasthenia gravis, sarcoidosis (uveoparotid fever), osteopetrosis (bone overgrowth and sclerosis with marrow loss and frequent fractures)

Source: Adapted from Refs. 1, 2, 8, 17–20, 33, 42–46, 48, 50, 60, 74, 142.

zoster oticus, is characterized by an acute peripheral facial palsy associated with varicelliform lesions involving the ipsilateral external ear, external auditory canal, neck, or soft palate. There is often involvement of some combination of other cranial nerves (V, VIII, IX, X) and upper cervical branches (C2, C3, C4), with associated symptoms of otalgia, dysacusis, unilateral hearing loss, tinnitus, and vertigo (8,9). While earlier descriptions of herpes zoster oticus and its associations with lesions of cranial nerves VII and VIII were described by German authors from 1887 (Gruber) to 1904 (Körner), Hunt was the first to postulate that this syndrome represented a specific inflammation in the geniculate ganglion, analogous to the then recognized herpetic infections of posterior spinal and trigeminal ganglia (6,10), and the first to organize the syndrome as a "new and distinct clinical entity," and thus it bears his name (6). Hunt classified the syndrome clinically into three groups: (1) herpes zoster auricularis (involving the auricle and external auditory canal); (2) herpes zoster auricularis with facial palsy; and (3) herpes zoster auricularis with facial palsy and auditory symptoms (6). The third group was subsequently refined in his 1908 manuscript as occurring with either hypoacusis alone or in a Meniere's complex of symptoms (tinnitus, deafness, vertigo, nystagmus, vomiting, and dysequilibrium) (7). Hunt proposed a cone-shaped "geniculate zoster zone" involving the auricle, concha, external auditory canal, and tympanum as a cutaneous pattern of geniculate zoster infection, and that the trigeminal (Gasserian), geniculate, acoustic, glossopharyngeal, vagal, and second, third, and fourth cervical ganglia could be regarded as a ganglionic series or chain as they are of the same embryonal origin (i.e., neural crest), and thus are represented by a contiguous system of cutaneous zones from face to ear to palate to head and neck (6,7). Hunt also proposed subgroups of the herpetic syndrome, labeled

Table 2 Infectious Etiologies of Facial Palsy

Adenovirus	Measles virus (rubeola)
Botulism (*Clostridium botulinum*)	Meningitis
Cat scratch disease	Mucormycosis
Coxsackie virus (A,B)	Mumps virus
Cytomegalovirus (CMV)	Mycoplasma
Dengue fever	Otitis media (acute, chronic)
Diphtheria	Osteomyelitis
Encephalitis	Parotitis/Parotid abscess
Enterovirus 70 (acute hemorrhagic conjunctivitis)	Petrositis
Epstein-Barr virus (EBV)	Poliomyelitis (viral)
Gnathostomiasis	Pontine abscess
Hepatitis B/Delta virus coinfection	Rubella virus
Herpes simplex virus (HSV-1, HSV-2)	Syphilis
Human herpesvirus 6 (HHV-6)	Tetanus (*Clostridium tetani*)
Human immunodeficiency virus (HIV)	Toxoplasmosis
Influenza virus A,B	Trichinosis (*Trichinella spiralis*)
Kawasaki disease	Tuberculosis (TB) (*Mycobacterium tuberculosis*)
Leprosy (*Mycobacterium leprae*)	Postvaccination (DPT)
Lyme disease (*Borrelia burgdorferi*)	Varicella-zoster virus (VZV)
Malaria	chickenpox, zoster
Mastoiditis	Ramsay Hunt syndrome

Source: Adapted from Refs. 1–4, 17–20, 30, 33, 34, 40, 41, 43–67, 69–73, 75, 76, 97, 122, 124–223.

as "herpes facialis," "herpes auricularis," "herpes occipitocollaris," and "herpes cephalicus" (6,7).

PATHOPHYSIOLOGY

Acute Idiopathic Peripheral Facial Palsy

The anatomical and physiological basis for acute facial nerve dysfunction have been debated for well over a century. In cases of AIPFP, the primary disease is likely a secondary ganglionitis of the central nervous system with motor nerve palsy, with facial muscle weakness caused by inflammation and autoimmune demyelination of the facial nerve (5). This appears to be the final common pathway for facial nerve dysfunction resulting from numerous possible etiologies.

Ramsay Hunt Syndrome

For herpes zoster oticus, Hunt proposed a mechanism by which the other cranial nerves and cervical branches are affected: each has an anatomical neural connection to the facial (VII) nerve and its ganglion (6). For example, cranial nerve V connects via the greater and lesser petrosal nerves, which pass to Meckel's and the otic ganglia, respectively; similarly, cranial nerve IX connects via Jacobson's nerve; and cranial nerve X connects via its small auricular branch (6). He also suggests parenthetically that these relationships form a basis for "reflected" (i.e., referred) pain (6). Histopathological changes characteristic of Ramsay Hunt syndrome have been seen on postmortem studies, consisting of widespread lymphocytic infiltration along the course of the facial nerve and other affected cranial nerves (11). Also seen are changes in middle ear mucosa near the facial canal, consisting chiefly of perivascular inflammation with lymphocytes, plasma cells, macrophages, and osteoclasts, and VZV-specific antigens found by immunofluorescence methods in the cytoplasm and nucleus of elliptically shaped and round cells (11). In 1934, Maybaum and Druss described the pathological abnormalities in the geniculate ganglion in the Ramsay Hunt syndrome consisting of mild degenerative changes with cytoplasmic shrinkage, pyknosis, nuclear absence, and ganglionic infiltration with lymphocytes and plasma cells, as well as perivascular lymphocytic cuffing (12). There is also lymphocytic infiltration in the endoneurial and perineurial tissues with variable degrees of degeneration of facial, cochlear, and vestibular nerves (13). In chronic Ramsay Hunt syndrome with no return of facial nerve function after one year, biopsy of the labyrinthine segment of cranial nerve VII has revealed a sharp line of demarcation between sclerotic nerve proximal to and necrotic nerve distal to the meatal foramen area of the fallopian canal (14), forming a "physiological bottleneck" in which the cranial nerve VII fibers may be "strangulated in the presence of inflammatory edema" (15).

CLINICAL PRESENTATION

Incidence

The incidence of AIPFP is between 20 and 30 per 100,000 population, with the former figure more often reported (1,16–18). Recurrence rates for AIPFP are approximately 10–15% (5,8,19,20). The incidence of Ramsay Hunt syndrome is 2–3 per 100,000 population, approximately one-tenth the incidence of AIPFP (16). While more common in adults (in various studies, most patients are over 20 years of age and at least 50% are 50–69 years of age) (21,22), Ramsay Hunt syndrome has been reported in children as young as 6 months of age (23). In a series by May in 1981, 170 cases of facial palsy in children were reported, of which 4 cases were associated with Ramsay Hunt syndrome (24).

Facial Nerve Dysfunction

The clinical presentation of a lower motor neuron type of paresis or paralysis of the facial nerve involves dysfunction of muscles innervated by its five main peripheral branches (temporal, zygomatic, buccal, mandibular, and cervical) (see Fig. 1) and therefore results in weakness of forehead wrinkling, of eye closure, of mouth retraction, and of platysmal contraction, as well as evidence of flattening of the ipsilateral nasolabial fold. In addition, depending on the site of the lesion along the course of the facial nerve, additional ipsilateral symptoms of decreased or absent lacrimation, decreased salivation, hyperacusis, and dysgeusia involving the anterior two thirds of the tongue may be seen (2,5,20,25–28) (see Fig. 2). Topographic diagnosis of facial nerve dysfunction is based on the motor, sensory, and secretory deficits elicited by careful examination and is dependent upon the site and extent of the lesion. It is interesting to note here, however, that topographic localization of the lesion(s) involved in facial palsy may be misleading secondary to the possibility of demyelination at multiple sites from the brainstem to the periphery and the possibility of "skip areas" where demyelination is not found (5). There is bilateral involvement of facial palsy in 0.3–2.0% of cases (17,18) due to the etiological agents listed in Table 3. A viral prodrome may precede the onset of facial palsy (24,29–31), and with Bell's palsy, other cranial nerves may be clinically involved as well, with resultant facial numbness or pain or weakened muscles of mastication (trigeminal nerve), dysacusis, tinnitus, or vertigo (vestibulocochlear nerve), dysphagia or pharyngeal pain (glossopharyngeal nerve), dysphonia (vagus nerve), or numbness or pain in the upper cervical (C2, C3, C4) dermatomes (5,8,20,24,31–33).

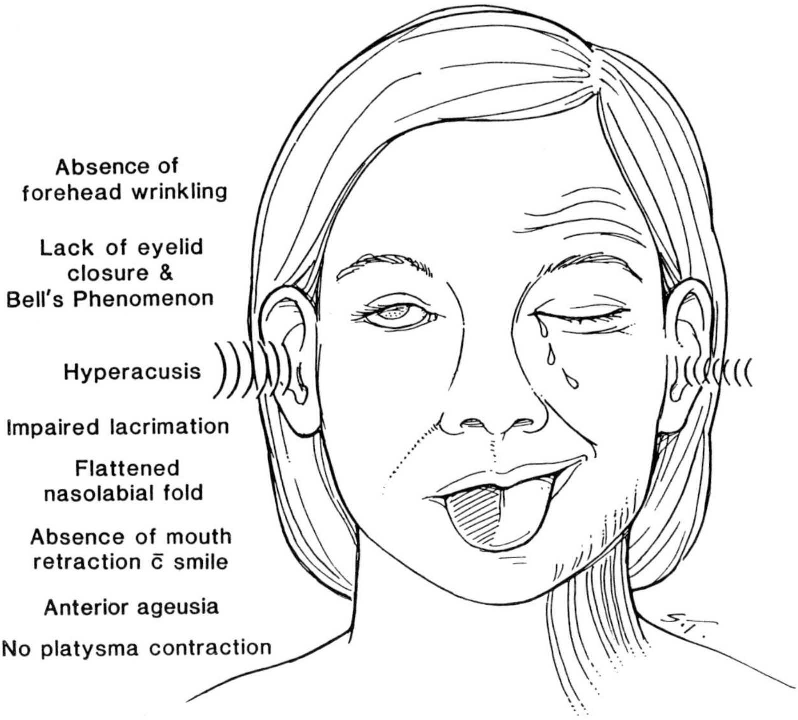

Figure 1 **Clinical presentation of a lower motor neuron facial paralysis.**

Ramsay Hunt Syndrome

The clinical presentation of Ramsay Hunt syndrome is that of an acute peripheral facial palsy in association with varicelliform lesions of the auricle, external auditory canal, tympanum, pre- or postauricular areas, palate, or neck regions (6,7). However, a small minority of patients with Ramsay Hunt syndrome will not have vesicular lesions of VZV infection while demonstrating seroconversion to VZV, an entity described as *zoster sine herpete* (1). There are other associated symptoms and signs referable to the multiple cranial nerve and ganglion involvement (including otalgia, dysacusis, unilateral hearing loss, tinnitus, vertigo, nystagmus, dysphagia, vomiting, or dysequilibrium) (7,34,35). In most cases of Ramsay Hunt syndrome, vesicles and facial weakness appear concurrently (in 25%, vesicles precede facial weakness), external ear vesicles are found in 90% of patients, maximal facial weakness occurs usually within 1 week (but may occur as late as 3 weeks), and complete facial hemiparalysis is twice as common as incomplete paralysis (36).

A minority of patients diagnosed with Ramsay Hunt syndrome may have some type of immunocompromised state due to immunosuppressive therapy, HIV infection (37,38), Hodgkin's disease, non-Hodgkin's lymphoma, hematological malignancy, bronchogenic carcinoma, bladder carcinoma, or nasopharyngeal carcinoma (39). Other disorders that may be associated with Ramsay Hunt syndrome include systemic lupus erythematosus (39), diabetes mellitus (39) (although one study of 625 patients with Bell's palsy and 124 patients with Ramsay Hunt syndrome revealed a significant association of hypertension and diabetes mellitus with Bell's palsy but no significant association of either with Ramsay Hunt syndrome) (40) and meningococcal meningitis (41). Due to the small number of cases of children with Ramsay Hunt syndrome, it

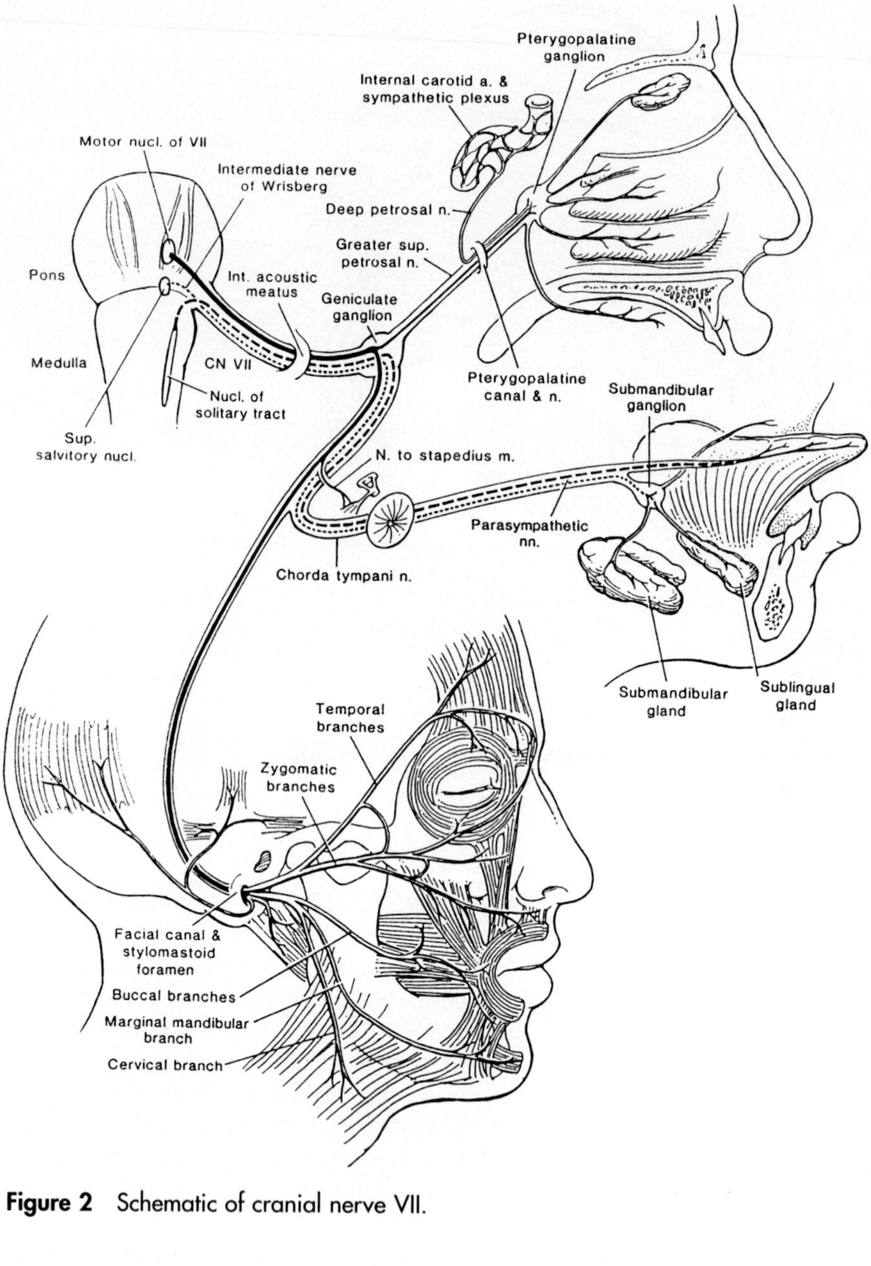

Figure 2 Schematic of cranial nerve VII.

is not possible to determine if disease associations occur more frequently in children than in adults (41).

DIFFERENTIAL DIAGNOSIS

The differential diagnosis of acute peripheral facial palsy is quite extensive (see Table 1): categories include infectious, congenital/birth, traumatic, inflammatory, metabolic, toxic, neoplastic, iatrogenic, and idiopathic. There are numerous infectious etiologies of peripheral facial

Table 3 Infectious Etiologies of Bilateral Facial Palsy

Spirochetal	Viral
Lyme disease (*Borrelia burgdorferi*)	Arbovirus
syphilis (*Treponema pallidum*)	Coxsackievirus
Bacterial	Encephalitis
Abscess, intracranial	Epstein-Barr virus
Diphtheria	Herpes simplex virus
Leprosy	Influenza virus
Leptospirosis	Meningitis
Mastoiditis	Mumps virus
Meningitis	Poliomyelitis
Mycoplasma	Varicella-zoster virus
Otitis media	Parainfectious
Tetanus	Acute inflammatory demyelinating
Tuberculosis	polyradiculoneuropathy (Guillain-Barré
Parasitic	syndrome)
Malaria	
Trichinosis	

Source: Refs. 9, 29, 32, 33, 76, 82, 87, 93, 98, 107, 115, 131, 142, 143, 146.

palsy (see Table 2), of which one of the most common today is Lyme disease. Several reviews of the differential diagnosis of acute peripheral facial palsy have been published, and the reader is referred to these sources for further information on noninfectious causes of facial palsy (2,17,20,42–46).

Specific etiologies of acute facial palsy may be determined by increases in pathogen-specific antibody titers, pathogen-specific DNA hybridization tests, complement fixation (CF) tests, radioimmunoassays (RIAs), enzyme-linked immunosorbent assays (ELISAs), and cultures (see below). However, positive test results should not be accepted as inferring absolute causality, as some pathogens (e.g., herpes simplex virus) may remain dormant in a host until the host encounters internal or external stressors (such as an unrelated infection), which in turn may activate replication of the previously dormant pathogen, thereby appearing as if it were responsible for the acute facial palsy. In some studies, control groups without facial palsy had equally high incidences of antibodies to herpes simplex virus as those with facial palsy (32,47,48).

Leading the list of infectious etiologies for causing acute "idiopathic" peripheral facial palsy (i.e., Bell's palsy) is herpes simplex virus, although there is as yet no consensus or irrefutable confirmation of its role in AIPFP (1,5,24,29,32,47–67).

DIAGNOSIS

Facial Palsy

The diagnosis of acute peripheral facial palsy is made on clinical grounds as outlined above. The cornerstone of diagnosis, therefore, is a careful history and examination, with subsequent investigations directed by clinical suspicions and a knowledge of the vast differential of etiological possibilities and discriminating characteristics of each. The history should include special attention to antecedent risk factors and recent symptoms of illness (including immunosuppression), medication use, recent immunizations, history of trauma, history of tick exposure (or of exposure to endemic areas), history of previous facial palsy, family history of facial palsy, possibility of pregnancy, time course of development of facial weakness (slow progression over several weeks is not seen with AIPFP and should prompt an investigation for benign or malignant tumors) (20,30). The physical and neurological examinations should include special attention to such areas as skin, dysmorphic features, mucous membranes (including palate), parotid gland, tympanic membranes and external auditory canals, systemic signs of infection, functioning of cranial nerves other than the facial nerve, and those nonmotor functions of the facial nerve previously mentioned (20,30).

Investigations

Investigations in patients with acute peripheral facial palsy may be divided into those that should typically be performed in all patients and those that are reserved for patients with an atypical history, examination, or disease course, in whom diagnosis of an etiology may be more challenging. Those studies appropriate for all patients presenting with acute peripheral facial palsy include fasting blood sugar, complete blood count with differential, and erythrocyte sedimentation rate. In areas endemic for Lyme disease, a serological test for *B. burgdorferi* antibodies is included in the initial laboratory evaluation. Audiometric testing, radiographic evaluation of temporal bony areas, and electrodiagnostic studies utilizing evoked electromyography (EEMG) should be performed where indicated (20,30,68). The list of more specific studies reserved for selected circumstances is much more extensive and includes such laboratory tests as lumbar puncture with cerebrospinal fluid (CSF) examination (for meningitis, encephalitis, Guillain-Barré syndrome, multiple sclerosis, or meningeal carcinomatosis), angiotensin-converting enzyme level, serum and urine calcium, and serum globulin (for sarcoidosis), glucose tolerance test or glycosylated hemoglobin (for diabetes mellitus), peripheral blood smear (for malaria), HIV antibody testing, monospot test or heterophil antibody titer (for infectious mononucleosis), antinuclear antibody test and rheumatoid factor (for collagen vascular disorders), fluorescent treponemal antibody (for syphilis), hepatitis screens, heavy metal screen, toxicology, and volatile screens (for such toxins as ethanol), urine and fecal exams (for porphyria or botulism), cold agglutinins (for mycoplasma), skin testing or sputum stains and cultures (for *Mycobacterium tuberculosis*), antibodies to *Trichinella* (for trichinosis), serum antibodies to *Toxoplasma*, carboxyhemoglobin levels (for carbon monoxide poisoning), bone marrow examination (for leukemia or lymphoma), and lymph node biopsy with Warthin-Starry staining (for cat scratch disease) (2,20).

Other investigations may include edrophonium (Tensilon) testing (for myasthenia gravis), electronystagmography (if vertigo or other vestibular complaints exist), chest radiographs, temporal bone tomography, and magnetic resonance imaging (MRI) with gadolinium-DTPA contrast (see below) (8,20,30).

Acute Idiopathic Peripheral Facial Palsy

Herpes simplex virus or varicella zoster virus may be identified as the etiology in some patients with presumed AIPFP by determination of rising serum antibody titers, with the ELISA test more sensitive in some studies than the CF tests (4,32,48,49,57,58,60,61,64,69–76). However, the utility of testing for herpes simplex virus routinely in acute peripheral facial palsy patients is debatable at the present time.

Cerebrospinal fluid studies in patients with AIPFP are suggestive of an abnormality in the blood-brain barrier with pleocytosis and/or local immunoglobulin (IgA, IgG, and IgM) synthesis within the central nervous system (CNS) (occurring in approximately 25% of AIPFP patients) (49).

Ramsay Hunt Syndrome

The minimum clinical findings of otalgia, ipsilateral facial palsy, and varicelliform periauricular lesions are usually sufficient to make the presumptive diagnosis of Ramsay Hunt syndrome (6,8,77). Definitive diagnosis of varicella zoster virus (VZV) infection can be made by isolation and characterization of the virus, by detection of specific viral antigens, or by DNA hybridization techniques (78). Alternatively, specific serum VZV-IgA antibody titers (determined by immunoperoxidase assay) are seen to be elevated early in the course of Ramsay Hunt syndrome, and anticomplement immunofluorescent antibody titration may be useful for diagnosing VZV in Ramsay Hunt syndrome (78,79). In the cerebrospinal fluid of patients with Ramsay Hunt syndrome, intrathecal VZV-specific IgG synthesis, manifested by an increase in the CSF/serum IgG ratio, is detectable as long as 4 months after the onset of disease, at which time all other CSF parameters are normal (49). Viral cultures in human fibroblast of kidney cell tissue cultures may also be obtained from swabs of open cutaneous vesicles to confirm the diagnosis of VZV infection (77).

MRI Findings

Magnetic resonance imaging (MRI) with gadolinium-DTPA (Gd-DTPA) contrast enhancement is useful in the evaluation of acute peripheral facial palsy to look for cerebellopontine angle, brainstem, posterior cranial fossa, or temporal bone area lesions (80–82).

MRI with Gd-DTPA may demonstrate enhancement in the distal internal auditory canal and labyrinthine segment of cranial nerve VII in AIPFP (8) (see Fig. 3) and, additionally, enhancement in the cochlea, cochlear nerve, and vestibular nerve in patients with Ramsay Hunt syndrome (82–84). This enhancement occurs presumably by disruption of the blood-brain barrier with leakage of Gd-DTPA "in the endoneurium through blood vessels (82). There is no significant correlation between intensity or pattern of facial nerve enhancement on MRI with Gd-DTPA, the severity or duration of disease, or the patient's prognosis for recovery (85). The lesions of Ramsay Hunt syndrome as seen by Gd-DTPA–enhanced MRI may mimic intracanalicular acoustic neuromas (86–88).

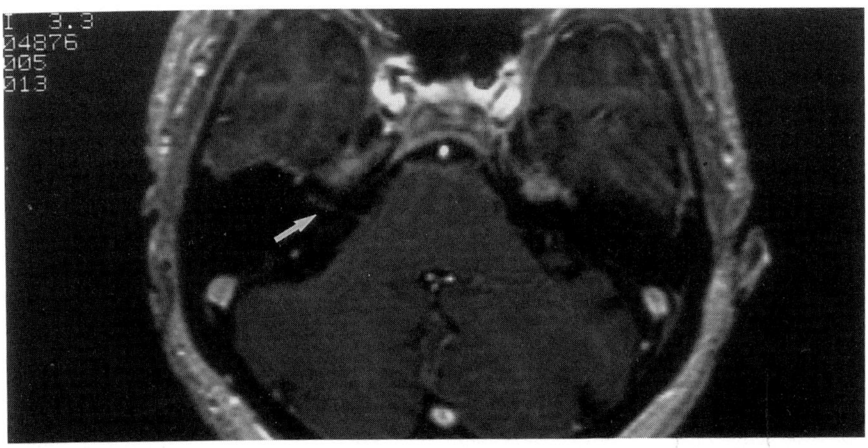

Figure 3 Axial T_1-weighted MR scan with gadolinium-DTPA demonstrates contrast enhancement of the facial nerve (cranial nerve VII) on the right [white arrow] as it exits the pons at the cerebellopontine angle.

Electrophysiology

Afferent Systems Tests

Electrophysiological studies may be used to determine the extent of involvement of the cranial nerves in acute peripheral facial palsy, including the Ramsay Hunt syndrome. Disorders of audition may be studied by electrocochleography, pure-tone audiometry, and brainstem auditory evoked responses (BAERs). Some studies suggest that the cochlea is the site of abnormality responsible for hearing loss in Ramsay Hunt syndrome (89), while other studies indicate that both cochlear and retrocochlear involvement are responsible (10,90). BAER studies in Ramsay Hunt patients characteristically show prolongation of latencies of waves III and V, with preservation of wave I, suggesting retrocochlear involvement (90), and may be used to validate signs of clinical auditory improvement during recovery (91). Pure-tone audiograms often confirm sensorineural hearing loss suggested by clinical exam in Ramsay Hunt syndrome, with speech frequency loss by audiogram correlating more with clinical auditory symptoms than does high-frequency loss (10,92). Electronystagmography (ENG) may reveal absence of caloric response on the ipsilateral side in Ramsay Hunt syndrome patients with vestibular symptoms and signs (93).

Efferent (Motor) Systems Tests

Electromyography EMG), evoked electromyography (EEMG), nerve excitability testing (NET), and electroneuronography (ENOG) are all useful tests in following recovery of facial nerve function by providing an index of nerve injury severity as evidenced by the proportion of motor fibers affected (8).

EMG. Electromyography (EMG) performed within the first 2 weeks of the course of acute peripheral facial palsy may be misleading as sparse residual motor units may be seen early, suggesting a favorable outcome, even though severe injury to large portions of fibers at risk for degeneration continues, resulting in a less favorable outcome. EMG is useful for following reinnervation or persistent degeneration in cases of prolonged paralysis (8).

EEMG. Evoked electromyography (EEMG) records the compound muscle action potential to a supramaximal stimulus using surface electrodes and compares affected to unaffected sides. Facial EEMG is most reliable during the initial phase of accelerated denervation (in the first 2–3 weeks after onset) and when clinically correlated may provide an accurate prognostic guide relatively early in the disease course, and thus is felt to be the most accurate electrophysiological means of determining prognosis in facial nerve dysfunction (8,94). Absence of any EEMG response on serial tests strongly suggests a tumor and neuroimaging and/or nerve exploration should be considered in such a case (94).

NET. Nerve excitability testing (NET) using a nerve stimulator also compares responses of the involved side with the uninvolved side. This test may be falsely negative in the first 48–72 h of acute peripheral facial palsy secondary to the required progression time of intratemporal to extratemporal segmental cranial nerve VII involvement. It is best used as a screening method to determine which patients require further evaluation (8).

ENOG. Electroneuronography (ENOG) is approximately equivalent in prognostic value to NET (although ENOG is more precise and quantitative) and is thus best used as a screening method (95).

TREATMENT

With the exception of the Ramsay Hunt syndrome and those other identifiable infectious causes of acute peripheral facial palsy that require specific antibiotic treatment (see Table 2), therapy for Bell's palsy (AIPFP) may include any or all of the following: (1) steroid (glucocorticoid) therapy;

(2) nerve decompression; (3) antiviral (acyclovir) therapy; (4) supportive measures to prevent secondary injury (i.e., bacterial superinfection, ophthalmological injury, aspiration); or (5) rehabilitation therapies.

(Other infectious causes of acute peripheral facial palsy that are treatable are covered in other chapters in this textbook.)

Glucocorticoids

The use of glucocorticoids (e.g., oral prednisone) for early treatment of AIPFP has been a topic of considerable controversy for over 40 years. There remains to date a paucity of well-designed, controlled, double-blinded, randomized prospective studies of steroid use versus placebo in the treatment of AIPFP. While numerous studies report a benefit with steroid therapy (5,8,24, 31,50,96–104) and others claim no proven benefit (67,105–107), still others maintain that the data are presently inconclusive as to whether or not steroids are efficacious (30,67,68,108–112). Glucocorticoid therapy is thought to be beneficial by an anti-inflammatory mechanism, through which edema and host cytokines and other mediators of inflammation are minimized (8,50,67). The use of steroid therapy in Ramsay Hunt syndrome has been suggested to reduce the risk of denervation, to lessen the risk of synkinesis, to prevent the progression from incomplete to complete paralysis, to hasten recovery, and to decrease the risk of postherpetic neuralgia (8).

If the decision is made to use steroid therapy in AIPFP, the recommended dosage of oral prednisone is 1 mg/kg/day, in two divided doses, with reexamination of the patient on day 5 or 6 of paralysis. If paralysis is incomplete, the prednisone dose is then tapered daily to zero over the next 5 days. If facial paralysis is complete, prednisone is continued at the same dosage for 10 days more, then tapered daily to zero over 5 days (5,24,31). Steroid doses are tapered instead of abruptly discontinued to avoid rebound inflammation, which can lead to further denervation (5,8,24,31). The recommended dosage of oral prednisone used in the treatment of Ramsay Hunt syndrome is 1 mg/kg/day, given in two or three divided doses, for 7–10 days duration, then tapered daily to zero over the next 7–10 days (5,8,77,101). Side effects of short-term glucocorticoid therapy include hyperglycemia, fluid and electrolyte disturbances, GI irritation, CNS effects (psychosis), and increased risk of infection, all of which are decreased in frequency by dividing doses and rapidly tapering off steroids when possible (8). Steroid therapy should be avoided in those who are immunosuppressed or who have ophthalmic involvement of herpes lesions (8,97,103).

Facial Nerve Decompression Surgery

Facial nerve decompression surgery remains an option for treatment of peripheral facial palsy, but should be reserved for a very select few patients. In the 1930s decompression surgery was performed on the distal facial nerve at the stylomastoid foramen, while in the 1940s and 1950s surgery was directed at the segment of the facial nerve between the geniculate ganglion and the stapedial branch. By the 1960s the segment between the stapedial branch and the chorda tympani was targeted, and in the 1970s and 1980s decompression of the meatal and labyrinthine segments through a middle cranial fossa approach was advocated, an approach still in favor today (5). Consideration for nerve decompression surgery should be based on the clinical course of paralysis and the electrographic findings, reserving surgery for select cases in which the EEMG amplitude on the affected side is no more than 10% that of the unaffected side, when the EEMG study is performed within the first 2 weeks of onset of paralysis (8). Surgical decompression beyond 2 weeks' disease duration has shown no benefit in either AIPFP or Ramsay Hunt syndrome (5,95). Trials to better delineate the efficacy of and indications for facial nerve decompression surgery are ongoing (30,77,97,113).

Acyclovir

Numerous studies have indicated that acyclovir (9-[2-hydroxyethoxymethyl] guanine), a synthetic purine nucleotide analog, when instituted early in the course of Ramsay Hunt syndrome, is efficacious in treating the VZV infection resulting in substantially greater functional return, earlier recovery of facial nerve function, reversal of sensorineural hearing loss, decreased duration of pain, and decreased duration of viral shedding, and in immunocompromised patients, decreased viral dissemination (8,96,114–118). The efficacy of acyclovir in treatment of AIPFP remains more controversial, however, since the role of such viruses as HSV-1 or HSV-2 in AIPFP is less clear. Although some advocate using acyclovir for AIPFP (5), others maintain that the data are insufficient to show efficacy at this time (8,24,108,112). Acyclovir must first be phosphorylated by the herpes virus–infected cells containing virus-encoded thymidine kinase (TK) before assuming an active form; thus, acyclovir is effective against replicating virus only, leaving uninfected host cells and those in which virus is dormant unaffected (118). The TKs of VZV are less sensitive to acyclovir than those of herpes simplex virus (HSV), thus requiring a higher acyclovir dosage for treatment of VZV (118). Intravenous acyclovir is preferred to oral acyclovir to treat Ramsay Hunt syndrome, with a dosage of 10 mg/kg IV every 8 h for 7 days (8,118). One recent study suggests that treatment of acute herpes zoster may be effectively completed with oral acyclovir for 7 days, but this did not include patients with the Ramsay Hunt syndrome (119). There has been no evidence to support the use of oral acyclovir to provide any further benefit after completion of a course of parenteral acyclovir for the Ramsay Hunt syndrome (118). The incidence of toxicity with acyclovir therapy is low and includes renal toxicity (drug crystallizing in glomeruli in patients with decreased GFR) (118), hepatic toxicity (increased alkaline phosphatase) (118), bone marrow depression (120), and local injection site phlebitis (117).

Supportive Measures to Prevent Secondary Injury

In acute peripheral facial nerve palsy, analgesics should be used as needed for pain (121), although prednisone therapy alone often obviates the need for additional analgesics (5,24,31). Protective care of the eye, which can neither close to protect itself nor lacrimate to lubricate itself adequately, is most important. Shielding the eye with eyeglasses reduces the risk of mechanical injury and air-drying, and instillation of ophthalmic lubricants (artificial tears in the daytime, ointments at night while sleeping) prevents drying and exposure keratitis (8,24,110,112). Some patients with severe facial paralysis may require tarsorraphy or canthopexy to protect the exposed eye (5,8), and selective injection of the levator palpebrae superioris muscle on the affected side with botulinum toxin is reported to be a successful alternative to surgical eyelid closure (107). Closed patching of the eye during sleep may increase the risk of corneal abrasion by unopposed action of the levator palpebrae during sleep (8). The varicelliform cutaneous lesions of the periauricular areas and external auditory canal may, upon crusting and opening, become secondarily infected (i.e., cellulitis), requiring antibiotic therapy (77). When cranial nerves IX and X are involved, as evidenced by varicelliform lesions of the palate, pharynx, and larynx, impaired gag reflex, dysphagia with solids or liquids, or hoarseness, there is a considerable risk of aspiration. Modified barium swallow, speech therapy assessment, and ENT referral may be indicated, with consideration of enteral supplementation via nasogastric or orogastric tube until the dysphagia improves or resolves.

Rehabilitation Therapies

Speech and audiology therapy may assist with articulation, chewing, swallowing, and compensation for unilateral hearing loss in selected patients. Muscle retraining with EMG feedback is used with highly motivated patients who have synkinesis following facial nerve recovery (8). Electrical stimulation of paralyzed muscles as a form of physiotherapy has been shown to retard ingrowth of neurofibrils to the motor endplate and thus may be detrimental to reinnervation recovery (5,24,122).

NEUROLOGICAL COMPLICATIONS AND SEQUELAE

The prognosis of facial paralysis in patients with Ramsay Hunt syndrome has been reported to be worse overall than in patients with AIPFP, with approximately 50–78% of patients with Ramsay Hunt syndrome showing poor or incomplete recovery (8,40,95,101, 117,118), while approximately 70–80% of those with AIPFP have a full recovery, with only 5–10% experiencing a poor outcome and 10–15% showing incomplete recovery (30,50,107,110). Patients with Ramsay Hunt syndrome are more apt to develop denervation during the disease course than are patients with AIPFP (95). The small number of reported cases in children limits prognostication (21,40). The association of severe pain (5), hyperacusis, impaired lacrimation, and pain of an aural, anterior facial, or radicular character all imply a worse prognosis for recovery by some reports (24). Recovery of hearing is often poor in Ramsay Hunt syndrome patients when associated with advanced age, retrocochlear hearing loss, male gender, vertigo, and speech frequency hearing loss (10). Electrodiagnostic procedures (i.e., EEMG) are helpful in predicting recovery from facial nerve dysfunction. Within the first 3 weeks of the disease course, an EEMG response of 0–20% will usually predict an incomplete return of facial function, while an EEMG response of at least 60% will predict a return to normal facial function. Furthermore, serial EEMG after several weeks has little value in predicting final recovery of facial function (94). Other studies maintain that accurate prognosis cannot be determined prior to day 21 of the disease course as electrical tests can deteriorate in Ramsay Hunt syndrome after day 14 (101). There appears to be a trend toward more recovery of facial function in those patients with complete paralysis who show clinical signs of recovery within the first 6 weeks of the disease course (8). Chances for complete recovery appear to be augmented by early, accurate diagnosis and subsequent early institution of treatment.

Summary Table of Diagnosis and Treatment

A. Clinical diagnosis of acute peripheral facial palsy with:
   1. History (special attention to recent or concurrent illnesses, medications, recent immunizations, trauma, previous facial palsies, pregnancy, time course of disease, family history, etc.)
   2. Neurological and ancillary examinations (special attention to dysmorphic features, skin, mucous membranes, systemic infectious signs, parotid gland, tympanic membranes and external auditory canals, other cranial nerve functions, etc.)

B. Investigations:
   1. All patients:
      Fasting blood glucose
      Complete blood count with differential
      Erythrocyte sedimentation rate
   2. Consider:
      Audiometric testing
      Radiographic evaluation of temporal bony areas (x-ray/CT/MR)
      EEMG (evoked EMG)

3. Labs in selected patients:
   Lyme serology
   ACE level, serum and urine calcium, and serum globulin (sarcoidosis)
   Antinuclear antibody test and rheumatoid factor (collagen vascular disorders)
   Bone marrow examination (leukemia or lymphoma)
   Carboxyhemoglobin levels (carbon monoxide poisoning)
   Cold agglutinins (mycoplasma)
   Fecal exam for Clostridium (tetanus)
   Fluorescent treponemal antibody test (syphilis)
   Glycosylated hemoglobin or glucose tolerance testing (diabetes mellitus)
   Heavy metal screen
   Hepatitis screens
   HIV antibody test
   Lumbar Puncture/CSF exam (meningitis)
   Monospot test (infectious mononucleosis)
   Peripheral blood smear (malaria)
   TB skin/sputum testing
   Toxicology and volatile screens
   Toxoplasma antibodies
   Trichinella antibodies (trichinosis)
   Urine porphyrins (porphyria)
4. Ancillary tests in selected patients:
   Schirmer lacrimation testing
   ENG (electronystagmography)
   Lymph node biopsy (with special stains)
   MRI with gadolinium
   Edrophonium (Tensilon) test
   Chest radiography
   Temporal bone tomography
5. Treatment:
   a. Glucocorticoids:
      Prednisone (oral) 1 mg/kg/day in two or three divided doses.
      Patient is reexamined on day 5 or 6:
      i. If paralysis is incomplete, the prednisone dose is tapered daily to zero over the next 5 days.
      ii. If facial paralysis is complete, prednisone is continued at the same dosage for 10 days more, then tapered daily to zero over 5 days.
   b. Protective care of the eye:
      i. Awake: Eyeglasses
         Artificial tears:
         - Cellufresh 0.5%
         - Celluvisc 1%
         - Lacri-lube Solution
         - Tears Naturale II
         - Tears Naturale Free
      ii. Asleep: Convex eye shield
         Ophthalmic Ointments (qhs)
         - Lacri-lube NP

Lacri-lube SOP
Refresh PM

c. Acyclovir (if Ramsay Hunt Syndrome):
10 mg/kg IV every 8 h for 7 days

d. Facial nerve decompression surgery:
In select cases based on the EEMG amplitude on the affected side

REFERENCES

1. Morgan M, Nathwani D. Facial palsy and infection: the unfolding story. Clin Infect Dis 1992; 14: 263–271.
2. May M, Klein S. Differential diagnosis of facial nerve palsy. Otolaryngol Clin North Am 1991; 24(3):613–645.
3. Inamura H, Aoyagi M, et al. Viral infection in acute peripheral facial palsy investigation in Yamagata Prefecture. Acta Otolaryngol (Stockh) 1988; 446:23–26.
4. Kukimoto N, Ikeda M, et al. Viral infections in acute peripheral facial paralysis nationwide analysis centering on CF. Acta Otolaryngol (Stockh) 1988; 446(suppl):17–22.
5. Adour KK. Medical management of idiopathic (Bell's) palsy. Otolarygnol Clin North Am 1991; 24(3):663–673.
6. Hunt JR. On herpetic inflammations of the geniculate ganglion. A new syndrome and its complications. J Nerv Ment Dis 1907; 34:73–96.
7. Hunt JR. A further contribution to the herpetic inflammations of the geniculate ganglion. Am J Med Sci 1908; 136:226–241.
8. Niparko J, Mattox D. Bell's palsy and herpes oticus. In: Johnson R, Griffin J, eds. Current Therapy in Neurologic Disease, 4th ed. St. Louis: BC Decker, 1993:355–361.
9. Cozzi P, Talano J. Excessive salivation as an anginal equivalent: a sequela to Ramsay Hunt syndrome. Am J Med 1991; 91:201–220.
10. Wayman D, Pham H, et al. Audiological manifestations of Ramsay Hunt syndrome. J Laryngol Otol 1990; 104:104–108.
11. Yanagihara N, Kurata T. Middle ear mucosa in Ramsay Hunt syndrome. Ann Otol Rhinol Laryngol 1990; 99:359–362.
12. Maybaum J, Druss J. Geniculate ganglionitis (Hunt's syndrome). Clinical features and histopathology. Arch Otolaryngol 1934; 19:574–581.
13. Etholm B, Schuknecht H. Pathological findings and surgical implications in herpes zoster oticus. Adv Otorhinolaryngol 1983; 31:184–190.
14. Jackson C, Hyams V. Pathologic findings in the labyrinthine segment of the facial nerve in a case of facial paralysis. Ann Otol Rhinol Laryngol 1990; 99:327–329.
15. Fisch U. Surgery for Bell's palsy. Arch Otolaryngol 1981; 107:1–11.
16. Yanagihara N. Incidence of Bell's palsy. Ann Otol Rhinol Laryngol 1988; 97:4.
17. Steenerson R. Bilateral facial paralysis. Am J Otol 1986; 7(2):99–100.
18. Sherwen P, Thong N. Bilateral facial nerve palsy: a case study and literature review. J Otolaryngol 1987; 16(1):28–33.
19. Mamoli B, Neumann H, Ehrmann L. Recurrent Bell's palsy: etiology, frequency, prognosis. J Neurol 1977; 216:119–125.
20. May M. Differential diagnosis by history, physical findings, and laboratory results. In: May M, ed. The Facial Nerve. New York: Thieme Inc., 1986:181–216.
21. Devriese P. Facial paralysis in cephalic herpes zoster. Ann Otol Rhinol Laryngol 1968; 1101–1119.
22. Heathfield KWG, Mee A. Prognosis of the Ramsay Hunt syndrome. Br Med J 1978; 1:343–344.
23. O'Neill H. Herpes zoster auris ('geniculate ganglionitis'). Arch Otolaryngol 145; 42:309–326.
24. Adour KK, Hetzler D. Current medical treatment for facial palsy. Am J Otol 1984; 5(6):499–502.
25. Miehlke A. Typical sites of facial-nerve lesions. Arch Otolaryngol 1969; 89:148–152.

26. Möller F. Critical viewpoints on the pathogenesis in Bell's palsy. Acta Neurol Scand 1967; 43: 228–238.
27. DeMyer W. Neuroanatomy. Malvern, PA: Harwal Publishing Company, 1988.
28. Moore K. Clinically Oriented Anatomy, 2d ed. Baltimore: Williams and Wilkins, 1985:818–832.
29. Korczyn A, Swirski R, Henig E. Bell's palsy and viral infections. Eur Neurol 1973; 10:191–196.
30. Gantz B. Idiopathic Facial Paralysis. Curr Ther Otolaryngol Head Neck Surg 1987; 3:62–66.
31. Adour KK. Diagnosis and management of facial paralysis. N Engl J Med 1982; 307(6):348–351.
32. Adour KK, Bell D, Hilsinger R. Herpes simplex virus in idiopathic facial paralysis (Bell palsy). JAMA 1975; 233(6):527–530.
33. May M, Fria T, et al. Facial paralysis in children: differential diagnosis. Otolaryngol Head Neck Surg 1981; 89:841–848.
34. Benninger M. Acyclovir for the treatment of idiopathic vocal fold paralysis. Ear Nose Throat J 1992; 71:207–208.
35. Engstrom H, Wohlfart G. Herpes zoster of the seventh, eighth, ninth and tenth cranial nerves. Arch Neurol Psychiat 1949; 62:638–652.
36. Devriese P, Moeskev W. The natural history of facial paralysis in herpes zoster. Laryngoscope 1988; 98:776–779.
37. Mishell J, Applebaum E. Ramsay-Hunt syndrome in a patient with HIV infection. Otolaryngol Head Neck Surg 1990; 102:177–179.
38. Morris M, Prasad S. Otologic disease in the acquired immunodeficiency syndrome. Ear Nose Throat J 1990; 69:451–453.
39. Chang C, Woo E, et al. Herpes zoster and its neurological complications. Postgrad Med J 1987; 63: 85–89.
40. Yanagihara N, Hyodo M. Association of diabetes mellitus and hypertension with Bell's palsy and Ramsay Hunt syndrome. Ann Otol Rhinol Laryngol 1988; 97:5–7.
41. Bjerkhoel A, Hyden D. Ramsay-Hunt syndrome in a preschool infant. ORL 1989; 51:251–254.
42. Gorman J, Nagler B, Botton J. Facial diplegia and its causes. Virginia Med 1977; (Aug):544–546.
43. Linthicum, Jr. F. Facial nerve paralysis in children. Otolaryngol Clin North Am 1974; 7(2):433–436.
44. Rontal E, Sigel M. Bilateral facial paralysis. Laryngoscope 1972; 82(4):981–982.
45. Hora J, Elwell R. Facial diplegia. Arch Otolaryngol 1966; 83:53–55.
46. Browder JP. Facial paralysis in children. Ear Nose Throat J 1978; 57:6–12.
47. Jannetta P, Bissonette D. Bell's palsy: a theory as to etiology. Laryngoscope 1978; 88:849–854.
48. Thomsen J, Barfoed C. Idiopathic facial palsy—viral, hereditary, or both? Arch Otorhinolaryngol 1979; 222:109–112.
49. Weber T, Jürgens S, Lüer W. Cerebrospinal fluid immunoglobulins and virus-specific antibodies in disorders affecting the facial nerve. J Neurol 1987; 234:308–314.
50. McGovern F, Estevez J. Current concepts in the etiology and pathology of Bell's palsy. Virginia Med 1983; 110:544–546.
51. Wilson J. Bell's palsy and herpes simplex. Br Med J 1978; 2(6138):704.
52. Juel-Jensen B. Bell's palsy and herpes simplex. Br Med J 1978; 1(6104):49.
53. Juel-Jensen B. Bell's palsy and herpes simplex. Br Med J 1977; 2(6094):1086.
54. Juel-Jensen B. Bell's palsy and herpes simplex. Br Med J 1978; 2(6142):953–954.
55. Grout P. Bell's palsy and herpes simplex. Br Med J 1977; 2(6090):829–830.
56. Ross C. Bell's palsy and herpes simplex. Br Med J 1978; 2(6142):953–954.
57. Vahlne A, Edström S, et al. Bell's palsy and herpes simplex virus. Arch Otolaryngol 1981; 107:79–81.
58. Lewis B, Morris C. Bell's palsy and herpes-simplex infection. Lancet 1976; 1(7950):100.
59. Vassallo L, Galea-Debono A. Aetiology of Bell's palsy. Lancet 1972; 2(773):383.
60. Djupesland G, Berdal P, et al. Viral infection as a cause of acute peripheral facial palsy. Arch Otolaryngol 1976; 102:403–406.
61. Djupesland G, Berdal P, et al. The role of viral infection in acute peripheral facial palsy. Acta Otolaryngol 1975; 79:221–227.
62. Ghonim M, Gavilan C, Sarria M. Bilateral simultaneous Bell's palsy. ORL 1988; 50:269–272.

63. Vahlne A, Edström S, et al. Possible association of herpes simplex virus infection with demyelinating disease. Scand J Infect Dis 1985; 47(suppl):16–21.
64. Smith M, Scott G, et al. Herpes simplex virus and facial palsy. J Infect 1987; 15:259–261.
65. Steven N, Nathwani D. Clin Inf Dis 1993; 16:181.
66. Spruance S. Bell palsy and herpes simplex virus. Ann Intern Med 1994; 120(12):1045–1046.
67. Hyden D, Roberg M, et al. Acute "idiopathic" peripheral facial palsy: clinical, serological, and CSF findings and effects of corticosteroids. Am J Otolaryngol 1993; 14(3):179–186.
68. Manning J, Adour KK. Facial paralysis in children. Pediatrics 1972; 49(1):102–108.
69. Vest C, Munneke J, Smith R. Herpes zoster oticus. Postgrad Med 1979; 65(4):143–150.
70. Mertens T, Thomas J, et al. Peripheral facial palsy and viral infections—findings and problems. Med Microbiol Immunol 1982; 171:77–83.
71. Mair I, Flugsrud L. Peripheral facial palsy and herpes zoster infection. J Laryngol Otol 1976; 90(4): 373–379.
72. Berg R, Forsgren M, Schiratzki H. Acute facial palsy. Acta Otolaryngol 1976; 81:462–467.
73. Mair I, Traavik T. Peripheral facial palsy and viral replication. Acta Otolaryngol 1983; 95:528–531.
74. Djupesland G, Degre M, et al. Acute peripheral facial palsy—part of a cranial polyneuropathy? Arch Otolaryngol 1977; 103:841–844.
75. Njoo F, Wertheim-vanDillen P, Devriese P. Serology in facial paralysis caused by clinically presumed herpes zoster infection. Arch Otorhinolaryngol 1988; 245:230–233.
76. Tomita H, Tanaka M, et al. An ELISA study on varicella-zoster virus infection in acute peripheral facial palsy. Acta Otolaryngol (Stockh) 1988; 446(suppl):10–16.
77. Hirsch B. Infections of the external ear. Am J Otolaryngol 1992; 13:145–155.
78. Hadar T, Tovi F, et al. Detection of specific IgA antibodies to varicella zoster virus in serum of patients with Ramsay Hunt syndrome. Ann Otol Rhinol Laryngol 1990; 99:461–465.
79. Shigeta S, Baba M, et al. Importance of anticomplement immunofluorescence antibody titration for diagnosing varicella-zoster virus infection in Bell's palsy. J Clin Pathol 1986; 39:1254–1258.
80. LaBagnara, Jr. J, Jahn A, et al. MRI findings in two cases of acute facial paralysis. Otolaryngol Head Neck Surg 1989; 101:562–565.
81. Li J, Xiong L, Jinkins J. Gadolinium-enhanced MRI in a patient with AIDS and the Ramsay-Hunt syndrome. Neuroradiology 1993; 35:269.
82. Yanagida M, Ushiro K, et al. Enhanced MRI in patients with Ramsay-Hunt's syndrome. Acta Otolaryngol (Stockh) 1993; 500(suppl):58–61.
83. Canellas R, Torres C, et al. Ramsay-Hunt syndrome and high resolution 3DFT MRI. J Comput Assist Tomogr 1993; 17:495–497.
84. Osumi A, Tien R. MR findings in a patient with Ramsay-Hunt syndrome. J Comput Assist Tomogr 1990; 14:991–993.
85. Korzec K, Sokol S, et al. Gadolinium-enhanced MRI of the facial nerve in herpes zoster oticus and Bell's palsy: clinical implications. Am J Otol 1991; 12:163–168.
86. Anderson R. Ramsay Hunt syndrome mimicking intracanalicular acoustic neuroma on contrast-enhanced MR. AJNR 1990; 11:409.
87. Daniels D, Czervionke L, Millen S. MR findings in the Ramsay Hunt syndrome. AJNR 1988; 9:609.
88. Han M, Jabour B, et al. Nonneoplastic enhancing lesions mimicking intracanalicular acoustic neuroma on gadolinium-enhanced MR images. Radiology 1991; 179:795–796.
89. Kusakari J, Takeyama M, et al. Studies with electrocochleography and auditory brainstem response in Ramsay Hunt syndrome. Acta Otolaryngol (Stockh) 1988; 446(suppl):81–84.
90. Abramovich S, Prasher D. Electrocochleography and brainstem potentials in Ramsay Hunt syndrome. Arch Otolaryngol Head Neck Surg 1986; 112:925–928.
91. Iragui V. Auditory dysfunction in Ramsay Hunt syndrome. J Neurol Neurosurg Psychiat 1986; 49: 824–826.
92. Hiraide F, Kakoi H, et al. Acute profound deafness in Ramsay Hunt syndrome. Acta Otolaryngol (Stockh) 1988; 456(suppl):49–54.
93. Longridge N. Recurrent vestibulopathy: support for a viral etiology. J Otolaryngol 1989; 18:99–100.

94. Silverstein H, McDaniel A, Hyman S. Evoked serial electromyography in the evolution of the paralyzed face. Am J Otol 1985; (suppl):80–87.
95. Kanzaki J. Electrodiagnostic findings in the early stages of Bell's palsy and Ramsay-Hunt's syndrome. Acta Otolaryngol (Stockh) 1988; 446(suppl):42–46.
96. Feldman S, Ford M, Briggaman R. Herpes zoster and facial palsy. Cutis 1988; 42:523–524.
97. Crabtree J. Herpes zoster oticus and facial paralysis. Otolaryngol Clin North Am 1974; 7(2):369–373.
98. Austin J, Peskind S, et al. Idiopathic facial nerve paralysis: a randomized double blind controlled study of placebo versus prednisone. Laryngoscope 1993; 103:1326–1333.
99. Merren M. Bell's palsy (2 cases). Am J Otol 1992; 13(5):488.
100. Adour KK, Wingerd J, et al. Prednisone treatment for idiopathic facial paralysis (Bell's palsy). N Engl J Med 1972; 287(25):1268–1272.
101. Robillard R, Hilsinger, Jr. R, Adour KK. Ramsay Hunt facial paralysis: clinical analyses of 185 patients. Otolaryngol Head Neck Surg 1986; 95:292–297.
102. Wolf SM, Wagner, Jr., JH, et al. Treatment of Bell's palsy with prednisone: a prospective randomized study. Neurology 1978; 28:158–161.
103. Devriese PP. Prednisone in idiopathic facial paralysis (Bell's palsy). Otol Rhinol Laryngol 1977; 39: 257–271.
104. Teverner D, Cohen SB, Hutchinson BC. Comparison of corticotrophin and prednisolone in treatment of idiopathic facial paralysis (Bell's palsy). Br Med J 1971; 4:20–22.
105. May M, Wette R, et al. The use of steroids in Bell's palsy: a prospective controlled study. Laryngoscope 1976; 86:1111–1122.
106. Taverner D. Cortisone treatment of Bell's palsy. Lancet 1954; 2:1052–1054.
107. Bateman D. Facial palsy. Br J Hosp Med 1992; 47(6):430–431.
108. Hughes GB. Facial Nerve Study Group—1990 meeting minutes. Am J Otol 1991; 12:69–70.
109. Burgess L, Yim D, Lepore M. Bell's palsy: the steroid controversy revisited. Laryngoscope 1984; 94:1472–1476.
110. Louis S. Medical treatment for Bell's palsy. In: Rubin L, ed. Reanimation of the Paralyzed Face: New Approaches. St. Louis: Mosby, 1977:201–203.
111. Stankiewicz JA. A review of the published data on steroids and idiopathic facial paralysis. Otol Head Neck Surg 1987; 97:481–486.
112. Morgenlander JC, Massey EW. Bell's palsy: ensuring the best possible outcome. Postgrad Med 1990; 88(5):157–164.
113. Britton BH. Present-day concepts of surgical treatment for Bell's palsy. In: Rubin L, ed. Reanimation of the Paralyzed Face: New Approaches. St. Louis: Mosby, 1977:204–210.
114. Inamura H, Aoyagi M, et al. Effects of aciclovir [sic] in Ramsay Hunt syndrome. Acta Otolaryngol (Stockh) 1988; 446(suppl):111–113.
115. Stafford W, Welch AR. The use of acyclovir in Ramsay Hunt syndrome. J Laryngol Otol 1986; 100:337–340.
116. Hall SJ, Kerr AG. Acyclovir in herpes zoster oticus. Lancet 1985; 8437:1103.
117. Uri N, Meyer W, et al. Herpes zoster oticus: treatment with acyclovir. Ann Otol Rhinol Laryngol 1992; 101:161–162.
118. Dickens JRE, Smith JT, Graham SS. Herpes zoster oticus: treatment with intravenous acyclovir. Laryngoscope 1988; 98:776–779.
119. Wood M, Johnson R, et al. A randomized trial of acyclovir for 7 days or 21 days with or without prednisolone for the treatment of acute herpes zoster. N Engl J Med 1994; 330:896–900.
120. Bean B, et al. Adverse effects of high-dose intravenous acyclovir in ambulatory patients with acute herpes zoster. J Infect Dis 1985; 2:362–365.
121. Rathore M, Friedman A, et al. Herpes zoster oticus. Am J Dis Child 1991; 145:722.
122. Jansen JKS, Lomo T, et al. Hyperinnervation of skeletal muscle fibers: dependence on muscle activity. Science 1973; 181:559–561.
123. Traavik T, et al. Peripheral facial palsy and coincidental cytomegalovirus infection or reactivation. Scand J Infect Dis 1983; 15:233–238.
124. Olsen K. Facial nerve paralysis. Postgrad Med 1984; 76:95–97,100–102,105.

125. Yalaburgi S, Mistry P. Bell's palsy—varicella zoster and meningitis. J Laryngol Otol 1977; 91(12):1073–1075.
126. Leeming R. Varicella-zoster virus and facial palsy. J Laryngol Otol 1976; 90(4):365–371.
127. Murthy VK, Sawhney IMS, et al. Isolated facial palsy in chickenpox. J Neurol Neurosurg Psychiatry 1984; 47:754–755.
128. Walters BNJ, Redman CWG. Bell's palsy and cytomegalovirus mononucleosis in pregnancy. J R Soc Med 1984; 429–430.
129. Terasawa K, Ichinose E, et al. Neurological complications in Kawasaki disease. Brain Dev 1983; 5:371–374.
130. Davis L, Sperry S. Bell's palsy and secondary syphilis: CSF spirochetes detected by immunofluorescence. Ann Neurol 1978; 4:378–380.
131. Krol TC, Mullen GM. Herpes zoster with facial paralysis. Arch Neurol 1980; 37:391–392.
132. Trigeminal zoster producing facial paralysis and postural hypotension. Br Med J 1976; 1(6002): 131–132.
133. Ernster J. Bilateral facial nerve paralysis associated with mycoplasma pneumonia infection. Ear Nose Throat J 1984; 63:585–590.
134. Economou P. Hemiparesis and Bell's palsy following brachial plexus herpes zoster. JAMA 1984; 252(8):1012.
135. Murphy M, Brenton D, et al. Locked-in syndrome caused by a solitary pontine abscess. J Neurol Neurosurg Psychiatry 1979; 42:1062–1065.
136. Weintraub M. Bilateral facial palsy—a rare presentation of infectious mononucleosis. Clin Pediatr 1977; 16(12):1158–1159.
137. Shoji H, Hirose K, et al. A case of facial diplegia following herpes zoster ophthalmicus. Eur Neurol 1980; 19:327–329.
138. Jain M, Khanijo S, Sharma N. Motor spastic paraplegia and unilateral infranuclear facial palsy complicating tetanus. Br Med J 1982; 285:477–478.
139. Verduijn P, Bleeker J. Secondary syphilis of the facial nerve. Arch Otolaryngol 1982; 108:382–384.
140. Bomholt A. Facial palsy in lymphocytic meningoradiculitis (Bannwarth's syndrome). Arch Otolaryngol 1984; 110:763–764.
141. Golding D. Bell's palsy and infectious mononucleosis. Lancet 1973; 2(829):621.
142. Alberti P, Biagioni E. Facial paralysis in children: a review of 150 cases. Laryngoscope 1972; 82(6): 1013–1020.
143. Duff TB. Parotitis, parotid abscess and facial palsy. J Laryngol Otol 1972; 86(2):161–165.
144. Grose C. Facial palsy and infectious mononucleosis. Arch Otolaryngol 1974; 99:309.
145. Martin G, Weintraub M. Brachial neuritis and seventh nerve palsy—a rare hazard of DPT vaccination. Clin Pediatr 1973; 12(8):506–507.
146. Shoji H, Hirose K, et al. A case of peripheral facial palsy following varicella. J Neurol 1975; 209: 149–150.
147. McGovern F. Facial paralysis. Arch Otolaryngol 1972; 96:92.
148. Michel R, Pope, Jr. T, Patterson C. Infectious mononucleosis, mastoiditis, and facial paralysis. Arch Otolaryngol 1975; 101:486–489.
149. Mishra M, Sinha BN. Facial palsy in tetanus. Br Med J 1972; 3(824):475–476.
150. Achari A. Facial palsy in tetanus. Br Med J 1973; 3(879):543–544.
151. Faden A. Neurological sequelae of malignant external otitis. Arch Neurol 1975; 32:204–205.
152. Pollack M, Grose C, Friend H. Measles associated with Bell [sic] palsy. Am J Dis Child 1975; 129:747.
153. Chandler JR. Pathogenesis and treatment of facial paralysis due to malignant external otitis. Ann Otol 1972; 81:648–658.
154. Chandler JR. Malignant external otitis and facial paralysis. Otolaryngol Clin North Am 1974; 7(2): 375–383.
155. Farquharson RG. Cephalic tetanus. Proc R Soc Med 1972; 65(10):875–876.
156. Grose C, Henle W, et al. Primary Epstein-Barr infections in acute neurologic disorders. N Engl J Med 1975:292(8):392–395.
157. McGovern F. Facial nerve paralysis in herpes oticus. Virg Med Monthly 1975; 102(8):609–613.

158. Jachuck SJ, et al. A brainstem syndrome associated with Mycoplasma pneumoniae infection—a report of two cases. Postgrad Med J 1975; 51:475–477.
159. Redston RH. The aetiology of Bell's palsy in relation to age. Med J Aust 1972; 2:81–82.
160. Caruso VG. Facial paralysis from Lyme disease. Otolaryngol Head Neck Surg 1985; 93:550–553.
161. Sheriff DS. Another cause of facial nerve palsy. Postgrad Med 1985; 77(5):54.
162. Kleiman MB, Passo MH. Incomplete Kawasaki disease with facial nerve paralysis and coronary artery involvement. Ped Inf Dis J 1988; 7(4):301–302.
163. DelSette M, Caponnetto C, et al. Unusual neurological manifestations of Lyme disease: a case report. Ital J Neurol Sci 1989; 10:455–456.
164. Klar A, Gross-Kieselstein E, et al. Bilateral Bell's palsy due to Mycoplasma pneumoniae infection. Israel J Med Sci 1985; 21(8):692–694.
165. Kamitsuka M, Feldman K, Richardson M. Facial paralysis associated with otitis media. Ped Inf Dis 1985; 4(6):682–684.
166. Henderson P, Baldone S. Facial nerve palsy secondary to acute otitis media. J Am Osteopath Assoc 1989; 89:207–210.
167. Einhaeupi K, Pfister HW. Facial palsy in Bannwarth's syndrome: a tick-borne spirochetosis. Arch Otolaryngol 1985; 111:557.
168. Asbrink E, Olsson I, et al. Facial palsy. Arch Otolaryngol 1985; 111:349.
169. Glasscock M, Pensak M, et al. Lyme disease: a cause of bilateral facial paralysis. Arch Otolaryngol 1985; 111:47–49.
170. Mohanaruban K, Fisher DJH. A combination of cranial and peripheral nerve palsies in infectious mononucleosis. Postgrad Med J 1986; 62:1129–1130.
171. Lambert PR, Ruth RA, Hodges AV. Meningitis and facial paresis. Arch Otolaryngol Head Neck Surg 1987; 113:1101–1103.
172. Jonsson L Stiernstedt G, Thomander L. Tick-borne Borrelia infection in patients with Bell's palsy. Arch Otolaryngol Head Neck Surg 1987; 113:303–306.
173. Andrews J, Abemayor E, et al. Parotitis and facial nerve dysfunction. Arch Otolaryngol Head Neck Surg 1989; 115:240–242.
174. Yaniv E, Avedillo H. Facial paralysis due to primary tuberculosis of the parotid gland. Int J Ped Otorhinolaryngol 1985; 9:195–196.
175. Takahashi H, Nakamura H, et al. Analysis of fifty cases of facial palsy due to otitis media. Arch Otorhinolaryngol 1985; 9:163–168.
176. Jagoda A, Riggio S, Burguieres T. Cephalic tetanus: a case report and review of the literature. Am J Emerg Med 1988; 6:128–130.
177. Krejcova H, Bojar M, et al. Otoneurological symptomatology in Lyme disease. Adv Oto-Rhino-Laryngol 1988; 42:210–212.
178. Watson MG, Murty GE. Lyme disease facial palsy. Br Med J 1989; 299:975.
179. Markby DP. Lyme disease facial palsy: differentiation from Bell's palsy. B Med J 1989; 299:605–606.
180. Andersson J, Sterner G. A 16-month-old boy with infectious mononucleosis, parotitis and Bell's palsy. Acta Paediatr Scand 1985; 74:629–632.
181. Clark JR, et al. Facial paralysis in Lyme disease. Laryngoscope 1985; 95:1341–1345.
182. Wiselka M, Nicholson K, et al. Acute infection with HIV associated with facial nerve palsy and neuralgia. J Infect 1987; 15:189–190.
183. Shone GR, Stewart S. Facial paralysis in parotitis. Br J Surg 1985; 72:902.
184. Premachandra DJ, Radcliffe G. Bilateral facial nerve palsy following secretory otitis media. J Laryngol Otol 1989; 103:685.
185. Cargnel A, Davoli C, et al. Case report: seventh cranial nerve paralysis with myokymia during acute co-infection with hepatitis B and delta viruses. J Med Virol 1988: 25:245–247.
186. Schielke E, Pfister HW, Einhäupl KM. Peripheral facial nerve palsy associated with HIV infection. Lancet 1989: 1(8637):553–554.
187. Belec L, Georges AJ, et al. Peripheral facial paralysis indicating HIV infection. Lancet 1988; 2(8625): 1421–1422.

188. Olsson I, Engervall K, et al. Tick-borne borreliosis and facial palsy. Acta Otolaryngol (Stockh) 1988; 105:100–107.
189. Bjerkhoel A, Carlsson M, Ohlsson J. Peripheral facial palsy caused by the Borrelia spirochete. Acta Otolaryngol (Stockh) 1989; 108:424–430.
190. Lopez-Lozano JJ, Garcia Merino JA, Liaño H. Bilateral facial paralysis secondary to trichinosis. Acta Neurol Scand 1988; 78:194–197.
191. Lewis DW, Clancy RR. Peripheral facial palsy. Acta Paediatr Scand 1986; 75:172–174.
192. Schon F, O'Dowd L, et al. Tetanus: delay in diagnosis in England and Wales. J Neurol Neurosurg Psychiatry 1994; 57:1006–1007.
193. Watanabe Y, Ikeda M, et al. A case report of facial nerve palsy associated with chickenpox. J Laryngol Otol 1994; 108:767–768.
194. Werra R. Bell's palsy and Lyme disease. Am Family Phys 1990; 41(4):1090.
195. Heininger U, Ries M, et al. Simultaneous palsy of facial and vestibular nerve in a child with Lyme borreliosis. Eur J Ped 1990; 149:781–782.
196. Lee PYC, Drysdale AJ. Tuberculous otitis media: a difficult diagnosis. J Laryngol Otol 1993; 107:339–341.
197. Edmond, Jr. C, Antoine G, et al. A case of facial diplegia associated with acute bilateral otitis media. Int J Pediatr Otorhinolaryngol 1990; 18:257–262.
198. Wilborn F, Schmidt C, et al. A potential role for human herpesvirus type 6 in nervous system disease. J Neuroimmunol 1994; 49:213–214.
199. Grundfast KM, Guarisco JL, et al. Diverse etiologies of facial paralysis in children. Int J Pediatr Otorhinolaryngol 1990; 19:223–239.
200. Halperin JJ, Golightly M, et al. Lyme borreliosis in Bell's palsy. Neurology 1992; 42:1268–1270.
201. Eggenberger ER. Facial palsy in Lyme disease. N Engl J Med 1993; 328(21):1571.
202. Ovesen J. Bilateral facial palsy caused by the Borrelia spirochete. Acta Otolaryngol (Stockh) 1992; 492(suppl):115–116.
203. Jacobsson M, Nylén O, Tjellström A. Acute otitis media and facial palsy in children. Acta Paediatr Scand 1990; 79:118–120.
204. Park MS, Lee HY, et al. Facial nerve paralysis associated with Kawasaki disease. Yonsei Med J 1991; 32(3):279–282.
205. Harker L, Pignatari S. Facial nerve paralysis secondary to chronic otitis media without cholesteatoma. Am J Otol 1992; 13(4):372–374.
206. Patey O, Ollivaud L, et al. Unusual neurologic manifestations occurring during Dengue fever infection. Am J Trop Med Hyg 1993; 48(6):793–802.
207. McCue J, Pepe J. A rare cause of facial nerve paralysis. Hosp Pract 1990; 25(5A):17.
208. Bance M, Rutka J. Speculation into the etiologic role of viruses inn the development of Bell's palsy and disorders of inner ear dysfunction: a case history and review of the literature. J Otolaryngol 1990; 19(1):46–49.
209. Rutter MJ, Currie AR, et al. Acute otitis media and facial palsy. NZ Med J 1992; 105(945):459.
210. Gallagher PG. Facial nerve paralysis and Kawasaki disease. Rev Infect Dis 1990; 12(3):403–405.
211. Orobello P. Congenital and acquired facial nerve paralysis in children. Otolarygnol Clin North Am 1991; 24(3):647–652.
212. Taylor L, Parsons-Smith G. Infectious mononucleosis, deafness, and facial paralysis. J Laryngol Otol 1969; 83(6):613–616.
213. Mendonca D. A case of infectious mononucleosis presenting with a bilateral facial palsy. J Laryngol Otol 1971; 85(9):981–982.
214. Beardwell A. Facial palsy due to mumps virus. Br J Clin Pract 1969; 23:37–38.
215. O'Duffy JD, Carney JA, Deodhar S. Behçet's disease: report of 10 cases, 3 with new manifestations. Ann Intern Med 1971; 75:561–570.
216. Vaz FA, Ulson CM, et al. Cervical adenitis due to acquired tuberculosis, with partial peripheral paralysis of the face in the newborn. Helv Paediatr Acta 1967; 22:572–578.
217. Fondu P, DeMeuter F. Facial palsy, a manifestation of acquired toxoplasmosis. Helv Paediatr Acta 1969; 24:208–211.

218. Korcyzn AD. Aetiology of Bell's palsy. Br Med J 1971; 4(785):491–492.
219. El-Ebiary HM. Facial paralysis: a clinical study of 580 cases. Rheum Phys Med 1971; 11:100–110.
220. Dinapoli RP, Thomas JE. Neurologic aspects of malignant external otitis: report of three cases. Mayo Clin Proc 1971; 46(5):339–344.
221. Goodwin MR. Complicated acute mastoiditis treated conservatively. NY State J Med 1969; 69: 594–598.
222. Blatt IM, Freeman JA. Bell's palsy II: pathogenetic mechanism of idiopathic peripheral facial paralysis. Transact Am Acad Ophthalmol Otolaryngol 1966; 70:381–397.
223. Rowland LP. Injury to cranial and peripheral nerves: seventh (facial) nerve. In: Rowland LP, ed. Merritt's Textbook of Neurology, 8th ed. Philadelphia: Lea and Febiger, 1989:422–425.

19

Poliomyelitis and Postpolio Syndrome

Robert M. Pascuzzi
Indiana University School of Medicine, Indianapolis, Indiana

INTRODUCTION

Although new cases of paralytic poliomyelitis are now rare in the United States, in some underdeveloped countries in which wild polio virus has not been eradicated, polio is a significant cause of paralytic illness. In the United States, as recently as the 1950s, poliomyelitis was a prominent cause of paralysis in children and adults. Even though polio has been largely eradicated, in some countries the survivors of polio infection have residual disabilities, and some have postpolio syndrome.

HISTORY

Poliomyelitis has been considered to be the last of the great childhood plagues. Paul (1) reviewed the early history of polio, citing examples from 3000 years ago depicted on Egyptian murals. Reports in the 1700s and 1800s described an illness tending to affect children and characterized by fever and residual paralysis, eventually referred to as infantile paralysis. Landmark work by Landsteiner and Popper in 1908 showed that paralytic polio was caused by an infectious virus that could be transmitted to monkeys (1). An understanding of the disease and the pursuit of a vaccine was provided by the work of Enders et al., who developed the capability of growing polio virus in tissue culture (2). The development of polio vaccines by Salk (3) and Sabin (4) represents a triumph of twentieth-century medical research, as well as an intriguing saga of science, social issues, politics, and dynamic individuals (5).

The name poliomyelitis derives from the Greek *polios*, meaning gray, reflecting the involvement of the anterior horn gray matter in the spinal cord.

PATHOPHYSIOLOGY

Poliomyelitis is a generalized viral infection with an affinity for lower motor neurons (6). The poliovirus is a single-stranded RNA enterovirus belonging to the picornavirus group (7). There are three polioviruses (numbered 1, 2, and 3), which have antigenic differences. The three types of poliovirus have been completely sequenced, their crystallographic appearance is known, and the cellular receptors have been identified (7). The poliovirus receptor is an integral membrane protein with structural features of the immunoglobulin superfamily of proteins (8). Poliovirus receptor is present in high concentration on lower motor neuron cell bodies in the spinal cord and brain stem. The route of entry of the poliovirus into the central nervous system (CNS) may be from the blood, or alternatively, it may be transported from the muscle through the peripheral nerve. In addition, Leon-Monzon et al. studied the poliovirus receptor on human muscle fiber, noting that the receptor is rapidly upregulated in muscle fibers undergoing degeneration and is located in the end-plate region (9,10). Therefore, poliovirus could bind to receptor located at the muscle endplate during the acute infection, travel transynaptically to the motor nerve terminal, and then through retrograde transport reach the anterior horn of the spinal cord. This theory offers an explanation for the association between intramuscular injections and poliomyelitis (so-called provocation paralysis; see below).

EPIDEMIOLOGY

The epidemiology of polio infection has been extensively reviewed by Horstmann (11). Prior to vaccines, the natural infection was widespread. Infection was endemic in regions having poor sanitation. Infants were exposed to the virus early and developed immunity. In infancy the illness was usually benign and only rarely produced paralysis. Endemic infection decreased in this century as a result of improved hygiene and sanitation in developed countries. Therefore, a large population of unexposed children and young adults became vulnerable to sporadic and epidemic infection. The poliovirus is extremely infectious but usually benign, with 90–95% of cases being asymptomatic. In 4–8% of cases there is a nonspecific viral syndrome. Only 1–2% of cases are associated with paralysis. The potential for paralysis increases with age. In children, paralysis occurs in 1 of 1000 cases compared with 1 of 75 in adults (11). The paralytic rate also varies with the virulence of the strain of poliovirus.

Wild poliovirus enters the body by the oral route, replicates in lymphoid tissue of the pharynx and ileum, and spreads regionally to lymphoid tissue. Viremia may follow, which is associated with a "minor illness" (see below). Viremia leads to infection of the CNS.

Poliovirus has a predilection of anterior horn cells. Suggested mechanisms for this specificity include the presence and density of poliovirus receptors on the cell's surface, and the spread of virus along nerve fiber pathways (12). The virus replicates within anterior horn cells, and these cells develop a reduced metabolic rate. Poliovirus titers increase in the CNS prior to paralysis. Oral and fecal shedding of virus occurs within 24 h of initial exposure. By 5 days close contacts also excrete the virus.

The pathological findings of acute paralytic polio consist of inflammation of meninges and anterior horn with loss of spinal and bulbar motor neurons (13). Less prominent abnormalities involve the cerebellar nuclei, reticular formation, thalamus, hypothalamus, cortical neurons, and dorsal horn.

CLINICAL PRESENTATION AND CLINICAL COURSE

Following initial exposure there is an incubation period of 1–5 days prior to the onset of the "minor illness," which is characterized by malaise, myalgias, and low-grade fever, usually lasting 1–3 days. These symptoms usually resolve spontaneously, but some patients proceed to develop more severe symptoms, labeled the "major illness" (11,14).

The "major illness," which begins 7–14 days after initial infection, is characterized by fever, headache, stiff neck, and back pain, typical for viral meningitis. These symptoms resolve spontaneously in about half of cases without further incident. In the remaining cases paralysis develops acutely or subacutely on the second to fifth day of the major illness, often with associated intense myalgia, shooting pain, and hyperesthesia. Asymmetrical weakness evolves over several hours to several days and involves legs more commonly than arms, with cranial muscles less often affected. Severe bulbar (oropharyngeal) weakness occurs in 10–15% of paralytic cases. Ophthalmoplegia is rare but is most likely to occur in cases with oropharyngeal involvement. Nystagmus may be present. Muscle atrophy appears within the first week or two of paralysis. Dysautonomia produces cardiac arrhythmias, blood pressure instability, and impaired bladder and bowel function. Sensory loss is uncommon. Mental status is relatively unaffected, although anxiety, confusion, and stupor may occur. Acute mortality is usually from respiratory or bulbar involvement. When paralysis occurs, about 10% die during the acute illness. Those who survive the acute illness usually regain function in partially paralyzed muscles. Roughly half gain full functional recovery, and the others possess long-term residual weakness, often in a single limb. Improvement begins in weeks and reaches a plateau by 6 months.

LABORATORY STUDIES

Cerebrospinal fluid (CSF) abnormalities are suggestive of inflammation as would be seen during viral meningitis or encephalitis (15). Pleocytosis, usually 20–300 white blood cells/mm^3, may initially be neutrophilic, but by 72 h becomes predominantly lymphocytic. The cell count is highest just prior to paralysis and drops within the first 2 or 3 weeks after the onset of weakness. The cerebrospinal fluid total protein concentration increases in the first few weeks, but typically does not exceed 200 mg/dl.

Nerve conduction studies are usually normal, although the compound muscle action potentials may have low amplitude (16). Needle examination shows a reduced number of voluntary motor unit potentials in the initial phase of paralysis, and fibrillation is present at about 3 weeks. In subsequent months, as the patient improves, the motor units become markedly enlarged ("giant motor units") reflecting the reinnervation of denervated muscle fibers. As reinnervation occurs, fibrillation largely disappears.

Poliovirus can be cultured from the stool in 90% of patients by 10 days. Demonstration of a rise in antibody titer to polio virus (or other enteroviruses) in convalescent serum may be helpful in confirming the diagnosis, especially in the minority of cases in which poliovirus is not cultured from the stool. Poliovirus is difficult to culture from spinal fluid.

DIFFERENTIAL DIAGNOSIS

The differential diagnosis includes the spectrum of disorders that produce acute or subacute paralysis. Guillain-Barré syndrome will usually present with a more symmetrical paralysis associated with a mild sensory disturbance, cytoalbuminological dissociation in the CSF, and slowing of motor and sensory nerve conduction velocities. Myasthenia gravis, botulism, and transverse myelitis can be distinguished on clinical, laboratory, and electrophysiological grounds. Myasthenia gravis usually presents with chronic fluctuating weakness involving ocular, bulbar, and limb muscles without clinical or laboratory evidence for viral meningitis. Botulism typically presents as acute descending paralysis beginning in the ocular and bulbar muscles. Botulism is associated with anticholinergic signs including large pupils, dry mouth, and constipation (ileus), and there are no spinal fluid abnormalities. Transverse myelitis typically presents with an acute symmetrical paraparesis or quadriparesis with associated inflammatory spinal fluid abnormalities. The presence of a discrete sensory level on the trunk and associated bladder and bowel disturbance distinguishes this condition from paralytic polio.

When considering polio as a diagnosis, the physician should carefully explore the patient's immunization history, including time and type of polio vaccination, recent travel history, and household contacts having recent vaccination. Stool culture for poliovirus will usually confirm the clinical suspicion. Abnormal spinal fluid, although nonspecific, will provide evidence for a meningomyelitis. Electrophysiological studies should help distinguish between polio, Guillain-Barré syndrome, myasthenia gravis, and other motor unit diseases. Acute and convalescent poliovirus antibody titers should be obtained, particularly if stool culture is normal and alternative diagnoses have been ruled out. Suspected cases should be reported to the State Board of Health and the Centers for Disease Control (CDC) in Atlanta. Patients with acute polio in the United States should be screened for immunodeficiency, particularly hypogammaglobulinemia.

TREATMENT

Management is largely supportive with particular emphasis on pulmonary stability, with a low threshold for intubation and mechanical ventilation, and observation in an intensive care setting. Criteria for intubation and mechanical ventilation include the following: forced vital capacity below 12 ml/kg, forced vital capacity in adults below 1 L, or significant subjective dyspnea. Early and aggressive physical and occupational therapy is indicated, along with optimal nutritional support and management of the common complications of immobility. Intense musculoskeletal pain during the acute illness should be treated with analgesics.

PREVENTION

During the polio epidemic in North America from 1952 to 1954, the incidence of new cases was 15 per 100,000. After the initial success of Salk's inactivated polio vaccine in the Francis field trial of 1954, the vaccine was approved for widespread use in the United States (17). Following extensive immunization, by 1963 the incidence of new cases dropped to 0.4 per 100,000. The last confirmed case of paralytic polio from domestic wild virus in the United States occurred in 1979 (CDC, personal communication). Domestic wild virus has been essentially eradicated from the United States and other developed countries as a result of widespread vaccination.

The inactivated polio vaccine (IPV) or Salk vaccine uses three antigenic types of poliovirus grown in cell culture and inactivated with formalin and is administered by injection. The Sabin trivalent oral poliomyelitis vaccine (TOPV) is attentuated live virus grown in cell culture.

The current polio vaccines are among the safest of all vaccines currently in use. An early vaccine incident in 1955 (referred to as the "Cutter incident") caused by inadequate inactivation of the virus in one lot of the Salk vaccine produced 55 cases of paralysis in 400,000 vaccinated individuals (18,19). The current Salk vaccine (IPV) has not been reported to cause paralytic polio.

Paralytic polio is a rare complication of the current oral vaccine. Nyowane et al. analyzed vaccine-associated paralytic polio in the United States from 1973 to 1984 and found that paralysis from TOPV occurred in one per 520,000 of the first vaccination doses compared with one per 12.3 million subsequent doses (20). More recent data from the CDC indicate that one case of paralytic polio occurs for every 2.5 million doses of TOPV in the United States; the greatest risk is from the initial dose, with paralysis occurring at a rate of one in every 700,000 doses distributed (21). Household and community contacts may all be exposed to TOPV and to the potential for paralytic polio. Most new cases of paralytic polio in developed countries (in which modern vaccination is used) are from exposure by recipients or their household contacts to the TOPV. Possible mechanisms for vaccine-associated paralysis include loss of attenuation of the live virus, genetic instability with viral mutation (particularly in the type 3 strain), and change in viral antigens.

The last confirmed case of paralytic polio from domestic wild-type virus in the United States occurred in 1979. Confirmation is based on isolation of poliovirus from stool and, using molecular methods, determining Type 1, 2, 3, and wild versus vaccine virus. Between 1980 and 1989 the CDC confirmed 80 cases of paralytic polio in the United States (about 8 per year) (21). Thirty cases occurred in the recipients of the vaccine; all had paralytic illness begin 4–30 days after vaccination. Another 32 were household contact cases occurring 4–60 days after the recipient's vaccination, and 4 were community contacts. In 14 patients there was a predisposing immunodeficiency, most often hypogammaglobulinemia (21). When stool culture, vaccination history, and serology do not support poliovirus infection, there may be a different virus such as coxsackievirus, echovirus, or other enteroviruses, producing the clinical picture of paralytic polio.

The World Health Organization is committed to the global eradication of polio by the year 2000. Wright et al (22) recently updated the progress of this program. Since 1974 when vaccination (including polio) in developing countries was estimated at less than 5%, immunization programs have been implemented to such an extent that in 1991, 85% of children worldwide were estimated to be receiving three doses of TOPV in the first year of life. Eradication of polio is more challenging than elimination of smallpox, since polio infection is usually asymptomatic and the virus is transmitted enterally, complicating case identification and containment. Smallpox vaccine is heat stable, single dose, and leaves an identifiable mark, but TOPV is heat labile, loses potency after one day at room temperature, and requires repeated doses for adequate effect.

Comprehensive immunization and surveillance programs in the Americas have produced a steady decline in stool specimens positive for wild poliovirus—only 15 cases of confirmed poliomyelitis were reported in the Americas in 1990 and no cases have been reported since 1991.

Worldwide immunization is estimated to have prevented 442,000 new cases of paralytic polio in 1990. Nonetheless, 116,000 new cases of paralytic polio occurred worldwide in 1990 because of inadequate immunization in developing countries, particularly in Africa, India, and Asia. TOPV is generally preferred over IPV because of low cost, ease of administration, superiority in conferring intestinal immunity, and ability to infect (and therefore immunize) household and community contacts. In countries with endemic poliomyelitis, TOPV is recommended at birth and at 6, 10, and 14 weeks of age (22). When a suspected case occurs, children under 5 years of age living in the area should receive a dose of TOPV with a follow-up dose 4–6 weeks later, regardless of their prior immunization status.

The immunogenicity and efficacy of TOPV have been questioned since occasional outbreaks of poliomyelitis occurred in developing countries in spite of high immunization rates (23). Seroconversion rates following vaccination have been variable. A World Health Organization survey of seroconversion in children receiving TOPV in 15 developing countries revealed 70–90% mean conversion rates for the three poliovirus types (23).

Even when widespread vaccination has taken place, occasional outbreaks have occurred. An outbreak in Taiwan occurred in 1980 in spite of a 90% vaccination rate with TOPV (24). Finland

Table 1 Recommendations in the United States for Poliomyelitis Vaccination (through 1996)

1. All immunologically normal infants and young adults up to age 18 years should receive one of the following schedules: (a) inactivated poliovirus vaccine (IPV) at ages 2 and 4 months, and trivalent oral polio virus (TOPV) at age 12–18 months, and at age 4–6 years; (b) IPV at ages 2 months, 4 months, 12–18 months, and 4–6 years; (c) TOPV at 2 months, 4 months, 6–18 months, and 4–6 years. While each of these schedules is acceptable, and parents and providers may choose among them, the ACIP routinely recommended schedule (a) (the sequential schedule).
2. People over age 18 years are not routinely vaccinated (many have been exposed earlier in life; the risk of paralysis from TOPV is greater in adults).
3. Immunocompromised children should receive (IPV).
4. Children with household contacts who are immunosuppressed should receive IPV.
5. Adults traveling to countries where polio is common:
   if previously vaccinated should receive an extra dose of whichever vaccine was originally used.
   if not previously vaccinated should receive IPV.

Source: Ref. 28.

was the site of a small epidemic in 1985, even though there was a nearly 100% IPV vaccination rate (25). In 1987 an epidemic occurred in adults in Israel due to changeover from TOPV to IPV (26).

Serial administration of both IPV and TOPV has been successful in Scandinavia and is being recommended in the United States beginning in 1997 (27,28).

Beginning in 1997, in order to decrease the occurrence of vaccine-associated paralytic poliomyelitis, the Advisory Committee on Immunization Practices has suggested a preferred sequential childhood schedule of two doses of IPV followed by two doses of TOPV, with the expectation of reducing the frequency of vaccine-associated paralysis by at least 50–75% (Table 1) (28). Individuals over age 18 in the United States are not routinely vaccinated, since many are likely to have been exposed earlier in life, and the risk of paralysis from the TOPV is higher in adults. If an unvaccinated adult is planning to travel to a region in which wild polio exists, then vaccination is advised using the IPV or, more recently, "enhanced potency" inactivated vaccine (E-IPV). Adults with prior vaccination who are traveling to countries where polio is common should get at least one dose of either TOPV (if they originally received this type of vaccination) or IPV. The E-IPV is also recommended for immunocompromised patients. Those children who have immunosuppressed household contacts should also receive E-IPV for their vaccination (28).

INTRAMUSCULAR INJECTIONS AND VACCINE-ASSOCIATED POLIOMYELITIS

Strebel et al. observed a strong association between multiple intramuscular injections and vaccine-associated paralytic poliomyelitis in Rumanian children (29). For decades it has been suggested (although poorly documented) that the limb or limbs most vigorously exercised or traumatized (including the use of IM shots) before or at the onset of poliomyelitis tend to be the limbs most severely paralyzed (so-called "provocation paralysis") (30,31). Illa et al. investigated the role of muscle and the participation of the poliovirus receptor in the transport of the poliovirus from muscle to motor neuron, noting the upregulation of receptors in muscle fibers undergoing degeneration (as might occur from IM injections or vigorous exercise) (9,10). Such an increase in receptors might explain the phenomenon of "provocation paralysis." The viremia that follows

TOPV may allow virus to enter and bind to motor end-plates of muscle bearing poliovirus receptors. The virus may travel transsynaptically from the end-plate region to intramuscular nerve terminals, and through retrograde transport to the regional anterior horn cells in the spinal cord (32).

NEUROLOGICAL SEQUELAE: THE POSTPOLIO SYNDROME

The National Health Survey estimated that 640,000 people living in the United States in 1987 had paralytic polio during the epidemics of the 1940s and 1950s (33). About 50% of these patients recovered completely, and the other 50% had residual weakness. All of these individuals are at risk for the postpolio syndrome. Several recent comprehensive reviews summarize the growing interest in postpolio syndrome (34–36).

HISTORY OF POSTPOLIO SYNDROME

In 1875 Raymond (37) presented a case of a 19-year-old with progressive limb weakness and atrophy superimposed on an illness, presumed to be polio, which occurred at age 6 years. Charcot analyzed the case and suggested that a previous disease of the spinal cord might produce susceptibility to later spinal dysfunction. Cornil and Lepine in 1875 described a patient with progressive weakness and atrophy at age 17 years, many years after acute poliomyelitis (38). Charcot speculated on the relationship between old polio and late progressive weakness.

Zilkha (39) from Guy's Hospital in London reviewed a series of patients with motor neuron disease at Queen's Square from 1948 to 1962, emphasizing those with a slow prolonged course. In 1962, he described 11 patients who had polio prior to age 6 years with residual weakness who developed new slowly progressive weakness 20–40 years later. Fasciculations were prominent. It is of interest that about half of those patients had extensor toe signs. He stated, "the subsequent development of disease of the motor neuron in those patients with a previous history of poliomyelitis, usually 25 years before, is related to the occurrence of that earlier disease" (39).

In 1969 Campbell et al. (40) reported five patients with late progressive weakness occurring about four decades after paralytic polio. They emphasized the relatively benign clinical course and frequent skeletal deformities.

In 1972 Mulder et al. (41) from the Mayo Clinic examined the question of whether "late progression of poliomyelitis" is "forme fruste amyotrophic lateral sclerosis" by reviewing the cases of 34 patients who had a remote history of polio, partial recovery of function, at least 10 years of stability, and subsequent progressive neuromuscular weakness. The very slow rate of progression differentiated these patients from those with ALS, but the authors suggested that ALS could be caused by an insult (viral) early in life with manifestations of motor impairment three to four decades later.

Anderson et al. (42) investigated loss of ambulation in nine patients with old polio, emphasizing frequent falls, recurrent joint pain, and benefits of bracing.

CLINICAL FEATURES OF POSTPOLIO SYNDROME

The reports cited above delineate the principal features of the postpolio syndrome: slowly progressive weakness and atrophy beginning two to four decades after paralytic polio, fatigue and decreased endurance, and musculoskeletal pain (39–42).

The late development of progressive weakness and atrophy has been called postpoliomyelitis progressive muscular atrophy (PPMA) by Dalakas et al. (43,44). Patients with PPMA commonly experience muscle cramps, myalgias, and fasciculations. Weakness in the postpolio syndrome tends to involve those muscles with the greatest residual weakness from the original illness. On occasion, new, progressive weakness is reported in muscles that were previously spared.

Sonies and Dalakas (45) studied bulbar function in 32 patients with postpolio syndrome, 14 of whom had new symptoms of dysphagia. Only 12 had bulbar involvement in the original illness. All but one of 32 patients had oropharyngeal dysfunction shown by oral motor examination, fluoroscopy, or ultrasound studies. Four patients who had serial studies demonstrated deterioration over several years. These observations suggest that patients with postpolio syndrome frequently have symptomatic or asymptomatic oropharyngeal dysfunction that is potentially progressive. Periodic assessment of swallowing in postpolio patients may help to identify those with progressive bulbar dysfunction who are at risk for aspiration. Management should involve simple changes in swallowing position, use of mechanical soft diet, and consultation with a therapist familiar with neuromuscular dysphagia (45).

Late progressive symptoms from pulmonary insufficiency may occur. Sleep apnea can take several forms. Central apnea is presumed to be from residual dysfunction of brain-stem neurons, and obstructive apnea may be from oropharyngeal weakness or musculoskeletal deformities. Nocturnal hypoventilation from residual or new diaphragm weakness may also occur (46).

The distribution and frequency of late progressive symptoms were surveyed by Codd et al. (47), who reported that 22% of Olmsted County polio patients complained of new symptoms. Among those having new symptoms, 70% reported new weakness, 66% joint discomfort, 46% muscle pain, and 50% cramps. Symptoms tended to be associated with exertion. Windebank et al. (48) selected 50 subjects from 247 survivors of old polio in Olmsted County for comprehensive prospective evaluation of history, examination, and electrophysiology. Of these 50 subjects, 64% had new muscle pain, weakness, or fatigue, and in 18% these symptoms led to a change in lifestyle or activity. New complaints were not related to present age or interval since polio. Electrophysiological studies were similar in patients with and those without new symptoms. New symptoms were usually in a lower limb and in limbs most severely affected by the original paralytic illness. Elevation of creatine kinase was observed in some subjects with new symptoms. Those 50 patients were followed prospectively for 5 years with serial clinical and electrophysiological studies; no evidence for progressive muscle weakness was observed, suggesting that progressive muscle atrophy and weakness may be uncommon, and that the majority of postpolio symptoms result from degenerative joint disease, mechanical causes, and other factors (48a).

The frequency of late progression among survivors of acute polio is unclear. Schmutzhard et al. (49) found that only 16% of 50 patients had evidence of late progressive symptoms 28–32 years after the acute illness. Codd et al. (47) found that 22% complained of new symptoms, whereas Dalakas and Illa (44) and Windebank et al. (48) noted new symptoms in the majority of their patients.

Dalakas et al. (43) observed several factors to be associated with earlier age of onset of postpolio syndrome, including severity of the acute paralytic disease, older age at time of the acute illness, and severity of residual weakness.

New weakness progresses at an extremely slow rate. Using the Medical Research Council scale, Dalakas et al. (43) estimated a loss of neuromuscular function of about 1% per year.

Neurological examination shows lower motor neuron deficits including asymmetrical atrophy, fasciculations, and weakness. Sensation is normal. Although extensor toe signs are occasionally reported, their presence should trigger an aggressive search for alternative diagnoses.

Laboratory studies reveal occasional elevation of creatine kinase. Most reports have noted relatively normal spinal fluid, but Dalakas detected oligoclonal immunoglobulin G (IgG) bands in three of five patients with PPMA (50). Nerve conduction studies are normal except for low amplitude of the motor responses. Electromyography (EMG) shows giant voluntary motor unit potentials and occasional mild fibrillation. The muscle biopsy shows nonspecific chronic neurogenic changes, most notably fiber type grouping. Perimysial and perivascular lymphocytic infiltration are occasionally present (43).

Caution is advised in making the diagnosis of postpolio syndrome. Any patient having a history of old polio who develops new neurological symptoms should be thoroughly evaluated for causes other than postpolio syndrome. Postpolio syndrome should be a diagnosis of exclusion after ruling out other motor unit diseases. Patients with old polio who develop new neuromuscular symptoms from peripheral neuropathy, myositis, myasthenia gravis, and spinal cord tumor can mimic the clinical picture of postpolio syndrome. I have not seen patients who later developed ALS, although this is in the differential diagnosis (41). Patients with old polio are susceptible to development of entrapment neuropathies, particularly carpal tunnel syndrome, ulnar neuropathy at the elbow, and peroneal neuropathy. Degenerative joint disease, nonspecific effects of aging, and depression may be factors in functional decline in patients with old polio. Some patients overreact to the publicity surrounding postpolio syndrome, and present with anxiety and psychosomatic symptoms.

MANAGEMENT

Therapy is best individualized according to the patient's particular symptoms. Patient education, emphasizing the tendency for symptoms to be chronic with extremely slow progression, will provide reassurance and a realistic outlook. Many patients with old polio have the mistaken notion that they will inevitably develop new, progressive symptoms with a high likelihood of rapidly progressive disability. Those patients with pain and weakness due to degenerative joint disease should be evaluated by a specialist in physical medicine and rehabilitation in order to plan an optimal program of physical therapy, occupational therapy, and, on occasion, orthopedic surgery. Bracing and reduced workload will help some patients. Medication for pain of degenerative arthritis and myalgia should be considered. A neurologist should follow the patient periodically to monitor symptoms and function and should remain alert to the possibility of focal entrapment neuropathies, localized joint deterioration, oropharyngeal and pulmonary insufficiency, and unrelated neurological disease.

One small study reported reduction in subjective fatigue in eight of nine patients with postpolio syndrome following treatment with amantadine 100 mg twice daily (51). Subsequently, Stein et al. performed a 6-week prospective placebo-controlled, double-blind study of amantadine on fatigue, which showed no significant difference compared with placebo (52). Trojan and Cashman suggested the benefit of cholinesterase inhibitors in the management of fatigue (53). High-dose prednisone has been tested and shown to be of no benefit (54).

PATHOGENESIS

The mechanism of late progressive weakness is unknown, but several hypotheses have been formulated. Cashman et al. prospectively studied clinical features, EMG, and muscle histological appearances in 18 patients with old polio, 13 of whom had new symptoms (55). Those with new symptoms reported new atrophy (9 of 13) and fatigue (10 of 13). Old denervation was present on EMG and muscle biopsy, but "active denervation" on EMG (fibrillation or abnormal jitter on single fiber EMG) and biopsy findings of active denervation were present in nearly all patients, regardless of the presence or absence of new symptoms. They concluded that extensive reinnervation of denervated muscle fibers is followed by late denervation of reinnervated fibers (55).

Electrophysiological studies by Wiechers and Hubbell (56) suggest that in postpolio syndrome motor neurons are unstable, with constant denervation and repair of the motor unit. As the result of such observations, Dalakas et al. have proposed that chronic overwork by surviving motor neurons produces an inability to maintain the metabolic demands of their distal nerve terminals, leading to late denervation and progressive weakness (44).

Since varicella zoster and other neurotropic viruses can exist in a dormant state in the nervous system for many years prior to reactivation, it is logical to consider a similar mechanism in postpolio syndrome. There is no direct evidence that poliovirus stays dormant in the human CNS and later reactivates. Several observations provide indirect evidence that either inflammation or infection may occur in some patients with late progression. Pezeshkpour and Dalakas (57) studied long-term changes in the spinal cord of eight patients with old polio, five with stable deficits, and three with new progressive symptoms. All polio cases showed loss of motor neurons, atrophic motor neurons, reactive gliosis, and, more surprisingly, mild to moderate parenchymal and perivascular inflammation. These findings were present in the spinal cord and in patients with and without late progressive symptoms.

Although Dalakas (50) found oligoclonal IgG bands in spinal fluid from three of five patients, others have not. Salazar-Gruesco et al. (58) performed isoelectric focusing studies on serum and spinal fluid from 21 patients with old polio, 13 of whom had late progression, and found none with oligoclonal IgG bands. They found polyclonal antipolio virus antibody in serum and spinal fluid from 19 patients with old polio, but in only one was there evidence for intrathecal antibody production. Sharief et al. (59) reported oligoclonal IgM bands directed against poliovirus in spinal fluid in 58% of 36 patients with postpolio syndrome; they found no such bands in 67 controls (including 13 patients with old polio without postpolio syndrome and 18 with ALS). Quantitative studies suggested increased intrathecal production of IgM antibodies to poliovirus only in patients with postpolio syndrome. Such observations have yet to be confirmed.

As with other late-onset progressive neurological disorders, the concept of a normal death rate of neurons superimposed on a depleted pool of viable cells (in this case from remote polio infection) can be applied to PPMA. Some studies suggest that age-related reduction in spinal cord motor neurons does not become significant until the seventh decade (and would therefore not explain symptoms that progress at younger ages) (60). Kawamura et al. (61, 62), who counted the number of anterior horn cells and motor axons at different levels in normal human spinal cord, suggested that age-related reduction begins by the third decade. They estimated a reduction rate of about 5–6% per decade (close to the estimate by Dalakas of a 1% per year reduction in neuromuscular function) (43). It remains plausible that age-related attrition of motor neurons is a significant factor in late progressive weakness, at least in some patients.

Fetell et al. (63) suggested the existence of a "benign" syndrome of cramps and fasciculations beginning decades after poliomyelitis, without progressive weakness and atrophy (for at least 3 years of observation).

The relationship between poliomyelitis and subsequent development of ALS has been disputed for several decades (40). Using data from the Mayo Clinic, Armon et al. (64) explored the relationship between old polio and subsequent development of ALS. They concluded that ALS occurred less frequently in polio patients, raising the possibility of a protective effect of polio infection. Presently there is no firm evidence that old polio infection predisposes the patient to subsequent development of ALS.

By remaining assiduous with worldwide vaccination programs, and vigilant in the evaluation of patients with acute flaccid paralysis, wild-type poliomyelitis will be completely eliminated over the next few years. This triumph of twentieth century medical research wil represent the first global eradication of a neurological disorder in the history of humankind!

ACKNOWLEDGMENT

Mrs. Linda Hagan assisted with the preparation of this manuscript.

REFERENCES

1. Paul JR. A History of Poliomyelitis. New Haven, CT: Yale University Press, 1971.
2. Enders JR, Weller TH, Robbins FC. Cultivation of the Lansing strain of poliomyelitis virus in cultures of various human embryonic tissues. Science 1949; 109:85–87.
3. Salk JE, Bennett BL, Lewis LJ, et al. Studies in human subjects on active immunization against poliomyelitis. I. A preliminary report of experiments in progress. JAMA 1953; 151:1081.
4. Sabin AB. Properties and behavior of orally administered attenuated poliovirus vaccine. JAMA 1957; 164:1216–1223.
5. Smith, JS. Patenting the Sun: Polio and the Salk Vaccine. New York: W. Morrow, 1990.
6. Bodian D. Emerging concept of poliomyelitis infection. Science 1955; 12:105–108.
7. Brown RH. Molecular biology of poliovirus—a review. In: Munsat TL, ed. Post-polio Syndrome. Boston: Butterworth-Heinemann, 1991:9–21.
8. Mendelsohn CL, Wimmer E, Racaniello VR. Cellular receptor for poliovirus: molecular cloning, nucleotide sequence, and expression of a new member of the immunoglobulin superfamily. Cell 1989; 56:855–865.
9. Leon-Monzon ME, Illa I, Dalakas MC. Expression of poliovirus receptor in human spinal cord and muscle. Ann NY Acad Sci 1995; 753:48–57.
10. Illa I, Leon-Monzon M, Agboatwalla M, et al. Role of the muscle in acute poliomyelitis infection. Ann NY Acad Sci 1995; 753:58–66.
11. Horstmann DM. Epidemiology of poliomyelitis and allied diseases 1963. Yale J Biol Med 1963; 36: 5–26.
12. Brown RH, Johnson D, Ogonowski M, Weiner HL. Type 1 human poliovirus binds to human synaptosomes. Ann Neurol 1987; 21:64–70.
13. Bodian D. Poliomyelitis: pathologic anatomy. In: Poliomyelitis: Papers and Discussions Presented at the First International Poliomyelitis Conference. Philadelphia: Lippincott, 1949:62–84.
14. Horstman DM. Clinical aspects of polio. Am J Med 1945; 6:592–605.
15. Merritt HH, Fremont-Smith F. The Cerebrospinal Fluid. Philadelphia: WB Saunders, 1937:130–134.
16. So Yt, Olney RK. AAEM case report #23: acute paralytic poliomyelitis. Muscle Nerve 1991; 14:1159–1164.
17. Francis TM, Korns RF, Voight RB, et al. An evaluation of the 1954 poliomyelitis vaccine trials [summary report]. Am J Public Health 1955; 45(5,part 2):1–63.
18. Nathanson N, Langmuir AD. The Cutter incident: poliomyelitis following formaldehyde-inactivated poliovirus vaccination in the United States during the spring of 1955. I. Background. Am J Hyg 1963; 78:16–28.
19. Nathanson N, Langmuir AD. The Cutter incident: poliomyelitis following formaldehyde-inactivated poliovirus vaccination in the United States during the spring of 1955. II. Relationship of poliomyelitis to Cutter vaccine. Am J Hyg 1963; 78:20–60.
20. Nyowane BM, Wassilak SGF, Orenstein WA, et al. Vaccine-associated paralytic poliomyelitis. United States: 1973 through 1984. JAMA 1987; 257:1335–1340.
21. Strebel PM, Sutter RW, Cochi SL, et al. Epidemiology of poliomyelitis in the United States one decade after the last reported case of indigenous wild virus-associated disease. Clin Infect Dis 1992; 14: 568–579.
22. Wright PF, Kim-Farley RJ, DeQuadros CA, et al. Strategies for the global eradication of poliomyelitis by the year 2000. N Engl J Med 1991; 325:1774–1779.
23. Patriarca PA, Wright PF, John TJ. Factors affecting the immunogenicity of oral poliovirus vaccine in developing countries: review. Rev Infect Dis 1991; 13:926–930.
24. Kim-Farley RJ, Rutherford G, Lichfield P, et al. Outbreak of paralytic poliomyelitis, Taiwan. Lancet 1984; 888:1322–1324.

25. Hovi T, Houvilainen A, Kuronen T, et al. Outbreak of paralytic poliomyelitis in Finland: widespread circulation of antigenically altered poliovirus type 3 in a vaccinated population. Lancet 1986; 2:1427–1432.
26. Poliomyelitis—Israel. MMWR 1988; 37:624–625.
27. McBean AM, Modlin JF. Rationale for the sequential use of inactivated poliovirus vaccine and live attenuated poliovirus vaccine for routine poliomyelitis immunization in the United States. Ped Infect Dis J 1987; 6:881–887.
28. Update on adult immunization. Recommendations of the Immunization Practices Advisory Committee (ACIP). MMWR 1997; 46(2):35–39.
29. Strebel PM, Ion-Nedelcu N, Baughman, AL et al. Intramuscular injections within 30 days of immunization with oral poliovirus vaccine—a risk factor for vaccine-associated paralytic poliomyelitis. N Engl J Med 1995; 332:500–506.
30. Ross RT. Letter to the editor. N Engl J Med 1995; 333(1):63.
31. Sabin AB. Pathogenesis of poliomyelitis infection: Reappraisal in the light of new data. Science 1956; 243:1450–1455.
32. Dalakas MC, Illa, I, Leon-Monzon M. Intramuscular injections and vaccine-associated poliomyelitis. N Engl J Med 1995; 333:62.
33. National Health Survey. Prevalence of Selected Impairments (series 10). Washington, DC: U.S. Department of Health and Human Services 1981; 134:5.
34. Halstead LS, Wiechers DO, eds. Research and clinical aspects of the late effects of poliomyelitis. Birth Defects 1987; 23(4).
35. Munsat TL. Post-polio syndrome. In: Munsat TL, ed. Post-Polio Syndrome. Boston: Butterworth-Heinemann, 1991.
36. Dalakas MC, Bartfeld H, Kurland LT, eds: The post-polio syndrome: advances in the pathogenesis and treatment. Ann NY Acad Sci 1995; 753.
37. Raymond M. Paralysie essentielle de l'enfance, atrophy musculaire consecutive. C R Soc Biol 1875; 27:158.
38. Cornil V, Lepine R. Sur un cas de paralysie generale spinale anterieure subaigue, suivi d'autopsie. Gaz Med Paris 1875; 4:127–129.
39. Zilkha KJ. Discussion on motor neurone disease. Proc R Soc Med 1962; 55:1028–1029.
40. Campbell AMG, Williams ER, Pearce J. Late motor neuron degeneration following poliomyelitis. Neurology 1969; 19:1101–1106.
41. Mulder DW, Rosenbaum RA, Layton DD. Late progression of poliomyelitis or forme fruste amyotrophic lateral sclerosis? Mayo Clin Proc 1972; 47:756–761.
42. Anderson AD, Levine SA, Gellert H. Loss of ambulatory ability in patients with old anterior poliomyelitis. Lancet 1972; 2:1061–1063.
43. Dalakas MC, Elder G, Hallet M, et al. A long-term follow-up study of patients with post-poliomyelitis neuromuscular symptoms. N Engl J Med 1986; 314:959–963.
44. Dalakas M, Illa I. Post-polio syndrome: concepts in clinical diagnosis, pathogenesis, and etiology. Adv Neurol 1991; 56:495–511.
45. Sonies BC, Dalakas MC. Dysphagia in patients with post-polio syndrome. N Engl J Med 1991; 324:1162–1167.
46. Fisher DA. Sleep-disordered breathing as a late effect of poliomyelitis. Birth Defects 1978; 23:115–120.
47. Codd MB, Mulder DW, Kurland LT, et al. Poliomyelitis in Rochester, Minnesota, 1935-1955: epidemiology and long-term sequelae: a preliminary report. In: Halstead LS, Wiechers DO, eds. Late Effects of Poliomyelitis. Miami: Symposia Foundation, 1985:121–134.
48. Windebank AJ, Litchy WJ, Daube JR, et al. Late effects of paralytic poliomyelitis in Olmsted County, Minnesota. Neurology 1991; 41:501–507.
48a. Windebank AJ, Litchy WJ, Daube JR, Iverson RA. Lack of progression of neurological deficit in survivors of paralytic polio: A five-year prospective population-based study. Neurology 1996; 46:80–84.
49. Schmutzhard E, Kraft S, Berek K, et al. Letter to the editor. N Engl J Med 1991; 325:1108.
50. Dalakas MC. New neuromuscular symptoms in patients with old poliomyelitis: a three-year follow-up study. Eur Neurol 1986; 25:381–387.

51. Dunn MG. Post-polio fatigue treated with amantadine. Arch Neurol 1991; 48:570.
52. Stein DP, Dambrosia JM, Dalakas MC. A double-blind, placebo-controlled trial of amantadine for the treatment of fatigue in patients with the post-polio syndrome. Ann NY Acad Sci 1995; 753:296–302.
53. Trojan DA, Cashman Neil R. Anticholinesterases in post-polio syndrome. Ann NY Acad Sci 1995; 753:285–295.
54. Dinsmore S, Dambrosia J, Dalakas MC. A double-blind, placebo-controlled trial of high-dose prednisone for the treatment of post-poliomyelitis syndrome. Ann NY Acad Sci 1995; 753:303–313.
55. Cashman NR, Maselli R, Wollmann RL, et al. Late denervation in patients with antecedent paralytic poliomyelitis. N Engl J Med 1987; 317:7–12.
56. Wiechers DO, Hubbell SL. Late changes in the motor unit after acute poliomyelitis. Muscle Nerve 1981; 4:524–528.
57. Pezeshkpour GH, Dalakas MC. Long-term changes in the spinal cords of patients with old poliomyelitis. Arch Neurol 1988; 45:505–508.
58. Salazar-Gruesco EF, Grimaldi LME, Roos RP, et al. Isoelectric focusing studies of serum and cerebrospinal fluid in patients with antecedent poliomyelitis. Ann Neurol 1989; 26:709–713.
59. Sharief MK, Hentges R, Ciardi M. Intrathecal immune response in patients with the post-polio syndrome. N Engl J Med 1991; 325:749–756.
60. Tomlinson BE, Irving D. The numbers of limb motor neurons in the human lumbosacral cord throughout life. J Neurol Sci 1977; 34:213–219.
61. Kawamura Y, Okazaki H, O'Brien P, Dyck PJ. Lumbar motor neurons of man: 1) Number of diameter histogram of alpha and gamma axons of ventral root. J Neuropathol Exp Neurol 1977; 36:853–860.
62. Kawamura Y, O'Brien P, Okazaki H, Dyck PJ. Lumbar motor neurons of man II: The number and diameter distribution of large and intermediate diameter cytons in "motorneuron columns" of spinal cord of man. J Neuropathol Exp Neurol 1977; 36:861–870.
63. Fetell MR, Smallberg G, Lewis LD, et al. A benign motor neuron disorder: delayed cramps and fasciculation after poliomyelitis or myelitis. Ann Neurol 1982; 11:423–427.
64. Armon C, Daube JR, Windebank AJ, Kurland LT. How frequently does classic amyotrophic lateral sclerosis develop in survivors of poliomyelitis? Neurology 1990; 40:172–174.

20

Guillain-Barré Syndrome

Robert M. Pascuzzi
Indiana University School of Medicine, Indianapolis, Indiana

INTRODUCTION

Guillain-Barré syndrome (GBS) is considered to be the prototype "postinfectious" neurological disorder. The majority of patients describe an antecedent febrile illness, followed in days or weeks by the development of ascending paralysis, which appears to be on the basis of an acute inflammatory peripheral neuropathy. Although most skilled neurologists recognize GBS when they see it, the disorder is heterogeneous and diverse in its antecedent events, clinical presentations, and natural course. Even the name is diverse, with GBS, Landry–Guillain-Barré–Strohl syndrome, acute inflammatory demyelinating polyradiculoneuropathy (AIDP), and acute inflammatory neuropathy all being synonymous.

HISTORY

Octave Landry is credited with the earliest description of what has come to be recognized as Guillain-Barré syndrome (1). In 1859 Landry reported a condition, which he called "acute ascending paralysis," describing a patient who had a febrile illness in the springtime followed by the development of sensory symptoms within 2 months. One month later the patient developed subacute progressive inability to walk (due to leg weakness), respiratory failure, and death. Landry pointed out that bowel and bladder function were spared, that sensory involvement was mild, and that muscles would respond to faradic electrical stimulation. The patient had an autopsy, but this apparently did not include the peripheral nerves. Landry reviewed four other cases from his own experience, and five from the medical literature. He emphasized the absence of central nervous system symptoms or signs, the occasional presence of muscle cramps, occasional relapsing course, and the tendency for a favorable outcome. He also noted that two of the cases occurred after an acute illness, two were associated with menstrual irregularities, one was postpartum, and one possibly associated with syphilis. Westfall, in 1876, referred to this condition as "Landry's ascending paralysis."

Then, in 1916, Guillain, Barré, and Strohl reported two soldiers who developed an acute paralysis associated with loss of muscle stretch reflexes (2). They emphasized the presence of elevated cerebrospinal fluid (CSF) protein concentration with a normal cell count (albumino-cytological dissociation). Their report did not recognize Landry's prior observations. Guillain, Barré, and Strohl stated in their original paper that the illness:

> is characterized by motor difficulties, loss of the deep tendon reflexes with preservation of cutaneous reflexes, paresthesias with slight impairment of objective sensation, muscle tenderness, slight alteration in nerve conduction and electromyographic patterns, and a remarkable increase in cerebrospinal fluid albumin in the absence of a cellular reaction (albumino-cytologic dissociation).

While the general clinical observations are attributed to Guillain and Barré, Andre Strohl was probably responsible for the electrophysiological aspects. Guillain and Barré further developed their concept of the disease in subsequent publications including the text *Travaux Neurologiques DeGuerre* in 1920 (3). Strohl's name was largely eliminated in the subsequent publications by Guillain and Barré.

Death from respiratory failure remained a common outcome until the late 1940s when the development of intensive care units and mechanical ventilation allowed for an overall reduction in mortality from GBS.

Additional landmarks in clinical thinking on Guillain-Barré syndrome include the observation by C. Miller Fisher of a variant associated with ophthalmoplegia, ataxia, and areflexia published in 1956 (4).

PATHOPHYSIOLOGY

In 1949 the classic clinical pathological correlations were first reported by Haymaker and Kernohan (5). In 50 cases of what was called "Landry-Guillain-Barré syndrome" they noted predominant inflammatory abnormalities in the anterior spinal roots. Since inflammatory cells were not present in more distal segments of peripheral nerves until late in the illness, they described the disorder as a "polyradiculoneuropathy." The subsequent seminal neuropathological study by Asbury et al. in 1969 described findings in 19 patients, noting abundant lymphocytic infiltration in spinal roots and nerves, leading them to conclude that "the pathologic hallmark of idiopathic polyneuritis is a perivascular mononuclear inflammatory infiltrate" (6).

INFLAMMATORY DEMYELINATING NEUROPATHY

The pathology is classically that of a mononuclear inflammatory infiltrate in the endoneurium and myelin sheath. Patchy segmental multifocal demyelination is present along peripheral nerves, including nerve roots, while the axons themselves are relatively spared except in more severe cases. Inflammatory infiltrates are comprised of lymphocytes, monocytes, and occasional plasma cells and tend to be perivascular. Less commonly, polymorphonuclear leukocytes are seen. The abnormalites are prominent around ventral roots and in the plexus and proximal nerve trunks, but in some cases are present to an equal or greater extent distally along peripheral nerves. Similar inflammatory abnormalities can also be seen in dorsal roots and autonomic ganglia. In occasional patients there is axonal degeneration; in such cases, degeneration of anterior horn cells and dorsal root ganglia cells can be present, suggesting chromatolysis. While most of the pathology is found in the peripheral nervous system, occasional case reports demonstrate perivascular inflammation in the central nervous system. A few weeks after the onset of demyelination, Schwann cells are noted to proliferate. Several weeks later, as inflammation resolves, remyelination becomes evident.

Animal models resembling GBS were developed as early as 1955 by Waksman and Adams (7). Experimental allergic neuritis (EAN) depends on the sensitivity of the P2 protein of peripheral nerve myelin and closely resembles human GBS in terms of clinical, electrophysiological, and pathological features. However, in humans there is no clear evidence that the primary inflammatory attack is directed at the P2 protein (8,9). A second animal model, galactocerebroside neuritis, involving antibodies against galactocerebroside, has been developed in rabbits. This animal model is not as similar pathologically as EAN, since the cellular component of the nerve attack is not demonstrable. In addition, antigalactocerebroside antibodies are not present in human GBS.

Clearly, GBS is an inflammatory or immune-mediated condition. While most of the pathological observations have emphasized lymphocyte-mediated delayed hypersensitivity as a possible mechanism, there is also evidence to suggest the role of circulating autoantibodies directed against the myelin sheath (8–10). Perhaps GBS is a syndrome with a variety of immunological mechanisms to account for an acute or subacute peripheral neuropathy.

Campylobacter jejuni INFECTION, GBS, AND AXONAL GBS

In 1984 Kaldor and Speed reported serological evidence for *Campylobacter jejuni* infection in 38% of a group of GBS patients from Australia (11). Subsequent reports supported this association, including that of Vriesendorp et al. (12), in which 15% of 58 GBS patients showed evidence of recent *Campylobacter* infection. Enders et al. (13) noted a similar association. Rees and Hughes (14) found *Campylobacter jejuni* in stool samples of 11% of GBS patients, along with serological abnormalities in an additional 5 of 36 patients. Of the 25% of patients overall who had either stool culture or serological evidence for *Campylobacter* infection, most had experienced diarrhea as an antecedent illness. In these series, there was a tendency for patients to have predominantly an axonal neuropathy as opposed to a demyelinating neuropathy, as well as the presence of IgG anti-GM1 ganglioside antibodies.

While GBS is typically a demyelinating neuropathy, there is a subgroup of patients having clinical, electrophysiological, and pathological features indicating primarily an axonal injury, as opposed to loss of the myelin sheath. Feasby et al. in 1986 noted a subgroup of GBS patients who had electrophysiological findings of axonal degeneration, usually with severe paralysis and relatively slow recovery, and pathological changes in two cases indicating axonal degeneration without demyelination, and called this variant "axonal GBS" (15,16). There has been disagreement about whether this represents an axonal variant of GBS or whether it represents a truly distinct type of peripheral neuropathy.

Griffin et al. reported four patients who died 7–60 days after the onset of clinically diagnosed GBS (17). Two of these patients had serological evidence for recent *Campylobacter jejuni* infection. Autopsy findings in three patients studied 7–18 days after onset of symptoms showed ongoing Wallerian degeneration of ventral and dorsal root fibers and also peripheral nerves with relatively mild demyelination or lymphocytic infiltration. Macrophages were present in the periaxonal space of myelinated internodes, and occasional intraaxonal macrophages were present as well. The patients studied 60 days after the onset of symptoms showed extensive loss of large fibers in roots and peripheral nerves, and only mild demyelination and remyelination. These carefully studied cases confirm that GBS, as defined clinically, can be associated with a severe sensorimotor neuropathy in which the predominant lesion involves axons of motor and sensory fibers, and that an axonal form of GBS can follow *Campylobacter jejuni* infection (17–19). A pure motor acute axonal neuropathy, a frequent cause of paralysis in China, has also been associated with antiganglioside antibodies (19,20).

One theory for the association between *Campylobacter* infection and GBS is based on the lipopolysaccharide coat, which is rich in glycoconjugates. This lipopolysaccharide coat has similarities to human glycoconjugates, and it may be that antibodies generated against the lipopolysaccharide coat cross-react with glycoconjugates on peripheral nerves. Therefore, it may be that there is a shared epitope between the *Campylobacter* organism and human peripheral nerves (17), or so-called "molecular mimicry" (21).

Illa et al. reported axonal GBS in seven patients beginning 5–15 days after parenteral injection of gangliosides (22). These patients had high titers of IgG GM1 antibodies with specificity for motor nerve terminals. Studies by Yuki et al. (23–26) indicate that the neuroepitope could be GM1 ganglioside or GD1a ganglioside. The Fisher variant of GBS has been associated with antibodies against GQ1b gangliosides (26–28). Therefore, it may be that glycolipids or glycoproteins having epitopes similar to GM1 or GD1a are the immunological attack site in the axonal forms of GBS (17).

CLINICAL FEATURES

Guillain-Barré syndrome is the most common cause of acute nontraumatic generalized paralysis in young adults, with an annual incidence of 1.2 cases per 100,000 in developed countries. It can affect any age group from children to the elderly, although epidemiological studies suggest that there is a peak in young adults and a second smaller peak in the fifth to seventh decades. It occurs in males slightly more often than in females.

ANTECEDENT EVENTS

A variety of antecedent events have been noted to precede the development of acute ascending paralysis. Ropper et al. prospectively studied GBS patients at Massachusetts General Hospital, noting that 49% had a prior upper respiratory tract infection, 10% had a diarrhea illness, and 3% had some form of pneumonia (10,29). In 3% of cases, Epstein-Barr virus infection was implicated, and cytomegalovirus infection occurred in 3%. Generalized malaise was noted in 3%, and another 3% had miscellaneous associated antecedent events including Hodgkin's disease, surgery, systemic lupus, or vaccination. In 27% of patients, there was no prior identifiable illness or antecedent event (29). Other reported associations with GBS have included viral hepatitis, mycoplasma, Lyme disease, and sarcoidosis. Reports of GBS in the setting of HIV infection suggest a stronger association than would be expected by chance occurrence (30). *Campylobacter jejuni* infection as a cause of an acute diarrhea illness can be associated with subsequent GBS, as described above. Vaccinations have occasionally been implicated. Widespread public attention and notoriety occurred with the swine flu vaccination program in 1975 due to the suggestion of an increased incidence of GBS associated with the vaccine.

SYMPTOMS AND SIGNS

Usually the patient experiences an acute respiratory or gastrointestinal illness, which lasts for several days and then resolves. This is followed in 1–2 weeks by the development of "ascending paralysis." Typically, the legs are involved initially, and within a few days, the arms. Although described as an ascending paralysis, the weakness is usually about as marked in proximal limb muscles as in distal muscles. Patients will often present with a complaint of difficulty walking, trouble arising from a chair, going up or down stairs, or simply instability of gait. Weakness tends to progress, usually over a course of 1–3 weeks. On occasion, patients have a fulminant rapidly progressive course in which paralysis becomes maximal within 1 or 2 days. Overall, about 50% of patients with GBS reach maximal weakness by 1 week, 70% by 2 weeks, and 80% by 3 weeks into the course of the illness. While symptoms are predominantly motor, patients commonly have mild paresthesias or mild objective sensory deficits on exam, particularly those involving position and vibration sense. Limb weakness is relatively symmetrical, and there is symmetrical loss of the muscle stretch reflexes. About one third of patients develop respiratory involvement requiring mechanical ventilation, and 50% develop cranial nerve involvement, which is most often facial weakness. One half of patients develop oropharyngeal weakness, and 10–20% some degree of ocular involvement. About 50% of patients develop autonomic dysfunction (including fluctuations of blood pressure, heart rate, ileus, or urinary retention). After the progression of weakness stops, patients tend to plateau for 2–4 weeks and then slowly recover. The recovery is such that by 6 months into the course of illness, 85% of patients are ambulatory. In 3% of cases there is recurrence of the paralytic illness, although some of these patients may have instead a chronic inflammatory neuropathy, as opposed to recurrent GBS.

Overall, the mortality from the acute illness is reported to be 2–5%. About 50% of patients have some degree of long-term residual symptomatic abnormality. Fifteen to twenty percent of patients have residual motor weakness at one year, and 5% remain severely disabled. This generally favorable natural history is the standard basis against which any therapeutic modality must be compared.

LABORATORY STUDIES

Within the first few days most patients typically develop an abnormal spinal fluid profile, with a high CSF protein concentration in the absence of a pleocytosis (albumino-cytological dissociation). Glucose concentration is normal, as are cultures. The elevation of CSF protein concentration is presumed to result from an increased permeability of the blood-CSF barrier. In the first day or two, the CSF protein concentration is commonly normal. In Ropper's series, 34% of patients had normal CSF protein concentrations when measured in the first week, while in the second week only 18% were normal. Serial CSF studies may be necessary to demonstrate an abnormality. Up to 5–10% of GBS patients may have a lymphocytic pleocytosis with as many as 100 WBC/mm^3. In patients with a CSF pleocytosis, the possibility of GBS associated with HIV infection, Lyme disease, or sarcoidosis should be considered.

About 5% of GBS patients have abnormal liver function tests. Occasionally, patients demonstrate increased muscle enzymes as is seen with many forms of acute denervation. In severe or sudden cases of paralysis, stool cultures for *Campylobacter jejuni* may be positive, and many of these patients have associated anti-GM1 antibodies in serum.

Electromyography and nerve conduction studies can document the presence of a peripheral neuropathy which is of a demyelinating type (31–35). A demyelinating neuropathy tends to produce very slow nerve-conduction velocities, dispersed compound muscle action potentials (CMAP), and multifocal conduction block. Early on, the abnormalities on nerve conduction studies may be limited to very prolonged F-waves. Because the neuropathy is typically of a demyelinating type with sparing of the axons, there is usually relatively little fibrillation on electromyography needle exam. In the first few days, the nerve-conduction studies may be normal or only mildly abnormal. The electrophysiological abnormalities tend to lag behind the clinical examination. Severe reduction in the CMAP amplitude may predict the long-term outcome. Miller et al. showed that CMAP amplitudes less than 10% of normal were associated with a less favorable long-term prognosis (36). Similarly, the North American Guillain-Barré study group noted worse prognosis associated with CMAP amplitude less than 20% of normal.

Such observations are not universally accepted, as Triggs found that 50% of patients with severely reduced CMAP amplitudes were clinically normal at one year (37).

FISHER'S SYNDROME

In 1956 C. Miller Fisher reported "an easily recognizable syndrome ... characterized among other features by total external ophthalmoplegia, severe ataxia and loss of the tendon reflexes" (4). This well-recognized variant of GBS has been given the eponym of Fisher's syndrome and accounts for approximately 5% of the cases of acute GBS in most series. Patients typically present with diplopia followed within several days by ataxia or clumsiness of the limbs. Some patients describe dizziness. Over the first week of neurological symptoms, patients usually develop hypoactive or absent muscle stretch reflexes. One half of patients describe paresthesias. Occasionally, other cranial nerves are involved, resulting in oropharyngeal or facial weakness. About one third of patients develop associated severe limb weakness with respiratory failure. The ophthalmoplegia evolves over 1–3 days and is usually severe or complete and relatively symmetrical. Most patients have ptosis. Pupillary function tends to be normal. The presence of ataxia has raised the question of cerebellar involvement. There may be intention tremor, suggesting a cerebellar deficit. Some patients have unsteadiness, lightheadedness, or dizziness. However, vertigo, nystagmus, cerebellar dysarthria, and scanning speech are usually absent. Patients with Fisher's syndrome most often have an elevated spinal fluid protein concentration, but they are more likely than typical GBS patients to have normal CSF. The electrophysiological studies show mild slowing of nerve-conduction velocities compared with typical GBS, and are more likely to be normal in the limbs than in GBS.

DIFFERENTIAL DIAGNOSIS

The differential diagnosis includes the spectrum of illnesses causing acute or subacute paralysis. Spinal cord compression, transverse myelitis, and spinal cord infarction should be considered. Peripheral neuropathies from a variety of causes can mimic GBS including critical illness polyneuropathy; various toxins including nitrofurantoin, chemotherapeutic drugs, and heavy metal poisoning, such as arsenic and thallium; autoimmune inflammatory diseases such as systemic lupus and polyarteritis nodosa; meningoradiculitis as can be seen with Lyme disease, HIV infection, carcinomatous meningitis, and sarcoidosis; a paraneoplastic acute peripheral neuropathy; acute intermittent porphyria; and diphtheria. Hypokalemic periodic paralysis, myasthenia gravis, botulism, and poliomyelitis should also be considered.

RECOMMENDED LABORATORY EVALUATION OF GBS

The patient who presents with an acute or subacute paralytic syndrome resembling GBS should have the following laboratory studies considered in every case:

1. If there is evidence pointing to a focal spinal cord lesion the patient should have emergent magnetic resonance imaging (MRI) scan of the appropriate level of the spine. The presence of focal spinal pain, a discreet sensory level, prominent bladder and bowel dysfunction, paraparesis without arm involvement, or selective areflexia in the legs with normal reflexes in the arms should all mandate careful exclusion of a myelopathy by performing an emergency MRI scan.
2. Cerebrospinal fluid should be analyzed for evidence of a myelitis as well as for the

albumino-cytological dissociation typical for GBS. If the spinal fluid is sampled within the first few days and is normal, a repeat study a week or two into the illness may be helpful if the diagnosis remains unclear.

3. Appropriate blood work includes CBC, electrolytes, and liver and renal function tests. With regard to underlying conditions which can mimic or be associated with GBS, serum tests for an autoimmune inflammatory disease such as systemic lupus and polyarteritis nodosa should be done. All patients should be screened for HIV infection, and selected patients screened for Lyme disease and sarcoidosis.
4. Urine collection for acute intermittent porphyria is indicated.
5. Tests for hypokalemic periodic paralysis, myasthenia gravis, botulism, poliomyelitis, and diphtheria depend on the clinical evidence and suspicion and are not necessary in every patient.
6. Heavy metal poisoning can produce an acute or subacute peripheral neuropathy. In patients with a predominantly axonal form of GBS, heavy metal screens should be obtained, particularly for arsenic and thallium. Similarly, patients with pancytopenia, elevated liver function tests, and a history suggestive of a systemic illness should also be carefully screened for heavy metal poisoning. Patients with recurrent episodes of acute neuropathy should also be carefully screened for toxins.
7. When the antecedent illness is gastrointestinal syndrome with diarrhea, stool cultures and serological studies may reveal evidence of *Campylobacter jejuni*.
8. Screening for infection from Epstein-Barr virus, cytomegalovirus, and hepatitis virus as well as *Mycoplasma pneumoniae* should be considered.
9. A careful review of the patient's prior medication list for any potentially neurotoxic drug, such as nitrofurantoin, may lead to a diagnosis of drug-induced toxic neuropathy, as might a history of recent cancer chemotherapy. Megadose vitamin exposure, particularly pyridoxine, should also be considered.

MANAGEMENT

All patients with suspected GBS should be hospitalized for vigilant monitoring due to the high risk of respiratory failure and need for intubation and mechanical ventilation. Baseline spirometry, including forced vital capacity (FVC) and oximetry, should be obtained. Indications for intubation include an FVC dropping below 12 ml/kg or, in a normal-sized adult, FVC falling below 1 L. Patients who are subjectively dyspneic or look to be struggling to breathe should be intubated, even if their forced vital capacity is above these levels. In general, one should err on the side of early intubation rather than late. A simple bedside estimate of FVC can be made by having the patient count out loud. If the patient can take a maximal inspiration and then can count up to 25, the FVC is probably about 2 L. A patient who can count up to 10 probably has about a 1 L FVC.

The cornerstone of treatment is that of meticulous general medical support. There should be a low threshold for putting the patient in an intensive care unit. All patients who are having progression of their weakness should be in an intensive care unit. The common complications of GBS include respiratory failure, dysautonomia (especially cardiac arrhythmias, which may occur in 5% of cases), pneumonia, bladder dysfunction, pain, depression, phlebitis, pulmonary embolus, and SIADH. Further complications from immobility and bedrest include decubiti, secondary compression neuropathy such as ulnar neuropathy and peroneal neuropathy, and the psychiatric sequelae associated with a prolonged immobilizing stay in the intensive care unit. Intense back and limb pain improve with corticosteroids.

IMMUNOTHERAPY

Corticosteroids

To date there have been no studies that demonstrate the effectiveness of corticosteroids in the treatment of GBS. There have been retrospective nonrandomized studies, along with several small prospective randomized studies, which have shown no clear benefit (38). The use of high-dose intravenous methylprednisolone, as reported by Hughes, has also shown no benefit (39).

Plasma Exchange

In 1978, Brettle et al. first reported the benefits of plasma exchange in the treatment of GBS (40). Several large randomized trials have subsequently demonstrated benefit of plasma exchange in treating GBS (41–45). The North American GBS Study Group (42,43), the French (45), and the Swedish (41) studies have all shown comparable benefit. In the North American GBS Study Group, the total volume of exchange was 200 ml/kg over 1–2 weeks, or about four to five exchanges of 3.5–4 L on average (42). There was no clear difference in the occurrence of complications in the plasma exchange versus the control group. The time to improve one clinical grade, which was defined as coming off the ventilator or being able to walk, decreased by 50% in the plasma exchange group (19 vs. 40 days in the untreated group). The percent of patients who were improved at one month, and also the average clinical grade, was about 15–20% better in the plasma exchange group than in the control group. In addition, the time to regain independent walking was decreased by about 40% in the plasma exchange group (53 vs. 85 days in the untreated patients). No benefit was shown in this study when plasma exchange was started later than 2 weeks from onset of symptoms, leading to the suggestion that it be used as early as possible when the diagnosis is made (42). About 10% of patients are found to "rebound" and they often improve with repeat plasma exchange.

Intravenous Immunoglobulin

High-dose intravenous immunoglobulin (IVIG) was initially reported to be beneficial in GBS by Kleyweg et al. in 1988 (46). In 1992, the Dutch GBS Study Group reported a prospective randomized trial comparing IVIG with plasma exchange (47). In their study, IVIG was given at a dose of 0.4 g/kg per day for 5 days and was shown to be as beneficial as plasma exchange. The IVIG-treated patients showed a significantly shorter time to improve one disability grade, and somewhat fewer complications occurred in the IVIG group. Smaller series have suggested the greater possibility of clinical worsening during and following IVIG treatment (48), along with an increase in the relapse rate of patients following treatment with IVIG (48,49). Interestingly, the plasma exchange group in the Dutch study had outcome results similar to the control group (untreated group) of the North American Plasma Exchange Trial. More recently, Bril et al. (50) prospectively compared IVIG with plasma exchange in the treatment of 50 patients with GBS. Standard outcome measures did not differ between the two groups. Sixty-one percent of the plasma exchange–treated patients and 69% of the IVIG patients improved by one disability grade at one month. The complication rate was found to be somewhat higher in the plasma-exchange group. They concluded that the efficacy of IVIG in the treatment of GBS is similar to that of plasma exchange, and that it can be used with safety. There was no difference in the relapse rate between the two therapies. This compares with the Dutch GBS Study Group, which reported 34% improvement of one disability grade within one month of receiving plasma exchange (47), compared with 53% in those receiving IVIG and the reported 59% improvement rate of the plasma exchange–treated patients in the North American trial (42). Brill et al. also noted an increased frequency of complications in the plasma-exchange group, including pneumonia, venous thrombosis, and line sepsis, compared with the IVIG group (19 vs. 5). In the Dutch GBS study, 68 complications were noted in the plasma-exchange group compared with 39 in the IVIG group. An ongoing prospective multicenter trial may clarify the potential value and role of combination therapy.

In general, IVIG is considered relatively safe. Mild side effects including headache, nausea, myalgia, fever, or chills are reported in 1–15% of patients (51–55). However, there are sporadic anecdotal reports of more severe complications including transmission of hepatitis C (56), acute renal failure (57), nephrotic syndrome, stroke (58,59), myocardial infarction (60,61), aseptic meningitis (62–64), and reversible encephalopathy with cerebral vasospasm (65). Toxicity may be a result of sucrose toxicity, allergic phenomena, and effects of the high protein concentration on blood viscosity.

Presently, there is evidence to support the use of either plasma exchange or IVIG within the first week or two in the treatment of GBS. Current data do not provide an indication of one therapy being clearly superior to the other. Ongoing comparative trials should help clarify the role each will play in the management of future patients.

ACKNOWLEDGMENT

Mrs. Linda Hagan kindly helped prepare this manuscript.

REFERENCES

1. Landry O. Note sur la paralysie ascendante aigue. Gaz Hebd 1859; 5:472–474.
2. Guillain G, Barré JA, Strohl A. Sur un syndrome de radiculo-nevrite avec hyperalbuminose du liquide cephalo-rachidien sans reaction cellulaire. Remarques sur les caracteres clinques et graphiques des reflexes tendineux. Bulletins et memories de la societe medicale des hopitaux de Paris. Paris: Masson et Cie 1916; 40:1462–1470.
3. Guillain G, Barré JA. Travaux Neurologiques de Guerre. Paris: Masson et Cie, 1920.
4. Fisher CM. An unusual variant of acute idiopathic polyneuritis (syndrome of ophthalmoplegia, ataxia and areflexia.) N Engl J Med 1956; 255:57–65.
5. Haymaker W, Kernohan JW. The Landry-Guillain-Barré syndrome. A clinicopathologic report of fifty fatal cases and a critique of the literature. Medicine 1949; 28:59–141.
6. Asbury AK, Arnason BG, Adams RD. The inflammatory lesion in idiopathic polyneuritis. Medicine 1969; 48:173–215.
7. Waksman BH, Adams RD. Allergic neuritis: an experimental disease of rabbits induced by the injection of peripheral nervous tissue and adjurants. J Exp Med 1955; 102:213–235.
8. Hartung HP, Pollard JD, Harvey GK, Toyka KV. Immunopathogenesis and treatment of the Guillain-Barré syndrome—part I. Muscle Nerve 1955; 18:137–153.
9. Hartung HP, Pollard JD, Harvey GK, Toyka KV. Immunopathogenesis and treatment of the Guillain-Barré syndrome—part II. Muscle Nerve 1955; 18:154–164.
10. Ropper AH. The Guillain-Barré syndrome. N Engl J Med 1992; 326:1130–1136.
11. Kaldor J, Speed BR. Guillain-Barré syndrome and *Campylobacter jejuni*: a serological study. Br Med J 1984; 288:1867–1870.
12. Vriesendorp FJ, Mishu B, Blaser M, Koski CL. Serum antibodies to GM1, peripheral nerve myelin, and *Campylobacter jejuni* in patients with Guillain-Barré syndrome and controls: correlation and prognosis. Ann Neurol 1993; 34:130–135.
13. Enders U, Karch H, Toyka KV, et al. The spectrum of immune responses to *Campylobacter jejuni* and glycoconjugates in Guillain-Barré syndrome and in other neuroimmunological disorders. Ann Neurol 1993; 34:136–144.
14. Rees JH, Hughes RAC. *Campylobacter jejuni* and Guillain-Barré syndrome. Ann Neurol 1994; 35(2):248.

15. Feasby TE, Gilbert JJ, Brown WF, et al. An acute axonal form of Guillain-Barré polyneuropathy. Brain 1986; 109:1115–1126.
16. Feasby TE, Hahn AF, Brown WF, et al. Severe axonal degeneration in acute Guillain-Barré syndrome: evidence of two different mechanism? J Neurol Sci 1993; 116:185–192.
17. Griffin JW, Li CY, Ho TW, Tian M, Gao CY, et al. Pathology of the motor-sensory axonal Guillain-Barré syndrome. Ann Neurol 1996; 39:17–28.
18. Griffin JW, Li CY, Ho TW, et al. Guillain-Barré syndrome in northern China: the spectrum of neuropathologic changes in clinically defined cases. Brain 1995; 118:577–595.
19. Ho TW, Mishu B, Li CY, et al. Guillain-Barré syndrome in northern China: relationship to *Campylobacter jejuni* infection and anti-glycolipid antibodies. Brain 1995; 118:597–605.
20. McKhann GM, Cornblath DR, Griffin JW, et al. Acute motor axonal neuropathy: a frequent cause of acute flaccid paralysis in China. Ann Neurol 1993; 33:333–342.
21. Oomes PG, Jacobs BC, Hazenberg MPH, Banffer JRJ, van der Meché FGA. AntiGM_1 IgG antibodies and *Campylobacter* bacteria in Guillain-Barré syndrome: evidence of molecular mimicry. Ann Neurol 1995; 38:170–175.
22. Illa I, Ortiz N, Gallard E, Juarez C, Grau JM, Dalakas MC. Acute axonal Guillain-Barré syndrome with IgG antibodies against motor axons following parenteral gangliosides. Ann Neurol 1995; 38:218–224.
23. Yuki N, Taki T, Takahashi M, et al. Penner's serotype 4 of *Campylobacter jejuni* has a lipopolysaccharide that bears a GM1 ganglioside epitope as well as one that bears a GD1a epitope. Infect Immun 1994; 62:2101–2103.
24. Yuki N, Yamada M, Sato S, et al. Association of IgG anti-GD1a antibody with severe Guillain-Barré syndrome. Muscle Nerve 1993; 16:642–647.
25. Yuki N, Yoshino H, Sato S, Miyatake T. Acute axonal polyneuropathy associated with anti-GM1 antibodies following *Campylobacter jejuni* enteritis. Neurology 1990; 40:1900–1902.
26. Willison HJ, Veitch J, Patterson G, Kennedy PGE. Miller Fisher syndrome is associated with serum antibodies to GQ1b ganglioside. J Neurol Neurosurg Psychiatry 1993; 56:204–206.
27. Yuki N, Sato S, Tsuji S, et al. Frequent presence of anti-GQ1b antibody in Fisher's syndrome. Neurology 1993; 43:414–417.
28. Willison HJ, Veitch J. Immunoglobulin subclass distribution and binding characteristics of anti-GQ1b antibodies in Miller Fisher syndrome. J Neurochem 1994; 50:159–165.
29. Ropper AH, Wijdicks, EFM, Truax BT. Guillain-Barré Syndrome. Philadelphia: F.A. Davis, Publishers, 1991.
30. Cornblath DR, McArthur JC, Kennedy PGE, Witte AS, Griffin JW. Inflammatory demyelinating peripheral neuropathies associated with HTLV III infection. Ann Neurol 1987; 21:32–40.
31. Albers JW, Donofrio PD, McGonagle TK. Sequential electrodiagnostic abnormalities in acute inflammatory demyelinating polyradiculoneuropathy. Muscle Nerve 1985; 8:528–539.
32. Albers JW, Kelly JJ Jr. Acquired inflammatory demyelinating polyneuropathies: clinical and electrodiagnostic features. Muscle Nerve 1989; 12:435–451.
33. Eisen A, Humphreys P. The Guillain-Barré syndrome. A clinical and electrodiagnostic study of 25 cases. Arch Neurol 1974; 30:438–443.
34. McLeod JG. Electrophysiological studies in the Guillain-Barré syndrome. Ann Neurol 1981; 9(suppl): 20–27.
35. Olney RK, Aminoff MJ. Electrodiagnostic features of the Guillain-Barré syndrome: the relative sensitivity of different techniques. Neurology 1990; 40:471–475.
36. Miller RG, Peterson GW, Daube JR, Albers JW. Prognostic value of electrodiagnosis in Guillain-Barré syndrome. Muscle Nerve 1988; 11:769–774.
37. Triggs WJ, Cros D, Gominak SC, Zuniga G, Beric A, et al. Motor nerve inexcitability in Guillain-Barré syndrome. Brain 1992; 115:1291–1302.
38. Hughes RAC, Newsom-Davis JM, Perkin GD, Pierce JM. Controlled trial of prednisolone in acute polyneuropathy. Lancet 1978; (October 7):750–753.
39. Guillain-Barré Syndrome Steroid Trial Group. Double-blind trial of intravenous methylprednisolone in Guillain-Barré syndrome. Lancet 1993; 341:586–590.
40. Brettle RP, Gross M, Legg NJ, Lockwood M, Pallis C. Treatment of acute polyneuropathy by plasma exchange. Lancet 1978; 2(8099):1100.

41. Osterman PO, Lundemo G, Pirskanen R, et al. Beneficial effects of plasma exchange in acute inflammatory polyradiculoneuropathy. Lancet 1984; 2(8415):1296–1299.
42. The Guillain-Barré Syndrome Study Group. Plasmapheresis and acute Guillain-Barré syndrome. Neurology 1985; 35:1096–1104.
43. McKhann GM, Griffin JW, Cornblath DR, et al. Plasmapheresis and Guillain-Barré syndrome: analysis of prognostic factors and the effect of plasmapheresis. Ann Neurol 1988; 23:347–353.
44. French Cooperative Group on Plasma Exchange in Guillain-Barré Syndrome. Efficiency of plasma exchange in Guillain-Barré syndrome: role of replacement fluids. Ann Neurol 1987; 22:753–761.
45. French Cooperative Group on Plasma Exchange in Guillain-Barré syndrome. Plasma exchange in Guillain-Barré syndrome: one-year follow-up. Ann Neurol 1992; 32:94–97.
46. Kleyweg RP, van der Meche FGA, Meulstee J. Treatment of Guillain-Barré syndrome with high-dose gammaglobulin. Neurology 1988; 38:1639–1641.
47. van der Meche FGA, Schmitz PIM, Dutch Guillain-Barré Study Group. A randomized trial comparing intravenous immune globulin and plasma exchange in Guillain-Barré syndrome. N Engl J Med 1992; 326:1123–1129.
48. Castro LHM, Ropper AH. Human immune globulin infusion in Guillain-Barré syndrome: worsening during and after treatment. Neurology 1993; 43:1034–1036.
49. Irani DN, Cornblath DR, Chaudry V, Borel C, Hanley DF. Relapse in Guillain-Barré syndrome after treatment with human immune globulin. Neurology 1993; 43:872–875.
50. Bril V, Ilse WK, Pearce R, Dhanani A, Sutton D, et al. Pilot trial of immunoglobulin versus plasma exchange in patients with Guillain-Barré syndrome. Neurology 1996; 46:100–103.
51. Mokrzycki MH, Kaplan AA. Therapeutic plasma exchange: complications and management. Am J Kidney Dis 1994; 23:817–827.
52. Rodnitzky RL, Goeken JA. Complications of plasma exchange in neurologic patients. Arch Neurol 1982; 39:350–354.
53. Bouget J, Chevret S, et al. Plasma exchange morbidity in Guillain-Barré syndrome: results from the French prospective, double-blind, randomized, multicenter study. Crit Care Med 1993; 21:651–658.
54. Thornton CA, Ballow M. Safety of intravenous immunoglobulin. Arch Neurol 1993; 50:135–136.
55. Duhem C, Dicato MA, Ries F. Side-effects of intravenous immune globulins. Clin Exp Immunol 1994; 97(suppl 1):79–83.
56. Bjoro K, Froland SS, Yun Z, Samdal HH, Haaland T. Hepatitis C infection in patients with primary hypogammaglobulinemia after treatment with contaminated immune globulin. N Engl J Med 1994; 331:1607–1611.
57. Tan E, Hajinazarian M, Bay W, Neff J, Mendell JR. Acute renal failure resulting from intravenous immunoglobulin therapy. Arch Neurol 1993; 50:137–139.
58. Silbert PL, Knezevic WV, Bridge DT. Cerebral infarction complicating intravenous immunoglobulin therapy for polyneuritis cranialis. Neurology 1992; 42:257–258.
59. Steg RE, Letkowitz DM. Cerebral infarction following intravenous immunoglobulin therapy for myasthenia gravis. Neurology 1994; 44:1180–1181.
60. Woodruff RK, Grigg AP, Firkin FC, Smith IL. Fatal thrombotic events during treatment of autoimmune thrombocytopenia with intravenous immunoglobulin in elderly patients. Lancet 1986; 328:217–218.
61. Dalakas MC. High-dose intravenous immunoglobulin and serum viscosity: risk of precipitating thromboembolic events. Neurology 1994; 44:223–226.
62. Scribner CL, Kapit RM, Phillips ET, Rickles NM. Aseptic meningitis and intravenous immunoglobulin therapy. Ann Intern Med 1994; 121:305–306.
63. Sekul EA, Cupler EJ, Dalakas MC. Aseptic meningitis associated with high-dose intravenous immunoglobulin therapy: frequency and risk factors. Ann Intern Med 1994; 121:259–262.
64. DeVlieghere FC, Peetermans WE, Vermylen J. Aseptic granulocytic meningitis following treatment with intravenous immunoglobulin. Clin Infect Dis 1994; 18:1008–1010.
65. Voltz R, Rosen FV, Yousry T, Beck J, Hohlfeld R. Reversible encephalopathy with vasospasm in a Guillain-Barré syndrome patient associated with intravenous immunoglobulin. Neurology 1996; 46:250–251.

21

Postinfectious Neurological Syndromes

Lauren B. Krupp
State University of New York at Stony Brook, Stony Brook, New York

INTRODUCTION

The spectrum of neurological complications following viral and bacterial infection ranges from subtle behavioral changes to paraplegia, coma, and death. Among the postinfectious neurological syndromes reviewed in this chapter are postinfectious and postvaccinal encephalomyelitis, neurological complications associated with varicella-zoster virus (VZV) infections, post–Lyme disease syndromes, and chronic fatigue syndrome (CFS). Several specific postinfectious neurological disorders including acute cerebellar ataxia, transverse myelitis, and toxic encephalopathy are also briefly summarized.

DEFINITION

Postinfectious neurological disorders refer to those conditions that have a clear temporal relationship to infection or immunization but are thought *not* to result from primary neural tissue invasion by the organism. The etiology of such disorders may include an autoimmune pathogenesis or reactivation of latent infection.

POSTINFECTIOUS ENCEPHALOMYELITIS

A variety of terms have been used for postinfectious encephalomyelitis. Names that refer to the clinical disease include parainfectious, postexanthematous, and postvaccinal encephalomyelitis (167). Names that refer to the pathology include acute disseminated encephalomyelitis (ADEM) (167,168,252) perivascular myelinoclasis (182), perivenous encephalitis (88), and demyelinating encephalomyelitis. Other proposed terms refer to pathogenic mechanisms: immune-mediated encephalomyelitis (109), and hyperergic encephalomyelitis (62).

Pathogenesis

Postinfectious encephalomyelitis is believed to be immune mediated. This is supported by the fact that there is a lag phase between the infection itself and the onset of the postinfectious syndrome and by the failure to demonstrate infectious agents in neural tissue or within the intrathecal compartment.

The neuropathology of postinfectious encephalomyelitis consists of grayish discoloration along veins and characteristic lesions in the cerebral white matter, brain stem, and spinal cord. A central histological finding is mononuclear infiltration around small veins accompanied by lipid-laden macrophages and demyelination. Consistent with a presumed immune attack against myelin, there is concordant loss of myelin-associated glycoprotein and myelin basic protein (49,70,112,143). In the hyperacute or necrotizing cases, the brain is often swollen and congested and there may be petechial hemorrhages. These cases may have an intense fibrinoid vascular necrosis and perivascular edema (2,223).

Pathological findings similar to those of postinfectious encephalomyelitis have been described in the brains of monkeys inoculated with normal brain tissue homogenate (194,195) and are seen in experimental allergic encephalomyelitis (EAE) (1987). The shared pathological findings for postinfectious encephalomyelitis and EAE support the postulated autoimmune etiology of the human disorder.

Despite careful investigation of postmeasles encephalitis cases, no signs of measles virus have been found in the CNS and intrathecal measles antibody production is absent (111,112). Early in postmeasles encephalomyelitis, myelin basic protein (MBP) is released into the cerebrospinal fluid (CSF), suggesting it is the target of an immune attack (77). Almost half of postmeasles encephalomyelitis cases studied show a lymphoproliferative response to myelin basic protein (113). The vigorous immune response to CNS white matter, in particular MBP, is consistent with an autoimmune etiology. An increased lymphocyte proliferative response to myelin basic protein has also been observed in postvaccinal encephalomyelitis (91) and in cases following VZV or rubella infections.

Epidemiology

Worldwide, the most common agents that trigger postinfectious encephalomyelitis are viruses, particularly those that cause exanthematous illnesses. These include measles (1:1000 cases), VZV (< 1:10,000), rubella (< 1:20,000), and in previous eras, vaccinia (1:63 to 1:300,000). Other viruses on rare occasions have been associated with postinfectious encephalomyelitis (31,111, 167). They include influenza, mumps, Epstein Barr virus (EBV), cytomegalovirus (CMV), and enteroviruses. In addition to these identified agents, nonspecific upper respiratory tract infections, presumably due to ubiquitous but unidentified agents (such as respiratory syncytial virus or adenovirus), can also be responsible. Nonviral agents, such as *Mycoplasma pneumoniae*, have also been implicated (47,131). The necrotizing form of the disease is most frequently associated with nonspecific upper respiratory infections (111). Influenza-A virus has been linked to a few cases.

A syndrome similar to postinfectious encephalomyelitis occurs following vaccination for smallpox (49), rabies (90,91,195), and following other vaccines (177). Encephalopathy has been noted following immunization with pertussis (36,80) but not diphtheria or tetanus toxoids (218). The last case associated with smallpox vaccination in the United States was in 1978 and is now of only historical interest (195).

Clinical Features

The clinical features of postinfectious encephalomyelitis are shown in Table 1. The disorder is most common in children (92%), but may also be seen in adults (8%) (11).

The disease usually appears within 1–3 weeks of acute illness or immunization. The subsequent neurological syndrome shows no correlation with the severity of the preceding infection (109–111,167,168).

The clinical features of postinfectious encephalomyelitis have been best described for measles virus as the inciting agent (110,112,113,152). Measles remains a major health problem worldwide even in developed countries (95). Most postmeasles encephalomyelitis patients are between 3 and 10 years of age (67,113). Nonspecific initial manifestations of postinfectious encephalomyelitis include fever, anorexia, myalgia, and headache. More severe initial symptoms are seizures (47%) and stupor (45%), which may progress to coma (167). Alterations in behavior, delirium, nausea, vomiting, and meningismus are also frequent signs and symptoms. Focal findings including hemiplegia occur in 12% and may be associated with stroke (167). In a review of cases between 1928–1954, the overall mortality rate was 24% (167). However, in a series of 19 cases from Peru in the 1980s there were no deaths (113). The other postinfectious encephalitis syndromes have characteristics similar to those of postmeasles cases.

Cases of recurrent postinfectious encephalomyelitis (multiphasic disseminated encephalomyelitis) have been grouped into two types. In one, subsequent attacks are stereotypic; in the other, multiple episodes differ in clinical presentation (117,183). Unusual clinical manifestations of postinfectious or postvaccinal encephalomyelitis include alternating hemiparesis (117) and encephalomyeloradiculopathy (160).

In the acute necrotizing form of the disease, the course of illness tends to be more fulminant. This more severe form of postinfectious encephalomyelitis has been referred to by a variety of terms including acute necrotizing hemorrhagic encephalopathy (1), acute hemorrhagic leukoencephalitis (110), Hurts disease, and hemorrhagic immune-mediated encephalomyelitis (88). In these patients, symptom onset is sudden and there is rapid neurological deterioration to coma. Most patients die within 5 days, and survivors have severe neurological deficits.

Diagnostic Tests

The CSF abnormalities in postinfectious encephalomyelitis are nonspecific. CSF may be under increased pressure, show increased protein concentration (usually less <1 g), moderate lymphocytosis, and occasionally elevated myelin basic protein. In the necrotizing form of the disease, the CSF may contain predominantly neutrophils and occasionally red blood cells. In approximately one-third of cases, CSF is entirely normal (167). The EEG often shows generalized or diffuse slowing (167,243) but may be normal.

Typical computed tomography (CT) findings are bilateral lesions of low attenuation in the periventricular, frontal, and parietal white matter (154,227). Less commonly, hypodense lesions are present in the basal ganglia and thalamus (51). Clinical correlation between neurological examination and CT appearance is variable. There may be a delay between the onset of the

Table 1 Clinical Features of Postinfectious Encephalomyelitis

Preceding antigenic exposure (usually a brief viral illness) with a 1- to 3-week latency before the neurological syndrome
Latent period followed by the acute onset of multifocal or diffuse CNS dysfunction
Potential for major clinical recovery

clinical syndrome and the appearance of CT abnormalities (154). Relapsing-remitting cases have been described in which deterioration was associated with multifocal white matter lesions and remission was associated with radiographic improvement (234). Contrast CT may show ring enhancement, as well as nodular, heterogeneous, periventricular, or gyral enhancement patterns (227).

MRI is more sensitive than CT (9,18,26,27,50,64,182). MRI frequently reveals multiple hyperintense lesions on T_2-weighted images in the supratentorial and infratentorial white matter, which are usually asymmetrical, nonhemorrhagic, and lack mass effect (7). Little is usually seen on T_1-weighted images except for occasional low-signal areas. Lesions may also be present on MRI in the diencephalon, brain stem, and posterior fossa (9,40). Acute lesions may enhance with gadolinium (26,232). Occasionally lesions are large, have mass effect, and mimic focal tumors (124).

Clinical correlation with MRI is variable. Patients with few or no neurological findings may have multiple MRI lesions (182). However, clinical improvement may be associated with shrinkage of the lesions. Persistent MRI abnormalities have been reported as long as 3 years after clinical recovery (182).

Differential Diagnosis

It can be difficult to differentiate postinfectious encephalomyelitis from acute infectious meningitis or viral encephalitis. One distinguishing characteristic of the postinfectious syndrome is the presence of a latent period between clinical infection and subsequent neurological disease.

At times the distinction between postinfectious encephalomyelitis and the first attack of multiple sclerosis (MS) may be challenging. A recent history (within the past 3 weeks) of infection or vaccination is typical of postinfectious encephalomyelitis. Decreased level of consciousness, delirium, stupor, and coma are characteristic features of postinfectious encephalomyelitis, but are extremely rare in MS. Seizures occur in approximately 50% of postinfectious patients, but are present in less than 10% of patients with MS and are even more unlikely at disease onset. While postinfectious syndromes are usually monophasic, MS in approximately 85% of cases has a relapsing and remitting course.

The CSF and MRI abnormalities in postinfectious neurological syndromes and MS often overlap (117,125). While both MS and postinfectious syndromes have white matter lesions best seen on T_3-weighted images, deep gray matter lesions involving caudate, thalami, globus pallidus, and putamen are more often associated with postinfectious encephalomyelitis. Lesions that are extensive and outline the cortical mantle are also more characteristic of postinfectious encephalomyelitis (125).

In the more severe (hemorrhagic) form of postinfectious encephalomyelitis, CSF shows a predominance of polymorphonuclear leukocytes with red blood cells, and neuroimaging shows hemorrhagic lesions (190), neither of which are seen in MS. Nonetheless, distinguishing the first attack of MS from a mild case of postinfectious encephalomyelitis may only be possible from the subsequent clinical course.

Treatment

Many of the major viruses implicated in postinfectious syndromes are preventable through active immunization programs. In developed countries this has led to a marked decrease in the frequency of postinfectious encephalomyelitis due to measles, mumps, and rubella. The use of rabies vaccines not grown in CNS tissue has also helped prevent postinfectious neurological complications, as has the end of vaccinia as an infectious disease.

For postinfectious encephalomyelitis, no specific therapy is proven as effective. Corticosteroids are commonly used based on anecdotal data (3), their anti-inflammatory and immunosuppressive effects, and the premise that they are beneficial in EAE and MS. A common treatment regimen is 3–5 days of intravenous methylprednisolone, followed by an oral prednisone taper. There are, however, some nonrandomized studies and one randomized study that have been unable to document any benefit from steroid therapy (225,244).

There are several reports that plasmapheresis benefits patients who fail to respond to corticosteroids or who have particularly fulminant disease (118,176,222). In these cases there seemed to be a temporal relationship between pheresis and clinical improvement, so that this is a reasonable treatment to offer in more severe cases. Intravenous immune globulin has not been beneficial in postinfectious CNS syndromes (111). Supportive measures include control of body temperature, seizures, and increased intracranial pressure; assisted ventilation; and precautions to avoid skin breakdown and complicating infections. Such treatment can be rewarding, since many patients make dramatic recoveries.

NEUROLOGICAL COMPLICATIONS OF VARICELLA ZOSTER VIRUS

VZV is one of seven human DNA herpesviruses. Primary infection causes chickenpox (varicella), a disease primarily in children, and reactivation causes shingles (herpes zoster), a disorder most common in the elderly. VZV can produce a diverse group of neurological conditions affecting both the central and the peripheral nervous systems.

Primary infection with VZV generally occurs via inhalation, with subsequent infection of the reticular endothelium and viremia. Viremia leads to infection of the skin and the emergence of the chickenpox lesions. Cutaneous infection is presumably followed by retrograde axonal transport of virus into the sensory ganglia (101). Viremia may also directly produce infection of the ganglia. In situ hybridization in a child who died of progressive varicella revealed a pattern consistent with blood borne seeding of the ganglia (39).

Although there are no good animal models for VZV and the virus is difficult to study in vitro (39), the site of latency within sensory trigeminal and thoracic ganglia is suggested by the identification of viral DNA and RNA in neurons of these ganglia (71,56).

Many of the neurological syndromes associated with VZV are due to reactivation of the virus from its latent state. This applies not only to syndromes associated with shingles (zoster) but also for some associated with chickenpox (varicella). Other neurological complications of VZV may result from autoimmune factors.

Neurological Complications Associated with Varicella (Chickenpox)

The most frequent neurological complications of varicella are shown in Table 2.

Acute Cerebellar Ataxia

Acute cerebellar ataxia occurs in 25–35% of neurological complications with varicella when not associated with the acquired immunodeficiency syndrome (AIDS). Symptoms usually appear after the rash, but in some cases may precede the eruption of the vesicles (73,180). In one series of postvaricella patients, 47% had cerebellar syndromes (167). Increased intracranial pressure, papilledema, and findings that mimic a posterior fossa mass lesion may develop (73). Most patients recover, though some residual cerebellar signs may persist. Several studies suggest that viral reactivation may also contribute to pathogenesis.

Table 2 Neurological Complications Following Varicella (Chickenpox)

Acute cerebellar ataxia
Toxic encephalopathy (Reye's syndrome)
Encephalomyelitis
Cerebral vasculitis
Myelitis
Guillain-Barré syndrome

Toxic Encephalopathy

A postinfectious encephalopathy syndrome has been associated with varicella. It is pathologically distinct from encephalomyelitis in that there is no inflammation or demyelination. When the encephalopathy is accompanied by liver failure, it is part of Reye's syndrome (193).

Encephalomyelitis and Vasculopathy

In the era of AIDS, VZV encephalitis cases have become increasingly more frequent (4,76). The pathology is predominantly a vasculopathy involving small and large vessels. Seizures, alterations in mental status, and focal deficits are among the clinical presentations. Brain imaging reveals infarctions of varying sizes in the gray and white matter. Deep-seated ischemic or demyelinating white matter lesions are often present (4).

A syndrome of delayed vasculopathy and infarction has been described in a number of children (25,54,116,145,208). Patients developed symptoms of stroke 1–9 months following the rash of chickenpox.

Other Neurological Syndromes Associated with Varicella

Transverse myelitis accounts for approximately 3% of postvaricella neurological complications. Myelitis typically occurs within one week of the rash. There is a sensory level in about half the cases (122). CSF usually shows mild pleocytosis. Guillain-Barré syndrome (GBS) may also follow varicella. It is indistinguishable from idiopathic GBS.

Neurological Complications Associated with Zoster

Zoster has a distinct epidemiology from varicella. It is largely a disease of the elderly or immunosuppressed (101). Zoster-associated syndromes are best understood in relation to the factors leading to viral reactivation.

Viral reactivation is likely to be related to changes in the host cellular immune response. Impaired cellular immunity, as measured by declining in vitro peripheral lymphocyte response to VZV, occurs in the elderly and has been used to explain the increased incidence of zoster with aging (39). That patients with AIDS and other immunodeficient states are at increased risk for zoster underscores the importance of immune competence in preventing zoster (191). Common neurological syndromes associated with zoster are shown in Table 3.

Acute and Postherpetic Neuralgia

Clinical Features. Zoster is usually idiopathic, but in 10% an identifiable risk factor (malignancy, radiation treatment, chemotherapy, or trauma) can be determined. Pain, itching, and paresthesia usually precede the rash. Eruption of the rash may be associated with systemic symptoms (malaise, lymphadenopathy). Pain is most severe in the dermatomal distribution of the rash and generally disappears in several weeks. Pain which persists >4 weeks is considered to be PHN (226). PHN patients can be separated into clinically distinct groups: those with continuous

Table 3 Neurological Syndromes Associated with Herpes Zoster

Acute neuralgia
Postherpetic neuralgia (PHN)
Segmental motor weakness (radiculitis)
Cranial neuropathy
Vasculopathy and infarction
Encephalomyelitis
Myelitis
Guillain-Barré syndrome

pain localized to a region of sensory loss, and those in whom pain on touch is the main sensory abnormality (198).

In patients over 60, 30–50% may develop PHN following zoster (87). In one prospective study, age over 80 and severe pain at onset were significant risk factors for PHN (87).

Pathogenesis of Pain. The pathophysiological changes that produce PHN are unclear. In one postmortem case the dorsal horn of the thoracic spinal cord from T_4 to T_8 was atrophic on the affected side (236). It has been postulated that pain is due to preferential loss of large inhibitory afferent myelinated fibers leading to diminished inhibition of smaller segmental pain sensitive fibers (67,236). Increased nociceptive transmission by dorsal horn neurons may also play a role (236).

Treatment. Current therapy for *acute zoster* is acyclovir (800 mg orally 5 times daily for 7 days) or famciclovir (500 mg orally 3 times daily for 7 days) (67,231). Parenteral acyclovir (5–10 mg/kg every 8 h for 5–7 days) is similarly effective. Treatment of the acute infection does not appear to prevent PHN (57,102,166). However, some but not all studies suggest that in acyclovir-treated patients compared to placebo, postherpetic neuralgia is less frequent in the first 3 months. A randomized double-blind placebo-controlled trial with famciclovir for acute herpes zoster significantly decreased the duration of PHN by approximately 2 months (231). Hence, famciclovir may be more effective than acyclovir in shortening the duration of PHN.

Once PHN develops, the pain is generally responsive to amitriptyline (elavil) in a dose of 25–50 mg 2–3 times daily. Pain relief has been correlated with amitriptyline dose (163). Other tricyclic antidepressants such as desipramine (norpramine) (127) or nortriptyline (pamelor) are also beneficial. In patients with lancinating pain, carbamazepine (tegretol), baclofen (lioresal), pimozide (orap) (67), or parenteral lidocaine may be effective (200). In addition to systemic therapies, topical treatment with capsaicin (zostrix) or lidocaine can be tried (14,199,235).

Segmental Weakness (Radiculitis)

A syndrome of limb weakness occurs in association with zoster and has been well described since the nineteenth century (122). Thoracic segments (51%) are most often involved, although the cervical (19%) and lumbar regions (18%) may also be affected (188,228). In 90% of cases, muscle paralysis occurs within the dermatome affected by the rash. Once weakness develops it rapidly progresses within hours to several days. Cervical involvement has led to diaphragmatic paralysis (217). Overall, the prognosis of segmental weakness following zoster is excellent, and 75% of patients recover completely.

Cranial Neuropathy

All cranial nerves may be affected, but the facial nerve is most frequently involved (Ramsay Hunt syndrome). In Ramsay Hunt syndrome, facial paralysis occurs ipsilateral to otic zoster and is associated with symptoms of auricular pain, herpetic rash, hyperacusis, vertigo, and tinnitus. Vesicles may appear along the pinna or external auditory canal. Hearing loss may occur. In a series of 153 Ramsay Hunt cases evaluated with audiograms, 19% developed hearing loss attributable to the infection (237). Loss of hearing was most frequent in patients with vertigo and auricular pain (237).

Pure ocular complications of zoster may occur with involvement of the ophthalmic division of the trigeminal nerve. They include conjunctivitis, keratitis, scleritis, retinitis, and glaucoma. Other cranial nerves may also be affected by zoster. However, involvement of the ninth, tenth, and eleventh cranial nerves is rare.

Cerebral Infarction

A well-recognized complication of zoster is cerebral vasculopathy and infarction (19,30,55,94, 115,188,211). The syndrome develops within a few days to 6 months after zoster. Most cases are due to zoster involvement of the ophthalmic division of the trigeminal nerve [zoster ophthalmicus (HZO)] and involve the ipsilateral middle cerebral artery with resultant hemispheric infarction (19,94). However, cerebral infarction may occur after thoracic zoster (188), mandibular zoster (185), and zoster oticus (Ramsay Hunt syndrome) (115). Cervical zoster has been associated with brain-stem infarction (211). MRI has demonstrated infarction in the basal ganglia and thalamus following HZO (25). Occasionally there is delayed hemorrhage rather than ischemic infarction, presumably due to necrotizing vasculitis or to aneurysm formation (171). Angiography typically shows irregular narrowing of the cerebral arteries consistent with vasculopathy (19,65,94). Although the middle cerebral artery is most commonly affected, other vessels may be involved (63). CSF may reveal oligoclonal bands, lymphocytic pleocytosis, and elevated protein concentration, or it may be normal.

The likely pathogenesis is viral reactivation with spread into the cerebral vasculature, possibly by way of the trigeminal nerve. Consistent with this hypothesis is the identification of viral particles by electron microscopy in vasculitic lesions, immunohistochemical localization of VZV antigens in smooth muscle cells of affected middle cerebral arteries, and viral isolation (5,52,55). On the other hand, the delayed onset of the syndrome and occasional histological findings of lymphocytic infiltration suggest that immune-mediated mechanisms may also be important.

Treatment consists of parenteral acyclovir. Some authors also advocate concurrent use of high-dose steroids. Recurrent strokes have been reported but are uncommon. Although poor outcome or death may occur, the majority of patients recover.

Other Syndromes

Zoster has been associated with myelitis, encephalitis, and encephalomyelitis (6,96,97,167). These syndromes occur more often in patients with AIDS and other diseases associated immunosuppression.

SPECIFIC POSTINFECTIOUS NEUROLOGICAL SYNDROMES

Most of the neurological syndromes described in association with measles, varicella, or zoster may also occur after other infections. Several specific postinfectious neurological syndromes and their etiological agents are reviewed below.

Acute Ataxia

Acute cerebellar ataxia is a frequent complication of many viral infections. Although most commonly associated with varicella, it may develop after any upper respiratory flulike illness or

Table 4 Infections Preceding Acute Cerebellar Ataxia

VZV	Mumps
Measles	Rubella
Enterovirus	Epstein-Barr virus
Coxsackie A 2,4,7,9	Mycoplasma pneumoniae
Coxsackie B 1 -6	
Echo virus 6,9	
Enterovirus 71	
Poliovirus 1,3	

other infection. The infectious agents most often associated with acute ataxia are shown in Table 4. Patients usually recover fully.

Toxic Encephalopathy

Toxic encephalopathy occurs after nonspecific upper respiratory tract infections, varicella, rubella, pertussis, gastrointestinal infections, and pneumonia. The hallmarks are increased intracranial pressure, acute brain swelling, fever, and no evidence of inflammation or demyelination. The classic toxic encephalophy is Reye's syndrome. The diagnostic criteria for Reye's syndrome are listed in Table 5.

The main clinical features of Reye's syndrome are the rapid development of irritability, nausea, vomiting, confusion, and coma. There is increased intracranial pressure, sympathetic overactivity, and, in severe cases, decorticate and decerebrate posturing. Due to an increased association between aspirin use and Reye's syndrome, the FDA advises avoiding giving aspirin to children with viral illness (82,103). Laboratory abnormalities consist of elevated serum ammonia, increased levels of transaminases, and prolonged prothrombin times. The CSF is under increased pressure but is otherwise normal. Liver biopsy can confirm the diagnosis but is usually not necessary.

The primary site of injury is the mitochondria of multiple organs, and particularly the liver (178). There is depressed mitochondrial enzyme activity (20). It has been suggested that metabolic abnormalities and elevated serum ammonia interact synergistically with injured CNS mitochondria to produce encephalopathy and cerebral edema (92). As there is no pathological evidence of demyelination or inflammation, autoimmune factors are not considered to be etio-

Table 5 Diagnostic Criteria for Reye's Syndrome

Antecedent viral illness
Latent interval (several days) before onset of vomiting
Diffuse encephalopathy
Elevation (>3-fold) of serum alanine, aminotransferase (ALT, SGPT), and aspartate aminotransferase (AST, SGOT)
Prolonged prothrombin time
Elevated serum ammonia
Normal CSF examination
No other explanation for hepatic and cerebral abnormalities

Source: Ref. 19.

Table 6 Antecedents Associated with Acute Transverse Myelitis

VZV	*Mycoplasma pneumoniae*
Measles	Typhoid fever
Echovirus-2	Pertussis
Epstein-Barr virus	Upper respiratory tract infection
Hepatitis B	

logically important. Treatment includes management of raised intracranial pressure, hydration with hypertonic fluids with 10% dextrose if hypoglycemia is present, fresh frozen plasma to correct coagulopathy, and cooling blankets and acetaminophen suppositories as needed for hyperthermia. Intravenous L-carnitine is used to prevent a secondary carnitine deficiency. Neomycin and lactulose can be used to treat hyperammonemia.

Transverse Myelitis

Acute transverse myelitis may follow infection from a variety of infectious agents, some of which are listed in Table 6. Cases have also occurred following vaccination for rabies or rubella. The thoracic cord is most frequently involved. MRI may show areas of increased signal within the cord on T_2-weighted images and occasionally cord swelling. Recovery is variable (108,197). Differences between postinfectious myelitis and transverse myelopathy associated with MS include a lower frequency of oligoclonal bands in the cerebrospinal fluid in postinfectious myelitis and a clinical syndrome of ascending spinal cord dysfunction in postinfectious myelitis (108).

POST–LYME DISEASE SYNDROMES

Lyme disease is a multisystem disorder caused by the tick-transmitted spirochete *Borrelia burgdorferi* (12,212). Lyme disease is the most common vectorborne infection in the United States, with a steady rise in the number of cases reported to the Centers for Disease Control and Prevention (CDC), with over 13,000 cases reported by 43 states to the CDC in 1994 (24).

Although there are a number of problematic issues related to diagnosis and management in the early and late stages of infection, "post-Lyme syndrome" has become a controversial example of a postinfectious syndrome. Some of these patients are believed to have persistent *B. burgdorferi* infection for months to years; others may be suffering from immune changes secondary to the infection, which are not responsive to antibiotic therapy. Lack of guidelines have led to costly and at times inappropriate treatment (58,214).

Clinical Features

There are three categories of patients who are labeled with either chronic Lyme disease or post-Lyme syndrome:

1. The clearest category involves patients who can be considered to have had a posttreatment or post-Lyme syndrome. These are patients who have had clear-cut Lyme disease, received standard and presumably appropriate treatment, but have continued to experience symptoms months to years after antibiotics. Persistent symptoms experienced by these treated patients have been extensively documented (9,42,43,138,161,172,207,213).

2. The second category involves seropositive patients (without a prior history of Lyme disease), who have nonspecific complaints not explained by alternative diagnoses.
3. The third category includes seronegative patients (for the most part from endemic areas) without a history of Lyme disease, who have similar nonspecific complaints that are unexplained by alternative diagnoses.

Because the relationships between Lyme disease and patients in categories (2) and (3) are purely speculative, only patients from category (1) are reviewed here. The major clinical problems in post-Lyme syndrome are listed in Table 7.

Primary neurological features of post-Lyme syndrome are cognitive complaints and headache. These problems differ from patients with early disseminated infection, in whom meningitis, radiculitis, and severe encephalitis are more common (192). Frequent nonneurological symptoms include arthralgias and myalgias. Fibromyalgia may be a problem for some patients (50,209). Minor clinical features include dizziness, mood changes, paresthesias, photophobia, sleep disturbance, and hearing problems.

Post-Lyme syndrome patients assessed in a population-based study had significantly more fatigue, concentration and memory difficulties, irritability, arthralgias, and sensory and sleep complaints compared to their case controls (213). On the average, these patients had been treated for Lyme disease 6 years earlier. In a retrospective review of 215 patients with treated Lyme disease, more than half continued to experience fatigue, arthralgias, cognitive complaints, and other symptoms an average of 3 years after their antibiotic treatment (8).

Persistent fatigue was noted in as many as 21–62% of patients following treatment of late disease (42). Fatigue at the onset was an associated risk factor for persistent fatigue after treatment. Ceftriaxone therapy was more effective than penicillin in preventing persistent fatigue (42).

In a study by Krupp et al. in which 15 treated Lyme patients were evaluated for persistent cognitive impairment months after completion of antibiotic therapy, 60% had objective evidence of mild encephalopathy on neuropsychological testing (138). Problems with verbal memory and attention were the most common findings. These cognitive deficits are similar to those noted in other studies of chronic or untreated Lyme patients (84,119,151).

Varying degrees of psychiatric disturbance are common (68,69,83,133). Although many patients have elevated depressive symptoms, the majority do not satisfy DSM-IV criteria for current major depression (68). Rare cases of severe psychiatric syndromes including psychosis, panic attacks, and severe anxiety disorders associated with *B. burgdorferi* infection have been described, but most resolve following antibiotic treatment (60,61,196).

Evaluation and Treatment

In post-Lyme syndrome, in contrast to early or late infection, CSF is usually acellular and intrathecal anti–*B. burgdorferi* antibody production is absent. Unlike other postinfectious neuro-

Table 7 Clinical Features of Post-Lyme Syndrome

Persistent severe fatigue
Fibromyalgia
Mild encephalopathy
Headache
Mood disturbance/Depressive symptoms

logical syndromes, post-Lyme syndrome often lacks a latent period. Instead, certain symptoms that were variably present during the early or late clinical disease continue to persist even after other signs of Lyme disease subside.

The most important issue in post-Lyme syndrome is to determine whether active infection from *B. burgdorferi* remains. Currently there is no established marker of persistent infection. While intrathecal antibody synthesis is used by the CDC as evidence of CNS infection, this finding may be absent during active infection (38,44,205) or may persist after completion of antibiotic therapy and does not necessarily reflect continued infection (86). Experimental studies using PCR, antigen detection in CSF, or lymphocyte proliferation measures have been proposed as potential markers of active infection, but these are still under investigation (37,38,44,153). In patients in whom all serological markers of infection are absent and in whom an adequate course of antibiotic therapy has been completed, there is no rationale for a second course of antibiotic therapy. Problems such as fatigue can be addressed symptomatically.

Prior to symptomatic therapy, other potential etiologies for fatigue, headache, or cognitive loss should be excluded. For example, in patients with fatigue complaints, other etiologies such as hypothyroidism, sleep disturbance, anemia, or affective disorders should be considered (139). In cases in which no other underlying cause other than the past Lyme disease can be identified and in which there are no signs of active infection, a symptomatic approach is useful. Fatigue can be treated with a multimodality program including reassurance, improved sleep hygiene, and in some cases medication such as mild stimulants (134,238). In patients with associated symptoms of depression, antidepressants such as fluoxetine (prozac) or protriptyline (vivactil) may be beneficial. Fibromyalgia may respond to mild physical therapy programs and often is helped by tricyclic antidepressant medication such as amitriptyline or nortriptyline. There is no specific treatment for cognitive impairment. Some patients are helped by cognitive rehabilitation. The majority of patients recover spontaneously.

CHRONIC FATIGUE SYNDROME

CFS is a genuine but poorly understood illness. This disorder has been the subject of much controversy in the lay and medical community. Many infectious agents have been suggested as the etiological agent, but no one organism has emerged as the primary causative organism. Current opinion is that a variety of agents may trigger a postinfectious syndrome of persistent fatigue in a susceptible host.

Pathogenesis

Interest in the study of fatigue as a potential infectious disorder was galvanized in the United States by reports during the mid-1980s of patients with chronic fatigue and multiple somatic complaints with elevated Epstein-Barr virus (EBV) antibody titers (53,81,100,221,230). Subsequent studies suggested EBV was not necessary to the illness (89,224). Elevated antibody titers to a variety of viral agents were found in CFS patients including antibodies to herpes, cytomegalovirus, enterovirus, and measles virus (53,81,100,169,230,242). While at one time there was much interest in retrovirus (45) and HHP-6 (1,43) as potential etiologies, no single virus has been identified as the cause of CFS, and many individual agents have been excluded as an etiological organism including retrovirus, HHP-6, enterovirus, and hepatitis C virus (41,15, 130,126). Despite the lack of a direct link between a specific viral agent and CFS, the finding of increased antibodies to a variety of viruses suggested that a generalized immunological dysfunction might accompany CFS (128,141).

While CFS is not associated with changes in the overall number of B cells, (79,128) relative elevations in specific subsets of B cells and decreases in IgG subclasses, and increased circulating immune complexes have been described (173). Defects in natural killer (NK) cell activity and reductions in the number of NK cells have been reported by some (28,128,150,162,186) but not others (141). An increase in the number of cell adhesion markers on NK cells was noted in a study of 40 consecutively evaluated CFS patients who fulfilled CDC criteria (229).

Other T-cell abnormalities in CFS include increased expression of activation markers (particularly on CD8 cells), a hypoactive response to mitogenic stimulation (220), and increases in adhesion molecules on CD4+ T cells. Monocyte/macrophage abnormalities include changes in surface receptors, phagocytic ability, and response to interferon. Cytokine abnormalities in CFS include increased levels of transforming growth factor β (TGFβ), increased in vitro synthesis of IL-2 and gamma-interferon, and elevated concentrations of an interferon-induced leukocyte enzyme, 2′,5′-oligoadenylate synthetase (32). An animal model of fatigue found increased serum TGFβ levels compared to control animals (33).

While immune studies often show conflicting results, the most consistent theme is that CFS is associated with a state of immune activation. However, similar immune changes have been noted in major depression (13,59,106,215) and sleep deprivation (107). Hence, the specificity of the immune abnormalities in CFS still needs to be established.

Other pathophysiological investigations have explored abnormalities in the cardiovascular response as an explanation for CFS. One study found CFS patients differed from controls in their cardiovascular response during an upright tilt-table test (17). The authors concluded that CFS is associated with neurally mediated hypotension. Similar findings were reported by another research group, who used EKG spectrum analysis in CFS patients and controls to quantify vagal activity (210). The results showed significant reductions in vagal activity in the CFS patients. Although these findings are interesting, they are also difficult to interpret. Several factors could be responsible for the cardiovascular changes seen in these patients, including mechanoreceptor overstimulation, cardiac deconditioning, and/or medications taken as a result of the CFS disorder. Another possible contributing factor is decreased sympathetic drive from central (brain-stem) neuradrenergic neurons (175). Further research is needed to help clarify the relationship between neurally mediated hypotension and CFS.

Definition and Clinical Features

The current definition for CFS used in the United States evolved from one initially designed for research purposes (96) to a less restrictive definition (66). Both the original and current definitions define CFS as a condition of severe fatigue, present for at least 6 months and not explained by other medical disorders. The revisions require that patients with specific psychiatric diagnoses and certain postinfectious fatigue syndromes be excluded, while patients with selected confounding diagnoses be included (93,142,157,158,203). It has been suggested that the evaluation for CFS include tender-point examination (241), screening for psychiatric disorder (using self-report instruments) (66), and reliable measures of fatigue (137). The current defining inclusion and exclusion criteria recommened for CFS (66) are specified below in Table 8.

Individuals who may be classified as CFS despite the presence of concurrent problems include those with fibromyalgia and those with postinfectious fatigue such as patients with either Lyme disease with persistent fatigue after appropriate antibiotic therapy or brucellosis with persistent fatigue after appropriate antibiotic therapy. Concurrent nonpsychotic and nonmelancholic depression, somatoform disorders, or generalized anxiety disorder/panic disorder do not necessarily exclude the diagnosis of CFS.

Table 8 Inclusion and Exclusion Critieria for CFS

Inclusion criteria:

1. The fatigue must be of new onset (not a lifelong problem), not due to ongoing exertion, not alleviated by rest, and result in substantial reduction of previous occupational, educational, social, or personal activities. It is advised that the levels of fatigue be measured with a self-report instrument that assesses performance and subjective aspects.
2. There must be four or more of the following symptoms, all of which must have been persistent or recurred during 6 or more consecutive months of illness and must not have predated the fatigue:
   a) memory or concentration problems severe enough to interfere with day-to-day functioning
   b) sore throat
   c) tender cervical or axillary lymph nodes
   d) muscle pain
   e) multijoint pain without joint swelling or redness
   f) headaches of a new type
   g) unrefreshing sleep
   h) postexertional malaise lasting more than 24 h

Specific exclusions:

1. Active medical disorders that can cause fatigue (such as untreated hypothyroidism, sleep apnea, medication side effects)
2. Incomplete resolution or past disorders, which may cause chronic fatigue (treated malignancy, unresolved hepatitis B or C virus infection)
3. Past or current major depressive disorder with psychotic or melancholic features, bipolar affective disorders, schizophrenia of any subtype, delusional disorders of any subtype, dementias of any subtype, anorexia nervosa, or bulimia nervosa
4. Alcohol or substance abuse within 2 years before the onset of chronic fatigue and at any time afterward

Epidemiology

In primary care clinics, fatigue defined "as a major problem of more than one month" was noted in one study among 19% of men and 28% of women (132). Other studies of patients in primary care clinics report a similar high prevalence (129,144). The prevalence of CFS is significantly lower. In a prospective cohort study of HMO members, the prevalence of prolonged fatigue was 1775–6321 per 100,000; the frequency of CFS was 75–267 per 100,000 (22). Based on different exclusionary criteria, others have found a prevalence of CFS of 0.3–1.0% (10,148).

Psychiatric and Psychological Studies

The frequency of psychiatric disorders in CFS range from 21 to 86% (93,121,142,157,179,140). The variability may be due in part to the clinical setting in which the patients are evaluated (specialty center vs. primary care environments, the criteria for patient selection, and the nature of the psychiatric assessment). Depression, somatization disorder, anxiety disorder, and dysthymia are the most frequent comorbid psychiatric disorders (93,121,179).

Mood changes in CFS may be secondary to fatigue, chronic illness factors, or relate to social stigma associated with the disorder and lack of available treatment. However, when the frequency of psychiatric illness in CFS is compared to other chronic medical disorders, including those with severe fatigue (such as MS, rheumatoid arthritis, or diabetes), CFS patients have more frequent current and lifetime psychiatric diagnoses (179,69,93). However, CFS patients compared to patients with major depression show less psychological distress (179).

While some would argue that these findings suggest that CFS is another form of primary psychiatric illness (98), it can also be argued that psychological vulnerability may predispose some individuals to prolonged recoveries from viral infection. The early work suggesting this relationship were prospective studies of military personnel at risk for developing the Asian flu (104,105). Imboden et al. noted that elevated scores of depression and loss of morale on the MMPI were associated with delayed recovery from the flu. Canter et al. (29) noted that elevated MMPI scores were associated with a higher incidence of hypersensitivity reactions to prophylactic inoculation.

A landmark study by Cohen et al. (34) showed that levels of stress prior to inoculation with live viruses were associated with susceptibility to clinical syndromes of several upper respiratory infection viruses. Three-hundred and ninety-four volunteers were exposed to one of several viruses that produce upper respiratory infection. A psychological stress index was created by combining three separate stress scales, and the association between the stress index and outcome was examined. There was a linear rise in the proportion of subjects infected and clinical evidence of the "a cold" as stress levels increased. Similarly the proportion of subjects with colds was notably less at the lower stress levels (under 30% had colds) compared to the highest levels (where about 45% had colds). These findings suggest that psychological factors and stress may predispose to the development of CFS. A study of family practice clinic attendees found postviral fatigue was associated with increased psychological stress and attributional style (35). Thus, psychological vulnerability, attributional style, and coping are important mechanisms contributing to the development of CFS. The psychological and immune findings suggest that an individual with elevated stress and poor coping skills may also have associated immune perturbations, which in conjunction with an external insult, such as a viral infection, lead to a prolonged illness associated with severe fatigue.

Neurological Findings

Routine neurological exam is typically normal (136). The results of neuropsychological testing indicate that CFS patients may have mild memory impairment, as well as possible deficits in the speed of information processing (46,75,140,165) and attention (189,204). Complex tests of attention as measured by the PASAT (78) and other measures (189,204) may be abnormal. Memory disturbance has been associated with conceptual tasks involving encoding and retrieval (75). Memory problems are not associated with specific measures of disease activity, laboratory abnormalities, or physical findings but have been associated with depressive symptoms (140). In our experience, CFS patients perform relatively well on computerized tests of mental speed (L. B. Krupp and D. Polina, unpublished data) and on standardized neuropsychological batteries. This is in contrast to patients with chronic medical disorders such as Lyme disease or MS (69,140), who perform poorly on such tests.

Event-related potential (ERP) markers of attention to relevant visual stimuli were normal in CFS patients despite systematic increases in response times to these stimuli (202). These results suggest that the CFS-related impairments may be limited to response-related processes.

Neuroradiological findings in CFS include nonspecific focal areas of increased T_2 signal abnormalities in the subcortical and cerebellar white matter on magnetic resonance (MR) (174,206). Abnormalities on SPECT involving both white and grey matter have been noted. The extent to which these abnormalities are specific for CFS is unclear.

Some CFS patients have sleep disorders as assessed by polysomnography. Difficulties in initiating or maintaining sleep, abnormalities in sleep wave physiology (with alpha-wave intrusion) and poor sleep efficiency have been reported (21,135,159,170,240). Among chronically fatigued patients evaluated in specialized centers, 30–81% are found to have sleep disorders on polysomnography. Specific sleep disorders noted in several studies have included sleep apnea, narcolepsy, periodic leg movement disorder, or excessive daytime somnolence (22,135).

No significant differences between CFS patients and healthy controls have been found on muscle testing (146,147). During a series of maximal isometric contractions, peak force fell in CFS patients and controls by approximately the same amount (147). Measures of intracellular metabolism and muscle neurophysiology during maximum voluntary contraction of the tibialis anterior muscle were also not significantly different in patients and controls (123). At the present time, no peripheral motor control abnormality has been found in CFS (201,216). Whether central motor pathways are affected as suggested by some studies requires further investigation (204).

Therapy for CFS

Pharmacological therapies for CFS have largely focused on treatment of one or another proposed pathogenic hypothesis. Initially the possibility that CFS was related to persistent viral infection led to a treatment trial with acyclovir (219). No improvement with drug was noted over the placebo response. Immunoglobulin therapy has been attempted with conflicting results. One study demonstrated no significant benefit (181), while another using a special subset of CFS patients did show improvement (149). In the United States, most CFS centers do not advocate parenteral immunoglobulin therapy for CFS. Treatments that have been tried and are not superior to placebo include folic acid and cyanocobalamin extract from bovine liver (120) and intravenous multivitamin preparations.

Several treatment studies have focused on the high frequency of depressive symptoms in CFS (155). Various antidepressants have been used with reported success (74). Nonpharmacological approaches including cognitive-behavioral therapy have also been attempted (23,64). Cognitive approaches to CFS therapy have focused on restoring illness predictability and control. Future trials using sensitive and theoretically based outcome measures are necessary to clarify these results.

REFERENCES

1. Ablashi DV, Zombetta C, Lease C, et al. Human herpes virus-6 in chronic fatigue syndrome (CFS). In: Rozee KR, ed. Proceedings of the Chronic Fatigue Workshop (Toronto, 1989). Can Dis Week 1991; 17(suppl):33–37.
2. Adams RD, Cammermeyer J, Denny-Brown D. Acute necrotizing hemorrhagic encephalopathy. J Neuropathol Exp Neurol 1949; 8:1–29.
3. Allen JR. Treatment of measles encephalitis with adrenal steroids. Pediatrics 1957; 20:87–91.
4. Amlie-Lefond C, Kleinschmidt-DeMasters BK, Mahalingam R, Davis LE, Gilden DH. The vasculopathy of varicella-zoster virus encephalitis. Ann Neurol 1995; 37:784–790.
5. Andiman WA, White-Greenwald M, Tinghitella T. Zoster encephalitis: isolation of virus and measurement of varicella-zoster-specific antibodies in cerebrospinal fluid. Am J Med 1982; 73:769–772.
6. Appelbaum E, Kreps SI, Sunshine A. Herpes zoster encephalitis. Am J Med 1962; 32:25–31.
7. Araki Y, Kohmura E, Nakamura H, et al. MR imaging of acute disseminating encephalomyelitis. Radiation Med 1993; 11:263–266.
8. Asch ES, Bujak DI, Weiss M, Peterson MGE, Weinstein A. Lyme disease: an infectious and postinfectious syndrome. J Rheumatol 1994; 21:454–461.
9. Atlas SW, Grossman RI, Goldberg HI, et al. MRI diagnosis of acute disseminated encephalomyelitis. J Comp Ass Tomogr 1986; 10:798–801.
10. Bates DW, Schmitt W, Buchwald D, Ware NC, Lee J, Thoyer E, Kornish RJ, Komaroff AL. Prevalence of fatigue and chronic fatigue syndrome in a primary care practice. Arch Intern Med 1993; 153:2759–2765.
11. Behan PO. Postviral neurologic syndromes. Br Med J 1983; 287:853–854.

12. Benach JL, Bosler EM, Hanrahan JP, et al. Spirochetes isolated from the blood of two patients with Lyme disease. N Engl J Med 1983; 308:740–742.
13. Bennett T, Cohen H, Cohen S. Depression and immunity: a meta-analytic review. Psych Bull 1993; 113:472–486.
14. Bernstein JE, Korman NS, Bickers DR. Topical capsaicin treatment of chronic postherpetic neuralgia. J Am Acad Dermatol 1989; 21:265–270.
15. Bode L, Komaroff AL, Ludwig N. No serologic evidence of Borna disease virus in patients with CFS. Clin Infect Dis 1992; 15:1049–1052.
16. Boe J, Solberg CO, Saeter T. Corticosteroid treatment for acute meningoencephalitis: a retrospective study of 346 cases. Br Med J 1965; 1:1094–1095.
17. Bou-Holaigah I, Rowe PC, Kan J, Calkins H. The relationship between neurally mediated hypotension and the chronic fatigue syndrome. JAMA 1995; 274:961–967.
18. Boulloche J, Parain D, Mallet E, et al. Postinfectious encephalitis with multifocal white matter lesions. Neuropediatrics 1989; 20:173–175.
19. Bourdette DN, Rosenberg NL, Yatsu FM. Herpes zoster ophthalmicus and delayed ipsilateral cerebral infarction. Neurology 1983; 33:1428–1432.
20. Brown RD, Forman DT. The biochemistry of Reye's syndrome. Crit Rev Clin Lab Sci 1982; 17: 247–297.
21. Buchwald D, Pascualy R, Bombardier C, and Kith P. Sleep disorder inpatients with chronic fatigue. Clin Infect Dis 1994; 18(suppl 1):S68–72.
22. Buchwald D, Umali P, Umali J, Kith P, Pearlman T, Komaroff A. Chronic fatigue and the chronic fatigue syndrome: prevalence in a Pacific Northwest health care system. Ann Intern Med 1995; 123:81–88.
23. Butler S, Chalder T, Ron M, Wessely S. Cognitive behavior therapy in chronic fatigue syndrome. J Neurol Neurosurg Psychiatry 1991; 54:153–159.
24. CDC. Lyme disease—United States, 1994. MMWR 1995; 44(24):459–462.
25. Caekebeke J, Boudewyn Peters AC, et al. Cerebral vasculopathy associated with primary varicella infection. Arch Neurol 1990; 47:1033–1035.
26. Caldemeyer KS, Harris TM, Smith RR, Edwards MK. Gadolinium enhancement in acute disseminated encephalomyelitis. J Comp Ass Tomogr 1991; 15:673–675.
27. Caldemeyer KS, Smith RR, Harris TM. MRI in acute disseminated encephalomyelitis. Neuroradiology 1994; 36:216–220.
28. Caligiuri M, Murray C, Buchwald D, Levine H, Cheney P, Peterson D, Kamaroff AL, Ritz J. Phenotypic and functional deficiency of natural killer cells in patients with chronic fatigue syndrome. J Immunol 1987; 139:3306–3313.
29. Canter A, Cluff LE, Imboden JB. Hypersensitive reactions to immunization inoculations and antecedent psychological vulnerability. J Psychosom Res 1972; 16:99–101.
30. Cavaletti G, Boglium G, Tagliabue M. MRI evaluation of a case of herpes zoster ophthalmicus with delayed contralateral hemiplegia. Ital J Neurol Sci 1990; 11:297–300.
31. Centers for Disease Control. Measles encephalitis—United States 1972–1979. MMWR 1981; 30:362–364.
32. Chao CC, Janoff EN, Hu S, Thomas K, Gallagher M, Tsang M, Peterson PK. Altered cytokine release in peripheral blood mononuclear cell cultures from patients with the CFS. Cytokine 1991; 3:292–298.
33. Chao CC, DeLa Hunt M, Hu S, Close K, Peterson PK. Immunologically mediated fatigue: a murine model. Clin Immun Immunopath 1992; 64:161–165.
34. Cohen S, Tyrrell AJ, Smith AP. Psychological stress and susceptibility to the common cold. N Engl J Med 1991; 325:606–612.
35. Cope H, David A, Pelosi A, Mann A. Predictors of chronic "postviral" fatigue. Lancet 1994; 344: 864–868.
36. Cowan LD, Griffin MR, Howson CP, et al. Acute encephalopathy and chronic neurological damage after pertussis vaccine. Vaccine 1993; 11:1371–1379.
37. Coyle PK, Deng Z, Schutzer SE, Belman AL, Krupp LB, Luft B. Detection of *Borrelia burgdorferi* antigens in cerebrospinal fluid. Neurology 1993; 3:1093–1097.

38. Coyle PK, Schutzer SE, Deng Z, Krupp LB, Belman AL, Benach JL, Luft BJ. Detection of *Borrelia burgdorferi* specific antigen in antibody-negative cerebrospinal fluid in neurologic Lyme disease. Neurology 1995; 45:2010–1015.
39. Croen KD, Straus SE. Varicella-zoster virus latency. Ann Rev Microbiol 1991; 45:265–282.
40. Cusmai R, Bertini E, Di Capua M, et al. Bilateral, reversible, selective thalamic involvement demonstrated by brain MR and acute severe neurological dysfunction with favorable outcome. Neuropediatrics 1994; 25:44–47.
41. Dale JK, DiBisceglie AM, Hoornagle JH, et al. Chronic fatigue syndrome: Lack of association with hepatitis C virus infection. J Med Virol 1991; 34:119–121.
42. Dattwyler RJ, Halperin JJ, Volkman DJ, et al. Treatment of late Lyme borreliosis—randomized comparison of ceftriaxone and penicillin. Lancet 1988; 1:1191–1194.
43. Dattwyler RJ, Volkman DJ, Conaty SM, Platkin SP, Luft BJ. Treatment of early Lyme borreliosis, a randomized trial comparing amoxicillin plus probenecid to doxycycline in patients with erythema migrans. Lancet 1990; 336:1404–1406.
44. Dattwyler RJ, Volkman DJ, Luft BJ, Halperin JJ, Thomas J, Golightly MG. Seronegative Lyme disease. N Engl J Med 1988; 319:1441–1446.
45. DeFreitas E, Hilliard B, Cheney PR, et al. Retroviral sequences related to human T-lymphotropic virus type II in patients with chronic fatigue immune dysfunction syndrome. Proc Natl Acad Sci USA 1991; 88:2922–2926.
46. DeLuca J, Johnson SK, Beldowicz D, Natelson BH. Neuropsychological impairments in chronic fatigue syndrome, multiple sclerosis, and depression. J Neurol Neurosurg Psychiatr 1995; 58:38–43.
47. Den Heijer JC, Peters ACB, Van Gemert GW. Postinfectious meningoencephalitis complicating *Mycoplasma pneumoniae* in a child. J Neurol Neurosurg Psychiatr 1986; 49:600–602.
48. DeVivo DC. Reyes syndrome. Neurol Clin North Am 1985; 3:95–115.
49. Devries E. Postvaccinial Perivenous Encephalitis. A Pathological Anatomical Study on the Place of Postvaccinial Perivenous Encephalitis in the Group Encephalitis. Amsterdam, Elsevier 1960.
50. Dinerman H, Steere AC. Lyme disease associated with fibromyalgia. Ann Intern Med 1992; 117: 281–285.
51. Donovan MK, Lenn NJ. Postinfectious encephalomyelitis with localized basal ganglia involvement. Pediatr Neurol 1989; 5:311–313.
52. Doyle PW, Gibson G, Dolman CL. Herpes zoster ophthalmicus with contralateral hemiplegia: Identification of cause. Ann Neurol 1983; 14:84–85.
53. DuBois R, Seeley JK, Brus I, Sakamoto K, Ballow M, Harada S, Bechtold TA, Pearson G, Purtilo, DT. Chronic mononucleosis syndrome. South Med J 1984; 77:1376–1382.
54. Eda I, Takashima S, Takeshita K. Acute hemiplegia with lacunar infarct after varicella infection in childhood. Brain Dev 1983; 5:494–499.
55. Eidelbert D, Sotrel A, Horoupian DS, et al. Thrombotic cerebral vasculopathy associated with herpes zoster. Ann Neurol 1986; 19:7–14.
56. Epperson LW, Whitaker JN, Kapila A. Cranial MRI in acute disseminated encephalomyelitis. Neurology 1988; 38:332–333.
57. Esman V, Geil SP, Kroon S, et al. Prednisone does not prevent post-herpetic neuralgia. Lancet 1987; July 18:126–129.
58. Ettestad PJ, Campbell GL, Welbel SF, Genese CA, Spitalny KC, Marchetti CM, Dennis DT. Biliary complications in the treatment of unsubstantiated Lyme disease. J Infect Dis 1995; 171:356–361.
59. Evans DL, Folds JD, Petitto JM, et al. Circulating natural killer cell phenotypes in men and women with major depression. Arch Gen Psychiatry 1992; 49:388–395.
60. Fallon BA, Nields JA, Parsons B, Liebowitz MR, Klein DF. Psychiatric manifestations of Lyme borreliosis. J Clin Psychiatry 1993; 54:263–268.
61. Fallon BA, Nields, JA. Lyme disease: A neuropsychiatric illness. Am J Psychiatry 1994; 151:1571–1583.
62. Ferraro A, Roizin. Hyperergic encephalomyelitides following exanthematic diseases, infectious diseases and vaccination. J Neuropathol Exp Neurol 1957; 16:423–445.

63. Filloux F, Townsend J. Herpes zoster ophthalmicus with ipsilateral cerebellar infarction. Neurology 1985; 35:1531.
64. Friedberg F, Krupp LB: A comparison of cognitive behavioral treatment for chronic fatigue syndrome and primary depression. Clin Infect Dis 1994; 18(suppl 1):105–110.
65. Freyer DG, Crane R, Margolis MT. Angiographic changes in intracranial arteritis of ophthalmic herpes zoster. Ann Neurol 1984; 15:311–312.
66. Fukuda K, Straus SE, Hickie I, Sharpe MC, Dobbins JG, Komaroff A. The chronic fatigue syndrome: a comprehensive approach to its definition and study. Ann Intern Med 1994; 121:953–959.
67. Galer BS. Portenoy R. Acute herpetic and postherpetic neuralgic clinical features and management. Mt Sinai S Med 1991; 58:257–266.
68. Gaudino E, Coyle PK, Doscher C, Krupp LB. Neuropsychiatric profile of post-Lyme syndrome. Neurology 1994; 44(suppl):A376.
69. Gaudino EA, Geisler MW, Preston T, Coyle PK, Masur DM, Krupp LB. Neuropsychiatric differences between chronic Lyme disease and chronic fatigue syndrome. Neurology 1995; 45(supp):A166.
70. Gendelman HE, Wolinsky JS, Johnson RT, et al. Measles encephalomyelitis: lack of evidence of viral invasion of the central nervous system and quantitative study of demyelination. Ann Neurol 1984; 15:353–360.
71. Gilden DH, Rozenman Y, Murray R, et al. Detection of varicella-zoster virus nucleic acid in neurons of normal human thoracic ganglia. Ann Neurol 1987; 22:377–380.
72. Goldenberg DL, Simms RW, Geiger A, Komaroff AL. High frequency of fibromyalgia in patients with chronic fatigue seen in a primary care practice. Arthritis Rheum 1990; 33:381–387.
73. Goldston AS, Millichap JG, Miller RH. Cerebellar ataxia with preeruptive varicella. Am J Dis Child 1963; 106:197–200.
74. Goodnick PJ, Sandoval R. Psychotropic treatment of chronic fatigue syndrome and related disorders. J Clin Psychiatry 1993; 54:13–20.
75. Grafman J, Schwartz V, Dale JK, Scheffers M, Houser C, Straus SE. Analysis of neuropsychological functioning in patients with chronic fatigue syndrome. J Neurol Neurosurg Psychiatry 1993; 56: 684–689.
76. Gray F, Belec L, Lescs MC, et al. Varicella-zoster virus infection of the central nervous system in the acquired immune deficiency syndrome. Brain 1994; 117:987–999.
77. Griffin DE, Ward BJ, Jauregui E, et al. Immune activation in measles. N Engl J Med 1989; 320:1667–1672.
78. Gronwall DM. Paced auditory serial-addition task: a measure of recovery from concussion. Percept Motor Skills 1977; 44:367–373.
79. Gupta S, Vayuvegula B. A comprehensive immunological analysis in chronic fatigue syndrome. Scand J Immunol 1991; 33:319–327.
80. Halperin SA, Marrie TJ. Pertussis encephalopathy in an adult: case report and review. Rev Infect Dis 1991; 13:1043–1047.
81. Halpin D, Wessely S. VP-1 antigen in chronic post-viral fatigue syndrome. Lancet 1989; 1:1028–1029.
82. Halpin TJ, Holzhauer FJ, Campbell RJ, et al. Reye's syndrome and medication use. JAMA 1982; 248:687–691.
83. Halperin JJ, Krupp LB, Golightly MG, Volkman DJ. Lyme borreliosis-associated encephalopathy. Neurology 1990; 40:1340–1343.
84. Halperin JJ, Pass HL, Anand AK, Luft BJ, Volkman DJ, Dattwyler RJ. Nervous system abnormalities in Lyme disease. Ann NY Acad Sci 1988; 539:24–34.
85. Hamblin TJ, Hussain J, Akbar AN, Tang YC, Smith JL, Jones DB. Immunological reason for chronic ill health after infectious mononucleosis. Br Med J 1983; 287:85–88.
86. Hansen K, Lebach AM. Lyme neuroborreliosis: a new sensitive diagnostic assay for intrathecal synthesis of *Borrelia burgdorferi*-specific immunoglobulin G, A, and M. Ann Neurol 1991; 30: 197–205.
87. Harding SP, Lipton JR, Wells JCD: Natural history of herpes zoster ophthalmicus: predictors of postherpetic neuralgia and ocular involvement. Br J Ophthalmol 1987; 71:353–358.

88. Hart M. Hemorrhagic and perivenous encephalitis: a clinical-pathological review of 38 cases. J Neurol Neurosurg Psych 1957; 38:585–591.
89. Hellinger WC, Smith TF, Van Scoy RE, et al. Chronic fatigue syndrome and the diagnostic value of antibody to Epstein-Barr virus early antigen. JAMA 1988; 260:971–972.
90. Hemachudha T, Phanuphak P, Johnson RT, et al. Neurological complications of Semple-type rabies vaccine: Clinical and immunologic studies. Neurology 1987; 37:550–556.
91. Hemachudha T, Griffin DE, Giffels JJ, et al. Myelin basic protein as an encephalitogen in encephalomyelitis and polyneuritis following rabies vaccination. N Engl J Med 1987; 316:369–374.
92. Heubi JE, Partin JC, Partin JS, et al. Reye's syndrome: current concepts. Hepatology 1987; 7:155–164.
93. Hickey I, Lloyd A, Wakefield D, Parker G. The psychiatric status of patients with the CFS. Br J Psychiatry 1990; 156:534–540.
94. Hilt DC, Buchholz D, Krumholz A, et al. Herpes zoster ophthalmicus and delayed contralateral hemiparesis caused by cerebral antitis: diagnosis and management approaches. Ann Neurol 1983; 14:543–553.
95. Hilton E, Kozarsky P, Smith M, et al. Status of immunity to tetanus, measles, mumps, rubella and polio among US travelers. Ann Intern Med 1991; 115:32–33.
96. Holmes GP. Defining the chronic fatigue syndrome. Rev Infect Dis 1991; 13(suppl 1):S53–55.
97. Hogan EL, Krigman MR. Herpes zoster myelitis: evidence for viral invasion of spinal cord. Arch Neurol 1973; 29:309–313.
98. Holland R. Chronic fatigue syndrome. Correspondence. Can Med Assoc J 1989; 140:1016.
99. Holmes GP, Kaplan JE, Gantz, et al. Chronic fatigue syndromes: a working case definition. Ann Intern Med 1988; 108:385–389.
100. Holmes GP, Kaplan JE, Stewart JA, Hunt B, Pinsky PF, Schonberger LB. A cluster of patients with a chronic mononucleosis-like symptoms. JAMA 1987; 257:2297–2302.
101. Hope-Simpson RE. The nature of herpes zoster: a long-term study and a new hypothesis. Proc R Soc Med 1965; 58:9–20.
102. Huff JC, Drucker JL, Clemmer A, et al. A randomized trial of acyclovir for 7 days or 21 days with and without prednisolone for treatment of acute herpes zoster. N Engl J Med 1994; 330:896–900.
103. Hurwitz ES, Nelson DB, Davis C, et al. National surveillance for Reye syndrome: a five-year review. Pediatrics 1982; 70:895–900.
104. Imboden JB, Canter A, Cluff LE. Convalescence from influenza. Arch Intern Med 1961; 108:393–399.
105. Imboden JB, Canter A, Cluff LE, Trevor RW. Brucellosis: psychologic aspects of delayed convalescence. Arch Intern Med 1959; 103:406–444.
106. Irwin M, Patterson T, Smith T, Caldwell C, Brown SA, Gillin JC, Grant I. Reduction of immune function in life stress and depression. Biol Psychiatry 1990; 27:22–30.
107. Irwin M, Mascovich A, Gillin JC, Willoughby R, Pike J, Smith TL. Partial sleep deprivation reduces natural killer cell activity in humans. Psychosom Med 1994; 56:493–498.
108. Jeffrey DR, Mandler RN, Davis LE. Transverse myelitis. Retrospective analysis of 33 cases, with differentiation of cases associated with multiple sclerosis and parainfectious events. Arch Neurol 1993; 50:532–535.
109. Johnson KP, Wolinsky JS, Ginsberg AH. Immune mediated syndromes of the nervous system related to virus infections. In: Vinken PJ, Bruyn GW, Klawans HL, eds. Handbook of Clinical Neurology New York: Elsevier, 1978.
110. Johnson RT. The pathogenesis of acute viral encephalitis postinfectious encephalomyelitis. J Infect Dis 1987; 155:359–364.
111. Johnson RT, Griffin De. Postinfectious encephalomyelitis. In: Kennedy PGE, ed. Infections of the Nervous System. London: Butterworths, 1987.
112. Johnson RT, Griffin DE, Gendelman HE. Postinfectious encephalomyelitis. Sem Neurol 1985; 5: 180–190.
113. Johnson RT, Griffin DE, Hirsch RL, et al. Measles encephalomyelitis—clinical and immunologic studies. N Engl J Med 1984; 310:137–141.
114. Josephs SF, Henry B, Balachandran N, et al. HHV-6 reaction in chronic fatigue syndrome. Lancet 1991; 337:1346–1347.

115. Joy JL, Carolo JR, Velez-Borros JR. Cerebral infarction following herpes zoster: the enlarging clinical spectrum. Neurology 1989; 30:1640.
116. Kamholz J, Tremblay G. Chickenpox with delayed contralateral hemiparesis caused by cerebral angiitis. Ann Neurol 1985; 18:358–360.
117. Kahn S, Yaqub B, Poser C, Al Deeb S, Bohlega S. Multiphasic disseminated encephalomyelitis presenting as alternating hemiplegia. J Neurol Neurosurg Psychiatry 1995; 58:467–470.
118. Kanter DS, Horensky D, Sperling RA, et al. Plasmapheresis in fulminant acute disseminated encephalomyelitis. Neurology 1995; 45:824–827.
119. Kaplan RF, Meadows ME, Vincent LC. Memory impairment and depression in patients with Lyme encephalopathy: comparison with fibromyalgia and nonpsychotically depressed patients. Neurology 1992; 42:1263–1267.
120. Kaslow JE, Rucker L, Onishi R. Liver extract folic acid-cyanocobalamin vs placebo for chronic fatigue syndrome. Arch Intern Med 1989; 149:2501–2503.
121. Katon W, Buchwald DS, Simon GE et al. Psychiatric illness in patients with chronic fatigue and those with rheumatoid arthritis. J Gen Intern Med 1991; 6:277–285.
122. Kennedy PGE. Neurological complications of varicella-zoster virus. In: Kennedy PGE, ed. Infections of the Nervous System. London: Butterworths, 1987.
123. Kent-Braun JA, Sharma KR, Weiner MW, Massie B, Miller RG. Central basis of muscle fatigue in chronic fatigue syndrome. Neurology 1993; 43:125–131.
124. Kepes JJ. Large focal tumor-like demyelinating lesion of the brain: Intermediate entity between multiple sclerosis and acute disseminated encephalomyelitis. Ann Neurol 1993; 33:18–27.
125. Kesselring J, Miller D, Robb S, et al. Acute disseminated encephalitis. MRI findings and the distinction from multiple sclerosis. Brain 1990; 113:291–302.
126. Khan AS, Heneine WM, Chapman LE, et al. Assessment of a retrovirus sequence and other possible risk factors for the chronic fatigue syndrome in adults. Ann Intern Med 1993; 118:241–245.
127. Kishore-Kumar R, Max MB, Schafer SC. Desipramine relieves postherpetic neuralgia. Clin Pharmacol Ther 1990; 47:305–312.
128. Klimas NG, Salvato FR, Morgan R, Fletcher MA. Immunologic abnormalities in CFS. J Clin Microbiol 1991; 28:1403–1410.
129. Klonoff DC. CFS. Clin Infect Dis 1992; 15:812–823.
130. Komaroff AL, Wang SP, Lee J, Grayston JT. No association of chronic chlamydia pneumoniae infection with CFS. J Infect Dis 1992; 165:184.
131. Kornips HM, Verhagen WI, Prick MJ. Acute disseminated encephalomyelitis probably related to a *Mycoplasma pneumoniae* infection. Clin Neurol Neurosurg 1993; 95:59–63.
132. Kroenke K, Wood DR, Mangelsdorff AD, Meier NJ, Powell JB. Chronic fatigue in primary care: prevalence, patient characteristics, and outcome. JAMA 1988; 260:929–934.
133. Krupp LB. Fatigue in Lyme borreliosis. In: Coyle PK, ed. Lyme Disease. St. Louis: Mosby Year Book, 1993:196–203.
134. Krupp LB, Coyle PK, Doscher C, et al. Fatigue therapy in multiple sclerosis: results of a double-blind, randomized, parallel trial of amantadine, pemoline, and placebo. Neurology 1995; 45:1956–1961.
135. Krupp LB, Jandorf L, Coyle PK, Mendelson WB. Sleep in chronic fatigue syndrome. J Psychosom Res 1993; 37:325–331.
136. Krupp LB, Lagenbach L, Fernquist L, et al. Neurological evaluation in chronic fatigue syndrome. Ann Neurol 1990; 28:251.
137. Krupp LB, LaRocca NC, Muir-Nash J, Steinberg AD. The fatigue severity scale. Application to patients with multiple sclerosis and systemic lupus erythematosus. Arch Neurol 1989; 46:1121–1123.
138. Krupp LB, Masur D, Schwartz J, et al. Cognitive functioning in late lyme borreliosis. Arch Neurol 1991; 48:1125–1129.
139. Krupp LB, Mendelson WB, Friedman R. An overview of chronic fatigue syndrome. J Clin Psychiatry 1991; 52:403–410.
140. Krupp LB, Sliwinski M, Masur D, Friedberg F, Coyle PK. Cognitive functioning and depression in patients with chronic fatigue syndrome and multiple sclerosis. Arch Neurol 1994; 51:705–710.

141. Landay AL, Jessop C, Lennette ET, et al. Chronic fatigue syndrome: clinical condition associated with immune activation. Lancet 1991; 338:707–711.
142. Lane TJ, Manu P, Matthews DA. Depression and somatization in the chronic fatigue syndrome. Am J Med 1991; 91:335–344.
143. Levine S, Sowinski R. Hyperacute allergic encephalomyelitis. Am J Pathol 1973; 73:247–260.
144. Lewis G, Wessely S. The epidemiology of fatigue: more questions than answers. J Epidemiol Commun Health 1992; 46:92–97.
145. Liu GT, Holmes GL. Varicella with delayed contralateral hemiparesis detected by MRI. Pediatr Neurol 1990; 6:131–134.
146. Lloyd AR, Gandevia SC, Hales JP. Muscle performance, voluntary activation, twitch properties, and perceived effort in normal subjects and patients with chronic fatigue syndrome Brain 1991; 114:85–98.
147. Lloyd AR, Hales JP, Gandevia SC. Muscle strength, endurance and recovery in the post-infection fatigue syndrome. J Neurol Neurosurg Psychiatry 1988; 51:1316–1322.
148. Lloyd AR, Hickie I, Boughton CR, et al. Prevalence of chronic fatigue syndrome in an Australian population. Med J Aust 1990; 153:522–528.
149. Lloyd A, Hickie I, Wakefield D, Boughton CR, Dwyer J. A double-blind, placebo-controlled trial of intravenous immunoglobulin therapy in patients with chronic fatigue syndrome. Am J Med 1990; 89:561–568.
150. Lloyd AR, Wakefield D, Boughton CR, Dwyer JM. Immunological abnormalities in the CFS. Med J Austr 1989; 151:122–124.
151. Logigian EL, Kaplan RF, Steere AC. Chronic neurologic manifestations of Lyme disease. N Engl J Med 1990; 21:1433–1437.
152. Lucas J. An account of uncommon symptoms succeeding the measles; with additional remarks on the infection of measles and smallpox. London Med J 1790; 11:325–331.
153. Luft BJ, Steinman CR, Neimark HC, Muralidhar B, Rush T, Finkel MK, Kunkel M, Dattwyler RJ. Invasion of the central nervous system by Borrelia burgdorferi in acute disseminated infection. JAMA 1992; 267:1364–1367.
154. Lukes SA, Norman D. Computed tomography in acute disseminated encephalomyelitis. Ann Neurol 1983; 13:567–572.
155. Lynch S, Seth R, Montgomery S. Antidepressant therapy in the chronic fatigue syndrome. Br J Gen Pract 1991; 41:339–342.
156. Mahalingam B, Wellish M, Wolf W, et al. Latent varicella-zoster viral DNA in human trigeminal and thoracic ganglia. N Engl J Med 1990; 323:627–631.
157. Manu P, Matthews DA, Lane TJ. The mental health of patients with a chief complaint of chronic fatigue. Arch Intern Med 1988; 148:2213–2217.
158. Manu P, Matthews DA, Lane TJ. Panic disorder among patients with chronic fatigue. South Med J 1991; 34:451–456.
159. Manu P, Lane TJ, Matthews DA, Castriotta RJ, Watson RK, Abeles M. Alpha-delta sleep in patients with a chief complaint of chronic fatigue. South Med J 1994; 37:465–470.
160. Marrie TJ, Purdy RA, Johnston BL, et al. Encephalomyeloradiculopathy of infectious or parainfectious etiology—a new entity? Clin Infect Dis 1995; 20:945–953.
161. Massarotti EM, Luger SW, Rahn D, et al. Treatment of early Lyme disease. Am J Med 1992; 92: 396–403.
162. Masuda A, Nozoe S, Matsuyama T, Tanaka H. Psychobehavioral and immunological characteristics of adult people with chronic fatigue and patients with chronic fatigue syndrome. Psychosom Med 1994; 56:512–516.
163. Max MB, Schafer SC, Culnane M, et al. Amitriptyline but not lorazepam relieves postherpetic neuralgia. Neurology 1988; 38:1427–1432.
164. McCombe PA, Chalk JB, Searle JW, et al. Progressive encephalomyelitis with rigidity: a case report with magnetic resonance imaging findings. J Neurol Neurosurg Psych 1989; 52:1429–1431.
165. McDonald E, Cope H, David A. Cognitive impairment in patients with chronic fatigue: a preliminary study. J Neurol Neurosurg Psychiatry 1993; 56:812–815.

166. McKendrick MW, McGill JI, White JE. Oral acyclovir in acute herpes zoster. Br Med J 1986; 293: 1529–1532.
167. Miller HG, Stanton JB, Gibbons JL. Parainfectious encephalomyelitis and related syndromes. Q J Med 1956; 25:427–505.
168. Miller HG, Stanton JB, Gibbons JL. Acute disseminated encephalomyelitis and related syndromes. Br Med J 1957; 668–672.
169. Miller NA, Carmichael HA, Calder BD. Antibody to coxsackie B virus in diagnosing postviral fatigue syndrome. Br Med J 1991; 302:140–143.
170. Morriss R, Sharpe M, Sharpley A, Cowen PJ, Hawton K, Morris J. Abnormalities of sleep in patients with the chronic fatigue syndrome. Br Med J 1993; 306:1161–1164.
171. Mossuto-Agatiello L, Iovine C, Kniahynicki C. Herpes zoster ophthalmicus and delayed ipsilateral intracerebral hemorrhage. Neurology 1987; 37:1264–1265.
172. Nadelman RB, Luger SW, Frank E, et al. Comparison of cefuroxime axetil and doxycycline in the treatment of early Lyme disease. Ann Intern Med 1992; 117:273–280.
173. Natelson BH, Ellis SP, Braonain PJ, DeLuca J, Tapp WN. Frequency of deviant immunological test values in chronic fatigue syndrome patients. Clin Diag Lab Immunol 1995; 2:238–240.
174. Natelson BH, Cohen JM, Brassloff I, Lee HJ. A controlled study of brain magnetic resonance imaging in patients with the chronic fatigue syndrome. J Neurol Sci 1993; 120:213–217.
175. Natelson BH, Cheu J, Pareja J, Ellis SP, Policastro T, Findley TW. Randomized, double-blind, controlled placebo-phase in trial of low dose phenelzine in the chronic fatigue syndrome. Psychopharmacology (in press).
176. Newton R. Plasma exchange in acute post-infectious demyelination. Dev Med Child Neurol 1981; 23:538–543.
177. Ohtaki E, Murakami Y, Komori H, et al. Acute disseminated encephalomyelitis after Japanese B encephalitis vaccination. Pediatr Neurol 1992; 8:137–139.
178. Partin JC, Schubert WK, Partis JS. Mitochondrial ultrastructure in Reye's syndrome (encephalopathy and fatty degeneration of the viscera). N Engl J Med 1971; 285:1339–1343.
179. Pepper C, Krupp LB, Friedberg F, Doscher C, Coyle PK. Comparison of psychiatric characteristics in chronic fatigue syndrome, multiple sclerosis, and depression. J Neuropsychiatry Clin Neurosci 1993; 5:1–7.
180. Peters ACB, Versteeg J, Bots GTAM, et al. Varicella and acute cerebellar ataxia. Arch Neurol 1978; 35:769–771.
181. Peterson PK, Shepard J, Macres M, Schench C, Crosson J, Rechtman D, Lurie N. A controlled trial of intravenous immunoglobulin G in CFS. Am J Med 1990; 89:554–560.
182. Poser C. Magnetic resonance imaging in asymptomatic disseminated vasculomyelinopathy. J Neurol Sci 1989; 94:69–77.
183. Poser C, Roman G, Emery E. Recurrent disseminated vasculomyelinopathy. Arch Neurol 1978; 35: 166–170.
184. Puchhammer-Stockl E, Popow-Kraupp T, Heinz FX, et al. Detection of varicella-zoster virus DNA by polymerase chain reaction in the cerebrospinal fluid of patients suffering from neurological complications associated with chicken pox or herpes zoster. J Clin Microbiol 1991; 29:1513–1516.
185. Pullicino P, Fava S. Recurrent cerebral infarction and central retinal artry occlusion following mandibular zoster. J Can Sci Neurol 1991; 18:105.
186. Rasmussen AK, Nieslsen H, Andersen V, Barington T, Bendtzen K, Hansen MB, Nielsen L, Pedersen BK, Wiik A. Chronic fatigue syndrome—a controlled cross-sectional study. Ugeskr Laeg 1994; 156:6836–6840.
187. Ravkina L, Harib I, Manovitch Z, et al. Hyperacute experimental allergic encephalomyelitis in rhesus monkeys as a model of acute necrotizing hemorrhagic encephalomyelitis. J Neurol 1979; 221: 113–125.
188. Rawlinson WD, Cunningham AL. Contralateral hemiplegia following thoracic herpes zoster. Med J Aust 1991; 155:344–346.
189. Ray C, Phillips L, Weir W. Quality of attention in chronic fatigue syndrome: Subjective reports of

everyday attention and cognitive difficulty, and performance on tasks of focused attention. J Clin Psychol 1993; 32:357–364.
190. Reich H, Lin SR, Goldblatt D. Computerized tomography in acute hemorrhagic leukoencephalopathy: a case report. Neurology 1979; 29:255–258.
191. Reichman RC. Neurologic complications of varicella-zoster infections: herpes zoster-varicella infections in immunosuppressed patients. Ann Intern Med 1978; 89:375–388.
192. Reik L, Steere AC, Bartenhagen NH, Shope RD, Malawista SE. Neurologic abnormalities of Lyme disease. Medicine 1979; 58:281–294.
193. Reye RDK, Morgan G, Baral J. Encephalopathy and fatty degeneration of the viscera: a disease entity in childhood. Lancet 1963; 2:749–752.
194. Rivers TM, Sprent DH, Berry GP. Observations on attempts to produce acute disseminated encephalomyelitis in monkeys. J Exp Med 1933; 58:39–54.
195. Rockoff A, Spigland I, Lorenstein B, et al. Postvaccinial encephalomyelitis without cutaneous vaccination reaction. Ann Neurol 1979; 5:99–101.
196. Roelcke U, Barnett W, Wilder-Smith E, et al. Untreated neuroborreliosis: Bannwarth's syndrome evolving into acute schizophrenia-like psychosis. J Neurol 1992; 129–131.
197. Ropper AH, Poskanzer DC. The prognosis of acute and subacute transverse myelopathy based on early signs and symptoms. Ann Neurol 1978; 4:451–459.
198. Rowbotham MC, Fields HL. Post-herpetic neuralgia: the relation of pain complaint, sensory disturbance and skin temperature. Pain 1989; 39:129–144.
199. Rowbotham MC, Fields HL. Topical lidocaine reduces pain in post herpetic neuralgia. Pain 1989; 38:297–301.
200. Rowbotham MC, Reisner-Keller LA, Fields HL. Both intravenous lidocaine and morphine reduce the pain of post herpetic neuralgia. Neurology 1991; 41:1024–1028.
201. Rutherford OM, White PD. Human quadriceps strength and fatiguability in patients with post viral fatigue. J Neurol Neurosurg Psychiatry 1991; 54:961–964.
202. Scheffers MK, Johnson R Jr, Grafman J, Dale JK, Straus SE. Attention and short-term memory in CFS patients. Neurology 1992; 42:1667–1675.
203. Schluederberg A, Strauss SE, Peterson P, Blumenthal S, Domaroff AL, Spring SB, et al. NIH conference chronic fatigue syndrome research. Definition and medical outcome assessment. Ann Intern Med 1992; 117:325–331.
204. Schmaling KB, DiClementi JD, Cullum CM, Jones JF. Cognitive functioning in chronic fatigue syndrome and depression: a preliminary comparison. Psychosomat Med 1994; 56:383–388.
205. Schutzer SE, Coyle PK, Belman AL, et al. Sequestration of antibody to *Borrelia burgdorferi* in immune complexes in seronegative Lyme disease. Lancet 1990; 1:312–315.
206. Schwartz RB, Garada BM, Kamaroff AL, Tice HM, Gleit M, Jolesz FA, Holman BL. Detection of intracranial abnormalities in patients with chronic fatigue syndrome: comparison of MR imaging and SPECT. Am J Roentgen 1994; 162:935–941.
207. Shadick NA, Phillips CB, Logigian EL, Steere AC, Kaplan RF, Berardi VP, Duray PH, Larson MG, Wright EA, Ginsburg KS, Katz JN, Liang MH. The long-term clinical outcomes of Lyme disease. Ann Intern Med 1994; 121:560–567.
208. Shuper A, Vining EP, Freeman JM. Central nervous system vasculitis after chickenpox—cause or coincidence? Arch Dis Child 1990; 65:1245–1248.
209. Sigal LH. Experience with the first one hundred patients referred to a Lyme disease referral center. Am J Med 1990; 88:577–581.
210. Sisto SA, Tapp W, Drastal S, Bergen M, DeMasi I, Cordero D, Natelson B. Vagal tone is reduced during paced breathing in patients with the chronic fatigue syndrome. Clin Autonom Res 1995; 5: 139–143.
211. Snow BJ, Simcock JP. Brainstem infarction following cervical herpes zoster. Neurology 1988; 38:1331.
212. Steere AC, Grodzicki RL, Kornblatt AN, et al. The spirochetal etiology of Lyme disease. N Engl J Med 1983; 08:733–740.

213. Steere AC, RE Levin, et al. Treatment of Lyme arthritis. Arthritis Rheum 1994; 37(6):878–888.
214. Steere AC, Taylor E, McHugh GL, Logigian EL. The overdiagnosis of Lyme disease. JAMA 1993; 269:1812–1816.
215. Stein M, Miller AH, Trestman RL. Depression, the immune system, and health and illness. Arch Gen Psychiatry 1991; 48:171–177.
216. Stokes MJ, Cooper RG, Edwards RT. Normal muscle strength and fatigability in patients with effort syndromes. Br Med J 1988; 297:1014–1017.
217. Stowasser M, Cameron J, Oliver WA. Diaphragmatic paralysis following cervical herpes zoster. Med J Aust 1990; 153:555–556.
218. Stratton KR, Johnson-Howe C, Johnston RB. Adverse events associated with childhood vaccines other than pertussis and rubella; summary of a report from the institute of medicine. JAMA 1994; 271:1602–1605.
219. Straus SE, Dale JK, Tobi M, Lawley T, Preble O, Blaese RM, Hallahan C, Henle W. Acyclovir treatment of the CFS: lack of efficacy in a placebo-controlled trial. N Engl J Med 1988; 319:1692–1698.
220. Straus SE, Fritz S, Dale JK, Gould B, Strober W. Lymphocyte phenotype and function in the chronic fatigue syndrome. J Clin Immunol 1993; 13:30–40.
221. Straus SE, Tosato G, Armstrong G, Lawley T, Preble OT, Henle W, Davey R, et al. Persisting illness and fatigue in adults with evidence of Epstein-Barr virus infection. Ann Intern Med 1985; 102:7–16.
222. Stricker RB, Miller RG, Kiprov DD. Role of plasmapheresis in acute disseminated (postinfectious) encephalomyelitis. J Clin Apheresis 1992; 7:173–179.
223. Suchowersky O, Sweeney VP, Berry K, Bratty PJA. Acute hemorrhagic leukoencephalopathy: a clinical, pathological, and radiological correlation. Can J Neurol Sci 1983; 10:63–67.
224. Sumaya CV. Serologic and virologic epidemiology of Epstein-Barr virus: relevance to CFS. Rev Infect Dis 1991; 13(S):S19–25.
225. Swanson BE. Measles meningoencephalitis: a summary of 24 cases treated at Grasslands over a ten-year period. Am J Dis Child 1956; 12:272–275.
226. Tenser RB. Herpes simples and herpes zoster. Nervous system involvement. Neurol Clin 1984; 2: 215–240.
227. Thajeb P, Chen ST. Cranial computed tomography in acute disseminated encephalomyelitis. Neuroradiology 1989; 31:8–12.
228. Thomas JE, Howard FM. Segmental zoster paresis—a disease profile. Neurology 1972; 22:459–466.
229. Tirelli U, Marotta G, Improta S, Pinto A. Immunological abnormalities in patients with chronic fatigue syndrome. Scand J Immunol 1994; 40:601–608.
230. Tobi M, Morag A, Ravid Z, Chowers I, Feldman-Weiss V, Michaeli Y, Ben-Chetrit E, et al. Prolonged atypical illness associated with serological evidence of persistent Epstein-Barr virus infection. Lancet 1982; 1:61–64.
231. Tyring GS, Barbarash RA, Nahlik JE, et al. Famciclovir for the treatment of actue Herpes Zoster: Effects on acute disease and postherpetic neuralgia. A randomized double-blind, placebo-controlled trial. Ann Intern Med 1995; 123:89–96.
232. van der Meyden CH, de Villiers JF, Middlecote BD, et al. Gadolinium ring enhancement and mass effect in acute disseminated encephalomyelitis. Neuroradiology 1994; 36:221–223.
233. Walker RJ, Gammal TE, Allen MB. Cranial arteritis associated with herpes zoster. Radiology 1973; 107:109–110.
234. Walker RWH, Gawler J. Serial cerebral CT abnormalities in relapsing acute disseminated encephalomyelitis. J Neurol Neurosurg Psych 1989; 52:1100–1102.
235. Watson CPN, Evans RJ, Watt VR. Postherpetic neuralgia and topical capsaicin. Pain 1988; 33: 333–340.
236. Watson CPN, Morshead C, Van der Kooy D, et al. Post-herpetic neuralgia: post-mortem analysis of a case. Pain 1988; 34:129–138.
237. Wayman DM, Pham HN, Byl FM, et al. Audiological manifestations of Ramsay Hunt syndrome. J Laryngol Otol 1990; 104:104–108.

238. Weinshenker BG, Penman M, Bass B. A double-blind, randomized, crossover trial of pemoline in fatigue associated with multiple sclerosis. Neurology 1992; 42:1468–1471.
239. Weller TH, Witton HM. The etiologic agents of varicella and herpes zoster. Serologic studies with the viruses propagated in vitro. J Exp Med 1958; 108:869–890.
240. Whelton CL, Salit I, Moldofsky H. Sleep, EBV infection, musculoskeletal pain, and depressive symptoms in CFS. J Rheumatol 1992; 19:939–943.
241. Wolfe F, Smythe HA, Yunus MB, Bennett RM, Bombardier C, Goldenberg DL, Tugwell P, et al. American College of Rheumatology 1990 criteria.
242. Yousef G, Bell EJ, Mann GF, et al. Chronic enterovirus infection in patients with post-viral fatigue syndrome. Lancet 1988; 1:146–148.
243. Ziegler DK. Acute disseminated encephalitis. Arch Neurol 1966; 14:476–488.
244. Ziegra SR. Corticosteroid treatment for measles encephalitis. J Pediatr 1961; 59:322–323.

22

Brain Abscess

David P. Fritz and Paul B. Nelson
Indiana University School of Medicine, Indianapolis, Indiana

HISTORY

The father of brain abscess management is William Macewen. His textbook published in 1893 set forth the principle of surgical drainage of cerebral abscess (1). Walter Dandy proposed the method of "tapping" in an attempt to minimize damage to surrounding brain when open drainage was attempted (2).

Recent advances in antimicrobial therapy and imaging techniques have lowered the mortality of this once dreaded disease. The single most important development in the diagnosis and management of brain abscess is the availability of CT scanning for both initial evaluation as well as subsequent follow-up (3).

INCIDENCE

The incidence of brain abscess is estimated at 4–13 per million people per year (4–6). The incidence appears to be decreasing due at least in part to better treatment of chronic otitis media (4,6). Brain abscess is fairly evenly distributed across age groups. The male:female ratio is fairly constant, ranging from 2:1 to 4:1.

ETIOLOGY

The etiology of the majority of brain abscesses can be divided into three groups: (1) contiguous spread from adjacent foci of infection, (2) hematogenous spread from distant foci of infection, and (3) trauma/postcraniotomy. Table 1 lists the etiology of brain abscess from several series from different areas of the world. Otitis media or sinusitis are the most common contiguous infections associated with brain abscess formation. Eighteen to 70% of brain abscesses are caused by

Table 1 Etiology of Brain Abscess

No. of patients	Country	Etiology (%) Contiguous	Hematogenous	Trauma	Other	Unknown	Ref.
400	China	70	17	3	0	10	7
50	India	48	30	2	0	20	8
200	Denmark	31	28	17	9	15	9
71	England	56	18	11	6	9	11
140	China	37	16	4	2	41	25
39	Switzerland	23	28	5	5	39	33
102	United States	19	25	24	11	21	67

contiguous spread of infection from otitis media, sinusitis, dental, or scalp infections (7–10). A marked decrease in the number of abscesses caused by contiguous spread of infection from 70% to 17% has been seen over the past 40 years in China (7,11). This decrease has been attributed to the better treatment of otitis media over this 40-year period.

As stated above, brain abscess of otogenic origin appears to be decreasing in frequency due to better treatment of acute and chronic forms of otitis media and mastoiditis (8,10). There are, however, still recent reports of brain abscesses that are primarily secondary to chronic otitis media. Kulah et al. found 73% of brain abscess secondary to chronic ear infection in 19 patients (12). Chronic suppurative otitis media with an associated cholesteatoma is the most common antecedent in patients with brain abscess secondary to ear pathology (13–16). Patients with chronic suppurative otitis media with mucosal disease (but not cholesteatoma) as well as those that have previously undergone mastoidectomy are also at risk of developing brain abscess (15). The rate of developing a brain abscess in a patient with chronic otitis media is about 1/3500 per year to 1/10,700 per year. A 30-year-old with chronic otitis media has about a 1/200 lifetime risk of developing an intracranial abscess. Acute otitis media is implicated 8–14 times less often than chronic otitis media as the etiology of brain abscess (15,17,18).

Brain abscess due to sinusitis also appears to be decreasing in frequency. Sinusitis is associated with 0.5–20% of all brain abscesses (11,19). The majority of cases appear in the 10- to 30-year-old age group (20–22). In a recent study, 24 of 649 patients admitted for sinusitis developed complications, 11 of which were brain abscesses (22). Sphenoid sinusitis is the least common location for sinusitis, but is the most common type of sinusitis to be associated with an intracranial complication as a result of septic thrombosis of the nearby cavernous sinus with local extension of infection (23,24). Overall, pan sinusitis is the most common type of sinusitis associated with the formation of a brain abscess. A brain abscess due to sinusitis is most often located in the frontal lobe (22).

Odontogenic brain abscesses are rare, with a reported incidence of 0–13% (7,10,11,19,25). These abscesses are usually associated with a dental procedure performed within the previous 4 weeks (26) and may be associated with cavernous sinus thrombosis (27). The brain abscess may be distant from the mouth. There is a report of four patients who developed a homonymous hemianopsia from an occipital lobe abscess. Three of the patients' abscesses grew oral flora, and all four of the patients had a history of dental work in the 2–4 weeks before the development of symptoms. No other source for brain abscess was detectable in any of the four patients (28).

The face, scalp, and skull are rarely cited as the source of infection leading to brain abscess formation. Penetrating skin infections and osteomyelitis of the skull account for about 1% of all brain abscesses (7,11). Brain abscess has been reported following halo usage (29), dog bites, and rooster pecking to the skull (30–32). Infections of the face are the most common cause of septic thrombosis of the cavernous sinus, which in turn is associated with local formation of a brain abscess (27).

Brain abscess due to hematogenous spread of infection was reported as the etiology in 30% of cases in two recent studies (8,33). Included in this category are brain abscess caused by pulmonary infections, heart disease, or other infections associated with bacteremia (including wound, skin, abdominal, and pelvic infections, osteomyelitis, and cholecystitis). Table 2 lists the frequency of pulmonary infections, congenital heart disease, and sepsis resulting in brain abscess formation in several series.

Congenital cyanotic heart disease is the most common cause of brain abscess in children, with a tetralogy of Fallot as the underlying abnormality in the majority of cases (34,35). Other less frequent cardiac anomalies associated with brain abscess formation include ventricular septal defects, patent foramen ovale, transposition of the great arteries, and patent ductus arteriosus. The incidence of brain abscess in the population of patients with congenital heart disease ranges from 2 to 6% (36–38). A combination of factors increases the risk of brain abscess in those with congenital heart disease. These factors include bypass of the pulmonary capillary bed and therefore its filtering ability for infectious particles in the systemic circulation, polycythemia (which can increase the risk of thrombotic occlusion of cerebral vessels leading to ischemic infarction and areas of encephalomalacia and necrosis, which are more susceptible to bacterial seeding), and hypoxia (34).

A lung abscess is the most common pulmonary infection associated with brain abscess formation (19,39). Bronchiectasis and pneumonia are also predisposing conditions for brain abscess formation. Cystic fibrosis has only rarely been implicated as the cause of a brain abscess (40).

Pulmonary arteriovenous malformations (AVMs) are also associated with brain abscess, but differ from other pulmonary etiologies in that the AVMs are not the actual source of infection, but rather the conduit through which infection is passed from another source, much like the process allowing for the spread of infection in congenital cyanotic heart disease. Five to six percent of patients with pulmonary AVMs will develop brain abscesses. A review of the literature found that 51 of 53 cases of brain abscess secondary to pulmonary AVMs were associated with the Rendu-Osler-Weber syndrome (hereditary hemorrhagic telangiectasia) (41). It is reasonable to consider prophylactic antibiotics in patients with pulmonary AVMs who are undergoing dental or other invasive procedures (associated with transient bacteremia) to decrease the risk of brain abscess formation (42).

There are many less common sources of hematogenous spread of infection. Brain abscess is a known complication of infective endocarditis. The acute form of infective endocarditis is more commonly associated with brain abscess than the subacute form. The development of brain abscess seems to depend upon the degree and duration of bacteremia, the virulence of the

Table 2 Sources of Hematogenous Acquired Brain Abscess

Pulmonary	44%
Congenital heart disease	36%
Sepsis	20%

Source: Refs. 7, 9, 19, 33, 54, 67.

infecting organism, and the number of septic emboli (43). Brain abscess has been reported following esophageal dilatation (44) as well as following endoscopic injection sclerotherapy (19,45).

Trauma is the etiology of between 2 and 25% of brain abscesses (7,9,11,33). The rate of brain abscess formation following penetrating craniocerebral injuries in Vietnam was 3–17% (46–48). One study of 1221 patients from the Vietnam war with penetrating craniocerebral injuries found the incidence of posttraumatic brain abscess to be 3%. Several risk factors for future development of brain abscesses were identified. Gunshot wound victims were three times more likely than fragment-injured victims to develop a brain abscess. An altered level of consciousness immediately following the injury was a risk factor for subsequent abscess formation. The presence of retained bone fragments and cranial wound complications, especially CSF fistulas, increased the risk of abscess formation. Forty-six percent of abscesses presented within 7–21 days of the initial injury and 70% within the first month (46).

Intracranial pressure monitors, halo usage (29), dog bites (30,31), rooster pecking (32), and intracranial foreign bodies, such as toothpicks, have been associated with brain abscess formation (49). The episode of head trauma can be many years prior to the development of a brain abscess, as evidenced by the diagnosis of brain abscess secondary to retained glass fragment in the brain from trauma 10 years prior to development of the abscess (50). Brain abscess formation in an embolized arteriovenous malformation has been reported, thought secondary to the presence of the embolic agent acting as a nidus for infection (51).

The rate of brain abscess following clean neurosurgery is about 6–7 per 10,000 cases (52). Prophylactic preoperative antibiotic therapy has been instrumental in decreasing the incidence of brain abscess formation as a complication of a neurosurgical procedure.

LOCATION

Brain abscesses most commonly develop in the frontal, parietal, and temporal lobes. The frequency with which the frontal lobe, the parietal lobe, and the temporal lobe are reported as the site of a brain abscess is about equal, and one of these areas is the reported site in 47% of cases. The cerebellum is involved in 6–29% of cases. The occipital lobe is only involved in 1–11% of cases (7,8,11,33,39,53,54). The location of an abscess is frequently related to its etiology. Sinusitis is associated with frontal lobe abscesses. Otitis is associated with temporal lobe and cerebellar abscesses. Metastatic lesions typically occur in the middle cerebral artery distribution. The brain stem, thalamus, basal ganglia, and pituitary are only very rarely involved. Abscesses in these areas are usually of a hematogenous origin. They are usually smaller upon presentation and are more commonly associated with hydrocephalus (55).

The majority of brain abscesses are solitary. Multiple abscesses are most commonly associated with hematogenous spread, but may be due to any etiology (11,53,56,57).

Pituitary abscesses may arise in the presence or absence of a pituitary tumor. These abscesses may be associated with headache, fever, visual loss in the form of a bitemporal hemianopsia, and occasionally meningitis (58,59).

STAGES OF DEVELOPMENT

Brain abscesses evolve through four stages of development. The pathological stages and the CT scan findings have been well described in dogs after intracerebral inoculation with alpha-hemolytic streptococci, and in turn correlated with disease in humans (60,61). The four stages are early and late cerebritis and early and late capsule formation.

The first stage is an early cerebritis (days 1–3), characterized histologically as an area of inflammation that is poorly demarcated from surrounding brain tissue. In this stage, no frank pus is present, but some soft and/or necrotic brain is seen. CT scan reveals an area of low density, with variable amount of ring enhancement.

The second stage of late cerebritis from days 4–9 is characterized histologically by the appearance of fibroblasts and a reticulin matrix. Some pus is present at this stage. This stage has a well-formed ring of enhancement on CT scan. The enhancement will diffuse into the center of the lesion if a delayed scan is obtained.

Early capsule formation, the third stage (days 10–13), is characterized histologically by an increase in new blood vessel formation with migration of fibroblasts into a well-formed layer of the developing capsule. There are focal areas of mature collagen present in the capsule. Frank pus is present at this time. The appearance of this stage on CT scan resembles that of the late cerebritis stage.

Late capsule formation occurs around day 14 or later and is characterized histologically by the appearance of a mature collagen capsule surrounding the necrotic center of the abscess. Also present is a zone of gliosis surrounding the capsule. Frank pus is present at this time. The appearance of this stage on CT scan resembles that of the appearance of the late cerebritis stage and that of early capsule formation. Delayed postcontrast scans, however, fail to reveal diffusion of contrast into the center of the lesion.

Brain abscess formation as described above after intracerebral inoculation of canine brain with alpha-hemolytic streptococci may be modified slightly by different microorganisms. In a model of *Bacteroides fragilis* and *Staphylococcus epidermidis* brain abscess, the same stages of abscess formation were observed but there was delayed and incomplete encapsulation of the abscess cavity. In addition, these abscesses were more prone to rupture into the ventricular system (62). This suggests that different organisms may produce abscesses, which may appear different at any given stage by pathological examination or CT scanning.

BACTERIOLOGY

The bacteriology of brain abscess varies with geographical location, etiology or predisposing conditions, and time period. Virtually any bacteria may cause a brain abscess, but certain bacteria are more frequently isolated. *Streptococcus* species, specifically *Streptococcus milleri*, is probably the most common bacterial species isolated, and aerobic or microaerophilic streptococci are isolated, either singly or in mixed culture, from 23–46% of abscesses. Also commonly isolated are various *Bacteroides* species, found in approximately 13–28% of isolates. Six to 17% of isolates from brain abscesses include *Staphylococcus aureus*, *Proteus* species, diphtheroids (both aerobic and anaerobic), other *Streptococcus* species (both aerobic and anaerobic), and *Haemophilus* species (25,53,63,64).

The bacteria found in a particular brain abscess can be predicted by the location of the abscess, which in turn is influenced by the etiology of the abscess. Temporal lobe abscesses are most frequently secondary to chronic infections of the ear, and the bacteria most typically found in these abscesses include *Bacteroides* sp., streptococci, *Enterobacteriaceae*, and gram-negative aerobic bacilli, most notably *Proteus* sp. (53,63,65). Brain abscesses due to chronic otitis media frequently yield cultures that grow multiple organisms (53). Frontal lobe abscesses are usually caused by chronic sinusitis and frequently yield *Streptococcus milleri* in pure culture. The majority of abscesses secondary to trauma or craniotomy are caused by *S. aureus* (46,63). Brain abscess from hematogenous spread is secondary to the organism from the primary site. *Streptococcus milleri* is again frequently isolated.

Aspergillus, *Candida*, *Cryptococcus neoformans*, *Blastomyces dermatitidis*, other fungi, and protozoa and helminths are increasingly the etiological organisms of brain abscess. The most common of these is *Toxoplasma gondii*, which is the most frequent causative organism of a focal mass lesion in patients with human immunodeficiency virus (HIV) infection.

A brain abscess in an immunocompromised individual is due to different organisms than a brain abscess in an immunocompetent individual. T-lymphocyte mononuclear phagocytic cell defects occur in patients on chronic immunosuppressive therapy, those with lymphoma, lymphocytic leukemia, solid organ and bone marrow transplantation, and acquired immunodeficiency syndrome (AIDS). The organisms most commonly isolated from brain abscess in these patients are *Toxoplasma gondii*, *Nocardia asteroides*, *Aspergillus* sp., *Candida* sp., and *Cryptococcus neoformans*. Neutrophil defects occur in patients treated with cytotoxic chemotherapy and those with chronic granulomatous disease of childhood or myeloperoxidase deficiency. The most common organisms recovered from brain abscesses in these patients are *Enterobacteriaceae*, *Pseudomonas aeruginosa*, and fungi such as *Aspergillus*, Zygomycetes, and *Candida*. Patients with T-lymphocyte mononuclear phagocytic cell dysfunction secondary to AIDS are unique when compared with patients with this defect but without AIDS. Brain abscess in AIDS patients is usually due to *T. gondii*, *C. neoformans*, *Listeria*, *Mycobacterium* sp., *Candida*, or *Aspergillus*. Other lesions on CT or MRI, which may mimic brain abscess in patients with AIDS, are multifocal leukoencephalopathy and primary CNS lymphoma.

Meticulous culture technique definitely increases the yield of positive cultures from brain abscess cavities. Positive culture results reported in the literature range from 58% (7) to 100% (63) with a general range of 70–90%. De Louvois et al. utilized meticulous technique in achieving a perfect positive culture technique (63). This included culturing all specimens within 16 h of collection (most were cultured within 5 h) and specific culture techniques for both aerobes and anaerobes. Several studies cite more positive anaerobic cultures and mixed cultures at the end of their investigation when compared with the beginning. This is likely secondary to increasingly meticulous technique, which includes more attention to anaerobic culturing (4,64). It is often thought that it is more difficult to obtain a positive culture in patients who are on antibiotics at the time the culture is obtained, but several studies dispute this (9,25,53,63,64,67).

CLINICAL PRESENTATION

The clinical presentation of a brain abscess is quite variable. The signs and symptoms are either due to the mass effect of the lesion or the infectious nature of the disease process or both. The classic triad of fever, headache, and focal neurological deficit is present in less than 50% of patients (68). Table 3 lists various signs and symptoms of brain abscess and the frequency of each at the time of presentation. Fever is reported in 40–75% of patients in most series. In the absence of fever, many brain abscesses are mistaken as tumors. Less common findings described only sporadically include ataxia in 9–19% of patients, hemianopsia in 13%, aphasia in 3–12%, unilateral mydriasis in 21%, paresthesias in 4–7%, and nystagmus in 19% (4,7,8,9,19). These

Table 3 Frequency of Various Symptoms and Signs of Brain Abscess

Symptom	Frequency (%)	Symptom	Frequency (%)
Headache	64–97	Hemiparesis	9–44
Fever	42–75	Seizures	13–33
Vomiting	35–85	Papillaedema	6–56
Meningitis	18–49	Ataxia	9–14

findings become more apparent later in the course of the disease when compared to the initial presentation (4). The duration of symptoms prior to presentation ranges from hours to 6 weeks, but the majority present within 7–11 days from onset of symptoms (19,39). With the frequent use of CT and MRI to aid in the evaluation of patients with presumed neurological disease, a diagnosis is made and treatment begun before many of the other symptoms appear.

At the time of presentation, patients are commonly placed into one of four groups based on the initial level of consciousness. Level A refers to patients who are fully awake and alert and oriented, level B to those who are drowsy and disoriented but respond to commands, level C to those responding only to painful stimulation, and level D to those patients who are comatose with no response to stimulation (69).

DIAGNOSIS

The diagnosis of brain abscess is usually made after obtaining a cranial CT or MRI that reveals the classic ring-enhancing lesion. The cranial CT with and without contrast is probably the simplest, most sensitive test for the detection of brain abscess. The precontrast scan reveals an area of decreased density surrounded by edema. The postcontrast scan reveals a ring-enhancing lesion (Fig. 1). The ring is generally thin and homogeneous, slightly thicker on the cortical side than on the ventricular side. This serves to differentiate brain abscess from other lesions such as high-grade astrocytomas, metastatic tumors, and areas of ischemic infarction. Determining the age of the abscess can be estimated from the rate of diffusion of contrast material into the center of the lesion, as described earlier in this chapter.

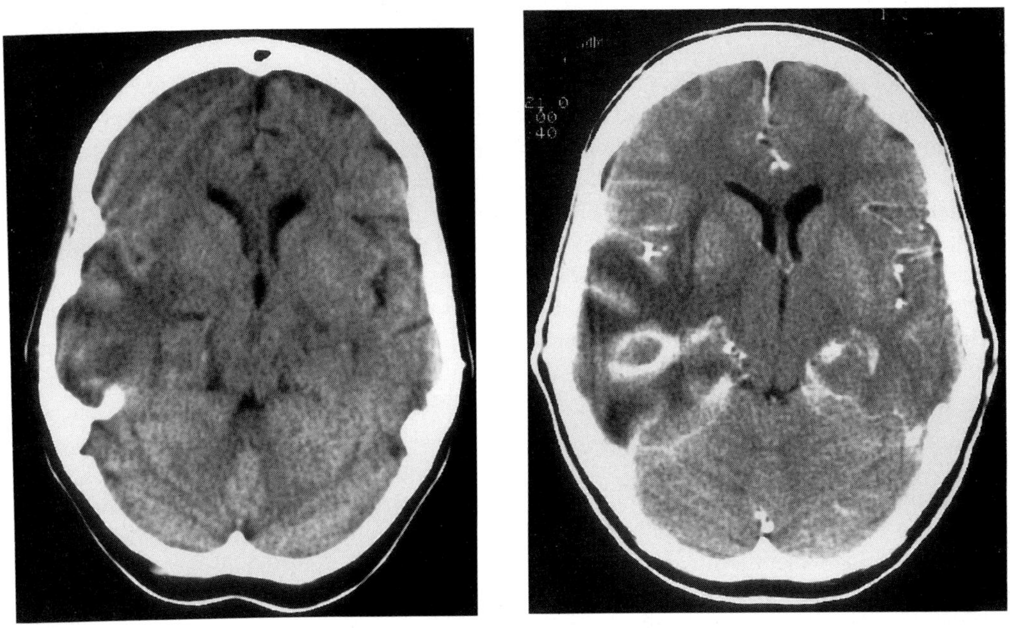

(a) (b)

Figure 1 (a) Noncontrast CT of a brain abscess showing an area of hypodensity in the right temporal lobe. (b) Contrast-enhanced CT of same patient. Note ring enhancement and intense surrounding edema.

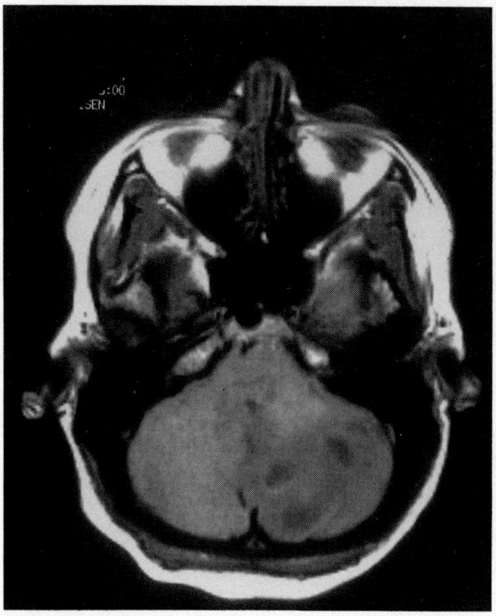

(a)

Figure 2 (a) T_1-weighted MR image of cerebellar abscess, which shows central hypodensity with a nearly isointense capsular rim. (b) T_2-weighted MR image of same patient showing large area of increased signal representing abscess and surrounding edema. (c) Gadolinium-enhanced T_1-weighted MR image of same patient showing ring enhancement of the abscess capsule.

MRI is a useful adjunctive study to CT scanning, much as it is in the evaluation of brain tumors, etc. In the early cerebritis stage, T_1- and T_2-weighted images will reveal an area of hypointensity and hyperintensity, respectively, both with indistinct margins. In the encapsulation space, T_1 images will demonstrate a lesion of low intensity centrally with the capsule being iso- to hyperintense. T_2 images reveal a high-intensity center, with a hypointense rim with surrounding hyperintense signal representing edema. T_1 images with gadolinium enhancement will show an enhancing capsule if the abscess is mature enough (Fig. 2).

The white blood cell (WBC) count is elevated in 50% of adults with brain abscess and 67–83% of children (70,71). The erythrocyte sedimentation rate (ESR) is elevated in 48–65% of patients. The ESR may be lower in patients with brain abscess with underlying congenital cyanotic cardiac disease. One study examined the ESR in patients with brain abscess based on the presence or absence of congenital cyanotic heart disease and found it elevated in 20 and 89% of patients, respectively.

Measurement of the C-reactive protein (CRP) concentration has been determined to be useful in diagnosing brain abscess, especially when brain tumor is in the differential diagnosis. In one study, seven to nine patients with abscess had elevated CRP levels, for a sensitivity of 78%. All 11 tumors in this series had low CRP levels. Higher CRP levels correlated with abscesses still in the cerebritis stage. It is important to note that CRP is a nonspecific marker of inflammation and is elevated in any form of infection, so that it is plausible for a patient with a tumor and a concomitant infection to have an elevated level. It has been suggested that CRP levels can be followed serially to determine the adequacy of treatment (72).

Indium-111–labeled WBC scans are useful for detecting foci of infection in many areas of the

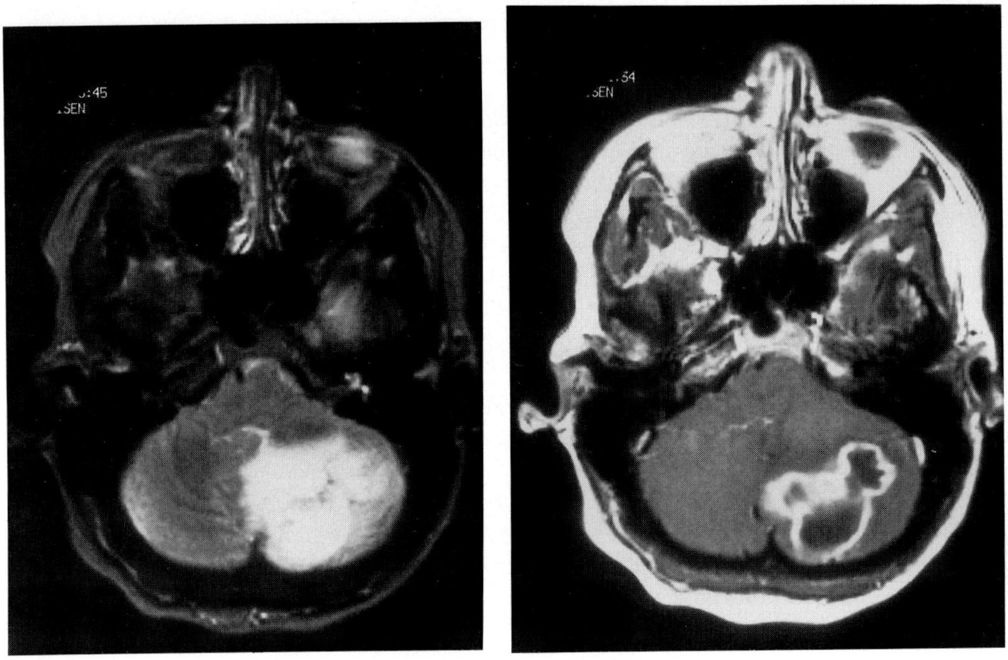

(b) (c)

body, including the brain. The sensitivity and specificity of this technique are between 80–100%. The utility of this study appears to be in the distinction between abscess and tumor, both of which may have similar features on CT scanning. False-positive results are thought secondary to leukocyte infiltration into tumors, especially tumors with severe necrosis, which in turn leads to an inflammatory response. False-negative results are associated with prior treatment with antibiotics or steroids (73–76). In one series, small numbers of patients on steroids who initially had negative scans had positive scans after steroid therapy was decreased or discontinued (77). Steroid therapy should be discontinued for 48 h prior to scanning to improve the sensitivity of this technique (76). A newer agent than Indium-111 that may be used to tag leukocytes is 99mTc-hexamethylproplyeneamine oxime (99mTc-HMPAO). The 99mTc-HMPAO appears to give very similar results to and may be easier to obtain than Indium-111 (76,77).

Historically, before the advent of computed tomography and magnetic resonance imaging, angiography, ventriculography, electroencephalography, and even plain films were frequently utilized to help obtain a diagnosis and locate the lesion. Angiography localized the lesion in 73–100% of cases (7,8,11,19,39,69) and appeared to localize lesions best in the temporal lobe when compared with the frontal or parietal lobes (69). Ventriculography produced similar results, localizing the abscess in 84–100% of cases (7,11,39,69). This modality had higher success rates for abscesses located in the posterior fossa and parietal lobes, followed by the frontal lobes and temporal lobes. Electroencephalography was abnormal in 60–100% of cases (7,8,11,19,39). Slow wave foci over the lesion, seizure activity, or diffuse encephalopathic patterns were seen. Plain films of the skull were useful in 15–41% of cases, mainly by demonstrating shift of a calcified pineal gland (7,39).

Lumbar puncture (LP) is seldom used today for the diagnosis of a brain abscess due to the availability of CT and MRI and the risk of cerebral herniation. The results of the LP are usually nonspecifically abnormal. An elevated opening pressure is found in the majority of patients, an elevated CSF WBC count in 14–82%, an increased protein concentration in 33–71%, and positive cultures in 6–22%. The etiological organism can rarely be identified from CSF cultures obtained by lumbar puncture. Positive cultures are usually associated with rupture of the abscess into the ventricular system. The benefits and risks of performing a lumbar puncture in a patient in whom an abscess is possible must be carefully considered. A lumbar puncture may cause brain herniation. The rate of neurological decline in abscess patients in the 2 days following lumbar puncture ranges from 1 to 29%, the average being 15% (56 of 368 patients) (8,11,39,69). When a cranial CT or MRI demonstrates a brain abscess, specimens for smear and culture should be obtained by a neurosurgical procedure.

TREATMENT

The treatment of brain abscess is directed at the drainage of pus or extirpation of the abscess, the systemic administration of antibiotics, and treatment of the primary source of infection (11). Very rarely a brain abscess may be managed with medical treatment alone.

Almost all brain abscesses are treated with some form of surgical therapy. Surgical therapy allows for the diagnosis of brain abscess to be made, provides material for the identification of the causative organism, and decreases the mass effect associated with the abscess. Options for the surgical management of brain abscess are either complete extirpation of the abscess or aspiration of the abscess cavity with or without placement of a drainage catheter into the abscess cavity. It is impossible to determine which method is "best" as no randomized trial has ever been undertaken to determine the efficacy of each treatment in comparison with other methods. In some instances, combinations of these therapies must be utilized, such as extirpation of a recurrent abscess that has already been aspirated on one or more occasions. Three other methods—tapping, marsupialization, and the migration method of Kahn, have been described but are mainly of historical interest (78).

Aspiration is performed through a burr hole and may be done either freehand or under stereotactic guidance. The advantage of aspiration over extirpation is that it allows for the recovery of purulent material for the identification of the causative organism and has a lower morbidity than that of invasive craniotomy. There is also a lower risk of seizures with aspiration than with complete excision of the abscess. The disadvantages of aspiration include the need for repeat procedures, especially in cases of multiloculated abscesses and abscesses secondary to a foreign body, and when the capsule is adherent to the dura, falx, or the base of the skull (supposedly preventing collapse of the abscess). Abscesses secondary to a foreign body may never heal without complete removal of the abscess and the foreign body. Failure of the aspiration method leads to craniotomy for excision of the abscess (8,11,79).

CT- or MRI-guided stereotactic aspiration of an abscess is becoming more common and the procedure of choice for initial management of the majority of intracranial abscesses. Stereotactic aspiration is definitely the procedure of choice for deep-seated abscesses and abscesses in eloquent areas of the brain. Several small series and case reports support the use of this technique in situations where minimal damage to surrounding tissue can be tolerated (80–83). Recommendations for the use of this technique include (1) initial aspiration of 50–60% of the estimated volume of the abscess, (2) external drainage of an abscess cavity with initial diameter greater than 30 mm, and (3) a poor neurological or medical condition that would be a contraindication to excision (84). Some experts agree with external drainage and think it should be used in all but the smallest lesions (85,86), while others suggest that there is never a need for external drainage (87). After aspiration, the abscess cavity may or may not be irrigated with antibiotic solution (84), and if an external drainage tube is placed, this may be irrigated with antibiotic solution as well (86).

The initial stereotactic technique may fail due to excessive or suboptimal drainage at the time of the initial aspiration, systemic disease, or exacerbating systemic conditions (84).

The complete excision of a brain abscess is favored by some. The advantages of excision include early decompression, definitive removal of the offending lesion from the parenchyma of the brain, and decreased hospital stay and amount of time required for antimicrobial therapy. Disadvantages of excision include the damage to surrounding parenchyma incurred during the removal process and the requirement that the abscess be firmly encapsulated to allow complete removal without spillage of the contents into the surrounding parenchyma. A slightly higher rate of seizures occurs following excision compared with aspiration (8,11,39,88).

Occasionally, excision may be required for rapid decompression or for complete cure of a cerebral abscess, such as those that are secondary to foreign bodies, those due to fungi, and abscesses that fail to resolve despite repeated aspirations and antibiotics. Abscesses secondary to *Nocardia* species usually require complete extirpation to cure. The presence of gas within the abscess cavity is an indication for excision of the abscess as this may represent a persistent extracranial communication. Excision is then performed as well as attempted closure of the abnormal communication (89).

Medical management alone, without surgical intervention, is generally reserved for patients who have medical problems increasing the risk of surgery, lesions inaccessible to surgery, multiple abscesses, or concomitant meningitis (90). Few patients respond to medical therapy alone; there are, however, a few case reports of brain-stem abscesses treated successfully with antibiotics (91,92). With the advent of stereotactic neurosurgery, fewer abscesses are truly inaccessible. After purulent material is obtained for Gram's stain and culture, treatment is initiated with broad-spectrum intravenous antibiotics and occasionally steroids and/or mannitol. The response of the abscess to medical therapy alone is determined by serial neurological examinations and serial CT or MRI scanning. Surgery must be considered if the patient's condition continues to worsen despite maximal therapy.

Multiple brain abscesses are occasionally treated with medical management alone. A recently proposed treatment algorithm suggests stereotactic aspiration or excision of the largest lesion or the most symptomatic lesion in order to obtain a histological diagnosis. If the diagnosis of brain abscess is confirmed, then stereotactic aspiration or excision of all abscesses greater than 2.5 cm and/or those causing significant mass effect should be performed followed by broad-spectrum antibiotics for at least 6–8 weeks. Follow-up CT or MRI scans are obtained every 2 weeks or sooner if the clinical condition deteriorates. Any enlarging abscesses are then aspirated or excised. This is continued until a course of antimicrobial therapy is completed and the abscesses are resolving. Neuroimaging is performed monthly until all abscesses have resolved. Excision is recommended for abscesses requiring more than two aspirations (57).

The treatment of brain abscess in immunocompromised patients usually proceeds as it does in immunocompetent patients. Biopsy/aspiration of the lesion for confirmation of diagnosis and to obtain culture material is indicated, after which the treatment algorithm outlined above is followed.

In patients with AIDS, the treatment algorithm may be modified, as approximately one third to two thirds of focal CNS lesions in AIDS patients will be due to *Toxoplasma gondii*. The remainder may be almost equally divided into those due to lymphoma followed by progressive multifocal leukoencephalopathy, *C. neoformans*, *L. monocytogenes*, *Mycobacterium* sp., *Candida*, and *Aspergillus*. In an AIDS patient with an enhancing lesion or lesions on CT/MRI, it is reasonable to try a 7- to 10-day course of treatment for toxoplasmosis. If the patient continues to deteriorate, or if follow-up scans reveal no response to treatment, then biopsy/aspiration is indicated. A biopsy is probably also indicated for nonenhancing lesions in these patients (93,94).

ANTIBIOTICS

Regardless of the type of surgical therapy used for brain abscess, antibiotics will always be a part of the therapy (Table 4). Antibiotics are chosen on the basis of not only their activity against the infecting organism but also their penetration into CSF and the abscess cavity and their effectiveness in the acidic environment found in most cavities. Traditionally, penicillin G and chloramphenicol were the mainstay of treatment. With the development of other antibiotics, new regimens have evolved that extend the coverage and minimize the potential side effects of chloramphenicol.

Many studies have been performed that measure antibiotic concentration in normal brain and in abscess cavities. Chloramphenicol obtains a concentration ninefold higher in brain parenchyma than in serum (95), yet concentrations in abscess cavities are erratic (96,97). Vancomycin, moxalacatam, cefotetan, cefotaxime, and penicillin achieve sufficient concentration in abscess cavities to promote eradication of the infection (96,98–100). Clindamycin has poor penetration into traumatized monkey brain tissue in experimental studies (101). Penicillin, ampicillin, and cephaloridin are inactivated by brain abscess pus, whereas streptomycin and fusidic acid are not (102). Aminoglycosides have poor penetration into CSF and brain tissue, even in the presence of inflammation. For this reason, the use of aminoglycosides should be restricted to

Table 4 Antimicrobial Therapy of Brain Abscess

Organism	Antibiotic
Streptococci	Third-generation cephalosporin
	or
	Penicillin G
	20–24 million units/day (IV)
Bacteroides sp.	Metronidazole
	500 mg q 6 h IV (adult)
	7.5 mg/kg q 8 h IV (child)
Staphylococci	
methicillin-sensitive	Nafcillin
	2 g q 4 h IV
methicillin-resistant	Vancomycin
	2 g/day IV (adult)
	40–60 mg/kg/day (child)
Toxoplasma gondii	Pyrimethamine
	100–200 mg loading dose and 50–75 mg/day orally for 3–6 weeks
	plus
	Sulfadiazine
	4–6 g/day (orally)
	or
	Clindamycin
	1200 mg q 6 h IV
Cryptococcus neoformans	Amphotericin B
Aspergillus sp.	0.5–1.0 mg/kg/day
Candida sp.	or
	Liposomal amphotericin B
	3 mg/kg/day: increase to 15 mg/kg/day

second-line therapy (103). Sulfonamides appear to have good penetration through the blood-brain barrier even in the absence of inflammation. When coupled with trimethoprim, the activity is enhanced.

The combination of vancomycin, a third-generation cephalosporin, and metronidazole provides the broadest antibacterial coverage possible and is recommended for empiric therapy. Vancomycin is indicated for staphylococci including methicillin-resistant strains as well as other gram-positive organisms. The addition of metronidazole provides coverage for anaerobes. Empiric therapy is based on the most likely infecting organism predicted by predisposing factors or underlying condition. If the patient has no history of trauma or surgery, then the probability that the abscess is due to methicillin-resistant staphylococci is very low, and therefore vancomycin is not required. In this circumstance, a third-generation cephalosporin, such as cefotaxime or ceftriaxone, combined with metronidazole should provide sufficient coverage. The combination of cefotaxime and metronidazole has been specifically studied and has been found efficacious in the treatment of brain absces (104). The final culture results and sensitivities can help narrow the antibiotic coverage. However, it must be kept in mind that abscesses are frequently polymicrobial and that unless meticulous culture methods are utilized, bacteria may be present in the abscess that will not grow in the final culture. If this is suspected, it is necessary to continue broad-spectrum antibiotics until the abscess has resolved (for example, anaerobes are often present in an abscess of otitic origin but are difficult to grow in culture). The choice of antibiotics can also be dictated by the etiology of the infection. For example, an abscess associated with sinusitis is most often due to a species of streptococci susceptible to penicillin G alone. Otitic abscesses have a number of causative organisms, including anaerobes (specifically *Bacteroides* sp.), and broader coverage is necessary. In most cases, treatment with antibiotics should continue for at least 6–8 weeks or longer in cases where resolution of the abscess is slow.

The use of corticosteroids in the treatment of brain abscess remains controversial. Steroids should be used to treat vasogenic cerebral edema surrounding the abscess, to decrease mass effect, and to decrease raised intracranial pressure. Steroid therapy may also be detrimental in that steroids decrease the penetration of antibiotics into brain tissue by decreasing inflammation and stabilizing the blood-brain barrier, thus preventing diffusion of antibiotics into the infected brain. In animal models, steroids decrease the concentration of certain antibiotics in both normal and infected brains (105). The effect of steroid therapy on outcome is difficult to ascertain because, in general, steroids are used more often in patients with worse neurological conditions and outcome is generally worse (as would be expected as prognosis is related to initial neurological condition) (9,19).

PROGNOSIS

The mortality of brain abscess has decreased significantly in the last 20 years due to the development and widespread use of CT and MRI as well as better antimicrobial agents and improved culturing techniques. Mortality rates in recent series of brain abscess, in which CT scanning was performed, ranged from 0 to 14% (3,8,9,10,25,67,106). Mortality is most closely associated with the condition of the patient when the diagnosis is made (8,25,106,107). Increased age, male sex, decreased mental status on admission, and a pulmonary source of the abscess were all statistically significant predictors of mortality in one study (19).

Neurological sequelae of brain abscess is again correlated with the condition of the patient at the time of the initial presentation. Most patients that are awake and alert at the time of presentation have a favorable outcome (10,67,107). Few studies quantitate the actual numbers of specific complications. Seizures occur in 10–15% of survivors (9,19,67). In general, seizures are more common in patients undergoing excision than those managed with aspiration (11,39,88).

SUMMARY

A CT or MRI scan should be done immediately in any case of a suspected infectious mass lesion. If a mass lesion is present on scan, but is not clearly an abscess, then a CRP concentration or an Indium-111 or a 99mTc-HMPAO–tagged white blood cell scan may be obtained to help establish the diagnosis of brain abscess. Once the diagnosis of brain abscess has been made, or is in the differential, a stereotactic aspiration of the abscess (the largest or most accessible in a patient with multiple abscesses) should be performed to confirm the diagnosis, obtain material for culture, and relieve mass effect. Occasionally, craniotomy may be required for rapid decompression and diagnosis. Broad-spectrum antimicrobial therapy should be initiated. The decision as to which antimicrobial agents to use is based on the location and presumed etiology of the abscess (Table 4). Steroids are used only when necessary to reduce vasogenic edema associated with the abscess. Serial CT or MRI scans are obtained every 2 weeks. Scans should be obtained immediately if the clinical condition deteriorates. Abscesses that enlarge or do not become smaller may need repeat stereotactic aspiration or extirpation. Extirpation should be used in any abscess thought secondary to a retained foreign body and in most abscesses due to *Nocardia*. Antibiotics should be continued for 6 weeks after the last aspiration. Antibiotics may be stopped sooner if extirpation is carried out. Rarely, only medical therapy may be used if the patient has adverse risk factors to surgery.

REFERENCES

1. Macewen W. Pyogenic Infective Diseases of the Brain and Spinal Cord. Meningitis, Abscess of Brain, Infective Sinus Thrombosis. Glasgow: J. Maclehose & Sons, 1893.
2. Dandy WE. Treatment of chronic abscess of the brain by tapping. J Am Med Assoc 1926; 87:1477–1478.
3. Rosenblum ML, Hoff JT, Norman D, Weinstein PR, Pitts L. Decreased mortality from brain abscesses since advent of computerized tomography. J Neurosurg 1978; 49:658–668.
4. Nicolosi A, Hauser WA, Musicco M, Kurland LT. Incidence and prognosis of brain abscess in a defined population: Olmsted County, Minnesota, 1935–1981. Neuroepidemiology 1991; 10:122–131.
5. Clayman GL, et al. Intracranial complications of paranasal sinusitis: a combined institutional review. Laryngoscope 1991; 101:234–239.
6. Carey ME, et al. Follow-up study of 103 American soldiers who sustained a brain wound in Vietnam. J Neurosurg 1974; 41:542–549.
7. Nielsen H, Byldensted C, Harmsen A. Cerebral abscess: aetiology and pathogenesis, symptoms, diagnosis and treatment; a review of 200 cases from 1935–1976. Acta Neurol Scand 1982; 65: 609–622.
8. Yang SY, Zhao CS. Review of 140 patients with brain abscess. Surg Neurol 1993; 39:290–296.
9. Mampalam TJ, Rosenblum ML. Trends in the management of bacterial brain abscesses: a review of 102 cases over 17 years. Neurosurgery 1988; 23:451–458.
10. Svanteson B, Nordstrom CH, Rausing A. Non-traumatic brain abscess: epidemiology, clinical symptoms and therapeutic results. Acta Neurochirurg 1988; 94:57–65.
11. Yang SY. Brain abscess: a review of 400 cases. J Neurosurg 1981; 55:794–799.
12. Kulah A, Ozatik N, Topcu I. Otogenic intracranial abscesses. Acta Neurochirurg 1990; 107:140–146.
13. Mathews TJ, Marus G. Oteogenic intradural complication: a review of 37 patients. J Laryngol Otol 1988; 102:121–124.
14. Gower D, McGuirt WF. Intracranial complications of acute and chronic infectious ear disease: a problem still with us. Laryngoscope 1983; 93:1028–1033.
15. Browning GG. The unsafeness of 'safe' ears. J Laryngol Otol 1984; 98:23–26.
16. Nalbone VP, Kuruvilla A, Gacek RR. Otogenic brain abscess: the Syracuse experience. Ear Nose Throat J 1992; 71:238–242.

17. Nunez DA, Browning GG. Risks of developing an otogenic intracranial abscess. J Laryngol Otol 1990; 104:468–472.
18. Wright JLW, Grimaldi PMGB. Otogenic intracranial complications. J Laryngol Otol 1973; 87:1085–1096.
19. Chun HC, et al. Brain abscess: a study of 45 consecutive cases. Medicine 1986; 65:415–431.
20. Bradley PJ, Manning KP, Shaw MDM. Brain abscess secondary to paranasal sinusitis. J Laryngol Otol 1984; 98:719–725.
21. Chalstrey S, Pfleiderer AG, Moffat DA. Persisting incidence and mortality of sinogenic cerebral abscess: a continuing reflection of late clinical diagnosis. J Roy Soc Med 1991; 84:193–195.
22. Clayman GL, et al. Intracranial complications of paranasal sinusitis: a combined institutional review. Laryngoscope 1991; 101:234–239.
23. Teed RW. Meningitis from the sphenoid sinus. Arch Otolaryngol 1938; 28:589–619.
24. Lew D, et al. Sphenoid sinusitis: a review of 30 cases. N Engl J Med 1983; 309(19):1149–1154.
25. Richards J, et al. Microbiology, chemotherapy and mortality of brain abscess in Newcastle-upon-Tyne between 1979 and 1988. Scand J Infect Dis 1990; 22:511–518.
26. Hollin SA, Hayashi H, Gross SW. Intracranial abscesses of odontogenic origin. Oral Surg 1967; 23: 277–293.
27. DiNubile MJ. Septic thrombosis of the cavernous sinuses. Arch Neurol 1988; 45:567–572.
28. Wohl TA, et al. Hemianopsia from occipital lobe abscess after dental care. Am J Ophthalmol 1991; 112:689–694.
29. Williams FH, Nelms DK, McGaharan KM. Brain abscess: a rare complication of halo usage. Arch Phys Med Rehabil 1992; 73:490–492.
30. Klein DM, Cohen ME. Pasteurella multocida brain abscess following perforating cranial dog bite. J Pediatr 1978; 92:588–589.
31. Alpert G, Sutton LN. Brain abscess following cranial dog bite. Clin Pediatr 1984; 23:580.
32. Berkowitz FE, Jacobs DWC. Fatal case of brain abscess caused by rooster pecking. Pediatr Infect Dis J 1987; 6:941–942.
33. Lakshmi V, Rao RR, Dinakar I. Bacteriology of brain abscess—observations on 50 cases. J Med Microbiol 1993; 38:187–190.
34. Yang SY. Brain abscess associated with congenital heart disease. Surg Neurol 1989; 31:129–132.
35. Kagawa M, et al. Brain abscess in congenital cyanotic heart disease. J Neurosurg 1983; 58: 913–917.
36. Brandt M, et al. Brain abscess in children with congenital heart disease. Adv Neurosurg 1981; 9:86.
37. Fischbein CA, et al. Risk factors for abscess in patients with congenital heart disease. Am J Cardiol 1974; 34:97.
38. Newton EJ. Haematogenous brain abscess in cyanotic congenital heart disease. Q J Med 1956; 25:201.
39. Samson DS, Clark K. A current review of brain abscess. Am J Med 1973; 54:201–210.
40. Kline MW. Brain abscess in a patient with cystic fibrosis. Pediatr Infect Dis 1985; 4(1):72–73.
41. Momma F, et al. Brain abscess associated with congenital pulmonary arteriovenous fistula. Surg Neurol 1990; 34:439–441.
42. Mohler ER, et al. Cerebral abscess associated with dental procedure in hereditary haemorrhagic telangiectasia. Lancet 1991; 338:508–509.
43. Lerner PI. Neurologic complications of infective endocarditis. Med Clin North Am 1985; 69(2): 385–399.
44. Algoed L, et al. Brain abscess after esophageal dilatation for stenosis. Clin Neurol Neurosurg 1992; 94:169–172.
45. Kumar P, et al. Pyogenic meningitis and cerebral abscesses after endoscopic injection sclerotherapy. Am J Gastroenterol 1991; 86:1672–1674.
46. Rish BL, et al. Analysis of brain abscess after penetrating craniocerebral injuries in Vietnam. Neurosurgery 1981; 9:535–541.
47. Carey ME, et al. Follow-up study of 103 American soldiers who sustained a brain wound in Vietnam. J Neurosurg 1974; 41:542–549.
48. Dinakar I, Rao SB. Post-traumatic brain abscess. J Postgrad Med 1971; 17:137–141.

49. Vandertop WP, et al. Recurrent brain abscess due to an unexpected foreign body. Surg Neurol 1992; 37:39–41.
50. Gordon SB, Sharma BS, McKinstry CS, Fannin TF. Brain abscess ten years after penetrating glass injury to the skull. Ulster Med J 1992; 61:116–118.
51. Mourier KL, et al. Pyogenic parenchymatous and nidus infection after embolization of an arterio-venous malformation. Acta Neurochirurg 1993; 122:130–133.
52. Tenney JH. Bacterial infections of the central nervous system in neurosurgery. Infect Dis Central Nervous System 1986; 4:91–114.
53. Pit S, Jamal F, Cheah F. Microbiology of cerebral abscess: a four-year study in Malaysia. J Trop Med Hygiene 1993; 96:191–196.
54. McClelland CJ, Craig BF, Crockard HA. Brain abscesses in Northern Ireland: a 30 year community review. J Neurol Neurosurg Psychiatry 1978; 41:1043–1047.
55. Lutz TW, Landolt H, Wasner M, Gratzl O. Diagnosis and management of abscesses in the basal ganglia and thalamus: a survey. Acta Neurochirurg 1994; 127:91–98.
56. Rousseaux M, Lesoin F, Destee A, Jomin M, Petit H. Developments in the treatment and prognosis of multiple cerebral abscesses. Neurosurgery 1985; 16:304–308.
57. Mamelak AN, Mampalam TJ, Obana WG, Rosenblum ML. Improved management of multiple brain abscesses: a combined surgical and medical approach. Neurosurgery 1995; 36:76–86.
58. Domique JN, Wilson CB. Pituitary Abscesses: report of seven cases and review of the literature. J Neurosurg 1977; 46:601–608.
59. Nelson PB, Haverkos H, Martinez A, Robinson N. Abscess formation within pituitary tumors. Neurosurgery 1983; 12:331–333.
60. Britt RH, Enzmann DR, Yeager AS. Neuropathological and computerized tomographic findings in experimental brain abscess. J Neurosurg 1981; 55:590–603.
61. Britt RH, Enzmann DR. Clinical stages of human brain abscesses on serial CT scans after contrast infusion. J Neurosurg 1983; 59:972–989.
62. Britt RH, Enzmann DR, Placone RC, Obana WG, Yeager AS. Experimental anaerobic brain abscess: computerized tomographic and neuropathological correlations. J Neurosurg 1984; 60:1148–1159.
63. deLouvois J, Gortvai P, Hurley R. Bacteriology of abscesses of the central nervous system: a multicentre prospective study. Br Med J 1977; 2:981–984.
64. Puthucheary SD, Parasakthi N. The bacteriology of brain abscess: a local experience in Malaysia. Trans R Soc Trop Med Hygiene 1990; 84:589–592.
65. de Louvois J. The bacteriology and chemotherapy of brain abscess. J Antimicrob Chemother 1978; 4:395–413.
66. Armstrong D. Central nervous system infections in the immunocompromised host. Infection 1984; 12(suppl 1):S58–S64.
67. Seydoux CH, Francioli P. Bacterial brain abscesses: factors influencing morality and sequelae. Clin Infect Dis 1992; 15:394–401.
68. Wispelwey B, Scheld WM. Brain abscess. Semin Neurol 1992; 12:273–278.
69. Garfield J. Management of supratentorial intracranial abscess: a review of 200 cases. Br Med J 1969; 2:7–11.
70. Saez-Llorens XJ, Umann MA, Odio CM, McCracken GH, Nelson JD. Brain abscess in infants and children. Pediatr Infect Dis J 1989; 8:449–458.
71. Aebi C, Kaufmann F, Schaad UB. Brain abscess in childhood—long-term experiences. Eur J Pediatr 1991; 150:282–286.
72. Hirschberg H, Bosnes V. C-reactive protein levels in the differential diagnosis of brain abscesses. J Neurosurg 1987; 67:358–360.
73. Bellotti C, Aragno MG, Medina M, Viglietti AL, Oliveri G, Ettorre F, Barrale S, Camuzzini G. Differential diagnosis of CT-hypodense cranial lesions with indium-111-oxime-labeled leukocytes. J Neurosurg 1986; 64:750–753.
74. Rehncrona S, Brismar J, Holtas S. Diagnosis of brain abscesses with indium-111-labeled leukocytes. Neurosurgery 1985; 16:23–26.

75. Kock-Jensen C, Andersen BB, Sogaard I. Leucocyte scanning—a valuable tool in diagnosing cerebral abscess—a survey. Acta Neurochirurg 1986; 83:121–124.
76. Grimstad IA, Hirschberg H, Rootwelt K. 99mTc-hexamethylpropyleneamine oxime leukocyte scintigraphy and C-reactive protein levels in the differential diagnosis of brain abscesses. J Neurosurg 1992; 77:732–736.
77. Schmidt KG, Rasmussen JW, Frederiksen PB, Kock-Jensen C, Pedersen NT. Indium-111-granulocyte scintigraphy in brain abscess diagnosis: limitations and pitfalls. J Nuclear Med 1990; 31:1121–1127.
78. Stephanov S. Surgical treatment of brain abscess. Neurosurgery 1988; 22:724–730.
79. Ohaegbulam SC, Saddeqi NU. Experience with brain abscesses treated by simple aspiration. Surg Neurol 1980; 13:289–291.
80. Rajshekhar V, Chandy MJ. Successful stereotactic management of a large cardiogenic brain stem abscess. Neurosurgery 1994; 34:368–371.
81. Nauta HJW, Contreras FI, Weiner RL, Crofford MJ. Brain stem abscess managed with computed tomography-guided stereotactic aspiration. Neurosurgery 1987; 20:476–480.
82. Jamjoom ZAB. Solitary brainstem abscess successfully treated by microsurgical aspiration. Br J Neurosurg 1992; 6:249–254.
83. Fujino H, Kobayashi T, Goto I, Nagata E, Shima F. Cure of a man with solitary abscess of the brainstem. J Neurol 1990; 237:265–266.
84. Kondziolka D, Duma CM, Lunsford LD. Factors that enhance the likelihood of successful stereotactic treatment of brain abscesses. Acta Neurochirurg 1994; 127:85–90.
85. Bidzinski J, Koszewski W. The value of different methods of treatment of brain abscess in the CT era. Acta Neurochirurg 1990; 105:117–120.
86. Hasdemir MG, Ebeling U. CT-guided sterotactic aspiration and treatment of brain abscesses—an experience with 24 cases. Acta Neurochirurg 1993; 125:58–63.
87. Stapleton SR, Bell BA, Uttley D. Stereotactic aspiration of brain abscesses: is this the treatment of choice? Acta Neurochirurg 1993; 121:15–19.
88. Westcombe DS, Dorsch NWC, Teo C. Management of cerebral abscess in adolescents and adults—experience in the CT-scan era. Acta Neurochirurg 1988; 95:85–89.
89. Young RF, Frazee J. Gas within intracranial abscess cavitites: an indication for surgical excision. Ann Neurol 1984; 16:35–39.
90. Rosenblum ML, Hoff JT, Norman D, Edwards MS, Berg BO. Nonoperative treatment of brain abscesses in selected high-risk patients. J Neurosurg 1980; 52:217–225.
91. Carpenter JL. Brain stem abscesses: cure with medical therapy, case report, and review. Clin Infect Dis 1994; 18:219–226.
92. Ruelle A, Zerbi D, Zuccarello M, Andrioli G. Brain stem abscess treated successfully by medical therapy. Neurosurgery 1991; 28:742–746.
93. Schmidek HH, Sweet WH. Operative Neurosurgical Techniques. 3rd ed. Philadelphia: WB Sanders 1995:1681–1688.
94. Levy ML, Bredesen DE, Rosenblum ML. Neurological manifestations of the acquired immunodeficiency syndrome (AIDS): Experience at UCSF and review of the literature. J Neurosurg 1985; 62:475–495.
95. Kramer PW, Griffith RS, Campbell RL. Antibiotic penetration of the brain—a comparative study. J Neurosurg 1969; 31:295–302.
96. de Louvois J, Gortvai P, Hurley R. Antibiotic treatment of abscesses of the central nervous system. Br Med J 1977; 2:985–987.
97. Black P, Graybill JR, Charache P. Penetration of brain abscess by systemically administered antibiotics. J Neurosurg 1973; 38:705–709.
98. Levy RM, Gutin PH, Baskin DS, Pons VG. Vancomycin penetration of a brain abscess: case report and review of the literature. Neurosurgery 1986; 18:632–636.
99. Yamamoto M, Jimbo M, Ide M, Tanaka N, Umebara Y, Hagiwara S. Penetration of intravenous antibiotics into brain abscesses. Neurosurgery 1993; 33:44–49.
100. Sjolin J, Eriksson N, Arneborn P, Cars O. Penetration of cefotaxime and desacetylcefotaxime into brain abscesses in humans. Antimicrob Agents Chemother 1991; 35:2606–2610.

101. Picardi JL, Lewis HP, Tan JS, Phair JP. Clindamycin concentrations in the central nervous system of primates before and after head trauma. J Neurosurg 1975; 43:717–720.
102. de Louvois J, Hurley R. Inactivation of penicillin by purulent exudates. Br Med J 1977; 1:998–1000.
103. Everett ED, Strausbaugh LJ. Antimicrobial agents and the central nervous system. Neurosurgery 1980; 6:691–714.
104. Sjolin J, Lilja A, Eriksson N, Arneborn P, Cars O. Treatment of brain abscess with cefotaxime and metronidazole: prospective study on 15 consecutive patients. Clin Infect Dis 1993; 17:857–863.
105. Kourtopoulos H, Holm SE, Norrby SR. The influence of steroids on the penetration of antibiotics into brain tissue and brain abscesses. An experimental study in rats. J Antimicrob Chemother 1983; 11:245–249.
106. Alderson K, Strong AJ, Ingham HR, Selkon JB. Fifteen-year review of the mortality of brain abscess. Neurosurgery 1981; 8:1–6.
107. Lunardi P, Acqui M, Ferrante L, Mastronardi L, Fortuna A. Non-traumatic brain abscess. Neurosurg Rev 1993; 16:189–196.

23

Cranial Epidural Abscess and Cranial Subdural Empyema

Scott Shapiro
Indiana University School of Medicine, Indianapolis, Indiana

CRANIAL EPIDURAL ABSCESS

History

Reports of intracranial suppuration date back as early as the second century A.D. when Galen used trephination and trepanation to drain pus collected under the skull (1). In 1885, MacEwen reported success with drainage of cranial epidural abscess (2). However, the operative mortality rate in the preantibiotic era was substantial (3). With the advent of antibiotics and advanced imaging, this infection has become easily curable.

Pathophysiology

The cranial epidural abscess is reportedly rare (4). Normally the dura is closely applied to the inner cranium and there is no epidural space. A cranial epidural abscess develops between the dura and the inner table of the skull (Fig. 1). Hematogenous spread as a cause of cranial epidural abscess is extremely rare (5). A more common mechanism for bacteria to enter into the epidural space is from cranial (calvarial) osteomyelitis. An epidural abscess complicating paranasal sinusitis develops in the frontal area (6–8). An epidural abscess complicating otitis media or mastoiditis develops in the temporoparietal region (9). Less often, an epidural abscess can occur from a sinusitis infecting the perforating veins that traverse the bone without an associated osteomyelitis (10). Trauma, especially open depressed skull fractures involving the nasal sinuses, can lead to osteomyelitis/epidural abscess (11). At the present time, the most common cause of cranial epidural abscess is elective craniotomy and secondary infection of the wound, bone flap, and epidural space (4,6,11). The reported incidence of epidural abscess after clean craniotomy is

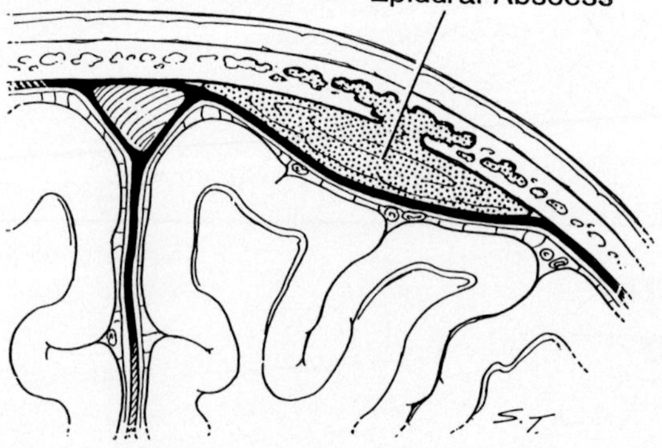

Figure 1 **A cranial epidural abscess develops between the dura and the inner table of the skull.**

0.4–1.8% (4,12). There are rare reports of halo or skull tong erosion with cranial osteomyelitis/ epidural abscess formation (13). Since the dura is such an effective barrier, the epidural abscess is usually contained locally and any neurological symptoms are due to mass effect. Approximately 10% of epidural abscesses are associated with a subdural empyema (14).

Microbiology

Most cases of cranial epidural abscess complicating trauma or surgery are due to *Staphylococcus aureus* and coagulase-negative staphylococci (6,11,12). Abscesses complicating sinusitis are often due to hemolytic and microaerophilic streptococci, aerobic staphylococci, and anaerobic organisms. An organism can be cultured in 89% of cases (12). There is an increasing incidence of cranial epidural abscess due to aerobic gram-negative bacilli, perhaps as a result of the increasing number of patients with cancer, diabetes, and chronic obstructive lung disease who are at increased risk for infection due to these organisms (13–16).

Clinical Findings

Headache is the primary complaint. A low-grade fever may be present. The area involved is usually tender, erythematous, and swollen. Nuchal rigidity may be present. There is typically no evidence of a neurological deficit. If the abscess is large enough to cause mass effect, than obtundation, hemiparesis, and/or a disturbance of language may be present.

Diagnostic Evaluation

Plain x-rays that demonstrate paranasal sinusitis, mastoiditis, or calvarial erosion may be helpful (14). The CT scan without and with contrast will show the enhancing epidural collection of pus if it is large enough (17) and any associated osteomyelitis of the calvarium with bone erosion (14). MRI scan is more sensitive than CT scan for demonstrating an epidural abscess (18–21). The MRI scan is superior in its ability to detect extracerebral fluid collections, since it is free from bony artifacts adjacent to the inner table of the skull. The epidural fluid will be of higher signal intensity on both T_1- and T_2-weighted images than that of CSF in the ventricles. In addition, the dura appears as a thin, low-intensity line, separating the epidural abscess from the parenchyma. Following gadolinium administration, there is significant enhancement of the dura.

When an epidural abscess develops at a craniotomy site, it is quite easy to needle a burr hole or the subgaleal area for aspiration of purulent material for culture. An intravenous angiocatheter can be used and the inner needle removed after the burr hole is penetrated.

Treatment

The primary treatment is surgical debridement followed by intravenous antibiotics. In cases complicating paranasal sinusitis, the infected, exposed sinus must be drained, exenterated, and packed to avoid recurrence. Removal of the osteomyelitic bone is recommended. Gross epidural pus should be irrigated away. The granulation tissue adherent to the dura should be scraped away. In cases of subgaleal/epidural abscess complicating a craniotomy, there are no firm recommendations available on what to do with the bone flap. In the majority of cases, the flap is removed and a cranioplasty performed 6 months to 1 year after the infection has resolved (12,14). It is possible to autoclave the flap and replace it immediately or in a delayed fashion and have a successful outcome. Cranioplasty can consist of rib, split thickness cranium, or nebcin impregnated methacrylate (12,14,22). Given the apparent relationship between poor antibiotic selection and worse outcome, the selection of empiric antimicrobial therapy before organism identification should cover aerobic streptococci, staphylococci, and anaerobes (Table 1) (12,14). In those cases complicating a craniotomy, vancomycin should be added for coverage of methicillin-resistant staphylococci (12).

Prognosis

In most series, no mortality or neurological morbidity has occurred in the management of cranial epidural abscess. Recurrence of infection is the primary complication following cranioplasty (12,14,22).

Table 1 Antimicrobial Therapy

Organism	Adult	Dosing interval	Child	Dosing interval
Staphylococcus aureus				
methicillin-sensitive	Nafcillin 9–12 g/day	4 h	Naficillin 200 mg/kg/day	4 h
methicillin-resistant	Vancomycin 2 g/day	12 h	Vancomycin 40–60 mg/kg/day	12 h
Streptococci	Penicillin G 20–24 miU/day	4 h	Penicillin G 250,000–400,000 U/kg/day	4–6 h
Gram-negative bacilli	Ceftriaxone 4–6 g/day	12 h	Ceftriaxone 80–100 mg/kg/day	12 h
	or		or	
	Cefotaxime 8–12 g/day	4 h	Ceftotaxime 200 mg/kg/day	6 h
	or		or	
	Ceftazidime 6 g/day	8 h	Ceftazidime 125–150 mg/kg/day	8 h
Anaerobes	Metronidazole 600 mg/day	8 h	Metronidazole 22.5 mg/kg/day	8 h
	or		or	
	Chloramphenicol 4 g/day	6 h	Chloramphenicol 100 mg/kg/day	6 h

CRANIAL SUBDURAL EMPYEMA

Pathophysiology

Empyema refers to an infection within a preexisting normal space (Fig. 2). The subdural space is a potential space between the dura mater and the arachnoid. The arachnoid, in theory, would be the inner barrier, but it is not a strong barrier and subdural empyema always breaches the arachnoid and even causes subpial infection (14). The subdural space has no barriers so the infection can extend throughout the supratentorial and infratentorial compartments. The primary etiology of subdural empyema in the older literature was otitis media (23–28). The primary etiology of subdural empyema at the present time is paranasal sinusitis. Septic thrombophlebitis from sinusitis, mastoiditis, or otitis extends to the subdural space causing the empyema. Superficial infection of the scalp and skull can also lead to subdural empyema. Subdural empyema can complicate elective craniotomies. Most subdural empyemas are supratentorial with 3% in the infratentorial space (29).

Microbiology

Aerobic and anaerobic streptococci are the organisms cultured most often from subdural empyemas. Staphylococci, *Proteus mirabilis*, *Bacteroides fragilis* and other nonstreptococcal anaerobes, and *Pseudomonas* sp. are cultured less often (23–29). Mixed infections are not uncommon.

Clinical Presentation

Acute subdural empyema is a neurosurgical emergency in most cases. The patient appears acutely ill with headache, fever, chills, and nuchal rigidity (23–29). In children and adults, the triad of

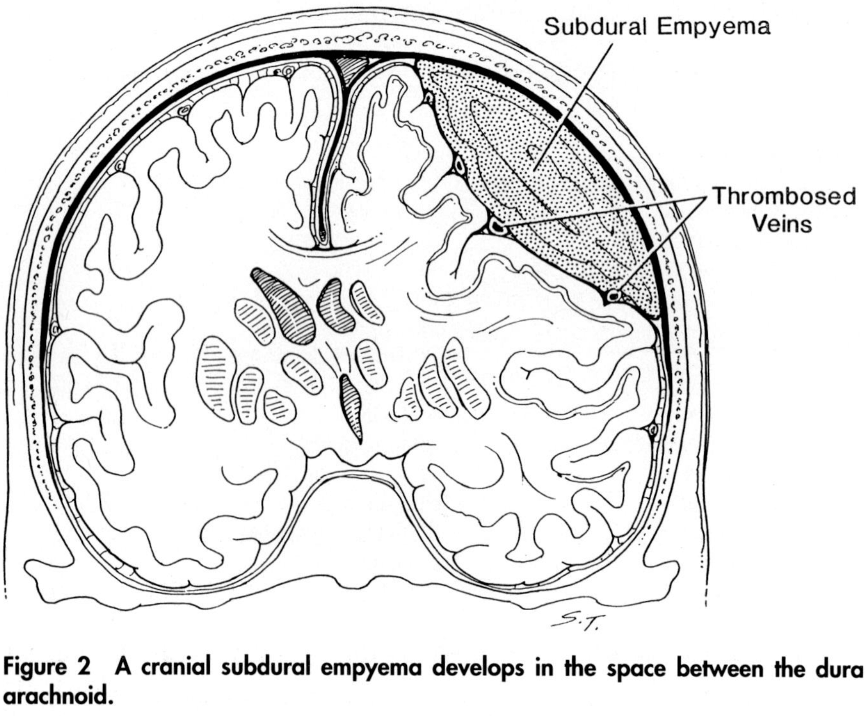

Figure 2 A cranial subdural empyema develops in the space between the dura mater and the arachnoid.

sinusitis, fever, and an acute neurological deficit warrants immediate investigation for a subdural empyema. Paranasal sinusitis, when the predisposing condition, is often associated with periorbital edema and erythema. The headache is initially localized to the side of the infection. The headache becomes increasingly more severe and is followed by a change in the level of consciousness. A decreased level of consciousness due to increased intracranial pressure is present in at least 55% of cases of subdural empyema. Neurological deficits are due to mass effect from the subdural collection and to cortical vein thrombophlebitis. Hemiparesis, a disturbance in language, and cranial nerve palsies are reported in 39% of cases (23–29). Seizures (usually focal) occur in 30–60% of cases. Status epilepticus develops in only about 8% of cases. Rarely, cortical vein thrombophlebitis progresses to complete superior sagittal sinus thrombosis.

Diagnostic Evaluation

A lumbar puncture is dangerous in the setting of subdural empyema associated with increased intracranial pressure. Plain skull films can demonstrate paranasal sinusitis or mastoiditis, but are rarely helpful. CT scan without and with contrast may demonstrate a hypo- or isodense extra-axial collection (Fig. 3) as well as evidence of fluid in or opacification of the sinuses (25). However, negative CT scans have been reported in 10–30% of patients with symptomatic subdural empyemas (29–32). MRI is significantly better than CT for imaging subdural empyemas (18–21). MRI is superior in its ability to detect extracerebral fluid collections, since it is free from streak artifacts from the bony calvarium. Even small subdural empyemas are visible as crescentic fluid collections, often with mass effect, along the surface of the brain. MRI may differentiate between benign subdural effusions and infected subdural empyemas by virtue of the shortened T_1 relaxation times of purulent fluid in comparison to CSF. Direct visual inspection of a subdural empyema will show fluid of mildly increased signal intensity on T_1- and markedly increased signal intensity on T_2-weighted images compared to that of CSF in the ventricles. A subdural effusion is isointense to CSF on T_1- and T_2-weighted images. MRI can differentiate subdural empyema from a chronic hematoma more readily than CT. On CT, both entities appear as hypodense collections, whereas on MRI, hematomas are more hyperintense than empyemas. Cerebral angiography can be helpful in difficult cases by demonstrating displacement of vessels away from the inner table of the skull, mass effect, and vessel narrowing/occlusion on the surface (33,34).

Treatment

Successful treatment is dependent on early diagnosis, surgical drainage, and intravenous antibiotics. Surgical drainage can be accomplished by either craniotomy or multiple burr holes (23–26,35). Accumulation of pus in the posterior part of the subdural space has been described for over 40 years and must be addressed at the time of surgery. The subdural space should be irrigated with both bacitracin irrigation and vancomycin irrigation. Drains can be left in the subdural space allowing for both further drainage of purulent fluid after surgery and antibiotic irrigation. This is not mandatory. Regardless of whether or not drains are left in the subdural space, it is not uncommon to have to reoperate in a few days for further irrigation and drainage of loculated pockets of pus. Thus, frequent CT scans or MRI scans are important in evaluating resolution of infection. Sinusitis, if present, requires exenteration and packing of the sinus.

Intravenous antibiotics are given for at least 2 weeks and typically for 4–6 weeks. The empiric selection of antibiotics must cover aerobic and anaerobic streptococci, staphylococci, and gram-negative bacilli (Table 1). Bok et al. recommend a regimen of three intravenous antibiotics consisting of penicillin G (6 million U q 6 h adults, 400,000 U/kg/day for children/infants), chloramphenicol (1 g q 6 h adults, 100 mg/kg/day for infants/young children), and metronidazole

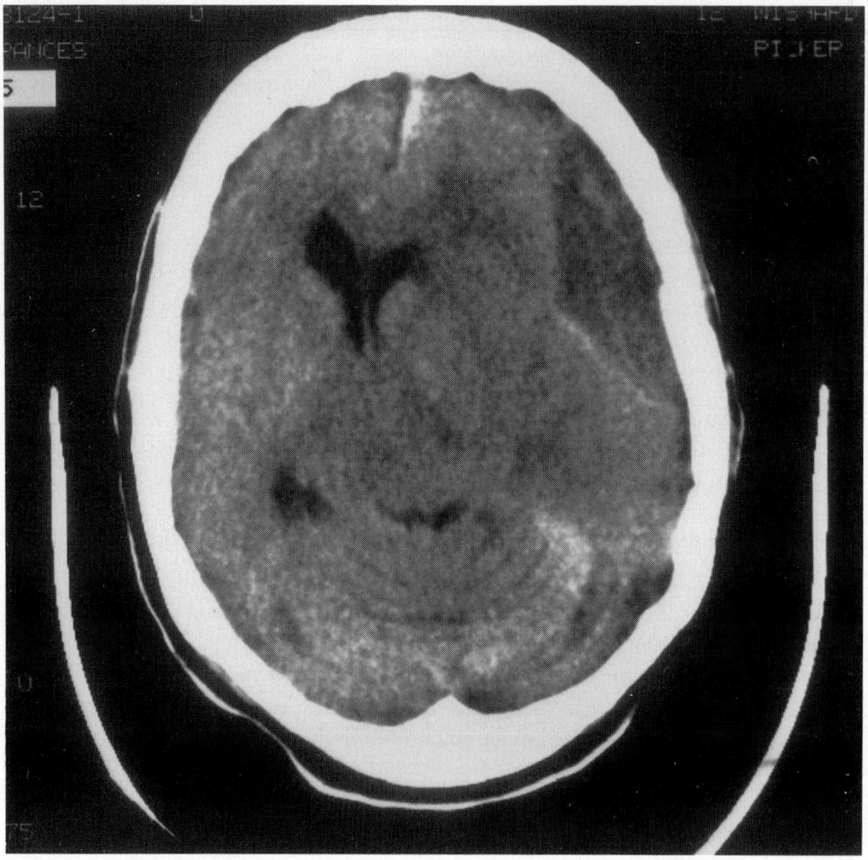

Figure 3 CT scan demonstrating cranial subdural empyema producing a mass effect with midline shift and effacement of the lateral ventricle.

(200 mg q 8 h adults, 7.5 mg/kg q 8 h infants/young children) (24). Oral antibiotic therapy can be substituted for intravenous antibiotic therapy after week 4 to complete a 6-week course of therapy. Close follow-up after antibiotic therapy is completed is mandatory for at least 3 months. One report has documented antibiotic treatment alone for a few select patients with subdural empyema (36). This is not recommended unless underlying medical illness makes surgery a prohibitive risk.

Prognosis

At the present time, the mortality rate is between 8–35%. There appears to be a strong correlation between outcome and the preoperative Glasgow coma scale. The combined mortality and severe disability rate for the GCS 3–7 group is 33% as compared to 11% for the GCS 8–11 group and 2% for the GCS 12–15 group. Overall, neurological deficits, including chronic seizure disorder requiring anticonvulsant therapy, occur in 14–20%.

REFERENCES

1. Horrax G. Neurosurgery—an historical sketch. In: De Bakey ME, Spurling RG, eds. American Lectures in Surgery. Springfield, IL: Charles C Thomas, 1952.
2. MacEwen W. Pyogenic Infective Diseases of the Brain and Spinal Cord. New York: The Macmillian Co., 1893.
3. Webster J, Gurdjian E. Collective review: the surgical management of intracranial suppuration. Methods in diagnosis and management, and report of 23 cases of civilian and 33 cases of military. Surg Gynecol Obstet Suppl Int Abstr Surg 1950; 90:209–235.
4. Wright RL. Postoperative Craniotomy Infections. Springfield, IL: Charles C Thomas, 1966.
5. Dandy WE. Surgery of the Brain. Hagerstown, MD: Prior, 1945.
6. French L, Chou S. Osteomyelitis of the skull and epidural abscess. In: Gurdjian ES, ed. Cranial and Intracranial Suppuration. Springfield, IL: Charles C Thomas, 1969:59–72.
7. Maxwell J. Acute suppurative frontal sinusitis: intracranial complications. Ann Otol Rhinol Laryngol 1950; 59:451–460.
8. Skillern R. Extradural abscess complicating frontal sinusitis. Ann Otol Rhinol Laryngol 1992; 31:997–1006.
9. Lund W. A review of 50 cases of intracranial complications from otogenic infection between 1961 and 1977. Clin Otolaryngol 1978; 3:495–501.
10. Brunner H. Pachymeningitis externa (extradural abscess). In: Brunner H, ed. Intracranial Complications of Ear, Nose and Throat Infections, section II, Clinical Aspects. Chicago: Year Book Publishing Co, 1946:89–110.
11. Davidson R. Intracranial epidural suppuration: the occult empyema. Neurosurgery 1982; 11:390–394.
12. Hlavin M, Kaminski H, Fenstermaker R, White R. Intracranial suppuration: a modern decade of postoperative subdural empyema and epidural abscess. Neurosurgery 1994; 34:974–981.
13. Tindall G, Flanagan J, Nashold B. Brain abscess and osteomyelitis following skull traction: a report of 3 cases. Arch Surg 1959; 79:638–641.
14. Renaudin J. Cranial epidural abscess and subdural empyema. In: Wilkins R, Rengachary S, eds. Neurosurgery. New York: McGraw-Hill, 1985:1961–1963.
15. Yoshikawa T, Chow A, Guze L. Role of anaerobic bacteria in subdural empyema. Report of four cases and review of 327 cases from the English literature. Am J Med 1975; 58:99–104.
16. Guentzel M. Escherichia, Klebsiella, Enterobacter, Serratia, Citrobacter, and Proteus. In: Baron S, ed. Medical Microbiology. Menlo Park, CA: Addison-Wesley, 1986:495–506.
17. Lott T, El Gammal T, Dasilva R, Hanks D, Reynolds J. Evaluation of brain and epidural abscesses by computed tomography. Radiology 1977; 122:371–376.
18. Weingarten K, Zimmerman R, Becker R, et al. Subdural and epidural empyemas: MR imaging. Am J Neuroradiol 1989; 10:81.
19. Bydder G, Steiner R, Young I, et al. Clinical NMR imaging of the brain: 140 cases. Am J Neuroradiol 1982; 3:459.
20. Davidson H, Steiner R. Magnetic resonance imaging in infections of the central nervous system. Am J Neuroradiol 1985; 6:499.
21. Brant Zawadzki M, Kelly W, Kjos B, et al. Magnetic resonance imaging and characterization of normal and abnormal intracranial cerebrospinal fluid spaces: initial observations. Neuroradiol 1985; 27:3.
22. Shapiro S. Cranioplasty, vertebral body replacement, and spinal fusion with tobramycin-impregnated methylmethacrylate. Neurosurgery 1991; 28:789–791.
23. Bannister G, Williams B, Smith S. Treatment of subdural empyema. J Neurosurg 1967; 26:41–45.
24. Bok A, Peter J. Subdural empyema: burr holes or craniotomy? J Neurosurg 1993; 78:574–578.
25. Hitchcock E, Andread A. Subdural empyema: a review of 29 cases. J Neurol Neurosurg Psychiatr 1964; 27:422–434.
26. Kaufman D, Miller M, Steibigel N. Subdural empyema: analysis of 17 recent cases and review of the literature. Medicine 1975; 54:485–498.
27. Renaudin J, Frazee J. Subdural empyema—importance of early diagnosis. Neurosurgery 1980; 4:477–479.

28. Smith H, Hendrick E. Subdural empyema and epidural abscess in children. J Neurosurg 1983; 58: 392–397.
29. Borovich B, Johnston E, Spagnuolo E. Infratentorial subdural empyema: clinical and computerized tomography findings. J Neurosurg 1990; 72:299–301.
30. Dunker R, Khakoo M. Failure of computed tomographic scanning to demonstrate subdural empyema. JAMA 1981; 246:1116–1118.
31. Luken M, Whelan M. Recent diagnostic experience with subdural empyema. J Neurosurg 1980; 52:764–771.
32. Wortzman D, Tucker W, Finlayson D, McPhedran R, Gershater R. Subdural empyema with negative CT scan: a case report. Can J Neurol Sci 1980; 7:67–69.
33. Kim K, Weinberg P, Magidson M. Angiographic features of subdural empyema. Radiology 1976; 118:621–625.
34. Wilkins R, Goree J. Interhemispheric subdural empyema: angiographic appearance. J Neurosurg 1970; 32:459–462.
35. Gurdjian E, Webster J. Modern surgical treatment of acute subdural abscess. Arch Surg 1948; 57: 411–426.
36. Leys D, Destee A, Petit H, Warof P. Management of subdural intracranial empyemas should not always require surgery. J Neurol Neurosurg Psychiatry 1986; 49:635–639.

24

Spinal Epidural Abscess and Spinal Subdural Empyema

Scott Shapiro
Indiana University School of Medicine, Indianapolis, Indiana

SPINAL EPIDURAL ABSCESS

Historical Perspective

The first recorded descriptions of spine infections were those in Hippocrates' textbooks on tuberculous spondylitis written between the fourth century B.C. and the first century A.D. (1). Sir Percival Pott's description of paralysis in association with tuberculosis of the spine in the eighteenth century led to the eponym "Pott's paraplegia" (2). The first report of an acute infection in the spinal epidural space was in 1796 (3). The name peripachymeningitis was given to this condition in 1853 (4). In 1901, Barth reported the first successful operation with recovery (4). Schick proposed the name of this condition be changed from peripachymeningitis to pachymeningitis externa in 1909 (4). Both names are actually histologically incorrect, as the infection is not of the meninges, but of the tissues of the epidural space (4). Dandy described in detail the cadaveric dissection of the epidural space and related the autopsy findings to the clinical findings in a landmark paper (4). This study included 25 cases of acute abscesses with frank pus and 10 cases of chronic granulation tissue. From Dandy's description of the latter came the concept of chronic epidural abscess. The collective mortality rate in Dandy's report was 83%. In 1945, Grant reported that antibiotics and surgery reduced the mortality to 25% for nontuberculous spinal epidural infections (5). In 1975, Baker reported a further decrease in mortality to 18% (6).

Pathophysiology and Anatomy

An epidural abscess develops most often by either direct extension of a contiguous infection or by metastasis through the bloodstream from a distant infection (4,6–8). In approximately 10% of cases, epidural abscess arises as a direct complication of lumbar puncture, spinal surgery, or spinal anesthesia (9).

Approximately 50% of epidural abscesses are the result of hematogenous spread of infection from distant foci of infection to the epidural space (4,6,9–13). Distant foci that are the source of bacteremia leading to epidural infection include skin/soft tissue infections, pharyngeal abscess, dental abscess, pulmonary infections (pneumonia, bronchiectasis), pelvic inflammatory disease, phlebitis, otitis media, sinusitis, urinary tract infections, and bacterial endocarditis. There may also be hematogenous spread of infection to the vertebral bodies or disc causing discitis/osteomyelitis with subsequent extension into the spinal epidural space (13,14). Intravenous drug abuse is an increasing cause of pyogenic epidural abscess with or without discitis and or osteomyelitis (6,12,15). Infection of the epidural space has been reported to occur from direct extension of infection from decubitus ulcers, psoas abscesses, infected abdominal wounds, pharyngeal abscess, and pulmonary and mediastinal abscesses (8,12).

Immunosuppression from chronic disease, chemotherapy, corticosteroid therapy, or the acquired immunodeficiency syndrome (AIDS) is present in approximately 50% of cases of spinal epidural abscesses (6,9,16). Diabetes mellitus is the most common underlying medical condition in spinal epidural abscess reported in 12.8–33% of patients. Chronic renal failure requiring dialysis has been reported in as many as 12% of cases of spinal epidural abscess, and alcoholism is an associated condition in 10% of cases. Malignancy, chemotherapy, and chronic corticosteroid therapy may increase the risk of bacteremia or spinal deformities that may predispose to the development of an epidural abscess. Intravenous drug abuse and AIDS are becoming increasingly more common as the reported predisposing conditions for spinal epidural abscess formation (16).

The spinal epidural space is only a real space dorsal to the spinal cord and the spinal nerve attachments (4). Ventral to the spinal cord, the dura is closely adherent to the bones of the vertebrae and their ligaments from the first cervical to the second sacral vertebrae. The epidural space is filled with fat and loose areolar tissue containing the epidural veins (Fig. 1). In the cervical region the epidural space consists of only a few strands of fibrous tissue and almost no fat between the laminae and dura. The epidural space really begins to appear at the seventh cervical vertebra and gradually deepens along the thoracic vertebrae, attaining a depth of about 0.5–0.75 cm between the fourth and eighth thoracic vertebrae. The space tapers again and becomes shallow between the eleventh thoracic vertebra and second lumbar vertebrae. Over the remaining lumbar and the first and second sacral vertebrae, the epidural space attains its greatest depth. The fat and loose areolar tissues are embedded with blood vessels and offer a foothold for bloodborne infection (Fig. 2). There is no barrier for this infection to spread both rostrally and caudally throughout the epidural space. This explains why most acute epidural abscesses that arise from hematogenous seeding from a remote site of infection involve the dorsal epidural space in the thoracic, lumbar spine and lower cervical spine and encompass, on average, 3 spinal segments and as many as 13 segments (6,8,9,12).

Anterior epidural abscesses occur primarily in association with vertebral osteomyelitis or a contiguous site of infection. Fortunately, these are usually confined to one or two segments and do not extend rapidly rostrally and caudally along the length of the spinal epidural space, as is typical of epidural abscesses that are dorsal to the spinal cord (3,9).

The pathophysiology of spinal cord dysfunction in association with spinal epidural abscess has been described in a rabbit model (17,18). In the presence of an epidural abscess, the changes in spinal cord white matter included vacuolization, loss of myelin, and axonal swelling. The gray matter of the spinal cord was relatively preserved. There was no microscopic evidence of thrombosis or vasculitis in the major blood vessels supplying the spinal cord, and histopathological changes were more consistent with direct compression of neural tissue than with infarction in the group with mild and moderate cord compression with paraplegia. In the group with severe cord compression, vessel occlusion and infarction were observed. Histopathological changes were more consistent with direct compression of neural tissue than with infarction in cases of

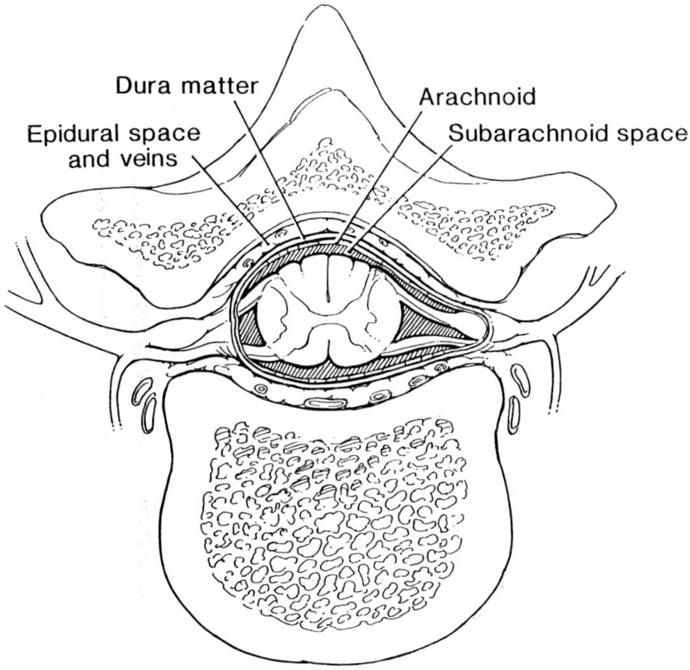

Figure 1 Schematic cross-section of a normal spine and spinal cord demonstrating the epidural space and subarachnoid space.

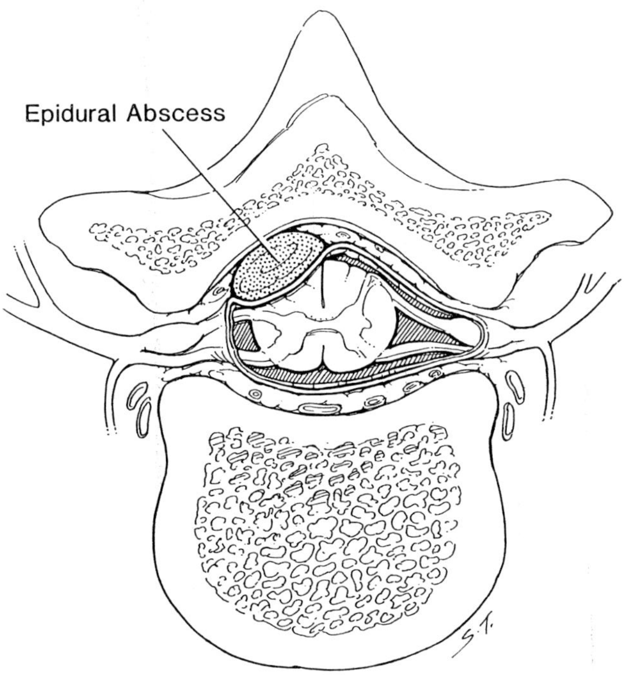

Figure 2 Schematic cross-section of a spinal epidural abscess posterior to the spinal cord.

minimal and moderate spinal cord compression with paraplegia. A few human autopsy reports on patients who died from spinal epidural abscesses with cord compression have demonstrated thrombophlebitis and cord infarction (6,8). Obviously, as in most cases of acute and rapidly progressive spinal cord compression, subsequent recovery is directly related to the rapidity of surgical decompression.

Several reports have correlated the duration of infection and the gross appearance at operation or autopsy. There is a very early presuppurative phase in which the inflammatory lesion is characterized by an epidural mass of swollen, red, friable fat without any gross pus (19). In patients who have had symptoms for less than 2 weeks, gross pus with varying amounts of red granulation tissue has been identified (6,7,9,14,19). Above and below the level of pus, the epidural fat may undergo a reactive change and appear swollen and necrotic (7). In patients with symptoms of longer duration, granulation tissue is often identified on the dura. There frequently are small beads of pus embedded in the granulation tissue (6,7,9,14,19). In delayed cases with symptoms for 150 days or longer, grayish-white granulation tissue or maturing fibrous tissue has been found.

Epidemiology

Most cases of spinal epidural abscess occur in adults with a mean age of 57 years (range 2–81 years) (9). A spinal epidural abscess is rare in children under the age of 12 years (20). The male-to-female ratio is 1:1 (9). The incidence of spinal epidural abscess is reported to be 0.2–2.8 patients per 10,000 hospital admissions (6).

Microbiology

Acute pyogenic epidural abscesses in the older literature were almost exclusively due to *Staphylococcus aureus*. In more recent reports, *S. aureus* accounts for approximately 60% of acute pyogenic epidural abscesses. There is an increasing incidence of gram-negative aerobic bacilli, aerobic streptococci, and anaerobes. A tuberculous spinal epidural abscess is usually associated with vertebral osteomyelitis. Other etiological organisms of epidural abscess include *Brucella* sp., *Actinomyces* sp., *Nocardia*, *Cryptococcus neoformans*, *Blastomyces dermatitidis*, and *Aspergillus* sp.

Clinical Presentation

The triad of fever, back pain, and spine tenderness is the most common presentation of an acute epidural abscess. Spine pain is present in at least 90%. An initial wrong diagnosis is made in approximately 50% of cases, so a high index of suspicion is necessary to make the diagnosis expeditiously. Nuchal rigidity can be present. Patients who present acutely and who have had symptoms for less than 2–3 weeks generally have a better-defined syndrome than do patients with more chronic disease.

Neurological findings and the rate of neurological deterioration can be quite variable, ranging from hours to weeks to months, but most cases progress rapidly in less than 24 h. If the site of infection is thoracic, an intercostal radiation of pain is possible. If the site of infection is in the lumbar area, "root pain" manifesting as lumbar or sacral radiculopathy may be present. Spinal cord dysfunction characterized by paraparesis with a sensory level and sphincter disturbance occurs in 45–50% of patients by the time the diagnosis is made. Complete paraplegia is a less common complication occurring in 17% of cases. The diagnosis needs to be made before neurological deterioration occurs.

There appear to be two basic rates of progression. In the acute presentation of a spinal epidural abscess, there is an average of 5 days of symptoms at the time of presentation; neurological deterioration can occur in just a few short hours, making diagnosis imperative. In the chronic presentation of a spinal epidural abscess, there is an average of 6.7 weeks of symptoms at the time of presentation. Neurological deterioration in this group is much slower.

Diagnostic Evaluation

An acute epidural abscess is usually due to hematogenous seeding of the epidural space, and patients with an acute presentation more often have a systemic illness than those with a chronic presentation. The peripheral leukocyte count averages 13,400–22,000 in most reports. The erythrocyte sedimentation rate is almost always elevated. The analysis of the cerebrospinal fluid (CSF) is consistent with a parameningeal focus of infection with a minimal pleocytosis (<150 WBCs/mm^3), slight elevation in protein concentration, and a normal glucose concentration. CSF cultures are positive in 17%. Blood cultures are positive in 60% of acute epidural abscesses.

Plain radiographs are usually obtained, but rarely helpful unless discitis or osteomyelitis is present with disc space collapse and bone erosion or pathological compression fracture. Historically, myelography with or without computerized tomography (CT) scan was the diagnostic tool of choice. Plain CT scans can demonstrate an extradural mass, but plain CT has a high false-negative rate. Nuclear bone scans can be positive, but are not very helpful for preoperative evaluation. The magnetic resonance imaging (MRI) scan is now the imaging study of choice. MRI is noninvasive and is able to image the degree of cord compression as well as the rostral and caudal extent of the abscess. Areas of epidural space infection have isointense signal intensity on T_1-weighted images (Fig. 3) and high signal intensity on T_2-weighted images. There is enhancement of the lesion following the administration of the MRI contrast agent, gadolinium diethylenetriamine pentaacetic acid (Gd-DTPA) (Fig. 4). The MRI scan should be done emergently in the middle of the night if the clinical presentation is suggestive of an epidural abscess. False-negative MRI studies can result from the following:

1. Patient movement in the scanner can severely degrade the image, making it nondiagnostic.
2. CSF is of high signal intensity on a T_2-weighted image, and thus there is little contrast between CSF and the abscess.

A myelogram/CT scan should be performed in patients with negative MRI scans if an epidural abscess is a possibility.

In the presence of discitis/osteomyelitis and a small contained epidural abscess (Fig. 5), a CT-guided needle biopsy and culture is an option, especially if the patient is neurologically normal.

Treatment

An acute epidural abscess must be treated emergently. Traditional management has been surgery for abscess drainage and culture, followed by 4–6 weeks of intravenous antibiotic therapy, which is then followed by 2–3 months of oral antibiotic therapy. Because pyogenic acute epidural abscesses are usually posterior, a laminectomy is the surgical procedure of choice. Although involvement of a long length of the vertebral canal by an inflammatory mass lesion may appear to be a relative contraindication to surgery, skip laminectomies can be used to successfully drain an extensive abscess. The wound should be closed over extradural drains. The drain can be used for antibiotic irrigation if so desired. Reoperation for irrigation and debridement is sometimes necessary. The previous practice of leaving the wound open and packing it is no longer recommended. In children, laminoplasty or small skip laminotomies with drainage is a preferable option in order to avoid spinal deformity.

When the abscess is secondary to vertebral osteomyelitis/discitis and the pathology is in the anterior space, an anterior approach may be necessary. Cervical discitis with a contained anterior

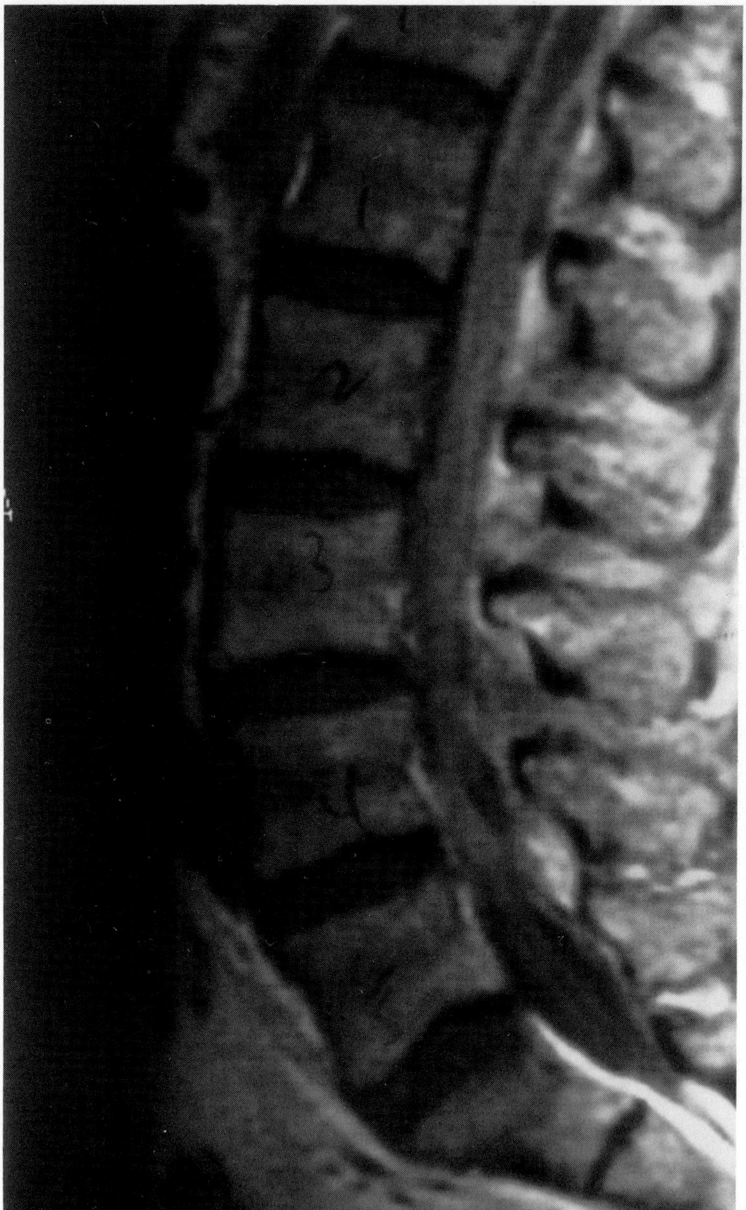

Figure 3 Sagittal T_1-weighted MRI scan shows a spinal epidural abscess posterior to the cord at L1.

epidural abscess can be treated with an anterior cervical discectomy, with or without fusion, and drainage of the abscess. Thoracic and lumbar discitis with a contained anterior epidural abscess can be operated on from an anterior approach via a thoracotomy, via a retroperitoneal approach, or by a posterior approach via a laminectomy. Severe osteomyelitis with vertebral body collapse and anterior epidural abscess should be managed with an anterior operation including vertebrectomy, abscess drainage, and vertebral body reconstruction with autologous iliac crest. A prevertebral drain should be left in for a few days. Successful bone grafting with or without instrumenta-

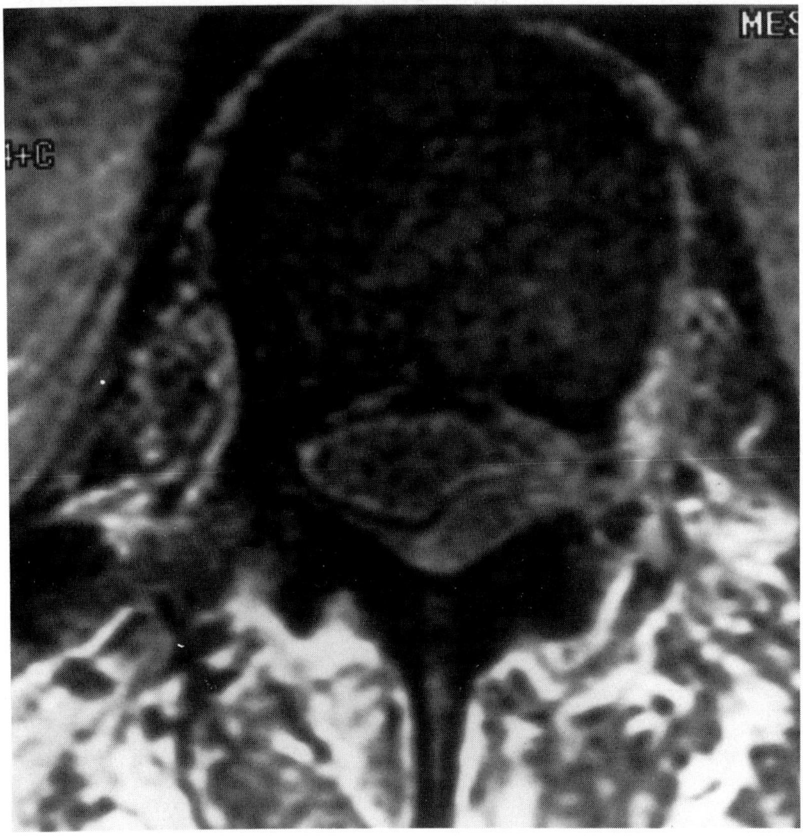

Figure 4 Axial MRI shows a spinal epidural abscess posterior to the spinal cord with cord compression.

tion in the presence of infection can be done following anterior discectomy or vertebrectomy. Laminectomy alone for anterior space epidural abscess is, for the most part, not therapeutically successful.

Most surgeries for tuberculous spinal epidural abscess are anterior surgeries, due to the fact that in the majority of cases, tuberculous epidural abscess is due to extension of infection from vertebral osteomyelitis or discitis. The most common indications for surgery of tuberculous spinal epidural abscess are neurological deficit and progressive spinal deformity (21–23). The mainstay of treatment for tuberculous spinal epidural abscess is antituberculous chemotherapy, including isoniazid (INH) and rifampin with the addition of pyrazinamide or ethambutol and streptomycin in HIV-positive individuals (21–23). HIV-negative individuals are usually treated with a combination of INH, rifampin, and pyrazinamide. Ethambutol may need to be added as well. Multiple antituberculous agents are indicated because of the potential for resistance to a single agent. A 6- to 24-month course of treatment is recommended, with the longer course being used in cases with concomitant bone involvement.

Some recent reports have documented successful nonoperative management of pyogenic spinal epidural abscess (9,36,37). Criteria for nonsurgical treatment of spinal epidural abscess include the following: (1) poor surgical risk, (2) the absence of a significant neurological deficit, and (3) complete paralysis for more than 3 days (36). Identification of the infecting organism via

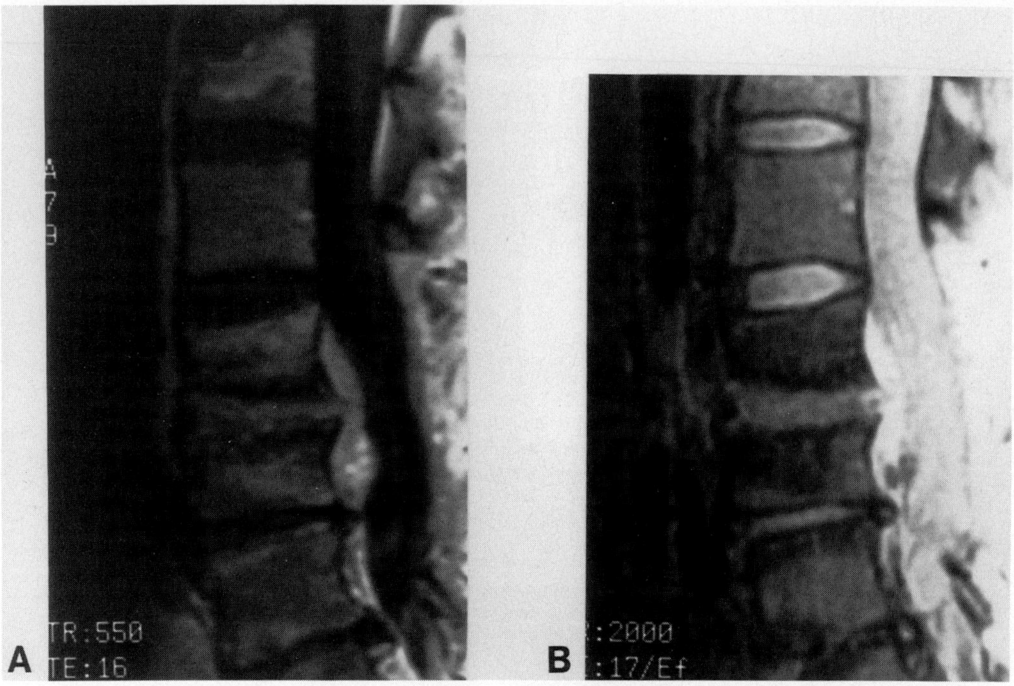

Figure 5 (A) T_1-weighted sagittal MRI of an IV drug user with discitis/osteomyelitis of the L3-L4 disc space and vertebral bodies with an anterior epidural abscess. (B) T_2-weighted sagittal MRI of the same patient.

blood cultures or CT-guided needle biopsy is necessary. Intravenous antibiotic therapy is continued for 4–6 weeks, followed by oral antibiotic therapy for an additional 2–12 weeks. Serial MRI scans are used to monitor the resolution of the abscess. Nonoperative management is best suited for those patients who are neurologically normal when the diagnosis is made.

Treatment for fungal spinal epidural abscess consists of surgery, as previously discussed, and antifungal therapy (24–29). Intravenous amphotericin B with or without flucytosine is the recommended antifungal treatment. Because most patients with fungal epidural abscess are immunocompromised, treatment failure or relapse is common. In patients with AIDS, the goal is suppression of the disease and not cure.

Prognosis

Reported mortality rates for pyogenic epidural abscess in recent years range from 7 to 22% (6,9,12,16). The vast majority of patients that die from epidural abscess have severe paralysis and overwhelming sepsis at presentation, in addition to the risk factors previously discussed. If the patient is diagnosed and treated when ambulatory, then there is a greater than 90% chance of survival with intact ambulation. The prognosis for neurological recovery depends on the duration and severity of the neurological deficit. In Heusner's series, patients with paresis of less than 36 h duration had a complete recovery (8). No patient in that series with complete paralysis for more than 48 h recovered significant function (8).

SPINAL SUBDURAL EMPYEMA

Historical Perspective

Spinal subdural empyema (subdural abscess) is rare. Most of our knowledge is based on a small number of case reports (38–43).

Pathophysiology

A recent or concurrent bacterial infection is commonly present. A dermal sinus tract with connection to the skin and dura may result in a spinal subdural empyema, or the etiology may be hematogenous spread of infection to the spinal subdural space from a distant infection, trauma, or previous spine surgery. *Staphylococcus aureus* is the most common etiological agent.

Clinical Presentation

Systemic signs such as fever and chills are common. Spinal pain (as is typical of spinal epidural abscess) may be absent, making diagnosis more difficult. Signs of spinal cord compression develop very rapidly (Fig. 6), and then the diagnosis must be made and treatment initiated. A high index of suspicion is necessary to make the diagnosis in a patient with fever and signs of rapidly progressive spinal cord compression. Usually the spinal neurological deficit will ascend if left untreated.

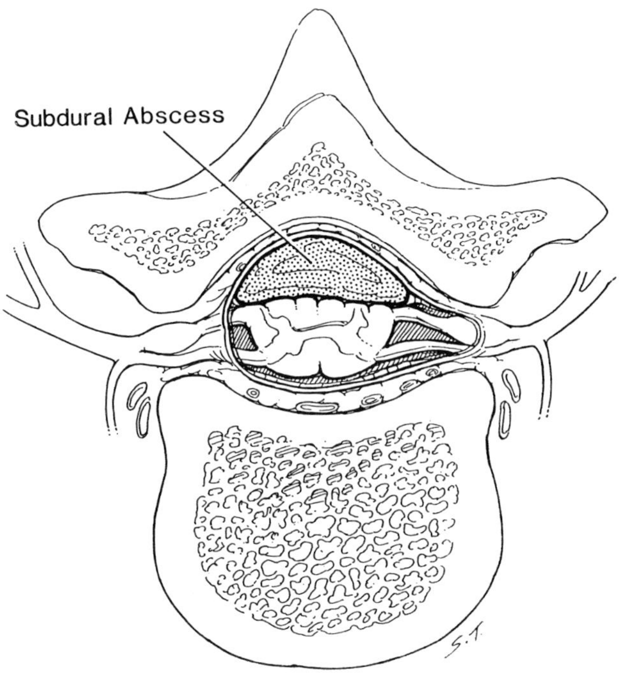

Figure 6 Schematic cross-section demonstrating a subdural abscess with spinal cord compression.

Diagnostic Evaluation

The CSF is usually abnormal, with findings compatible with meningitis. The CSF glucose concentration is decreased, the protein concentration is increased, and there is a pleocytosis. Plain x-rays are usually of no help. A myelogram will reveal an intradural extramedullary block. MRI scan can demonstrate the infection.

Treatment

A spinal subdural empyema is a surgical emergency in most instances. A laminectomy and dural incision with drainage is necessary. Extensive irrigation with bacitracin and another antibiotic, such as vancomycin or gentamicin, is recommended. Rarely a subdural empyema and spinal cord abscess occur together. The dura should be closed primarily. A lumbar subarachnoid drain is usually not necessary, but an extradural drain is often useful. Intravenous antibiotics are necessary for 4–8 weeks and often longer. Oral antibiotic therapy can be substituted at 6–8 weeks and continued for a longer period as necessary.

Prognosis

As previously mentioned, the duration and severity of the neurological deficit is the most important prognostic factor. Early surgery prior to complete paralysis can lead to recovery. Because the blood vessels of the spinal cord are directly exposed to the infection, thrombophlebitis may develop earlier and more severely than in spinal epidural abscess.

REFERENCES

1. Adams F. The Genuine Works of Hippocrates. Vols. 1, 2. New York: Wood, 1886.
2. Pott P. Remarks on That Kind of Palsy of the Lower Limbs Which Is Frequently Found to Accompany a Curvature of the Spine and Is Supposed to Be Caused by It, Together with Its Method of Cure. London: Johnson J, 1779:1–84.
3. Hancock D. A study of 49 patients with acute spinal extradural abscess. Paraplegia 1973; 10:285–288.
4. Dandy W. Abscesses and inflammatory tumors in the spinal epidural space (so called pachymeningitis externa). Arch Surg 1926; 13:477–494.
5. Grant F. Epidural spinal abscess. JAMA 1945; 128:509–511.
6. Baker A, Ojemann R, Swartz M, Richardson E. Spinal epidural abscess. New Engl J Med 1975; 293:463–468.
7. Browder J, Meyers R. Pyogenic infections of the spinal epidural space. A consideration of the anatomic and physiologic pathology. Surgery 1941; 10:296–308.
8. Heusner A. Nontuberculosis spinal epidural infections. N Engl J Med 1948; 239:845–854.
9. Danner R, Hartman B. Update of spinal epidural abscess: 35 cases and review of the literature. Rev Infect Dis 1987; 9:265–274.
10. Guerrero I, Slap G, MacGregor R, Lawner P, Ruggeri S, Gennarelli T. Anaerobic spinal epidural abscess; case report. J Neurosurg 1978; 48:465–469.
11. Hulme A, Dott N. Spinal epidural abscess. Br Med J 1954; 1:64–68.
12. Kaufman D, Kaplan J, Litman N. Infectious agents in spinal epidural abscesses. Neurology 1980; 30: 844–850.
13. Messer H, Lenchner G, Brust J, Resor S. Lumbar spinal abscess managed conservatively: case report. J Neurosurg 1977; 46:825–829.
14. Russell N, Vaughn R, Morley T. Spinal epidural infection. Can J Neurol Sci 1979; 6:325–328.
15. Jabbari B, Pierce J. Spinal cord compression due to pseudomonas in a heroin addict; case report. Neurology 1977; 27:1034–1037.

16. Hlavin M, Kaminski H, Ross J, Ganz E. Spinal epidural abcess: a ten year perspective. Neurosurgery 1990; 27:177–184.
17. Feldenzer J, McKeever P, Schaberg D, Campbell J, Hoff J. Experimental spinal epidural abscess: a pathophysiological model in the rabbit. Neurosurgery 1987; 20:859–867.
18. Feldenzer J, McKeever P, Schaberg D, Campbell J, Hoff J. The athogenesis of spinal epidural abscess: microangiographic studies in an experimental model. J Neurosurg 1988; 69:110–114.
19. Corradini E, Turney M, Browder E. Spinal epidural infection. NY State J Med 1948; 48:2367–2370.
20. Baker C. Primary spinal epidural abscess. Am J Dis Child 1971; 121:337–339.
21. Konstam P, Blesovsky A. The ambulant treatment of spinal tuberculosis. J Bone Joint Surg 1967; 49(B):668–673.
22. Liefso R, Weaver P, Harder E. Tuberculous spondylitis in adults. J Bone Joint Surg 1985; 67(A):1405–1413.
23. Medical Research Council Working Party on Tuberculosis of the Spine. A controlled trial of six month and nine month regimens of chemotherapy in patients undergoing radical surgery for tuberculosis of the spine in Hong Kong. Tubercle 1986; 67:243–259.
24. Awad I, Bax J, Petersen J. Nocardial osteomyelitis of the spine with epidural spinal cord compression—a case report. Neurosurgery 1984; 15:254–256.
25. Siao P, McCabe P, Yagnik P. Nocardial spinal epidural abscess. Neurology 1989; 39:996.
26. Ganado W, Craig A. Brucellosis myelopathy. J Bone Joint Surg 1958; 40(A):1380–1388.
27. Gehweiler J, Capp M, Chick E. Observation on the roentgen patterns in blastomycosis of bone: a review of cases from the blastomycosis cooperative study of the Veterans Administration and Duke University Medical Center. AJR 1970; 108:497–510.
28. Diamond R. Cryptococcus neoformans. In: Mandell G, Douglas R, Bennet J, eds. Principles and Practice of Infectious Diseases. 3rd ed. New York: Churchill Livingstone, 1990:1980–1989.
29. Holmes P, Osterman D, Tullos H. Aspergillus discitis. Report of two cases and review of the literature. Clin Orthop 1988; 226:240–246.
30. Pritchard D. Granulomatous infections of bones and joints. Orthop Clin North Am 1975; 6:1029–1047.
31. Gardner R, Cammisa F, Eismont F, Green B. Nongranulomatous spinal epidural abscesses. Orthop Trans 1989; 13:562–563.
32. Koppel B, Tuchman A, Mangiardi J, et al. Epidural spinal infection in intravenous drug abusers. Arch Neurol 1988; 45:1331–1337.
33. Angtuaco E, McConnell J, Chadduck W, Flanigan S. MR imaging of spinal epidural sepsis. AJR 1987; 149:1249–1253.
34. Bertino R, Porter B, Stimac G, Tepper S. Imaging spinal osteomyelitis and epidural abscess with short T1 inversion recovery (STIR). AJNR 1988; 9:563–564.
35. Erntell M, Holtas S, Norlin K, et al. Magnetic resonance imaging in the diagnosis of spinal epidural abscess. Scand J Infect Dis 1988; 20:323–327.
36. Leys D, Lesoin F, Viaud C, et al. Decreased morbidity from acute bacterial spinal epidural abscesses using computed tomography and nonsurgical treatment in selected patients. Ann Neurol 1985; 17: 350–355.
37. Mampalam T, Rosegay H, Andrews B, et al. Nonoperative treatment of spinal epidural infections. J Neurosurg 1989; 71:208–210.
38. Dacey R, Winn H, Jane J, Butler A. Spinal subdural empyema: report of two cases. Neurosurgery 1978; 3:400–403.
39. Heindel C, Ferguson J, Kumarasamy T. Spinal subdural empyema complicating pregnancy: case report. J Neurosurg 1974; 40:654–656.
40. Negrin J, Clark R. Pyogenic subdural abscesses of the spinal meninges: report of two cases. J Neurosurg 1952; 9:95–100.
41. Schnegg J, Glauser M, de Tribolet N. Infection of a lumbar dermonid cyst by an anaerobic peptococcus. Acta Neurochir (Wein) 1981; 58:127–129.
42. Wright R. Infections of the spine and spinal cord. In: Youmans J, ed. Neurological Surgery. 2d ed. Philadelphia: Saunders, 1982:3449–3458.
43. Fraser R, Ratzan K, Wolpert S, Weinstein L. Spinal subdural empyema. Arch Neurol 1973; 28:235–238.

25

Cerebrospinal Fluid Shunt Infections

Joel C. Boaz
Indiana University School of Medicine, Indianapolis, Indiana

For centuries hydrocephalus has been a disfiguring, neurologically devastating, and generally fatal disease. The availability of ventricular shunting over the last 40 years has enabled us to forget this. In a detailed study of untreated hydrocephalics from 1938 to 1957, the likelihood of an untreated hydrocephalic neonate surviving to adulthood was 20–23%. The average IQ of survivors was 69, with only 73% of survivors "educable" (IQ > 50). Thirty-four of 81 were severely handicapped or incapacitated (1). One year later (2), a 5-year study that compared shunted and nonshunted hydrocephalics showed a 10-year survival of 61% with shunting vs. 22% without (2). Fifty-four percent were predicted to be competitive (IQ > 75) with shunt vs. 6% without. These dramatic accomplishments with early ventriculoatrial (VA) shunts have continued to improve with better technique and technology.

Although a variety of ingenious methods have been utilized for treatment of hydrocephalus, their relatively high morbidity and failure rates have led to the virtual abandonment of nonshunt methods such as choroid plexectomy (3), cauterization of the choroid plexus (4), or carotid ligation (5). Improvement in stereotactic and endoscopic technology has rendered third ventriculostomy a viable alternative for obstructive hydrocephalus (6), but ventricular shunting remains the mainstay in the treatment of hydrocephalus.

In 1952 Nulsen and Spitz described the successful performance of a ventriculojugular shunt utilizing a valve apparatus comprised of two one-way valves in series with a chamber between preventing reflux of blood from fouling the system (7). Along with the subsequent use of a distal slit valve by Pudenz (8), the treatment of hydrocephalus was revolutionized. These two valves are the forerunners of our current proximal and distal valves, respectively. For the next 15–20 years, VA shunts held sway. Initial efforts at ventriculoperitoneal (VP) shunting were confounded by high rates of early fibrosis distally or cysts in the peritoneum (9), but a recognition of the dangers of VA shunts including pulmonary emboli, pulmonary hypertension, pericardial tamponade (10), shunt nephritis (11), and the need for frequent revisions, along with the availability of silastic

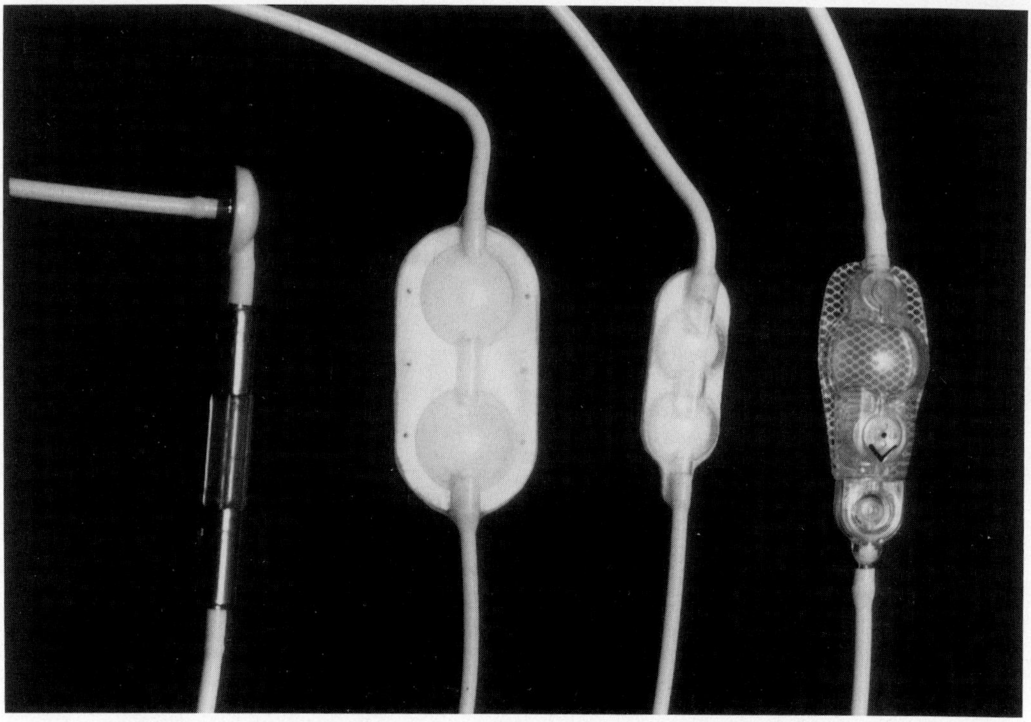

Figure 1 Proximal Holter valve, two double-bubbles (for distal slit valves), proximal Delta valve.

shunt material, led to a resurgence of ventriculoperitoneal shunting (12). Several studies have demonstrated advantages of VP over VA shunts (13–16), and the ventriculoperitoneal shunt is currently used more than 90% of the time for the treatment of hydrocephalus. Current shunt systems are composed of a ventricular catheter with or without reservoir for access, a valve to regulate rate of flow—proximal (behind the ear) or distal (peritoneal)—and a distal peritoneal or atrial catheter (Fig. 1).

Despite the fact that ventricular shunts represent one of the major advances in neurosurgery, like all man-made devices they are fraught with potential problems. Mechanical obstructions, disconnections and malfunctions are statistically the most common complications (17). These are usually easily remedied and entail short hospital stays. Shunt infections, on the other hand, are associated with long hospital stays, substantial expense, and serious morbidity or mortality. It behooves us to diligently study infection and its therapy and prevention to optimize the care of the hydrocephalic patient.

RISK FACTORS FOR SHUNT INFECTION

The reported rates of infection of ventricular shunts generally range from 5 to 15% (16,18–29). This is expressed as an operative infection rate (infections per procedure) rather than a case rate (infections per shunt device or infections per patient). To use this method of reporting implies that the risk of developing a shunt infection is directly related to the operative procedures themselves, an assertion that will be justified later.

Infection rates appear to be decreasing over time, and even within given institutions improvements are not uncommon. Forrest experienced a 16% infection rate in his first 150 cases, but this decreased to 8% for the next 300 (19). Nulsen and Becker (20), Shurtleff et al. (27), and Spanu et al. (23) all describe similar decreases (about 50%) in infection rates over the respective periods of study. The reasons for these decreases are certainly multifactorial and complicate the analysis of specific factors.

Factors influencing the infection rate are important to examine both to understand the pathophysiology of shunt infections and to reduce their frequency. In a review of the 25-year experience with shunting at Johns Hopkins, it was determined that the attending neurosurgeon was the single most important factor in the incidence of shunt infections (30). Individual rates varied from 1.8 to 50%, and there was a clear trend for lower infection rates among the surgeons who performed the most procedures (30). Lund-Johansen et al. reported an 11.5% infection rate in operations performed by residents and a 2.2% infection rate in operations performed by specialists (31). Length of operation may correlate with higher risk of infection. Two studies found trends toward higher infection rates with longer surgeries (19,32). Raimondi et al. experienced a 17.7% infection rate with three-piece systems and a 7.3% rate with one-piece systems (29). All things being equal, experience, speed, and simplicity are critical to minimize the risk of shunt infection.

Many studies have looked at the impact of the etiology of the hydrocephalus on the risk of shunt infection. The majority have found no dramatic differences in risk of infection based on the etiology of the hydrocephalus, but conflicting results are reported with respect to myelomeningocele, with some studies demonstrating an increased rate for myelomeningoceles (21,27,33), some a lower rate (34), and some no difference (16,32,35,36).

Perhaps the most universally identified risk factor in shunt patients is young age (25,30,36–38). In some studies young age was the only significant risk factor identified (25,38). Unfortunately, the age below which the rate is higher has varied widely from 4 months (25) to 4 years (30), with the typical designation around 6 months (36,38). Neonates and premies may be at particularly high risk (39). One reason suggested for the high infection rate in infants is their relatively deficient immune system (36). Maternal IgM is not transferred across the placenta, maternal IgG levels decrease well before the infant's IgG levels become sufficient, and neonatal complement levels are low (36). These factors could explain the high rates of shunt infection in young infants. Alternatively, immunoglobulins and complement may not be protective against shunt colonization (38); instead, the higher skin densities of *Staphylococci* in neonates and the higher prevalence of multiple antibiotic resistance, adherent strains, and single biotypes (40) may explain the higher rates of shunt infection in young infants (38).

Despite the acknowledged higher incidence of shunt malfunctions or complications (particularly severe ones) in VA vs. VP shunts (13–16), the evidence that the infection rates are higher for VA shunts is less clear. Some papers describe a higher rate of infection with VA shunts (13,15), but most claim a very similar rate (16,24). In one series, VP shunts were consistently more prone to infection than VA shunts, perhaps due to the larger surface area involved in prepping and draping (28).

One frequent caveat is that patients with skin lesions, poor skin condition, or sites of preexisting infection at the time of surgery are at high risk of infection (23,36,41,42). If shunt procedures can be postponed until such problems are cleared up, the risks can be minimized.

CLINICAL PRESENTATION

Shunt infections present in a variety of ways, but generally soon after shunt placement or revision. According to Schoenbaum's classical description, 70% of infections present within 2 months of the last surgical procedure and 78% within 4 months (24). This pattern of early presentation of shunt infection has held up in other series (21,29,32). This temporal inhomogeneity in the frequency of presentation is suggestive that the bacteria are introduced at the time of surgery and should lead one to have a higher index of suspicion for infection in the early postoperative period.

The single most frequent finding in shunt infections is fever (Table 1) (43). The fever may range from mild and intermittent to quite high. If a shunt infection is mistakenly diagnosed as an otitis or urinary tract infection and antibiotics are administered to treat the presumed cause, the fever may disappear only to recur when the medication is stopped.

Signs and symptoms of stiff neck, photophobia, and delerium are uncommon. Problems referable to the distal end of the shunt are more frequent, particularly with ventriculoperitoneal shunts. The most dramatic presentation is an acute abdomen with fever, abdominal pain, diffuse or local tenderness and sometimes rebound, anorexia, vomiting, and leukocytosis (44–46). Such patients would generally be taken for laparotomy if no shunt was present, but if due to shunt infection, such symptoms may resolve with externalization of the shunt (cutting down over the shunt in the chest or upper abdomen, slipping the catheter out of the body, and connecting it to an external drainage system) and administration of antibiotics. Cerebrospinal fluid (CSF) and peritoneal catheter culture should be sent for aerobic and anaerobic culture. *Staphylococcus aureus* is particularly common in such vicious abdominal infections and may be present without CSF pleocytosis. If the clinical picture does not improve, laparotomy may still be indicated, as a ruptured appendix may be to blame (47).

The abdominal presentation of shunt infection can also be much more subtle, with intermittent cramping, fleeting pains, or an abdominal malaise similar to that seen with hepatomegaly and splenomegaly of mononucleosis. This vague abdominal symptomatology is more common with indolent organisms such as *Propionibacter acnes* or *Staphylococcus epidermidis* (48). It may occur many months after shunt surgery has been performed.

Abdominal distention after ventriculoperitoneal shunting that persists or develops after the first few days (when it may be normal) can be a sign of CSF ascites with poor absorption of spinal fluid (49). The malabsorption has been ascribed to various factors (50), but should be considered infectious in etiology until proven otherwise; externalizing the shunt is preferable to implanting the distal end, which may be infected, into the vascular system as a VA shunt.

Shunt malfunction is a critical presentation of infection. This may be in the form of headaches, lethargy, vomiting, or paresis of upgaze in older patients or bulging fontanelle or excessive head growth in the infant. Early investigators reported frequent recurrent peritoneal obstructions in patients who then underwent multiple distal revisions (15). Such distal obstructions were ultimately recognized to be indicative of low-grade infection. In a retrospective study, shunt infections presenting as malfunction alone were more likely to be treated with medical therapy or no therapy directed specifically at infection than any other symptom complex. These two modes of therapy were demonstrably less effective than a surgical approach directed against a recognized infection (28).

Table 1 Presenting Symptoms in Shunt Infections

		Kontny			Walters	
	Odio	VA	VP	Forward	VA	VP
Fever	86%	100%	95%	79%		42%
Meningitis	20%	0%	29%	35%	0	2%
Abdominal symptoms	37%	0%	48%	33% (VP)	0	2%
Shunt malfunction	68%	14%	57%	NR	20%	25%
Wound infection	19%	NR	NR	26%	6%	29%

Deep wound infection or erythema or pus along the shunt tract is easily recognized. This mode of presentation will not be present in more than one third of cases, but can be readily identified as O'Brien's "external shunt infection," for which he advocated complete shunt removal and appropriate intravenous antibiotics (51). Occasionally a superficial stitch abscess or wound infection can be treated conservatively with antibiotics, but extension to or exposure of shunt hardware means that it is essentially doomed to be removed and must be recognized and surgically treated.

A particularly vexing problem is what to do with positive cultures of shunt hardware removed at the time of surgery in the absence of bacteria in the CSF and/or clinical evidence of infection, designated by Steinbok et al. as "asymptomatic bacteriological shunt contamination" (52). According to Steinbok et al., if these culture-positive shunts were truly identified in instances without any clinical evidence of infection, they were not associated with increased risk of future malfunction and therefore routine cultures should not be taken at surgeries for elective lengthening of a shunt or shunt disconnection (52). It should be noted, however, that signs of infection may be subtle (53) and shunt colonization should not be considered "asymptomatic" without careful consideration.

DIAGNOSIS

The sine qua non in the diagnosis of ventricular shunt infections is a positive spinal fluid culture from the shunt or a positive culture from shunt components. The key to prompt diagnosis is to have a high index of suspicion leading to an appropriate but not undue willingness to violate the system to obtain CSF for analysis and culture. A tap of the shunt itself prior to the initiation of antibiotic therapy should have a high yield—> 90% (24,54)—for a positive culture and is relatively safe (55). Lumbar puncture has a much lower yield (7–26%) (56), and positive blood cultures in VP shunt infections are the exception rather than the rule. Serum tests such as C-reactive protein or antistaphylococcal antibody titer (57) may be suggestive but are not definitive for infection (58) and should not determine therapy.

The two entities that shunt infections must be differentiated from are other infections and other malfunctions. The differential diagnosis of a febrile illness in a child includes pharyngitis, pneumonia, urinary tract infection, otitis, viral gastroenteritis, etc. Even a shunted child will have these afflictions more commonly than shunt infection and should be routinely evaluated by a pediatrician. Unexplained fevers, recurrent fevers, or early postoperative fevers must be investigated with respect to the shunt.

Shunt malfunctions are manifested by signs and symptoms of increased intracranial pressure. They can be divided into proximal or intracranial and distal infections involving the valve or peritoneal catheter. Along with clinical exam, a computed tomographic (CT) scan to document increased ventricular size is recommended. If a malfunction is felt to be proximal, surgical revision will be necessary to reestablish flow and no CSF will be available for preoperative analysis. Proximal malfunctions are rarely due to infection. Distal malfunctions, on the other hand, are frequently due to infection. An inflammatory sheath may surround the peritoneal catheter, and if this becomes distended with spinal fluid, a CSFoma may form. In either case, the distal resistance will be elevated. Prior to taking a patient to the operating room for distal revision, the possibility of infection should be investigated. A reservoir tap can be used to obtain CSF for cell count, Gram's stain, and culture. In cases with a distal slit valve, this can be combined with a "tap and flush" to possibly clear debris from the distal valve slits. If a traditional Holter or Hakim valve is present, a tap is performed below the proximal portion of the valve and Conray or Omnipaque is injected to check for sheathing distally (Fig. 2), which is almost always due to infection. Abdominal ultrasound or CT scan can delineate CSFomas or cysts (Fig. 3), which are

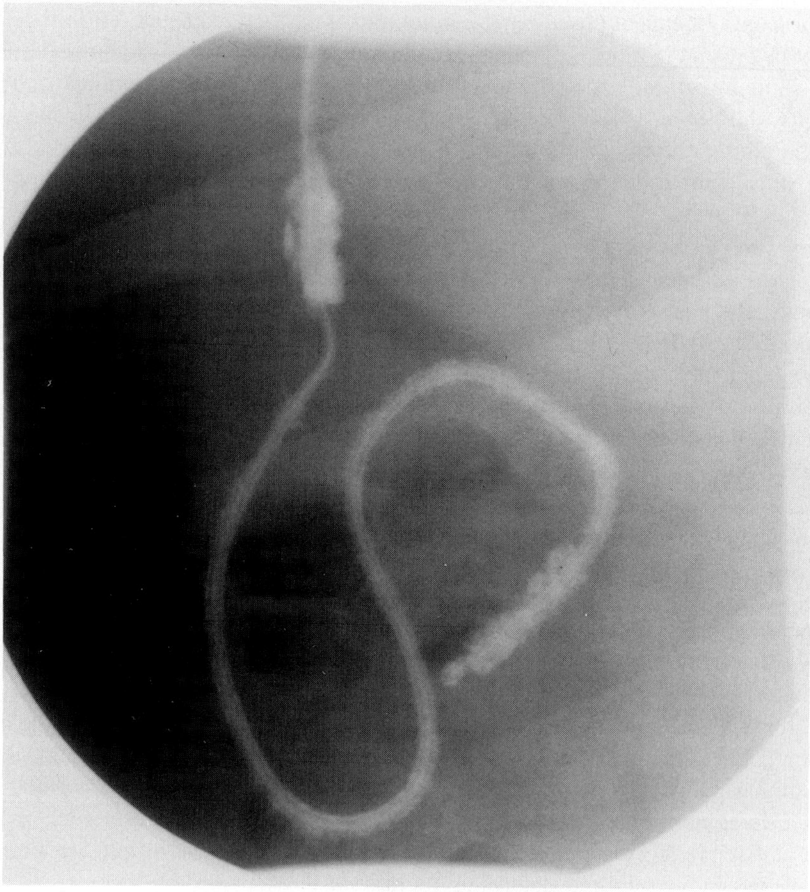

Figure 2 Shuntogram demonstrating distal sheathing due to infection.

very suggestive of infection. Laparoscopic or open resection of these cysts is not advocated (59), but, rather, they are managed by shunt externalization, culture, and antibiotic therapy.

BACTERIOLOGY

Coagulase-negative staphylococci are responsible for the majority of ventricular shunt infections. This was true in the early days of VA shunting (20,60–62) and continues to be true to the present (32,63). Most series report coagulase-negative staphylococci as the causative agent of 50–70% of shunt infections (16,24,29,30,33,37,64,65). Early studies designate these organisms as *Staphylococcus albus* (*albus* = white vs. *aureus* = yellow) on the basis of colony color and more recently as the familiar *S. epidermidis*. Taxonomists have subsequently expanded the classification of these organisms on the basis of colony morphology and pigment, biochemical reactions, cell wall composition, and substrate utilization, creating new species including *Staphylococcus capitis*, *warneri*, and *hominis* (66). Despite this confusing plethora of "new" bacteria, *S. epidermidis* remains the predominant organism found on the skin and in shunt infections (67). Other coagulase-negative staphylococci have been shown to cause shunt infection (67,68), but it is not clear that species designation is of any true significance in determining presentation, virulence,

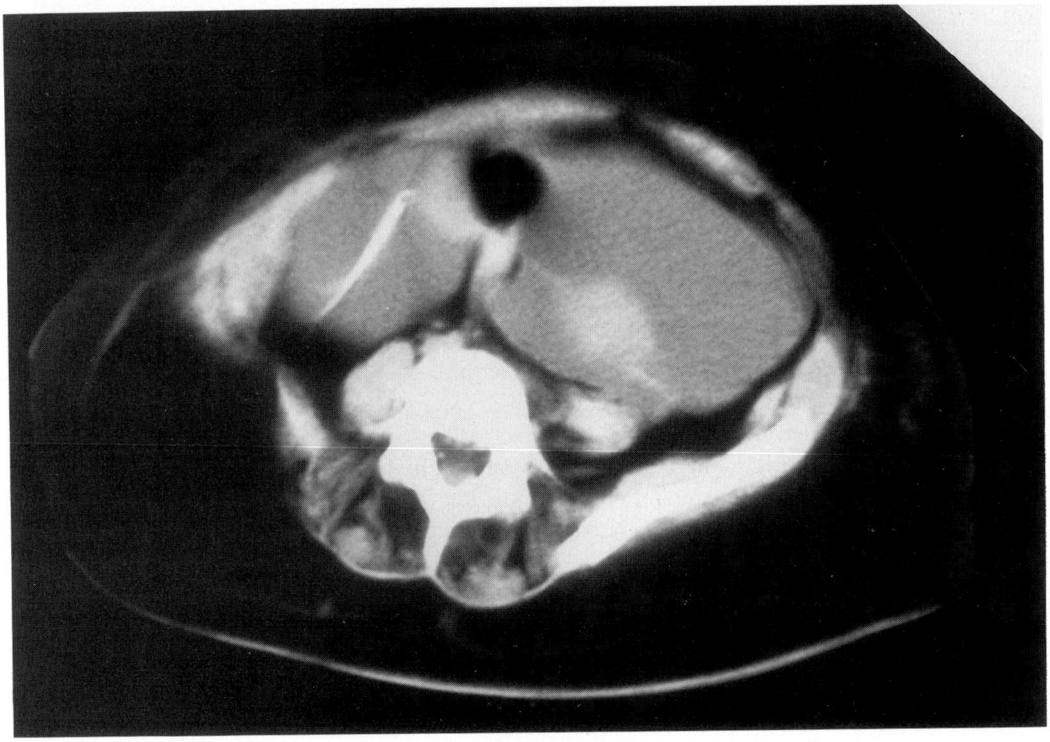

Figure 3 CT scan with CSFoma surrounding distal catheter.

or proper therapy of a coagulase-negative staphylococcal shunt infection (69). Even the potentially more clinically relevant characteristics of adhesion, slime production, and antibiotic resistance are not clearly helpful (70). These generally harmless skin organisms take on special significance in the presence of a foreign body, and their preeminence in shunt infection means that discussion of pathogenesis, prophylaxis, and plan for treatment is based largely on coagulase-negative staphylococci.

Coagulase-positive staphylococci or *S. aureus* has been the second most prevalent organism in shunt infections and is often associated with erythema or pus along the shunt tract, an acute abdomen, or high fever. The virulence of the clinical picture as well as clinical experience has caused some to be insistent on shunt removal in the treatment of *S. aureus* shunt infections (71).

Streptococci are relatively uncommon, with *Streptococcus viridans* being similar to coagulase-negative staphylococci in presentation and treatment. Enterococcus is seen on occasion in late infections, particularly in myelomeningoceles associated with a urinary or gastrointestinal source of infection.

Gram-positive rods of several types have been reported in shunt infections (72). *Listeria monocytogenes* shunt infection is likely due to *Listeria* meningitis in a patient with a preexisting VP shunt (73). *Corynebacterium jeikeium* is a relative newcomer frequently resistant to multiple antibiotics and tending to occur in the immunosuppressed or those who have been on antibiotic therapy (74). *Propionibacterium acnes* probably occurs most frequently in this group, and its occurrence is likely still underestimated (75). It may grow only on anaerobic media and may also present many months after shunt surgery with vague abdominal symptomatology or shunt malfunction. It would appear that this organism may exist in the relatively asymptomatic patient for as long as several years before problems arise and is also a possible contaminant in cultures, leading to doubts of its validity when cultured. In our institution, *Propionibacterium* has become second in frequency only to coagulase-negative staphylococci and approximately equal to *S. aureus* in occurrence.

Gram-negative bacilli may be responsible for shunt infections in up to 20% of cases. The route of infection in these cases is harder to delineate than with coagulase-negative staphylococci and may result from bowel perforation, bacteruria, or other predisposing factors. Frequent pathogens include *E. coli*, *Klebsiella*, *Proteus*, *Enterobacter*, and *Pseudomonas*. Gram-negative bacilli shunt infections had a mortality rate of 39% and a 78% risk of neurological sequelae in one series (76). A more recent study, however, demonstrated no mortality and only an 11% incidence of neurological sequelae (77). These authors stressed early diagnosis, immediate shunt removal with external ventricular drainage, and the superiority of third-generation cephalosporins over aminoglycosides in the treatment of these infections.

Haemophilus influenzae has been of particular interest in shunt infections (78–84). It was recognized early that this gram-negative organism might be eradicated with medical therapy alone (77). Other papers confirmed this (78,80,81), but some failures were encountered as well (79,82,83), stressing the need for excellent antibiotic selection and maintenance of shunt function during treatment.

Atypical mycobacteria have been demonstrated in at least one shunt infection (85) and, as expected, were quite difficult to eradicate. Fungal infections are uncommon and are generally caused by *Candida* (86,87) or *Cryptococcus* (88,89). The largest series of fungal infections involved eight premature babies, five of whom had received parenteral nutrition and been ventilated. Seven cultures grew *Candida* sp. and one culture grew *Torulopsis glabrata* (86). Three of eight CSF cultures obtained at the time of shunt placement grew fungus, but this positive culture was considered to be a contaminant. *Cryptococcus* sp. may infect existing VP shunts or could possibly be present at the time of placement, as this fungus may be responsible for cases of hydrocephalus without clear etiology.

PATHOGENESIS

Five mechanisms can be postulated for the colonization of ventricular shunts: introduction of bacteria at the time of shunt implantation or revision, hematogenous seeding of an existing shunt, spread to a shunt of a ventriculitis, infection of the shunt from the peritoneal cavity, or transcutaneous shunt infection via iatrogenic inoculation of the shunt or skin or wound breakdown.

The introduction of bacteria at the time of shunt surgery is felt to be the major cause of shunt infection for two reasons: (1) the organisms responsible for shunt infection are the same as organisms that can be cultured from the skin, and (2) the vast majority of shunt infections occur within the first few months after a surgical procedure (24).

The issue of where precisely the infecting organisms arise from (patient's skin, surgeon, airborne contamination) has been addressed by several studies. Bayston and Lari cultured the scalp, neck, and abdomen of 100 patients prior to ventricular shunt placement or revision (90). At the conclusion of the case, a velvet pad impression was taken of the wound prior to closure. Fifty-eight of 100 patients had organisms cultured from these impressions. Thirty-two of 58 organisms had been similarly recovered from the patient's skin preoperatively. Twenty-six of 58 positive cultures were of organisms not found on the patient preoperatively. The cases where cultures grew organisms found on the patient preoperatively had a approximately five times the number of colonies found in the cases that grew organisms not found on the patient preoperatively. Of the nine patients who subsequently developed shunt infection, seven had organisms that had been isolated from the patient, four before closure, three on the preoperative skin. The conclusions drawn were that it was not unusual for staphylococci to gain access to the surgical wound during shunt surgery and that most but not all of these organisms arose from the patient's skin (90). Shapiro preoperatively cultured the skin of 413 patients who underwent shunt surgery. In comparing the organisms subsequently isolated from the infected shunts, only 4 of 18 (22%) were identical to organisms previously isolated from the skin. Ten of 18 were typical skin organisms not found on the patient and presumably from the operating team or airborne contamination. Four of 18 were gram-negative rods with predisposing factors in each instance (25). Duhaime et al. placed Millipore filters on the patients' prepped skin under drapes, on top of the drapes, or on the instrument table. The highest percentage of positive cultures was found on the drapes (13.5%) rather than the instrument table (9.1%) or skin (2.1%). The conclusion drawn was that the major source of bacteria in the operating room was the surgical team (91). A compilation of data on perioperative wound contamination and subsequent shunt infections leads to the conclusion that most shunt infections are introduced at surgery and the organisms may arise from the patient, the surgical team, or airborne contamination.

Hematogenous seeding of other prosthetic devices long after their implantation is well documented. Although most total joint replacement infections probably arise at surgery (92) (as with shunts), a number of cases develop long after joint implantation in a previously asymptomatic patient after infection has been documented at another site with the same organism (93). Dental infections (94), bacterurias, other joint space infections (95), and pharyngitis (96) have all been reported in association with infection in prosthetic devices. Particularly convincing is the simultaneous infection of more than one artificial joint with the same organism.

Hematogenous infection of ventricular shunts is more controversial. With ventriculoatrial shunts, seeding of the atrial catheter by transient bacteremias arising from the intestinal tract or the skin has been postulated with resultant ascending infection (62). Nulsen and Becker's early admonition that the atrial catheter tip should be placed no lower than T6 on chest x-ray was based on the hypothesis that the catheter caused endocardial damage and thrombi predisposing to infections during bacteremia. A remarkable correlation between this infection rate and catheter position lends credence to their reasoning (20).

Others have argued against a hematogenous etiology based on the clustering of infections in the first 2 months following shunt surgery and the very comparable rates of infection for VP shunts and VA shunts despite the presumed higher risk of hematogenous seeding of the latter (24). A middle ground approach would admit that a certain percentage of infections arise beyond the first 2 months after insertion of the shunt and for VA shunts at least are presumed to be due to bacteremia (26).

Even with ventriculoperitoneal shunts, occasional cases are reported with bacteruria, with or without bacteremia documented, and concomitant VP shunt infection with the same organism (63,97,98). Although one could hypothesize a direct transperitoneal route for acquisition of the VP shunt infection, hematogenous spread of infection seems more likely.

Haemophilus influenzae has been isolated not infrequently from infected VA or VP shunts. Claims have been made that the frequency of *H. influenzae* infection in the CNS of shunted children is greater than one would expect in the general population. It is admitted, however, that no prospective study has been done to verify this. The timing of *H. influenzae* shunt infections is often quite delayed, sometimes years after shunt placement or revision has been performed. Even when the peritoneum is the distal terminus, blood cultures are often positive. These unusual features along with the not infrequent ability to sterilize the shunt in situ suggests that the mechanism of *H. influenzae* shunt infection differs from the usual perioperative contamination. The most plausible route of infection is from bloodstream to CSF to shunt, or a shunt infection originating as a ventriculitis. *Neisseria meningitidis* and *Streptococcus pneumoniae* have also been the etiological organism of shunt infections, again in a setting suggesting that the shunt infection is a complication of a primary ventriculitis.

Shunts can also be theoretically inoculated through the spinal fluid at open craniotomy. There is a high incidence of shunt infection after open surgery (99).

The peritoneal shunt catheter is at risk for contracting infection from ruptured appendix, bladder, or colonic perforation by the catheter itself. These complications may occur at any time and may result in particularly dangerous gram-negative or polymicrobial infections in the central nervous system. Ruptured appendix must be kept in mind when acute abdominal symptomatology occurs in the shunted patient (16,63), particularly if there is no improvement after shunt externalization (47), as fatal sepsis or ventriculitis may complicate delayed treatment. Bladder rupture is almost exclusively seen in the patient with neurogenic bladder and need for intermittent catheterization. The postaugmentation bladder of myelomeningoceles is at particular risk for rupture. These children may present with sepsis or shock and represent a urological emergency. The shunt is best externalized immediately. Gram-negative ventriculitis may still occur.

The shunt catheter is generally well tolerated by the abdomen and yet on occasion will perforate or enter the colon. Long lengths may be completely intraluminal (Fig. 4). Some have speculated that either a low-grade preexisting shunt infection (i.e., *Propionibacterium*, *S. epidermidis*) or a nonfunctional shunt without CSF dripping out is apt to become trapped by omentum or inflammatory tissue and secondarily erode into the colon. Subdural peritoneal shunts seem particularly prone to this (100,101), perhaps because they tend to stop draining after the subdural has resolved. The risk of infection in a shunt that is no longer functional is a good argument for removal of this type of shunt once the subdural has resolved (101).

A ventriculoperitoneal shunt may also be at risk of infection at the time of laparotomy. Many children with hydrocephalus will also have myelodysplasia, cerebral palsy, brain tumor, or other conditions which may necessitate laparotomy for Nissen fundoplication, gastrostomy tube, bladder augmentation, or urinary diversion. One group has reported VP shunt infection occurring with augmentation cystoplasty in 2 of 54 patients at risk (3.7%) (102). This concern has led some to routinely externalize a shunt for abdominal operations and to convert it (sometimes temporarily) to an atrial or pleural shunt (103). Pittman et al., on the other hand, experienced no shunt infections after 44 abdominal operations (104) and suggested that children with shunts can safely undergo abdominal operations with minimal risk to the shunt. How risky abdominal surgeries are for shunt infection and what the best method of dealing with the shunt at risk is, are topics of debate.

One final possible mechanism for introduction of bacteria into a shunt is by the transcutaneous route. Simple shunt taps for sampling of CSF are felt to be relatively safe (55) but must be done compulsively and with meticulous attention to detail (105). Injection of material into shunts, particularly radionuclides (106) or contrast material, must also be carefully considered. Poor planning of incisions (107) and use of high-profile devices in thin-skinned neonates may result in secondary shunt infection related to incisional breakdown or pressure sores (65).

After induction of bacteria by one of the five mechanisms discussed (most frequently operative contamination at the time of surgery), several factors conspire to make clinical infection more likely. Borges studied the function of human neutrophils and their interactions with glass slides and rods and then compared this to their interactions with shunt catheters in vitro (108). The white cells adhered very poorly to the shunt apparatus, and this contributed in part to the insufficient phagocytosis of *S. epidermidis*. The shunt apparatus also caused inappropriate exocytosis of myeloperoxidase, which suggested that intracellular killing could be negatively affected by the shunt as well (108).

With an implanted foreign body model (tissue cages in the subcutaneous space of guinea pigs),

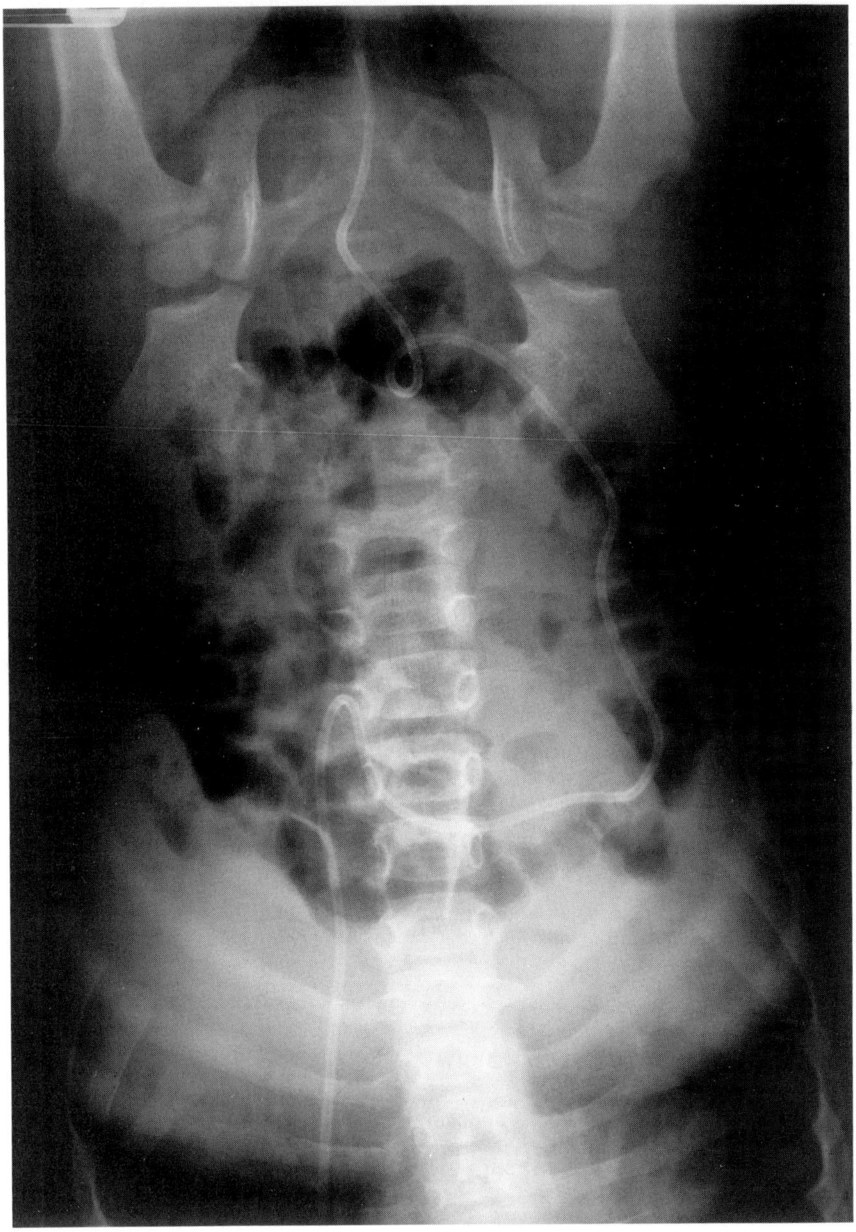

Figure 4 Shunt in colon, extending out of the rectum.

Zimmerli et al. reproduced Elek's classic demonstration that far fewer *S. aureus* organisms were necessary to elicit clinical infection in the presence than in the absence of a foreign body (109). They further showed that polymorphonuclear leukocytes from the vicinity of the foreign body demonstrated defective phagocytosis and defective intracellular killing compared to control cells. Opsonization of bacteria by tissue cage fluid decreased to low levels within the first day after infection (110). It would appear that foreign bodies such as shunts have direct effects on host defenses.

As long ago as 1972, a mucoid substance or slime had been identified on the walls of culture tubes of bottles used to culture *S. epidermidis* SIIA. Similar material isolated from infected shunts (stainable with alcian blue) could be demonstrated on the luminal surface of colonized shunt valves themselves. It was postulated that the slime encouraged infection by protecting the bacteria from lysozyme and antibiotics (111).

Subsequently it has been recognized that bacterial populations in nature exist in complex "biofilms." Surrounded by a glycocalyx of polysaccharide fibers, they may be well protected from shear forces, nutrient deprivation, and temperature changes (112,113). On the colonized foreign body such as a shunt, they may be likewise protected from antibiotics or phagocytosis (70). Biofilms have been identified on colonized vascular grafts, artificial joints, Foley catheters, breast implants, and cutaneous sutures (114,115).

The sequence of colonization of vascular catheters by *S. epidermidis* in vitro was studied with scanning electron microscopy (116). Initially solitary bacteria could be seen adhering to the catheter, particularly at pits or rough spots on the surface. These bacteria could be seen dividing and then ultimately, within a period of several hours, a thick slime encompassed the microcolonies (116). The initial adhesion of bacteria to shunt catheters during implantation may well be strongly dependent on hydrophobic interactions (117) and when modeled from a thermodynamic perspective will depend on the characteristics of the catheter, the bacteria, and the fluid at the interface (118). After the bacteria have established themselves on the catheter, the production of the extracellular slime keeps them firmly in place and protected from antibiotics or host defenses.

Studies of coagulase-negative staphylococci from vascular catheter–associated sepsis (119) as well as from shunt infections (67) demonstrated that these bacteria tended to produce slime and to be more adherent than skin isolates or contaminants. Shunt infections caused by slime-producing coagulase-negative staphylococci were far less likely to resolve without hardware removal than those caused by non–slime producers (120).

Bayston and Rodgers attempted to quantitate adherence and slime production and stressed that they are separate entities and that the former may correlate with infectivity and the latter with resistance to antibiotic therapy (70). If the success or failure of colonization of a shunt by bacteria does represent a "race for surface" (121) between the bacterial and host cells, perhaps infection rates can be modified by modification of shunt materials to make it less hospitable to the prokaryotes or more readily sheathed by the host.

TREATMENT

Intravenous or systemic antibiotic therapy is the mainstay of treatment of established ventricular shunt infections. Prior to consideration of antibiotics, a decision as to the fate of the hardware must be made. Three strategies regarding the shunt apparatus have been used: treatment of the shunt in situ with intravenous (and intraventricular) antibiotics, removal of the shunt with simultaneous replacement, and complete or partial shunt removal with delayed replacement.

A small prospective randomized study comparing the three methods of treatment was performed from 1975 to 1979 (122). Only 10 patients from each group were entered. All 30 patients had peritoneal ended shunts. Treatment of the shunt vigorously with intravenous and intraventricular antibiotics resulted in only 3 cures of 10 patients. Two of the remaining patients died. Shunt removal with immediate replacement resulted in 9 of 10 patients cured, and shunt removal with delayed replacement (with or without external drainage) led to cure of all 10 infections. An attempt was made in this study to ensure adequate doses and concentrations of antibiotics in the CSF and sufficient duration of therapy (122). Subsequent studies by the same authors confirmed the findings of very low cure rates with the in situ therapy (36%) and excellent cure rates with immediate replacement (85%) or delayed replacement (96%) (123).

As the previous data reflect the experience of only one investigator and very small numbers of patients, a more representative overview of success rates is afforded by a compilation of the experience of many institutions, which showed a cure rate of 36% with antibiotics alone, a 65% with immediate replacement, and 96% with delayed replacement with or without external ventricular drainage (EVD) (124). A more recent and very comprehensive review by Kaufman and McLone reported nearly identical percentages (64). Nevertheless, as the argument can be made that not all "antibiotics alone" or medical regimens used optimal routes or routines, that morbidity may be important in the overall success of a strategy (not simply "cure rate"), and that the ideal method of therapy may vary with the circumstances, each method will be discussed individually.

Robert McLaurin has been the most eloquent and persistent advocate of in situ or nonsurgical therapy for infected shunts (34,125–127). The rationale for attempting this would include a reluctance to sacrifice a venous channel for VA shunts and an avoidance of cerebral trauma, including increased intracranial pressure in the child with all shunt hardware removed, puncture porencephaly or hemorrhage if the ventricle is accessed percutaneously, or overdrainage or secondary infection in the case of external ventricular drainage.

Four of 11 shunt infections in VA shunts were cured with intravenous penicillin G in high doses (60). This modest success rate is still much higher than other early investigators could achieve. Intravenous methicillin was completely incapable of controlling VA shunt infections in one series. The addition of intraventricular methicillin led to temporary control of fever and symptomatology, but these recurred. Complete cure always required removal of the valve (128).

The utilization of intraventricular therapy has more recently been considered a "must" in treating shunt infections nonsurgically (126). Using compulsive regimens of intravenous and intraventricular antibiotics, a successful cure of shunt infections occurred in 11 of 19 patients (125). The intraventricular therapy (injected into the shunt) was felt to be mandatory due to failure of intravenous antibiotics to achieve satisfactory concentrations in the CSF (blood CSF barrier) or in the shunt hardware itself. Documentation of CSF antibiotic concentrations exceeding the minimum inhibitory concentration (MIC) are critical to cure shunt infections nonsurgically. Treatment courses consist of 2-week periods of intraventricular plus intravenous therapy followed by a third week of intravenous antibiotics alone. Only after two failures of such a regimen is nonsurgical therapy abandoned. The original shunts subjected to a nonsurgical regimen for treatment of infection were VA shunts. These shunts seem more attractive for this technique than VP shunts due to the desire to preserve vascular channels and the relatively short lengths of colonized catheter needing sterilization. Infection-related malfunctions of peritoneal shunts frequently necessitate partial replacements or revisions (127), blunting to some extent the benefits of "nonsurgical" therapy.

The second major method utilized for treating shunt infections is the replacement of the entire shunt at the same time the old shunt is removed, and generally in the same location as the original, in addition to antibiotic therapy. This method was described in six patients with ventriculoatrial shunts. All patients had *S. epidermidis* infections and had previously failed therapy with intravenous antibiotics alone. The benefits included preservation of the vascular channel, lack of morbidity associated with temporary lack of drainage, and avoidance of multiple surgical procedures. All six patients were cured with a 14-day course of intraventricular methicillin and a 14-day course of systemic methicillin/oxacillin (129).

The immediate replacement of the shunt for infected VA shunts has been advocated by investigators who demonstrated with serial blood cultures that the bacteremia could be eliminated in about 20 min. Antibiotics were administered intravenously for an additional 5 days at least. Excluding patients inappropriately treated, success was achieved in 21 of 23 patients (130).

It should be recognized that immediate replacement of the shunt is appropriate only if there are no organisms in the CSF. As with nonsurgical therapy, this method seems most applicable in VA shunts where a vascular channel is maintained and there is no large peritoneal surface left potentially infected.

The most frequent method of treating shunt infections currently is immediate shunt removal with delayed replacement. The recognition of the biofilm-encased colonies on microscopic examination suggests that infected foreign bodies must be removed. If the shunt is removed, three strategies can be used for management of the hydrocephalus. In some cases, particularly for babies with open fontanelles, no access has been inserted. Ventricular taps can be done for decompression, sampling CSF, or administering antibiotics. This is generally felt to be an unsatisfactory plan, subjecting the patient to the risks of uncontrolled intracranial hypertension, hemorrhage from transparenchymal ventricular puncture, or a puncture porencephaly. A second option is a subcutaneous reservoir, but this has the disadvantages of intermittent decompression, a sizable foreign body in a stagnant CSF space, and the need for surgical removal at the conclusion of therapy. This may be an attractive method for premature babies in whom external drainage carries high risks of secondary infection and electrolyte imbalance (39). A ventriculostomy is commonly used to drain CSF on a continual basis (131,132). The ventriculostomy is generally tunneled to decrease the risk of infection (133). The ventriculostomy can be placed at the existing burr hole or a separate site (i.e., frontal vs. parietal) at the time of shunt removal. The contralateral side is generally preserved for the replacement shunt. The tube is connected to a closed drainage bag with three-way stopcock and injection ports enabling the tubing to be clamped, CSF to be sampled or antibiotics to be injected. Drainage rate is determined by the difference in height between the head and the drip chamber.

As previously described, such a system has an excellent cure rate and is versatile. The hazards of this approach should not be underestimated. Catastrophic overdrainage will occur if the bag drops to the floor or the child is picked up and held above bag level. Electrolyte imbalances are another pitfall, with babies being at highest risk for hyponatremia and hypovolemia. CSF output must be monitored carefully and replaced cc for cc with normal saline. Unrecognized partial proximal obstruction may result in dangerous rises in ICP despite apparently good CSF output (132), and overdrainage in the face of large ventricles may result in subdural hematoma. CT scanning at intervals is recommended. CSF must be sampled frequently to monitor resolution of the infection. When the CSF is clear and sufficient time has elapsed for peritoneal sterility, the EVD is clamped, and after a contralateral shunt is placed at surgery, it is slid out and the exit site sutured closed.

A more conservative option is to externalize the existing shunt via a small incision under local anesthetic (63). This has the advantage of retaining a valve to decrease overdrainage, avoiding an operation, and enabling the shunt to be clamped and the ventricular size to be increased before any potential proximal procedure. The disadvantage is that for the time being the colonized hardware has not been removed but only "debulked." Cultures are monitored and, if persistently positive, intraventricular antibiotics may be added, the shunt converted to an EVD, or both.

The selection of antibiotics is made on the basis of likely and potential pathogens and modified when culture results are available. A bactericidal antibiotic is preferred to a bacteriostatic antibiotic (134). The majority of organisms involved in shunt infections are coagulase-negative staphylococci. Treatment with a penicillinase-resistant penicillin, such as methicillin, oxacillin, nafcillin, or cloxacillin, is recommended. Nafcillin is the preferred antibiotic because it achieves adequate CSF concentrations readily (136) and is not associated with the nephritis that can occur with methicillin (135). The other major option for treating staphylococcal shunt infections is vancomycin. This drug penetrates into the CSF poorly in the absence of inflammation (137,138), but even with the modest meningeal inflammation seen with shunt infection, comparable or superior penetration to the antistaphylococcal penicillins can be achieved (139). Rifampin can be given in combination with either nafcillin or vancomycin (140,141). The levels achieved in the CSF are many times the MIC in most cases, and rifampin may be the most active antibiotic against coagulase-negative staphylococci (140). Rifampin can be given orally but should not be used alone as resistance can develop rapidly to this antibiotic (140,141). Infections with gram-negative organisms are treated with a third-generation cephalosporin (77).

The addition of intraventricular antibiotics is considered mandatory for nonsurgical therapy and when immediate replacement of the shunt is planned. Vancomycin is the most frequently used antibiotic for intraventricular therapy of infections with gram-positive organisms. The dose is 5–20 mg once a day. Many investigators (143,144) report wide variation in the CSF levels achieved (not surprising, as some have external drainage and ventricular sizes vary considerably). Although high CSF concentrations have been achieved without apparent toxicity (145), CSF levels should be monitored closely as reports of CSF eosinophilia have led to concern of possible toxicity (146). The use of intraventricular vancomycin alone without systemic antibiotics (147) is considered radical and probably injudicious. The longest and most extensive experience with an intraventricular antibiotic is with gentamicin (148), which has good activity against gram-negative and gram-positive organisms. It is readily available preservative-free for intrathecal use and is favored by some who remain a bit leary of vancomycin.

SALVAGE SHUNTS

Currently the vast majority of ventricular shunts are peritoneal. Even following VP shunt infection, the peritoneum generally regains its absorptive capacity and the majority of replacement shunts can be put back into the peritoneal cavity (131). On some occasions a demonstrable lack of absorption, extensive adhesions, or fear of recurrent infection in the face of an augmented bladder will necessitate the use of an alternate distal terminus.

The VA shunt could logically be considered a candidate for a "salvage" shunt. Some of the unfortunate patients for whom VP shunts are no longer possible will also be inappropriate for VA shunts, such as those who require total parenteral nutrition through a central line, those with valvular cardiac disease, and those who are at high risk for recurrent bacteremia.

The ventriculopleural shunt was introduced into modern neurosurgical practice by Ransohoff in 1954 (149,150). The pleural surfaces absorb CSF very well, but these shunts may nevertheless be complicated by pleural effusions in up to 20% of cases. Effusions are most common in young children, and their frequency may be reduced by utilization of antisiphon devices (151). Infection rates are comparable to peritoneal shunts (152). The ventriculopleural shunt has been used with good success as a salvage shunt, but it should not be utilized in children under the age of 7 years or in patients with underlying pulmonary disease (bronchopulmonary dysplasia or scoliosis with restrictive disease). A high-resistance valve incorporating an antisiphon device is utilized in all patients.

Ventriculogallbladder shunting is another excellent alternative (153,154). All such shunts must incorporate a one-way valve to prevent bile reflux and should use low or very low pressure resistance in view of the intrinsic outlet resistance of the gallbladder itself. A straight metal connector is pushed at least 2 cm up the distal end of an open-ended peritoneal catheter, allowing the shunt to be securely pursestringed into the gallbladder's dome without kinking (Fig. 5) (153). Prior to consideration of such a shunt, an oral cholecystogram or nuclear function study should be performed. Seventy percent of ventriculogallbladder shunts continue functioning long-term (153), with low rates of infection and malfunction, particularly given the difficult subset of patients in whom they are used.

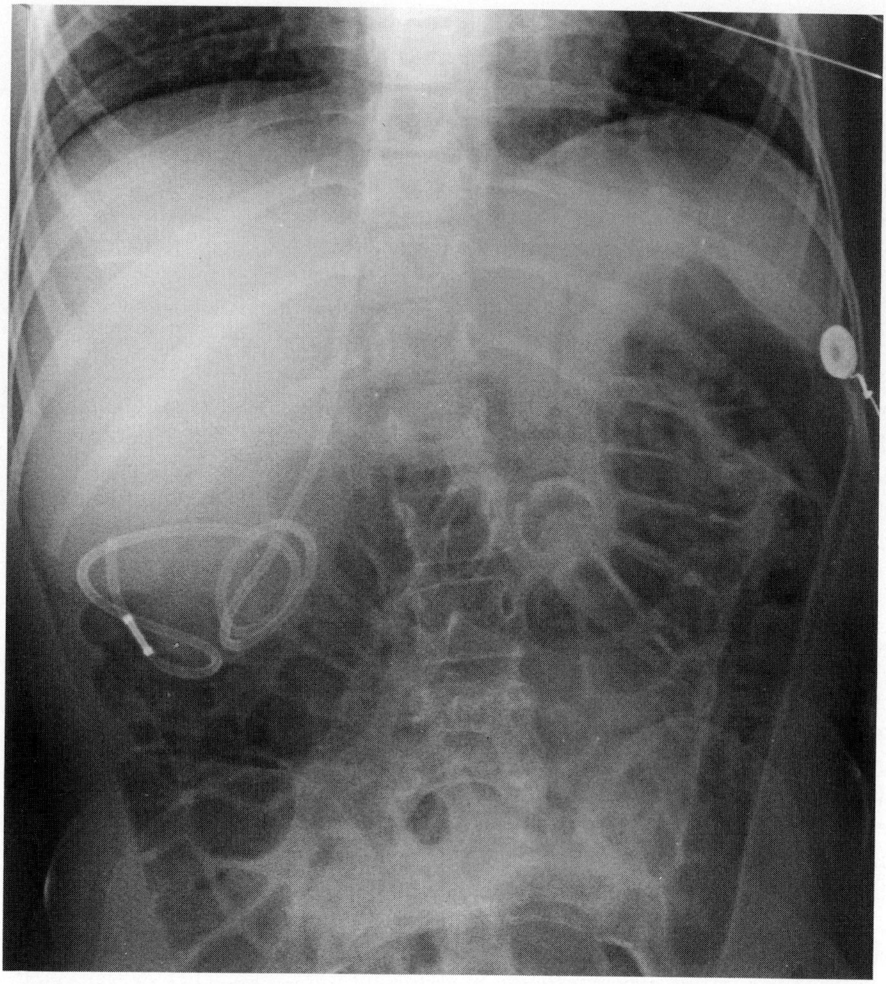

Figure 5 Ventriculogallbladder shunt.

On rare occasions a ventriculosubgaleal shunt may be of use as a temporary measure in a patient with a contraindication to tunneling across the neck due to eczema (42) or other skin condition or a fresh tracheostomy.

SEQUELAE

Early series reported mortality rates in cases of shunt infection in the range of 25% to 50% (20,24,35,155,156). Several factors have contributed to an overall reduction in mortality to approximately 6%, including better antibiotics, earlier recognition, and the lack of cardiac, pulmonary and renal complications associated with VA shunt infections since VP shunts have largely replaced VA shunts (30). Not all deaths are due to the infection; some result from the therapy.

Because most patients are infants or young children, it is hard to estimate how their intellectual or neurological function is affected by the shunt infection. A relatively homogeneous (or at least well-defined) group is available in myelomeningocele clinics. In a careful analysis of myelomeningocele children, it was not hydrocephalus or the presence of a shunt that correlated with poor IQ in spina bifida children, but rather a history of ventriculitis/shunt infection (157). In this study the IQ of nonshunted patients was 102, shunted patients 95, and shunted with a history of ventriculitis 75. The detrimental effect of shunt infection on IQ and the lack of correlation between ventricular size and intelligence in myelodysplastic children is evidence against a shunt procedure, the only indication of which is to improve the ventricular size on CT scan in otherwise asymptomatic children (158). In addition, there is a significantly increased incidence of seizure disorder in myelomeningoceles who have had a shunt infection (159).

PREVENTION

Substantial effort has been directed toward the prevention of shunt infections. The most quoted and emulated protocol is the Choux protocol, which is as follows: (1) two preoperative Betadine shampoos, (2) minimal shaving, (3) meticulous intraoperative skin preparation, (4) shunts scheduled first in the day with neonates first and no more than four shunt procedures a day, (5) expeditious surgical technique (20–40 min per case), a reduction of OR personnel with no scrub nurse present, experienced surgeon, adhesive drapes, simple shunts without connectors (6) wound irrigation with dilute betadine, (7) soaking of shunt components in gentamicin preimplantation, and (8) intravenous cloxacillin or oxacillin before the skin incisions. The use of the Choux protocol has been demonstrated to reduce the operative shunt infection rate from 7.8 to 0.17% (160). Kestle et al. were able to demonstrate a dramatic (70%) reduction in infection rate with a similar protocol (161). To reduce airborne or iatrogenic introduction of bacteria, the manipulation of overhead lights and the use of warming lights with convection currents should be avoided after the midportion of the skin prep. A change of the surgeon's and assistant's gloves prior to the handling of the prosthetic implant has been demonstrated to decrease the incidence of graft contamination in vascular surgery (162) and is a reasonable precaution for shunt surgery as well. Although plastic adhesive drapes are widely utilized, it is not clear that they reduce operative contamination (163) or postoperative infection (164). Ongoing modifications in draping systems continue to be made (165), and it is anticipated that these advances will decrease shunt infection rates in the future.

It is difficult to determine which of the various steps in these protocols is responsible for the reduction in infection rate. But because the reductions in infection rate appear to be dramatic (and more impressive than those achieved with intravenous antibiotics), it is important to scrutinize these regimens and attempt to exercise a comparable attention to detail.

In orthopedic surgery, hip and knee replacement infection rates were decreased tremendously by the performance of these surgeries in progressively "cleaner" air. Flow and filtration systems were refined and infection rates dropped accordingly (166,167). A surgical isolator, perhaps representing the ultimate in "clean air," has been utilized for shunt surgeries with reduction in overall infection rates from 19.7 to 7.4% (168).

Topical antibiotics are frequently used in neurosurgery (169), such as aminoglycosides (170) and bacitracin A, a bactericidal antibiotic that can also act as a detergent (171), rendering it both bactericidal (172,173) and able to prevent the adhesion of bacteria (169). Current practice is to use concentrations of bacitracin A of 50 U/cc (173) to 500 U/cc (22,27).

The use of prophylactic antibiotics administered intravenously or orally before shunt surgeries has been a topic of hot debate among neurosurgeons for decades. The rationale for use of such antibiotics is that even if bacteria are introduced at the time of surgery, they can be eliminated in many instances if high concentrations of antibiotics are present in the tissue or spinal fluid surrounding the device.

The role of prophylactic antibiotics in clean neurosurgical procedures was defined by a review of five randomized, placebo-controlled, double-blinded clinical trials comparing prophylactic antibiotics with placebo (174–179). Each of these studies demonstrated a statistically significant reduction in the rate of infection with prophylactic antibiotics (180). Antibiotic regimens varied from vancomycin and gentamicin (175,176) to cefazolin and gentamicin (177), vancomycin alone (178), or piperacillin (179). Subsequently a meta-analysis of craniotomies was carried out and showed benefit to prophylactic antibiotics in decreasing the rate of wound infection in craniotomies "about fourfold" for this subset of neurosurgical procedures. This led to the recommendation that future studies compare different antibiotic regimens rather than antibiotics versus placebo (181). Such comparisons between antibiotic regimens in an effort to optimize effectiveness while limiting toxicity are ongoing (182).

With ventricular shunts, the data are much less clear-cut. Several of the large and thorough reviews of ventricular shunt infection considered the effects of prophylactic antibiotics on infection rates (24,27,33). Some series have had somewhat lower rates of shunt infection in antibiotic-treated groups, but the differences are not statistically significant (24,27,33). A substantial reduction in infection rate with prophylactic antibiotics (5% vs. 20% untreated) was demonstrated in a retrospective analysis (183). A reduction in operative infection rate from 8 to 2.6% was reported using prophylactic methicillin (21). A progressive decrease in infection rate from 14 to 5% was reported with the use of topical oxacillin (98).

Unlike the studies of antibiotic prophylaxis in general neurosurgery, the prospective, randomized, double-blinded, placebo-controlled studies of efficacy in ventricular shunt surgery are not universally convincing. Whether this is due to the different bacterial pathogens, the peculiarities of foreign body infections, or both is difficult to say. Of the nine studies ultimately deemed "acceptable" by Haines (184), only two showed a significant effect of antibiotic prophylaxis on outcome (185), three could be categorized as demonstrating a trend toward efficacy (186,187), and four could not claim any efficacy (188–191). This is true despite the fact that eight of nine had lower infection rates in the antibiotic-treated group.

In order to circumvent the major difficulty with the studies (lack of sufficient numbers of patients to draw definite conclusions) and with the recognition that a large multicenter trial is unlikely to be forthcoming (192), two meta-analyses have recently been carried out (184,193). An analysis of 12 well-conducted studies suggested that the perioperative use of antibiotics in CSF shunt surgery reduced the risk of infection about 50% (193). A review of nine series found an approximately 50% reduction in infection rate with the use of prophylactic antibiotics (184). Although these two meta-analyses were very carefully performed, it is the position of the Infections in Neurosurgery Working Party of the British Society for Antimicrobial Chemotherapy that the varied "quality" of the component studies and the plethora of antibiotic agents and routes of administration used precluded a conclusion that prophylaxis was or was not efficacious (192). Others would assert that with scrupulous technique, prophylactic antibiotics are unnecessary (194).

If antibiotics are given, the most frequent agents used are antistaphylococcal penicillins (methicillin, oxacillin, nafcillin) (21,98,190,195,196) with or without the addition of gentamicin (188). Trimethoprim/sulfamethoxazole and rifampin are attractive antibiotics for prophylaxis (41,185,187,191) due to their intracellular killing potential, good CSF penetration (197), and oral route of administration. Vancomycin is rarely used despite its excellent gram-positive coverage, due to a concern for the emergence of resistant organisms, poor CSF penetration, and adverse effects (198) such as rash, hypotension, and respiratory problems particularly when under general anesthesia.

Ultimately it is anticipated that the polymers utilized for shunt manufacture can be modified or coated to make them less susceptible to bacterial adhesion (199). Antibiotics may also be incorporated for either short-term (200) or long-term release by prosthetic materials. Significant work has already been done on the impregnation of silicone elastomer with antibiotics (201,202) in anticipation of preventing their colonization with bacteria. Although our knowledge of ventricular shunt infections has increased, a great deal of work remains to be done.

REFERENCES

1. Laurence KM, Coates C. The natural history of hydrocephalus. Detailed analysis of 182 unoperated cases. Arch Dis Child 1962; 37:345–362.
2. Foltz EL, Shurtleff DB. Five-year comparative study of hydrocephalus in children with and without operation (113 cases). J Neurosurg 1963; 20:1064–1079.
3. Scarff JE. Treatment of hydrocephalus: an historical and critical review of methods and results. J Neurol Neurosurg Psychiatry 1963; 26:1–26.
4. Pudenz RH. The surgical treatment of hydrocephalus—an historical review. Surg Neurol 1981; 15: 15–26.
5. Davidoff LM. Treatment of hydrocephalus. Historical review and description of a new method. Arch Surg 1929; 18:1737–1762.
6. Hoffman HJ, Harwood-Nash D, Gilday DL. Percutaneous third ventriculostomy in the management of noncommunicating hydrocephalus. Neurosurgery 1980; 7:313–321.
7. Nulsen FE, Spitz EB. Treatment of hydrocephalus by direct shunt from ventricle to jugular vein. Surg Forum 1952; 2:399–403.
8. Pudenz RH, Russell FE, Hurd AH, Shelden CH. Ventriculo-auriculostomy. A technique for shunting cerebrospinal fluid into the right auricle. Preliminary report. J Neurosurg 1957; 14:171–179.
9. Jackson IJ, Snodgrass SR. Peritoneal shunts in the treatment of hydrocephalus and increased intracranial pressure. A 4-year survey of 62 patients. J Neurosurg 1955; 12:216–222.
10. Tsingoglou S, Eckstein HB. Pericardial tamponade by Holter ventriculoatrial shunts. J Neurosurg 1971; 35:695–699.
11. Finney HL, Roberts TS. Nephritis secondary to chronic cerebrospinal fluid-vascular shunt infection: "shunt nephritis." Child's Brain 1980; 6:189–193.
12. Ames RH. Ventriculo-peritoneal shunts in the management of hydrocephalus. J Neurosurg 1967; 27: 525–529.
13. Little JR, Rhoton AL, Mellinger JF. Comparison of ventriculoperitoneal and ventriculoatrial shunts for hydrocephalus in children. Mayo Clin Proc 1972; 47:396–401.
14. Ignelzi RJ, Kirsch WM. Follow-up analysis of ventriculoperitoneal and ventriculoatrial shunts for hydrocephalus. J Neurosurg 1975; 42:679–682.
15. Olsen L, Frykberg T. Complications in the treatment of hydrocephalus in children. A comparison of ventriculoatrial and ventriculoperitoneal shunts in a 20-year material. Acta Paediatr Scand 1983; 72: 385–390.
16. Keucher TR, Mealey J Jr. Long-term results after ventriculoatrial and ventriculoperitoneal shunting for infantile hydrocephalus. J Neurosurg 1979; 50:179–186.
17. Sainte-Rose C, Hoffman HJ, Hirsch JF. Shunt failure. Concepts Pediatr Neurosurg 1989; 9:7–20.
18. Illingworth RD, Logue V, Symon L, Uemura K. The ventriculocaval shunt in the treatment of adult hydrocephalus. Results and complications in 101 patients. J Neurosurg 1971; 35:681–685.
19. Forrest DM, Cooper DGW. Complications of ventriculo-atrial shunts. A review of 455 cases. J Neurosurg 1968; 29:506–512.
20. Nulsen FE, Becker DB. Control of hydrocephalus by valve-regulated shunt: infections and their prevention. Clin Neurosurg 1966; 14:256–273.
21. McCullough DC, Kane JG, Presper JH, Wells M. Antibiotic prophylaxis in ventricular shunt surgery. I. Reduction of operative infection rates with methicillin. Child's Brain 1980; 7:182–189.
22. Venes JL. Control of shunt infection. Report of 150 consecutive cases. J Neurosurg 1976; 45:311–314.
23. Spanu G, Karussos G, Adinolfi D, Bonfanti N. An analysis of cerebrospinal fluid infections in adults. A clinical experience of twelve years. Acta Neurosurg 1986; 80:79–82.

24. Schoenbaum SC, Gardner P, Shillito J. Infections of cerebrospinal fluid shunts: epidemiology, clinical manifestations, and therapy. J Infect Dis 1975; 131:543–552.
25. Shapiro S, Boaz J, Kleiman M, Kalsbeck J, Mealey J. Origin of organisms infecting ventricular shunts. J Neurosurg 1988; 22:868–872.
26. Shurtleff DB, Christie D, Foltz EL. Ventriculostomy-associated infection. A 12-year study. J Neurosurg 1971; 35:686–694.
27. Shurtleff DB, Stuntz JT, Hayden PW. Experience with 1201 cerebrospinal fluid procedures. Pediatr Neurosci 1985–86; 12:49–57.
28. Walters BC, Hoffman HJ, Hendrick EB, Humphreys RP. Cerebrospinal fluid infection. Influences on initial management and subsequent outcome. J Neurosurg 1984; 60:1014–1021.
29. Raimondi AJ, Robinson JS, Kuwamura K. Complications of ventriculo-peritoneal shunting and a critical comparison of the three-piece and one-piece systems. Child's Brain 1977; 3:321–342.
30. George R, Leibrock L, Epstein M. Long-term analysis of cerebrospinal fluid shunt infections. J Neurosurg 1979; 51:804–811.
31. Lund-Johansen M, Svendsen F, Wester K. Shunt failures and complications in adults as related to shunt type, diagnosis, and the experience of the surgeon. Neurosurgery 1994; 35:839–844.
32. Kontny U, Hofling B, Gutjahr P, Voth D, Schwarz M, Schmitt HJ. CSF shunt infections in children. Infection 1993; 21:89–92.
33. Odio C, McCracken GH, Nelson JD. CSF shunt infections in pediatrics. Am J Dis Child 1984; 138:1103–1108.
34. McLaurin RL. Infected cerebrospinal fluid shunts. Surg Neurol 1973; 1:191–195.
35. Anderson FM. Ventriculocardiac shunts. J Pediatr 1973; 82:222–227.
36. Renier D, Lacombe J, Pierre-Kahn A, Sainte-Rose C, Hirsch JF. Factors causing acute shunt infection. Computer analysis of 1174 operations. J Neurosurg 1984; 61:1072–1078.
37. Meirovitch J, Kitai-Cohen Y, Keren G, Fiendler G, Rubinstein E. Cerebrospinal fluid infections in children. Pediatr Infect Dis J 1987; 6:921–924.
38. Pople IK, Bayston R, Hayward RD. Infection of cerebrospinal fluid shunts in infants: a study of etiological factors. J Neurosurg 1992; 77:29–36.
39. Hahn YS, McLone DG, Raimondi AJ, Frisbie CL. Surgical outcome of preterm newborns with severe periventricular-intraventricular hemorrhage and posthemorrhagic hydrocephalus. Concepts Pediatr Neurosurg 1983; 4:66–80.
40. D'Angio CT, McGowan KL, Baumgart S, et al. Surface colonization with coagulase-negative *Staphylococci* in premature neonates. J Pediatr 1989; 114:1029–1034.
41. Viano JC, Tregnaghi M, Casagnas M, Suarez JC. Valvular infections in patients with hydrocephalus: preventive aspects. Child's Nerv Syst 1990; 6:397–399.
42. Steinbok P, Cochrane DD. Ventriculosubgaleal shunt in the management of recurrent ventriculoperitoneal shunt infection. Child's Nerv Syst 1994; 10:536–539.
43. Gardner P, Leipzig T, Phillips P. Infections of central nervous system shunts. Symposium on infections of the central nervous system. Med Clin North Am 1985; 69:297–314.
44. Hubschmann OR, Countee RW. Acute abdomen in children with infected ventriculoperitoneal shunts. Arch Surg 1980; 115:305–307.
45. Rekate HL, Yonas H, White RJ, Nulsen FE. The acute abdomen in patients with ventriculoperitoneal shunts. Surg Neurol 1979; 11:442–445.
46. Reynolds M, Sherman JO, McLone DG. Ventriculoperitoneal shunt infection masquerading as an acute surgical abdomen. J Pediatr Surg 1983; 18:951–954.
47. Hadani M, Findler G, Muggia-Sullam M, Sahar A. Acute appendicitis in children with a ventriculoperitoneal shunt. Surg Neurol 1982; 18:69–71.
48. Younger JJ, Simmons JCH, Barrett FF. Occult distal ventriculoperitoneal shunt infections. Pediatr Infect Dis 1985; 4:557–558.
49. Goodman GM, Gourley GR. Ascites complicating ventriculoperitoneal shunts. J Pediatr Gastroenterol Nutr 1988; 7:780–782.
50. Noh JM, Reddy MG, Brodner RA. Cerebrospinal fluid ascites following ventriculoperitoneal shunt. Report of a case and review of the literature. Mt Sinai J Med 1979; 46:475–477.

51. O'Brien M, Parent A, Davis B. Management of ventricular shunt infections. Child's Brain 1979; 5: 304–309.
52. Steinbok P, Cochrane DD, Kestle JRW. The significance of bacteriologically positive ventriculoperitoneal shunt components in the absence of other signs of shunt infection. J Neurosurg 1996; 84:617–623.
53. Fokes EC Jr. Occult infections of ventriculoatrial shunts. J Neurosurg 1970; 33:517–523.
54. Myers MG, Schoenbaum SC. Shunt fluid aspiration. An adjunct in the diagnosis of cerebrospinal fluid shunt infection. Am J Dis Child 1975; 129:220–222.
55. Noetzel MJ, Baker RP. Shunt fluid examination: risks and benefits in the evaluation of shunt malfunction and infection. J Neurosurg 1984; 61:328–332.
56. Drake JM, Sainte-Rose C. Shunt complications. In: Drake JM, Sainte-Rose C, eds. The Shunt Book. Ann Arbor, MI: Blackwell Science, 1995:121–192.
57. Bayston R. Microbial colonization of cerebrospinal fluid shunts. Med Lab Sci 1981; 38:259–267.
58. Walters BC. Cerebrospinal fluid shunt infection. Infections in neurological surgery. Neurosurg Clin North Am 1992; 3:387–401.
59. Bryant MS, Bremer AM, Tepas JJ III, Mollitt DL, Nquyen TQ, Talbert JL. Abdominal complications of ventriculoperitoneal shunts. Case reports and review of the literature. Am Surg 1988; 54:50–55.
60. Schimke RT, Black PH, Mark VH, Swartz MN. Indolent *Staphylococcus albus* or *aureus* bacteremia after ventriculoatriostomy. Role of foreign body in its initiation and perpetuation. N Engl J Med 1961; 264(6):264–270.
61. Morrice JJ, Young DG. Bacterial colonization of Holter valves: a ten-year survey. Dev Med Child Neurol 1974; 16(suppl 32):85–90.
62. Holt RJ. Bacteriological studies on colonized ventriculoatrial shunts. Dev Med Child Neurol 1970; 12(suppl 22):83–87.
63. Morissette I, Gourdeau M, Francoeur J. CSF shunt infections: a fifteen-year experience with emphasis on management and outcome. Can J Neurol Sci 1993; 20:118–122.
64. Kaufman BA, McLone DG. Infections of cerebrospinal fluid shunts. In: Scheld WM, Whitley RJ, Durack DT, eds. Infections of the Central Nervous System. New York: Raven Press, 1991:561–585.
65. Forward KR, Fewer HD, Stiver HG. Cerebrospinal fluid shunt infections. A review of 35 infections in 32 patients. J Neurosurg 1983; 59:389–394.
66. Kloos WE, Schleifer KH. Isolation and characterization of staphylococci from human skin. II. Descriptions of four new species: *Staphylococcus warneri*, *Staphylococcus capitis*, *Staphylococcus hominis*, and *Staphylococcus simulans*. Int J Syst Bacteriol 1975; 25:62–79.
67. Younger JJ, Christensen GD, Bartley DL, Simmons JCH, Barrett FF. Coagulase-negative staphylococci isolated from cerebrospinal fluid shunts: importance of slime production, species identification, and shunt removal to clinical outcome. J Infect Dis 1987; 156:548–554.
68. Torre D, Ferraro G, Fiori GP, Martegani R, Speranza F, Tambini R, Zeroli C. Ventriculoatrial shunt infection caused by *Staphylococcus warneri*: case report and review. Clin Infect Dis 1992; 14:49–52.
69. Christensen GD, Parisi JT, Bisno AL, Simpson WA, Beachey EH. Characterization of clinically significant strains of coagulase-negative staphylococci. J Clin Microbiol 1983; 18:258–269.
70. Bayston R, Rodgers J. Production of extra-cellular slime by *Staphylococcus epidermidis* during stationary phase of growth: its association with adherence to implantable devices. J Clin Path 1990; 43: 866–870.
71. Brown EM, Jones EM. Non-surgical management of CSF shunt infections. Eur J Pediatr Surg 1995; 5(suppl 1):26.
72. Rekate HL, Ruch T, Nulsen FE. Diphtheroid infections of cerebrospinal fluid shunts. The changing pattern of shunt infection in Cleveland. J Neurosurg 1980; 52:553–556.
73. Dominguez EA, Patil AA, Johnson WM. Ventriculoperitoneal shunt infection due to *Listeria monocytogenes*. Clin Infect Dis 1994; 19:223–224.
74. Greene KA, Clark RJ, Zabramski JM. Ventricular CSF shunt infections associated with *Corynebacterium jeikeium*: report of three cases and review. Clin Infect Dis 1993; 16:139–141.
75. Everett ED, Eickhoff TC, Simon RH. Cerebrospinal fluid shunt infections with anaerobic diphtheroids (*Propionibacterium* species). J Neurosurg 1976; 44:580–584.

76. Sells CJ, Shurtleff DB, Loeser JD. Gram-negative cerebrospinal fluid shunt-associated infections. Pediatrics 1977; 59:614–618.
77. Stamos JK, Kaufman BA, Yogev R. Ventriculoperitoneal shunt infections with gram-negative bacteria. Neurosurgery 1993; 33:858–862.
78. Rennels MB, Wald ER. Treatment of *Hemophilus influenzae* type b meningitis in children with cerebrospinal fluid shunts. J Pediatr 1980; 97:424–426.
79. Patriarca PA, Lauer BA. Ventriculoperitoneal shunt-associated infection due to *Hemophilus influenzae*. Pediatrics 1980; 65:1007–1009.
80. Lerman SJ. *Hemophilus influenzae* infections of cerebrospinal fluid shunts. J Neurosurg 1981; 54: 261–263.
81. Petrak RM, Pottage JC Jr., Harris AA, Levin S. *Hemophilus influenzae* meningitis in presence of a cerebrospinal fluid shunt. Neurosurgery 1986; 18:79–81.
82. Stern S, Bayston R, Hayward RJ. *Hemophilus influenzae* meningitis in the presence of cerebrospinal fluid shunts. Child's Nerv Syst 1988; 4:164–165.
83. Hellbusch LC, Penn RG. Cerebrospinal fluid shunt infections by unencapsulated *Hemophilus influenzae*. Child's Nerv Syst 1989; 5:315–317.
84. Hellbusch LC, Penn RG. Treatment of *Hemophilus influenzae* type b cerebrospinal fluid shunt infection with ceftriaxone and rifampin: case report. Neb Med J 1995; (2):27–29.
85. Chan K, Mann KS, Seto WH. Infection of a shunt by *Mycobacterium fortuitum*: case report. Neurosurgery 1991; 29:472–474.
86. Chiou CC, Wong TT, Lin HH, Hwang B, Tang RB, Wu KG, Lee BH. Fungal infection of ventriculoperitoneal shunts in children. Clin Infect Dis 1994; 19:1049–1053.
87. Gower DJ, Crone K, Alexander E Jr., Kelly DL Jr. *Candida albicans* shunt infection: report of two cases. Neurosurgery 1986; 19:111–113.
88. Walsh TJ, Schlegel R, Moody MM, Costerton JW, Salcman M. Ventriculoatrial shunt infection due to *Cryptococcus neoformans*: an ultrastructural and quantitative microbiological study. Neurosurgery 1986; 18:373–375.
89. Yadav SS, Perfect J, Friedman AH. Successful treatment of Cryptococcal ventriculoatrial shunt infection with systemic therapy alone. Neurosurgery 1988; 23:372–373.
90. Bayston R, Lari J. A study of the sources of infection in colonised shunts. Dev Med Child Neurol 1974; 16(suppl 32):16–22.
91. Duhaime A, Bonner K, McGowan KL, Schut L, Sutton LN, Plotkin S. Distribution of bacteria in the operating room environment and its relation to ventricular shunt infections: a prospective study. Child's Nerv Syst 1991; 7:211–214.
92. Charnley J. Postoperative infection after total hip replacement with special reference to air contamination in the operating room. Clin Orthoped 1972; 87:167–187.
93. Stinchfield FE, Bigliani LU, Neu HC, Goss TP, Foster CR. Late hematogenous infection of total joint replacement. J Bone Joint Surg 1980; 62-A:1345–1350.
94. Cruess RL, Bickel WS, vonKessler KLC. Infections in total hips secondary to a primary source elsewhere. Clin Orthoped 1975; 106:99–101.
95. D'Ambrosia RD, Shoji H, Heater R. Secondarily infected total joint replacements by hematogenous spread. J Bone Joint Surg 1976; 58-A:450–453.
96. Downes EM. Late infection after total hip replacement. J Bone Joint Surg 1977; 59-B:42–44.
97. Caesar RE, Scherz H, Bradley J, James HE. Cerebrospinal fluid shunt infection secondary to *Escherichia coli* bacteruria. Urology 1994; 44:288–290.
98. Klein DM. Comparison of antibiotic methods in the prophylaxis of operative shunt infections. Concepts Pediatr Neurosurg 1983; 4:131–141.
99. Naito H, Toya S, Shizawa H, et al. High incidence of acute postoperative meningitis and septicemia in patients undergoing craniotomy with ventriculoatrial shunt. Surg Gynecol Obstet 1973; 137:810–812.
100. Dan M, Spiegelmann R. Mixed bacterial subdural empyema complicating subdural peritoneal shunt. Acta Neurochirurg 1986; 81:77–78.
101. Korosue K, Tamaki N, Matsumoto S, Ohi Y. Intracranial granuloma as an unusual complication of subdural peritoneal shunt. J Neurosurg 1981; 55:136–138.

102. Kreder KJ, Webster GD, Oakes WJ. Augmentation cystoplasty complicated by postoperative ventriculoperitoneal shunt infection. J Urol 1990; 144:955–956.
103. Ahmed S, Simpson D. Re: Augmentation cystoplasty complicated by postoperative ventriculoperitoneal shunt infection. J Urol 1992; 147:171–172.
104. Pittman T, Williams D, Weber TR, Steinhardt G, Tracy T Jr. The risk of abdominal operations in children with ventriculoperitoneal shunts. J Pediatr Surg 1992; 27:1051–1053.
105. Sood S, Kim S, Ham SD, Canady AI, Greninger N. Useful components of the shunt tap test for evaluation of shunt malfunction. Child's Nerv Syst 1993; 9:157–162.
106. Uvebrant P, Sixt R, Bjure J, Roos A. Evaluation of cerebrospinal fluid shunt function in hydrocephalic children using ^{99m}Tc-DTPA. Child's Nerv Syst 1992; 8:76–80.
107. Sayers MP. Shunt complications. Clin Neurosurg 1976; 23:393–400.
108. Borges LF. Cerebrospinal fluid shunts interfere with host defenses. Neurosurgery 1982; 10: 55–60.
109. Elek SD, Conen PE. The virulence of *Staphylococcus pyogenes* for man: a study of the problems of wound infection. Br J Exp Pathol 1957; 38:573–586.
110. Zimmerli W, Waldvogel FA, Vaudaux P, Nydegger UE. Pathogenesis of foreign body infection: description and characteristics of an animal model. J Infect Dis 1982; 146:487–497.
111. Bayston R, Penny SR. Excessive production of mucoid substance in *Staphylococcus* SIIA: a possible factor in colonisation of Holter shunts. Dev Med Child Neurol 1972; 14(suppl 27):25–28.
112. Costerton JW, Geesey GG, Cheng KJ. How bacteria stick. Sci Am 1978; 238:86–95.
113. Costerton JW, Cheng KJ, Geesey GG, Ladd TI, Nickel JC, Dasgupta M, Marrie TJ. Bacterial biofilms in nature and disease. Ann Rev Microbiol 1987; 41:435–464.
114. Gristina AG, Costerton JW. Bacterial adherence to biomaterials and tissue. The significance of its role in clinical sepsis. J Bone Joint Surg 1985; 67-A:264–273.
115. Gristina AG, Price JL, Hobgood CD, Webb LX, Costerton JW. Bacterial colonization of percutaneous sutures. Surgery 1985; 98:12–18.
116. Peters G, Locci R, Pulverer G. Adherence and growth of coagulase-negative staphylococci on surfaces of intravenous catheters. J Infect Dis 1982; 146:479–482.
117. Hogt AH, Dankert J, deVries JA, Feijen J. Adhesion of coagulase-negative staphylococci to biomaterials. J Gen Microbiol 1983; 129:2959–2968.
118. Absolom DR, Lamberti FV, Policova Z, Zingg W, van Oss CJ, Neumann AW. Surface thermodynamics of bacterial adhesion. Appl Environ Microbiol 1983; 46:90–97.
119. Christensen GD, Simpson WA, Bisno AL, Beachey EH. Adherence of slime-producing strains of *Staphylococcus epidermidis* to smooth surfaces. Infect Immun 1982; 37:318–326.
120. Diaz-Mitoma F, Harding GKM, Hoban DJ, Roberts RS, Low DL. Clinical significance of a test for slime production in ventriculoperitoneal shunt infections caused by coagulase-negative staphylococci. J Infect Dis 1987; 156:555–560.
121. Gristina AG. Biomaterial-centered infection: microbial adhesion versus tissue integration. Science 1987; 237:1588–1595.
122. James HE, Walsh JW, Wilson HD, Connor JD, Bean JR, Tibbs PA. Prospective randomized study of therapy in cerebrospinal fluid shunt infection. Neurosurgery 1980; 7:459–463.
123. James HE, Walsh JW, Wilson HD, Connor JD. The management of cerebrospinal fluid shunt infections. A clinical experience. Acta Neurochirurg 1981; 59:157–166.
124. Yogev R. Cerebrospinal fluid shunt infections: a personal view. Pediatr Infect Dis 1985; 4:113–118.
125. McLaurin RL. Treatment of infected ventricular shunts. Child's Brain 1975; 1:306–310.
126. Wald SL, McLaurin RL. Cerebrospinal fluid antibiotic levels during treatment of shunt infections. J Neurosurg 1980; 52:41–46.
127. Frame PT, McLaurin RL. Treatment of CSF shunt infections with intrashunt plus oral antibiotic therapy. J Neurosurg 1984; 60:354–360.
128. Callaghan RP, Cohen SJ, Stewart GT. Septicaemia due to colonization of Spitz-Holter valves by staphylococci. Five cases treated with methicillin. Br Med J 1961; 1:860–863.
129. Perrin JCS, McLaurin RL. Infected ventriculoatrial shunts. A method of treatment. J Neurosurg 1967; 27:21–26.

130. Nicholas JL, Kamal IM, Eckstein HB. Immediate shunt replacement in the treatment of bacterial colonisation of Holter valves. Dev Med Child Neurol 1970; 12(suppl 22):110–113.
131. Mori K, Raimondi AJ. An analysis of external ventricular drainage as a treatment for infected shunts. Child's Brain 1975; 1:243–250.
132. Scarff TB, Nelson PB, Reigel DH. External drainage for ventricular infection following cerebrospinal fluid shunts. Child's Brain 1978; 4:129–136.
133. Chaparro, MJ, Pritz MB, Yonemura KS. Broviac ventriculostomy for long-term external ventricular drainage. Pediatr Neurosurg 1991–92; 17:208–212.
134. Barlig RWA, Selkon JB. The penetration of antibiotics into cerebrospinal fluid and brain tissue. J Antimicrob Chemother 1978; 4:203–227.
135. Everett ED, Strausbaugh LJ. Antimicrobial agents and the central nervous system. Neurosurgery 1980; 6:691–714.
136. Kane JG, Parker RH, Jordan GW, Hoeprich PD. Nafcillin concentration in cerebrospinal fluid during treatment of staphylococcal infections. Ann Intern Med 1977; 87:309–311.
137. Moellering RC Jr, Krigstad DJ, Greenblat DJ. Vancomycin therapy in patients with impaired renal function: a nomogram for dosage. Ann Intern Med 1981; 94:343–346.
138. Gump DW. Vancomycin for treatment of bacterial meningitis. Rev Infect Dis 1981; 3(suppl):S289–S292.
139. Schaad UB, Nelson JD, McCracken GH. Pharmacology and efficacy of Vancomycin for staphylococcal infections in children. Rev Infect Dis 1981; 3(suppl):S282–S288.
140. Ring JC, Cates KL, Belani KK, Gaston TL, Sveum RJ, Marker SC. Rifampin for CSF shunt infections caused by coagulase-negative staphylococci. J Pediatr 1979; 95:317–319.
141. Archer GL, Tenenbaum MJ, Haywood HB III. Rifampin therapy of *Staphylococcus epidermidis*. Use in infections from indwelling artificial devices. JAMA 1978; 240:751–753.
142. James HE, Wilson HD, Connor JD, Walsh JW. Intraventricular cerebrospinal fluid antibiotic concentrations in patients with intraventricular infections. Neurosurgery 1982; 10:50–54.
143. Reesor C, Chow AW, Kureishi A, Jewesson PJ. Kinetics of intraventricular Vancomycin in infections of cerebrospinal fluid shunts. J Infect Dis 1988; 158:1142–1143.
144. Wilson HD, Bean JR, James HE, Pendley MM. Cerebrospinal fluid antibiotic concentrations in ventricular shunt infections. Child's Brain 1978; 4:74–82.
145. Bayston R, Hart CA, Barnicoat M. Intraventricular vancomycin in the treatment of ventriculitis associated with cerebrospinal fluid shunting and drainage. J Neurol Neurosurg Psychiatry 1987; 50:1419–1423.
146. Grabb PA, Albright AL. Intraventricular vancomycin-induced cerebrospinal fluid eosinophilia: report of two patients. Neurosurgery 1992; 30:630–635.
147. Swayne R, Rampling A, Newsom SWB. Intraventricular vancomycin for treatment of shunt-associated ventriculitis. J Antimicrob Chemother 1987; 19:249–253.
148. Wen DY, Bottini AG, Hall WA, Haines SJ. The intraventricular use of antibiotics. Infections in neurological surgery. Neurosurg Clin North Am 1992; 343–354.
149. Ransohoff J. Ventriculo-pleural anastomosis in treatment of midline obstructed masses. J Neurosurg 1954; 11:295–301.
150. Ransohoff J, Shulman K, Fishman RA. Hydrocephalus. A review of etiology and treatment. J Pediatr 1960; 56:399–401.
151. Hoffman HJ, Hendrick EB, Humphreys RP. Experience with ventriculo-pleural shunts. Child's Brain 1983; 10:404–413.
152. Iosif G, Fleischman J, Chitkara R. Empyema due to ventriculopleural shunt. Chest 1991; 99:1538–1539.
153. West KW, Turner MK, Vane DW, Boaz J, Kalsbeck J, Grosfeld JL. Ventricular gallbladder shunts: an alternative procedure in hydrocephalus. J Pediatr Surg 1987; 22:609–612.
154. Stringel G, Turner M, Crase T. Ventriculo-gallbladder shunts in children. Child's Nerv Syst 1993; 9:331–333.
155. Nelson JD. Cerebrospinal fluid shunt infections. Pediatr Infect Dis 1984; 3(suppl):S30–S32.

156. Overton MC, Snodgrass SR. Ventriculo-venous shunts for infantile hydrocephalus. A review of five years' experience with this method. J Neurosurg 1965; 23:517–521.
157. McLone DG, Czyzewski D, Raimondi AJ, Sommers RC. Central nervous system infections as a limiting factor in the intelligence of children with myelomeningocele. Pediatrics 1982; 70:338–342.
158. Storrs BB. Ventricular size and intelligence in myelodysplastic children. Concepts Pediatr Neurosurg 1988; 8:51–56.
159. Chadduck W, Adametz J. Incidence of seizures in patients with myelomeningocele: a multifactorial analysis. Surg Neurol 1988; 30:281–285.
160. Choux M, Genitori L, Lang D, Lena G. Shunt implantation: reducing the incidence of shunt infection. J Neurosurg 1992; 77:875–880.
161. Kestle JRW, Hoffman HJ, Soloniuk D, Humphreys RP, Drake JM, Hendrick EB. A concerted effort to prevent shunt infection. Child's Nerv Syst 1993; 9:163–165.
162. Wooster DL, Louch RE, Krajden S. Intraoperative bacterial contamination of vascular grafts: a prospective study. Can J Surg 1985; 28:407–409.
163. Raahave D. Effect of plastic skin and wound drapes on the density of bacteria in operation wounds. Br J Surg 1976; 63:421–426.
164. Jackson DW, Pollock AV, Tindal DS. The value of a plastic adhesive drape in the prevention of wound infection. A controlled trial. Br J Surg 1971; 58:340–342.
165. Conn J Jr., Bornhoeft JW, Almgren C, Mucha DP, Olderman J, Patel K, Herring CM. In vivo study of an antimicrobial surgical drape system. J Clin Microbiol 1986; 24:803–808.
166. Charnley J, Eftekhar N. Postoperative infection in total prosthetic replacement arthroplasty of the hip-joint. With special reference to the bacterial content of the air of the operating room. Br J Surg 1969; 56:641–649.
167. Lidwell OM, Lowbury EJL, Whyte W, Blowers R, Stanley SJ, Lowe D. Effect of ultraclean air in operating rooms on deep sepsis in the joint after total hip or knee replacement: a randomised study. Br Med J 1982; 285:10–14.
168. Hirsch JF, Renier D, Pierre-Kahn A. Influence of the use of a surgical isolator on the rate of infection in the treatment of hydrocephalus. Child's Brain, 1978; 4:137–150.
169. Haines SJ. Topical antibiotic prophylaxis in neurosurgery. Neurosurgery 1982; 11:250–253.
170. Malis LI. Prevention of neurosurgical infection by intraoperative antibiotics. Neurosurgery 1979; 5:339–343.
171. Gower DJ, Gower VC, Richardson SH, Kelly DL Jr. Reduced bacterial adherence to silicone plastic neurosurgical prosthesis. Pediatr Neurosci 1985–86; 12:127–133.
172. Fischer PR, Gooch WM III, Walker ML, Storrs B. Bactericidal activities of five antibiotics during short-term exposure to coagulase-negative staphylococci. Antimicrob Agents Chemother 1984; 25:502–503.
173. Scherr DD, Dodd TA, Buckingham WW Jr. Prophylactic use of topical antibiotic irrigation in uninfected surgical wounds. A microbiological evaluation. J Bone Joint Surg 1972; 54A:634–640.
174. Haines SJ. Efficacy of antibiotic prophylaxis in clean neurosurgical operations. Neurosurgery 1989; 24:401–405.
175. Geraghty J, Feely M. Antibiotic prophylaxis in neurosurgery. A randomized controlled trial. J Neurosurg 1984; 60:724–726.
176. Shapiro M, Wald U, Simchen E, et al. Randomized clinical trial of intra-operative antimicrobial prophylaxis of infection after neurosurgical procedures. J Hosp Infect 1986; 8:283–295.
177. Young RF, Lawner PM. Perioperative antibiotic prophylaxis for prevention of postoperative neurosurgical procedures. A randomized clinical trial. J Neurosurg 1987; 66:701–705.
178. Blomstedt GC, Kytta J. Results of a randomized trial of vancomycin prophylaxis in craniotomy. J Neurosurg 1988; 69:216–220.
179. Bullock R, van Dellen JR, Ketelbey W, Reinach SG. A double-blind placebo-controlled trial of perioperative prophylactic antibiotics for elective neurosurgery. J Neurosurg 1988; 69:687–691.
180. Mollman HD, Haines SJ. Risk factors for postoperative neurosurgical wound infection. A case-control study. J Neurosurg 1986; 64:902–906.

181. Barker FG III. Efficacy of prophylactic antibiotics for craniotomy: a meta-analysis. Neurosurgery 1994; 35:484–492.
182. Pons VG, Denlinger SL, Guglielmo BJ, Octavio J, Flaherty J, Derish PA, Wilson CB. Ceftizoxime versus vancomycin and gentamicin in neurosurgical prophylaxis: a randomized, prospective, blinded clinical study. Neurosurgery 1993; 33:416–423.
183. Yu HC, Patterson RH Jr. Prophylactic antimicrobial agents after ventriculoatriostomy for hydrocephalus. J Pediatr Surg 1973; 8:881–885.
184. Haines SJ, Walters BC. Antibiotic prophylaxis for cerebrospinal fluid shunts: a metanalysis. Neurosurgery 1994; 34:87–92.
185. Blomstedt GC. Results of trimethoprim-sulfamethoxazole prophylaxis in ventriculostomy and shunting procedures. J Neurosurg 1985; 62:694–697.
186. Haines SJ, Taylor F. Prophylactic methicillin for shunt operations: effects on incidence of shunt malfunction and infection. Child's Brain 1982; 9:10–22.
187. Walters BC, Goumnerova L, Hoffman HJ, Hendrick EB, Humphreys RP, Levinton C. A randomized controlled trial of perioperative rifampin/trimethoprim in cerebrospinal fluid shunt surgery. Child's Nerv Syst 1992; 8:253–257.
188. Bayston R. Antibiotic prophylaxis in shunt surgery. Dev Med Child Neurol 1975; 17(suppl 35): 99–103.
189. Rieder MJ, Frewen TC, Del Maestro RF, Coyle A, Lovell S. The effect of cephalothin prophylaxis on postoperative ventriculoperitoneal shunt infections. Can Med Assoc J 1987; 136:935–938.
190. Schmidt K, Gjerris F, Osgaard O, Hvidberg EF, Kristiansen JE, Dahlerup B, Kruse-Larsen C. Antibiotic prophylaxis in cerebrospinal fluid shunting: A prospective randomized trial in 152 hydrocephalic patients. Neurosurgery 17:1–5.
191. Wang EEL, Prober CG, Hendrick BE, Hoffman HJ, Humphreys RP. Prophylactic sulfamethoxazole and trimethoprim in ventriculoperitoneal shunt surgery. JAMA 1984; 251(9):1174–1177.
192. Infection in Neurosurgery Working Party of the British Society for Antimicrobial Chemotherapy. Antimicrobial prophylaxis in neurosurgery and after head injury. Lancet 1994; 344:1547–1551.
193. Langley JM, LeBlanc JC, Drake J, Milner R. Efficacy of antimicrobial prophylaxis in placement of cerebrospinal fluid shunts: meta-analysis. Clin Infect Dis 1993; 17:98–103.
194. Gardner BP, Gordon DS. Postoperative infection in shunts for hydrocephalus: are prophylactic antibiotics necessary? Br Med J 1982; 284:1914–1915.
195. Weiss SR, Raskind R. Further experience with the ventriculoperitoneal shunt. Prophylactic antibiotics. Int Surg 1970; 53:300–303.
196. Ajir F, Levin AB, Duff TA. Effect of prophylactic methicillin on cerebrospinal fluid shunt infections in children. Neurosurgery 1981; 9:6–8.
197. Wang EEL, Prober CG. Ventricular cerebrospinal fluid concentrations of trimethoprim-sulphamethoxazole. J Antimicrob Chemother 1983; 11:385–389.
198. Odio C, Mohs E, Sklar FH, Nelson JD, McCracken GH Jr. Adverse reactions to vancomycin for CSF shunt procedures. Am J Dis Child 1984; 138:17–19.
199. Litsky W. Wanted: plastics with antimicrobial properties. Am J Public Health 1990; 80:13–15.
200. McDougal EG, Burnham SJ, Johnson G Jr. Rifampin protection against experimental graft sepsis. J Vasc Surg 1986; 4:5–7.
201. Bayston R, Milner RDG. Antimicrobial activity of silicone rubber used in hydrocephalus shunts, after impregnation with antimicrobial substances. J Clin Pathol. 1981; 134:1057–1062.
202. Bayston R, Grove N, Siegel J, Lawellin D, Barsham S. Prevention of hydrocephalus shunt catheter colonisation in vitro by impregnation with antimicrobials. J Neurol Neurosurg Psychiatry 1989; 52: 605–609.

26

Neurocysticercosis

Julio Sotelo
National Institute of Neurology and Neurosurgery of Mexico, Mexico City, Mexico

INTRODUCTION

Life Cycle of Taeniasis/Cysticercosis

Cysticercosis, a disease known to affect pork, has been known since ancient Greece. The first description in humans was made in 1550, and the name cysticercosis was given to the disease later by Laennec. It was not until the nineteenth century that the association between *Taenia solium* and cysticercus was discovered (1). Two hosts—humans and pigs—participate in the life cycle of *Taenia solium*. Humans are the only definitive host for the adult cestode *Taenia solium*, whereas both humans and pigs are intermediate hosts for the embryonic cestode cysticercus. In the usual cycle, humans harbor *Taenia* in the small intestine; taeniasis is acquired after ingestion of undercooked pork infected with cysticerci. Once in the intestine, the larva evaginates from the cyst, anchoring firmly to the wall of the first third of the small intestine and evolving within a few weeks from the metacestode to the adult *Taenia*. The adult cestode has a complex head with a globular scolex outfitted with four suckers and a crown of hooks in the center (Fig. 1), which are used to anchor itself to the intestinal wall. It has a large body, as long as 4 m, composed of several hundred proglottids; every day, a few gravid proglottids, each containing thousands of viable eggs, are released from the end of the *Taenia* body into the stools of the carrier, contaminating water, soil, and vegetation in places with deficient disposal of human feces. *Taenia solium* eggs are resistant to desiccation and can be viable even after several days of exposure to climatic changes. When pork, the natural intermediate host, with human feces containing the eggs of *T. solium* is ingested, cerebral and muscle cysticercosis will develop. In this way, the life cycle of the cestode is completed. However, humans can also act as intermediate hosts. The two main routes from which humans may acquire cysticercosis are ingestion of food contaminated with taenia eggs and self-contamination in *Taenia* carriers; the former is by far the most common form of transmission, as it is quite uncommon to find patients having both taeniasis and cysticercosis.

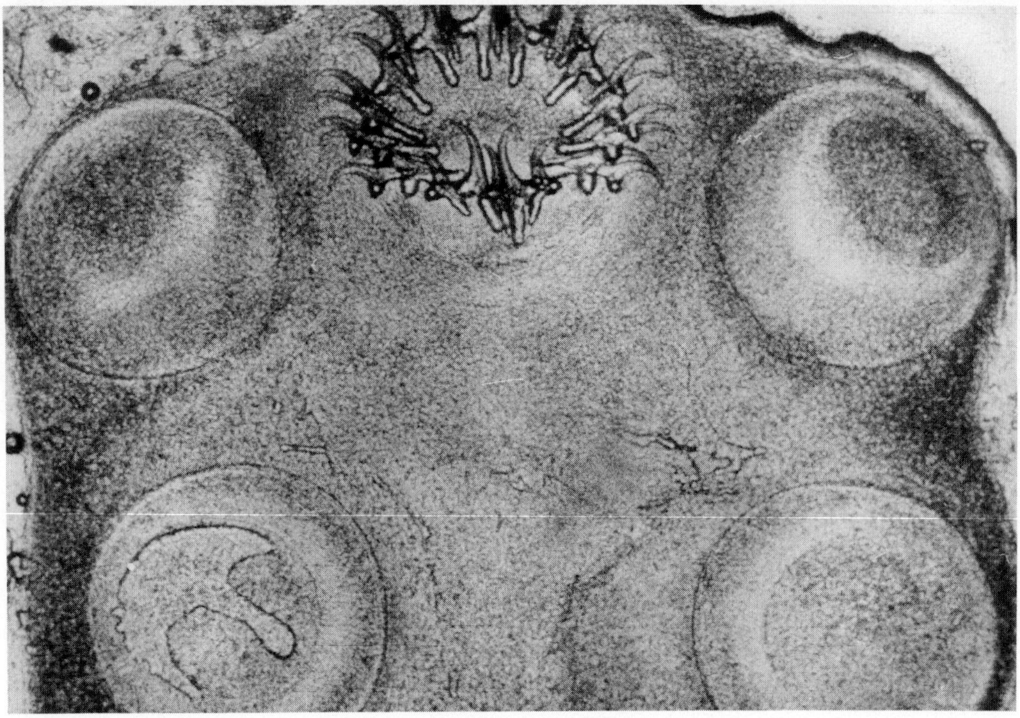

Figure 1 Rostellum from a cysticercus showing the typical features of *Taenia solium*, four suckers and a crown of hooks.

Airborne transmission of taenia eggs or autoinfestation by regurgitation of gravid proglottids into the stomach of taeniasis patients have also been proposed as possible mechanisms of infection; however, these are less likely to occur and have not been demonstrated.

Once in the stomach of the host, the taenia eggs lose their coat by action of gastric acid and hatch into oncospheres or hexacanth embryos; oncospheres cross the intestinal wall, enter the bloodstream, and are carried to the target organs, where after a period of about 2 months, the cysticercus develops (Fig. 1). The main target organs for cysticercus are the eye (Fig. 2), skeletal muscle, and the central nervous system; the latter is the most common area of severe infection. The cysticerci may lodge in the brain parenchyma, subarachnoid space, ventricular space, or spinal cord.

Epidemiology

The incidence of cysticercosis is highly variable in different areas of the same endemic country, depending on local background factors such as sociocultural status, sanitary implementation, porcine breeding methods, and agricultural systems. The precise incidence is not known, as the diagnosis of neurocysticercosis (NCC) cannot be made on clinical grounds alone; it depends largely on the findings on both neuroimaging studies (NIS) and immunodiagnostic tests in cerebrospinal fluid (CSF) (2) (Table 1). This presents obvious obstacles to epidemiological studies, as NIS are highly expensive for epidemiological use and lumbar puncture for CSF analysis cannot be practiced for population-based studies. Serum immunodiagnostic tests have a low sensitivity and specificity for the diagnosis of NCC, mainly due to the peculiarities of NCC

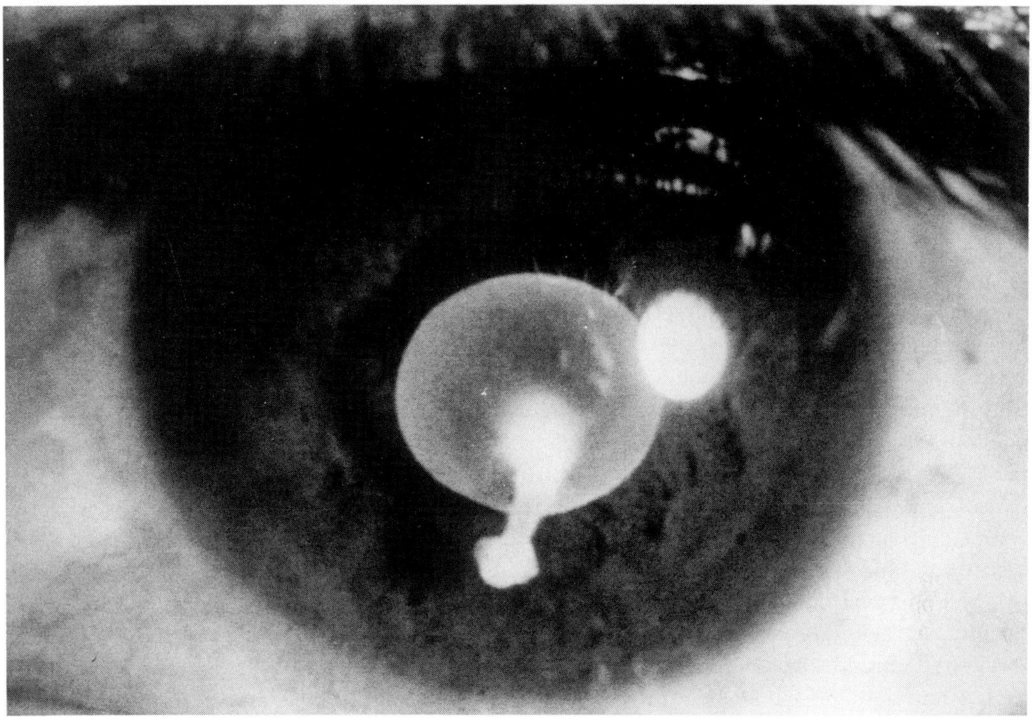

Figure 2 Cysticercus within the anterior chamber of the eye; the larva has evaginated from the cyst.

Table 1 Diagnosis and Therapy for Neurocysticercosis

	DIAGNOSIS
Clinical:	The diagnosis of neurocysticercosis should be contemplated in any patient with partial epilepsy, late-onset epilepsy, intracranial hypertension, or cognitive impairment who is a resident or immigrant from areas endemic for cysticercosis.
Imaging studies:	Computed tomography and magnetic resonance offer a clear visualization of active and inactive lesions as well as secondary complications such as hydrocephalus and infarctions. These studies are the framework for therapeutic decisions and prognosis.
Immunodiagnosis:	Specific antibodies against cysticercus antigens are found in cerebrospinal fluid of most patients with active forms of neurocysticercosis. ELISA, immunoblot, and complement fixation in CSF are reliable. The degree of pleocytosis and the protein concentration provides information on the degree of inflammation within the subarachnoid space for therapeutic decision making.
	RECOMMENDED THERAPY
Active lesions in brain parenchyma or subarachnoid space:	Albendazole 15 mg/kg/day in two doses for 8 days. For the first 4 days, dexamethasone 10 mg IM is recommended to decrease the inflammatory reaction due to the destruction of parasites. If lesions persist unchanged on CT or MR studies 3 months after therapy, praziquantel 50 mg/kg/day in two doses for 15 days is recommended. Simultaneous administration of steroids diminishes its cysticidal effectiveness.
Chronic arachnoiditis:	Surgical placement of a ventriculo-peritoneal shunt in cases of hydrocephalus. Prednisone 50 mg orally every other day in cases of chronic meningitis (as seen in CSF studies) or vasculitis (as seen in imaging studies). The length of therapy should be decided by follow-up studies. Cysticidal treatment.

rather than to technical limitations of the tests. A high proportion of healthy individuals from endemic areas have antibodies in serum, which give positive results to cysticerci antigens, and many patients with confirmed active NCC have negative results (3–5). Although of little value for individual diagnosis, serum immunodiagnostic tests provide information relative to the presence and distribution of the parasite in a given geographical area (6–10).

The above restrictions have made the demographic study of NCC difficult; however, NCC is considered to be the most common parasitic disorder of the central nervous system (11–13). Autopsy studies in general hospitals from endemic countries have shown an incidence of NCC in the general population as high as 4% for either the active disease form or inactive sequelae (11). In most cases, the disease was asymptomatic. In neurological centers of endemic countries, NCC ranks among the three most frequent neurological and neurosurgical disorders. For instance, in endemic countries, NCC is the most common cause of late-onset epilepsy, accounting for more than 50% of all cases (14,15). In most countries in Latin America (2,15–18), Asia (9,12,19,20), and Africa (21–23) and in some countries in Europe (24–27), NCC is a serious public health problem. Cysticercosis is almost absent in Muslim countries (28), as pork breeding is not part of their sociocultural lifestyle. In general terms, cysticercosis is present in areas that combine domestic pork breeding and deficient sanitary implementation, such as plantations irrigated with water contaminated with human feces, food handled by taenia carriers, or defecation in the open. In North America and some European countries, NCC was uncommon until recent decades, when massive immigration from endemic countries resulted in a sharp increase in its prevalence (25,29–32).

PATHOGENESIS AND PATHOLOGY

Immune Response

When a cysticercus invades the central nervous system, it can be exposed to a hostile environment. If the immune system recognizes the parasite, an appropriate inflammatory response will develop to overcome the infection. However, in many cases such a response develops slowly and fails to eliminate the parasite (Fig. 3); then, immune tolerance is developed, and the cysticercus may live almost unchanged for several years (Fig. 4). In contrast, in some patients a fast and intense immune reaction develops (Fig. 5), leading to acute destruction of cysticerci soon after entering the central nervous system; in those cases, the infection is overcome, but the brain tissue may be damaged as a result of this enhanced immune response, leaving as a permanent sequela a brain granuloma (Fig. 6) (33). Between the extremes of immune tolerance and hypersensitivity, there is a wide range of inflammatory responses induced by this complex host-parasite relationship, in which the host develops an immune reaction against the parasite while the parasite, by various mechanisms, evades immune surveillance (Fig. 7).

The mechanisms by which cysticerci elude the immune response are not understood, however, some hypotheses have been postulated (11,34), including (1) antigenic variation, (2) concomitant immunity, (3) molecular mimicry, and (4) active immunosuppression. Antigenic variation is a mechanism by which parasites change constantly the antigens presented to the immune afferents of the host; therefore, new antigens appearing on the surface of the parasite may escape an immune response developed against previous antigens. This mechanism has been demonstrated in trypanosomiasis and malaria (35), but not in cysticercosis; nevertheless, as the process of maturation of cysticerci is highly complex, antigenic variation is a plausible mechanism of immune evasion. Concomitant immunity has been documented in some cases of taeniasis where fully developed cysticerci are resistant to the immune response while young embryos are susceptible. In human cysticercosis, this mechanism could prevent reinfestation but avoid im-

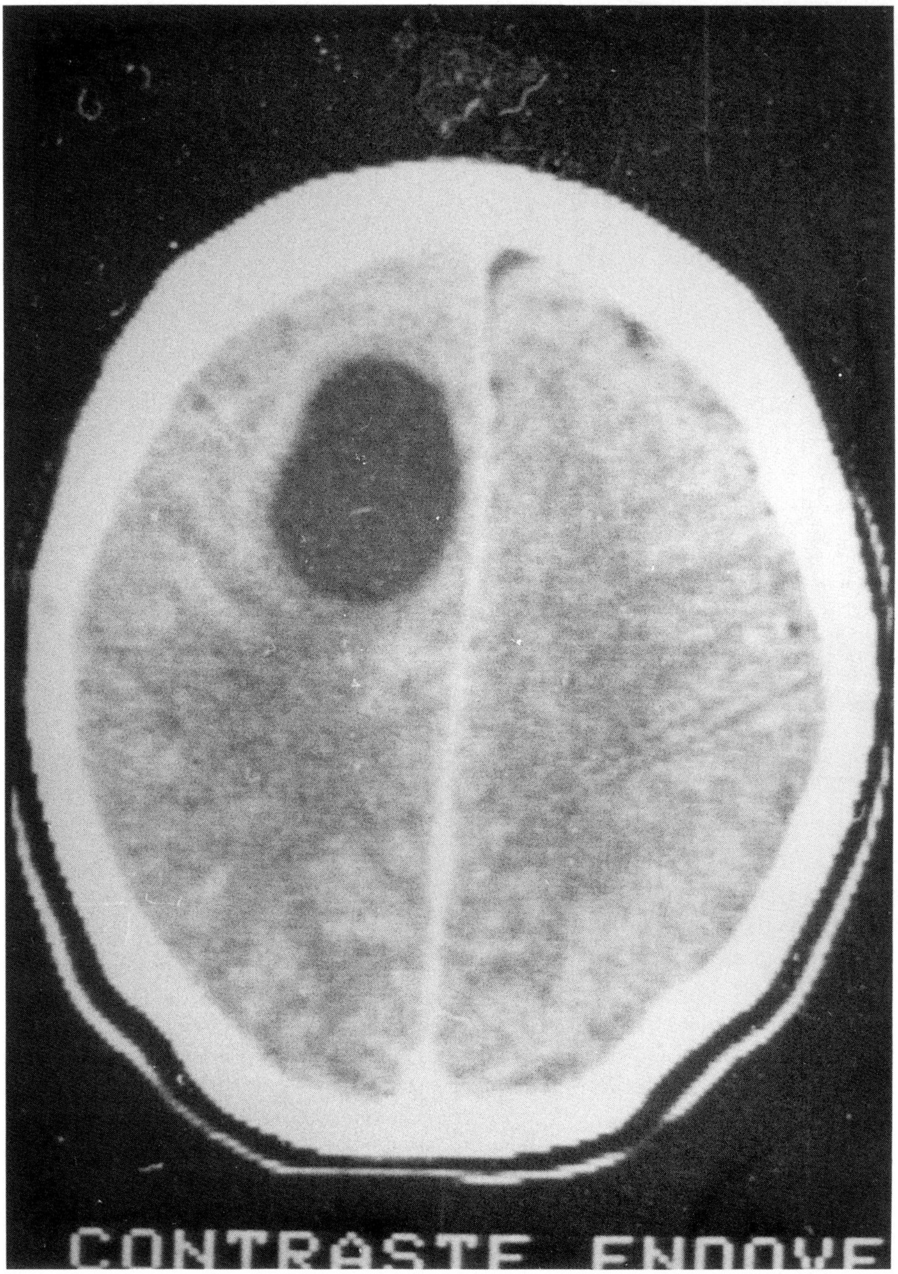

Figure 3 Contrasted CT showing a large cyst that has grown over a long period of time due to little or no immune response from the host, as seen by the absence of inflammation signs around the lesion.

mune recognition of mature cysts. Molecular mimicry consists of the active adherence of some molecules form the host to the surface of the parasite, so that it cannot be recognized as a foreign agent. This has been demonstrated in schistosomiasis, but some studies in cysticercosis have shown that attachment of HLA antigens from the host to the surface of some cysticerci induce even more inflammation than those without HLA covering (36). Active immunosuppression is

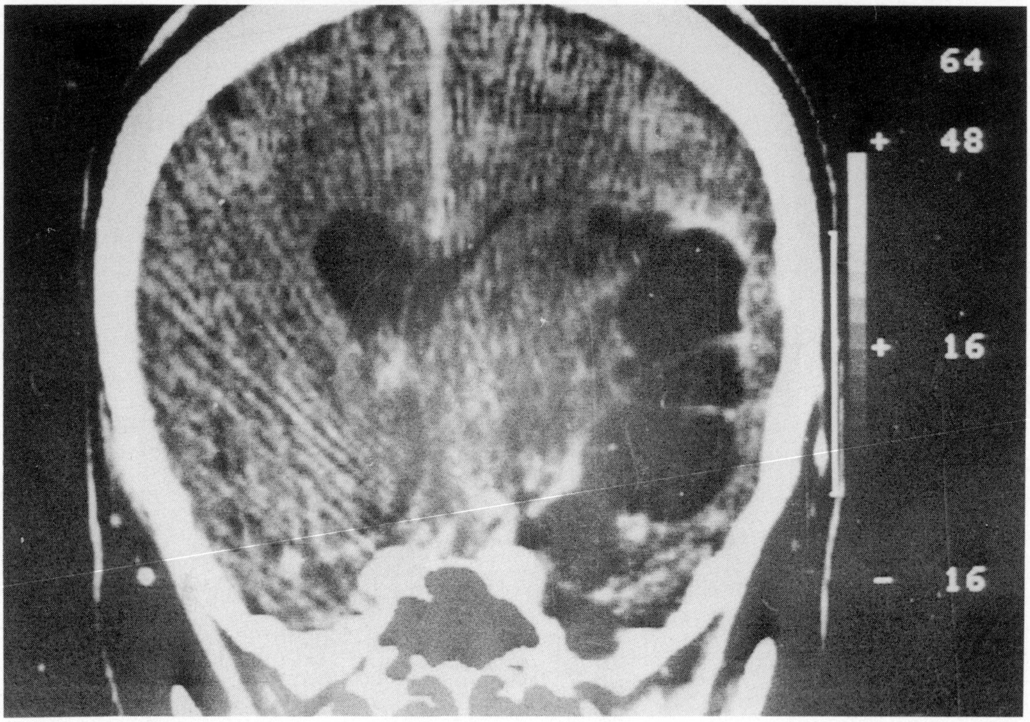

Figure 4 Coronal CT scan shows a clump of large cysticerci producing a mass effect with displacement of the frontal horn of the lateral ventricle.

induced by immunosuppressant substances released by the parasite. This mechanism seems to be important and is currently being studied in cysticercosis (37).

It appears that the interaction of several factors is responsible for the variable immune response to cysticercal infection of the CNS. One of these factors may be gender-related; the degree of inflammation secondary to parenchymal brain cysticercosis is greater in females than in males (38), whereas the degree of inflammation in meningeal cysticercosis is similar in males and females (39). There appears to be a gender-related factor within brain parenchyma that influences the immune response to the parasite, inducing either a more intense immune response in women or an active immunosuppression in men. There could also be an interaction between gender and HLA antigens of the host, as has been documented in other inflammatory and immune-mediated disorders of the CNS that are more frequent in women. Two histocompatibility antigens appear to be partly involved in the modulation of the immune response to cysticercosis: HLA-B28 and HLA-DQW2, the former as a risk antigen and the latter as a protective antigen. However, no differences between HLA antigens and host gender have been found (36).

Parenchymal Cysticercosis

When the parasite lodges in the brain parenchyma, histopathological changes vary from mild or minimal inflammation around the cysts to an intense reaction characterized by multiple foci of lymphocytes, plasma cells and eosinophils, perivascular infiltrates, edema, and reactive astrogliosis (33). The latter forms a thin capsule of fibrous tissue surrounding the cyst. With the passage of time, the capsule thickens. If the immune reaction is sufficiently intense, the parasite is

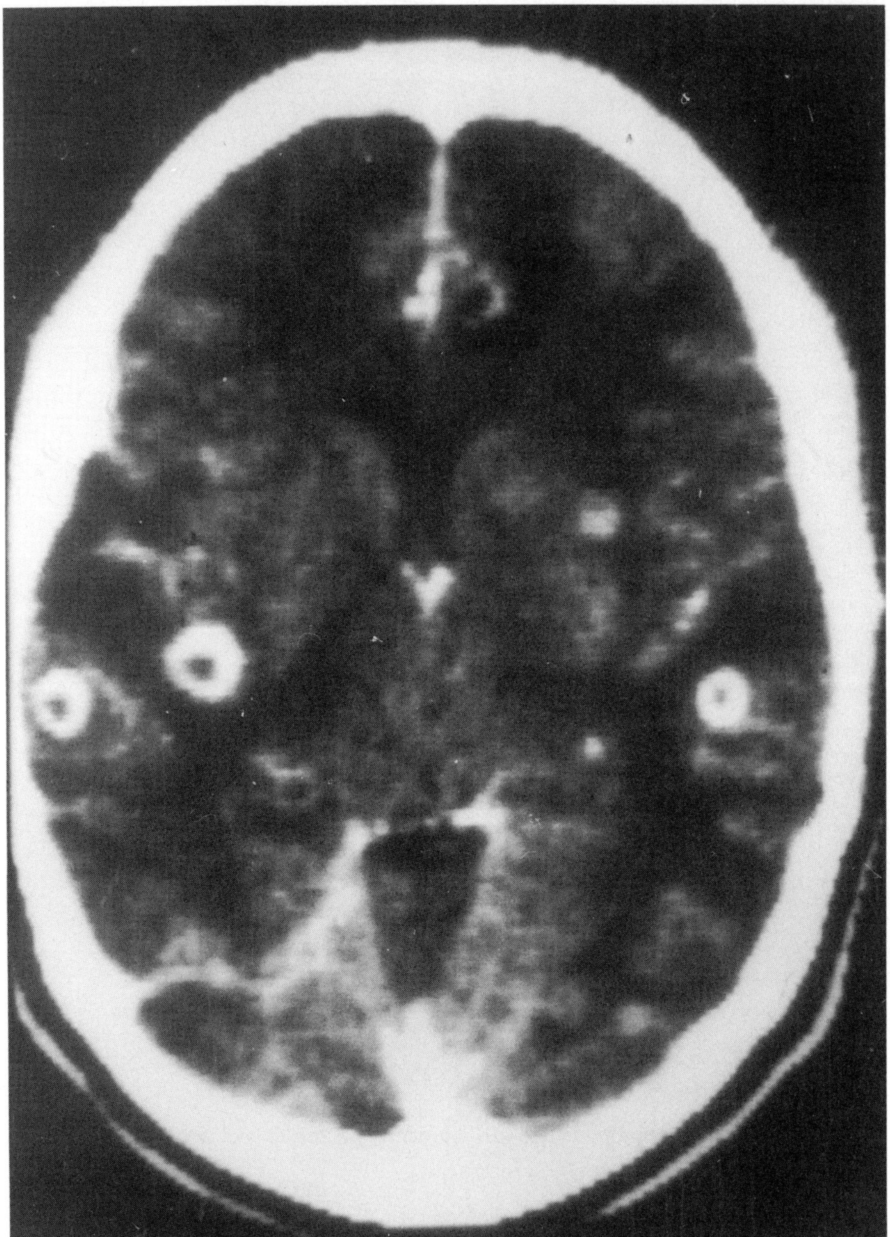

Figure 5 Cysticercotic encephalitis. Contrast-enhanced CT showing ringlike lesions due to intense inflammation around cysticerci and diffuse brain edema.

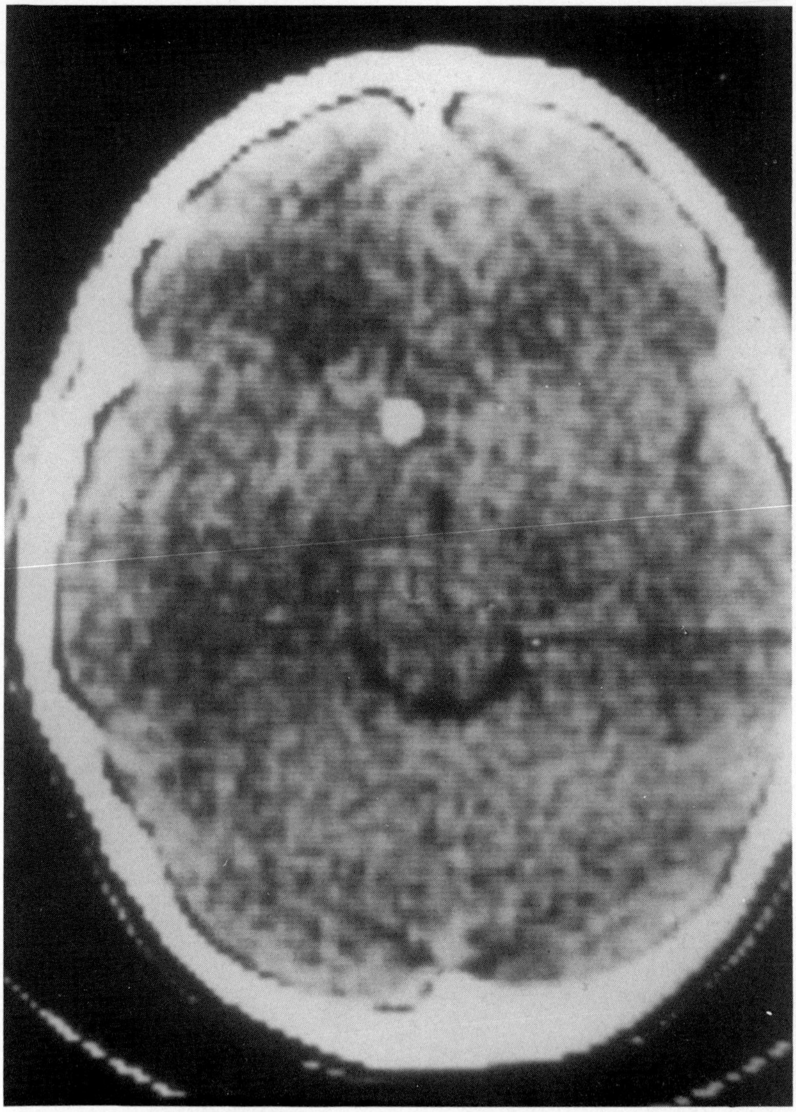

Figure 6 CT scan shows a parenchymal calcification, the common sequela of brain cysticercosis.

destroyed, and successive degenerative changes begin with hyaline transformation of the cystic fluid and destruction of the larva, followed by fragmentation of the cystic membrane and penetration of the parasite by macrophages and multinucleated cells. Afterward, the site where the cysts were located is replaced by a granuloma composed of astroglial and fibrous tissue. The granuloma subsequently becomes mineralized with deposits of calcium salts. In this way, a solid calcification can replace the fibrous granuloma. The process of calcification of the granuloma takes several years after the disappearance of the parasite. Each one of these histopathological stages of the lesions can now be clearly identified by NIS (40,41).

The number of cysticerci involved may vary from one isolated cyst to several hundred. In the general picture of parenchymal NCC, isolated benign lesions are more frequent than multiple

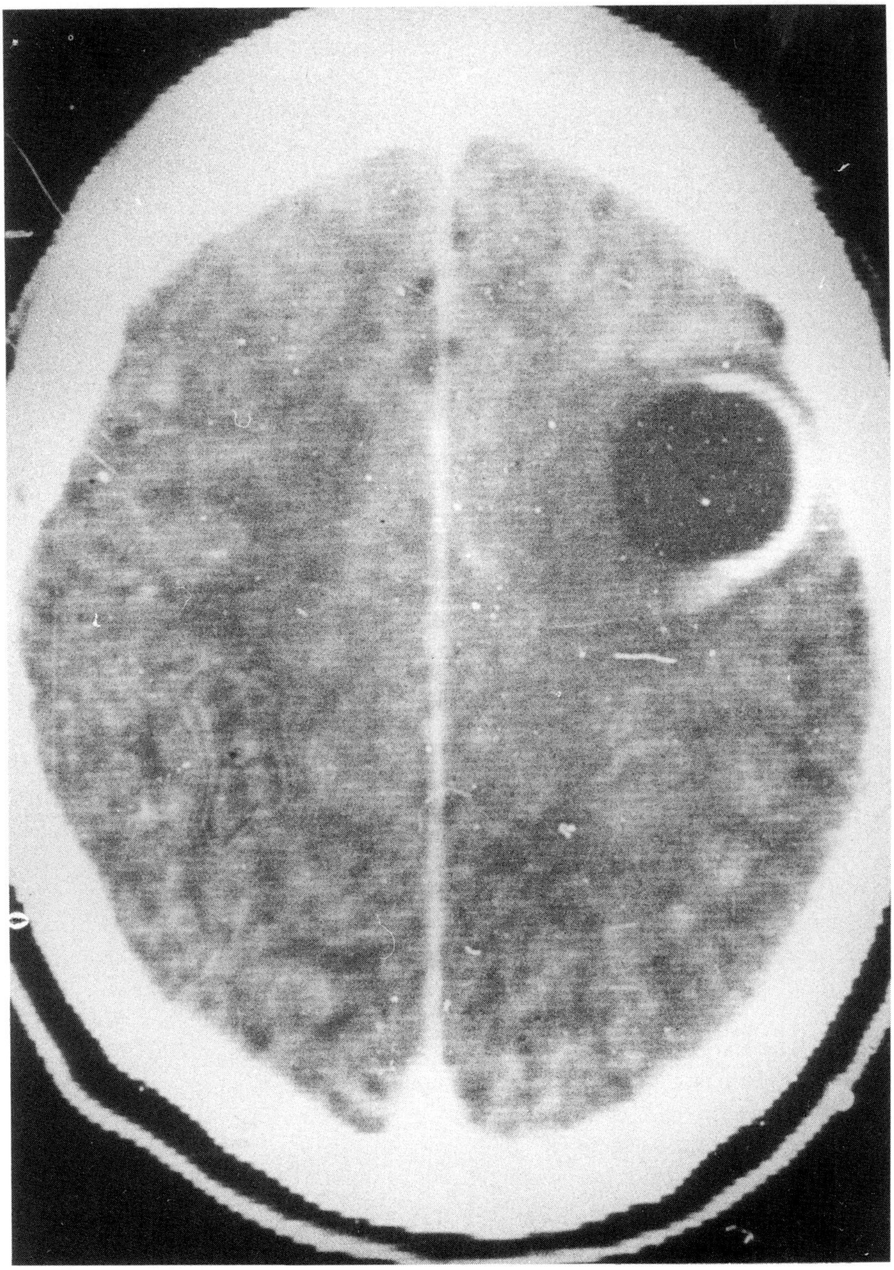

Figure 7 Parenchymal cysticercus showing on CT scan the variable immune response from the host. The right side of the cyst is surrounded by inflammation as seen by intense contrast enhancement, whereas the left side shows no inflammatory signs as evidence of immune tolerance.

lesions (2). They can be located anywhere in the brain parenchyma, but their most frequent locations are areas of rich vascularization, i.e., gray matter and basal ganglia. The natural history of the parasitic infection in the brain is closely related to the immune response from the host. In some cases, the cyst survives unchanged for several years as seen by serial NIS; in other cases, the cyst is destroyed within a few weeks, also documented by NIS. In this way, if the immune reaction from the host is strong, all histopathological stages of the lesion from the live cyst to the formation of a granuloma will be completed within 2 months; however, if the reaction is not strong enough or the parasite evades the immune system of the host, a chronic inflammation with persistence of the cyst will develop, making it almost impossible to predict whether the cyst will be destroyed by host mechanisms. NIS help somewhat to predict the natural history of lesions; if the cyst is surrounded by intense enhancement, the spontaneous elimination of the parasite is highly probable; in contrast, if no evidence of surrounding inflammation is found, a long persistence of active lesions can be predicted. The former picture is more frequent in children, whereas the latter is more frequent in adults (22).

Meningeal Cysticercosis

The pathophysiology of the lesions of cysticercosis is related to the location of the cysts. In meningeal cysticercosis, there is widespread inflammation and fibrosis of the arachnoid membranes with chronic meningitis that may last several years (39). The secondary complications of inflammation and fibrosis in the subarachnoid space are hydrocephalus and vasculitis, which represent the most severe and disabling complications of NCC (Fig. 8) (42). Hydrocephalus develops when chronic inflammation of the meninges interferes with the normal mechanisms of CSF absorption in the arachnoid granulations (24). Vasculitis is a frequent cause of brain infarctions secondary to occlusion of both large and small arteries (43). In cases of severe arachnoiditis at the base of the brain, the occlusion of brain-stem arteries is a frequent cause of death. Infarctions are also seen in small perforating arteries of the cerebral hemispheres, causing dementia.

The normal cysticercus is 0.5–1 cm in diameter (Fig. 9); however, when the cysts survive for long periods, they can grow to 10–15 cm (Fig. 4). These giant cysts, which are usually devoid of scolex, represent a hydatid degeneration of the parasite, in which the festooned cystic membranes continued growing in spite of the death of the metacestode. This explains why the histopathological features of giant cysts have the typical cysticercus membranes but the larva is not found. Furthermore, hydatid degeneration occasionally produces budlike processes giving the appearance of grapelike clumps of cysts. This mechanism of hydatid proliferation of membranes has been demonstrated in cysticerci from the helminth *Taenia crassiceps* (Fig. 10) (44). Formerly, cysticercosis was thought to be caused by two different forms of the parasite: racemose cysticercus and cellulose cysticercus, the latter being small cysts with larvae, the former being composed of clumps of large cysts devoid of larva. However, biochemical, immunological, and ultrastructural studies have shown that racemose and cellulose cysticerci represent different stages of the same parasite. Giant cysts are found mostly in areas with permissive space, such as the sylvian fissure and the subarachnoid space at the base of the skull.

Ventricular Cysticercosis

In ventricular cysticercosis there is usually a single cyst lodged inside the fourth ventricle, which produces a valve mechanism on the CSF transit and leads to subacute hydrocephalus with episodes of sudden increase of intracranial pressure related to movements of the head. If the cyst is detached from the ependymal lining, it does not induce inflammation, while in cases where the cyst adheres to the floor of the ventricle, intense inflammation with lymphocytic infiltrates

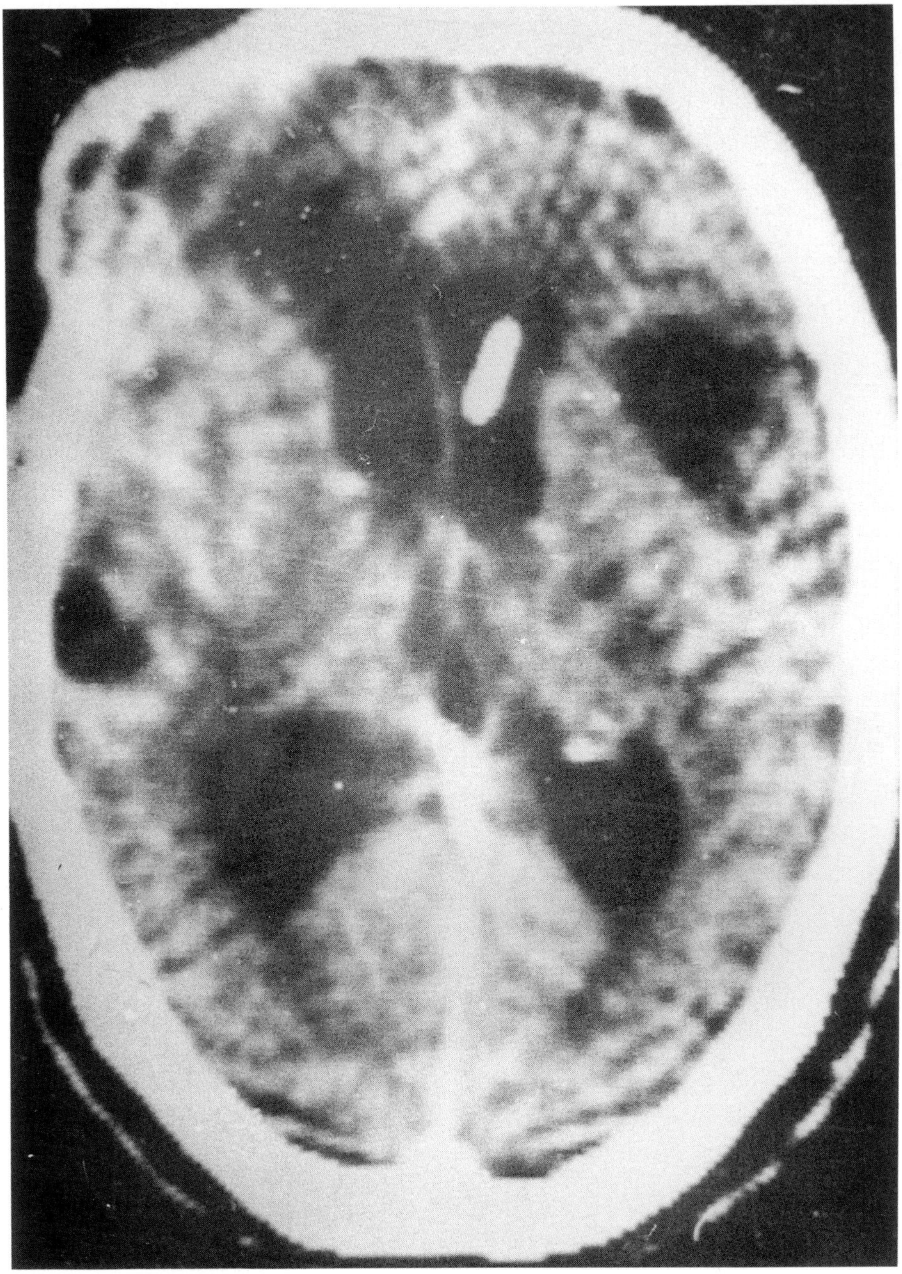

Figure 8 Fatal evolution of meningeal cysticercosis. CT scan shows the persistence of hydrocephalus despite a ventricular shunt, which was occluded due to the high concentration of cells and protein in the CSF. A surgical craniotomy is seen on the left with protrusion of brain parenchyma. Two large subarachnoid cysts are also seen.

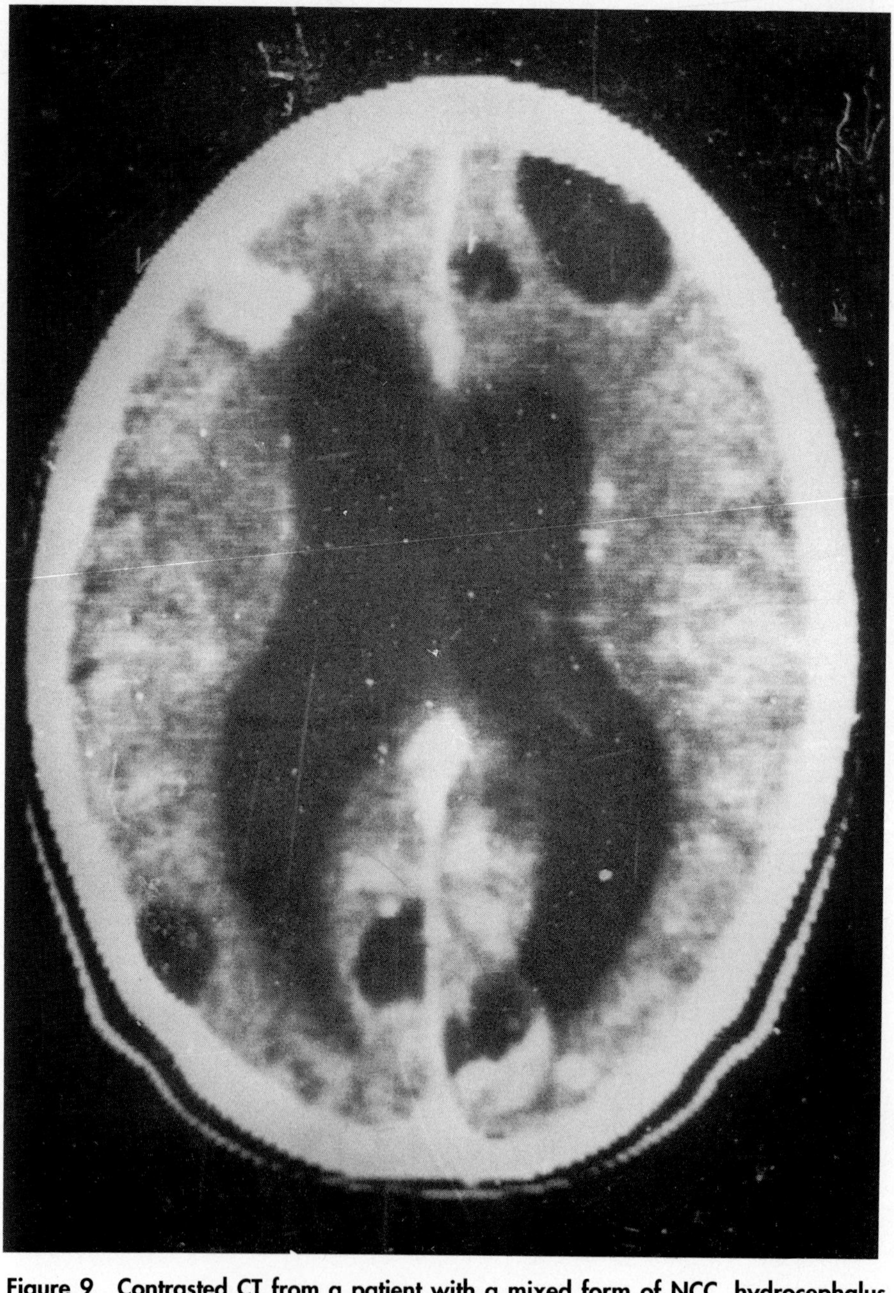

Figure 9 Contrasted CT from a patient with a mixed form of NCC, hydrocephalus secondary to arachnoiditis, calcifications, and parenchymal cysticerci.

develops. The plausible mechanism for the ventricular form of NCC (less than 1% of all cases) seems to be the initial arrival of the oncosphere at the choroid plexus of the ventricles via the bloodstream. Once in the ventricular cavities, the cysticercus quickly grows unchallenged by space resistance or tissue reaction, reaching a large size that prevents the passage of the parasite from the fourth ventricle to the subarachnoid space through the posterior foraminae. The first part

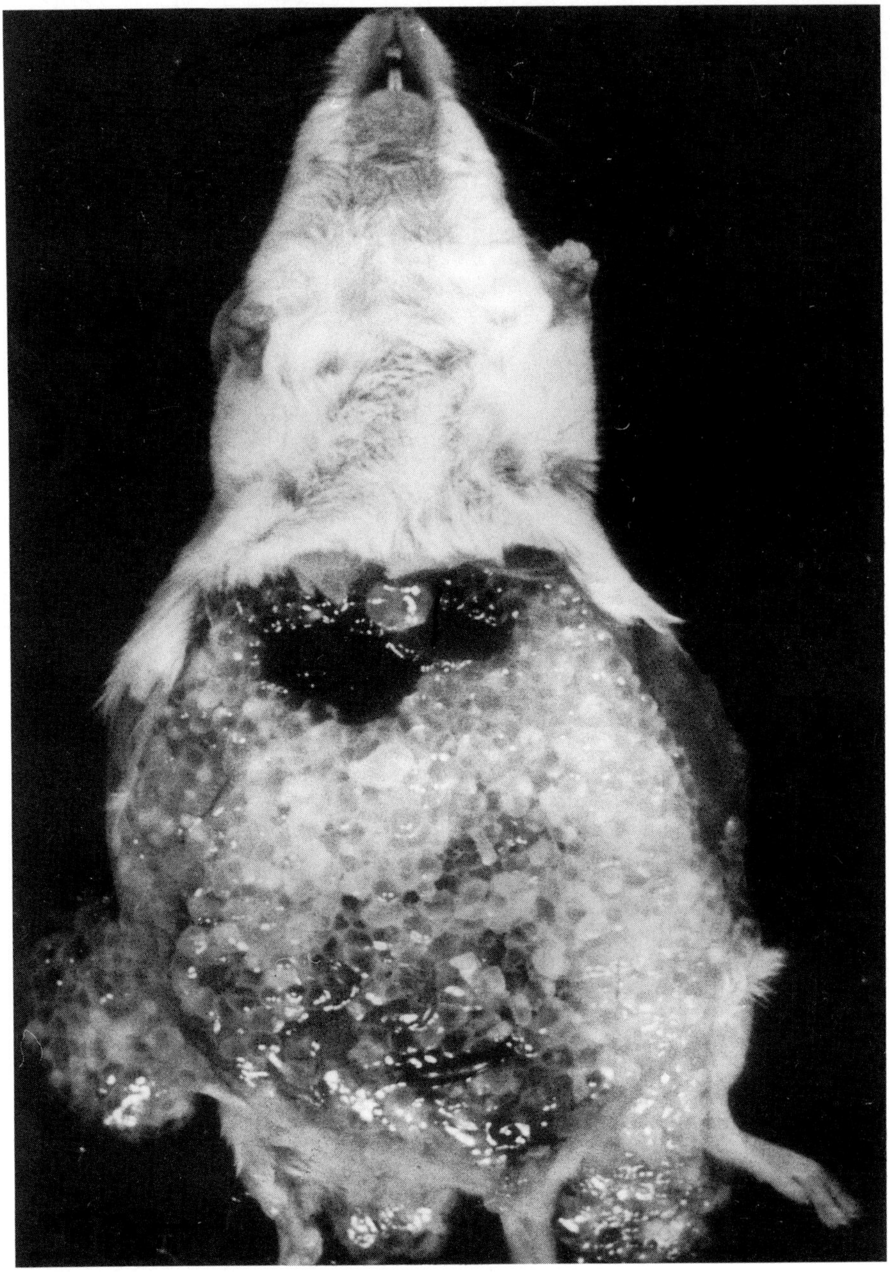

Figure 10 Two months after the intraperitoneal injection of 15 cysticerci of *Taenia crassiceps* in a BALB-C mice, several thousand cystercerci are obtained. Antigens from these parasites effectively replace those of *Taenia solium* cysticerci for immunodiagnosis of human cysticercosis in CSF; also, it provides unlimited amounts of antigens for studies on porcine vaccination.

of this mechanism also appears to be the source of both meningitis, which is a far more frequent form of NCC (around 30% of all cases), and cysticerci in the spinal canal (less than 1% of cases). In meningeal and spinal cord cysticercosis, although the arrival of the oncospheres is also through the choroid plexus, the passage of the parasites along the ventricles is fast, and the oncospheres reach the arachnoid membranes where they hatch and evolve into cysticerci.

CLINICAL ASPECTS

Neurocysticercosis can affect men or women at any age; however, the highest incidence is between the third and fourth decades of life. Age and gender are important for the clinicopathological features of the disease; NCC is far more frequent in adults than in children, and clinical expression is different in both age groups (2,22,31,45). In children, NCC is usually benign (31). The most frequent clinical manifestation of NCC in childhood is epilepsy. In a typical case, an otherwise healthy child presents with a seizure. Contrast-enhanced NIS demonstrate a single parenchymal cysticercus surrounded by edema and ringlike enhancement (22,46–48). On subsequent studies, the lesion will either spontaneously disappear or be replaced by a residual granuloma. When the lesion disappears, it is highly possible that the seizures will also disappear (24). For unknown reasons, other forms of NCC such as meningitis or ventricular cysts are rarely seen in children (45). Parenchymal cysticercosis in childhood is usually self-limited, and in most cases only a single lesion is found. A possible explanation for the infrequency of NCC in children could be that immunological barriers prevent the arrival of large number of cysticerci to the brain or to other locations such as the meninges or ventricular cavities. There is one exception—the location of a cysticercus within the eye is more frequent in children than in adults. In contrast to the pediatric experience with NCC, when the disease affects adults, the pathophysiology and clinical picture is complex and frequently severe (particularly meningeal cysticercosis) (2).

The incidence of NCC is similar for males and females (2,12,30), although the gender of the host influences the clinical expression of parenchymal cysticercosis. As demonstrated by NIS, women develop more intense inflammation around lesions than men. This becomes even more conspicuous in cysticercotic encephalitis, a rare parenchymal form of NCC characterized by diffuse and intense brain edema as a response of the host to a miliary invasion of the brain by cysticerci (Fig. 5). This deadly form of NCC is about seven times more frequent in young females than in males (11). In these cases, the clinical picture of encephalitis with visual disturbances, severe intracranial hypertension, and confusion or stupor is secondary to diffuse brain edema caused by the immune response rather than to the physical presence of several parasites in brain parenchyma. It is common to see other patients with several cysticerci scattered in the brain parenchyma, but with moderate or absent inflammatory reaction in whom the clinical picture is surprisingly mild despite a heavy parasitic burden (Fig. 11).

Clinical manifestations of NCC are related to several factors, the most important of which are the number of lesions, their biological stage, the location of cysts, and the degree of immune reaction developed by the host (2,24). A combination of these factors induce a great variety of neurological and psychiatric syndromes, and consequently, require an individualized therapeutic approach for almost every patient. The great variety of signs and symptoms that can be due to neurocysticercosis impedes its presumptive diagnosis on clinical grounds alone. NCC can express itself from a mild symptom such as headache, dizziness, or occasional seizures to a very severe neurological picture with intracranial hypertension or dementia.

In parenchymal brain cysticercosis, the most common manifestation is epilepsy, usually in the form of partial seizures with or without secondary generalization. In endemic areas, a parenchymal cyst or a granuloma are common findings in NIS in patients with epilepsy. A practical recommendation in endemic countries or in immigrants from endemic countries is the routine

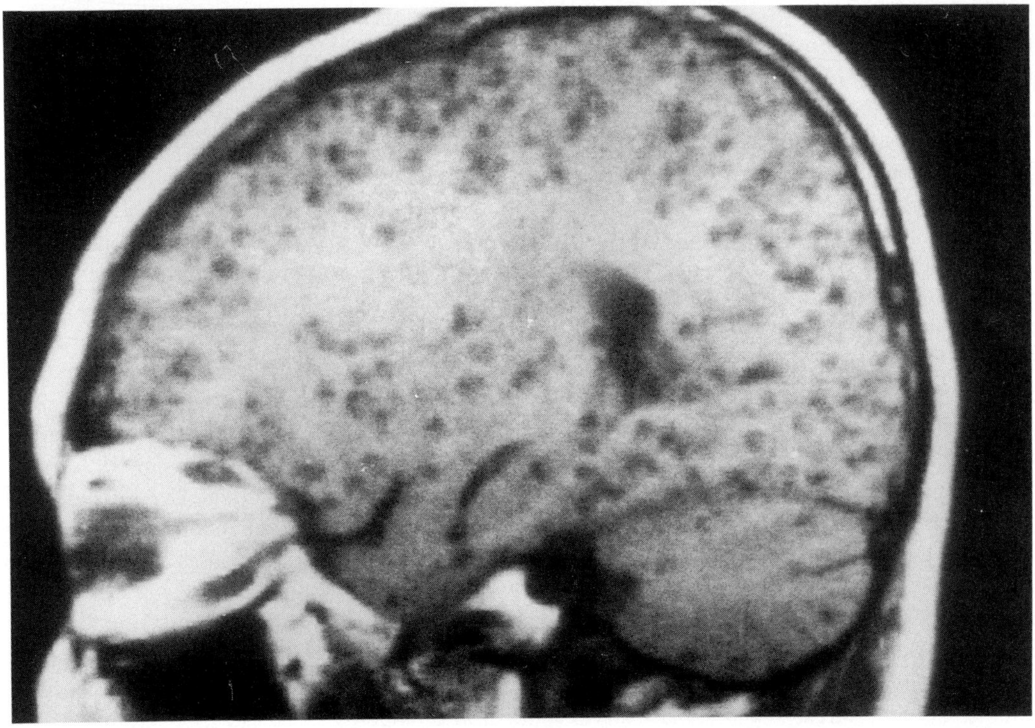

Figure 11 MR image from a patient with a milliar invasion of cysticerci in brain parenchyma. Countless cysticerci are seen in the cerebral hemispheres and cerebellum.

performance of NIS for diagnosis of NCC in any patient with partial seizures or with late-onset epilepsy (14). Sequelae of cysticerci in the form of parenchymal brain granulomas (Fig. 6) are present in more than 50% of patients with the diagnosis of NCC (14). In most cases, the clinical manifestation of parenchymal granulomas is epilepsy. Inactive forms of NCC such as granulomas and calcifications do not actually represent NCC but rather its sequelae. This point is important to stress to patients with a brain granuloma as a unique abnormality, in whom the incorrect diagnosis of NCC carries the psychological burden that the word cysticercosis implies.

Other symptoms of parenchymal cysticercosis include headache, which may be due to intracranial hypertension secondary to brain edema or to vasculitis. In vasculitis complicating NCC, the headache is similar to that produced by migraine. Another frequent presentation of parenchymal NCC is vague psychiatric symptomatology, which in a few cases becomes a complex psychosis. Before the advent of NIS, it was common to find long-term psychiatric hospital patients in whom the diagnosis of NCC was made by CSF analysis or even at autopsy. Cognitive deterioration and dementia are also manifestations of NCC, either due to diffuse parenchymal lesions, to several infarctions, or to chronic hydrocephalus. A rich variety of neurological signs and symptoms can also be caused by parenchymal cysticerci, which largely depend on the topography of the lesions. In this sense, NCC is similar to multiple sclerosis, where symptomatology and severity of the disease are related to the number and location of the lesions (2). The clinical picture of NCC is so varied that in neurological centers of endemic areas, the presumptive diagnosis of NCC is entertained in the initial medical notes of most neurological patients.

Meningeal cysticercosis is present in about 30% of patients with the diagnosis of NCC. The degree of inflammation in general terms is far more severe in meningeal cysticercosis than in any other form of NCC (Fig. 8) due to the intense and widespread immune response in the subarachnoid space, where local synthesis of immunoglobulins has been documented (49). More than 50% of patients with diffuse arachnoiditis develop subacute or chronic hydrocephalus. The main symptomatology in this group is due to increased intracranial pressure with headache, vertigo, vomiting, papilledema, mental deterioration, and gait disturbances. Chronic inflammation of the basilar meninges and surrounding brain stem may manifest with symptomatology related to dysfunction of cranial nerves from fibrotic entrapment in their arachnoidal sheaths. The most frequent symptoms of cranial nerve abnormalities are visual loss and diplopia. Vasculitis is another etiology of clinical symptomatology in chronic arachnoiditis. Vasculitis produces migrainelike syndromes and small infarctions in brain and brain stem secondary to inflammatory occlusive disease of the perforating arteries (43). Patients with chronic arachnoiditis who develop hydrocephalus in general have a poor prognosis with a fatality rate of more than 50% 2 years after diagnosis and severe neurological sequelae in another 25%. Inflammation is the major etiology of the pathophysiology of chronic meningitis, hydrocephalus, and vasculitis (42). Even in cases of severe arachnoiditis, most patients do not have hyperthermia or signs of meningeal irritation; therefore, the diagnosis of chronic meningitis is seldom proposed at clinical examination.

The most frequent location of subarachnoid cysticerci in which the parasites are either of a large size (10 cm or more) or assembled in clumps are the sylvian fissure, brain sulci, and basilar cisterns. In these locations, the cysts have a grapelike appearance on NIS, and the clinical picture is that of a tumorlike syndrome due to the large growth of the vesicles and compression of neighboring structures. When subarachnoid cysticercosis appears in the form of clumps rather than widespread cysticerci, inflammation in CSF is moderate, and the prognosis is far better than in those patients with diffuse chronic arachnoiditis. A rare location of arachnoid cysticerci is within the hypophysial fossa with compression of the pituitary body, producing a clinical picture of panhypopituitarism that frequently leads to the misdiagnosis of empty sella turcica. In most cases, the proper diagnosis is only made during surgery. Another symptom of an arachnoid cysticercus in this location is visual loss due to fibrotic entrapment of the optic nerve and chiasm (50).

Ventricular cysticercosis causes subacute or acute hydrocephalus. The most frequent location of the parasite is within the fourth ventricle. Most patients have Brun's sign, with intermittent episodes of sudden increases in intracranial pressure related to movements of the head in which the cyst produces a valve effect obstructing the flow of CSF (51). This may cause sudden death. The clinical symptomatology is explained by two pathophysiological mechanisms: (1) hydrocephalus with intracranial hypertension, which is usually more severe and life threatening than that caused by arachnoiditis because its development is acute or subacute precluding the compensatory mechanisms that take place when the development of hydrocephalus is slow (as in most cases of chronic arachnoiditis), and (2) dilatation and ependymitis of the fourth ventricle with signs of brain-stem dysfunction, such as paresis of oculomotor nerves and Parinaud's syndrome (52). Occasionally, the cysticercus is located either in the third or in the lateral ventricles. In the third ventricle it causes a clinical picture indistinguishable from that of a colloid cyst; in the lateral ventricles the cyst grows very large due to its permissive location and in most cases is asymptomatic, being revealed by NIS demonstrating asymmetrical dilatation of one lateral ventricle.

In the rare cases of cysticerci in the spinal cord parenchyma, the symptomatology is that of a neoplasm with signs of either total or partial spinal cord dysfunction. In cases of cysticerci located in the spinal canal, symptomatology is similar to that of a prolapsed disc or intraspinal tumor. In cases of intense trabecular fibrosis of the spinal canal, spastic quadriparesis develops (53).

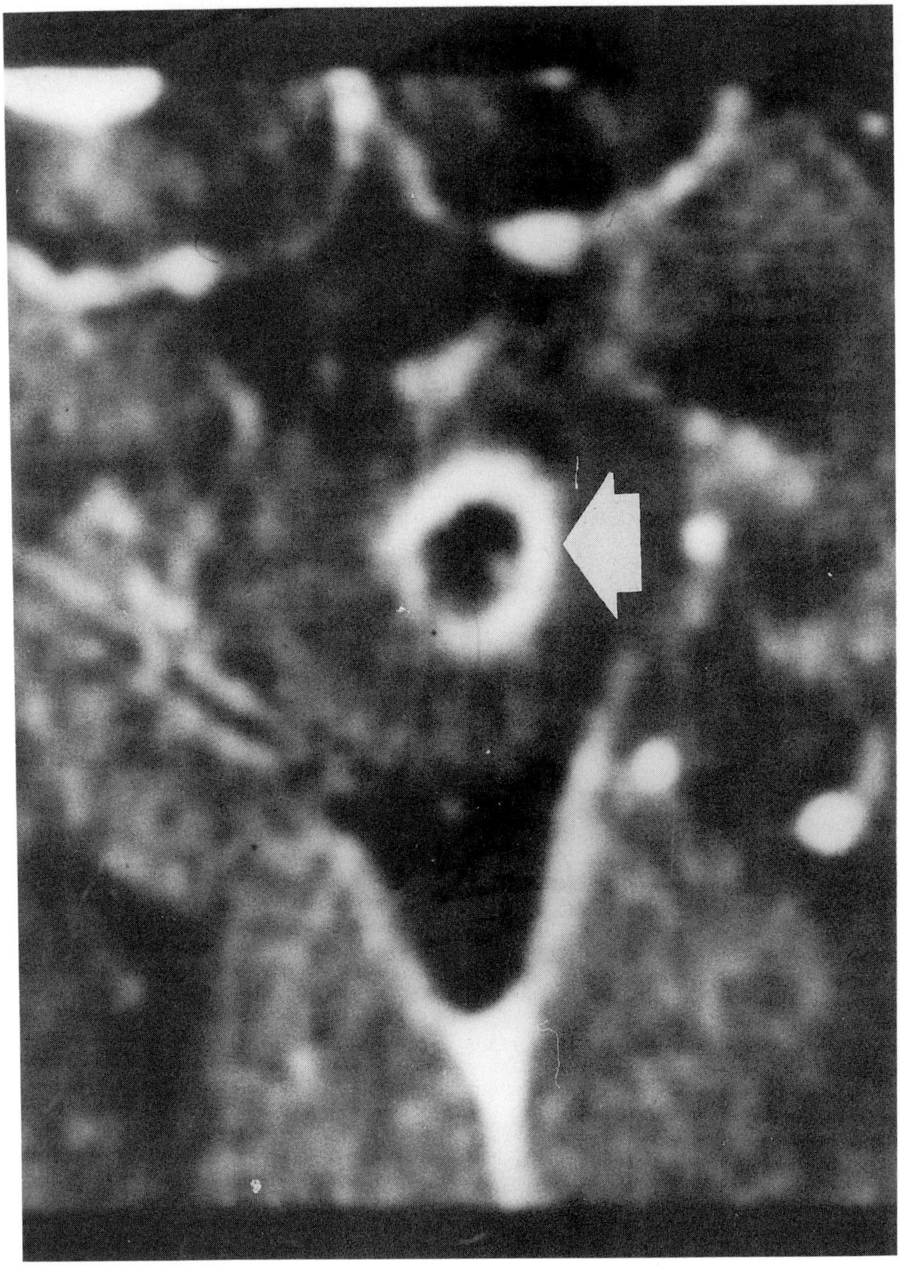

Figure 12 A single cysticercus may induce a severe neurological picture depending on its location; in this case the lesion was located in the mesencephalon (arrow), causing hemiplegia and lethargy. Total remission was obtained after albendazole therapy.

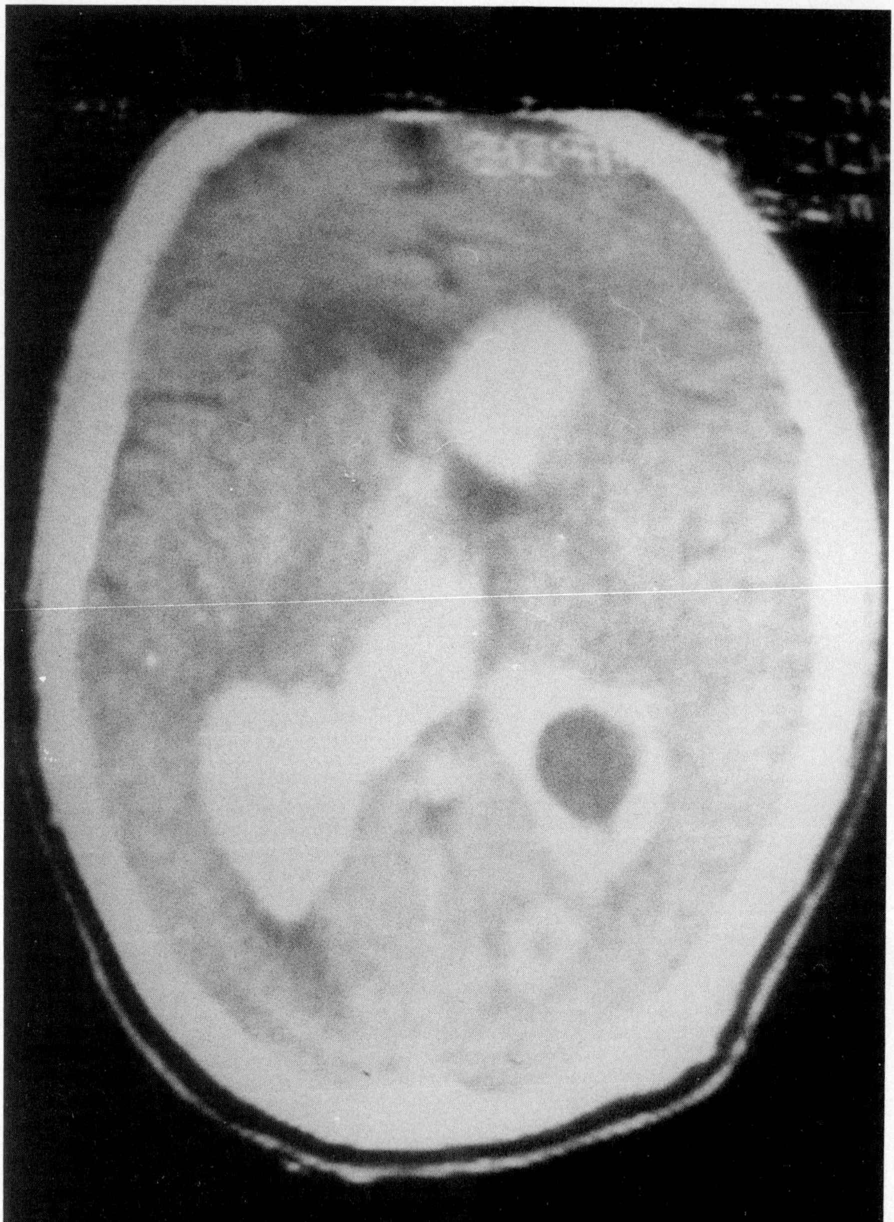

Figure 13 Ventricular cysticercus demonstrated by CT scan with intraventricular injection of metrizamide. A parenchymal cysticercus is also seen in the left occipital lobe.

The clinical presentation of NCC is very complex, not only because of number, location (Fig. 12), and variable inflammation of lesions, but also because more than 50% of patients have a combination of two or more forms of NCC. It is very common to find patients with a mixture of parenchymal plus meningeal or ventricular cysticercosis (Figs. 9 and 13). To make the possibilities of the clinical expression of NCC even more complex, some patients have only active forms of the disease with cysts and inflammation, while others have only inactive forms with granulomas and residual fibrosis. In the majority of cases, however, a combination of active and inactive forms of the disease are present (2).

DIAGNOSIS

Neuroimaging Studies

Imaging studies, computed tomography (CT) or magnetic resonance (MR) or both, must be performed in any patient in whom the diagnosis of NCC is possible (40,41) (Table 1). Since the advent of NIS, the diagnosis of NCC has been properly made and its clinicopathological features better defined (54). Before the advent of NIS, most cases of NCC were not detected and the diagnosis was primarily made during surgery performed for a presumptive diagnosis other than NCC. In endemic countries, many cases were detected at autopsy and occasionally through CSF studies; but the features and characteristics of the disease remained unknown. NIS now permit a fairly precise characterization of NCC, and together with CSF analysis, they are indispensable for the proper design of therapeutic strategies.

In parenchymal cysticercosis, plain NIS illustrate the presence, size, and characteristics of cysts, granulomas, calcifications, edema, and infarctions secondary to vasculitis (43). In addition, contrast-enhanced studies give valuable information about perilesional inflammation, which indirectly correlates with the degree of immune response of the host against the parasite (Figs. 4, 5, 7, and 11). Four types of parenchymal lesion due to cysticercosis have been described with NIS: cysts without contrast enhancement (no inflammation around the parasite), ringlike enhancement of cysts (indirect evidence of perilesional inflammation), granulomas with or without enhancement (these lesions are not visible on plain radiographs of the skull), and calcifications (also evident on skull radiographs). Serial CT studies of granulomas have demonstrated that it takes several years for a granuloma to become calcified. This is important due to the high incidence of granulomas; in fact, granulomas are the most common finding in NCC patients (Fig. 6). Small brain infarctions are seen on NIS in parenchymal or meningeal cysticercosis. When angiographic studies are performed, indirect signs of vasculitis are found with occlusion of small vessels and of the major arteries of the circle of Willis.

Magnetic resonance is a very valuable aid to CT scan, particularly for studies of the posterior fossa and basilar cisterns (Figs. 11 and 12), where CT has poor definition. MR clearly defines the anatomicopathological stage of the cysts. The vesicular fluid of live cysticercus has physical properties identical to those of the CSF on the T2 relaxation time. A very early sign of cyst death is hypointensity of the vesicular fluid on the T2 sequence when compared to CSF. This change in the appearance of the vesicular fluid represents the transformation of the cyst fluid due to cyst death into the colloidal stage. The appearance of the cyst on MR scan is very helpful particularly to evaluate the effectiveness of medical therapy. MR is also superior to CT for visualization of cerebral edema, ocular cysticercosis, cysticerci in periorbital area, spinal cysticercosis, clumps of subarachnoid cysticerci in basilar cisterns, and in some cases of ventricular cysticercus. However, MR is inferior to CT for detection of parenchymal granulomas and calcifications as these lesions on MR give only a weak hypointense signal. MR completes and in some instances increases the information obtained with CT for proper diagnosis and characterization of NCC (40,41,55).

Imaging studies also demonstrate hydrocephalus secondary to chronic arachnoiditis or to an intraventricular cyst (Figs. 8 and 9) (56). In some cases of hydrocephalus with circumferential enlargement of the fourth ventricle, the differential diagnosis between fourth ventricle cysticercus and ventriculitis secondary to chronic inflammation of posterior fossa and ventricular floor is difficult (51). When an intraventricular cysticercus is suspected, but not clearly demonstrated by NIS, a CT with injection of contrast medium into the ventricles (Fig. 13), usually through a ventricular shunt, might be necessary to confirm the diagnosis prior to surgery. Misdiagnosis in cases of ventriculitis is frequent and leads to unnecessary surgical procedures of the posterior fossa (51). In cases of cysticercosis of the spinal cord or the spinal canal, MR and myelography demonstrate the lesions.

Immunodiagnostic Tests

Analysis of cerebrospinal fluid is an indispensable study that completes the information obtained with NIS. The degree of the immune response is evaluated by the presence or absence of signs of inflammation in the CSF as demonstrated by an increase in the cell count ($>5/mm^3$), and protein concentration (>40 mg/dl). When no signs of inflammation are found in CSF, the disease is inactive, immune tolerance has developed, or the lesions are restricted to brain parenchyma without contact with the subarachnoid space. In cases of exclusive parenchymal NCC, the signs of inflammation in the CSF may be minimal or absent. In cases of ventricular cysticercosis, signs of inflammation in CSF are minimal to moderate. In cases of meningeal cysticercosis, the signs of inflammation are moderate to severe. In a study of CSF in 92 patients with meningeal cysticercosis, we found a mean of 140 mg/dl of protein and 80 mononuclear cells per cubic millimeter; however, the values for the protein concentration ranged from 45 to 1200 mg, and the cell count from 8 to 800 cells. Those patients with higher values had in the long term the worst prognosis (39). Pleocytosis is mostly composed of mononuclear cells, and eosinophils are present in about half of cases in a proportion of 1 to 10%. The presence of eosinophils in sediment, though not pathognomonic, is indirect evidence of NCC (2).

Immunodiagnostic tests in CSF are highly specific and sensitive due to the local production of anticysticercus antibodies within the subarachnoid space (49,57). The most common diagnostic tests for NCC in CSF are the enzyme-linked immunosorbent assay (ELISA) and the complement fixation test (CFT). In the experience of our laboratory, the ELISA has a 94% sensitivity and a 98% specificity, and the CFT has a 84% sensitivity with a 98% specificity for the diagnosis of NCC when inflammatory signs in CSF are present. These results were obtained with the ELISA using crude extracts of the membrane of cysts as antigen, the dilution of CSF 1:30, and the conjugate a mixture of antibodies to human IgG and IgM (58,59). The CFT was made with a microtest (60). Immunoblot analysis has been recently incorporated to NCC diagnosis; however, results are difficult to evaluate due to the complex antigenic composition of the parasite with hundreds of antigens, which give bizarre patterns of reactivity with antibodies from both NCC patients and healthy controls. These methods are useful as research tools for NCC, but impractical for everyday diagnosis, particularly in places with technical and economical restraints.

A major obstacle for obtaining access to immunodiagnostic assays for NCC is that laboratories that perform the tests are few and usually distant from localities where the testing is needed, and transportation of CSF to specialized laboratories is costly and difficult. To overcome these limitations, CSF can be stored in a piece of paper retaining its reactivity for the ELISA test almost unchanged for more than 2 months. One milliliter of CSF is placed in a 4×2 cm piece of white common paper, left to dry at room temperature, and mailed in an ordinary envelope to the reference laboratory, where the stored CSF will be rehydrated and the immunodiagnostic test performed. In this way, the transportation and testing of CSF is inexpensive and practical (59).

Another difficulty in the use of immunodiagnostic tests is the limited availability of cysticercus antigen; however, it has been shown that cysticerci antigens from the laboratory-adapted model of *Taenia crassiceps* in mice effectively replace the antigens of cysticerci from *T. solium* for the immunodiagnosis of human cysticercosis in CSF (58), thus providing an unlimited source of antigens for immunodiagnostic tests and their standardization (Fig. 10).

As the ELISA and the CFT are based on different principles for the measurement of humoral immunity to cysticercus antigens, both tests are highly useful for NCC diagnosis. Rather than one test replacing the other, they supplement each other, and their simultaneous use increases the possibility of diagnosis. Immunodiagnostic studies in CSF are also useful to distinguish inactive sequelae of NCC such as granulomas and calcifications, which, in the absence of active forms of the parasite, usually give negative CSF results. The immune test in CSF usually remains positive in cases successfully treated with an anticysticercus drug for a few months after the disappearance of cysts.

Immunodiagnostic tests in serum for NCC are a controversial issue. Some reports have claimed a high positive rate (6,61); however, the experience of many centers with expertise in NCC is that serum immunodiagnostic tests lack reliability for the diagnosis of NCC (3,5,18,57). Several factors might be responsible for their disappointing utility with the everyday diagnosis of NCC: in about 30% of healthy subjects from endemic areas, positive results in serum are obtained (3,5). Patients with asymptomatic muscle cysticercosis without brain involvement have positive results. Cross-reacting antibodies with several other parasitic diseases are also common (4,62). In addition, many patients with a confirmed diagnosis of parenchymal or ventricular NCC in whom CSF tests are positive have negative results in serum tests, particularly those cases with evidence by NIS of a weak or absent inflammatory response against the parasite, those with single lesions, or those with a local immune reaction restricted to the subarachnoid space without a parallel immune response in peripheral blood (49,63,64). It seems that the only practical use of serum immune tests for cysticercosis is for epidemiological studies on the number of individuals in contact with the parasite, but not for diagnostic purposes (5–8).

TREATMENT

Drug Treatment

Two drugs, a benzimidazole, albendazole (ALB), and an isoquinoline, praziquantel (PZQ), have strong cysticidal properties (65–69) (Table 1). The results of medical therapy are related to the location of cysts and the drug concentrations achieved in that location. The greatest benefit of cysticidal therapy is obtained for parenchymal cysticercosis and for clumps of cysticerci in subarachnoid space. The need for surgical extirpation of these cysticerci has sharply decreased during the last years, so that nowadays almost all cases of these forms of NCC are successfully treated with cysticidal drugs. In our experience, approximately 85% of parenchymal cysts are destroyed by a single course of albendazole and approximately 75% by a single course of praziquantel. These two drugs have different chemical and cysticidal properties. One drug may be effective in cases that have had a limited response to the other. The sequential use of one drug and then the other increases the possibility of successful elimination of parasites to more than 95% of parenchymal cysticerci. Drug therapy is effective even in large clumps of cysticerci. Although some of these cases might seem to be good candidates for surgery due to the large size of the cysts and their apparently easy surgical access, a trial of cysticidal therapy is recommended before attempting surgery (70,71). A few cases of large parenchymal or arachnoid cysticerci that did not seem to respond to medical treatment, as evidenced by persistence of the cystic cavity in NIS, were later demonstrated by surgery to be surrounded by a chronic thick capsule of fibrous collagen making a sort of hard cover that impedes the collapse of the cystic cavity after the destruction of the cysticercus.

A suggested therapeutic strategy for NCC is the administration of albendazole 15 mg/kg/day in two daily doses for 8 days (67,72,73); 3 months later, a repeat NIS will demonstrate the degree of therapeutic response by the disappearance or notorious shrinkage of cysts. If some cysts still persist unchanged, a second course of therapy could be attempted with praziquantel in doses of 50 mg/kg/day in three daily doses for 15 days. A higher dose of PZQ may improve its efficacy (69).

During the first few days of cysticidal therapy, headache, vomiting, seizures, or exacerbation of the neurological symptomatology may develop as reactions to drug therapy. Such adverse effects are not due to direct toxicity of either drug, as both ALB and PZQ are remarkably nontoxic in pharmacological studies and when administered to healthy volunteers. The adverse effects are due to an intense inflammatory response from the host to the acute death of the parasites and can be anticipated in patients harboring several cysts. Adverse reactions are intense in patients with many cysts, but moderate or null in patients with only one or two parasites. Nevertheless, the development of headache, usually within 3 days of the beginning of treatment, can be taken as a reliable prediction of treatment success. Then it is important to warn the patient about possible adverse reactions during treatment and what this represents in order to obtain the full cooperation of the patient and to avoid an early abandonment of treatment.

Administration of dexamethasone eliminates or ameliorates the adverse effects of cysticidal therapy; however, the simultaneous administration of dexamethasone and PZQ reduces the plasma concentration of the latter by 50%, decreasing its cysticidal effectiveness (74,75). Quite unexpectedly, it has also been demonstrated that, in contrast to PZQ, simultaneous administration of dexamethasone and ALB increases the plasma concentrations of ALB by 50% (76). Dexamethasone should not, if possible, be administered concomitantly with praziquantel, but it can be added safely to ALB therapy without lowering its cysticidal efficacy (50). An additional advantage of ALB is that it can be administered concomitantly with dexamethasone for the simultaneous therapy of cysticercosis and its associated inflammation.

Albendazole is slightly more effective than praziquantel, it is inexpensive, its length of therapy is shorter, and it can be administered concomitantly with steroids; thus, it seems logically the drug of first choice to begin the therapy of neurocysticercosis (77–79). In some studies, a reduction in the length of ALB therapy by 3 days has been proposed. In cases where diffuse and severe brain edema or vasculitis are present, as in cysticercotic encephalitis, initial therapy should be directed at the amelioration of the immune reaction with steroids and immunosuppressants such as azathioprine followed by cysticidal therapy (77).

For therapy of parenchymal cysticercosis, differentiation must be made between active and inactive forms of the parasite, such as granulomas and calcifications, which are inactive and permanent sequelae of a previous cysticerci. In inactive forms, no response to cysticidal therapy is to be expected.

Epilepsy is the most frequent clinical manifestation of parenchymal NCC and must be treated following the guidelines of the International League Against Epilepsy; however, in cases of seizures secondary to parenchymal cysts that are destroyed by drug therapy without leaving granulomas, the seizures remit within a short period of time (20,68), allowing early withdrawal of antiepileptic drugs. Epilepsy secondary to granulomas usually requires anticonvulsant therapy for several years, and in some cases the seizures are refractory to treatment.

Traditionally, therapy of ocular cysticercosis (Fig. 2) has been considered a surgical province, as early trials of treatment with praziquantel were unsuccessful (80). The possibility of a strong inflammatory reaction within the eye secondary to the destruction of the parasite led to recommendations of caution when attempting cysticidal therapy. Lozano-Elizondo and Barbosa-Horta recently obtained cure of six patients with ocular cysticercosis—four subretinal and two in the vitreous cavity—after 15 days of therapy with a combination of dexamethasone-albendazole. In the four subretinal cases, the lesions were reduced to a small chorioretinal scar. The cysts in the vitreous cavity were killed by the drug and then surgically removed; the procedure was easy as the parasite was immobile. Vision was improved in five of the patients (81).

Surgical Treatment

The treatment of hydrocephalus complicating NCC is a priority before cysticidal therapy is initiated. For hydrocephalus secondary to chronic arachnoiditis, a ventricular shunt is inserted (42,56,82). Once intracranial hypertension has been treated with the drainage of CSF through a ventricular shunt, medical therapy with cysticidal and anti-inflammatory drugs can be initiated; however, results of drug therapy are less effective for chronic arachnoiditis than for parenchymal cysticercosis. Although no controlled studies have been performed with cysticidal drugs for chronic arachnoiditis, it seems that periodical repetition of cysticidal therapy is most likely necessary (39).

Hydrocephalus secondary to a cyst obstructing the fourth ventricle may be resolved with a temporary ventricular shunt that could be removed after the ventricular cyst has been surgically extirpated and the normal CSF flow restored. As with ocular cysticercosis, therapy of ventricular cysticercosis has been primarily surgical (83); however, ALB achieves good concentrations in ventricular fluid. Successful drug therapy of ventricular cysticercosis has been reported in isolated cases (71,84), but controlled trials remain to be performed.

NEUROLOGICAL SEQUELAE

Neurocysticercosis may leave several disabilities. In general terms, the sequelae of NCC can be separated into lesions caused by parenchymal cysticercosis and those caused by meningeal cysticercosis.

Epilepsy is the most frequent sequela of parenchymal cysticercosis (2,15,68,84). In many cases of chronic epilepsy or late-onset epilepsy, NIS reveals a parenchymal brain calcification sequela of cysticercosis that did not produce clinical symptomatology during the active stages of the lesion, was asymptomatic for long periods of time, and presented as epilepsy several years after the destruction of the parasite. This explains why in endemic countries, NCC is the major etiology of late-onset epilepsy (14,15,85). In patients with acute seizures secondary to a single cyst surrounded by intense inflammation (46,47,85), the lesion is usually eliminated by the immune mechanisms of the host. In these cases, the natural history of the seizure disorder is towards remission. The majority of these children have only one or two seizures secondary to the acute infection. In adults, however, the natural history of the seizure disorder is far more complex and difficult to predict. The availability of cysticidal drugs has greatly improved the long-term prognosis of epilepsy secondary to parenchymal cysts. In serial studies, it has been demonstrated that cysticidal drugs not only result in faster elimination of cystic lesions, but can also result in a high cure rate of epilepsy (68). In general terms, when a cysticercus in brain parenchyma is left to its natural evolution and serial NIS demonstrate spontaneous disappearance over the following months or years, three out of every four cysts are replaced by a granuloma or a calcification (Fig. 6). In sharp contrast, most cystic lesions effectively destroyed by cysticidal therapy do not leave granulomas and the brain area that lodged the parasite heals, as demonstrated by a normal NIS at early follow-up (68). In many cases this can be seen within 3 months of cysticidal therapy. It has been demonstrated by clinical and epidemiological studies that the prognosis of seizures is closely related to the persistence of granulomas in brain parenchyma. This is another argument for early cysticidal therapy, which not only eliminates the parasites, but greatly diminishes their sequelae (68,78,86).

Hydrocephalus is the most common sequelae of meningeal cysticercosis; it also has the worst prognosis. The chronic presence of inflammation within the subarachnoid space with a high concentration of cells and protein in the CSF results in periodic occlusion of the valvular mechanisms of ventricular shunts and is the cause of frequent reinterventions, either to unclog the shunt or to change the device (Fig. 8). This type of complication makes the prognosis of meningeal cysticercosis poor in spite of cysticidal therapy (39,42).1 A new type of shunt devoid of a valve mechanism has shown promise for the surgical treatment of hydrocephalus secondary to NCC; however, its long-term performance is still unknown (82,87).

Cerebral infarctions secondary to arteritis are an etiology of mental deterioration and motor disability (43,88). These complications may be decreased by anti-inflammatory therapy with steroids, particularly in those cases with severe meningeal inflammation as demonstrated by CSF studies. In meningeal NCC, fibrotic nerve entrapment is a common etiology of abnormalities with amaurosis, diplopia, and cranial nerve dysfunction.

PREVENTION

Taenia may live in the human intestine for several years, liberating on a daily basis several thousand viable eggs; therefore, a single human host of taenia can be an extensive and lasting source of cysticercosis in the community. In most cases of taeniasis, the disease is asymptomatic. This explains why taeniasis is so rarely diagnosed, even in endemic areas of cysticercosis. The importance of taenia carriers has received little attention in public health strategies to control the spread of this disease. For instance, in surveys carried out among the general population from endemic areas, which have also included people with high educational levels, almost everyone knows what cysticercosis is; however, when asked about the form of transmission, the most frequent answer is that cysticercosis is acquired after eating pork meat infected with cysticerci. It is surprising for most people to learn the relationship of cysticercosis to the intestinal helminth and the transmission of the disease through any food contaminated with human feces. These deficiencies in public knowledge pose obstacles for its prevention by simple hygienic measures.

Eradication of NCC is possible, as has been shown in countries like Germany, which were once endemic for cysticercosis and have been free of the disease for more than 70 years, due to an improvement in living conditions and sanitary implementation. The disease is directly related to low socioeconomic and educational status. Several measures can be taken to interfere in the life cycle of taeniasis/cysticercosis, the most useful of which is massive health education programs of the population in endemic areas about the life cycle of the parasite. Through education, domestic measures can be taken, such as proper disposal of human feces, treatment of contaminated water prior to irrigation of vegetable plantations, compulsory search and treatment of taenia carriers, controlled methods of porcine breeding, and freezing of pork meat either before public distribution or domestically. Two days of freezing of contaminated pork meat kills the cysticerci (89). Although vaccine development with recombinant antigens is a future possibility for the control of endemic infectious diseases, its effectiveness in human parasitic disorders remains to be demonstrated. Vaccination of pigs, however, offers a viable possibility in order to interfere with the life cycle of the parasite (44,90).

REFERENCES

1. Nieto D. Historical notes on cysticercosis. In: Flisser A, Willms K, Laclete JP, Larralde C, Ridaura C, Beltrán F, eds. Cysticercosis: Present State of Knowledge and Perspectives. New York: Academic Press, 1982:1–7.
2. Sotelo J, Guerrero V, Rubio F. Neurocysticercosis: a new classification based on active and inactive forms: a study of 753 cases. Arch Intern Med 1985; 145:442–445.
3. Rosas N, Sotelo J, Nieto D. ELISA in the diagnosis of neurocysticercosis. Arch Neurol 1985; 43:353–356.
4. Larralde C, Montoya RM, Sciutto E, et al. Deciphering western blots of tapeworm antigens (Taenia solium, Echinococcus granulosus, and Taenia crassiceps) reacting with sera from neurocysticercosis and hydatid disease patients. Am J Trop Med Hyg 1989; 40:282–290.
5. Ramos-Kuri M, Montoya RM, Padilla A, et al. Immunodiagnosis of neurocysticercosis: disappointing performance of serology (enzyme-linked immunosorbent assay) in an unbiased sample of neurological patients. Arch Neurol 1992; 49:633–636.
6. Garcia HH, Gilman R, Martinez M, et al. The cysticercosis working group in Peru. Cysticercosis as a major cause of epilepsy in Peru. Lancet 1993; 341:197–200.
7. Willms K. Cestodes (tapeworms). In: Gorbach S, Bartlett JG, Blacklow NR, eds. Infectious Diseases. Philadelphia: W.B. Saunders, 1992:2021–2037.
8. Ciesielski S, Seed JR, Estrada J, et al. The seroprevalence of cysticercosis, malaria, and Trypanosoma cruzi among North Carolina migrant farmworkers. Public Health Rep 1993; 108:736–741.
9. Kong Y, Cho SY, Cho MS, et al. Seroepidemiological observation of Taenia solium cysticercosis in epileptic patients in Korea. J Korean Med Sci 1993; 8:145–152.
10. Michel P, Callies P, Raharison H, et al. Epidemiology of cysticercosis in Madagascar. Bull Soc Pathol Exot 1993; 86:62–67.
11. Del Brutto OH, Sotelo J. Neurocysticercosis: an update. Rev Infect Dis 1988; 10:1075–1087.
12. Gang-zhi W, Cun-jiang L, Jia-mei M, et al. Cysticercosis of the central nervous system: a clinical study of 1400 cases. Chinese Med J 1988; 101:493–500.
13. Sotelo J, Roman GC, Del Brutto OH. Cysticercosis. In: Remingtron JS, Swartz MN, eds. Current Clinical Topics in Infectious Diseases. Vol. 6. Cambridge: Blackwell Science, Inc. (in press).
14. Medina MT, Rosas E, Rubio F, et al. Neurocysticercosis as the main cause of late-onset epilepsy in Mexico. Arch Intern Med 1990; 150:325–327.
15. Placencia M, Shorvon SD, Paredes V, et al. Epileptic seizures in an andean region of Ecuador. Brain 1992; 115:771–782.
16. Flisser A. Neurocysticercosis in Mexico. Parasitol Today 1988; 4:131–137.
17. Villa AM, Monteverde DA, Rodriguez W, et al. Neurocysticercosis in a hospital of the city of Buenos Aires: study of 11 cases. Arq Neuropsiquiatr 1993; 51:333–336.
18. Spina-Franca A, Livramento JA, Machado LR. Cysticercosis of the central nervous system and cerebrospinal fluid. Immunodiagnosis of 1573 patients in 63 years (1929–1992). Arq Neuropsiquiatr 1993; 51:16–20.
19. Ohnishi K, Murata M, Nakane M, et al. Cerebral cysticercosis. Intern Med 1993; 32:569–573.
20. Rajshekhar V. Albendazole therapy for persistent, solitary cysticercus granulomas in patients with seizures. Neurology 1993; 43:1238–1240.
21. Geerts S. The taeniasis-cysticercosis complex in Africa. Meded Zitt K Acad Wet Bull Acad Sci Outre-Mer 1993; 38:245–264.
22. Morgado C, Gomes LB, de Campos JG. Neurocysticercosis. An imaging analysis of 35 cases. Acta Med Port 1994; 7:269–275.
23. Thomson AJ. Neurocysticercosis—experience at the teaching hospitals of the University of Cape Town. S Afr Med J 1993; 83:332–334.
24. Monteiro L, Almeida-Pinto J, Stocker A, et al. Active neurocysticercosis, parenchymal and extra-parenchymal: a study of 38 patients. J Neurol 1993; 241:15–21.
25. Bauer TM, Bruhwiler J, Aschwanden M, et al. Neurocysticercosis. Dtsch Med Wochenschr 1994; 119:175–179.

26. Vanista J, Lapkova E, Uhlikova M. Cysticercosis in the Czech Republic. Cesk Epidemiol Mikrobiol Immunol 1993; 42:187–189.
27. Dietrichs E, Tyssvang T, Aanonsen NO, et al. Cerebral cysticercosis in Norway. Acta Neurol Scand 1993; 88:296–298.
28. Aijaz F, Ahmed A. Cysticercosis in a Muslim woman. JPMA J Pak Med Assoc 1993; 43:23–24.
29. Earnest MP, Reller LB, Filley ChM, et al. Neurocysticercosis in the United States: 35 cases and a review. Rev Infect Dis 1987; 9:961–979.
30. McCormick GF, Zee C-S, Heiden J. Cysticercosis cerebri: review of 127 cases. Arch Neurol 1982; 39:534–539.
31. Mitchell WG, Crawford TO. Intraparenchymal cerebral cysticercosis in children: diagnosis and treatment. Pediatrics 1988; 82:76–82.
32. McCormick GF. Cysticercosis—review of 230 patients. Bull Clin Neurosci 1985; 50:76–101.
33. Escobar A. The pathology of neurocysticercosis. In: Palacios E, Rodríguez-Carbajal J, Taveras JM, eds. Cysticercosis of the Central Nervous System. Springfield, IL: Charles C Thomas, 1983:27–54.
34. Livramento JA, Machado LR, Spina-Franca A. Immunobiology of neurocysticercosis. In: Fejerman N, Chamoles NA, eds. New Trends in Pediatric Neurology. Amsterdam: Elsevier, 1993:307–312.
35. Turner M. Antigenic variation in the trypanosome. Nature 1982; 298:606–607.
36. Trejo V, Castro L, Granados G, et al. MHC Restriction mechanisms of immune response in human neurocysticercosis. Human Immunol 1988; 23:153–154.
37. Herrera LA, Santiago P, Rojas G, et al. Immune response impairment, gonotoxicity and morphological transformation induced by *Taenia solium* metacestode. Mutat Res 1994; 305:223–228.
38. Del Brutto OH, García E, Talamás O, et al. Sex-related severity of inflammation in parenchymal brain cysticercosis. Arch Intern Med 1988; 148:544–546.
39. Sotelo J, Marín C. Hydrocephalus secondary to cysticercotic arachnoiditis: a long-term follow-up review of 92 cases. J Neurosurg 1987; 66:686–689.
40. Rodríguez-Carbajal J, Palacios E. Infectious and parasitic supratentorial disorders. In: Taveras JM, Ferruchi JT, eds. Radiology-Diagnosis-Imaging Intervention. Philadelphia: Lippincott, 1986:207–217.
41. Gulati P, Jena AN, Tripathi RP, et al. MRI (magnetic resonance imaging) spectrum of epilepsy. J Indian Med Assoc 1994; 92:110–112.
42. Estañol B, Kleriga E, Loyo M, et al. Mechanisms of hydrocephalus in cerebral cysticercosis: implications for therapy. Neurosurgery 1983; 13:119–123.
43. Del Brutto OH. Cysticercosis and cerebrovascular disease: a review. J Neurol Neurosurg Psychiatry 1992; 55:252–254.
44. Sciutto E, Fragoso G, Trueba L, et al. Cysticercosis vaccine: cross protecting immunity with *T. solium* antigens against experimental murine *T. crassiceps* cysticercosis. Parasite Immunol 1990; 12:687–696.
45. Alcala H, Hernandez-Aguilar J, Davila G, et al. Neurocysticercosis in children: a study of 100 cases. In: Fukuyama Y, Kamoshita S, Ohtsuka C, Suzuki Y, eds. Modern perspectives of child neurology. Tokyo: Asahi Daily News Co., Ltd., 1991:73–93.
46. Chandy MJ, Rajshekhar V, Prakash S, et al. Cysticercosis causing single, small CT lesions in Indian patients with seizures. Lancet 1989; I:390–391.
47. Rajshekhar V, Haran RP, Prakash GS, et al. Differentiating solitary small cysticercus granulomas and tuberculomas in patients with epilepsy. J Neurosurg 1993; 78:402–407.
48. Byrd SE, Locke GE, Biggers S, et al. The computed tomographic appearance of cerebral cysticercosis in adults and children. Radiology 1982; 144:819–823.
49. Miller BL, Staugaitis SM, Tourtellotte WW, et al. Intra-blood-brain-barrier IgG synthesis in cerebral cysticercosis. Arch Neurol 1985; 42:782–784.
50. Santoyo H, Corona R, Sotelo J. Total recovery of visual function after treatment for cerebral cysticercosis. N Engl J Med 1991; 324:1137–1139.
51. Salazar A, Sotelo J, Martínez H, et al. Differential diagnosis between ventriculitis and fourth ventricle cyst in neurocysticercosis. J Neurosurg 1983; 59:660–663.
52. Keane JR. Cysticercosis: unusual neuro-ophthalmologic signs. J Clin Neuroophthalmol 1993; 13:194–199.
53. Kim KS, Weinberg PE. Spinal cysticercosis. Surg Neurol 1985; 24:80–82.

54. Suss RA, Maravilla KR, Thompson J. MR imaging of intracranial cysticercosis: comparison with CT and anatomopathologic features. AJNR 1986; 7:235–242.
55. Lotz J, Hewlett R, Alheit B, et al. Neurocysticercosis: correlative pathomorphology and MR imaging. Neuroradiology 1988; 30:35–41.
56. Zee CS, Segall HD, Destian S, et al. MRI of intraventricular cysticercosis: surgical implications. J Comput Assist Tomogr 1993; 17:932–939.
57. Katti MK, Chandramukhi A. Detection and characterization of circulating cysticercal antigens in human cerebrospinal fluid. Serodiagnosis Immunother Infect Dis 1990; 4:441–450.
58. Larralde C, Sotelo J, Montoya RM, et al. Immunodiagnosis of human cysticercosis in cerebrospinal fluid. Antigens from murine Taenia crassiceps cysticerci effectively substitute those from porcine Taenia solium. Arch Pathol Lab Med 1990; 114:926–928.
59. García E, Sotelo J. Storage of cerebrospinal fluid on paper. Lancet 1989; II:1046.
60. García E, Sotelo J. A new complement fixation test for the diagnosis of neurocysticercosis in cerebrospinal fluid. J Neurol 1991; 238:379–382.
61. Miller B, Goldberg MA, Heiner D, et al. A new immunologic test for CNS cysticercosis. Neurology 1984; 34:695–697.
62. Muhlschlegel F, Sygulla L, Frosch P, et al. Paramyosin of Echinococcus granulosus. cDNA sequence and characterization of a tegumental antigen. Parasitol Res 1993; 79:660–666.
63. Rubalcava MA, Sotelo J. Differences between ventricular and lumbar CSF in hydrocephalus secondary to cysticercosis. Neurosurgery (in press).
64. Fishman RA. Cerebrospinal Fluid in Diseases of the Nervous System. Philadelphia: W.B. Saunders, 1992.
65. Sotelo J, Escobedo F, Rodríguez-Carbajal J, et al. Therapy of parenchymal brain cysticercosis with praziquantel. N Engl J Med 1984; 310:1001–1007.
66. Leblanc R, Knowles KF, Melanson D, et al. Neurocysticercosis: surgical and medical management with praziquantel. Neurosurgery 1986; 18:419–427.
67. Sotelo J, Penagos P, Escobedo F, et al. Short course of albendazole therapy for neurocysticercosis. Arch Neurol 1988; 45:1130–1133.
68. Vázquez V, Sotelo J. The course of seizures after treatment for cerebral cysticercosis. N Engl J Med 1992; 327:696–701.
69. Bittencourt PRM, Gracia CM, Gorz AM, et al. High-dose praziquantel for neurocysticercosis: efficacy and tolerability. Eur Neurol 1990; 30:229–234.
70. Del Brutto OH, Sotelo J, Aguirre R, et al. Albendazole therapy for giant subarachnoid cysticerci. Arch Neurol 1992; 49:535–538.
71. Del Brutto OH, Sotelo J. Albendazole therapy for subarachnoid and ventricular cysticercosis. Case report. J Neurosurg 1990; 72:816–817.
72. Sánchez M, Suástegui R, González-Esquivel D, et al. Pharmacokinetic comparison of two albendazole dosage regimens in patients with neurocysticercosis. Clin Neuropharmacol 1993; 16:77–82.
73. Botero D, Uribe CS, Sanchez JL, et al. Short course albendazole treatment for neurocysticercosis in Columbia. Trans R Soc Trop Med Hyg 1993; 87:576–577.
74. Vázquez ML, Jung H, Sotelo J. Plasma levels of praziquantel decrease when dexamethasone is given simultaneously. Neurology 1987; 37:1561–1562.
75. Shandera WX, White AC Jr, Chen JC, et al. Neurocysticercosis in Houston, Texas. A report of 112 cases. Med Baltimore 1994; 73:37–52.
76. Jung H, Hurtado M, Medina MT, et al. Dexamethasone increases plasma levels of albendazole. J Neurol 1990; 237:279–280.
77. Del Brutto OH, Sotelo J, Roman G. Therapy for neurocysticercosis: a reappraisal. Clin Infect Dis 1993; 17:730–735.
78. Sotelo J, Del Brutto OH, Penagos P, et al. Comparison of therapeutic regimen of anticysticercal drugs for parenchymal brain cysticercosis. J Neurol 1990; 237:69–72.
79. Chotmongkol V. Treatment of neurocysticercosis with a two week course of albendazole. Southeast Asian J Trop Med Public Health 1993; 24:396–398.

80. Santos R, Chavarría M, Aguirre AE. Failure of medical treatment in two cases of intraocular cysticercosis. Am J Ophthalmol 1984; 97:249–250.
81. Lozano-Elizondo D, Barbosa-Horta S. Tratamiento con albendazol de la cisticercosis intraocular. Rev Mex Oftalmol 1990; 64:15–28.
82. Sotelo J, Rubalcava MA, Gomez-Llata S. A new shunt for hydrocephalus that relies on CSF production rather than on ventricular pressure: initial clinical experiences. Surg Neurol (in press).
83. Apuzzo MLJ, Dobkin WR, Zee C-S, et al. Surgical considerations in treatment of intraventricular cysticercosis: an analysis of 45 cases. J Neurosurg 1984; 60:400–407.
84. Allcut DA, Coulthard A. Neurocysticercosis: regression of a fourth ventricular cyst with praziquantel. J Neurol Neurosurg Psychiatry 1991; 54:461–462.
85. Del Brutto OH, Santibañez R, Noboa CA, et al. Epilepsy due to neurocysticercosis: analysis of 203 patients. Neurology 1992; 42:389–392.
86. Del Brutto OH. The use of albendazole in patients with single lesions enhanced on contrast CT. N Engl J Med 1993; 328:356–357.
87. Sotelo J. A new ventriculoperitoneal shunt for treatment of hydrocephalus. Experimental results. Eur J Biomed Technol RBM 1993; 15:1–6.
88. Monteiro L, Almeida J, Leite J, et al. Cerebral cysticercus arteritis: five angiographic cases. Cerebrovasc Dis 1994; 4:125–133.
89. Sotelo J, Rosas N, Palencia G. Freezing of infested pork muscle kills cysticerci. JAMA 1986; 256: 893–894.
90. Molinari JL, Soto R, Tato P, et al. Immunization against porcine cysticercosis in an endemic area in Mexico: a field and laboratory study. Am J Trop Med Hyg 1993; 49:502–512.

27

Rabies

Thiravat Hemachudha
Chulalongkorn University Hospital, Bangkok, Thailand

Although there is a broad range of pathogens that can cause acute viral encephalitis, rabies represents one of the most frequently recognized central nervous system (CNS) infections due to its typical and horrifying presentation and invariably fatal course. Rabies virus belongs to the *Lyssavirus* genus of the Rhabdovirus family. It is a strict neurotropic virus infection that can infect all mammals with nearly worldwide distribution. Different species have different levels of susceptibility, latency, and infectivity. Efficient transmission depends on the degree of aggression and efficiency of bites, as well as the amount of virus in salivary excretion. Rabies is the major cause of encephalitides in developing countries where the control of the dog population and immunization are not adequate. Among 35,000 annual human rabies deaths worldwide, most are attributable to dog bites (1). Rabies is a distant threat to humans in North America and Western Europe, where wildlife populations (e.g., bats, raccoons, foxes, skunks) are the major reservoirs. The number of rabies deaths in the United States significantly declined from approximately 50 in the 1940s and 1950s to an average of 2 per year during the following two decades (2,3). This paralleled the success of dog control programs, which then shifted the ecological balance of reservoirs from domestic animals to that of wild and sylvatic populations (4). Among the wildlife animals, bats have been responsible for most of the rabies deaths in the United States since 1980 (4). The number of cases of rabies may also have increased because of an increasing number of travelers to rabies-endemic areas and economic migrants. Physicians should be able to give proper advice in cases of both pre- and postexposure rabies prophylaxis and be able to diagnose and to differentiate rabies from other encephalitides.

HISTORY

Rabies was recognized thousands of years before the Christian era. The earliest record dates back to the period of Babylonian civilization (5,6). Rabies was described in the Laws of Eshnunna, circa 2000 B.C. The word *rabies* (Latin) is derived from *rabhas* (in Sanskrit), which means "to do violence." The disease is also called *Lyssa* or *Lytta* (in Greek) and *rage* (in French). Both names mean "madness," reflecting its characteristic clinical manifestation. The infectivity of saliva and even of urine of rabid dogs was suspected since the Roman times, and thus the disease was described as poisonous, for which the Latin word was *virus*. It was not until 1804 that transmission of infection by saliva was demonstrated. Burning or cupping of the wounds of those bitten by rabid dogs had been practiced since the first century and continued into the nineteenth century. Experiments during the last 100 years have confirmed the importance of appropriate wound care and of the use of locally applied virucidal agents as first aid treatment.

Virus spreading to the CNS by a neural route was postulated in 1769 by Morgagni based on the symptoms of paresthesias at the bite site before the onset of rabies. This mechanism of viral spread to CNS was also suggested by DiVesta and Zagari in 1889, who induced artificial infection in rabbits by direct inoculation of the virus into the nerve. However, it was Pasteur's ingenious experiment that for the first time in medical history demonstrated the CNS as a prime target and proved that the disease mainly affected the bulb that joined the spinal cord to the brain (6,7). Pasteur also showed that saliva was not the only source of virus, but that nervous tissue was also infectious, especially when inoculated beneath the dura mater. He discovered that the virulence of rabies increased with a fixed incubation period (7 days instead of several weeks) by serial subdural passage of the virus into rabbits. This is why it is referred to as a "fixed virus." Attenuation of the virus could be obtained by passing it from dog to monkey and then from monkey to monkey.

Rabies prophylaxis in humans became accepted in 1885, shortly after Pasteur had successfully immunized laboratory animals by serial subcutaneous injections beginning with avirulent and then increasingly virulent rabies-infected rabbit spinal cord preparations (6,7). Joseph Meister, a 9-year-old boy who had been bitten 14 times by a rabid dog, survived after receiving 13 injections of Pasteur's vaccine. Rabies vaccine made from animal nervous tissue has been used widely ever since. Pasteur's antirabies treatment saved the lives of countless victims, but it carried some serious neuroparalytic adverse effects. These were first documented in 1888 by Remlinger (6). Early studies indicated that these untoward effects were not caused by attenuated or inactivated rabies virus, but by "some component of the nerve substance" in the vaccine (8). This conclusion led Rivers and Schwentker to inoculate monkeys repeatedly with homogenates of normal rabbit brain, which resulted in the first induction of experimental allergic encephalomyelitis, a useful model in studying immune-mediated encephalitis and neuritis (9).

Modern cell culture rabies vaccine has proved itself to be close to an ideal immunogen based on its potency, few doses required, relative lack of side effects, and, most importantly, its efficacy. Human diploid cell rabies vaccine and heterologous (produced in mule) antirabies serum protected all but one of 45 persons who were bitten by rabid dogs and wolves in northern Iran in 1975 (10). Since then there have been safe and potent vaccines prepared in different cell cultures such as chick embryo and Vero cells. Due to the serious complications of nerve tissue vaccines that develop in approximately 1 in 400 vaccinated people (11,12) and the availability of safe and potent tissue culture rabies vaccines, in 1992 the World Health Organization (WHO) recommended limiting or abandoning the production and use of encephalitogenic brain tissue vaccines (13).

For postexposure prophylaxis in severely bitten cases, it became obvious that antirabies serum (purified rabies immune globulin nowadays) plus vaccine was more effective than an intensive course of vaccine alone. In 1954, a rabid wolf attacked 29 people in an Iranian village. Among the 17 persons treated with heterologous immune serum–inactivated brain tissue vaccine, only one died (versus 3 of 12 who received vaccine alone) (6,14). Due to unsatisfactory potency and serious side effects, the use of antirabies serum was soon replaced by a more potent and relatively safe equine and human rabies immune globulin.

Additional major events in rabies control include (1) the identification of pathognomonic Negri bodies, intracytoplasmic inclusions in 1903 (15), (2) the development of the mouse inoculation test (MIT) in 1935 (16), and (3) the fluorescent antibody test (FAT) in 1958 (17,18) for the diagnosis of infected brains. FAT remains the most practical and reliable diagnostic tool worldwide today (19,20). MIT continues to be useful as a confirmatory test for rabies in many countries, but has no role in the treatment decision because it requires at least 7 days to obtain results. More sensitive but sophisticated and expensive techniques include enzyme immunoassay, hybridization with DNA probes, and gene amplification technique by polymerase chain reaction (PCR) (21–23). These molecular methods with DNA fingerprinting and sequencing techniques, together with the use of monoclonal antibodies, led to the new era of rabies antigenic and genetic classifications (13,24–28).

Classical rabies virus and those isolated from terrestrial mammals and insectivorous and haematophagous bats constitute serotype 1. Rabies-related viruses are classified as serotype 2 (Lagos bat), serotype 3 (Mokola), serotype 4 (Duvenhage), and serotype 5 (European bat lyssavirus) or EBL 1 and 2, isolated from *Eptesicus serotinus* and Myotis bats, respectively (13). The public health significance of rabies-related viruses is minor, but may become a potential threat, especially in Africa (serotypes 2 to 4) and Europe (serotype 5) due to diagnostic difficulties and possible lack of efficacious vaccines (13,29).

The mass application of a potent single inoculation of rabies vaccine for dogs in the 1940s was an outstanding success in the control of rabies (6). Legally enforced canine rabies immunization, a practice of strict quarantine, and rigid control of stray dogs have brought canine rabies under control in North America and western Europe. However, rabies remains endemic in wildlife species and continues to pose a hazard due to its potential for incidental transmission to domestic animals and humans. Total eradication has been possible only in island populations (such as England, Japan, Australia, and New Zealand) (29). Recent progress led to the development of oral and parenteral poxvirus- and adenovirus-vectored recombinant and parenteral plasmid rabies vaccines that were successful in experimental studies in animals (30–33) and in humans (34). Oral immunization with modified live virus or recombinant vaccinia virus expressing the glycoprotein gene of rabies virus has proved to be effective in field trials in foxes (13,35,36). This is potentially applicable for use in dogs, especially in canine rabies endemic areas (almost all of Asia, Latin America, and Africa) (37).

PATHOPHYSIOLOGY

Rabies in humans worldwide is mostly caused by serotype 1 lyssavirus transmitted by means of bites or scratches from rabid dogs. In only rare circumstances is serotype 1 lyssavirus disease due to wildlife animal bites, especially those of hematophagous and insectivorous bats (29,38–44). The bullet-shaped rabies virus contains a single, nonsegmented RNA molecule of 11,932 nucleotides of negative polarity (45). Transcription of the genomic RNA template into complementary messenger RNA (mRNA) by RNA-dependent RNA polymerase is required before replication. Excessive accumulation of ribonucleoprotein in the cytoplasm results in the formation of Negri bodies (46).

Although rabies usually follows bite exposure, it can be acquired via aerosol exposure from aerosolized rabies virus in caves inhabited by rabid bats (47) and in laboratory accidents with infected aerosolized tissue (48,49). Transmission of rabies is also associated with handling and skinning of infected carcass (50,51), exposure of the conjunctiva, oral mucous membranes, genitalia, and skin abrasions to the saliva of rabid animals (52,53). A lick by a rabid animal is dangerous only if the skin is damaged (54). Human-to-human transmission other than corneal transplantation (55) has not been documented, although there is still a potential risk to the contact of patients with rabies since secretions are frequently virus-positive (56). The transplacental route has been rarely reported in humans (57), but is well recognized in cattle (58). Babies born to mothers with rabies encephalitis were found to be healthy (59,60). Rabies can also be transmitted in experimental animals through oral-nasal routes and tracheal instillation of virus (61,62).

Once rabies virus successfully penetrates the protective epithelium, it gains access to the CNS by retrograde axoplasmic flow at a rate of 8–20 mm/day (63–67). Neurectomy or leg amputation proximal to the inoculation site in mice and rats prevents rabies (68,69). It is the severity of the wound (transdermal bite with bleeding), particularly if deep enough to the muscle, at the area where muscle surfaces contain high densities of nicotinic acetylcholine receptor (nAchR) that determines the likelihood of developing rabies (13,70). The risk of rabies after a bite (5–80%) is about 50 times the risk after scratches (0.1–1%) (71). Binding of the virus glycoprotein to nAchR at the membrane of the muscle leads to a multiplication of virus in the muscle cells (72–75). The nAchR appears to be the rabies virus receptor (76–80). Rabies virus binding to nAchR is inhibited by α-bungarotoxin and d-tubocurarine. Sequence homology of amino acids between rabies viral glycoprotein and snake venom curaremimetic neurotoxins has also been demonstrated. Monoclonal antibodies to the α subunit of the nAchR and monoclonal antibodies against rabies virus (anti-idiotype antibodies) specifically block viral binding in vitro (81,82). Localization of virus to the muscles may lead to variable periods of delay, which in turn provides an opportunity for host immune clearance and for postexposure treatment (23,83,84). It remains unknown which factors—virus strain and concentration, inoculation route, genetic susceptibility or a prompt and effective host immune response—control the length of this period of delay (55,75,85).

After budding from plasma membranes of the muscle cells, virus or its genome is taken up into the unmyelinated nerve endings at the neuromuscular junctions or at the muscle spindles. Rabies virus reaches the CNS by retrograde axoplasmic flow, which can be prevented experimentally in mice by neurectomy and colchicine and vinblastine (63–69). Travel time from the peripheral nerve to CNS, therefore, is relatively constant and depends on the proximity of the lesion to the CNS. Upon reaching the dorsal root ganglion, rabies virus is able to multiply again. Viral replication may be recognized and attacked by immune effectors causing ganglioneuronitis (55,86). There is uncertainty about the relative involvement of sensory or motor pathways; however, motor nerve may be preferentially involved since classic prodromal symptoms of paresthesias and itch at the bite site, likely caused by ganglioneuronitis, have been observed in only one third of 100 cases. Furthermore, motor nerve is in close contact to neuromuscular junction, where virus antigen accumulation has been primarily observed.

In very rare circumstances, rabies virus may enter the nerve directly without prior replication in muscle, resulting in an extremely short incubation period. This was demonstrated in a man who had been bitten by a rabid dog with brachial plexus injury and died of rabies 5 days after the incident despite treatment with tissue culture vaccine and rabies immune globulin. This direct entry into the nerve has been confirmed by inoculating rabies virus into the anterior chamber of the eye of the rat (87) and also in a mouse model by inoculation of the masseter or of the forelimb muscles (88,89). The risk of rabies is very low from superficial wounds (71) (with no or only minute bleeding) even at areas of abundant nerve supply such as the face and hand, suggesting that direct entry into intradermal nerve from a superficial wound is unlikely.

Once rabies virus reaches the CNS, rapid amplification occurs in neuronal perikarya and virus disseminates via plasma membrane budding and direct cell-to-cell transmission or by transsynaptic propagation (73,90–92). Following stereotaxic inoculation into the striatum, rabies virus has been shown to travel by retrograde fast axonal transport (200–400 mm/day) (93). Neurons are the CNS cells selectively involved, although infection of astrocytes and glial cells in animals and humans has been reported (90,91,94–97). Glial cells are significantly less susceptible than neurons to rabies virus infection in vitro (98).

Early studies in rabies-infected mice demonstrated a selective vulnerability of the neuronal cells of the limbic system, especially the hippocampus, suggesting that virus localization to this area of the brain may account for the behavioral abnormalities of the disease (99,100). Subsequent studies in mice, however, had discrepant results, in that hippocampus contained a minimal amount or none of the rabies virus antigen in the early stage as determined by immunohistochemical techniques (101). Studies in skunks infected with skunk street rabies virus showed that areas that contained heavy accumulations were the motor nucleus of the vagus nerve, midbrain raphe, hypoglossal, and red nuclei (102). These street rabies virus–infected skunks manifested as furious rabies. All of this suggests that virus localization may not solely explain limbic symptomatology or the diversity of the clinical manifestations.

In human rabies, clinical and laboratory evidence suggests that functional changes and clinical manifestations (including mood and behavior, motor weakness, etc.) are due to a differential response of the various CNS regions (103). There is no correlation between the regional distribution of rabies viral antigen and clinical expression (encephalitic or paralytic) (97). The brain stem, thalamus, basal ganglion, cerebellum, and spinal cord are the areas mainly affected, as demonstrated by the presence of rabies antigen using avidin-biotin immunohistochemical technique. Patients in one series who had a survival time of 7 days or less had a greater amount of antigen-positive neurons in such structures (97). Moreover, minimal or no rabies viral antigen was found in hippocampus and neocortex. During the early phase of clinical rabies (within 72 h), serum cortisol levels were significantly elevated as compared to those with viral encephalitis other than rabies and others with immune-mediated encephalitis (103). This indicates early stimulation of limbic structures, including the hypothalamus, which may relate to the behavioral changes. None of these patients were comatose or in a state of circulatory collapse. No rabies viral antigen could be demonstrated in the hypothalamus of some of these patients studied. Involvement of the hypothalamo-pituitary-adrenal axis with adrenal hormone toxicity also resulted in wasting syndrome and lymphoid depletion in thymus, spleen, and lymph nodes in mice (104,105).

Clinical as well as subclinical seizures (as evidenced by abnormal paroxysmal high-amplitude sharp wave activity in electroencephalographic recordings) have been observed as early as 1 or 2 days after the onset of clinical symptoms (103,106). It is unlikely that these cortical discharges can be explained by the presence of virus in brain cortical cells at such an early period. Regional imbalance of neurotransmitters leading to neurophysiological abnormalities or remote effects from the actual site of virus replication, particularly in the brain stem, has been postulated (85,107,108).

Altered neurotransmitter metabolism in terms of a decrease in potassium-evoked 5-HT release in rabies virus–infected cortical synaptosomes and an increase in gamma-amino-*n*-butyric acid transport in infected primary cortical cultures has been reported (109,110). It has been shown that there are modifications in opiate and muscarinic acetylcholine and 5-HT1D receptor affinity in mouse neuroblastoma–rat glioma hybrid cells and in rabies-infected rat brain (111–113). Recent studies in rabies virus–infected dog brains during its early stage showed that muscarinic AchR binding was impaired only in hippocampus and brain-stem regions (114). It is not known whether alterations of certain neurotransmitter metabolism and receptor function are responsible for clinical diversity. Altered electrical activities and sleep pattern changes have been demonstrated in chronically implanted mice and cats infected with street and fixed rabies virus (115–117).

The presence and amount of virus in the CNS does not appear to determine the clinical and functional severity of the disease. Access of the virus to the CNS does not necessarily lead to rapid development of symptoms and death. High titers to virus in the brain and spinal cord can be found in animals long before clinical signs appear (118). Abortive rabies and recovery from clinical rabies with or without residua have been repeatedly reported in many species (118–127). As many as 20% of dogs recovered from rabies after developing clinical signs (128). The degree of muscarinic AchR function modifications in hippocampus was not dependent on the amount of virus (114). Rabies virus antigen was easily demonstrable by the immunofluorescent test in the frontal area of one paralytic patient who had quadriplegia and respiratory failure requiring ventilatory support and who was euphoric but conscious and rational at the time of biopsy, which was performed 19 days after the onset of the clinical illness (129). The mechanisms mediating this susceptibility/resistance are certainly complex and involve genetic, immunological, and virological factors.

Genetically resistant strains of mice demonstrate a restriction of viral replication within the CNS, which is in turn correlated with the early appearance of CNS-neutralizing antibody (130,131). CD8+ T cells appear to have no role in this murine resistance (132). Lymphoid depletion due to cortisol toxicity does not explain disease susceptibility since this was observed in both infected susceptible and resistant strains of mice (105). Adrenalectomy to decrease the cortisol level does not alter the development of neutralizing antibody or lethality. Virulence can also be determined by strain of virus. Fixed rabies virus injures neurons more extensively than street strains (133). Apathogenic rabies virus resulted from only one amino acid substitution at position 333 of the glycoprotein during an in vitro selection wilth antiglycoprotein monoclonal antibodies (134,135). Rate of cell-to-cell spread, number of infected neurons, and degree of cellular necrosis were much lower in the case of this apathogenic virus (136).

Successful clearance of rabies virus requires cooperation of both cellular and humoral immunity. Depletion of both T and B cells potentiates infection much more seriously than either one alone (137). Similarly, adoptive transfer in immunosuppressed animals with combined T and B cells soon after infection reduced mortality in more than either cell type alone (138). Cell-mediated cytotoxic response correlates with degree of survival in mice infected with rabies virus (139,140). Recovery in immunosuppressed mice correlates with the return of a cytolytic T-cell response (141,142).

In human rabies, multiple defects of immune responses or "immune paralysis" have been observed (Fig. 1) (103). Natural killer (NK) cells of rabies patients, examined during the first few days after the onset, are not fully stimulated although the number was normal (143). Moreover, NK cells could not be demonstrated in the brain of rabies patients (103). The process of activation, proliferation, and sequestration of NK cells may not occur in rabies patients and may reflect a naive condition. This may contribute to the rapid dissemination of virus. Only a minority (25%) of nonvaccinated rabies patients had neutralizing antibody in the serum (103,129,144). Development of the antibody does not correlate with survival, suggesting that it is not an insufficient antigenic mass that is responsible for the poor antibody response. Antibody was present as early as 3 days after onset of the first symptoms in one half of the patients. This suggests that the process of immune recognition and of antibody development at the inoculation sites or at the ganglion occurs earlier than the onset of clinical symptoms. Analysis of antibody response to different antigens of rabies virus showed an inefficient production of antibody to both glycoproteins and particularly, nucleocapsid antigens of rabies virus (144). Nucleocapsid antigen recognition is crucial for development of rabies-neutralizing antiglycoprotein antibody (31,145–148). Furthermore, there are defects in cell-mediated immune response and immune activation. Absence of cellular immunity to rabies virus and deficient production of soluble interleukin (IL)-2 receptor and IL-6 were noted in paralytic rabies patients (129,149). The effect of adrenal hormone toxicity on lymphoid depletion has been demonstrated in mice (105), however, elevated cortisol levels cannot explain this phenomenon in rabies patients. Elevated levels of serum cortisol have been found in both encephalitic (mean 49.45 μg/dl, $n = 22$) and paralytic rabies patients (mean 34.11 μg/dl, $n = 8$) (103).

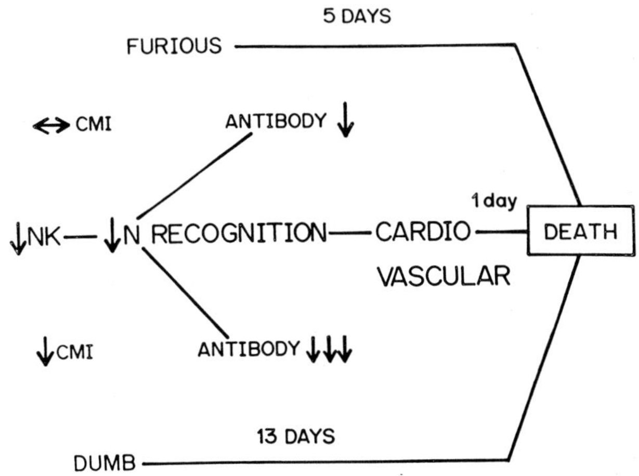

Figure 1 Defects of immune responses and immune-accelerated death in human rabies. Natural killer (NK) cells are not fully stimulated during the early stage. Defect in immune recognition to nucleocapsid (N) protein in addition to depressed cell-mediated immunity (CMI), particularly in the case of paralytic rabies, may be involved in the lack of or inefficient production of rabies virus–neutralizing antibody. Furious rabies patients have intact CMI and die faster (average of 5 days vs. 13 days in the case of paralytic rabies with depressed CMI) than paralytic rabies patients. Prime cause of rabies death is cardiovascular failure, which usually manifests during the last 24 h.

Immune responses in rabies patients also have a devastating role in accelerating disease course and influencing the clinical manifestations (Fig. 1) (129,149). Rabies patients with intact cellular immunity tend to present with encephalitic rabies and to die faster (average of 5 days). Those with an absence of a lymphocytic proliferation to rabies antigen and poor production of soluble IL-2 receptors and IL-6 survived longer (average of 13 days) in a paralytic form of rabies. This "early death" phenomenon has been shown in animal studies and suggests an immune role particularly of a T-lymphocyte dependency (150–155). It should be noted that rabies-infected humans and mouse with intact T-cell response have a similar rapid clinical course but differ in clinical expression (encephalitis in humans and paralysis in mouse). Moreover, an autoimmune process may also play a role since myelin basic protein cellular reactivity positive patients also die faster (129). Nevertheless, it is not clearly understood which mechanism(s) really mediates the neuronal functional derangements and death since inflammation and neuronal necrosis is usually scant even in the case of encephalitic rabies (55,97). Moreover, it remains puzzling how a neurotropic virus such as rabies with no viremia and no evidence of infection of circulating mononuclear cells causes immune paralysis.

The neuropathogenic effects may be mediated by cytokines. These cytokines may be produced either by activated circulating immune cells or by CNS cytokine-secreting cells in the brain stem where the virus resides. Nucleocapsid of the rabies virus is a superantigen thus able to powerfully stimulate the production of cytokines (156,157). However, serum levels of soluble IL-2 receptors in encephalitic rabies patients were comparable to those of nonrabies encephalitis and immune-mediated encephalitis (149). Nevertheless, it remains possible that the exogenous and locally produced cytokines in turn may initiate a breakdown of sphingomyelin and ceramide production with resultant apoptosis (158). In some cases where inflammation also exists, nitric oxide and excitotoxicity processes may also be responsible for neuronal damage (159). Rabies virus infection may alter neurotransmitter expression as previously shown in the cases of lymphocytic choriomeningitis virus (160) and Borna disease virus (161), thus inducing significant electrophysiological and sleep alterations (106,116,117,162). Recently, it has also been demonstrated that rabies infection modulates the expression of the immediate-early (*egr*-1, *jun* B, *c-fos*) and late response (encoding enkephalin) genes at particular regions of the brain (163). These gene products may render neurons more susceptible to viral replication.

Systemic immune dysfunction in human rabies may be affected by manipulation of the neuroendocrine control at the level of the hypothalamus-pituitary axis during the course of rabies infection. Immunocompetent cells contain a remarkable range of peptides, hormones, and receptors classically associated with neuronal tissue of endocrine cells (164). Peptides or hormones released from the neural axis can exert either inhibitory or stimulatory effects on activation, proliferation, migration, and secretion of various cell types including T, B, and NK cells and macrophages. Neural regulation of immune function is also possible through the sympathetic nervous system. Thymus, spleen, and lymph nodes are richly supplied by autonomic nerve fibers. The secretions of some of them can be regulated by catecholamines released at the autonomic nerve endings and from the adrenal medulla and by pituitary hormones.

Interactions among these three axes of infected neuron, altered neurotransmitter-peptide hormone, and immune acceleration-paralysis undoubtedly play a role in the complex but unique manifestations of human rabies.

Animal host and strain may not be the major determinant for clinical manifestations, although rabies after a vampire bat bite is almost always the paralytic form (40,41,43). A recent outbreak of human rabies in the Peruvian jungle transmitted by vampire bats, however, presented as the furious form (38). Furthermore, the same dog that transmitted paralytic rabies to one patient also caused classical encephalitic rabies in another (129). Characterization of rabies virus isolates that caused furious and dumb rabies in Thai dogs using panels of nucleoprotein (N) and glycoprotein (G)-specific monoclonal antibodies, and genetic analysis revealed an identical pattern (23). Furthermore, as mentioned above, localization of rabies viral antigen or degree of inflammation does not account for the two different clinical presentations, nor does the site of the bite (97,152). Unsuccessful immunization attempts, a widely quoted predisposing factor for paralytic rabies, were found in only five cases (personal experience of over 100 rabies patients, approximately one third with paralysis). This has also been the case in another report (165).

Centrifugal spread from the CNS along the autonomic nerves to peripheral organs, especially salivary glands, is an important component of a complete rabies cycle (166). Salivary excretion of virus can be detected up to 14 days before the development of clinical disease in dogs (128). Intermittent secretion of rabies virus also occurs in asymptomatic dogs and dogs that have recovered from clinical rabies (128,167). Peripheral tissues, such as nape of the neck and cornea, can serve as diagnostic materials (168). Since all neural and nonneural organs, except blood, are involved in the terminal phase, the organs of patients with neurological disease should not be used for transplantation (13). Six cases of rabies have been reported from transplantation of cornea from donors who died of undiagnosed rabies (4,55).

CLINICAL PRESENTATION AND CLINICAL COURSE

Not every rabid animal bite necessarily results in clinical rabies. Rabies mortality varies from 35 to 57% in unvaccinated bite victims (55). The risk of developing clinical rabies depends on the severity of the wound, regardless of the site and number, and the virus content of the saliva. Transdermal bites (especially with bleeding) at the head, face, neck, and hand carry the highest risk and are usually associated with a shorter incubation period; nevertheless, a bite on the leg or foot must be treated with the same urgency as bites elsewhere.

Clinical features of rabies differ in many aspects from other forms of encephalitis (55,103,129).

These can be classified into two separate types: encephalitic (furious) and paralytic (dumb) rabies. These two forms also differ in terms of the survival period. Once infection occurs, the clinical can be divided into five stages: the incubation period, the prodrome, the acute neurological phase, coma, and death or recovery.

Incubation Period

The incubation period for rabies is the most variable of all acute CNS infections. It is usually 1–2 months but may range from less than 7 days to 6 years (23,55,83,84). The cases with unusually long incubation periods (11 months, 4 and 6 years) as reported by Smith et al. (23), were migrants who came to the United States from Laos, the Phillippines, and Mexico. Isolates obtained from these cases were antigenically and genetically identical to those from the countries of origin. However, most cases with reported incubation periods exceeding one year may have been due to unrecognized or trivial exposure to bats or other animals. This is particularly true in rabies-endemic areas where frequent exposures are common. On the other hand, there may be no history of a bite (6% of 707 cases in Thailand between 1979 and 1985). There may have been an insignificant exposure, or exposure may have occurred so long before the onset of symptoms that it was not recognized by the patient.

Prodrome

The initial symtoms of rabies indicate the presence of virus in the CNS and dorsal root ganglion. The symptoms are usually vague and nonspecific in the form of fever, generalized muscular aching, and gastrointestinal symptoms. They are thus nondiagnostic and also occur in most patients who have been bitten but never develop the disease. Only the local symptoms at the bite site or a bitten extremity can be reliably used in diagnosis. There may be paresthesias, tingling, itching, or burning sensations starting at the wound, which then may gradually spread to involve the whole limb in a nonradicular pattern or the ipsilateral side of the face. Such local symptoms, although useful, must be interpreted with caution. Only an intense progressive local reaction that involves the whole limb is a reliable indicator of rabies. This "local prodrome" (paresthesias, itching, burning) may occur distant to the bite site (103). Two patients had a bite on the toes but developed severe itching in their ears as a prodrome. One of them tore his eardrum with a pencil trying to relieve these symptoms. Local symptoms are equally common in patients with encephalitic and paralytic rabies and may be seen in as many as 16–80% of the cases (30% in author's experience) (55,94,103,129,169–171).

Acute Neurological Phase

Within hours or a few days after the prodrome, rabies patients enter an acute neurological phase. Two thirds of the patients suffer from an encephalitic or furious form, and the remaining present with paralysis or a condition resembling Guillain-Barré syndrome (GBS). Patients with the furious presentation generally die within 7 days (average 5 days) after the clinical onset, although survival may be as long as 2–3 weeks. The average length of survival is 13 days in paralytic cases. The terms encephalitis and paralysis are used to emphasize that the symptoms and signs are indicative of cerebral hemispheric involvement in the former and of spinal cord and peripheral nerve involvement in the latter.

Encephalitic (Furious) Rabies

The earliest neurological abnormality in furious rabies is an intense anxiety reaction or nervousness that can be aggravated by internal (thirst or fear, etc.) or external (bright light, loud noise, etc.) stimuli. Fever is a constant finding and may appear during the prodromal phase. This is followed within hours by the typical furious rabies features. There are three major cardinal signs of furious rabies.

Fluctuating Consciousness. The mental status alternates between periods of progressively more severe agitation and periods of relative normalcy and depression. The patient abruptly becomes confused and disoriented without any warning (Fig. 2). This bizarre behavior usually lasts only for minute(s) and then abates. The patient then becomes lucid and cannot recall events. As the disease progresses, confusion becomes severe and may evolve to wild agitation and aggressiveness. Between these episodes of agitation, the patient is drowsy but arousable. The period of irritability is gradually succeeded by impaired consciousness and coma.

Phobic Spasms and Inspiratory Spasms. Aero- and hydrophobia occur in all patients with furious rabies; however, phobic spasms may not be present throughout all stages of the disease, especially once drowsiness and coma supervene. Aero- and hydrophobia can be demonstrated by blowing or fanning air on the face or chest wall of the patient and by encouraging the patient to swallow or merely offering a cup of water. This startle reaction results from spasms of the accessory respiratory muscles of the neck and diaphragm, followed by neck flexion or extension. Opisthotonos is extremely rare. Intermittent inspiratory spasms, which occur spontaneously every few minutes without inducing stimuli, replace the phobic spasms once the patient lapses into coma (Fig. 3). These inspiratory spasms actually may appear in the early stage but escape notice due to their nonintense character in the beginning and a relatively infrequent occurrence. The mechanism of these spasms has not been clearly delineated but may involve dysfunction of

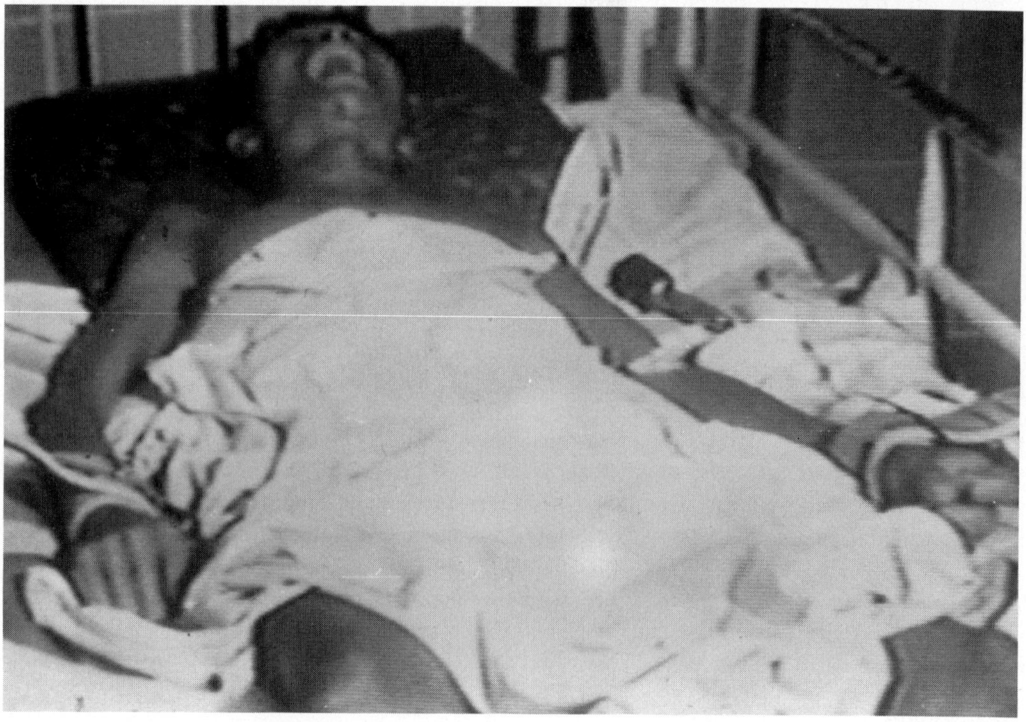

Figure 2 One of the characteristic features in patients with encephalitic rabies is alternating intervals of full comprehension, agitation, and confusion.

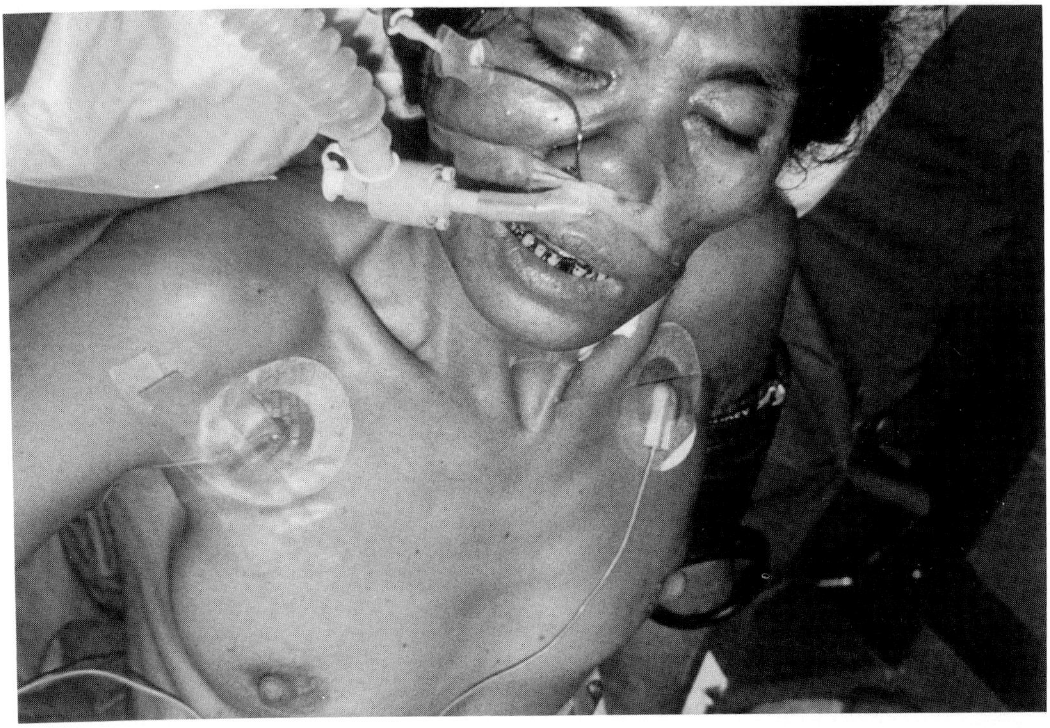

Figure 3 Although phobic signs no longer exist when the patient becomes obtunded and comatose, spontaneously occurring inspiratory spasms still continue.

limbic brain-stem structures. Selective infection of a specific brain-stem region (170) cannot explain this phenomenon since almost all neurons at such structures are rabies antigen positive (97). Paresis of palatopharyngeus muscles is rarely observed. Sensation of the soft palate and posterior pharyngeal wall remain intact with a preserved or a hyperactive gag reflex.

Signs of Autonomic Dysfunction. Hypersalivation is a unique feature, which persists to the preterminal phase (Fig. 4). Production of 1–1.5 liters of saliva in 24 h is not due to swallowing difficulties. During the confusional-agitation state, pupillary abnormalities such as fixed dilated or constricted pupils, anisocoria, localized (at the bitten limb) or generalized piloerection, neurogenic pulmonary edema, excessive sweating, priapism, as well as spontaneous ejaculation are occasionally observed. Horner's syndrome with unilateral anhidrosis was observed only in one case.

There are usually no detectable cranial nerve deficits, except, in rare cases, peripheral facial palsy, deafness, or oculomotor paresis. Seizures are rare in furious or dumb rabies, but may occasionally be seen in fully developed rabies or during the preterminal phase. However, an abnormal EEG with a paroxysmal pattern of spike and wave activity with no clinical signs of seizures may be seen as early as 1–2 days after the clinical onset of disease (103).

Acute hepatic porphyria with neuropsychiatric disturbances, such as psychosis, seizures, signs of autonomic dysfunction, and involvement of the peripheral nervous system, can be confused with rabies (55). Fluctuating consciousness is observed in both conditions, but phobic and inspiratory spasms are seen only in rabies. A family history of the disease, ingestion of porphyrinogenic agents, abdominal pain, and dark urine color with elevated δ-aminolevulinic acid and porphobilinogen, aid the diagnosis.

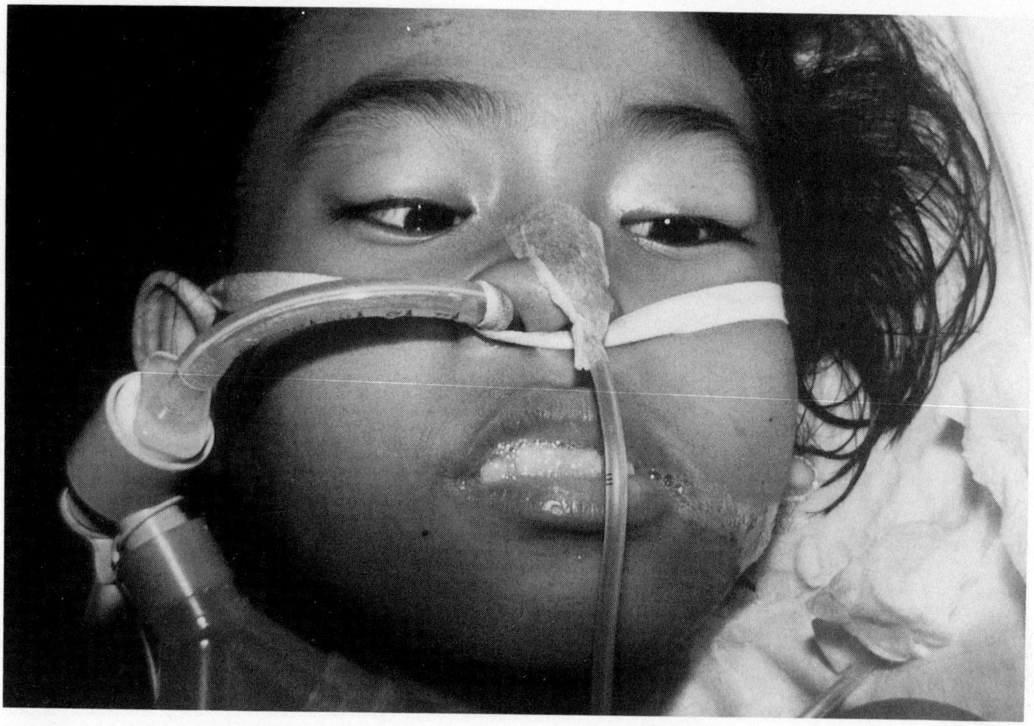

Figure 4 Hypersalivation, one of the autonomic stimulation signs, is a unique feature of furious rabies.

Other disease conditions mimicking rabies during the acute neurological phase include (1) intoxication by a variety of substances, such as atropinelike compounds, (2) cannabis, (3) alcohol withdrawal (delirium tremens), and (4) tetanus. Tetanus resembles rabies only in the form of reflex spasms. All patients with tetanus have a clear sensorium. Rabies patients do not have persistent rigidity or sustained contraction of axial musculature such as the jaw, neck, back, and abdomen, as seen in tetanus. Spasms in rabies predominantly involve accessory respiratory muscles and diaphragm, whereas in tetanus, spasms occur in muscles of axial structures. Opisthotonos is far more frequent in tetanus than in rabies (55).

In some parts of the world where nervous tissue (sheep, monkey, and mouse brain) rabies vaccines are still being used, allergic encephalomyelitis must be considered in the differential diagnosis. These "accidental" complications develop in approximately 1 of 400 vaccinees and appear between 6 and 14 days after the first injection in over 75% of affected individuals (11,12). Delayed onset and a picture of chronic progressive encephalitis have also been observed (172). Neither phobic spasms, paresthesias at bite sites, nor fluctuating consciousness are present in these postvaccination reactions. Guillain-Barré–like syndromes can be seen in both mature (sheep, monkey) and immature (suckling mouse) brain vaccinal complications, but are much more common in the latter (173,174).

Paralytic Rabies

This form of rabies is less readily diagnosed than the encephalitic form because of its lack of aggression and relative sparing of consciousness (Fig. 5). The major cardinal signs in furious rabies, described above, appear late and may be only mild in paralytic cases. Phobic spasms occur

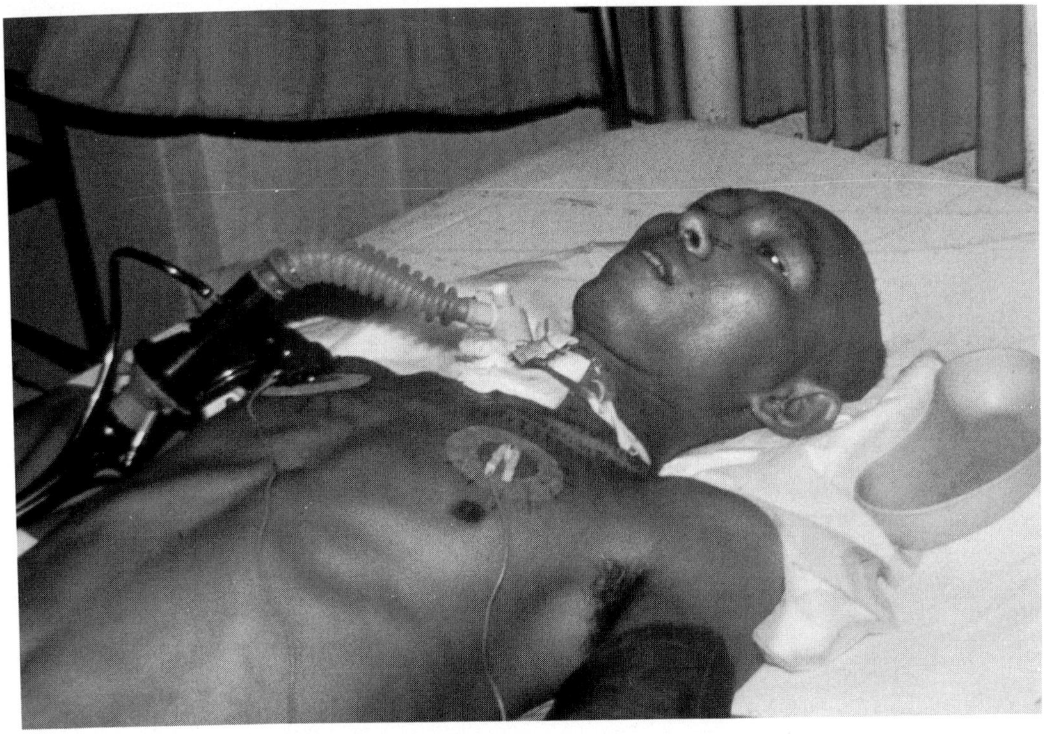

Figure 5 Patient with paralytic (dumb) rabies. Consciousness is relatively spared in this form despite severe weakness of the limbs and respiratory muscles.

in only one half of the patients; however, inspiratory spasms occur in all cases during the preterminal phase. Weakness usually starts in the bitten extremity and then progressively involves all limbs and pharyngeal and respiratory muscles. Bifacial paresis is as common as in sporadic GBS. In cases of facial bites, weakness may initially involve facial and oculomotor muscles of the same side; however, no correlation has been found between the development of paralytic rabies and the site of the bite (97). On rare occasions, presentation as an ascending myelitis with fasciculations and loss of joint position sense, as well as pinprick sensation to the thoracic level, has been observed (175).

The following may be useful in differentiating paralytic rabies from sporadic cases of GBS (55,103):

1. Fever is a constant finding in rabies (both forms) and tends to be more severe as the disease progresses. Fever is absent in GBS patients once weakness develops, unless there are complications such as aspiration pneumonia.
2. Sensory function is intact in all modalities (pinprick, vibration, and joint position) in paralytic rabies patients. Except for paresthesias at the site of the bite or in the bitten extremity, none of our rabies patients have had tingling sensations or numbness along distal extremities, as occurs in GBS cases.
3. Quadriparesis with predominant involvement of proximal muscles, loss of deep tendon reflexes, and urinary incontinence are universal findings in the early course of paralytic rabies. Urinary incontinence is unusual in GBS, especially during the early phase. Further-

more, proximal or distal muscles can be predominantly involved in equal proportion in GBS; however, weakness typically involves the distal musculature first.

4. Percussion myoedema is seen from the prodrome to the preterminal stage in paralytic rabies (176). This is best elicited by percussion of the chest, deltoid, and thigh regions with a tendon hammer, and consists of mounding of a part of muscle at the percussion site, which then flattens and disappears over a few seconds (Fig. 6). It is not seen in patients with sporadic GBS, encephalitic rabies, or in those who have neurological complications from rabies vaccination of nervous tissue origin. The myoedema sign can be seen in an extreme cachectic condition, hypothyroidism, hyponatremia, and renal failure. Myoedema during the late stage in rabies patients may be partly explained by severe hyponatremia from the syndrome of inappropriate secretion of antidiuretic hormone.

A distinction between paralytic rabies and brain tissue rabies vaccine–induced GBS is difficult. An absence of sensory deficits, fever, and urinary incontinence can be seen in vaccine-induced GBS. Inspiratory spasms with abnormal behavior may appear late in the course of paralytic rabies. Local symptoms at the bite site, myoedema, and signs of autonomic stimulation, especially hypersalivation, abnormal pupils, and piloerection, suggest paralytic rabies.

Asymmetrical weakness in an unimmunized patient in an epidemic setting suggests paralytic poliomyelitis. The Trinidad outbreak of paralytic rabies was initially thought to be poliomyelitis (40,41).

Coma

It is extremely difficult to diagnose rabies at this stage. The two forms of rabies are indistinguishable once the patient becomes comatose. Inspiratory spasms are the only helpful sign in diagnosis. Special attention is required to observe the spasms in comatose paralytic rabies patients, due to the generalized paralysis. In dumb rabies, alveolar hypoventilation and ventilatory failure develop before the patient becomes obtunded. In encephalitic rabies, abnormal breathing patterns and depression of consciousness appear simultaneously. Regular breathing, interspersed with inspiratory spasms, is replaced by tachypnea and then by apneustic respiration and terminally by ataxic breathing. In paralytic rabies, these patterns are not observed. Hypotension and sinus tachycardia, disproportionate to the fever, are evident in most cases although hydration is adequate. These are soon followed by severe sinus bradycardia or a nodal rhythm before death. Frequently, during the preterminal phase, there are arrhythmias of supraventricular origin, in the form of paroxysmal atrial tachycardia and a wandering atrial pacemaker, and premature ventricular ectopic beats. Myocarditis is likely to be an underlying mechanism based on postmortem findings and the presence of viral antigen in heart muscles (177,178), as well as failure to restore blood pressure with various inotropic drugs and a pacing device. Circulatory insufficiency is the prime cause of death. Aggressive attempts to save rabies patients must begin before hypotension develops. Hematemesis is seen in 30–60% of patients 6–12 h before death (51).

Treatment

Once clinical signs of rabies develops, there is no promising intervention to save life or lengthen survival. Patients should be sedated with appropriate tranquilizers. Neither interferon nor antiviral drugs such as vidarabine, tribavirin, and inosine pronobex or rabies polyclonal antibody or F(ab′)2 influence the course of rabies encephalitis or paralysis (103,179). These have been used either singly or in combination and via the systemic or the intrathecal route (interferon and antibody). Rabies virus–neutralizing monoclonal antibodies as well as polyclonal and monoclonal antibodies to internal viral proteins have been shown to inhibit virus spread from cell to cell

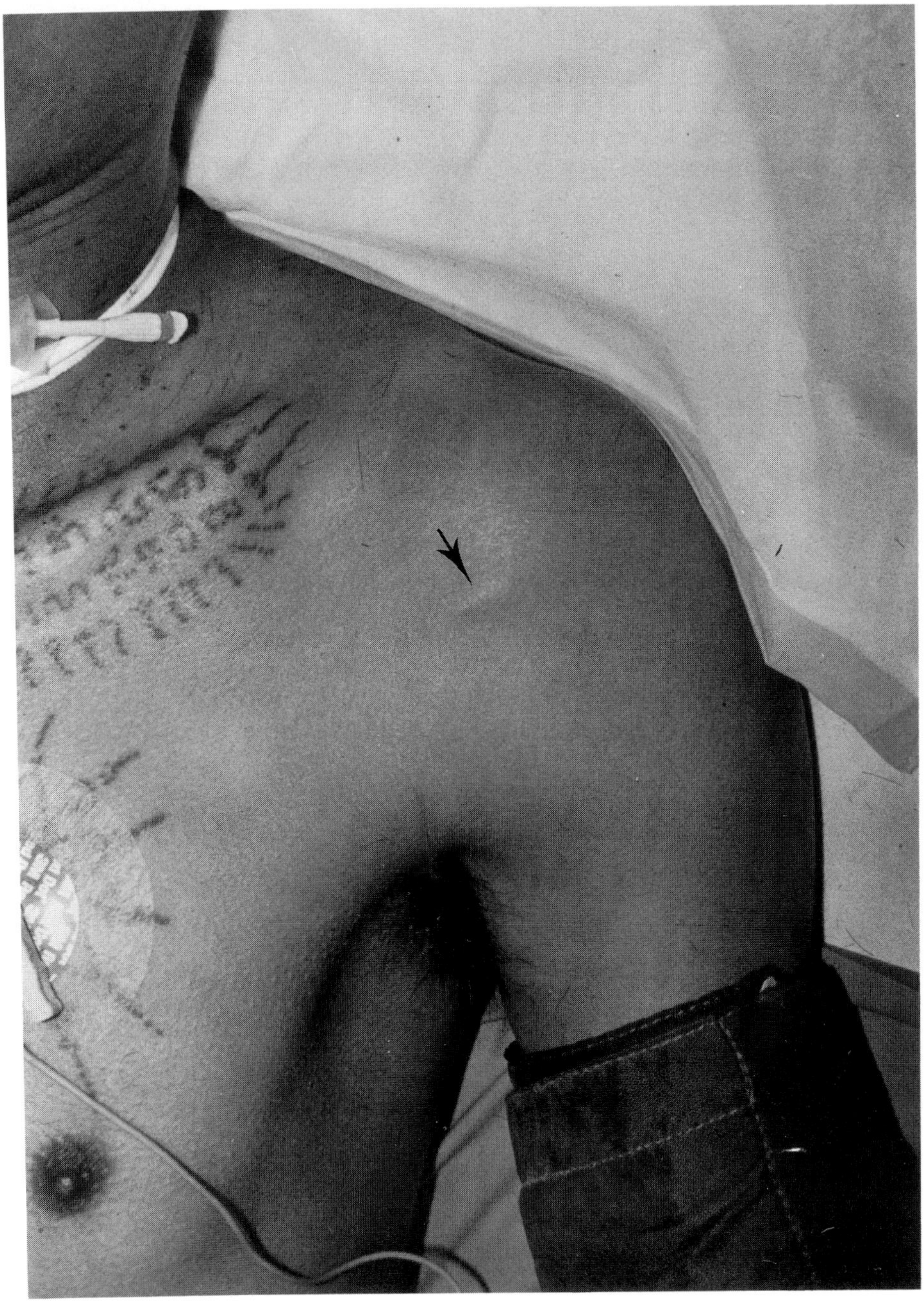

Figure 6 Myoedema in a patient with dumb rabies is demonstrated by percussion of the deltoid and consists of mounding of a part of the muscle (arrow) at the percussion site, which then flattens over a few seconds.

and to restrict rabies virus RNA transcription in vitro (180–182). A monoclonal antibody was able to clear virus from the CNS and protect rats against a lethal rabies infection in a postexposure experiment (182). Intrathecal vaccination with a live attenuated rabies virus after the clinical onset has been effective in dogs (183) but not in monkeys (184). Intensive life support should be offered when there is uncertainty of the diagnosis, particularly when the history of exposure is absent and clinical signs are considered atypical. If contamination from secretions occurs through the skin or mucous membranes, the individual should receive postexposure prophylaxis (13).

Recovery

Since 1972 there have been four documented recoveries from rabies (49,124,185,186). Diagnosis of the first three patients was based on very high rabies antibody concentrations in blood and CSF in serial observations, without definite evidence of intrathecal antibody synthesis or demonstration of viral antigen. Antibody concentrations were considered to be too high to be due to vaccine, but may also occur in cases with allergic encephalitis from nervous tissue vaccine (187). The first three patients (1972, 1976, 1977) received either pre- or postexposure prophylaxis with duck embryo or suckling mouse brain vaccine. Two of these three recoveries (1972,1976) had unusual clinical features of left-sided hemiparesis and a cerebello-striatal syndrome. Pyramidal weakness or cerebellar dysfunction has never been observed in any rabies patients in Thailand. The most recent case in Mexico (1994), who had postexposure prophylaxis with tissue culture rabies vaccinations, had high rabies antibody titers in both serum and CSF and positive oligoclonal bands. Only the third (1977) and fourth (1994) cases are considered true cases of rabies survival. None of these four cases demonstrated phobic spasms. It is not known whether different clinical features among these survivors (pyramidal weakness, cerebellar deficits, absence of phobic spasms) reflect different pathophysiological mechanisms or merely a manifestation of allergic encephalitis (especially in the first two patients).

DIAGNOSIS

At present there is no consistently reliable and sensitive technique for antemortem diagnosis of human rabies. Rabies antibody titers of low concentrations as determined by the rapid fluorescent focus inhibition test (RFFIT) in serum could be detected in only one fourth of the nonvaccinated rabies patients tested within 1–26 days after the onset of the disease. Rabies antibody in the CSF rarely develops but when it does appears after 7–10 days of illness (103). This is in contrast to patients with allergic encephalomyelitis from nervous tissue rabies vaccine (187). At the time of developing neurological complications, 95% have seroconversion of high rabies antibody titers during the first 14 days of the injection series as compared to 42% of uncomplicated recipients after 14 injections.

Rabies viral antigen may be detected by fluorescent antibody in corneal and salivary impressions and skin biopsies (13). These samples, once obtained, should be refrigerated immediately after collection and until the test is performed. Only a few rabies patients show fluorescent antibody positive results on skin biopsy at the nuchal area of the neck with hair follicles containing peripheral nerve during the early phase (103). The proportion of positive results tends to increase as the disease progresses (188). The sensitivity of the skin biopsy, nevertheless, is higher than the sensitivity of corneal and salivary impression smears (103).

Brain biopsy with Negri body detection by Seller's stain is of no value in antemortem diagnosis due to its poor sensitivity. Fluorescent antibody detection, regarded as the most sensitive test, may have a false-negative result in as many as one third of the patients when brain biopsy is performed during the first few days of the clinical illness (103). This may be due to a relative lack of viral antigen in the fronto-temporal region (97). This can be overcome by a technique of amplification of nucleocapsid gene, the polymerase chain reaction process, which allows detection of both rabies and rabies-related virus (21–23). Its efficacy has been demonstrated in fresh as well as decomposed infected dog and human brain samples (22). The whole polymerase chain reaction process, including reverse transcription, synthesis of cDNA from both mRNA and viral RNA, and DNA double amplification, can be accomplished within 24 h. This is also useful for detecting rabies virus genome in the CSF (189). However, high-quality collection and storage conditions (−70°C) and proper handling of the CSF specimens are extremely important and may affect the outcome.

Rabies virus may be isolated in mouse neuroblastoma cells from biopsied brain tissue and fluids, especially saliva and CSF (13). This cell culture isolation is sensitive and specific, and results are known within 5 days; however, all samples tested must be maintained frozen after collection with no preservatives. False-negative results may be obtained in decomposed brain samples (190). Intracerebral mouse inoculation is also useful for diagnosis using suckling mice that are less than 3 days old; however, at least a few weeks are required to obtain a result.

In the case of postmortem diagnosis where a full examination is not possible, brain tissue can be obtained by Silverman needle aspiration through a transorbital approach (S. Manutsathit, unpublished).

A high degree of awareness of the various clinical presentations of rabies as well as confirmation of the diagnosis by appropriate laboratory studies performed serially during the clinical course are requisites for early diagnosis. While a positive laboratory result is indicative of rabies, a single negative result does not rule out the possibility of rabies.

PREVENTION

Due to the seriousness of the disease, pre- and postexposure prophylaxis are of utmost importance. There is no seasonal predilection for rabies, and the incidence rate does not differ between urban and rural areas in canine rabies endemic countries. Any bite by dogs, cats, bats, or wild animals in any part of the world where there is wildlife or canine endemic or epizootic rabies is a potential exposure. This requires immediate postexposure therapy whenever killing of the biting animal and immediate brain examination by fluorescence microscopy cannot be done (13,55, 191). Treatment must be initiated but may be discontinued if the responsible dog or cat, but not other species, remains healthy throughout an observation period of 10 days. In all circumstances, the "provoked" or "unprovoked" behavior of the dog or cat is not applicable to the consideration of treatment initiation (13,192). Modification of this procedure would be indicated in a rabies-free area where animal bites are encountered.

Observation of the biting dog and postponement of treatment in a rabies-endemic area can be allowed in only three circumstances (193): (1) if there is a reliable history of dog vaccinations during the past 2 consecutive years (194); (2) if the dog has received good care from its owner with minimal risk of exposure; and (3) if there is a reasonable cause for being bitten such as feeding an unknown dog or stepping on its tail. Treatment must be initiated if the dog develops abnormal signs during this observation period.

The risk of acquiring rabies depends on the severity of the wound, regardless of the location and number (13,55). Even a single wound on the leg has the potential to cause rabies.

Postexposure treatment consists of immediate and repeated thorough cleansing of wounds with soap and water. This should be followed, whenever possible, with a cleansing solution of 70% ethanol or a solution of iodine. The wound should not be sutured. Tetanus prophylaxis and antibiotics should be given when indicated. Persons who have not received preexposure prophylaxis, or who have received pre- or postexposure treatment that utilized brain tissue–derived vaccine of unproven potency, should receive a complete postexposure course, including rabies immune globulin (RIG), as described for category III exposure (Tables 1 and 2). Treatment should be given to an exposed person regardless of the time interval since exposure, but usually is not required after a time interval of longer than a year.

All tissue culture rabies vaccines, human diploid cell, purified Vero cell, purified chick embryo cell, and purified duck embryo rabies vaccine are equally safe and effective and have been used interchangeably (each has a potency of more than 2.5 IU/dose). Any of these vaccines can be given by either intramuscular or intradermal injection (13,195).

Intramuscular (IM) schedule: One dose of vaccine is injected into the deltoid region or anterolateral thigh muscle of children on days 0, 3, 7, 14, and 30. Rabies vaccine should never be injected into the gluteal region. An abbreviated schedule (2-1-1) using two IM doses on day 0 and one each on days 7 and 21 can be used only if RIG is not also given (only in category II).

Intradermal (ID) schedule: An economically reduced dose, multiple site ID regimen (2-2-2-0-1-1) consists of 0.1 ml vaccine injected at each of two sites, either the forearm or the upper arm, on days 0, 3, and 7 and one dose at one site on days 30 and 90 (no injection on day 14) (13,195). This method is recommended only for clinics whose staff is experienced in intradermal administration and that have enough patients so that the remaining reconstituted vaccine is used up within 1 or 2 days. Separate syringes and needles must be used for each dose. The minimal potency of tissue culture vaccine proven to be efficacious in the postexposure situation by intradermal injection is 0.7 IU/ 0.1 ml (195).

Table 1 Guide for Postexposure Rabies Treatment[a]

Category	Type of contact[b]	Recommended treatment
I	Touching or feeding animal, licking over intact skin	None if reliable case history is available
II	Minor bites on uncovered skin, licks over broken skin, minor scratches, or abrasions with no bleeding	Administer vaccine immediately.[c] Stop treatment if animal (only dog or cat) remains healthy throughout observation period of 10 days or if animal is killed and found to be negative for rabies by fluorescent antibody test (FAT)
III	Single or multiple transdermal bites or scratches, licks over mucosa	Administer rabies immunoglobulin and vaccine immediately.[c] Stop treatment if animal (only dog or cat) remains healthy throughout observation period of 10 days or if animal is killed and found to be negative for rabies by FAT

[a]In any case where a reliable history cannot be obtained (e.g., small child, mentally retarded person) and there is the possibility that mucous membrane or trivial undetectable exposure may have occurred, immediate treatment should be considered. Since prolonged incubation periods have been noted, exposed persons who present for evaluation and treatment even months after having been bitten should be dealt with in the same manner as if the exposure had occurred recently.

[b]Contact with a suspected or confirmed rabid domestic or wild animal or animal unavailable for observation. Exposure to rodents, rabbits, and hares seldom if ever requires specific antirabies treatment.

[c]If an apparently healthy dog or cat in or from a low-risk area is placed in observation, the situation may warrant delaying initiation of treatment.

Source: Refs. 13, 55, 191.

Table 2 Schematic Diagram for Postexposure Rabies Treatment

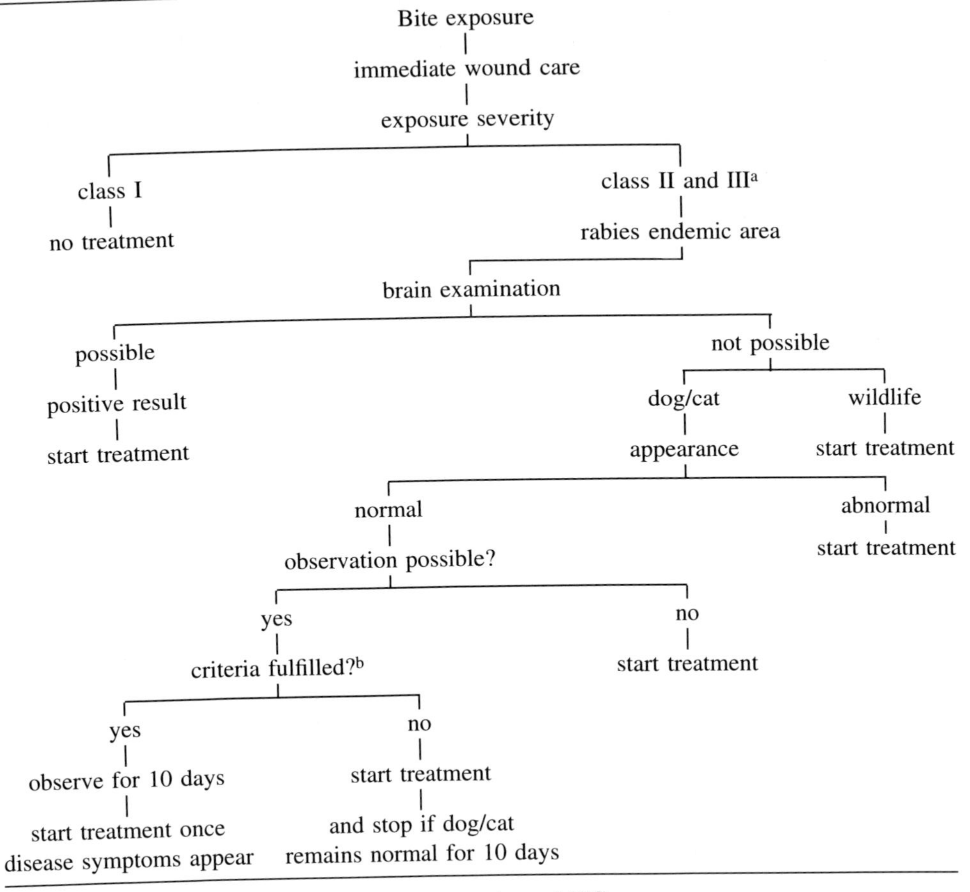

[a]Class II treatment = vaccine; class III treatment = vaccine and RIG.
[b]Criteria = (1) dog/cat receives good care with minimal exposure risk; (2) reliable history of dog/cat vaccination during the past 2 consecutive years; (3) good reason(s) to be bitten.

RIG should be given with the first dose of vaccine and no later than 7 days after the first dose of vaccine (if any delay occurs) to avoid interference with the active immune response from vaccination. As much human RIG (20 IU/kg) or equine RIG (40 IU/kg) as possible must be infiltrated in and around the wound, and the rest injected intramuscularly, deep into the buttock. Equine RIG has to be used with suitable precautions with prior skin testing. Human RIG carries negligible side effects, whereas equine RIG may have a small but definite risk of anaphylaxis and serum sickness–like reactions, which may appear within 1 week after administration. Corticosteroids should be avoided in this latter setting. Antihistamines and nonsteroidal anti-inflammatory agents are preferable.

Persons who have been previously vaccinated (either pre- or postexposure regimen) with tissue culture or purified duck embryo vaccine of proven potency should receive only two boosters on days 0 and 3 after reexposure with no RIG administration (13).

Preexposure immunization should be offered to persons at high risk of exposure, such as laboratory staff who work with rabies virus, veterinarians, animal handlers, wildlife officers, cave explorers, and others who live in or travel to areas where rabies is endemic. The primary immunization schedule consists of three intramuscular (one full dose) or intradermal (0.1 ml) injections on days 0, 7, and 28 in the deltoid area. A few days variation is acceptable. The WHO Rabies Advisory Committee recommends the following schedules for booster (one intramuscular dose or 0.1 ml intradermally at deltoid) (13):

Persons who work with live rabies should have their serum tested for rabies virus–neutralizing antibodies every 6 months. A booster dose should be administered when the titer falls below 0.5 IU/ml.

Persons at continued risk of rabies exposure, such as veterinarians and travelers to rabies-endemic regions, should have a serum sample tested for rabies virus–neutralizing antibodies every year. A booster should be administered when the titer falls below 0.5 IU/ml.

Unnecessary booster vaccination, especially when primary and booster immunizations are of different routes of administration (primary IM followed by ID booster or vice versa), may result in systemic hypersensitivity reactions (196).

ACKNOWLEDGMENTS

The author is indebted to Dr. Chansuda Wongsrichanalai for criticism and reviewing the manuscript and Miss Winita Prasertkul for preparing the manuscript. Clinical and research work was supported in part by grants from the Queen Saovabha Memorial Institute, The Thai Red Cross Society, and Chulalongkorn University Hospital and General Prayudh Charumani.

REFERENCES

1. WHO. World survey of rabies 28 (for year 1992). World Health Organization unpublished document WHO/Rabies/94.210,1992.
2. Held JR, Tierkel ES, Steele JH. Rabies in man and animals in the United States, 1946-65. Public Health Rep 1967; 82:1009–1018.
3. Anderson LJ, Nicholson KG, Tauxe RV, Winkler WG. Human rabies in the United States, 1960 to 1979: epidemiology, diagnosis, and prevention. Ann Intern Med 1984; 100:728–735.
4. Fishbein DB, Robinson LE. Rabies. N Engl J Med 1993; 25:1632–1638.
5. Baer GM, Bellini WJ, Fishbein DB. Rhabdoviruses. In: Fields BN, Knipe DM, eds. Virology. 2nd ed. New York: Academic Press, 1990:883–930.
6. Baer GM. The Natural History of Rabies. 2nd ed. Boca Raton, FL: CRC Press, 1991.
7. Hoenig LJ. Triumph and controversy. Pasteur's preventive treatment of rabies as reported in JAMA. Arch Neurol 1986; 43:397–399.
8. Stuart G, Krikorian KS. The neuro-paralytic accidents of anti-rabies treatment. Ann Trop Med Parasitol 1928; 22:327–377.
9. Rivers TM, Schwentker FF. Encephalomyelitis accompanied by myelin destruction experimentally produced in monkeys. J Exp Med 1935; 61:689–702.
10. Bahmanyar M, Fayaz A, Nour-Saleski S, Mohammadi M, Koprowski H. Successful protection of humans exposed to rabies infection. JAMA 1976; 236:2751–2754.
11. Hemachudha T, Griffin DE, Giffels JJ, Johnson RT, Moser AB, Phanuphak P. Myelin basic protein as an encephalitogen in encephalomyelitis and polyneuritis following rabies vaccination. N Engl J Med 1987; 316:369–374.
12. Hemachudha T, Phanuphak P, Johnson RT, Griffin DE, Ratanavongsiri J, Siriprasomsup W. Neurologic complications of Semple-type rabies vaccine: clinical and immunologic studies. Neurology 1987; 37:550–556.
13. WHO. 8th Report of the WHO Expert Committee on Rabies. Technical Report Series, No. 824, Geneva, 1992.

14. Habel K, Koprowski H. Laboratory data supporting the clinical trial of antirabies serum in persons bitten by a rabid wolf. Bull WHO 1955; 13:773–779.
15. Negri A. Beitrag zum Studium der Aetiologie der Tollwuth. Z Hyg Infektionskr 1903; 43:507–528.
16. Webster LT, Dawson JR Jr. Early diagnosis of rabies by mouse inoculation. Measurement of humoral immunity to rabies by mouse protection test. Proc Soc Exp Biol Med 1935; 32:570–573.
17. Kissling RE. The fluorescent antibody test in rabies. In: Baer GM, ed. Natural History of Rabies. Vol. 1. Orlando, FL: Academic Press, 1975:401–416.
18. Goldwasser RA, Kissling RE. Fluorescent antibody staining of street and fixed rabies virus antigens. Proc Soc Exp Biol Med 1958; 98:219–223.
19. Derakhshan I. Is the Negri body specific for rabies? Arch Neurol 1975; 32:75–79.
20. Bahmanyar M, Noorsalehi S, Fayaz A, Mohammad M. Light microscopical diagnosis of rabies. A reappraisal. Lancet 1978; 1:302–303.
21. Bourhy H, Sureau P. Laboratory Methods for Rabies Diagnosis. Paris: Institut Pasteur, 1991.
22. Kamolvarin N, Tirawatnpong T, Rattanasiwamoke R, Tirawatnpong S, Panpanich T, Hemachudha T. Diagnosis of rabies by polymerase chain reaction with nested primers. J Infect Dis 1993; 167:207–210.
23. Smith JS, Fishbein DB, Rupprecht CE, Clark K. Unexplained rabies in three immigrants in the United States: a virologic investigation. N Engl J Med 1991; 324:205–211.
24. Smith, JS. Rabies virus epitopic variation: use in ecologic studies. Adv Virus Res 1989; 36:215–253.
25. Smith JS, Orciari LA, Yager PA, Seidel HD, Warner CK. Epidemiologic and historical relationships among 87 rabies virus isolates as determined by limited sequence analysis. J Infect Dis 1992; 166: 296–307.
26. Smith JS. Monoclonal antibody studies in insectivorous bats of the United States. Rev Infect Dis 1988; 10(suppl 4):637–643.
27. Bourhy H, Kissi B, Lafon M, Sacramento D, Tordo N. Antigenic and molecular characterization of bat rabies virus in Europe. J Clin Microbiol 1992; 30:2419–2426.
28. Bourhy H, Kissi B, Tordo N. Molecular diversity of the Lyssavirus genus. Virology 1993; 194:70–81.
29. Brass DA. Rabies in Bats. CT: Livia Press, 1994.
30. Rupprecht CE, Kieney MP. Development of a vaccinia-rabies glycoprotein recombinant virus vaccine. In: Campbell JB, Charlton KM, eds. Rabies. MA: Kluwer Academic Publishers, 1988:335–364.
31. Lodmell DL, Sumner JW, Esposito JJ, Bellini WJ, Ewalt LC. Raccoon poxvirus recombinants expressing the rabies virus nucleoprotein protect mice against lethal rabies virus infection. J Virol 1991; 65:3400–3405.
32. Campbell JB. Oral rabies immunization of wild life and dogs: challenges to the Americas. In: Rupprecht CE, Dietzschold B, Koprowski M, eds. Lyssavirus. Berlin: Springer-Verlag, 1994:245–266.
33. Xiang ZQ, Spitalnik S, Tran M, Wunner WH, Cheng J, Ertl HC. Vaccination with a plasmid vector carrying the rabies virus glycoprotein gene induces protective immunity against rabies virus. Virology 1994; 199:132–140.
34. Cadoz M, Strady A, Meignier B, Taylor J, Tartaglia J, Paoletti E, Plotkin S. Immunisation with canarypox virus expressing rabies glycoprotein. Lancet 1992; 339:1429–1432.
35. Brochier B, Kieny MP, Costy F, Coppens P, Bauduin B, Lecocq JP, Lanquet B, Chappuis G, Desmettre P, Afiademanyo K, Libois R, Pastoret P-P. Large-scale eradication of rabies using recombinant vaccinia-rabies vaccine. Nature 1991; 354:520–522.
36. Pastoret PP, Brochier B, copens P. Deliberate release of a recombinant vaccinia-rabies virus for vaccination of wild animals against rabies. Microb Rel 1993; 1:191–195
37. Haddad N, Ben Khelifa R, Matter H, Kharmachi H, Aubert MF, Wandeler A, Blancou J. Assay of oral vaccination of dogs against rabies in Tunisia with the vaccinal strain SADBern. Vaccine 1994; 12: 307–309.
38. Augusto LR, Percy MP, Edgar TV, Fishbein DB. Outbreak of human rabies in the Peruvian jungle. Lancet 1992; 339:408–411.
39. Acha PN. Epidemiology of paralytic bovine rabies and bat rabies. Bull Off Int Epizoot 1967; 67: 343–382.
40. Hurst EW, Pawan JL. A further account of the Trinidad outbreak of acute rabies myelitis. J Pathol Bacteriol 1932; 35:301–321.

41. Hurst EW, Pawan JL. An outbreak of rabies in Trinidad without history of bites and with the symptoms of acute ascending paralysis. Lancet 1931; 2:622–625.
42. Nehaul BBG. Rabies transmitted by bats in British Guiana. Am J Trop Med Hyg 1955; 43:550–553.
43. Verline JD, Li-Fo-Sjoe E, Veersteeg J, Decker SM. A local outbreak of paralytic rabies in Surinam children. Trop Geogr Med 1975; 27:137–142.
44. McCarthy TJ. Human depredation by vampire bats Desmodus rotundus following a hog cholera campaign. Am J Trop Med Hyg 1989; 40:320–322.
45. Tordo N, Poch O. Structure of rabies virus. In: Campbell JB, Charlton KM, eds. Rabies. MA: Kluwer Academic Publishers, 1988:25–45.
46. Gosztonyi G. Reproduction of Lyssaviruses: ultrastructural composition of Lyssavirus and functional aspects of pathogenesis. In: Rupprecht CE, Dietzschold B, Koprowski H, eds. Lyssaviruses. Berlin: Springer-Verlag, 1994:43–68.
47. Constantine DG. Rabies Transmission by Air in Bat Caves. United States Public Health Service Publication, 1967.
48. Winkler WG, Fashinell TR, Leffingwell L, Paxton H, Conomy JP. Airborne rabies transmission in a laboratory worker. J Am Med Assoc 1973; 226:1219–1221.
49. Rabies in a laboratory worker. MMWR 1977; 26:183.
50. Tariq WU, Shafi MS, Jamal S, Ahmad M. Rabies in man handling infected calf. Lancet 1991; 337:1224.
51. Kureishi A, Xu LZ, Wu H, Stiver HG. Rabies in China: recommendations for control. Bull WHO 1992; 70:443–450.
52. Babes V. Traite de la Rage. Paris: Bailliere et Fils, 1912:81–119.
53. Hattwick MAW, Gregg MB. The disease in man. In: Baer GM, ed. The Natural History of Rabies. New York: Academic Press, 1975:281–303.
54. Vibulbandhitkij S. Data from the rabies patients from Bumrasanaradura Hospital between 1971–1977. In: Thongcharoen P, et al., eds. Rabies. Bangkok: Aksarasamai, 1980:235–251.
55. Hemachudha T. Rabies. In: Vinken PJ, Bruyn GW, Klawans HL. Handbook of Clinical Neurology. Revised series. Amsterdam: Elsevier Science Publishers, 1989:383–404.
56. Helmick CG, Tauxe RV, Vernon AA. Is there a risk to contacts of patients with rabies? Rev Infect Dis 1987; 9:511–518.
57. Sipahioglu U, Alpaut S. Transplacental rabies in man. Mikrobiol Blt 1985; 19:95–99.
58. Martell MA, Ceronmontes F, Raulalcocer B. Transplacental transmission of bovine rabies after natural infection. J Infect Dis 1973; 127:291–293.
59. Lumbiganon P, Wasi C. Survival after rabies immunization in newborn infant of affected mother. Lancet 1990; 336:319.
60. Thongcharoen P. Prodrome and incubation period in human rabies. In: Thongcharoen P, et al., eds. Rabies. Bangkok: Aksarasamai, 1980:35–47.
61. Bell JF, Moore GJ. Susceptibility of carnivora to rabies virus administered orally. Am J Epidemiol 1971; 93:176–182.
62. Charlton KM, Casey GA. Experimental rabies in skunks: oral, nasal, tracheal and intestinal exposure. Can J Comp Med 1979; 43:168–172.
63. Bijlenga G, Heaney T. Postexposure local treatment of mice infected with rabies with two axonal inhibitors, colchicine and vinblastine. J Gen Virol 1980; 50:433–435.
64. Tsiang H. Evidence for an intraxonal transport of fixed and street rabies virus. J Neuropathol Exp Neurol 1979; 38:286–297.
65. Lycke E, Tsiang H. Rabies virus infection of cultured rat sensory neurons. J Virol 1987; 61:2733–2741.
66. Tsiang H, Ceccaldi PE, Lycke E. Rabies virus infection and transport in human sensory dorsal root ganglia neurons. J Gen Virol 1991; 72:1191–1194.
67. Tsiang H, Lycke E, Ceccaldi PE, Ermine A, Hirardot X. The anterograde transport of rabies virus in rat sensory dorsal root ganglia neurons. J Gen Virol 1989; 70:2075–2085.
68. Dean DJ, Evans WM, McClure RC. Pathogenesis of rabies. Bull WHO 1963; 29:803–811.
69. Baer GM, Shanthaveerppa TR, Bourne GH. The pathogenesis of street rabies virus in rats. Bull WHO 1968; 38:119–125.

70. Baer GM, Shaddock JH, Quirion R, Dam TV, Lentz TL. Rabies susceptibility and acetylcholine receptor. Lancet 1990; 335:664–665.
71. Hattwick MAW. Human rabies. Publ Health Rev 1974; 3:229–274.
72. Murphy FA, Bauer SP, Harrison AK, Winn WC. Comparative pathogenesis of rabies and rabies-like viruses. Viral infection and transit from inoculation site to the central nervous system. Lab Invest 1973; 28:361–376.
73. Charlton KM, Casey GA. Experimental rabies in skunks: immunofluorescent, light and electron microscopic studies. Lab Invest 1979; 41:36–44.
74. Charlton KM, Casey GA. Experimental rabies in skunks: persistence of virus in denervated muscle at the inoculation site. Can J Comp Med 1981; 45:357–362.
75. Charlton KM. The pathogenesis of rabies and other lyssaviral infections: recent studies. In: Rupprecht CE, Dietzschold B, Koprowski H, eds. Lyssaviruses. Berlin: Springer-Verlag, 1994:95–119.
76. Lentz TL, Benson RJJ, Klimowicz D, Wilson PT, Hawrot E. Binding of rabies virus to purified Torpedo acetylcholine receptor. Mol Brain Res 1986; 1:211–219.
77. Lentz TL, Burrage TG, Smith AL, Crick J, Tignor G. Is the acetylcholine receptor a rabies virus receptor? Science 1982; 215:182–184.
78. Lentz TL, Chester J, Benson RJJ, Hawrot E, Tignor GH, Smith AL. Rabies virus binding to cellular membranes measured by enzyme immunoassay. Muscle Nerve 1985; 8:336–345.
79. Lentz TL, Hawrot E, Wilson PT. Synthetic peptides corresponding to sequences of snake venom neurotoxins and rabies virus glycoprotein bind to the nicotinic acetylcholine receptor. Proteins: structure, function. Genet 1987; 2:298–307.
80. Lentz TL, Wilson PT, Hawrot E, Speicher DW. Amino acid sequence similarity between rabies virus glycoprotein and snake venom curaremimetic neurotoxins. Science 1984; 226:847–848.
81. Burrage TC, Tignor GH, Smith AL. Rabies virus binding at neuromuscular junctions. Virus Res 1985; 2:273–279
82. Hanham CA, Zhao F, Tignor GH. Evidence from the anti-idiotypic network that the acetylcholine receptor is a rabies virus receptor. J Virol 1993; 67:530–542.
83. Hemachudha T, Chutivongse S, Wilde H, Phanuphak P. Latent rabies. N Engl J Med 1991; 324:1890–1891.
84. McColl KA, Gould AR, Selleck PW, Hooper PT, Westbury HA, Smith JS. Polymerase chain reaction and other laboratory techniques in the diagnosis of long incubation rabies in Australia. Aust Vet J 1993; 70:84–89.
85. Rupprecht CE, Dietzschold B. Editorial: perspective on rabies virus pathogenesis. Lab Invest 1987; 57:603–606.
86. Yamamoto T, Ohtani S. Ultrastructural localization of rabies virus antigens in infected trigeminal ganglion of hamsters. Acta Neuropathol 1978; 43:229–233.
87. Kucera P, Dolivo M, Coulon P, Flamand A. Pathways of the early propagation of virulent and avirulent rabies strains from the eye to the brain. J Virol 1985; 55:158–162.
88. Shankar V, Dietzschold B, Koprowski H. Direct entry of rabies virus into the central nervous system without prior local replication. J Virol 1991; 65:2736–2738.
89. Coulon P, Derbin C, Kucera P, Lafay F, Prehaud C, Flamand A. Invasion of the peripheral nervous system of adult mice by the CVS strain of rabies virus and its avirulent derivative Av01. J Virol 1989; 63:3550–3554.
90. Iwasaki Y, Clark HF. Cell to cell transmission of virus in the central nervous system II. Experimental rabies in the mouse. Lab Invest 1975; 33:391–399.
91. Iwasaki Y, Ohtani S, Clark HF. Maturation of rabies virus by budding from neuronal cell membrane in suckling mouse brain. J Virol 1975; 15:1020–1023.
92. Perl DP. The pathology of rabies in the central nervous system. In: Baer GM, ed. The Natural History of Rabies. New York: Academic Press, 1975:236–272.
93. Gillet JP, Derer P, Tsiang H. Axonal transport of rabies virus in the central nervous system of the rat. J Neuropathol Exp Neurol 1986; 45:619–634.
94. Tangchai P, Yenbutr D, Vejjajiva A. Central nervous system lesions in human rabies. A study of 24 autopsy cases. J Med Assoc Thailand 1970; 53:471–488.

95. Matsumoto S. Electron microscopy of central nervous system infections. In: Baer GM, ed. The Natural History of Rabies. New York: Academic Press, 1975; 217–233.
96. Sung JH, Hayano M, Mastri AR. A case of human rabies and ultrastructure of the Negri body. J Neuropathol Exp Neurol 1976; 35:541–559.
97. Tirawatnpong S, Hemachudha T, Manutsathit S, Shuangshoti S, Phanthumchinda K, Phanuphak P. Regional distribution of rabies viral antigen in the central nervous system of human encephalitic and paralytic rabies. J Neurol Sci 1989; 92:91–99.
98. Tsiang H, Koulakoff A, Bizzini B. Neurotropism of rabies virus. J Neuropathol Exp Neurol 1983; 42:439–452.
99. Johnson RT. Experimental rabies: studies of cellular vulnerability and pathogenesis using fluorescent antibody staining. J Neuropathol Exp Neurol 1965; 24:662–674.
100. Johnson RT. Viral Infections of the Nervous System. New York: Raven Press, 1982.
101. Jackson AC, Reimer DL. Pathogenesis of experimental rabies in mice: an immunohistochemical study. Acta Neuropathol 1989; 78:159–165.
102. Smart NL, Charlton KM. The distribution of challenge virus standard rabies virus versus skunk street rabies virus in the brains of experimentally infected rabid skunks. Acta Neuropathol 1992; 84: 501–508.
103. Hemachudha T. Human rabies: clinical aspects, pathogenesis and potential therapy. In: Rupprecht CE, Dietzschold B, Koprowski H, eds. Lyssaviruses. Berlin: Springer-Verlag, 1994:121–143.
104. Torres-Anjel MJ, Volz D. Failure to thrive, wasting syndrome, and immunodeficiency in rabies: a hypophyseal/hypothalamic-thymic axis effect of rabies. Rev Infect Dis 1988; 10(suppl 4): 710–725.
105. Perry LL, Hotchkiss JD, Lodmell DL. Murine susceptibility to street rabies virus is unrelated to induction of host lymphoid depletion. J Immunol 1990; 144:3552–3557.
106. Hemachudha T, Tirawatnpong S, Phanthumchinda K. Seizures as the initial manifestation of paralytic rabies. J Neurol Neurosurg Psychiatry 1989; 52:808–810.
107. Tsiang H. Neuronal function impairment in rabies infected rat brain. J Gen Virol 1982; 61:277–281.
108. Tsiang H. An in vitro study of rabies pathogenesis. Bull Inst Pasteur 1985; 83:41–56.
109. Bouzamondo E, Ladogana A, Tsiang H. Alteration of potassium-evoked 5-HT release from virus-infected rat cortical synaptosomes. Neuroreport 1993; 4:555–558.
110. Ladogana A, Bouzamondo E, Pocchiari M, Tsiang H. Modification of tritiated gamma-amino-n-butyric acid transport in rabies virus-infected primary cortical cultures. J Gen Virol 1994; 75: 623–627.
111. Munzel P, Koschel K. Rabies virus decreases agonist binding to opiate receptors of mouse neuroblastoma-rat glioma hybrid cells 108-cc-15. Biochem Biophys Res Commun 1981; 10:1241–1250.
112. Koschel K, Munzel P. Inhibition of opiate receptor mediated signal transmission by rabies virus in persistently infected NG-108-15 mouse neuroblastoma-rat glioma hybrid cells. Proc Natl Acad Sci 1984; 81:950–954.
113. Ceccaldi PE, Fillion MP, Ermine A, Tsiang H, Fillion G. Rabies virus selectively alters 5-HT1 receptor subtypes in rat brain. Eur J Pharmacol 1993; 245:129–138.
114. Dumrongphol H, Srikiatkhachorn A, Hemachudha T, Kotchabhakdi N, Govitrapong P. Alteration of muscarinic cholinergic receptors in rabies viral-infected dog brains. J Neurol Sci 1996; 137:1–6.
115. Tsiang H. Interactions of rabies virus and host cells. In: Campbell JB and Charlton KM, eds. Rabies. MA: Kluwer Academic Publishers, 1988:67–100.
116. Gourmelon P, Briet D, Court L. Electrophysiological and sleep alterations in experimental mouse rabies. Brain Res 1986; 398:128–140.
117. Gourmelon P, Briet D, Clarenco D, Court L, Tsiang H. Sleep alterations in experimental street rabies virus infection occur in the absence of major EEG abnormalities. Brain Res 1991; 554:159–165.
118. Baer GM, Shantha TR, Bourne GH. The pathogenesis of street rabies virus in rats. Bull WHO 1968; 38:119–125.
119. Yasmuth C, Nelson KE, Laima T. Prevalence of abortive canine rabies in Chiangmai, Thailand. J Med Assoc Thailand 1983; 66:169–174.

120. Starr LE, Sellers TF, Sunkes EJ. Apparent recovery of dog from rabies. J Am Vet Med Assoc 1952; 121:296.
121. Stamm DD, Kissling RE, Edison ME. Experimental rabies infection in insectivorous bats. J Infect Dis 1956; 98:10–14.
122. Bell JF. Abortive rabies infection I. Experiment production in white mice and general discussion. J Infect Dis 1964; 114:249–257.
123. Bell JF. Latency and abortive rabies. In: Baer GM, ed. The Natural History of Rabies. New York: Academic Press, 1975:331–354.
124. Hattwick MAW, Weiss TT, Stechschulte CJ, Baer GM. Recovery from rabies. A case report. Ann Intern Med 1972; 76:931–942.
125. Doege TC, Northop RL. Evidence for inapparent rabies infection. Lancet 1974; 2:826–829.
126. Follmann EH, Ritter DG, Beller M. Survey of fox trappers in northern Alaska for rabies antibody. Epidemiol Infect 1994; 113:137–141.
127. Fekadu M, Baer GM. Recovery from clinical rabies of 2 dogs inoculated with a rabies virus strain from Ethiopia. Am J Vet Res 1980; 41:1632–1634.
128. Fekadu M. Pathogenesis of rabies virus infection in dogs. Rev Infect Dis 1988; 10(suppl 4): 678–683.
129. Hemachudha T, Phanuphak P, Sriwanthana B, Manutsathit S, Phanthumchinda K, Siriprasomsup W, Ukachoke C, Rasameechan S, Kaoroptham S. Immunologic study of human encephalitic and paralytic rabies. A preliminary study of 16 patients. Am J Med 1988; 84:673–677.
130. Lodmell DL, Ewalt LC. Pathogenesis of street rabies virus infections in resistant and susceptible strains of mice. J Virol 1985; 55:788–795.
131. Templeton JW, Holmberg C, Garber T. Genetic control of serum neutralizing antibody response to rabies vaccination and survival after a rabies challenge infection in mice. J Virol 1986; 59:98–102.
132. Perry LL, Lodmell DL. Role of CD 4+ and CD 8+ T cells in murine resistance to street rabies virus. J Virol 1991; 65:3429–3434.
133. Miyamoto K, Matsumoto S. The nature of the Negri body. J Cell Biol 1965; 27:677–682.
134. Dietzschold B, Wunner WH, Wiktor TJ, Lopes AD, Lafon M, Smith CL, Koprowski H. Characterization of an antigenic determination of the glycoprotein which correlates with pathogenicity of rabies virus. Proc Natl Acad Sci 1983; 80:70–74.
135. Seif I, Coulon P, Rollin PE, Flamand A. Rabies virulence: effect on pathogenicity and sequence characterization of rabies virus mutations affecting antigenic site III of the glycoprotein. J Virol 1985; 53:926–934.
136. Dietzschold B, Wiktor TJ, Trojanowski JQ, McFarlan RI, Wunner WH, Torres-Anjel WJ, Koprowski H. Differences in cell-to-cell spread of pathogenic and apathogenic rabies virus in vivo and in vitro. J Virol 1985; 56:12–18.
137. Miller A, Morse HC, Winkelstein J, Nathanson N. The role of antibody in recovery from experimental rabies I. Effect of depletion of B and T cells. J Immunol 1978; 121:321–326.
138. Mifune K, Takeuchi E, Napiorkowski PA, Yamada A, Sakamoto K. Essential role of T cells in the postexposure prophylaxis of rabies in mice. Microbiol Immunol 1981; 25:895–902.
139. Wiktor TJ, Doherty PC, Koprowski H. Suppression of cell mediated immunity by street rabies virus. J Exp Med 1977; 145:1617–1622.
140. Wiktor TJ. Cell mediated immunity and postexposure protection from rabies by inactivated vaccines of tissue culture origin. Dev Biol Stand 1978; 40:255–264.
141. Prabhakar BS, Fischman HR, Nathanson N. Recovery from experimental rabies by adoptive transfer of immune cells. J Gen Virol 1981; 56:25–31.
142. Smith JS. Mouse model for abortive rabies infection of the central nervous system. Infect Immun 1981; 31:297–308.
143. Panpanich T, Hemachudha T, Piyasirisilp S, Manutsathit S, Wilde H, Phanuphak P. Cells with natural killer activity in human rabies. Clin Exp Immunol 1992; 89:414–418.
144. Kasempimolporn S, Hemachudha T, Khawplod P, Manutsathit S. Human immune response to rabies nucleocapsid and glycoprotein antigens. Clin Exp Immunol 1991; 84:195–199.
145. Dietzschold B, Wang H, Rupprecht CE, Celis E, Tollis M, Ertl H, Heber-Katz E, Koprowski H.

Induction of protective immunity against rabies by immunization with rabies virus ribonucleoprotein. Proc Natl Acad Sci 1987; 84:9165–9169.
146. Sumner JW, Fekadu M, Shaddock JH, Esposito JJ, Bellini WJ. Protection of mice with vaccinia virus recombinants that express the rabies nucleoprotein. Virology 1991; 183:703–710.
147. Tollis M, Dietzschold B, Volia CB, Koprowski H. Immunization of monkeys with rabies ribonucleoprotein (RNP) confers protective immunity against rabies. Vaccine 1991; 9:134–136.
148. Fekadu M, Sumner JW, Shaddock JH, Sanderlin DW, Baer GM. Sickness and recovery of dogs challenged with a street rabies virus after vaccination with a vaccinia virus recombinant expressing rabies virus N protein. J Virol 1992; 66:2601–2604.
149. Hemachudha T, Panpanich P, Manutsathit S, Phanuphak P. Immune activation in human rabies. Trans R Soc Trop Med Hyg 1993; 87:106–108.
150. Smith JS, McClelland CL, Reid FL, Baer GM. Dual role of the immune response in street rabies virus infection of mice. Infect Immun 1982; 35:213–221.
151. Prabhakar BS, Nathanson N. Acute rabies death mediated by antibody. Nature 1981; 290:590–591.
152. Sugamata M, Miyazawa M, Mori S, Spangrude GJ, Ewalt LC, Lodmell DL. Paralysis of street rabies virus-infected mice is dependent on T lymphocytes. J Virol 1992; 66:1252–1260.
153. Weiland F, Cox JH, Meyer S, Dahme E, Reddehase MJ. Rabies virus neuritic paralysis: immunopathogenesis of nonfatal paralytic rabies. J Virol 1992; 66:5096–5099.
154. Iwasaki Y, Gerhard W, Clark HF. Role of the host immune response in the development of either encephalitic or paralytic disease after experimental rabies infection in mice. Infect Immunol 1977; 18:220–225.
155. Tignor GH, Shope RE, Gershon RK, Waksman BH. Immunopathologic aspects of infection with Lagos bat virus of the rabies serogroup. J Immunol 1974; 112:260–265.
156. Lafon M, Lafage M, Martinez-Arends A, Ramirez R, Vuillier F, Charron D, Lotteau V, Scott-Algara D. Evidence for a viral superantigen in humans. Nature 1992; 358:507–510.
157. Lafon M, Scott-Algara D, Marche PN, Cazenave PA, Jouvin-Marche E. Neonatal deletion and selective expansion of mouse T cells by exposure to rabies virus nucleocapsid superantigen. J Exp Med 1994; 180:1207–1215.
158. Obeid LM, Linardic CM, Karolak LA, Hannun YA. Programmed cell death induced by ceramide. Science 1993; 259:1769–1771.
159. Koprowski H, Zheng YM, Heber-Katz E, Fraser N, Rorke L, Fu ZF, Hanlon C, Dietzschold B. In vivo expression of inducible nitric oxide synthase in experimentally induced neurologic diseases. Proc Natl Acad Sci 1993; 90:3024–3027.
160. Lipkin WL, Battenberg ELF, Bloom FE, Oldstone MBA. Viral infection of neurons can depress neurotransmitter mRNA levels without histologic injury. Brain Res 1988; 451:333–339.
161. Lipkin WL, Carbone KM, Wilson MC, Duchala CS, Narayan O, Oldstone MBA. Neurotransmitter abnormalities in Borna disease. Brain Res 1988; 495:336–370.
162. Hantson P, Guerit JM, de Tourtchaninoff M, Deconinck B, Mahieu P, Dooms G, Aubert-Tulkens G, Brucher JM. Rabies encephalitis mimicking the electrophysiological pattern of brain death. A case report. Eur Neurol 1993; 33:212–217.
163. Fu ZF, Weihe E, Zheng YM, Schafer MKH, Sheng H, Corisdeo S, Rauscher FJ III, Koprowski H, Dietzschold B. Differential effects of rabies and borna disese viruses on immediate-early and late-response gene expression in brain tissues. J Virol 1993; 67:6674–6681.
164. Reichlin S. Mechanisms of disease: neuroendocrine-immune interactions. N Engl J Med 1993; 329:1246–1253.
165. Chopra JS, Banerjee AK, Murthy JMK, Pal SR. Paralytic rabies. A clinicopathological study. Brain 1980; 103:789–802.
166. Balachandran A, Charlton K. Experimental rabies infection of non-nervous tissues in skunks (Mephitis mephitis) and foxes (Vulpes vulpes). Vet Pathol 1994; 31:93–102.
167. Aghomo HO, Rupprecht CE. Further studies on rabies virus isolated from healthy dogs in Nigeria. Vet Microbiol 1990; 22:17–22.
168. Warrell MJ, Looareesuwan S, Manutsathit S, White NJ, Phuapradit P, Vejjajiva A, Hoke CH, Burke

DS, Warrell DA. Rapid diagnosis of rabies and post-vaccinal encephalitis. Clin Exp Immunol 1988; 71:229–234.
169. Johnson HN. Rabies virus. In: Horsfall FL, Tamm I, eds. Viral and rickettsial infections of man. Philadelphia: Lippincott, 1965:814–840.
170. Kaplan C, Turner GS, Warrell DA. Rabies: The Facts. 2nd ed. Oxford: Oxford University Press, 1986.
171. Wilson JM, Hettiarachchi J, Wijesuriya IM. Presenting features and diagnosis of rabies. Lancet 1975; 2:1139–1140.
172. Hemachudha T, Griffin DE, Johnson RT, Giffels JJ. Immunologic studies of patients with chronic encephalitis induced by postexposure Semple rabies vaccine. Neurology 1988; 38:42–44.
173. Hemachudha T, Griffin DE, Chen W, Johnson RT. Immunologic studies of rabies vaccination induced Guillain-Barre syndrome. Neurology 1988; 38:375–378.
174. Cabrera J, Griffin DE, Johnson RT. Unusual features of the Guillain-Barre syndrome after rabies vaccine prepared in suckling mouse brain. J Neurol Sci 1987; 81:239–245.
175. Phuapradit P, Manutsathit S, Warrell MJ, Warrell DA. Paralytic rabies: some unusual clinical presentations. J Med Assoc Thailand 1985; 68:105–110.
176. Hemachudha T, Phanthumchinda K, Phanuphak P, Manutsathit S. Myoedema as a clinical sign in paralytic rabies. Lancet 1987; 1:1210.
177. Warrell DA. The clinical picture of rabies in man. Trans R Soc Trop Med Hyg 1976; 701:188–195.
178. Metze K, Feiden W. Rabies virus ribonucleoprotein in the heart. N Engl J Med 1991; 324:1814–1815.
179. Warrell MJ, White NJ, Looareesuwan S, Phillips RE, Suntharasamai P, Chanthavanich P, Riganti M, Fisher-Hoch SP, Nicholson KG, Manutsathit S, Vannaphan S, Warrell DA. Failure of interferon alpha and tribavirin in rabies encephalitis. Br Med J 1989; 299:830–833.
180. Dietzschold B, Rupprecht CE, Tollis M, Lafon M, Mattei J, Wiktor TJ, Koprowski H. Antigenic diversity of the glycoprotein and nucleocapsid proteins of rabies and rabies related virus. Rev Infect Dis 1988; 10(suppl 4):785–798.
181. Lafon M, Lafage M. Antiviral activity of monoclonal antibodies specific for the internal proteins N and NS of rabies virus. J Gen Virol 1987; 68:3113–3123.
182. Dietzschold B, Kao M, Zheng YM, Chen ZY, Maul G, Fu ZF, Rupprecht CE, Koprowski H. Delineation of putative mechanisms involved in antibody-mediated clearance of rabies virus from the central nervous system. Proc Natl Acad Sci USA 1992; 89:7252–7256.
183. Baer GM, Shaddock JH, Williams LW. Prolonging morbidity in rabid dogs by intrathecal injection of attenuated rabies vaccine. Infect Immun 1975; 12:98–103.
184. Warrell MJ, Ward GS, Elwell MR, Tingpalapong M. An attempt to treat rabies encephalitis in monkeys with intrathecal live rabies virus RV675. Arch Virol 1987; 96:271–273.
185. Porras C, Barboza JJ, Fuenzalida E, Adaros HL. Recovery from rabies in man. Ann Intern Med 1976; 85:44–48.
186. Lucia Alvarez H, Ramon Fajardo V, Elvia Lopez M, Rina Pedroza F, Hemachudha T, Kamolvarin N, Gilberto Cortes C, Baer GM. Partial recovery from rabies in a nine-year-old boy. Ped Infect Dis J 1994; 13:1154–1155.
187. Hemachudha T, Khawplod P, Phanuphak P, Griffin DE. Enhanced antibody response to rabies virus in patients with neurologic complications following brain tissue-derived rabies vaccination. Asian Pac J Allergy Immunol 1989; 7:49–50.
188. Blenden DC, Creech W, Torres-Anjel MJ. Use of immunofluorescence examination to detect rabies virus antigen in the skin of human with clinical encephalitis. J Infect Dis 1986; 154:698–701.
189. Hemachudha T, Kamolvarin N, Tirawatnpong T, Tirawatnpong S, Panpanich T, Khawplod P, Wilde H, Chutivongse S. Ante- and postmortem diagnosis of rabies in man and animal by PCR using nested primers. Neurology 1992; 42(suppl 3):370.
190. Rudd R, Trimarchi CV. Development and evaluation of an in vitro virus inoculation procedure as a replacement for the mouse inoculation test in rabies diagnosis. J Clin Microbiol 1989; 27:2522–2528.
191. Hemachudha T, Wilde H. Rabies. In: Johnson RT, Griffin JW, eds. Current Therapy in Neurological Disease. 4th ed. St. Louis: Mosby Year Book, 1993:143–146.
192. Siwasontiwat D, Lumlertdaecha B, Polsuwan C, Hemachudha T, Chutivongse S, Wilde H. Rabies: Is

provocation of the biting dog relevant for risk assessment? Trans R Soc Trop Med Hyg 1992; 86:443.
193. WHO. Report of the symposium on rabies control in Asian countries. World Health Organization unpublished document WHO/Rab.Res/93.44, 1993.
194. Tepsumethanon W, Polsuwan C, Lumlertdaecha B, Khawplod P, Hemachudha T, Chutivongse S, Wilde H, Chiewbamrungkiat M, Phanuphak P. Immune response to rabies vaccine in Thai dogs: a preliminary report. Vaccine 1991; 9:627–630.
195. Chutivongse S, Wilde H, Supich C, Baer GM, Fishbein DB. Postexposure prophylaxis for rabies with antiserum and intradermal vaccination. Lancet 1990; 335:896–898.
196. Fishbein DB, Yenne KM, Dreesen DW, Teplis CF, Mehta N, Briggs DJ. Risk factors for systemic hypersensitivity reactions after booster vaccinations with human diploid cell rabies vaccine: a nationwide prospective study. Vaccine 1993; 11:1390–1394.

28

Cerebral Malaria

Kara K. Wools
Indiana University School of Medicine, Indianapolis, Indiana

HISTORICAL PERSPECTIVE AND BACKGROUND

Malaria

The term malaria came into use in the eighteenth century, based on the prevailing belief that the disease was caused by bad air surrounding swamps, marshes, and low-lying areas (1). Though the name is of relatively recent origin, malarial parasites have had a long association with humans. This position is supported by the parasites' high degree of host specificity and the presence of malaria-resistant blood polymorphisms, such as the Duffy negative blood type, hemoglobin S, and some of the thalasemias (2,3). Absence of malaria-associated blood polymorphisms in individuals native to the New World and the close association of human malaria parasites with those of African primates attests to the Old World origin of this disease (2).

Though accounts of intermittent fevers exist in the writings of ancient China, India, and Assyria, it is uncertain that these fevers were malaria (1,2,4). In the works attributed to Hippocrates (4th century B.C.), there are descriptions of several types of intermittent fevers; those described as quotidian, tertian, and quatrain are considered to be attributable to malaria. Hippocrates also describes the presence of splenomegaly in individuals residing in low-lying areas and marshes (5,6).

A significant discovery in the history of malaria was made in 1880 when Laveran, a French Army surgeon in Algeria, identified parasitic elements in the red blood cells of soldiers with fever (1,4). In the latter part of the nineteenth century, the associations between many human diseases and their insect vectors were identified, paving the way for Manson's hypothesis that the mosquito was responsible for malaria transmission. In 1897, Ross detected pigmented cysts in the stomach of an *Anopheles* mosquito (1). By 1898, Grassi, Bignami, and Bastianelli had described the malaria parasites' life cycle in the *Anopheles* mosquito. In 1900, Manson proved that malaria could be transmitted to healthy individuals through the bite of an infected mosquito (1,4).

The control of the mosquito during the early and mid part of the twentieth century eliminated endemic malaria from most of Europe, North America, and Australia (1,2). Despite control efforts, malaria continues to be endemic in most tropical and subtropical regions of the world, causing illness in 100–300 million people each year (7). The increase in international travel by Europeans and Americans has led to an increase in the number of cases of malaria seen by physicians in the United States and Europe and underscores the need for physician education in the prompt recognition and appropriate treatment of this disease.

Cerebral Malaria

Hippocrates described a disease manifesting as coma, which was generally fatal, occurring mostly in winter and attacking adults. This may be the first documentation of what we now know as cerebral malaria (5). Since Hippocrates' time, definitions of cerebral malaria have varied from author to author. The World Health Organization (WHO) currently defines cerebral malaria as "unarousable coma not attributed to any other cause in a patient with falciparum malaria" (8). In this chapter, the definition will be extended to include any alteration in mental status (delirium, stupor, coma, obtundation, etc.) or upper motor neuron signs in a patient with falciparum malaria that cannot be attributed to another cause (i.e., hypothermia, hypoglycemia, postictal state, central nervous system (CNS) depressants, secondary infection, etc.). Cerebral malaria, severe normocytic anemia, hypoglycemia, pulmonary edema, renal failure, shock, disseminated intravascular coagulation (DIC), repeated generalized convulsions, acidemia/acidosis, malarial hemoglobinuria, and parasitemia $> 5\%$ in a nonimmune patient are all considered severe manifestations of malaria.

CHARACTERISTICS OF THE PATHOGEN

Human malaria is caused by one of four species of *Plasmodia-falciparum*, *vivax*, *malaria*, or *ovale*. *P. falciparum* is responsible for 40–60% of malaria cases worldwide and has the highest per case mortality. All four species share a common vector and have very similar life cycles, which consist of an asexual phase (occurring in humans) and a sexual phase (occurring in mosquitoes). The asexual phase can be further subdivided into an exoerythrocytic stage and an erythrocytic stage. This chapter will concentrate on *P. falciparum* because it is the only species that causes cerebral malaria in humans.

Asexual Phase

P. falciparum is transmitted through the bite of the female *Anopheles* mosquito. In the process of taking a blood meal, it injects asexual parasitic forms known as sporozoites into the host's circulation. During the exoerythrocytic phase the sporozoites are transported to the liver, where they invade hepatocytes and develop into liver stage schizonts in 7–14 days. Each schizont contains 10,000–40,000 merozoites, which are eventually released into the circulation when the hepatocyte ruptures. In *P. falciparum* infections no dormant organisms remain in the liver at the time of schizont rupture; this differs from *P. vivax* and *P. ovale*. During the erythrocytic phase merozoites in the circulation invade erythrocytes, where they form trophozoites. The trophozoites go on to develop into erythrocytic-stage schizonts, which contain an average of 16 merozoites (7,9–12).

When the parasite reaches the trophozoite and schizont stage, knobs form on the outer membrane of infected erythrocytes. These knobs are composed of parasitic proteins, including *P. falciparum* erythrocyte membrane–associated proteins 1 and 2 (PF EMP1, PF EMP2) and *P. falciparum* histidine-rich protein 1 (Pf HRP1). Though not directly responsible for the cytoadherence of parasitized erythrocytes, the appearance of the knobs signals the period when infected cells begin to leave the peripheral circulation and sequester in the microvasculature (13). Sequestration occurs mostly in the microvasculature of the brain with lesser parasitic loads in the heart, liver, lung, kidney, and blood (14).

When the schizont has reached maturity, the erythrocyte ruptures, releasing merozoites into the circulation. The merozoites are then capable of infecting erythrocytes, thus continuing the cycle. The duration of the erythrocytic cycle determines the fever pattern in malaria. In *P. falciparum* infections, the cycle duration is 48 h. Unlike the other three species of *Plasmodia*, the *P. falciparum* cycle is not well synchronized, resulting in an erratic or continuous fever (7).

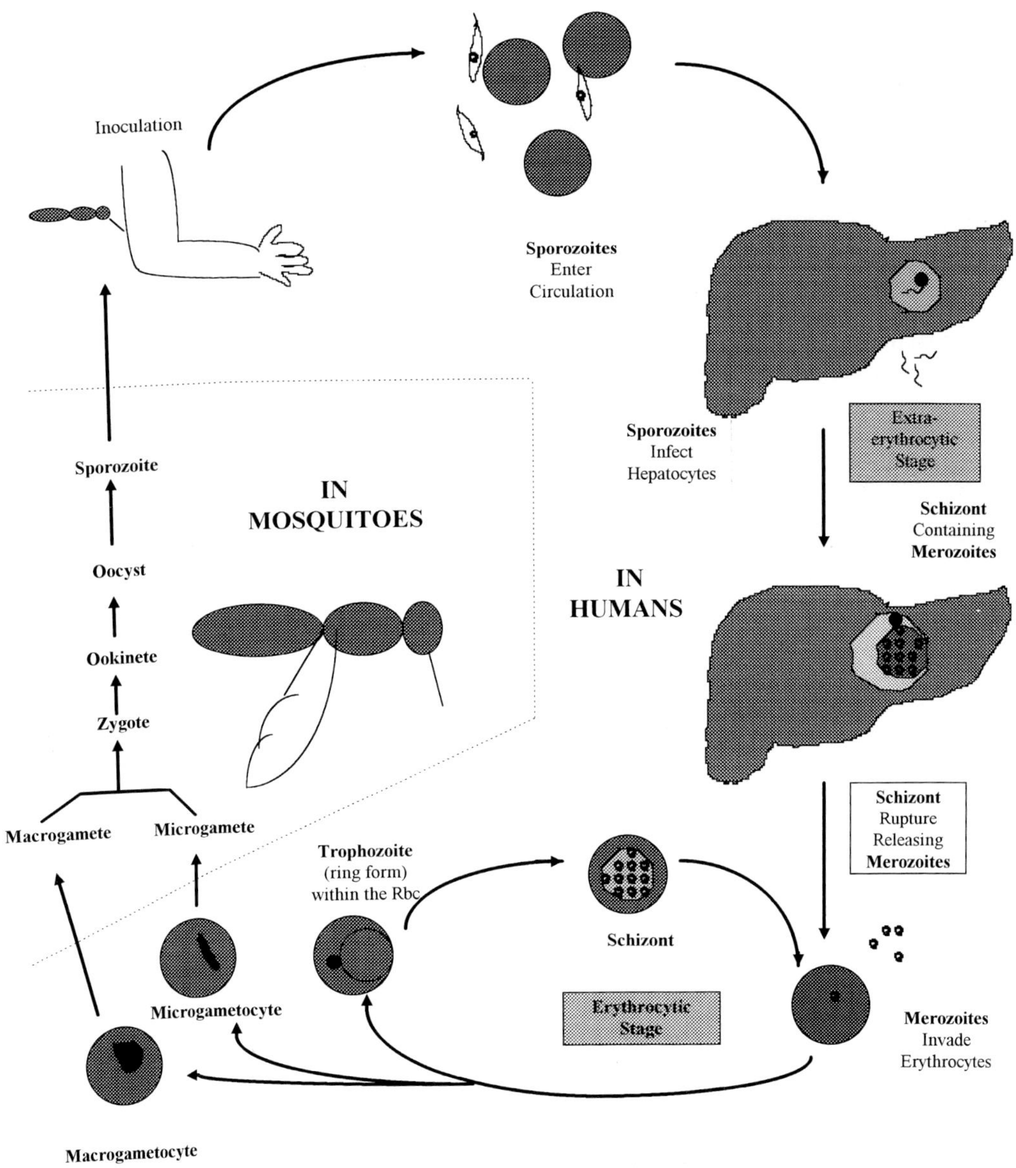

Figure 1 Simplified life cycle of *Plasmodium falciparum*.

Sexual Phase

Within the erythrocyte, merozoites may become gametocytes rather than develop into trophozoites. The two types of gametocytes—microgametocytes (male) and macrogametocytes (female)—require ingestion by an *Anopheles* mosquito in order to undergo further development. Once in the midgut of the mosquito, the gametocytes mature into gametes, which then fuse to become a zygote. The zygote matures to become an ookinete, which burrows between the epithelial cells of the stomach wall, encysts on the outer surface of the midgut, and becomes an oocyst. Sporozoites develop within the oocyst. Eventually the oocyst ruptures, liberating the sporozoites, which travel to the salivary glands of the mosquito. The mosquito is capable of transmitting disease and the cycle begins again (Fig. 1) (9–11).

EPIDEMIOLOGY

Vector control in the early and midportion of this century altered the epidemiology of *P. falciparum* malaria; however, it is still endemic in most of the world's tropical and subtropical areas, such as sub-Saharan Africa, Asia, and Latin America. The *Anopheles* mosquito continues to be the source of the vast majority of infections; however, malaria can also be transmitted through blood transfusions and intravenous injections with blood-contaminated needles.

The incidence of cerebral malaria in a population is determined by the population's immunity, which is in turn dependent on the prevalence and stability of malaria in the region. In areas where significant transmission of malaria occurs annually with little change from year to year (holoendemic areas), native adults rarely develop cerebral malaria (15). Those at risk for severe malaria in these areas are children from 1 to 4 years of age, previous residents returning after years abroad, new residents coming from nonendemic areas, residents who were maintained on chemoprophylaxis but have stopped, and pregnant women (Table 1) (16–19). Unstable endemicity is seen in regions where *P. falciparum* has recently been introduced or in areas where the incidence of malaria fluctuates radically from year to year. In such areas, all children and adults are at risk for the development of cerebral malaria. By definition, *P. falciparum* malaria seen in nonendemic areas is imported and the population, with few exceptions, lacks immunity. Those at highest risk for infection are travelers returning from endemic areas. Travelers returning from sub-Saharan

Table 1 Persons at Risk for Severe Malaria by Epidemiological Area

Epidemiological area	Persons at risk for severe malaria
Holoendemic	Children 1–4 years of age
	New residents (from nonendemic areas)
	Returning residents (from nonendemic areas)
	Residents stopping chemoprophylaxis
	Pregnant women
Unstable	All adults and children
Nonendemic	Travelers (from endemic areas)
	Sporadic[a,b]

[a]Airport malaria.
[b]Malaria in nontravelers infected via mosquitoes feeding on persons returning from endemic area.

Africa, Papua New Guinea, and the Solomon Islands are at highest risk for malaria. Travelers returning from India and Haiti are at intermediate risk, and travelers from Southeast Asia and Latin America are at low risk (20). Infected mosquitoes can be transported from endemic areas via airplane, leading to sporadic cases of malaria in persons residing near or working at European international airports (airport malaria) (21). Infrequent cases of malaria are seen in the United States in nontravelers as a result of native *Anopheles* mosquitoes transmitting infection from people coming from endemic areas (7,22,23). The pattern of endemicity may vary from region to region within a country.

PATHOPHYSIOLOGY

The pathophysiology of human cerebral malaria is poorly defined largely as a result of inadequate animal models for this disease. Theories often fall short of explaining characteristics of human cerebral malaria such as the low incidence of neurological sequela and the rapid reversal of symptoms after initiation of treatment (8,12). Current opinion favors a prominent role for cytoadherence and sequestration in the pathophysiology of cerebral malaria (8,12–14,24–27).

Microscopy of brain tissue from patients dying of cerebral malaria demonstrates perivascular ring hemorrhages and cerebral microvasculature packed with parasitized and nonparasitized erythrocytes. Electron-dense knobs projecting from the membrane of late-stage parasitized erythrocytes appear to be adherent to the endothelium of the cerebral microvasculature (27,28). In one autopsy series, patients who died from cerebral malaria had three times as many vessels containing infected erythrocytes and a higher percentage of tightly packed vessels (58.7% vs. 7.6%) than patients dying from noncerebral malaria (14). *P. falciparum* is the only species of human *Plasmodia* with cytoadherence and sequestration characteristics (29).

As noted previously, knobs containing parasitic proteins protrude from the outer membrane of the infected erythrocyte as the parasite matures. Knobs were originally thought to be required for cytoadherence since both developed at approximately the same time; however, with the discovery of knob negative cytoadherent strains, this does not appear to be the case (8,12,13,27). An erythrocyte outer membrane ligand and an endothelial cell receptor are required for cytoadherence (13). Three molecules present on endothelial cells—intracellular adhesion molecule (ICAM-1), CD 36, and thromboplastin—have been identified as receptors (30–32). Preferential sequestration in the brain may be secondary to increased receptor density within the cerebral microvascular bed, as compared to the systemic circulation, but further investigation is required to confirm this hypothesis.

In addition to endothelial adherence, parasitized erythrocytes are capable of binding uninfected erythrocytes (rosette formation) in vitro. The significance of this finding is unclear, as the capability of a strain to form rosettes does not always correlate with its cytoadherence capability (33). Thalassemic erythrocytes have a low capacity for rosette formation, as do erythrocytes containing Hgb SS or HgbAS, which have been exposed to low oxygen tension. As these hemoglobin types are known to be protective for cerebral malaria, the above findings provide circumstantial evidence that rosette formation plays a role in the pathophysiology of cerebral malaria (26).

Despite the body of evidence supporting endothelial cytoadherence and rosette formation as major participants in the development of cerebral malaria, no correlation between the strength of cytoadherence or rosette formation in vitro and the patients' clinical course has been found. It is probable that host factors, including antibody and cytokine production, are responsible for this discrepancy. The significant reduction of parasitemia in malaria patients treated with pooled African IgG led to the conclusion that antibodies modify disease (34). The question remains as to whether or not malaria-specific antibodies affect cytoadherence. Strain-specific antibodies to *P.*

falciparum have been shown to reverse cytoadherence in squirrel monkeys, and sera taken from patients with noncerebral malaria has the ability to disrupt rosette formation more often than sera from patients with cerebral malaria (24,35). This ability to disrupt rosette formation may be protective against cerebral malaria. However, there is no increase in mature asexual forms in the peripheral blood of patients treated with pooled immune IgG. This would be expected if the pooled antibody inhibited cytoadherence (34).

The association between high levels of cytokines and severe malaria has been documented in several studies (36–40). The glycosylphospatidylinositol moiety of *P. falciparum* has been proposed to be a tumor necrosis factor α (TNF)–inducing toxin (41). Elevated TNF levels have been found to correlate with hyperparasitemia, severe anemia, hypoglycemia, and young age (36). Cerebral malaria has been linked to elevated TNF levels in some clinical studies of malaria but not in others (36–40). Differences in findings reported from various studies may be a result of short TNF half-life. *P. berghei*–infected mice treated with antibody to TNF were protected against the development of cerebral malaria (42). It has been proposed that TNF promotes the disease process by upregulating the endothelial receptors, leading to increased parasite sequestration in the cerebral vasculature (38).

Parasitized erythrocytes are probably identified by the spleen as a result of their reduced deformability. Cytoadherence thus provides a developmental advantage for *P. falciparum* by preventing filtering by the spleen (12). The spleen is capable of modifying the cytoadherence properties of the parasite. Splenectomized squirrel monkeys have a mixture of mature and immature forms in the peripheral blood as compared to animals with spleens, who had mainly ring forms (immature forms), thus indicating reduced cytoadherence. In vitro experiments have confirmed that parasites taken from splenectomized animals have altered cytoadherence capabilities and are not able to bind to melanoma cells (35). These findings are consistent with the mixed peripheral parasitemia seen in asplenic patients (12).

Cytoadherence allows sequestration of metabolically active parasites in the cerebral microvasculature. It is hypothesized that these parasites alter the metabolic balance of the CNS microenvironment through competition for substrates. Parasite utilization of oxygen and glucose creates hypoxia and lactic acidosis and, as a consequence, coma. It is possible that the parasite also has a direct or a host-mediated toxic effect (29).

CLINICAL PRESENTATION

History

In nonendemic areas, *P. falciparum* malaria is frequently misdiagnosed during the initial physician visit (43,44). Clinicians practicing in nonendemic areas must maintain a high level of suspicion in order to prevent delay of treatment for a potentially life-threatening infection. As the patient presenting with fever and neuropsychiatric symptoms will be unable to provide a history, it is necessary to seek information from friends and relatives who have intimate knowledge of the patient's habits. A thorough history should include questions about drug use (intravenous, alcohol, and other), transfusions, location of residence, occupation, and travel (7,21,45,46).

If the patient has traveled within the last 2–3 years, questions should be expanded to elicit details of the patient's travel habits. Determination should be made as to whether or not a patient traveling to a nonendemic area has stopped in an endemic area. Malaria can be acquired during brief stopovers without disembarking from the plane. For patients who have traveled in malarious areas, it is necessary to know the complete travel itinerary, duration of stay, length of time elapsed since return, method of malaria prophylaxis, compliance with prophylaxis regimen, history of treatment for malaria, eating and drinking habits while abroad, vaccination, and exposure history

(45,46). A history of good compliance with a malaria prophylaxis regimen does not exclude the diagnosis of malaria (see Sec. X) (45).

Falciparum malaria requires a minimum of 8 days for incubation, with 95% of all infections presenting within 4 weeks of the last mosquito exposure (7,45). Untreated or partially treated infections are usually eliminated by the immune system within a year, but may infrequently persist for 2–3 years.

Signs and Symptoms

Adults may have systemic symptoms for several days prior to the development of cerebral malaria, whereas children usually develop cerebral symptoms within 2 days after the onset of systemic symptoms (8,47). An irregular and often continuous fever is present in the majority of patients, although some may be normo- or hypothermic. Rigors are present in only 10–30% of patients. Other symptoms include fatigue, diarrhea, vomiting, abdominal pain, anorexia, chest pain, cough, myalgias, and arthralgias (8,43,44,47,49). Cough is more frequently encountered in children than adults (8). Systemic signs of malaria include jaundice, retinal hemorrhages, and hepatosplenomegaly, with jaundice occurring more often in adults than in children (8,15,43, 44,47). Abnormal patterns of respiration may develop due to fever, hypoglycemia, acidosis, or pulmonary edema.

Neurological symptoms include headaches, convulsions, mental status changes, and rarely hemiparesis. Neurological signs may include any of the following: opisthotonos, decerebrate or decorticate posturing, upper motor neuron signs (such as ankle and patellar clonus) hypotonia, disorders of conjugate gaze, bruxism, coma, delirium, disorientation, restlessness, anxiety, hallucinations, delusions, and rarely focal signs such as hemiparesis (8,15).

Laboratory Findings

Hematological abnormalities are prominent in malaria. Hemolysis results in elevated bilirubin and lactate dehydrogenase levels as well as anemia. Leukocyte counts are usually normal but may be elevated or decreased, even in the absence of a secondary infection. Thrombocytopenia and coagulation abnormalities occur without the characteristic pathological abnormalities of platelet and fibrin deposition associated with DIC. In patients with renal involvement, an elevated creatinine and/or hemoglobinuria is present. Acid-base abnormalities may occur as a result of shock, pulmonary edema, or renal failure. Hyponatremia and other electrolyte abnormalities are present in some patients (8). Hypoglycemia is frequently found in children and pregnant women on presentation and in other patients after the initiation of quinine therapy (19,48,50).

Prognostic Indicators at Admission

In a study of 131 Malawian children with cerebral malaria, eight factors present at the time of admission were associated with a poor prognosis: (1) blood glucose $\leqslant$ 2.2 mmol/L, (2) parasitemia $> 10^6$ ring forms/μL (see laboratory diagnosis), (3) wbc $> 15 \times 10^9$/L, (4) a coma score of 0/5 (coma scale for young children, where 5 indicates that the child localizes and cries or speaks appropriately to painful stimuli, as well as watches or follows appropriately, and 0 indicates no motor or verbal response to pain and failure to watch or follow), (5) absent corneal reflexes, (6) decerebrate posturing, (7) convulsions, and (8) age under 3 years. Patients with four or more of these findings had a relative risk of 8.40 for an outcome of death or residual neurological deficits (47). The association between poor coma score, decerebrate posturing, hypoglycemia, and poor prognosis has been confirmed by other authors (51,52). Children with acidemia and/or an elevated creatinine have also been found to have a poorer chance of complete recovering than those without these findings (53). In adults, elevated levels of creatinine and/or bilirubin, hyperparasitemia, shizontemia, peripheral leukocytosis, and severe anemia have been found to be indicators of poor prognosis.

DIFFERENTIAL DIAGNOSIS

There are many diseases that can present with neuropsychiatric symptoms in patients returning from or residing in malaria-endemic areas (Table 2). Infectious diseases include African trypanosomiasis, typhoid fever, cholera, meningitis, viral encephalitis, and brain abscess. Like malaria, African trypanosomiasis can become symptomatic weeks to years after leaving an endemic area. Distinguishing features of African trypanosomiasis include a history of tsetse fly bite, lymphadenopathy, edema of the face and extremities, and rash. Positive parasite preps of blood, CSF, or lymph node aspirates confirm the diagnosis. Typhoid has an incubation period of 5–21 days and leukopenia and bradycardia as prominent features. A positive blood culture for *Salmonella typhi* is diagnostic for typhoid. Cholera can be differentiated from malaria by the pathognomonic profuse rice water diarrhea (55,56). Some authors support the practice of lumbar puncture in all patients presenting with suspected cerebral malaria in order to rule out bacterial meningitis. Others feel that the risk of complications from lumbar puncture outweigh the benefits and recommend empiric therapy for meningitis when indicated (57). Further details on the diagnosis of meningitis, viral encephalitis, and brain abscess can be found elsewhere in this volume.

The differential diagnosis of malaria also includes noninfectious disorders such as hypo/hyperglycemia, hyper/hyponatremia, uremia, hepatic encephalopathy, acute alcohol intoxication, delirium tremens, drug intoxication or withdrawal, brain tumor, stroke, head trauma, heat stroke, psychiatric illness, and eclampsia (15,46). Hypoglycemia is a frequent complication of *P. falciparum* infection, and as such the investigation for malaria should not be terminated with this finding. To aid in the diagnosis, initial laboratory evaluation should include CBC, glucose, electrolytes, BUN, creatinine, liver function tests, calcium, magnesium, and phosphorus. Tox and volatile screen, blood gas, and head CT should be done as clinically indicated.

LABORATORY DIAGNOSIS

Despite new developments in the diagnosis of malaria, microscopy (Fig. 2) remains the most common procedure used. It is easy to perform, inexpensive, and requires a minimum of equipment, and it is generally available even in remote areas. Both a thin and thick blood smear should be examined. The thick smear has the advantage of concentrating a large amount of blood for examination, but does not allow for speciation and is subject to greater observer variation in

Table 2 Differential Diagnosis of Cerebral Malaria

Infectious	Toxic/Metabolic	Other
Cerebral malaria	Hypo/Hyperglycemia	Brain tumor
Trypanosomiasis	Hyper/Hyponatremia	Stroke
Typhoid	Uremia	Trauma
Meningitis	Hepatic encephalopathy	Heat stroke
Viral encephalitis	Alcohol (acute intoxication or DTs)	Psychiatric illness
Brain abscess	Drug intoxication or withdrawal	Eclampsia
Cholera		

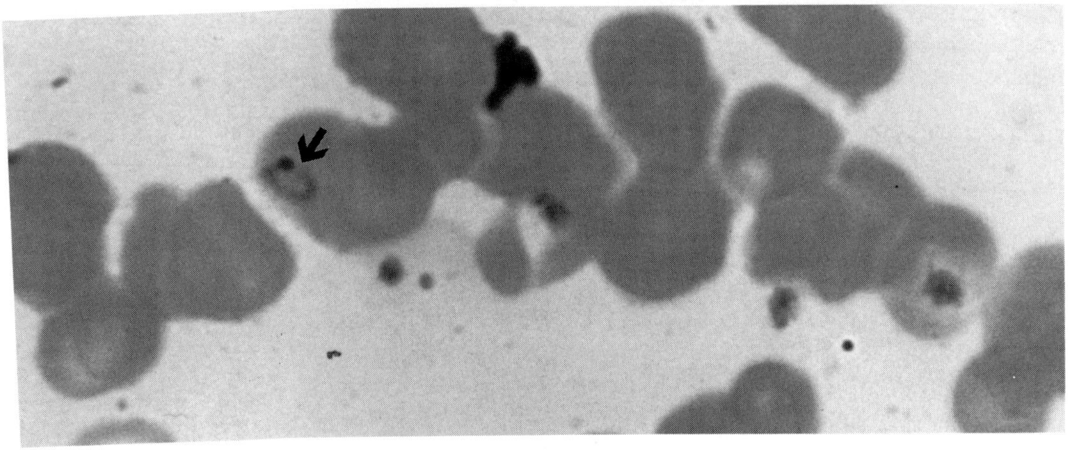

Figure 2 Blood smear demonstrating ring form (trophozoite) of *P. falciparum*.

results. Thin smears allow for parasite speciation and have less observer variability; however, with a thin smear, it is possible to miss low-level parasitemia because of the smaller quantity of blood examined. Quantitation of parasitemia can be done from both thick and thin blood smears. Accurate interpretation of a malaria slide requires an experienced observer. Results from a laboratory without expertise should be interpreted with caution. Blood smears should be done every 12–24 h for a period of 2–3 days (a minimum of three slides) in order to rule out malaria (Table 3) (11).

Another method for malaria detection is the quantitative buffy coat (QBC). This method uses centrifugation to concentrate infected cells and stains them with a fluorescent dye. Some studies have shown increased sensitivity with this method when compared to traditional microscopy, while others have shown decreased sensitivity and/or specificity (58–63). Serology for malaria is used in epidemiological studies and to screen blood supplies but has limited usefulness in the diagnosis of an acute infection (11,64). DNA and RNA probes, antigen capture assays, and PCR methods for malaria diagnosis are still in the experimental stages and are not currently available for clinical use (11,65–67).

THERAPY AND MANAGEMENT

Malaria therapy is dependent on the species of *Plasmodia*, the severity of disease, and the resistance patterns of the species in the area of acquisition. As *P. falciparum* is the only species

Table 3 Diagnostic Tests for Malaria

Test	Test frequency	Minimum number
Thick and thin blood smear or Quantitative Buffy Coat (QBC)	12–24 h	3

that causes cerebral malaria, which is considered a severe manifestation, the therapeutic recommendations discussed in this section are directed toward the treatment of severe *falciparum* malaria. Severe malaria is a medical emergency requiring prompt identification and treatment.

Management

Patients with cerebral malaria require intensive monitoring and dedicated nursing care and should be admitted to an intensive care unit when available. Routine care for coma patients including aspiration precautions, repositioning to prevent decubitus ulcers, prophylaxis of deep vein thrombosis, and nutritional supplementation should be provided. Fluid status should be monitored carefully.

Patients must be assessed and treated for other severe complications of *falciparum* malaria such as renal failure, pulmonary edema, severe normocytic anemia (Hct $< 15\%$ or Hgb < 5 g/dl), hypoglycemia, shock, DIC, recurrent generalized seizures, acidemia/acidosis, malarial hemoglobinuria, and hyperpyrexia. Renal failure as a result of acute tubular necrosis (ATN) is frequently seen in patients with severe *falciparum* malaria and should be managed with intravenous fluids and/or diuretics as indicated. Hemodialysis may be necessary in some patients. Pulmonary edema and acute respiratory distress syndrome may necessitate mechanical ventilation. Severe anemia should be treated with transfusion, but care should be taken not to overutilize transfusion, especially in countries where the blood supply is limited or where there is a risk of contaminated blood (8).

Hypoglycemia is a common finding in children and pregnant women with *falciparum* malaria. Quinine therapy can cause hypoglycemia in nonpregnant adults. Hypoglycemia can be treated with 50% dextrose 1–2 mg/kg followed by a continuous infusion of 10% dextrose for 4 h. If the glucose level stabilizes at 60 mg/dl, fluids can be changed to 5% dextrose. Blood glucose should be monitored every 6 h and evaluated promptly if the patient's clinical status deteriorates. Glucagon may be preferable to dextrose in patients with fluid overload, and glucose solutions per NG tube can be used when intravenous fluid solutions are not available (68).

DIC, acidemia, and shock suggests secondary bacterial infection, which should be evaluated with serial blood cultures and treated with broad-spectrum antibiotics. In patients with hemoglobinuria, adequate hydration with good urine output should be acheived in order to avoid pigment nephropathy. Fever may be controlled with antipyretics such as aspirin or acetaminophen. Seizure activity should be treated with anticonvulsants, and contributing metabolic abnormalities should be corrected. The use of prophylactic anticonvulsants in cerebral malaria may be beneficial. Deterioration in the coma score may be secondary to hypoxia, hypoglycemia, hyperpyrexia, convulsions, electrolyte disturbances, or severe anemia (7,8,68).

Antimalarial Therapy

Chloroquine therapy is no longer the antimicrobial agent of choice for severe *falciparum* malaria regardless of the antimicrobial resistance patterns of *P. falciparum* in the region of acquisition. In the United States, quinine is no longer available; therefore the standard of care for severe *falciparum* malaria is quinidine gluconate (Table 4). Cerebral malaria is treated with a loading dose of 10 mg/kg of IV quinidine gluconate over a period of 1–2 h followed by a continuous infusion of 0.02 mg/kg/min. Loading doses of quinine and quinidine are not recommended in patients who have received mefloquine, quinine, or quinidine in the 24 h prior to initiation of treatment. Plasma quinidine concentrations of 5–10 mg/liter are considered safe and effective. When the patient is able to take oral medication, therapy can be changed to one of the oral regimens described below to complete a total of 7 days of treatment from the initiation of intravenous therapy.

Table 4 Therapy for Cerebral Malaria

Drug therapy	Adult and pediatric loading dose	Adult and pediatric maintenance	Adult oral therapy	Child oral therapy	Total duration
Quinidine gluconate	10 mg/kg IV over 1–2 h	0.02 mg/kg/min continuous infusion	Quinine sulfate 650 mg q 8 h	Quinine sulfate 10 mg/kg q 8 h	7 days
Quinine gluconate	20 mg/kg IV over 4 h	10 mg/kg q 8 h	Quinine sulfate 650 mg q 8 h	Quinine sulfate 10 mg/kg q 8 h	7 days
plus					
Doxycycline[a,c,f]			100 mg q 12 h	—	7 days
or					
Tetracycline[a,c,f]			250 mg q 6 h	—	7 days
or					
Fansidar[b,d,e] (sulfadoxine-pyrimethamine)			3 tabs	Sulfadoxine 25 mg/kg Pyrimethamine 1.25 mg/kg	× 1 dose
or					
Clindamycin[f]			10 mg/kg q 12 h or 450 mg q 6 h	10 mg/kg q 12 h	3–5 days

[a]Contraindicated in pregnancy.
[b]Contraindicated in child < 1 month.
[c]Contraindicated in child < 8 years.
[d]Contraindicated in patients with sulfa allergy.
[e]Not recommended for malaria acquired in Southeast Asia or the Congo.
[f]Can be given IV if patient cannot swallow.

Side effects of quinidine include cinchonism (see below), hypoglycemia, arrhythmias, and cardiac conduction delays. Patients who have been on mefloquine in the preceding 2 weeks should be monitored closely for cardiac arrhythmias in an ICU setting where continuous blood pressure and cardiac monitoring can be done. For all patients, the use of telemetry to monitor for prolongation of the QT interval and widening of the QRS complex is recommended. Even though quinidine is a category C drug, most malariologists believe that the benefits of treating pregnant women with this drug far outweigh the risks to the fetus in severe malaria. To date, there have been no reports of quinidine resistance (69).

When practicing in a malaria-endemic area, an understanding of the treatment options suitable for that area is necessary. Outside the United States in areas where quinine is readily available and intensive care units are not, a regimen of quinine alone or quinine and tetracycline or doxycycline is frequently used. The recommended dosage of quinine in adults and children is 20 mg/kg IV loading dose given over 4 h followed by 10 mg/kg (infused over 4 h) IV every 8 h. Patients can be switched to an oral regimen of quinine and doxycycline when clinically improved to complete a total of 7 days of treatment. The recommended oral dose of quinine for adults is 650 mg every 8 h and for children, 10 mg/kg every 8 h. Plasma quinine concentrations of 10–15 mg/L are considered safe and effective.

Side effects of quinine include cinchonism, which is characterized by tinnitus, headache, nausea, vomiting, abdominal pain, blurred vision, transient loss of hearing, vertigo, and tremors. Cardiotoxicity is uncommon when quinine is given by a slow infusion. Glucose levels must be monitored in patients on quinine because a side effect of this drug is insulin release, resulting in hypoglycemia. Quinine is still classified as a category X drug, because its use in the past was associated with an increase in still births and preterm labor. Recent studies have not proven this to be true. The general opinion of malariologists is that the benefit of quinine therapy in pregnant patients infected with cerebral malaria exceeds the risk to the fetus. Quinine resistance has been reported from Southeast Asia (7,68,70).

Tetracycline or doxycycline should be added to the regimen in some geographic areas in order to achieve complete eradication of the parasite (for further information, please contact the CDC). Tetracyclines should be avoided in pregnant women and young children under 8 years of age. The recommended dose of doxycycline for adults is 100 mg po bid and for tetracycline is 250 mg po tid. If the patient is unable to take oral antibiotics for several days, tetracycline may be administered IV.

Combinations of quinine and clindamycin or fansidar (a combination of pyrimethamine and sulfadoxine) have also been used for malaria (70). Fansidar is not effective in treating malaria acquired in Southeast Asia or in the Congo. Fansidar is contraindicated in children younger than one month and in patients allergic to sulfa. Fansidar is listed as a category C drug in pregnancy with documented teratogenic effects in rats but no documented teratogenic effects in humans. Cost and benefit of its use in pregnancy must be individualized (68). When fansidar was used as a prophylactic agent, it was associated with severe cutaneous reactions such as Stevens-Johnson syndrome and toxic epidermolysis.

Artemisinin derivatives have been used in China for many centuries and are currently under investigation for the treatment of multidrug-resistant *P. falciparum*. Artemisinin derivatives appear to cause a rapid decrease in parasite load with a minimum of side effects. These antimalarial drugs are currently being used widely in China and other parts of Southeast Asia, but are not currently available in the United States (71–75).

Regardless of the antimalarial regimen chosen, clinical improvement should occur in 48–72 h with a 75% reduction in parasitemia by 48 h after the initiation of treatment. If clinical improvement does not occur in 72 h, consideration should be given to changing the therapeutic regimen.

Adjunct Therapy

Exchange transfusion has been recommended as adjunct therapy in patients with severe *falciparum* malaria. This procedure has been shown to cause a rapid decrease in the level of parasitemia, and uncontrolled series have shown improved clinical outcome in patients treated with this method. A prospective randomized controlled trial has not been done. The indications for exchange transfusion are not clear, nor is there a recommended volume of blood that should be exchanged. A reasonable approach is to consider exchange transfusion in patients with multi-organ failure who are not responding to conventional drug therapy. Exchange transfusion may be contraindicated in areas where the blood supply may be contaminated with HIV, hepatitis B, hepatitis C, *Treponema pallidum*, and/or *Plasmodia* and where screening is inadequate (76–80).

Corticosteroids were at one time recommended as adjunctive therapy in cerebral malaria. Prospective randomized controlled trials have shown no benefit to the use of steroids in cerebral malaria (81,82).

NEUROLOGICAL SEQUELAE

Neurological sequelae of cerebral malaria are uncommon in the adult population but occur in approximately 10% of children. Sequelae include hemiparesis, generalized hypotonia, inability to walk, generalized spasticity of limbs, cerebellar ataxia, persistent tremor, cortical blindness, and aphasia. In one study, 32 of 308 (12%) children with cerebral malaria had neurological sequelae. At an average follow-up of 6 months, 52% of these patients had completely recovered and 22% had shown some improvement in their neurological status. Long-term neurological complications such as epilepsy have been reported in patients with cerebral malaria (8,47,83,84).

PREVENTION

Malaria can be prevented by avoiding the bite of the *Anopheles* mosquito and by using chemoprophylaxis while traveling or residing in a malaria-endemic country. *Anopheles* mosquitoes bite during the period between dusk and dawn. Bites can be avoided by using bed nets treated with permethrin, closing windows before nightfall, spraying rooms with pyrethroid containing insect

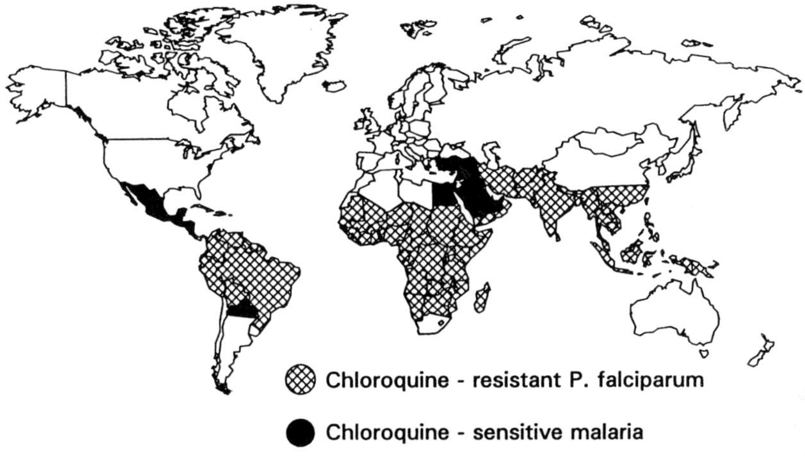

Figure 3 Distribution of malaria and chloroquine-resistant *P. falciparum*, 1994.

spray, wearing long sleeves, staying within enclosed areas during the evening and nighttime hours, and using *N,N*-diethylmethyltoluamide (DEET)–containing insect repellent. Recommendations for chemoprophylaxis vary with changing resistance patterns. Currently chloroquine-resistant *P. falciparum* exists in all countries, with the exception of the Dominican Republic, Haiti, Central America west of the Panama Canal, Egypt, and most countries in the Middle East (Fig. 3). Chloroquine is the recommended prophylactic agent for areas without resistant parasites. Mefloquine is the drug of choice for chemoprophylaxis in areas with chloroquine-resistant malaria. Doxycycline can be used as an alternative to mefloquine for prophylaxis in countries with chloroqine-resistant malaria. Doxycycline is not recommended for use in pregnant women or young children because it affects bone mineralization. The potential adverse effects of mefloquine in pregnancy and in children less than 15 kg are unknown; therefore it is currently not recommended for use in these populations. These recommendations are constantly changing; therefore, travelers to malaria-endemic areas should consult the CDC publication *Health Information for International Travel* (85).

REFERENCES

1. Bruce-Chwatt LJ. Essential Malariology. London: William Heinemann Medical Books Ltd, 1980.
2. Dunn FL. Malaria. In: Kiple KF, ed. The Cambridge World History of Human Disease. Cambridge: Cambridge University Press, 1993:855–861.
3. Boyd M. Historical Review. In: Boyd M, ed. Malariology 1. Philadelphia: W.B. Saunders Company, 1949:3–25.
4. Bispham W. Malaria. Baltimore: Williams and Wilkins Co., 1944.
5. Jones, WHS: Malaria and Greek History. Manchester: University Press, 1909.
6. Hippocrates. Medical Works. Trans: Chadwick J, Mann WN. Oxford: Blackwell Scientific Publications, 1950.
7. Hoffman SL. Diagnosis, treatment, and prevention of malaria. Med Clin North Am 1992; 76(6):1327–1353.
8. WHO. Sever and complicated malaria. Trans R Soc Trop Med Hyg 1990; 84(suppl 2):1–65.
9. Weatherly NF. Medical Protozoology. In: Joklik WK, Willett HP, Amos DB, eds. Zinsser Microbiology. Norwalk, CT: Appleton-Century-Crofts, 1984:1206–1229.
10. Dourado HV. Abdon NP. Martins SJ. Falciparum malaria: epidemiology in Latin America, biologic and clinical considerations, treatment and prophylaxis. Infect Dis Clin North Am 1994; 8(1):207–223.
11. Makler MT. Gibbins B. Laboratory diagnosis of malaria. Clin Lab Med 1991; 11(4):941–956.
12. White NJ. Pathophysiology. Clin Trop Med Com Dis 1986; 1(1):55–90.
13. Howard RJ. Malarial proteins at the membrane of Plasmodium falciparum-infected erythrocytes and their involvement in cytoadherence to endothelial cells. Prog Allergy 1988; 41:98–147.
14. Macpherson GG, Warrell MJ, White NJ, Looareesuwan S, Warrell Da. Human cerebral malaria: a quantitative ultrastructural analysis of parasitized erythrocyte sequestration. AJP 1985; 119(3): 385–401.
15. Marsden PD, Bruce-Chwatt LJ. Cerebral Malaria. Contemp Neurol Ser 1996; 12:29–44.
16. Greenwood BM, Bradley AK, Gerewood AM, et al. Mortality and morbidity from malaria among chidlren in a rural area of the Gambia, West Africa. Trans R Soc Trop Med Hyg 1987; 81:478–486.
17. McGregor IA. The significance of parasitic infection in terms of clinical disease: a personal view. Parasitology 1987; 94:S159–S178.
18. Looareesuwan S, White NJ, Karbwang J, Turner RC, Phillips RE, Kietinun S, Rackow C, Warrell DA. Quninine and severe falciparum malaria in late pregnancy. Lancet 1985; 2:4–8.
19. Nathwani D, Currie PF, Douglas JG, Green ST, Smith NC. Plasmodium falciparum malaria in pregnancy: a review. Br J Obstet Gynaecol 1992; 99:118–121.
20. Wyler DJ. Malaria chemoprophylaxis for the traveler. N Engl J Med 1993; 329(1):31–37.

21. Isaacson M. Airport malaria: a review. Bull WHO 1989; 67(60):737–743.
22. Ginsberg MM. Transmission of malaria in San Diego County, California. West J Med 1991; 154(4):465–466.
23. Anonymous. Mosquito-transmitted malaria—California and Florida, 1990. MMWR 1991; 40(6): 106–108.
24. Carlson J, Helmby H, Hill AVS, Brewster D, Greenwood BM, Wahlgren M. Human cerebral malaria: association with erythrocyte rosetting and lack of anti-rosetting antibodies. Lancet 1990; 336:1457–1460.
25. Sein KK, Maeno Y, Thuc HV, Anh TK, Aikawa M. Differential sequestration of parasitized erythrocytes in the cerebrum and cerebellum in human cerebral malaria. Am J Trop Med Hyg 1993; 48(4):504–511.
26. Carlson J, Nash GB, Gabutti V, Al-Yaman F, Wahlgren M. Natural protection against server Plasmodium falciparum malaria due to impared rosette formation. Blood 1994; 84(11):3909–3914.
27. Oo MM, Aikawa M, Than T, Aye TM, Myint PT, Igarashi I, Schoene WC. Human cerebral malaria: a pathological study. J Neuropathol Exp Neurol 1987; 46(2):223–231.
28. Aikawa M, Iseki M, Barnwell JW, Taylor D, Oo MM, Howard RJ. The pathology of human cerebral malaria. Am J Trop Med Hyg 1990; 43(suppl 2):30–37.
29. Goldring JD, Hommel M. Variation in the cytoadherence characteristics of malaria parasites: is this a true virulence factor. Mem Inst Oswaldo Cruz 1992; 87(suppl 3):313–322.
30. Roberts DD, Sherwood JA, Spitalnik SL, Panton LJ, Howard RJ, Dixit VM, Frazier WA, Miller LH, Ginsburg V. Thrombospondin binds falciparum malaria parsitized erythrocytes and may medicate cytoadherence. Nature 1985; 318:64–66.
31. Barnwell JW, Asch AS, Nachman RL, Yamaya M, Aikawa M, Ingravallo P. A Human 88KD membrane glycoprotein (CD36) functions in vitro as a receptor for cytoadherence ligand on Plasmodium falciparum-infected erythrocytes. J Clin Invest 1989; 84:765–772.
32. Berendt AR, Simmons DL, Tansey J, Newbold CI, Marsh K. Intercellular adhesion molecule-1 is an endothelial cell adhesion receptor for Plasmodium falciparum. Nature 1989; 341:57–59.
33. Hasler T, Handunnetti SM, Aguiar JC, van Schravendijk MR, Greenwood BM, Lallinger G, Cegielski P, Howard RJ. In viro rosetting, cytoadherence, and microagglutination properties of Plasmodium falciparum-infected erythrocytes from Gambian and Tanzanian patients. Blood. 1990; 76(9):1845–1852.
34. Sabchareon A, Burnouf T, Ouattara D, Attanath P, Bouharoun-Tayoun H, Chantavanich P, Foucault C, Chongsuphajaisiddhi T, Druilhe P. Parasitologic and clinical human response to immunoglobulin administration in falciparum malaria. J Trop Med Hyg 1991; 45(3):297–308.
35. David PH, Mommel M, Miller LH, Udeinya IJ, and Oligino LD. Parasite sequestration in Plasmodium falciparum malaria: spleen and antibody modulation of cytoadherence of infected erythrocytes. Proc Natl Acad Sci USA 1983; 80:5075–5079.
36. Shaffer N, Grau GE, Hedberg K, Davachi F, Lyamba B, Hightower AW, Breman JG, Nguyen-Dinh P. Tumor necrosis factor and severe malaria. JID 1991; 163:96–101.
37. Kwiatkowski D, Hill AVS, Sambou I, Twumasi P, Castracane J, Manogue KR, Cerami A, Brewster DR, Greenwood BM. TNF concentration in fatal cerebral, non-fatal cerebral, and uncomplicated Plasmodium falciparum malaria. Lancet 1990; 336:1201–1204.
38. Kern P, Hemmer CJ, Van Damme J, Gruss HJ, Dietrich M. Elevated tumor necrosis factor alpha and interleukin-6 serum levels as markers for complicated Plasmodium falciparum malaria. Am J Med 1989; 87:139–143.
39. Grau GE, Taylor TE, Moyneux ME, Wirima JJ, Vassalli P, Hommel M, Lambert PH. Tumor necrosis factor and disease severity in children with falciparum malaria. N Engl J Med 1989; 320(24):1586–1591.
40. Grau GE, Piguet PF, Lambert PH. Immunopathology of malaria: role of cytokine production and adhesion molecutes. Mem Inst Oswaldo Cruz 1992; 87(suppl 5):95–100.
41. Schofield L, Vivas L, Hackett F, Gerold P, Schwarz RT, Tachado S. Neutralizing monoclonal antibodies to glycosylphosphatidylinositol, the dominant TNF-α-inducing toxin of Plasmodium falciparum: prospects for the immunotherapy of severe malaria. Ann Trop Med Parasitol 993; 87(6):617–626.

42. Grau EG, Fajardo LF, Piguet PF, Allet B, Lamber PH, Vassalli P. Tumor necrosis factor (cachectin) as an essential mediator in murine cerebral malaria. Science 1987; 237:1210–1212.
43. McCaslin RI, Pikis A, Rodriguez WJ. Pediatric Plasmodium falciparum malaria: a ten-year experience from Washington, DC. Pediatr Infect Dis J 1994; 13:709–715.
44. Winters RA, Murray HW. Malaria—the mime revisited: fifteen more years of experience at a New York City teaching hospital. Am J Med 1992; 93:243–246.
45. Saxe SE, Gardner P. The returning traveler with fever. Infect Dis Clin North Am 1992; 6(2):427–439.
46. Gilles HM. Diseases of travelers returning from exotic areas. IM 1989; 10(6):71–97.
47. Molyneux ME, Taylor TE, Wirima JJ, Borgstein A. Clinical features and prognostic indicators in pediatric cerebral malaria: a study of 131 comatose Malawian children Q J Med 1989; 71(265):441–459.
48. Phillips RE, Solomon T. Cerebral malaria in children. Lancet 1990; 336:1355–1360.
49. Wiest PM, Opal SM, Romulo RL, Olds GR. Malaria in travelers in Rhode Island: a review of 26 cases. Am J Med 1991; 91:30–36.
50. Taylor TE, Molyneux ME, Wirima JJ, Fletcher KA, Morris K. Blood glucose levels in Malawian children before and during the administration of intravenous quinine for severe falciparum malaria. N Engl J Med 1988; 319(16):1040–1047.
51. Walker O, Salako LA, Scwunmi A, Thomas JO, Sodeine O, Bondi FS. Prognostic risk factors and post mortem findings in cerebral malaria children. Trans R Soc Trop Med Hyg 1992; 86(5):191–193.
52. Bondi FS. The incidence and outcome of neurological abnormalities in childhood cerebral malaria: along-term follow-up of 62 survivors. Trans R Soc Trop Med Hyg 1992; 86(1):17–19.
53. Taylor TE, Borgstein A, Molyneux ME. Acid-base status in pediatric Plasmodium falciparum malaria. Q J Med 1993; 86(2):99–109.
54. Niyongabo T, Deloron P, Aubry P, Ndarugirire F, Manirakiza F, Muhirwa G, Ndayiragije A, Brelivst JC. Prognostic indicators in adult cerebral malaria: a study in Burundi, an area of high prevalence of HIV infection. Acta Trop 1991; 56(1):299–305.
55. Gorbach SL, Bartlett JG, Blacklow NR, Infect Dis. Maguire JH, Hoff R. Trypanosoma. Philadelphia: W.B. Saunders Company, 1992:1984–1990.
56. Kirchhoff LV. Agents of African trypanosomiasis. In: Mandel GL, Bennett JE, Dolin R, eds. Infectious Diseases. 4th ed. New York: Churchill Livingstone, 1995:2450–2454.
57. Hall AP. Letters to the editor: cerebral malaria. Lancet 1991; 337:1281.
58. Kumar BK, Fadeel MA, Sehgal SC. Efficacy and limitations of QBC acridines orange staining as a routine diagnostic technique for malaria in developing countries. J Trop Med Hyg 1993; 96:245–248.
59. Anthony RL, Bangs MJ, Anthony JM, Purnomo. On-site diagnosis of Plasmodium falciparum, P. vivax, and P. malariae by using the quantitative buffy coat system. J Parasitol 1992; 78(6):994–998.
60. Bento A, Roche J, Molina R, Amela C, Alvar J. Application and evaluation of QBC malaria diagnosis in a holoendemic area. App Parasitol 1994; 35(4):266–272.
61. Gay F, Traore B, Zanoni J, Danis M, Gentilini M. Evaluation of the QBC system for the diagnosis of malaria. Sante 1994; 4(4):289–297.
62. Mak JW, Normaznah Y, Chiang GL. Comparison of the quantitative buffy coat technique with the conventional thick blood film technique for malaria case detection in the field. Singapore Med J 1992; 33(5):452–454.
63. Baird JK, Purnomo, Jones TR. Diagnosis of malaria in the field by fluorescence microscopy of QBC capillary tubes. Trans R Soc Trop Med Hyg 1992; 86(1):3–5.
64. Suzuki M. Malaria immunoepdemiology—a trial to link field study with basic science. Kaohsiung 1991; 7(5):224–232.
65. McLaughlin GL, Decrind C, Dayal-Drager R, Hassan-King M, Subramanian S, Greenwood BM. Optimization of a rapid nonisotopic DNA probe assay for Plasmodium falciparum in the Gambia. J Clin Microbiol 1991; 29(7):1517–1519.
66. Tirasophon W, Ponglikitmongkol M, Wilairat P, Boonsaeng V, Panyim S. A novel detection of a single Plasmodium falciparum in infected blood. Biochem Biophys Res Commun 1991; 175(1):179–184.
67. Beadle C, Long GW, Weiss WR, McElroy PD, Maret SM, Oloo AJ, Hoffman SL. Diagnosis of malaria by detection of Plasmodium falciparum HRP-2 antigen with a rapid dipstick antigen-capture assay. Lancet 1994; 343:564–568.

68. Hoffman SL. Treatment of malaria. Clin Trop Med Commun Dis 1986; 1(1):171–224.
69. Anonymous. Treatment with quinidine gluconate of persons with severe Plasmodium falciparum infection: discontinuation of parenteral quinine from CDC Drug Service. MMWR 1991; 10:21–23.
70. Wyler DJ. Malaria: overview and update. Clin Infect Dis 1993; 16(1):119–156.
71. Hien TT, White NJ. Qinghaosu. Lancet 1993; 341:603–608.
72. White NJ. Artemisinin: current status. Trans R Soc Trop Med Hyg 1994; 88(suppl 1):3–4.
73. Li G, Guo X, Fu L, Jian H, Wang X. Clinical trial of artemisinin and its derivatives in the treatment of malaria in China. Trans R Soc Trop Med Hyg 1994; 88(suppl 1):5–6.
74. Hien TT. An overview of the clinical use of artemisinin and its derivatives in the treatment of falciparum malaria in Viet Nam. Trans R Soc Trop Med Hyg 1994; 88(suppl 1):7–8.
75. Looareesuwan S. Overview of clinical studies on artemisinin derivatives in Thailand. Trans R Soc Trop Med Hyg 1994; 88(suppl 1):9–11.
76. Chiodini Pl, Somerville M, Salam I. Tubbs HR, Wood MJ, Ellis CJ. Exchange transfusion in severe falciparum malaria. Trans R Soc Trop Med Hyg 1985; 79(6):865–866.
77. Phillips P, Nantel S, Benny WB. Exchange transfusion as an adjunct to the treatment of severe falciparum malaria: case report and review. Rev Infect Dis 1990; 12(6):1100–1108.
78. Exchange transfusion in falciparum malaria. Lancet 1990; 335:324–325.
79. Chiodini PL, Hall AP. Controlled trial of exchange transfusion in falciparum malaria. Lancet 1990; 335:554.
80. Salord F, Allaouchiche B, Gaussorgues P, Boibieux A, Sirodot M, Gerard-Boncompain M, Biron F, Peyramond D, Robert D. Severe falciparum malaria (21 cases). Intensive Care Med 1991; 17:449–454.
81. Warrell DA, Looareesuwan S, Warrell MJ, Kasemsarn P, Intaraprasert R, Bunnag D, Harinasuta T. Dexamethasone proves deleterious in cerebral malaria. N Engl J Med 1982; 306(6):313–319.
82. Hoffman SL, Rustama D, Punjabi NH, Surampaet B, Sanjaya B, Dimpudus AJ, McKee KT, Paleologo FP, Campbell JR, Marwoto H, Laghlin L. High-dose dexamethasone in quinine-treated patients with cerebral malaria: a double-blind, placebo-controlled trial. J Infect Dis 1988; 158(2):325–331.
83. Carme B, Bouquety JC, Plassart H. Mortality and sequelae due to cerebral malaria in African children in Brazzaville, Congo. Am J Trop Med Hyg 1993; 48(2):216–221.
84. Brewster DR, Kwiatkowski D, White NJ. Neurological sequelae of cerebral malaria in children. Lancet 1990; 336:1039–1043.
85. CDC. Health Information for International Travel 1994. Atlanta: U.S. Department of Health for International Travel, 1994.

29

Neuroimaging of Central Nervous System Infections

Richard R. Smith
Indiana University School of Medicine, Indianapolis, Indiana

Infection of the central nervous system is increasing in frequency. This is partially due to the increased incidence of patients immunocompromised due to AIDS and organ transplantation. One other contributing factor relating to the increase in requests for neuroimaging of infection is the marked improvement in the ability to detect such infections and the need to follow serial scans for therapeutic purposes.

Although computer tomography (CT) represented a significant advance in neuroimaging, the introduction of magnetic resonance imaging (MRI) in the 1980s was particularly useful in the detection of intracranial and spinal infections (1–3). Although CT was useful in demonstrating larger, more prominent abnormalities such as large abscesses, MRI allowed the detection of small lesions. Additionally, the lack of bone artifacts and the multiplanar capabilities of MRI allowed abnormalities in the middle cranial fossa and posterior fossa to be imaged for the first time. Not only did MRI improve the detection of intracranial infection, it also improved the specificity. Utilizing MRI it is frequently possible to distinguish abscess from cystic neoplasm and to differentiate infected from noninfected subdural collections. One shortcoming of MRI is its inability to demonstrate small calcified lesions, such as those associated with TORCH infections or the calcifications of tuberculosis and cysticercosis.

Pre- and postcontrast CT images should be obtained if there is a possibility of an intracranial infection. Bone windows may be useful to evaluate adjacent paranasal sinuses or middle ear cavities and mastoid air cells. The standard MRI examination should consist of both T_1- and T_2-weighted images. A postcontrast T_1-weighted series should also be performed. Additional views may be useful. For example, coronal postgadolinium T_1-weighted images are the most sensitive images for the detection of abnormal meningeal enhancement. Coronal T_2-weighted images are most sensitive for the early detection of herpes encephalitis. Although there is an increased ability to detect calcification on gradient echo images, CT remains the procedure of choice (4). Additional pulse sequences such as MR venography or MR angiography may be helpful in evaluation of vascular complications associated with intracranial infection, such as dural sinus thrombosis.

MENINGITIS AND ITS COMPLICATIONS

Meningitis

The diagnosis of meningitis does not typically depend upon neuroimaging. Generally, the clinical history, physical examination, and laboratory examination of the CSF are sufficient to make the diagnosis. Neuroimaging, then, is typically reserved to evaluate the complications associated

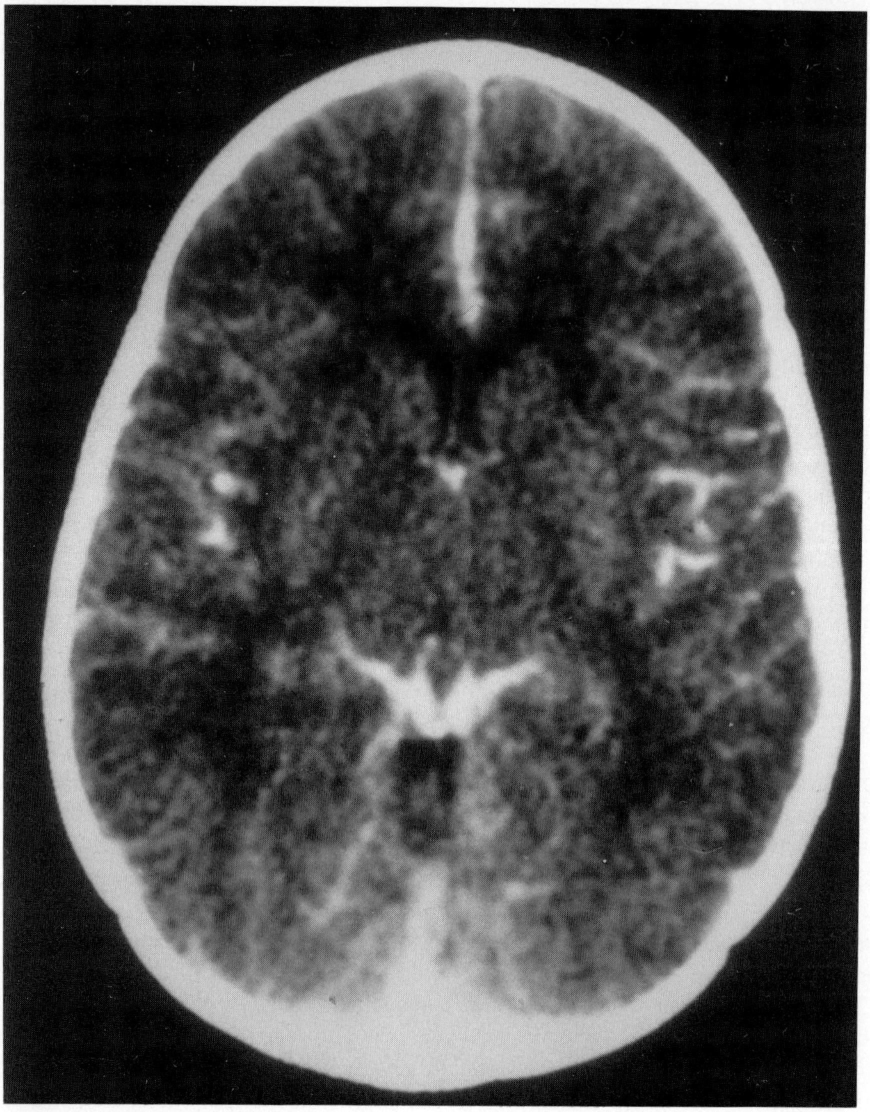

Figure 1 Meningitis. An enhanced axial CT image demonstrates an accentuated enhancement pattern in the sulci and anterior falx due to meningitis.

with meningitis, to evaluate direct extension from middle ear, sinus, and mastoid infections, or to aid in the evaluation of partially treated or clinically atypical infections. CT scanning may also be utilized to rule out an intracranial mass lesion before lumbar puncture. The imaging of meningitis is one area where MRI far exceeds the sensitivity of CT. The meninges on a typical contrast-enhanced CT scan show enhancement. This is usually seen along the falx and the tentorium. Enhancement of vessels in the sulci may be difficult to differentiate from purulent debris in the sulci. The convexity enhancement normally associated with the meninges on CT is typically not appreciated due to the adjacent dense bone. As a result, the detection of meningitis on CT is poor and in most cases the CT scan is normal, although in very florid cases the CT may be abnormal (Fig. 1) (5–7). On MRI, the meninges do not normally enhance with contrast, and as a result meningeal enhancement is pathological. Meningitis on MRI typically appears as a thin linear enhancement of the convexity meninges, falx, and tentorium (Fig. 2) (8,9). The more significant the infection, the more likely it is that all meningeal surfaces will enhance. Focal enhancement may be seen in less clinically severe cases or in cases associated with direct extension from a contiguous focus of infection (Fig. 3).

There are few reports prospectively evaluating the sensitivity of MRI in the detection of meningitis (10). Most reports suggest that the sensitivity of MRI for bacterial and tuberculous meningitis is high. The MRI scan is abnormal in less than 50% of viral and fungal meningitis cases.

The presence of meningeal enhancement is also not pathognomonic for meningitis. Abnormal meningeal enhancement can be due to any inflammatory process in the meninges, such as that due to craniotomy, head trauma, subarachnoid hemorrhage, carcinomatous meningitis, and sarcoidosis. In most cases, the differentiation from meningitis is easily made, whether that is based on the finding of a craniotomy site or the thick nodular enhancement associated with carcinomatous meningitis.

Complications

Prior to the advent of MRI, the diagnosis of meningitis on CT was frequently made based on the complications of this infection, such as communicating hydrocephalus. The complications associated with meningitis include the following (11):

1. Hydrocephalus—communicating or obstructive
2. Infarction
3. Venous or dural sinus thrombosis
4. Ventriculitis and choroid plexitis

Although other complications such as cerebritis and abscess may be associated with meningitis, these particular entities will be discussed under their own individual headings.

Hydrocephalus

Communicating hydrocephalus is a frequent complication of meningitis. The inflammatory exudate covering the surface of the brain obstructs the resorptive function of the pacchionian granulations. As a result there is dilatation of the ventricular and subarachnoid spaces (Fig. 4). Obstructive hydrocephalus develops when the inflammatory exudate impedes the flow of CSF through the ventricular pathways. On CT and/or MRI there is dilatation of the ventricular system proximal to the obstruction with decreased size of the ventricular system distally (Fig. 5).

Infarction

Cerebrovascular disease complicating meningitis may result in the occlusion of cerebral blood vessels, resulting in a large wedge-shaped infarction involving both the cortex and underlying

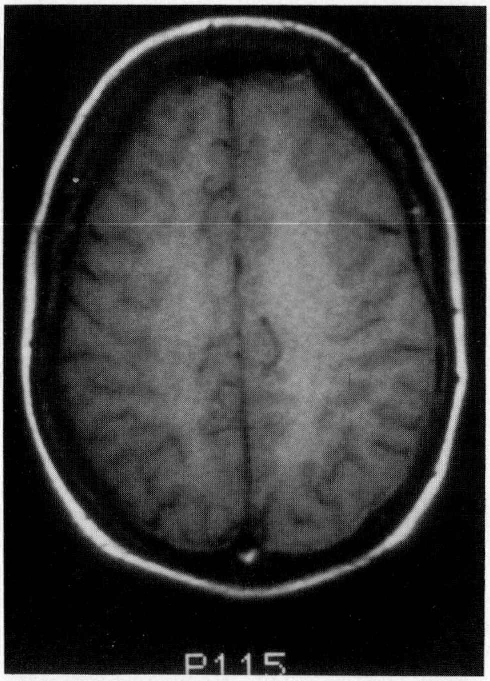

(A)

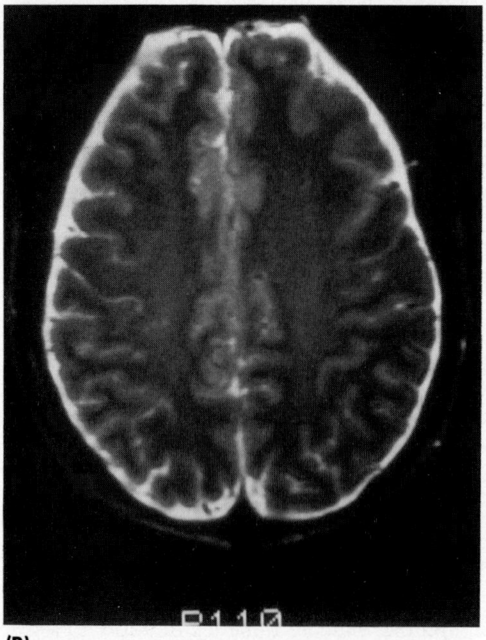

(B)

Figure 2 Meningitis. (A) and (B) are axial nonenhanced T_1- and T_2-weighted images, respectively. They are normal. Following intravenous contrast, axial (C) and coronal (D) images show abnormal convexity meningeal enhancement (arrows) as well as abnormal enhancement of the falx and tentorium (arrowheads).

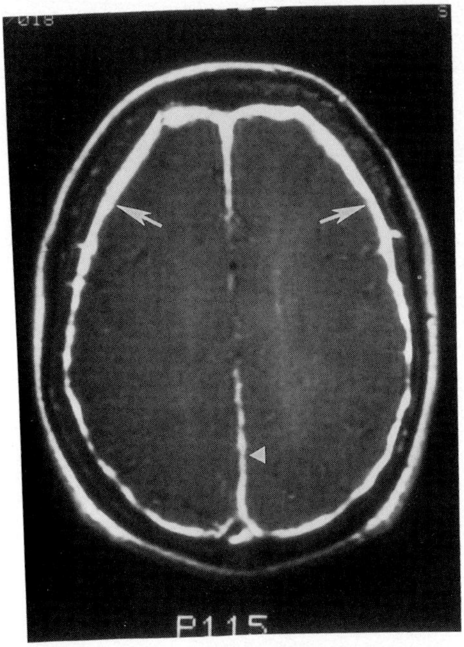

(C)

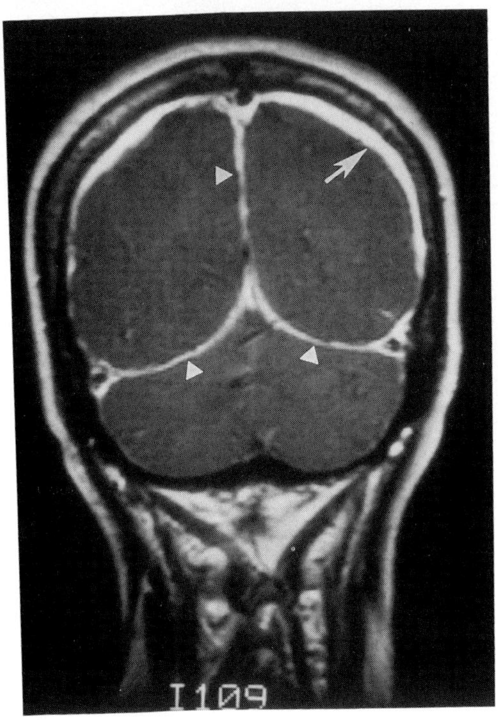

(D)

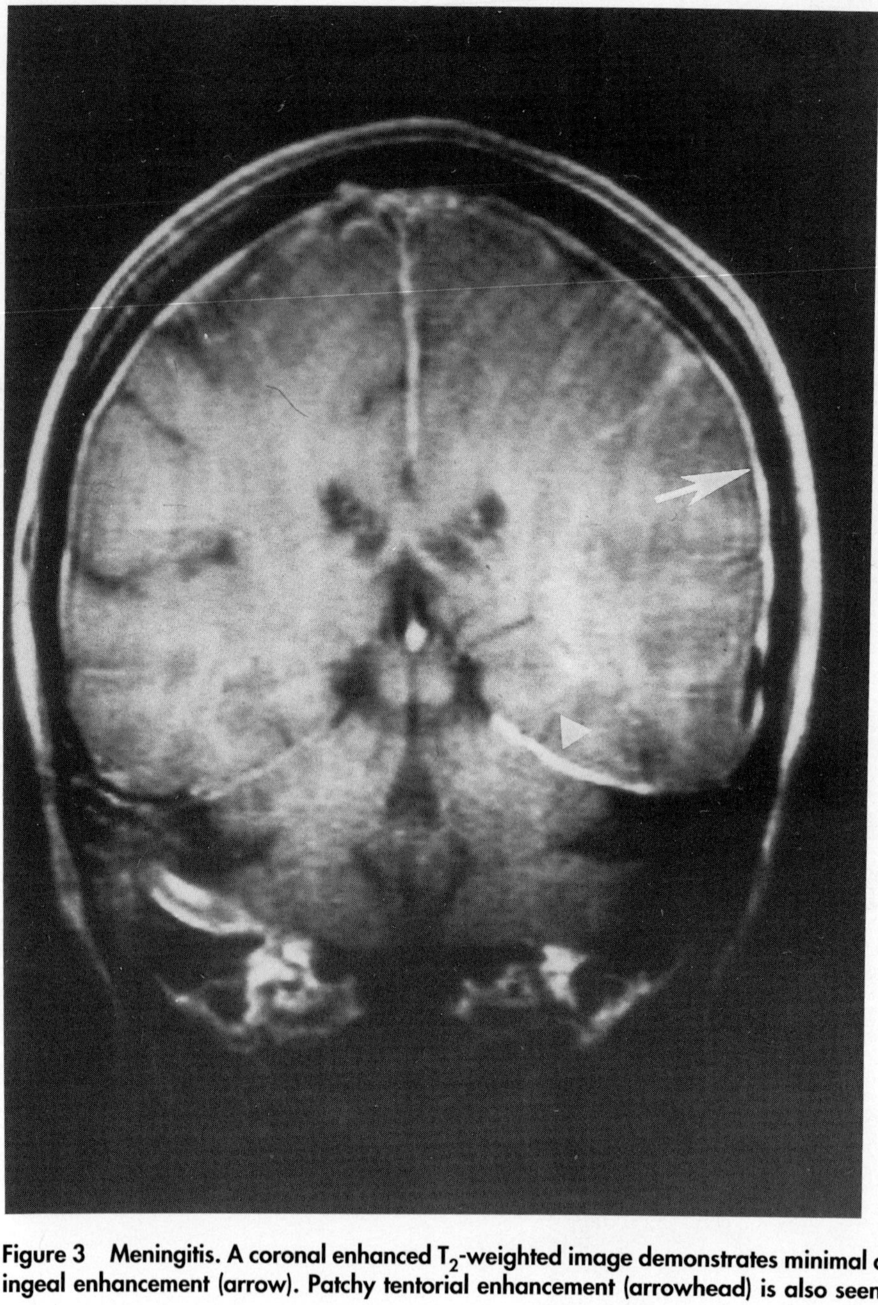

Figure 3 Meningitis. A coronal enhanced T_2-weighted image demonstrates minimal convexity meningeal enhancement (arrow). Patchy tentorial enhancement (arrowhead) is also seen.

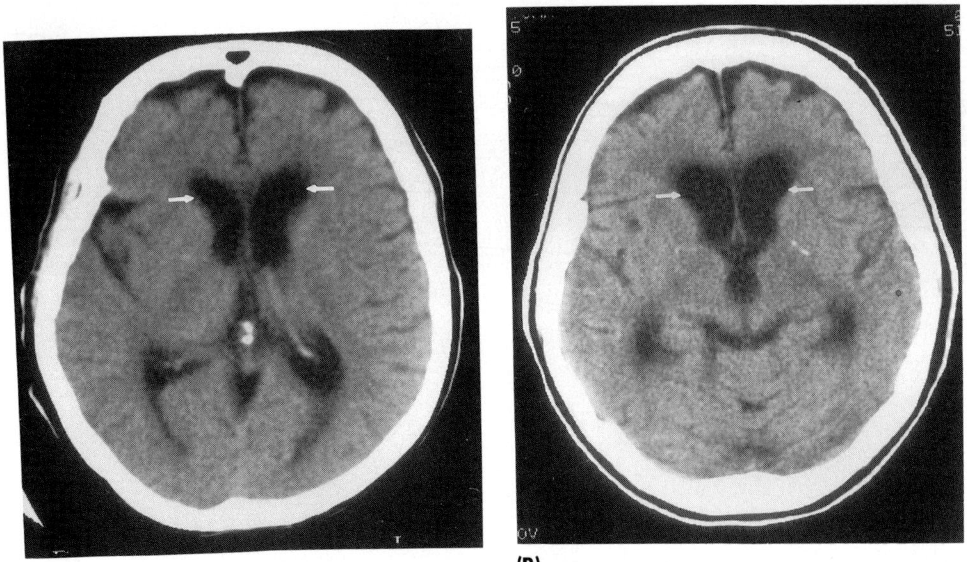

(A) (B)

Figure 4 Communicating hydrocephalus. An axial nonenhanced CT (A) at the time of presentation of meningitis demonstrates no abnormal ventricular enlargement (the lateral ventricular margins are marked by arrows). An axial nonenhanced CT (B) 2 weeks later shows moderate interval enlargement of the ventricular system with mild increased prominence of the sulcal space. This is consistent with mild communicating hydrocephalus.

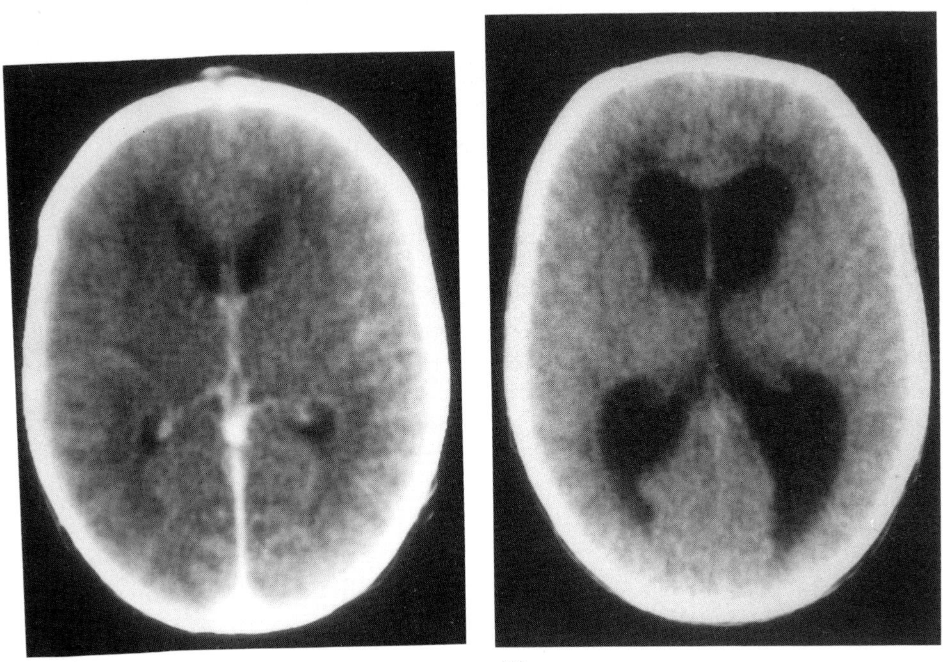

(A) (B)

Figure 5 Obstructive hydrocephalus. Axial CT images taken at the time of presentation (A) and 10 days later (B) show interval distention of the lateral ventricles with effacement of the cortical sulci. Other images demonstrated increased size of the third ventricle but a normal fourth ventricle consistent with inflammatory exudate obstructing the sylvian aqueduct.

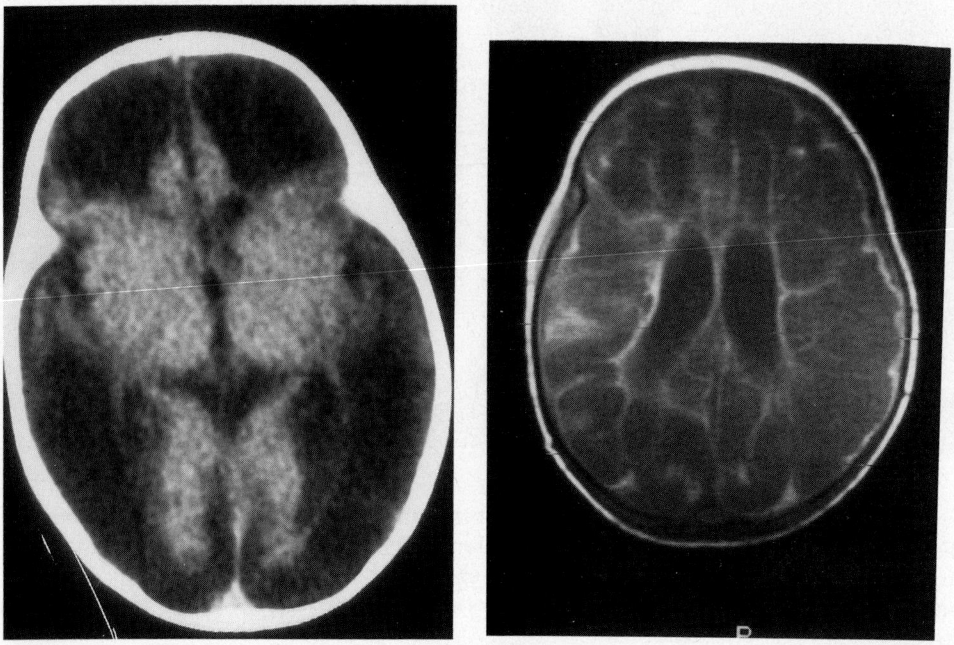

Figure 6 Infarction complicating meningitis. An axial nonenhanced CT image (A) demonstrates infarction in most of the cerebral cortex with sparing of the deep gray matter structures. An axial T_1-weighted image (B) shows diffuse infarction and multicystic encephalomalacia due to *Enterobacter sakoyaku* meningitis.

gray matter (Fig. 6) (12,13). An infarction will be hypodense with associated mass effect on CT. On T_2-weighted images, an acute infarction is hyperintense to adjacent brain and will also demonstrate mass effect.

Venous and Dural Sinus Thrombosis

Thrombosis of isolated cortical veins frequently leads to a venous infarction. Thrombosis of a dural sinus typically involves a much greater area of the brain. Venous infarction is hypodense on CT with associated hyperdense hemorrhage and mass effect. The presence of thrombosis may or may not be detectable on CT (14). On MRI, the area of venous infarction will be hypointense on T_1- and hyperintense on T_2-weighted images. Foci of hemorrhage are commonly seen. The signal intensity of the hemorrhage will depend upon the age of the hemorrhage. Acute hemorrhage is typically hypointense to brain on T_2-weighted images, while subacute blood is hyperintense on T_1-weighted images (15). Additionally, MRI is able to demonstrate dural sinus thrombosis. Instead of the usual dark flow void within the sinus, gray or bright signal intensity is seen within the dural sinus (16). MRI venography will demonstrate lack of flow within the involved sinus (Fig. 7).

Ventriculitis

Meningitis may be complicated by ventriculitis and choroid plexitis. Ventricular enlargement is an expected complication of meningitis, but in florid cases of ventriculitis there is so much surrounding edema that the ventricles may actually be decreased in size. On CT scanning, the ventricles are typically slightly irregular with decreased density in the periventricular white matter. Irregular enhancement is seen along the ventricular lining following contrast administration. On MRI, the periventricular white matter is hypointense on T_1- and hyperintense on T_2-weighted images. Pathological enhancement of the ventricular margins is identified (Fig. 8). Abnormal enhancement of the choroid plexus may also be present.

EPIDURAL AND SUBDURAL INFECTIONS

Epidural abscess is typically associated with the direct extension of infection from either middle ear or paranasal sinus and mastoid infection. Penetrating trauma may also be the etiology of an epidural abscess. An epidural abscess has the appearance of a biconvex or lens-shaped extra-axial collection. The dura, which is closely associated with the periosteum of the inner table, does not allow the purulent exudate to dissect freely, and as a result there is a collection of exudate creating the biconvex shape. On CT scanning, the collection is typically hypodense to brain but not as dark as CSF. Following contrast administration, the dura, which demarcates the medial aspect of the abscess, is displaced away from the convexity and shows significant enhancement (Fig. 9). The abscess contents do not enhance. Epidural abscess may be missed on CT because of adjacent bone artifacts. On MRI the epidural abscess is easily identified. The purulent exudate is seen to displace the dura medially. The dura is identified as a relatively thick dark band. This decreased signal intensity is due to the significant fibrous content of the dura. The purulent exudate is typically hypointense and hyperintense on T_1- and T_2-weighted images, respectively. It maintains a signal intensity between brain and CSF on the T_1-weighted images, but is as hyperintense as CSF on the T_2-weighted images. It is atypical to have an associated parenchymal abnormality since the dura is such a good barrier. Following gadolinium administration, the dura enhances significantly.

CT scanning is poor for the detection of spinal epidural abscess, but may demonstrate osteomyelitis. Postmyelogram CT is useful for demonstrating the mass effect upon the thecal sac, but the myelogram/CT is expensive and invasive. MRI is the procedure of choice for the detection of epidural spinal abscess (17,18). On T_1-weighted images, the involved marrow and disc space as well as the epidural space are hypointense. On T_2-weighted images, these same areas are very hyperintense. The dura is typically seen as a displaced black line between the epidural pus collection and the hyperintense thecal sac (Fig. 10). Following intravenous gadolinium administration, the margins of infection will enhance, although the purulent debris itself does not enhance. There will be abnormal thickening and enhancement of the inflamed dura. Percutaneous abscess aspiration is necessary for diagnosis of the infectious agent, but MRI is generally specific in terms of the simple diagnosis of discitis/osteomyelitis/epidural abscess.

Subdural collections may be infected or sterile. If the collection is infected, it is referred to as a subdural empyema, and if sterile, it is referred to as a subdural effusion. Because the subdural space is a potential space, a purulent fluid collection can diffuse throughout the space resulting in a crescenteric-shaped collection. A subdural effusion is typically isodense to CSF on CT scan (Fig. 11) and may be difficult to differentiate from a subdural hygroma or chronic subdural hematoma. On MRI, the collection is isointense to CSF on all imaging sequences (11). The adjacent brain is typically normal in signal intensity. The lack of blood products easily differentiates this collection from a chronic subdural hematoma.

The subdural empyema is also crescenteric in shape, but is generally slightly hyperdense to CSF on CT scan. The adjacent parenchyma is typically edematous and may show some patchy irregular enhancement. On MRI the subdural empyema is slightly greater than CSF signal intensity on T_1-weighted images and is as hyperintense as CSF on the T_2-weighted images (Fig. 12). The adjacent brain parenchyma may show some abnormal increased signal on the T_2-weighted images and some mild edema. The differentiation of subdural effusion and empyema is important. Subdural effusion is treated symptomatically and will resolve with appropriate treat-

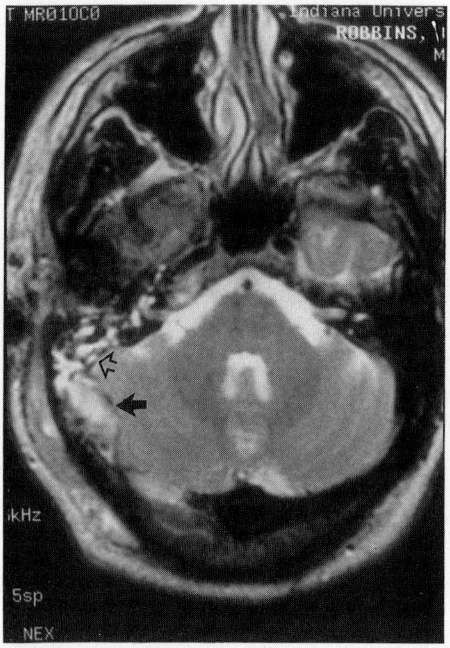

(A)

Figure 7 Dural sinus thrombosis. An axial T_2-weighted image (A) demonstrates an epidural abscess (closed arrow) in the right side of the posterior fossa. This was secondary to contiguous otomastoiditis (open arrow). A coronal enhanced T_1-weighted image (B) demonstrates the displaced dura (arrow) with the associated epidural abscess. Abnormal enhancement of the right tentorial leaflet is also appreciated. A coronal MR venogram reformat (C) demonstrates occlusion of the right transverse and sigmoid sinuses (arrow). The left side is normal.

ment of the underlying meningitis. When it develops as a complication of meningitis, subdural empyema is a neurosurgical emergency.

CEREBRITIS AND ABSCESS

Enzmann and colleagues divided the radiographic formation of an abscess into four stages: early cerebritis, late cerebritis, early capsule formation, and late capsule formation (19–21). Their work was done correlating the CT appearance with these stages of abscess formation in an animal model of experimental brain abscess. In the early cerebritis stage, CT shows focal low density with mass effect and typically patchy irregular enhancement. In the late cerebritis stage, a ring-enhancing lesion may be seen immediately following contrast administration. With delayed scanning, the contrast material appears to diffuse into the central portion of the lesion. Once in the abscess stage, there is central cyst formation and necrosis, which results in no delayed fill-in on the CT scan. During this stage, the contents of the abscess will be hypointense to brain. Occasionally the abscess capsule may be seen as an area of brain slightly hyperintense to the central necrosis and surrounding low-density edema. With contrast administration, there is ring enhancement of the abscess (Fig. 13). The walls of the abscess are typically thin and uniform with a smooth inner margin. If there is any asymmetrical thickening to the wall, it is on the side of the

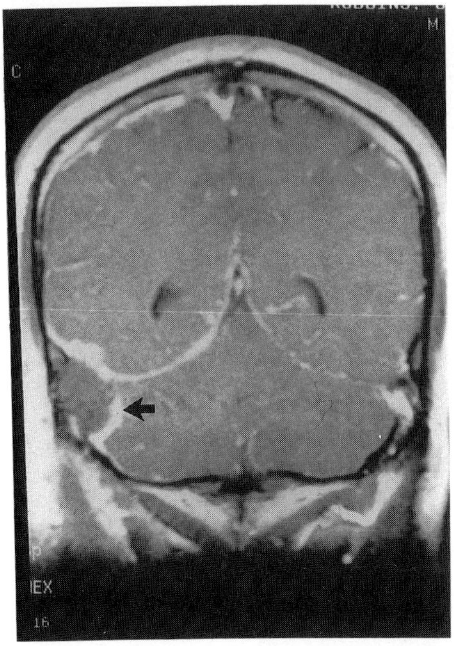

(B)

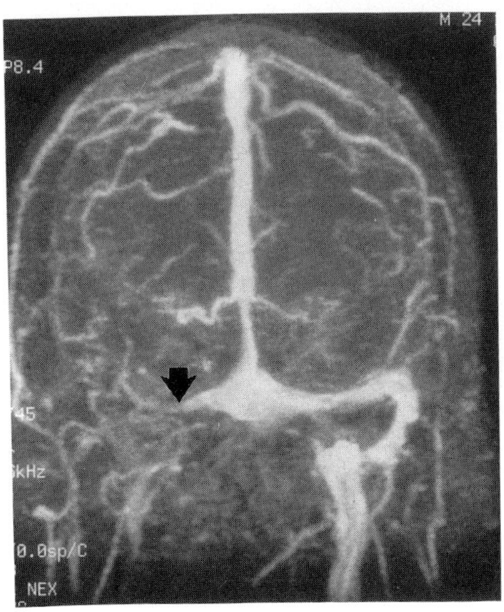

(C)

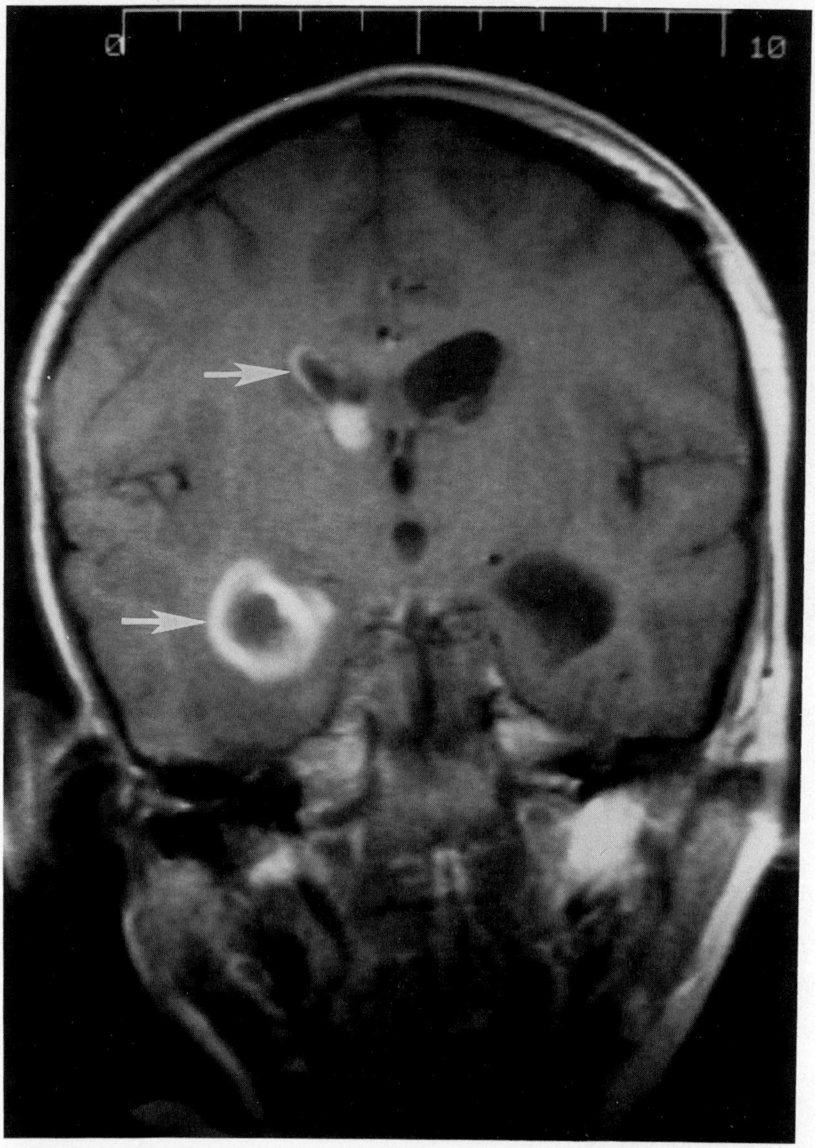

Figure 8 Ventriculitis. A coronal T_1-weighted image demonstrates enhancement along the margin of the right lateral ventricle including the frontal and temporal horns (arrows). Dilatation of the ventricular system consistent with hydrocephalus is also noted.

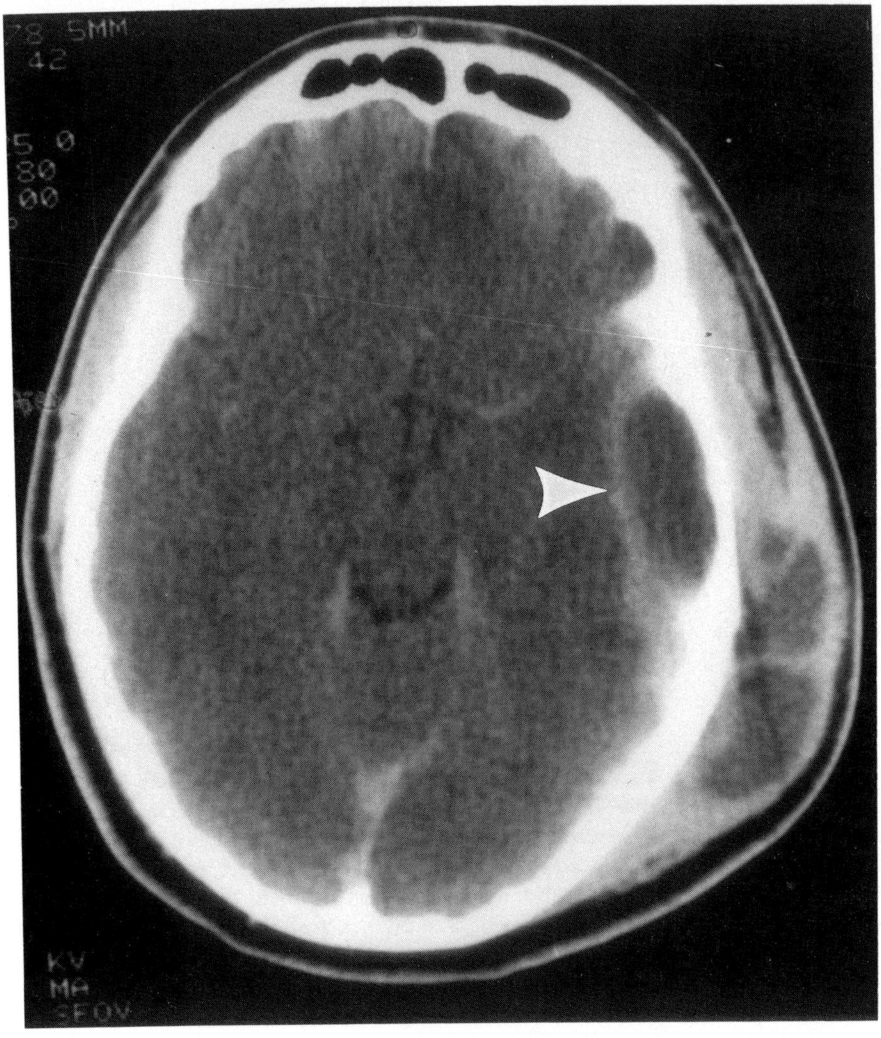

Figure 9 Cranial epidural abscess. An axial enhanced CT image demonstrates an epidural abscess in the left middle cranial fossa. The displaced dura is marked by an arrowhead. This was secondary to otitis media with infection in the petrous bone.

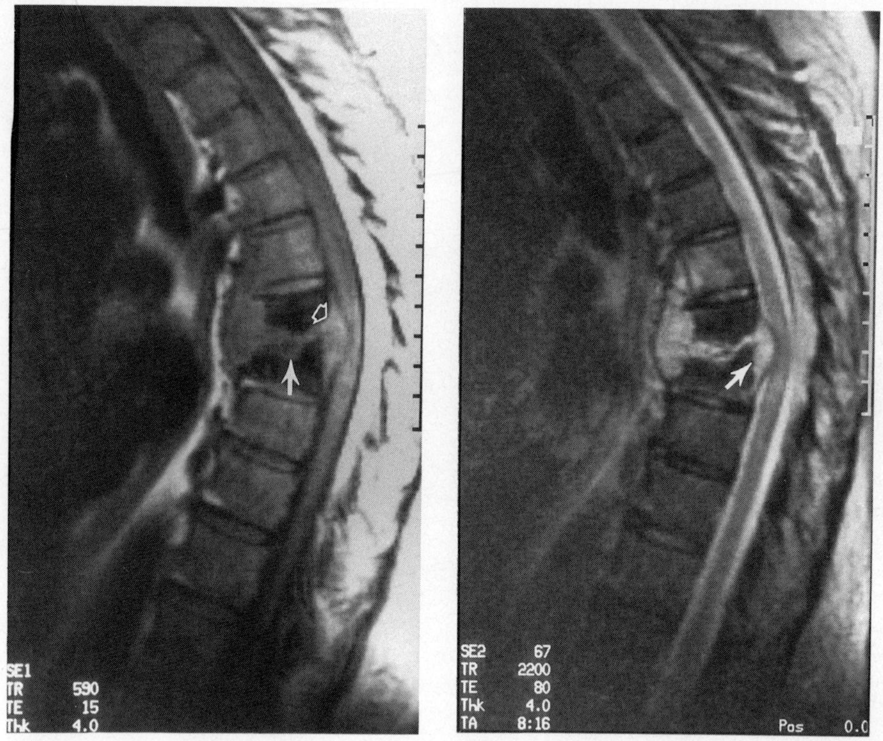

(A) (B)

Figure 10 Spinal epidural abscess. A sagittal T_1-weighted image of the thoracic spine (A) demonstrates decreased signal intensity in the T7 and 8 vertebral bodies. There is destruction of the intervertebral disc (closed arrow) consistent with discitis and osteomyelitis. The open arrow demonstrates the associated epidural abscess with cord compression. A sagittal T_2-weighted image (B) better demonstrates the epidural abscess. There is also a paraspinal component anterior to the same vertebral bodies. Postcontrast sagittal and axial T_1-weighted images (C,D) demonstrate the epidural abscess (arrow). On the axial image the compressed spinal cord is demarcated by the arrowhead.

abscess that is adjacent to the gray matter where there is increased blood flow and therefore an increase in capsule thickness.

On MRI, the cerebritis stage is evident as an area of low signal intensity of T_1- and hyperintense signal on T_2-weighted images. There is localized mass effect and patchy, irregular enhancement post gadolinium (Fig. 14). As the lesion progresses to an abscess, the capsule takes on some unique MRI characteristics (22,23). The capsule is frequently hyperintense on T_1- and hypointense on T_2-weighted images. Presumably this represents a paramagnetic effect that is related to the presence of free radicals within the abscess capsule that are formed due to the action of peroxidases. The central cavity is hypointense on T_1- and hyperintense on T_2-weighted images (Figs. 15,16). The surrounding edema has similar imaging characteristics. With contrast administration there is marked contrast enhancement of the abscess capsule.

As with meningitis, bacterial brain abscess can be secondary to hematogenous spread or direct extension of infection from a contiguous focus. An abscess due to paranasal sinus or middle ear disease is typically unifocal and relatively well localized. Lesions arising from hematogenous

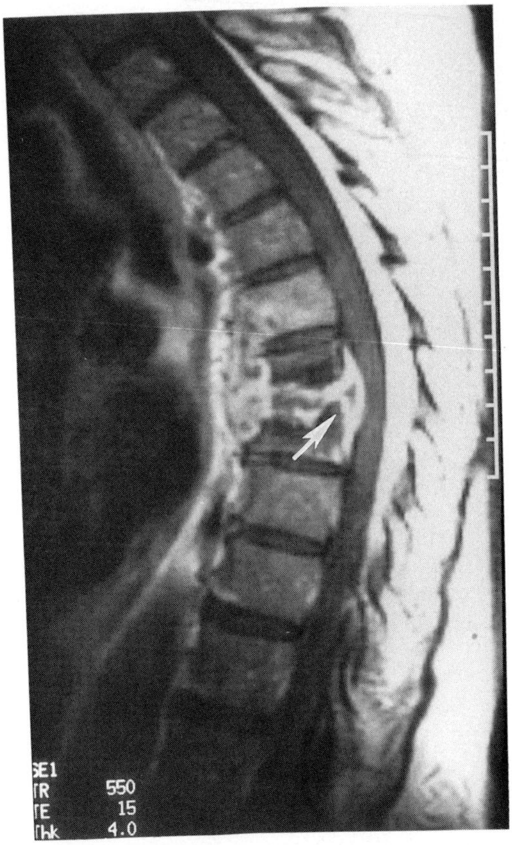

(C)

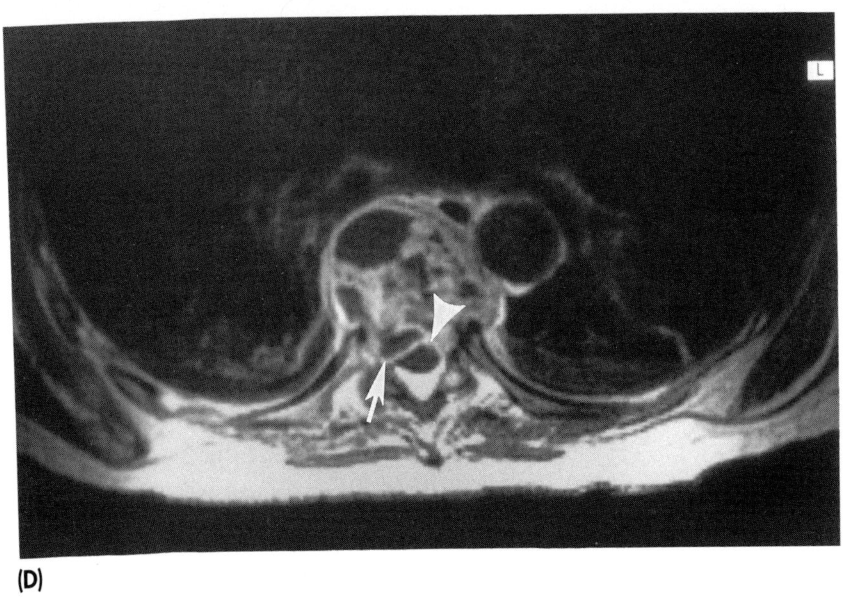

(D)

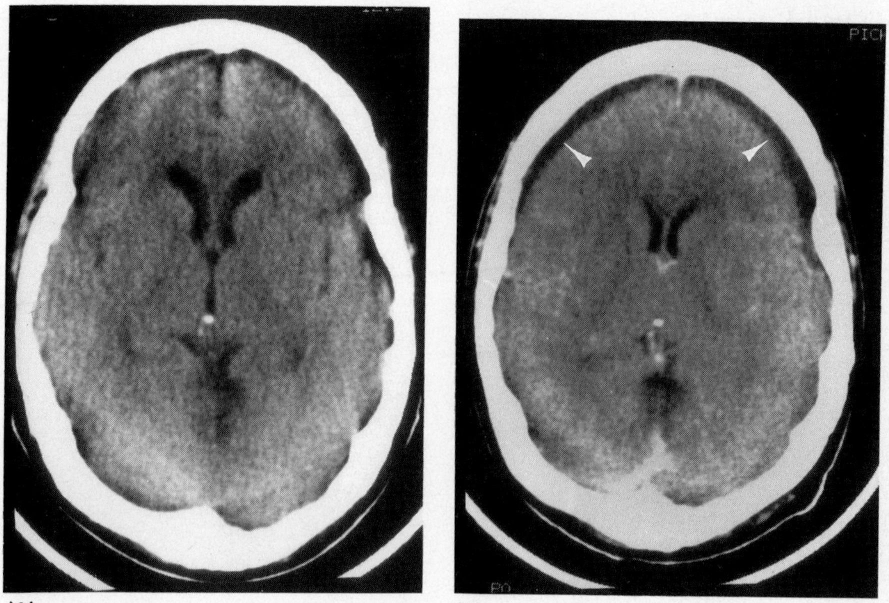

(A) (B)

Figure 11 Subdural effusion. An axial nonenhanced CT scan (A) taken at time of presentation of meningitis is normal. Seven days later, an enhanced CT (B) demonstrates the development of bilateral subdural effusions (arrowheads). The underlying brain is normal in intensity, although there is slight sulcal effacement.

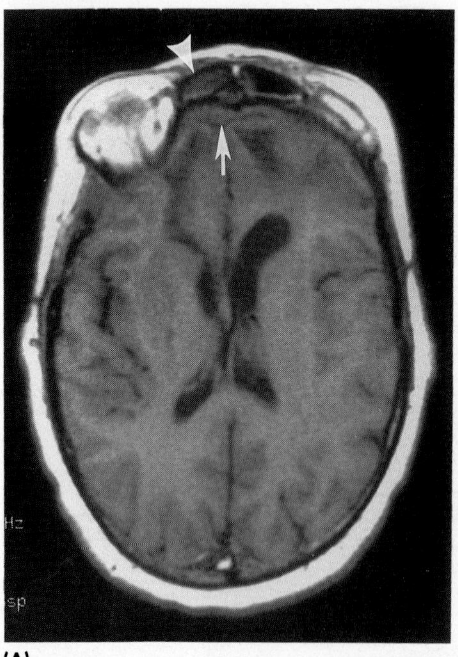

(A)

Figure 12 Subdural empyema. An axial T_1-weighted image (A) demonstrates opacification of the right frontal sinus (arrowhead). A subdural collection is present but difficult to identify adjacent to the frontal lobe tips (arrow). Abnormal low signal intensity is seen in the frontal lobes. An axial T_2-weighted image at a slightly lower level (B) demonstrates marked abnormal signal intensity in the

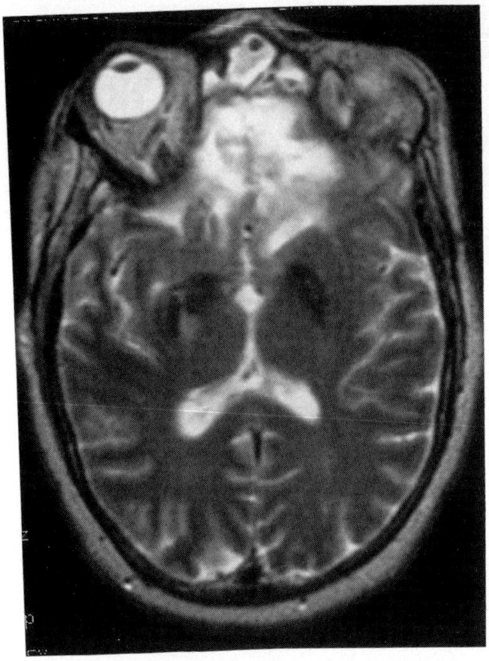

(B)

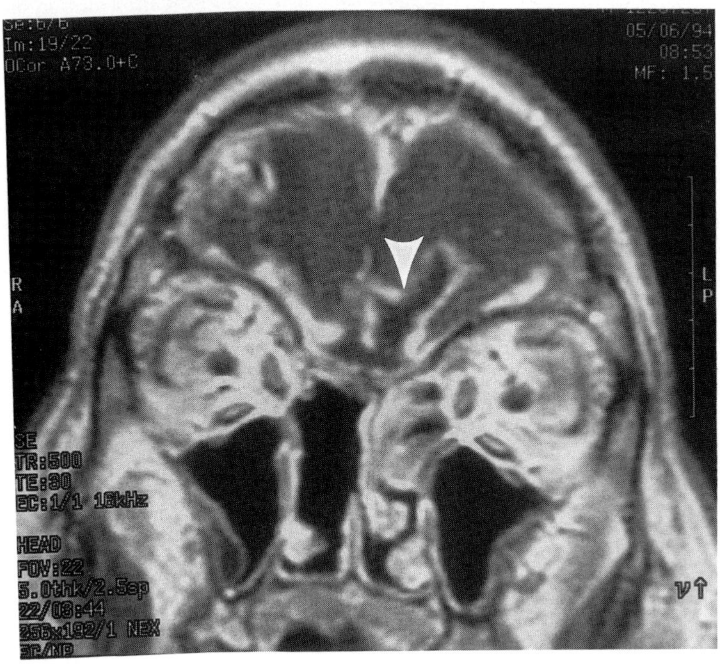

(C)

inferior frontal lobes as well as high-intensity opacification of the frontal sinuses. A coronal post-contrast T_1-weighted image (C) demonstrates the subdural empyema demarcated by the enhancing brain surface (arrowhead). The left ethmoid air cells are opacified. The right ethmoid air cells have been resected. This abscess was secondary to a contiguous paranasal sinus infection.

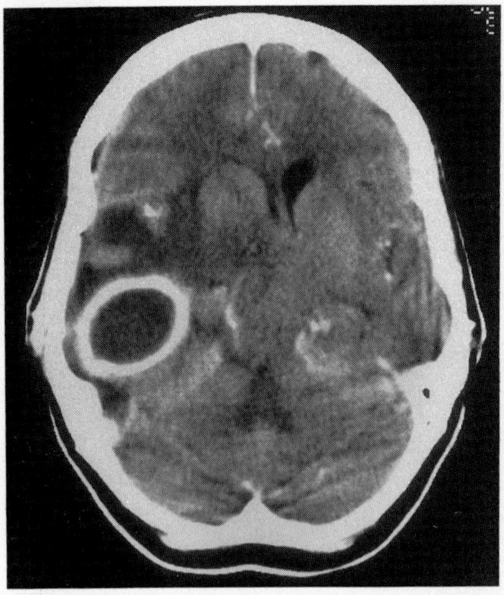

(A)

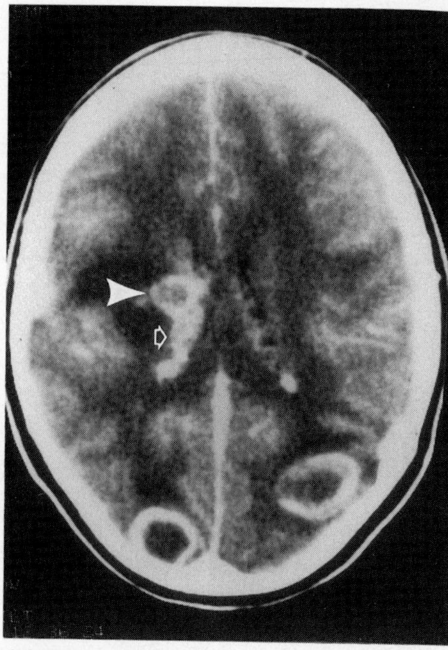

(B)

Figure 13 Cerebral abscess. An axial enhanced CT (A) demonstrates a ring-enhancing lesion in the right temporal lobe. The margins are thin and uniform. There is a smooth inner margin. Some surrounding vasogenic edema is noted. In a separate case, an axial enhanced CT scan (B) demonstrates multiple ring-enhancing abscesses. There is a small abscess along the ventricular margin on the right (arrowhead). Additionally, there is evidence of choroid plexitis on the right (open arrow).

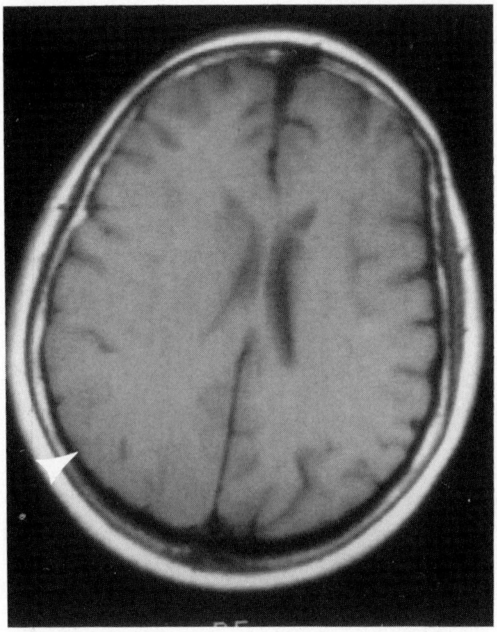

(A)

Figure 14 Cerebritis. An axial T_1-weighted image (A) demonstrates mass effect with sulcal effacement in the right parietal lobe (arrowhead). An axial T_2-weighted image (B) shows mass effect and

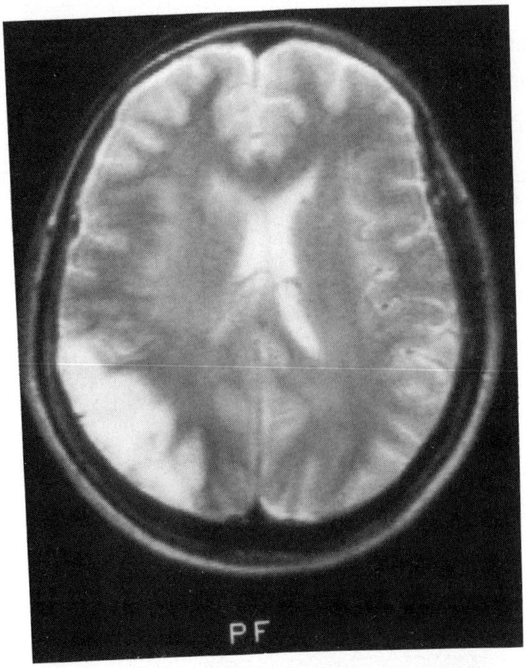

(B)

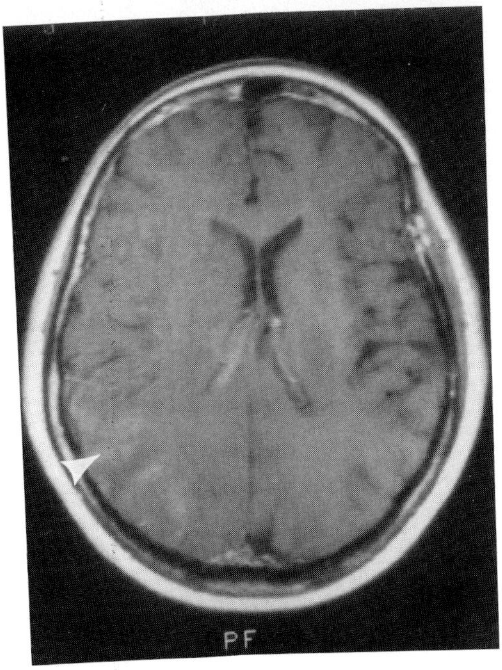

(C)

marked abnormal increased intensity in the right parietal lobe. A postcontrast T_1-weighted image (C) demonstrates patchy irregular enhancement (arrowhead).

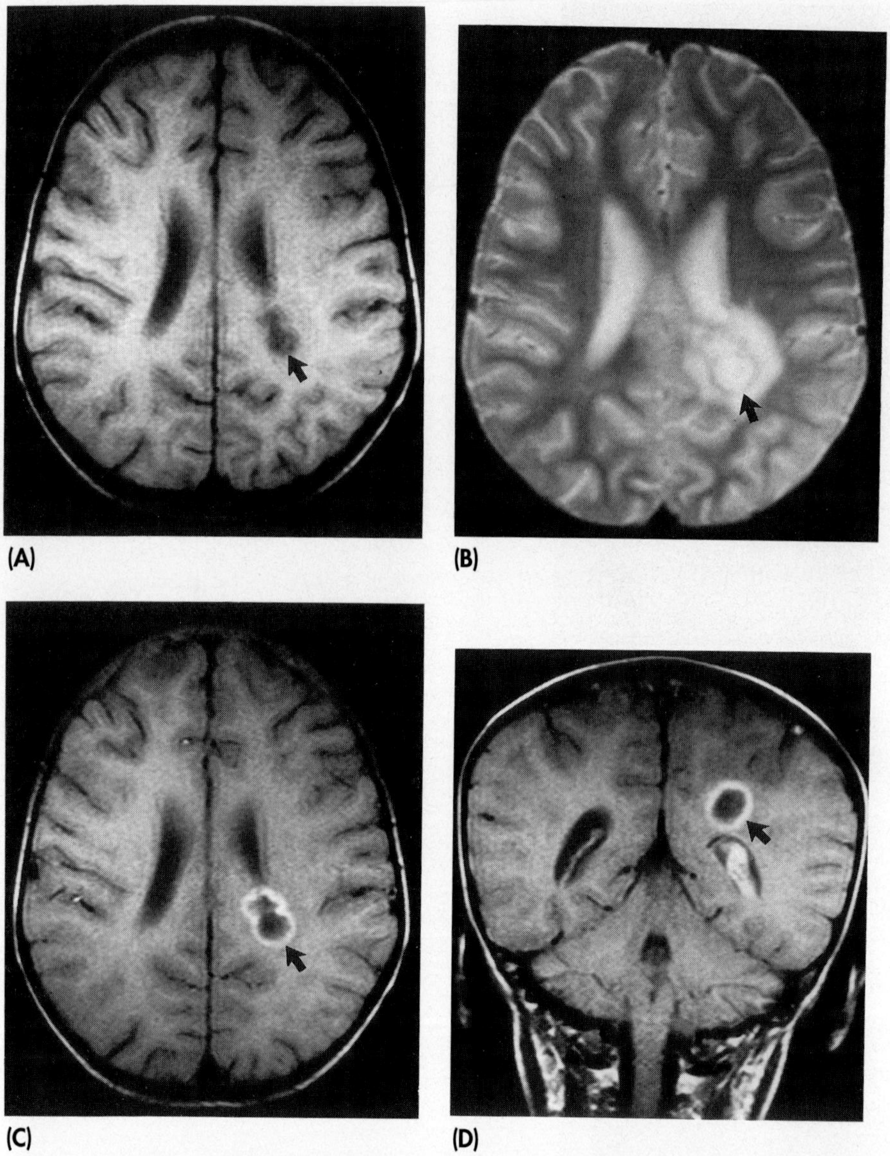

Figure 15 Cerebral abscess. Axial T_1 (A)- and T_2 (B)-weighted images demonstrate a necrotic lesion in the left periventricular region (arrow). There is surrounding edema identified on the T_2-weighted image. The capsule is slightly hypointense on the T_2-weighted image as well (arrow). Postcontrast axial and coronal T_1-weighted images (C,D) reveal a ring-enhancing lesion. The wall is relatively thin and uniform. There is a small daughter abscess seen anteriorly. The coronal image also demonstrates marked enlargement and enhancement of the left choroid plexus consistent with a choroid plexitis.

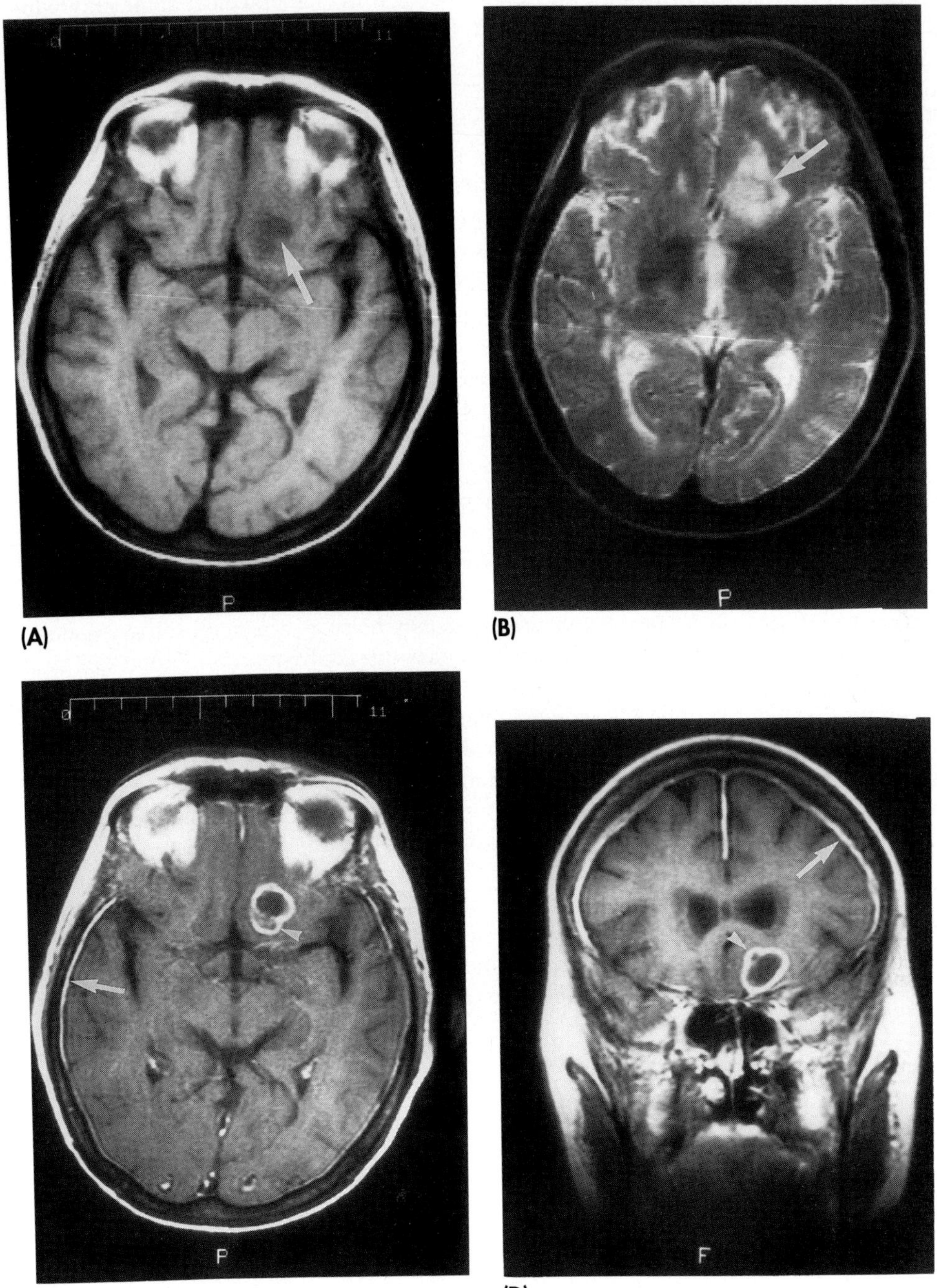

(A) (B) (C) (D)

Figure 16 Cerebral abscess. Axial T_1- and T_2-weighted images (A,B) demonstrate a necrotic focus in the inferior left frontal lobe (arrow). The capsular wall is hypointense on the T_2-weighted images, and there is surrounding hyperintense edema. Axial and coronal postcontrast T_1-weighted images (C,D) demonstrate a ring-enhancing lesion with a small daughter abscess seen superiorly and posteriorly (arrowhead). Note is made of convexity meningeal enhancement (arrows) as well as falcine enhancement, consistent with meningitis.

spread of infection are frequently multiple and tend to occur with their epicenter at the gray/white junction. In a significant number of cases no primary site is identified.

TUBERCULOSIS

Tuberculous meningitis has a propensity to involve the basal cisterns. The purulent exudate is typically thick and adherent. As a result, CT and MRI are quite sensitive to the detection of this infection. On CT, there may be loss of the normal CSF density in the suprasellar cistern and sylvian fissures (24). Following intravenous contrast administration, there is marked enhancement of the subarachnoid space and meninges. As with other forms of meningitis, complications such as hydrocephalus and infarction may occur. On MRI, the purulent exudate is seen as an altered signal within the CSF of the basal cisterns on both T_1- and T_2-weighted images (25). Marked enhancement is seen following gadolinium administration (Fig. 17). The degree of enhancement is generally greater on MRI than on CT, and the ability to visualize convexity enhancement as well as enhancement of the meninges in the posterior fossa is better on MRI than on CT.

The parenchymal infection takes the form of a tuberculoma. The imaging characteristics may depend on the size and age of the lesion. On computed tomography, the tuberculoma typically has a hypodense necrotic center, an isodense or slightly hyperdense capsular rim surrounded by low-density edema (26). Following contrast administration, there is enhancement of the tuberculoma capsule. In less well-established cases, the tuberculoma may be seen as a small solitary nodule. Because of the hematogenous origin of the infection, the lesions are frequently multiple and tend to occur at the gray/white junction. With chronicity or with successful treatment, calcification may be seen (Fig. 18). On MRI, the T_1-weighted images demonstrate hypointense signal in the central caseating necrosis as well as decreased intensity in the surrounding edema. The capsule wall is frequently isointense to minimally hyperintense to brain parenchyma. On T_2-weighted images, the central caseating region is typically hyperintense while the capsule is markedly hypointense, due to its fibrous nature (27,28). Surrounding hyperintense edema creates a targetlike lesion. Following intravenous contrast administration, there is enhancement of the capsular rim that is generally uniform, but may be thicker than that seen with other bacterial abscesses. As with CT, less well-established lesions may only be identified as areas of homogeneous focal nodular enhancement (Fig. 19). Calcification may be difficult to detect on MRI, although the possibility of gradient echo acquisitions can increase the sensitivity of MRI to calcific lesions (4).

VIRAL INFECTIONS

Herpes Encephalitis

Herpes encephalitis is the most common sporadic form of viral encephalitis. Because prognosis is directly related to the early institution of appropriate therapy, early diagnosis is critical. Herpes encephalitis is one infection where MRI has made a significant contribution to diagnosis. This is partly due to the lack of bone artifacts with resultant exquisite detailing of the anatomy of the temporal lobes as well as the multiplanar capabilities of MRI.

Herpes encephalitis may be caused by either the herpes simplex virus-1 (HSV-1) or the genital herpes simplex virus-2 (HSV-2). Most cases of herpes encephalitis are secondary to HSV-1. The less common HSV-2 encephalitis is usually a neonatal infection acquired during passage through an infected birth canal. Herpes encephalitis is frequently hemorrhagic and has a predisposition for the medial temporal lobes and insular cortex (29). The neonatal HSV infection is usually

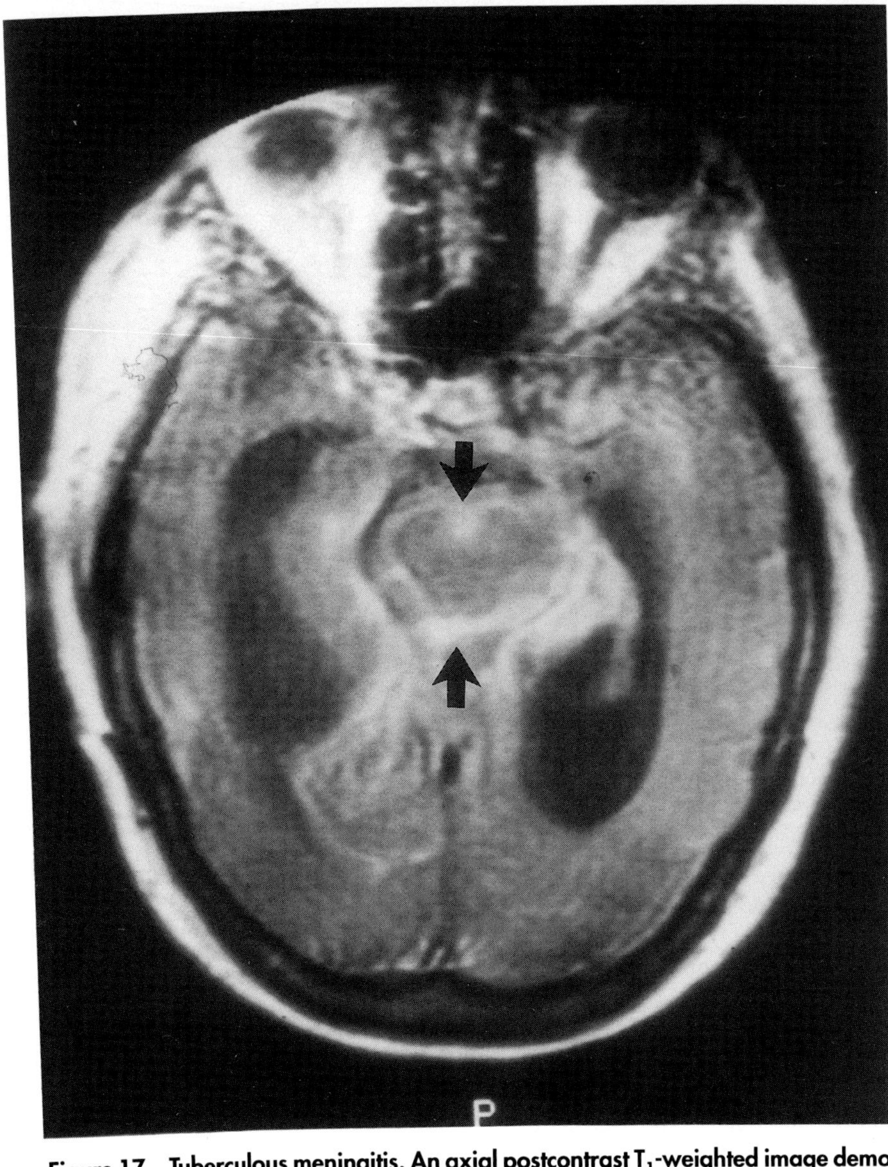

Figure 17 Tuberculous meningitis. An axial postcontrast T_1-weighted image demonstrates abnormal enhancement in the peri-mesencephalic and interpeduncular cisterns (arrows). Extension into the choroidal fissures is seen bilaterally. Enlargement of the lateral ventricles was due to communicating hydrocephalus.

disseminated in the brain, and although the temporal lobes may be involved, significant parietal and frontal lobe involvement is common.

The CT examination in herpes encephalitis is usually normal up to 5 days following the onset of symptoms (30,31). When positive, the CT shows decreased density in the temporal lobes (Fig. 20). Occasionally, foci of petechial or confluent hemorrhage may be seen. With contrast administration, there is a patchy irregular enhancement of the area of infection. The detection of herpes

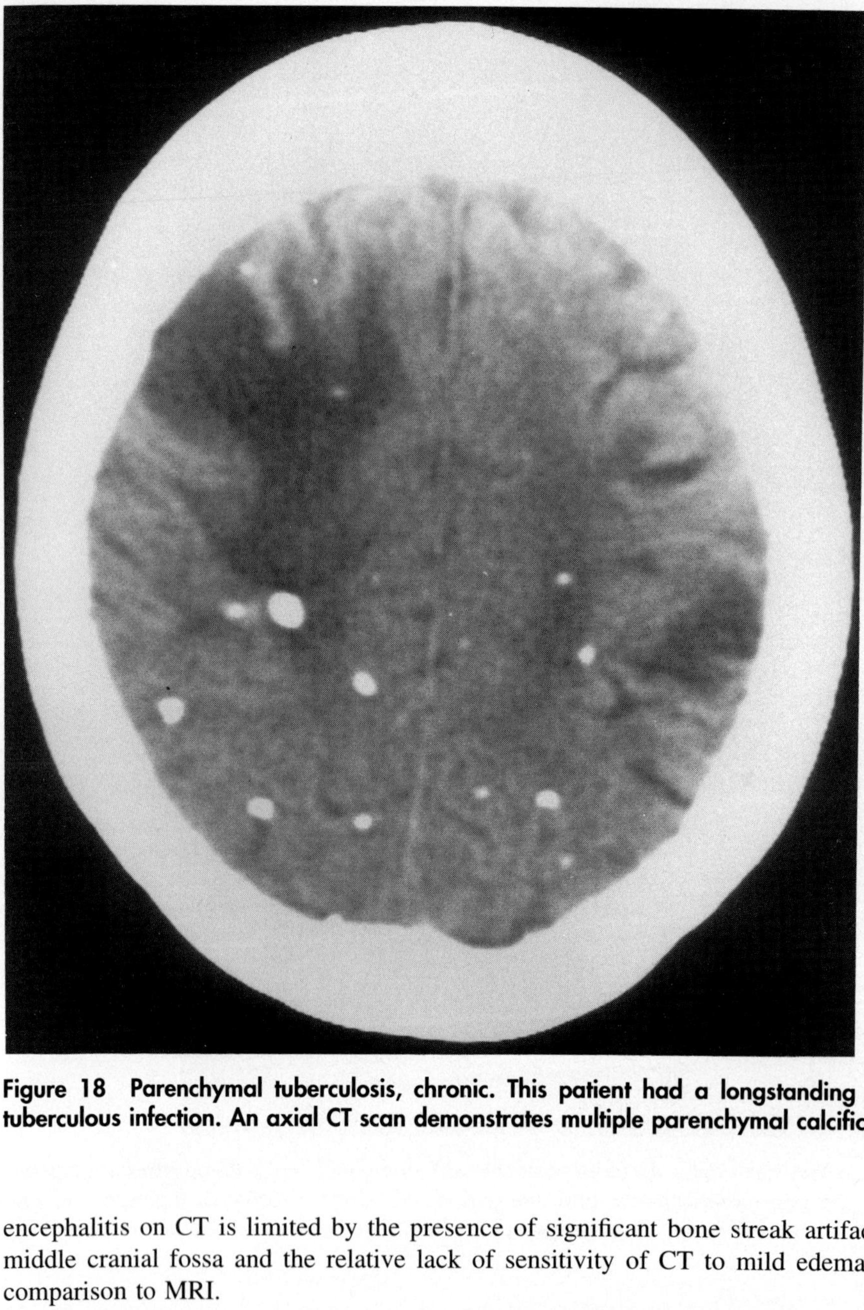

Figure 18 **Parenchymal tuberculosis, chronic. This patient had a longstanding history of prior tuberculous infection. An axial CT scan demonstrates multiple parenchymal calcifications.**

encephalitis on CT is limited by the presence of significant bone streak artifacts through the middle cranial fossa and the relative lack of sensitivity of CT to mild edematous lesions in comparison to MRI.

MRI is much more sensitive for the detection of herpes encephalitis in its early stages. Although T_1-weighted images may show mild early swelling of the medial temporal lobes, the T_2-weighted images demonstrate an abnormal hyperintense signal intensity in a bitemporal distribution (Fig. 21) (32,33). Foci of hemorrhage may be evident and if imaged early in the course of disease are probably representative of the presence of deoxyhemoglobin. As such, there may be petechial or confluent areas of decreased signal intensity on the T_2-weighted images. Occasionally, gradient echo images may be more sensitive in the detection of acute blood products than T_1- or T_2-weighted images. Following contrast administration, there is a patchy

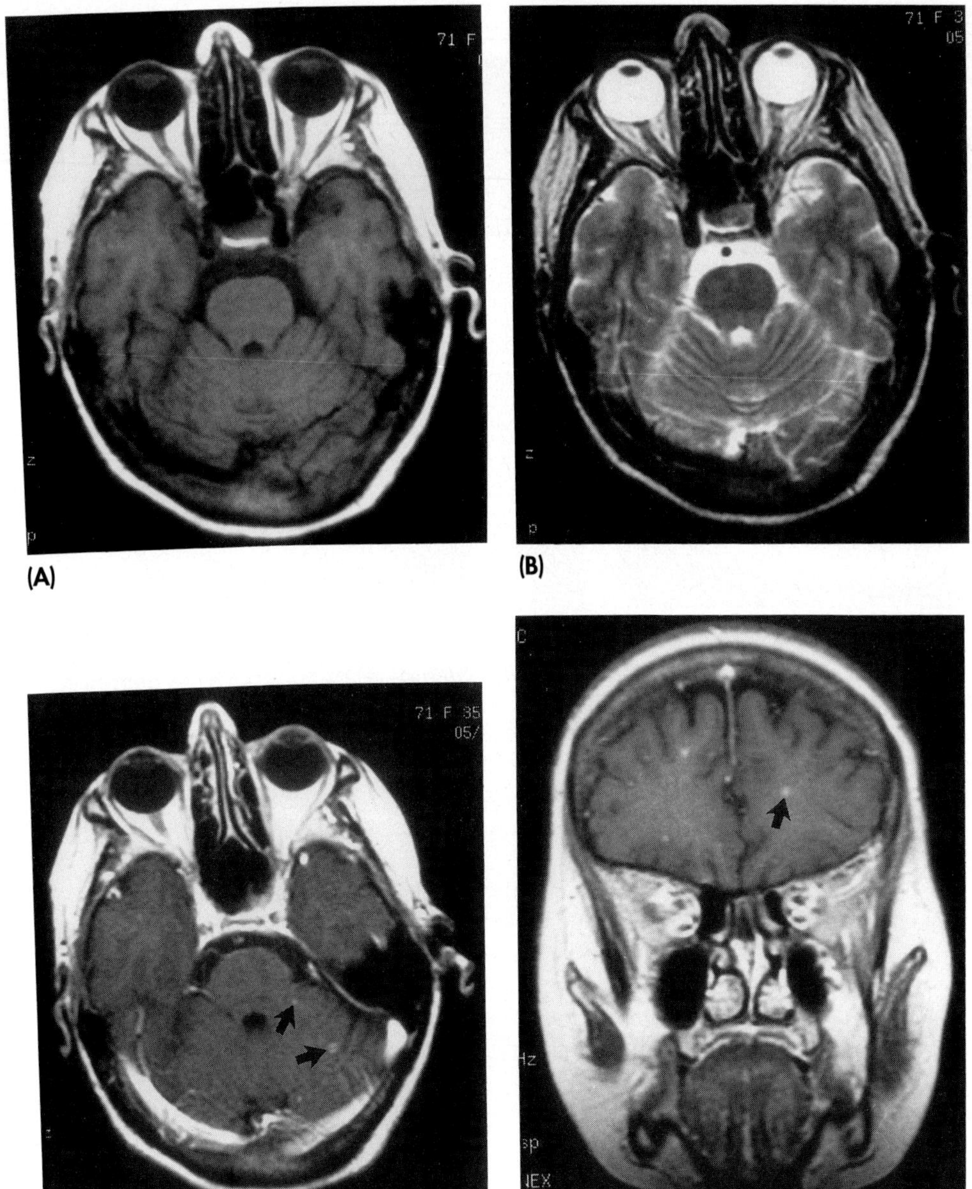

Figure 19 Parenchymal tuberculosis. Axial T_1- and T_2-weighted images (A,B) are normal. Postcontrast axial and coronal T_1-weighted images (C,D) demonstrate small punctate foci of abnormal enhancement (arrows) representing a hematogenous shower of tubercle bacilli from a lung infection.

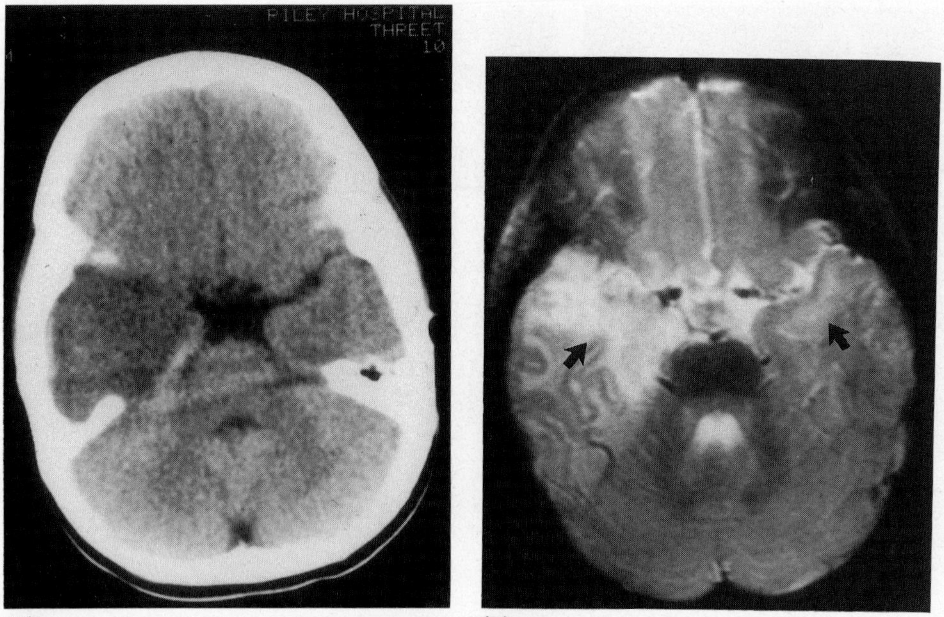

(A) (B)

Figure 20 Herpes encephalitis. An axial CT scan without contrast (A) demonstrates low density in the right temporal lobe consistent with herpes encephalitis. This image was obtained 3 days following the onset of symptomatology. An axial T_2-weighted image (B) obtained on the same day as the CT demonstrates the abnormal increased signal intensity in the right temporal lobe as well as small foci of infection in the left temporal lobe (arrows).

irregular enhancement in the involved areas. Since the signal abnormalities may remit following therapy, MRI may also be used to evaluate response to treatment (34). The appearance of neonatal HSV encephalitis on both CT and MRI may be subtle. Typically there are multifocal areas of edematous change with loss of gray/white differentiation (35). This may be difficult to differentiate from a meningitis or cerebritis. Antiviral therapy is important as the herpetic infection may move quickly through the brain resulting in multicystic encephalomalacia.

Acute Disseminated Encephalomyelitis

Acute disseminated encephalomyelitis (ADEM) is an autoimmune mediated demyelinating disease (36). It typically develops 1–3 weeks following a viral infection or vaccination. The hallmark of the lesion is multifocal demyelination. As such, MRI is of greater sensitivity in the detection of lesions associated with ADEM than is CT. If positive, the CT scan may show areas of decreased signal intensity in the periventricular and deep white matter, internal capsule, and pons. Rarely acute plaques may enhance on CT, similar to the acute enhancement of plaques in multiple sclerosis. MRI is the procedure of choice in the evaluation of this disease. Areas of demyelination are best seen on the T_2-weighted images. These are typically punctate and/or confluent areas of increased signal intensity on the T_2-weighted images in the periventricular and deep white matter (Fig. 22) (37,38). There is a propensity for involvement of the subcortical U fibers as well as the brain stem and brachium pontis. The lesions of ADEM may or may not be associated with subtle mass effect. Gadolinium administration may demonstrate peripheral enhancement along the

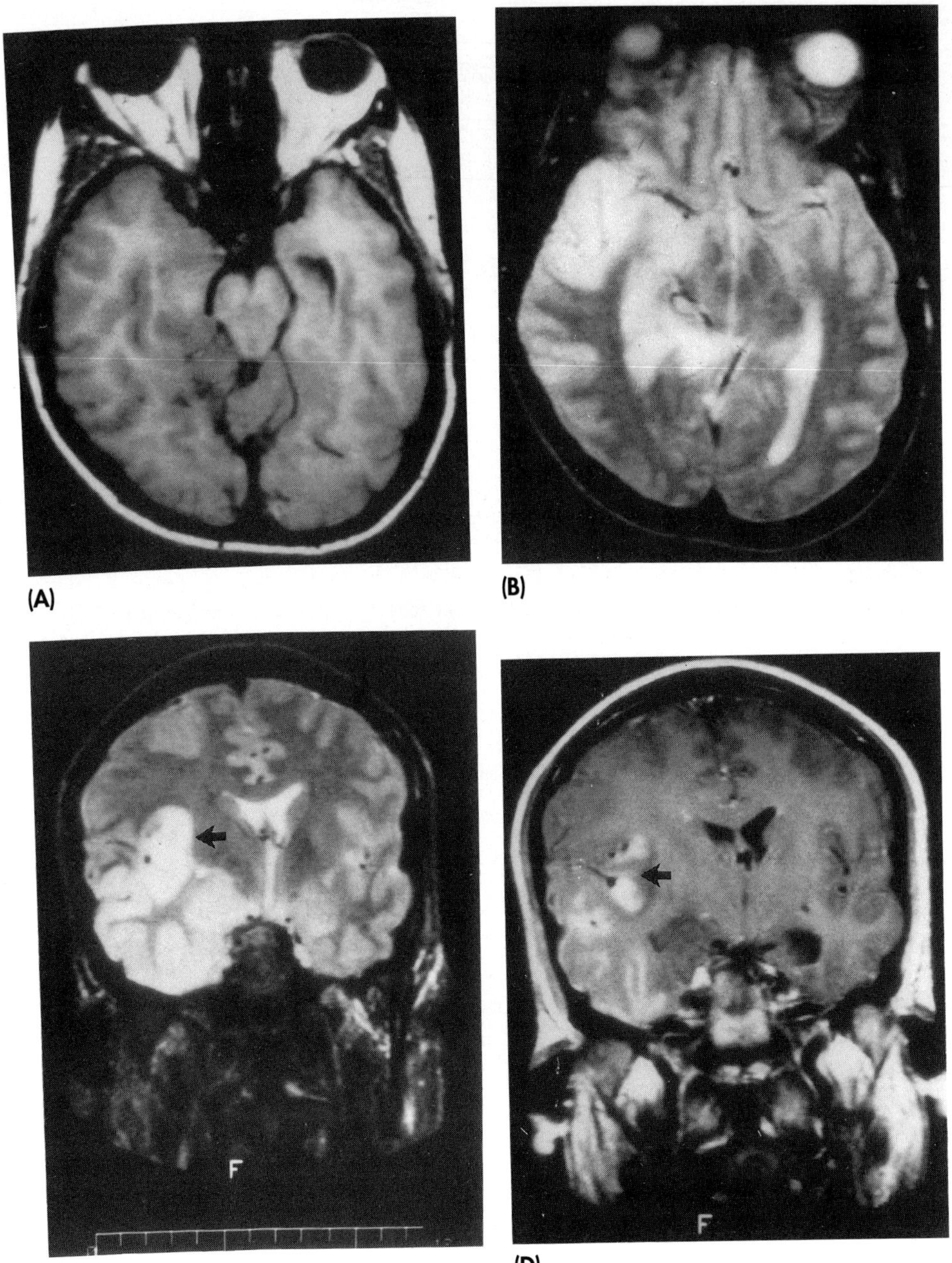

Figure 21 Herpes encephalitis. Axial T_1- and T_2-weighted images (A,B) demonstrate mass effect and abnormal signal intensity in the right temporal lobe, best seen on the T_2-weighted image. A coronal T_2-weighted image (C) demonstrates the abnormal signal intensity in the temporal lobe with extension into the insular cortex (arrow). A coronal postcontrast T_1-weighted image (D) shows patchy irregular enhancement predominately along the surface of the temporal lobe and insular cortex (arrow).

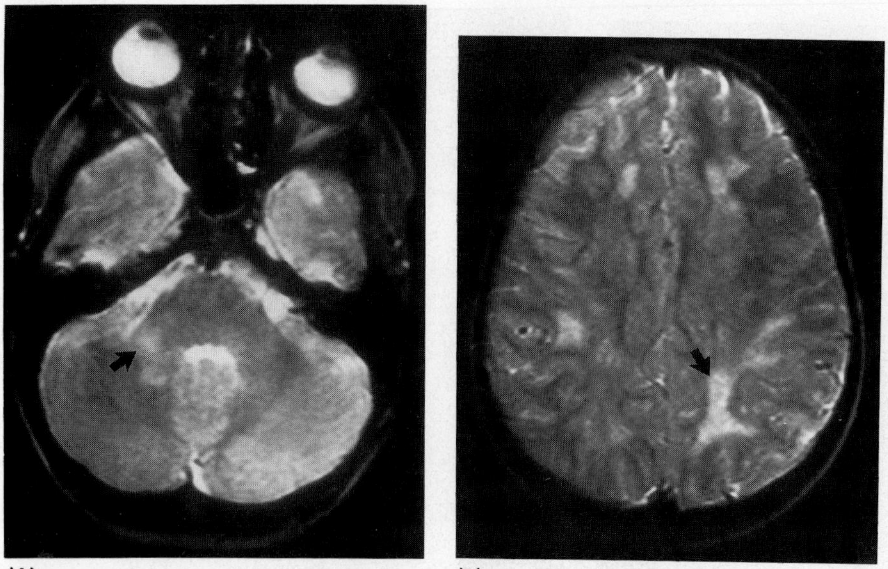

(A) (B)

Figure 22 ADEM. Axial T_2-weighted images demonstrate patchy irregular areas of increased signal intensity. In (A) there is a focus in the brachium pontis on the right (arrow). In (B) there are multiple areas of subcortical involvement, the largest marked by an arrow.

demyelinating edge in acute lesions. Follow-up studies performed on patients who have improved typically show resolution of the foci of demyelination.

Miscellaneous Viruses

Cytomegalovirus and rubella are two viral infections that make up part of the TORCH syndrome. Congenital cytomegalovirus (CMV) is associated with parenchymal periventricular brain calcifications (Fig. 23) (39). These small punctate subependymal calcifications are best detected on CT but may be identified on MRI if the calcifications are large or if gradient echo images are obtained. Rubella, another cause of congenital viral infection, may be associated with atrophic changes and occasionally some calcifications. Toxoplasmosis, a parasitic infection, will be discussed separately, but it is also associated with parenchymal calcifications in congenital cases.

FUNGAL INFECTIONS

Most cerebral fungal infections are secondary to immunodeficiency states from immunosuppressive therapy, cancer, or acquired immunodeficiency syndrome (AIDS). In most cases the CNS infection is the result of hematogenous dissemination from a distant site of infection. The pathological involvement may be meningeal, parenchymal, or both. The nature of the disease is in part determined by the type of infecting fungus. As Bazan et al. described, fungi that exist as yeasts (*Histoplasma capsulatum*) are able to penetrate deeply into the brain parenchyma and into the subarachnoid space (40), resulting in lesions that are seen as small foci of infection in the gray/white junction and meninges. Fungi that exist as pseudohyphae (*Candida*) cause arterial occlusions and microabscess formation. Fungi that infect the brain as hyphae (*Aspergillus*) obstruct large arteries, resulting in infarctions.

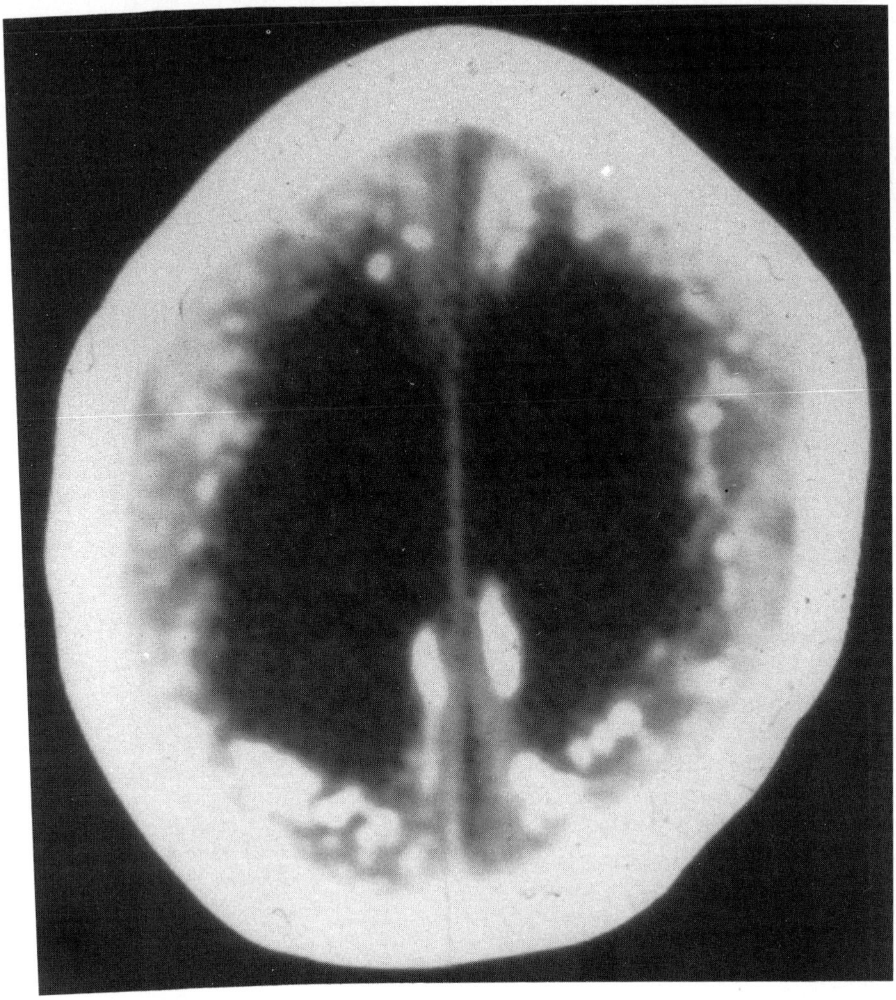

Figure 23 CMV, congenital. An axial nonenhanced CT scan demonstrates marked ventricular enlargement consistent with central atrophy. Multiple periventricular calcifications are identified.

MRI is the neuroimaging procedure of choice in the evaluation of fungal meningitis. There is little to differentiate fungal from viral meningitis on neuroimaging (10). The bacterial and tuberculous meningitides are associated with more prominent meningeal enhancement than fungal meningitis.

Fungal lesions associated with histoplasmosis may show little in the way of reactive vasogenic edema on T_2-weighted images. In fact, some small lesions may only be detected on postcontrast T_1-weighted images. These typically appear as small enhancing nodules at the gray/white junction and can be seen in the spinal cord as well (Fig. 24). The lesions of aspergillosis may be associated with hemorrhage from hemorrhagic septic infarction (41,42). In some cases, however, *Aspergillus* and *Candida* can grow as small enhancing nodules (Fig. 25).

In most cases of small nodular enhancing lesions, radiological identification of the infecting fungus cannot be made.

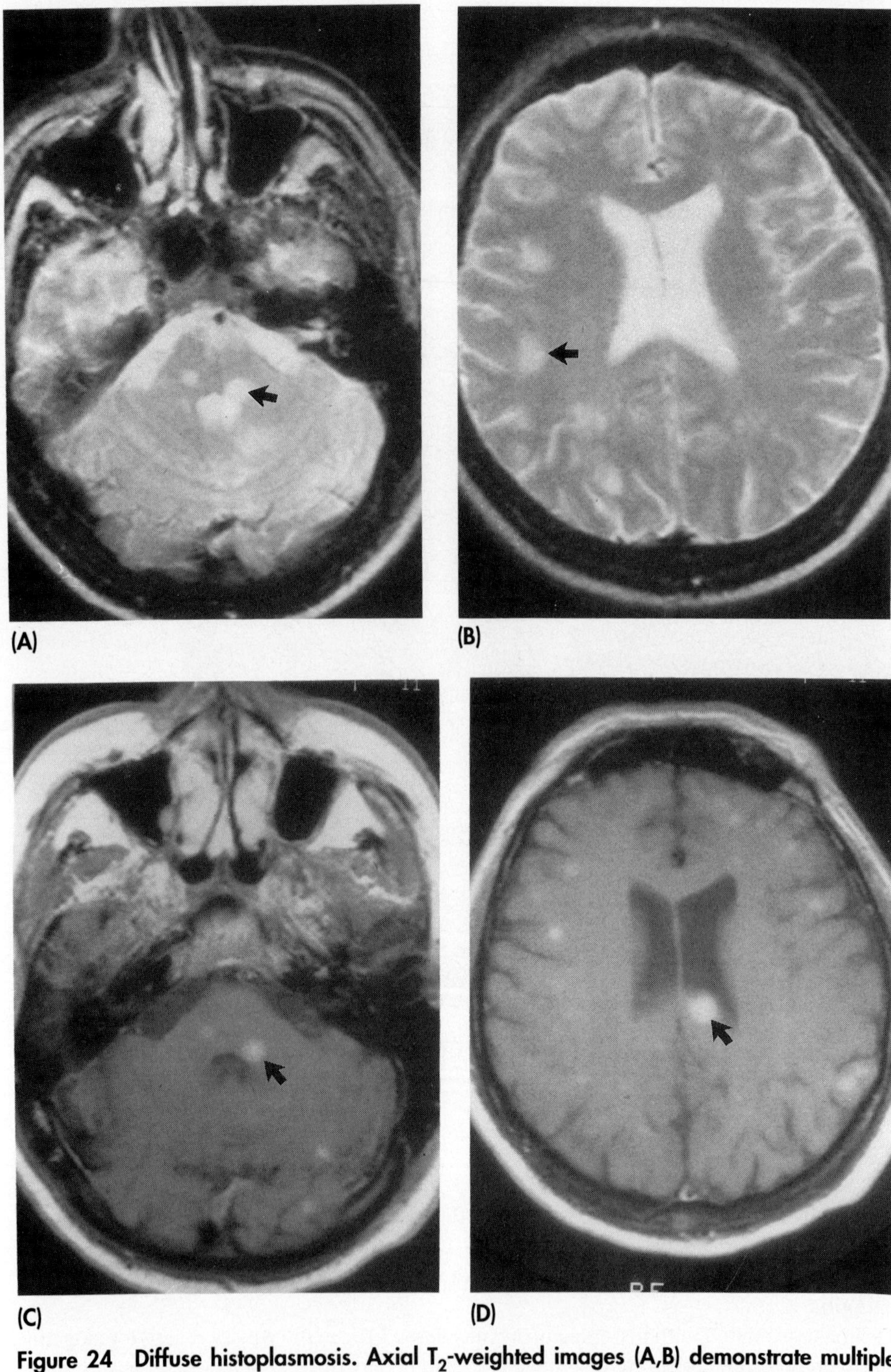

Figure 24 Diffuse histoplasmosis. Axial T_2-weighted images (A,B) demonstrate multiple areas of abnormal increased signal intensity in the brain stem, one marked with an arrow, and in the subcortical region in the supratentorial space, one marked by an arrow. Postcontrast axial T_1-weighted images (C,D) demonstrate a myriad of abnormal foci of enhancement. Some foci, such as the left pontine lesion (arrow), were identified on the T_2-weighted images. The callosal lesion (arrow) was not identified initially on the unenhanced images. Sagittal enhanced T_1-weighted images of the cervical and thoracic spine (E,F) demonstrate multiple cord histoplasmosis foci (black arrow). A small tonsillar abscess is seen on the cervical study (open arrow).

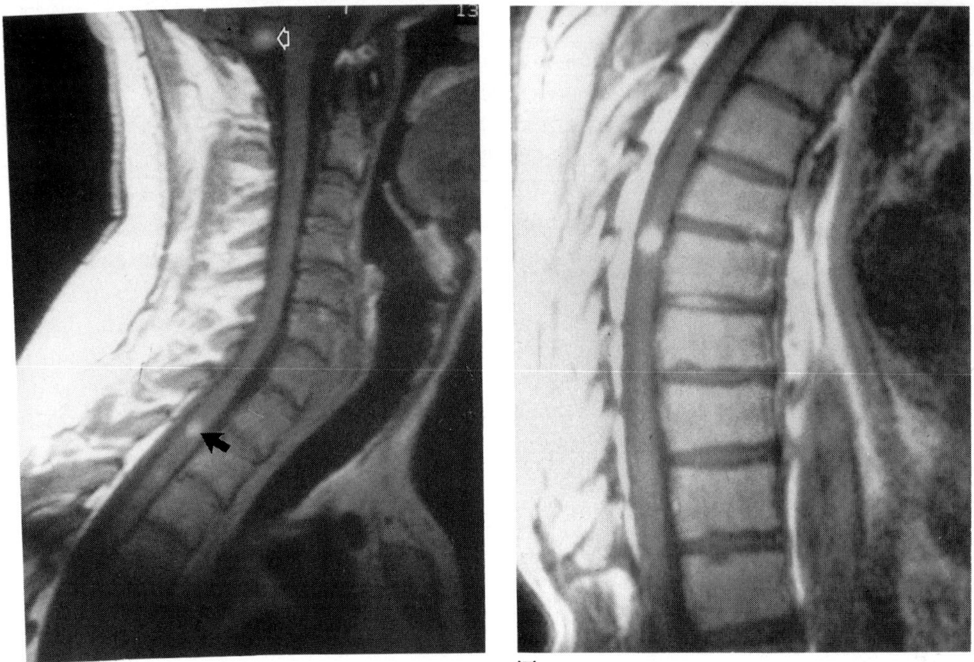

(E) (F)

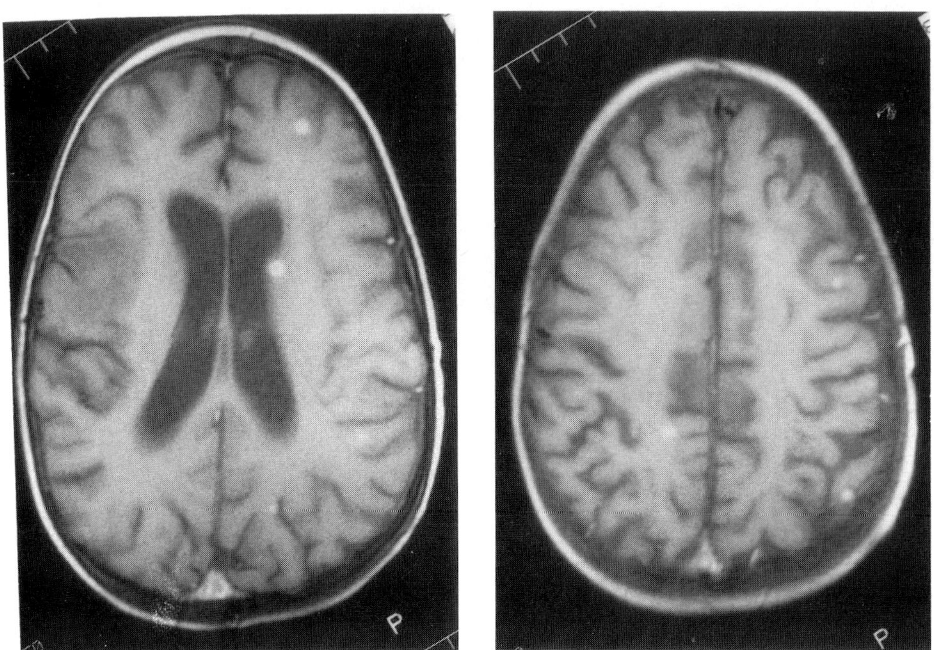

(A) (B)

Figure 25 Aspergillosis. Axial enhanced T_1-weighted images demonstrate multiple foci of punctate and ring-enhancing lesions. In most cases it will be difficult to differentiate one fungal infection from another by neuroimaging.

CYSTICERCOSIS

Infection caused by the larvae of *Taenia solium* results in cysticercosis. Cysticerci may develop in the brain parenchyma, the subarachnoid space, the ventricles, and/or the spinal canal. The appearance of the lesions of cysticercosis on CT and MRI is determined in part by the age of the infection and in part by the body's ability to encapsulate the parasite. The cysts may contain living or dead parasites. Inactive cysts calcify. Symptoms may not arise for several years after the primary infection. As with most other calcific lesions, cysticercosis calcifications will be best seen on CT (43). The lesions occur at the gray/white junction. They may or may not be associated with significant edema and mass effect. In contrast to the punctate calcifications seen in tuberculous and congenital viral infections, the calcifications in cysticercosis are typically cystic. Occasionally, some enhancement of the cyst wall can be seen, although this may be difficult to differentiate from the hyperdensity of the calcium itself on CT. The cysts that occur in the ventricles often have the same density as CSF, making their detection difficult. The development of hydrocephalus should be viewed with suspicion, however.

On MRI the cystic lesions have a low signal intensity like that of CSF. Occasionally, the scolex itself may be seen within the cyst. Hypointense edema and mass effect may also be seen on the T_1-weighted images. On the T_2-weighted images, the cysts have a high signal intensity with associated hyperintense edema (Fig. 26) (44,45). Following gadolinium administration, there is

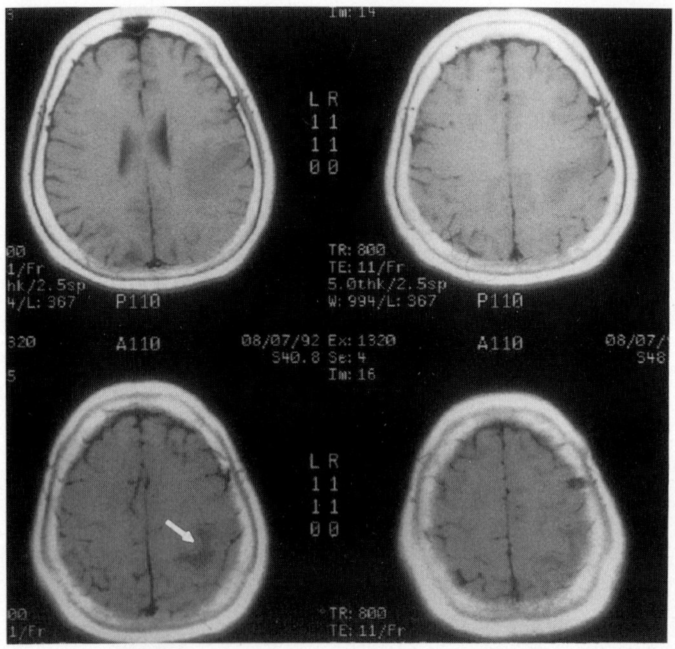

(A)

Figure 26 Cysticercosis. A series of axial T_1-weighted images (A) demonstrates low signal intensity and mass effect in the left temporal parietal lobe (arrow). T_2 axial images (B) demonstrate multiple foci of vasogenic edema. Target lesions are identified bilaterally (arrows). The central area is hyperintense consistent with the cystic contents. The capsule wall is hypointense due to its fibrous characteristics. Postconstrast T_1-weighted images (C) demonstrate ring enhancement of the cysticercosis capsules (arrows).

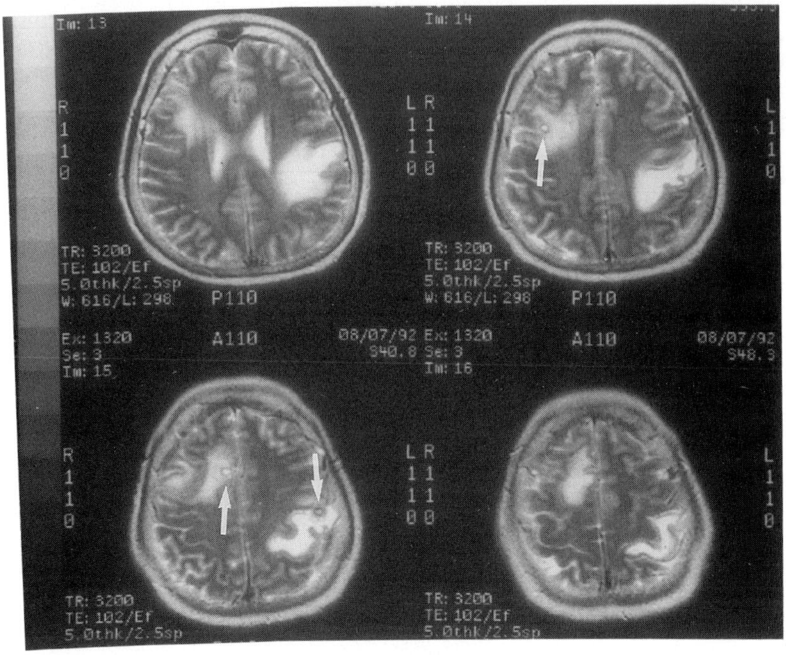
Im: 13
Im: 14
R 1 1 0
L R 1 1 1 1 0 0
L 1 1 0
TR: 3200
TE: 102/Ef
5.0thk/2.5sp
W: 616/L: 298
P110
Ex: 1320
Se: 3
Im: 15
A110
08/07/92
S40.8
Im: 16
S48.3
TR: 3200
TE: 102/Ef
5.0thk/2.5sp

(B)

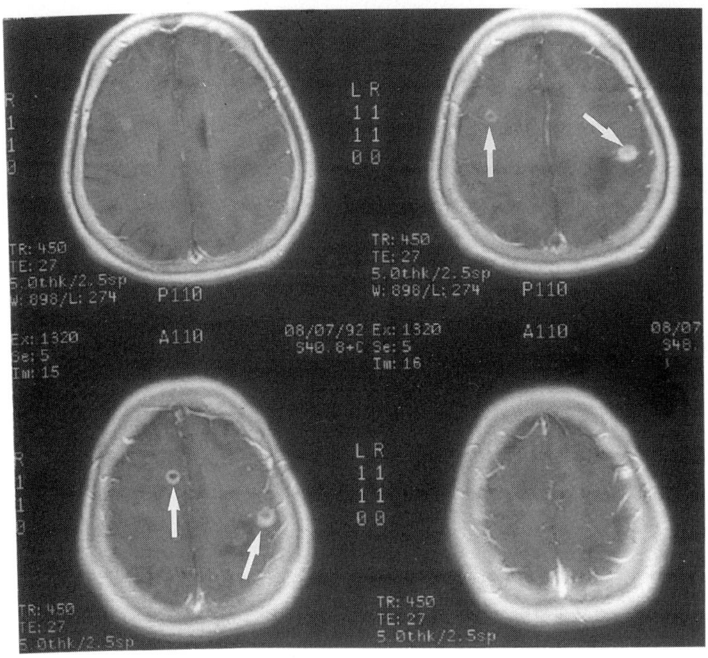
L R 1 1 1 1 0 0
TR: 450
TE: 27
5.0thk/2.5sp
W: 898/L: 274
P110
Ex: 1320
Se: 5
Im: 15
A110
08/07/92
S40.8+C
Im: 16
TR: 450
TE: 27
5.0thk/2.5sp

(C)

enhancement of the cyst wall. In the absence of the detection of calcification, the differentiation of lesions of cysticercosis from other metastatic or infectious diseases may be difficult. Intraventricular lesions are typically easily identified on T_1- and proton density–weighted images as rounded cysts of signal intensity higher than CSF (46). Intraventricular lesions may not be visualized on T_2-weighted images.

LYME DISEASE

Lyme disease is caused by a spirochete, *Borrelia burgdorferi*, which is endemic to the upper northeastern and midwestern United States and is transmitted by a tick bite. Neurological symptoms often occur months after the tick bite. The MRI abnormalities of Lyme disease are similar to those of multiple sclerosis or ADEM. There are typically low-density lesions in the periventricular and deep white matter on CT. On T_2-weighted images, the areas of abnormality are hyperintense and involve the periventricular and deep white matter as well as the subcortical U fibers (Fig. 27) (47). Involvement of the brain stem and brachium pontis is also common. Gadolinium enhancement of the lesions has not been described. Resolution of the MRI abnormalities is seen with treatment.

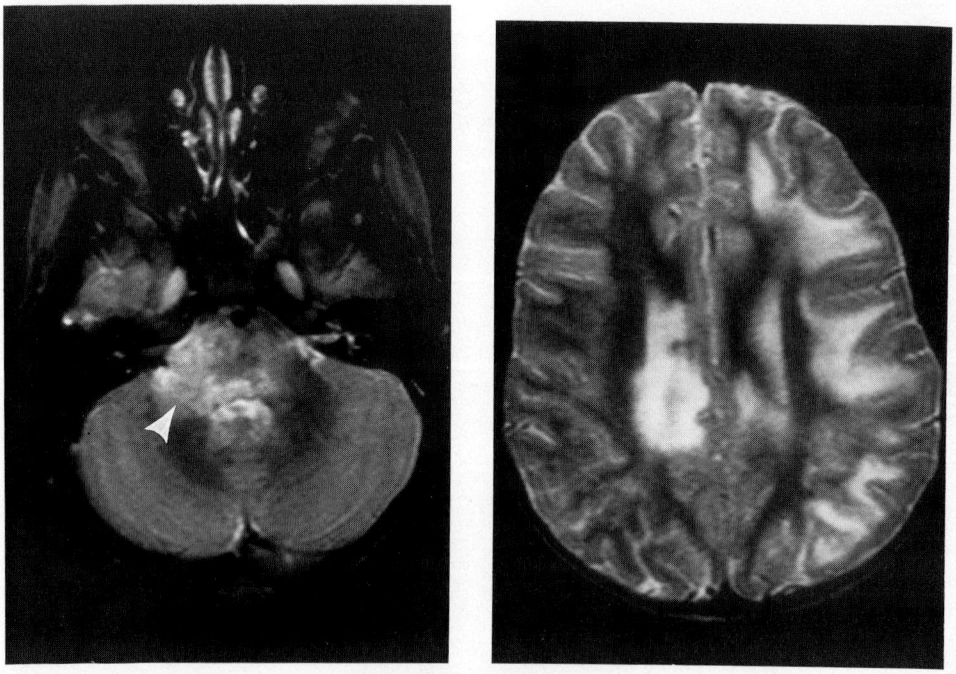

(A) (B)

Figure 27 Lyme disease. Axial T_2-weighted images demonstrate multiple areas of abnormal increased signal intensity. In the brain stem (A) there is an abnormal increased signal intensity extending into the brachium pontis (arrowhead). The supratentorial brain component (B) demonstrates multiple areas of subcortical involvement including involvement of the subcortical U fibers. Periventricular lesions are seen bilaterally.

ACQUIRED IMMUNODEFICIENCY SYNDROME

The radiological manifestations of AIDS can be broadly divided into four categories: cerebral atrophy, mass lesions, meningeal/ependymal disease, and white matter lesions.

Cerebral Atrophy

Cerebral atrophy is the most common neuroimaging abnormality seen in AIDS and usually represents a human immunodeficiency virus (HIV) cerebritis. It is characterized by an enlargement of the cortical sulci and the ventricles (Fig. 28) (48). Although the differentiation of atrophy and hydrocephalus is beyond the scope of this chapter, the lack of sulcal effacement and temporal horn dilatation excludes the possibility of an obstructive hydrocephalus. Communicating hydrocephalus typically will have a ventricular enlargement out of proportion to sulcal prominence. It is estimated that upwards of 50% of patients with cerebral atrophy and HIV infection will have the AIDS dementia complex.

Mass Lesions

A wide variety of mass lesions develop in the brains of patients with AIDS, for which the most common etiology if toxoplasmosis (49). Although toxoplasmosis is a disease that can be congenital in nature, most cases are in the immunosuppressed population. The parasitic infection is caused by the organism *Toxoplasma gondii*.

On noncontrasted CT studies, toxoplasmosis lesions are typically hypodense with associated vasogenic edema and mass effect (50). The lesions are frequently multiple. They have a slight propensity to occur in the region of the basal ganglia. Following contrast administration, the lesions demonstrate marked enhancement that may be of a ring-enhancing or solid nodular enhancement pattern.

On MRI, the lesions are hypo- and hyperintense on T_1- and T_2-weighted images, respectively (51). Occasionally, a small petechial hemorrhage is identified that may be dark on T_2-weighted images (deoxyhemoglobin) or bright on T_1-weighted images (methemoglobin). Following contrast administration, the lesions show a similar enhancement pattern to those on CT (Figs. 29,30). Occasionally, small cortical foci of nodular enhancement will be seen that cannot be appreciated on the unenhanced images. Typically antitoxoplasmosis treatment will be undertaken for any mass lesion in an AIDS patient. Biopsy is rarely performed unless the lesion fails to resolve with antitoxoplasmic chemotherapy. The anticipated response to therapy is a decrease in the size of the lesion, a decrease in the degree of enhancement, and a decrease in edema (Fig. 31).

The other major differential diagnostic consideration for a mass lesion with an appearance similar to toxoplasmosis in an AIDS patient is primary brain lymphoma (52,53). Unfortunately, in most instances, toxoplasmosis cannot be differentiated from lymphoma. The lesions of lymphoma may be multiple but are generally solitary. They have a slight propensity to be more peripherally placed than those of toxoplasmosis. The lesions can show ring or nodular enhancement and are associated with surrounding edema and mass effect. Toxoplasmosis and lymphoma may occur in the same patient. A mass lesion failing to respond to appropriate antitoxoplasmosis therapy should be biopsied to determine if it is a lymphoma. There may be some other imaging clues to the presence of lymphoma, however. Lymphoma may be minimally hyperdense on a noncontrasted CT. This is due to the high nuclear to cytoplasmic ratio and to the hypercellularity of the tumor. For the same reason, the lesions may be minimally hypointense to brain on T_2-weighted MRI images (Fig. 32). These findings can be helpful if identified, but are not present in the majority of cases.

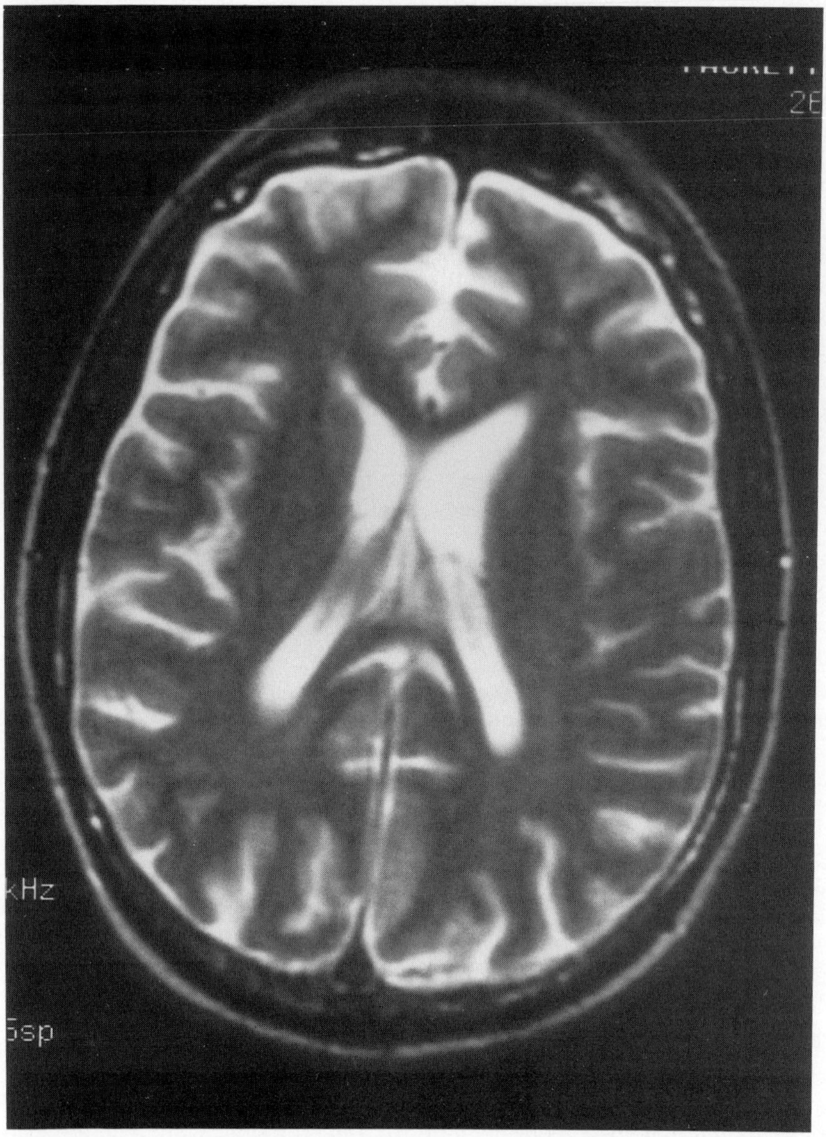

Figure 28 AIDS-related atrophy. An axial T_2-weighted image in a 26-year-old demonstrates ventricular and sulcal prominence consistent with atrophy. The patient clinically had mild dementia consistent with the AIDS dementia complex.

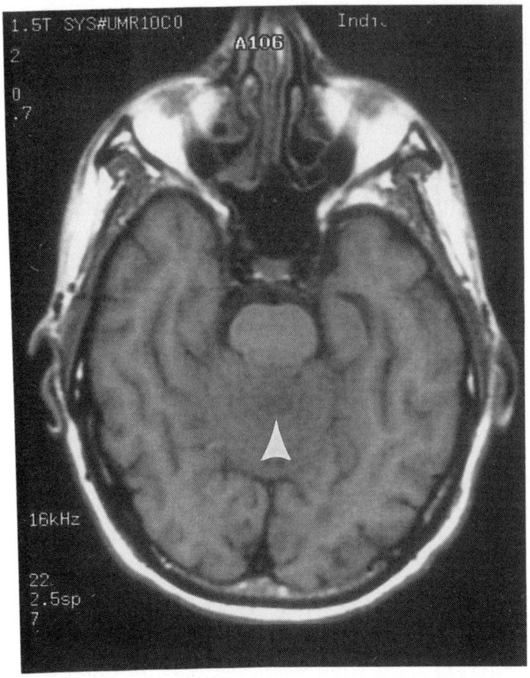

(A)

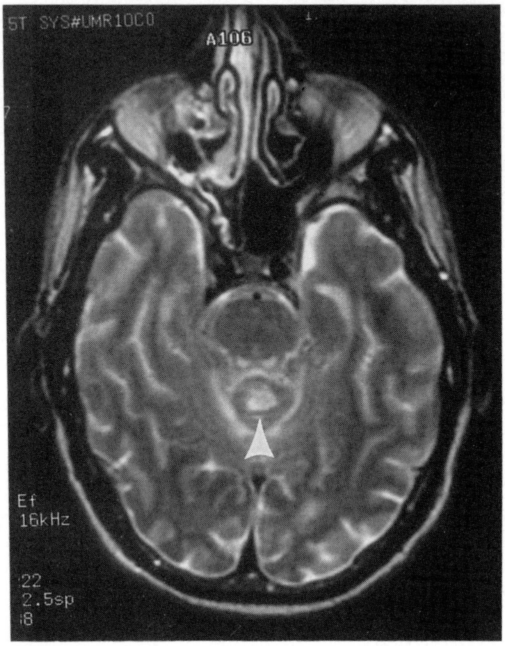

(B)

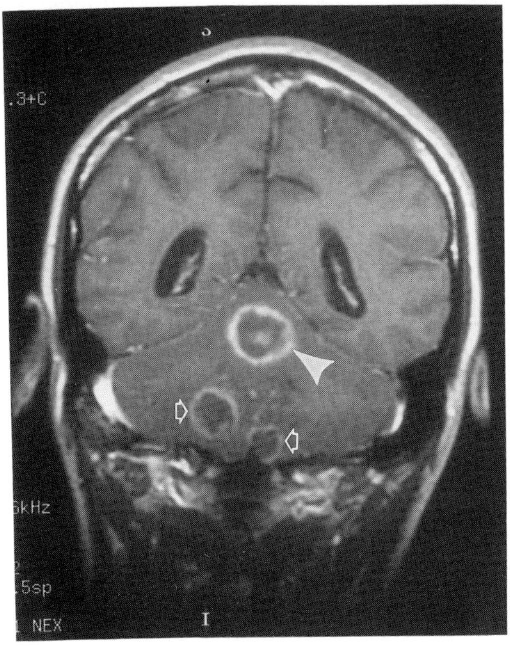

(C)

Figure 29 AIDS-related toxoplasmosis. An axial T_1-weighted image (A) demonstrates mass effect in the cerebellar vermis (arrowhead). An axial T_2-weighted image (B) demonstrates necrosis in the cerebellar vermis with associated mass effect and edema (arrowhead). A coronal postcontrast image (C) demonstrates a target lesion in the superior vermis (arrowhead). Two other ring-enhancing lesions, also toxoplasmosis foci, are identified lower in the cerebellum (open arrows).

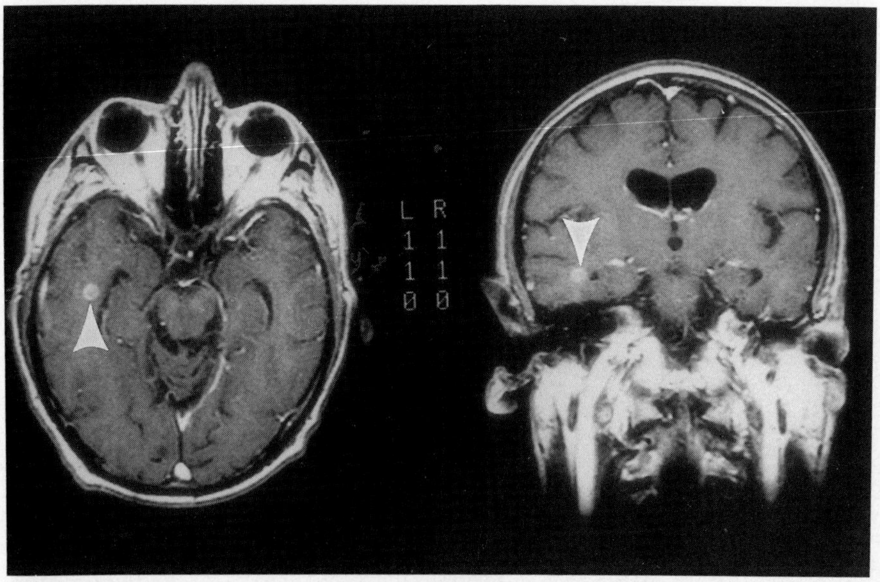

(A)

Figure 30 AIDS-related toxoplasmosis. Figure A is an axial and coronal postcontrast T_1-weighted series demonstrating a single small abnormal enhancing ring in the right temporal lobe. This was the only focus of infection seen and resolved with antitoxoplasmosis therapy. In many cases, the lesions are very small and punctate. Contrast administration will be mandatory for accurate detection. In a second case, a coronal postcontrast T_1-weighted image (B) demonstrates two large solidly enhancing foci, one in the basal ganglia, a relatively common location for toxoplasmosis, and one in the right temporal lobe (arrow). These images demonstrate the marked disparity in size and enhancement characteristics that can occur with AIDS-related toxoplasmosis.

Meningeal/Ependymal Disease

The most common meningeal pathogen in the AIDS patient is *Cryptococcus neoformans*. Cryptococcal infection may be difficult to visualize, even with contrast-enhanced MRI. There is minimal patchy meningeal enhancement along the base of the brain and in the sylvian fissure regions (Fig. 33). There may be abnormal signal intensity in the basal ganglia that may represent micro-abscesses that have extended along the lenticulostriate arteries or small infarctions associated with spasm or infiltration of these vessels (54). Ependymal disease or ventriculitis is most commonly due to cytomegalovirus. There is typically irregularity to the ventricular margins with abnormal signal intensity consistent with edema or both T_1- and T_2-weighted images. Following intravenous contrast enhancement, there is abnormal irregular enhancement of the ventricular and immediate periventricular regions (Fig. 34).

White Matter Lesions

White matter lesions in patients with AIDS can take the form of either diffuse or focal abnormalities. The diffuse abnormalities are frequently related to HIV cerebritis. As such, the white matter lesions are seen in association with central and cortical atrophy. The abnormal signal intensity is typically bilateral and roughly symmetrical (Fig. 35). It involves the periventricular and deep white matter in both the frontal and posterior aspects of the brain as well as the region

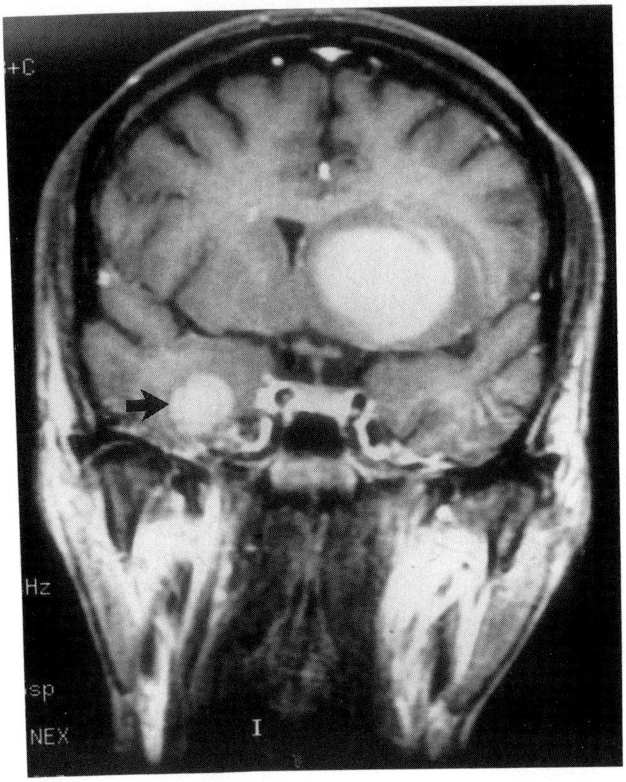

(B)

of the corona radiata. There is no mass effect, and enhancement is not seen. Similar lesions can be seen with CMV and other viral agents.

The most common focal white matter abnormality in patients with AIDS is progressive multifocal leukoencephalopathy (PML). This is an infection with a papova virus, the JC virus, which induces demyelination and leads to relatively rapid death. As with other demyelinating diseases, MRI is more sensitive in the detection of these lesions than is CT. On CT there may be minimal hypodensity in the white matter without evidence of mass effect or abnormal enhancement. The lesions are much better seen on MRI, particularly T_2-weighted images. On T_2-weighted images, the lesions are hyperintense and are seen generally bilaterally but in an asymmetrical pattern (Fig. 36) (55). The lesions have a propensity to be very peripherally located. The major area of involvement is in the subcortical U fibers and adjacent white matter. There is generally a relative sparing of the periventricular and particularly the periatrial regions. Mass effect is unusual, and although contrast enhancement has been reported, this is also an unusual finding.

CONCLUSION

With relatively few exceptions, MRI is the procedure of choice to image intracranial infection, and in most instances gadolinium administration will be required. Additionally, the multiplanar capability of MRI should be utilized to better identify lesions, particularly in the temporal lobes

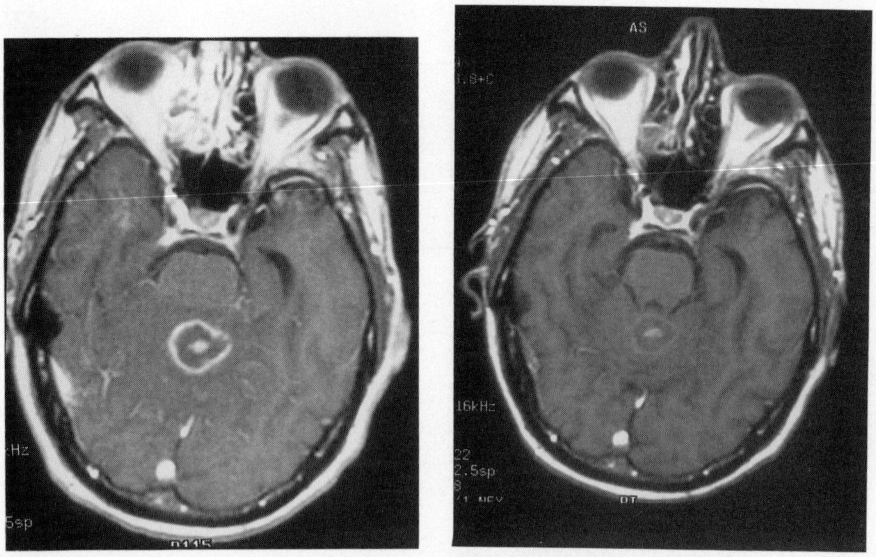

(A) (B)

Figure 31 AIDS-related toxoplasmosis pre- and posttreatment. An axial T_1-weighted image at diagnosis (A) demonstrates a target lesion in the superior vermis. Ten days following institution of antitoxoplasmosis therapy, an axial T_1-weighted image (B) demonstrates marked improvement in the size of the lesion and the degree of enhancement.

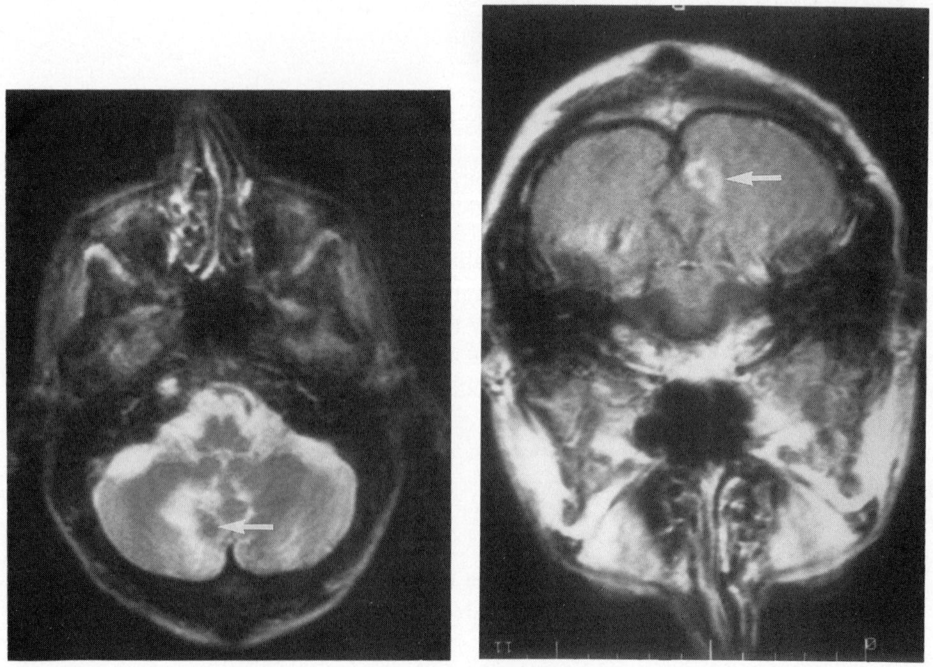

(A) (B)

Figure 32 AIDS-related lymphoma. An axial T_2-weighted image (A) demonstrates a focus of decreased signal intensity (arrow) surrounded by hyperintense edema in the right cerebellar hemisphere. Following intravenous contrast, a T_1-weighted image (B) demonstrates irregular ring enhancement of this lesion (arrow). Lymphoma may be ring or solidly enhancing. Some phase artifacts are seen in the anterior aspect of the posterior fossa.

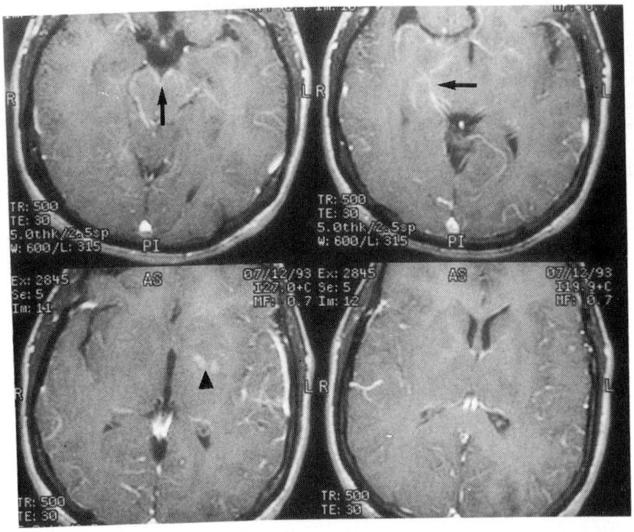

(A)

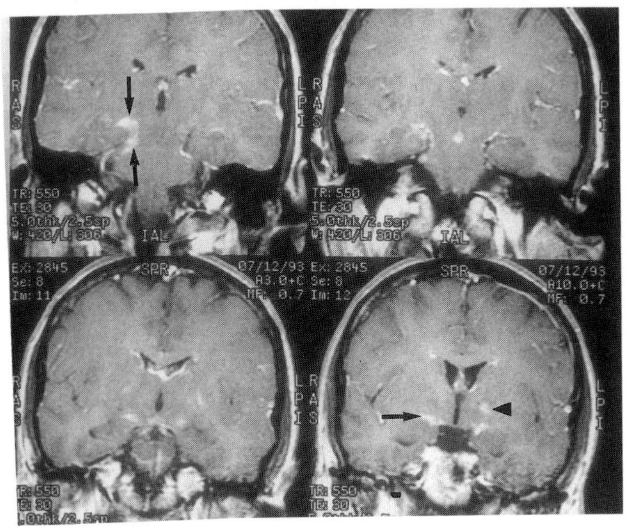

(B)

Figure 33 AIDS-related cryptococcal meningitis. Axial and coronal postcontrast T_1-weighted images (A and B, respectively) demonstrate abnormal enhancement in the basal meninges (arrows). This includes the perimesencephalic cistern, interpeduncular cistern, and extension into the choroidal fissures. Additionally there is some parenchymal enhancement in the left basal ganglia (arrowheads) that probably represents extension of the infection up along the lenticulo-striate vessels into the basal ganglia.

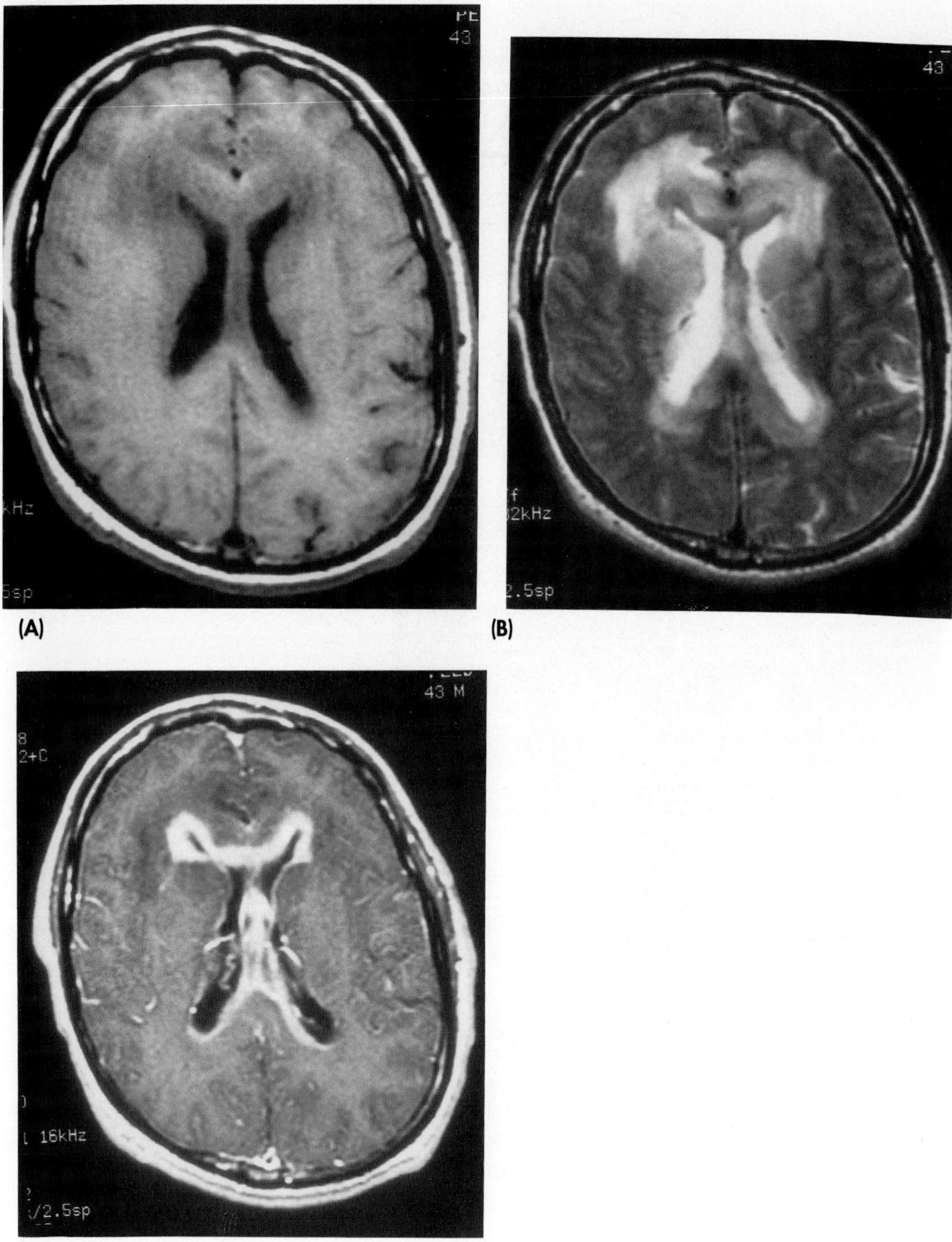

(A) (B) (C)

Figure 34 AIDS-related CMV ependymitis. Axial T_1- and T_2-weighted images (A,B) demonstrate irregularity of the lateral ventricular margins with abnormal signal intensity. A postcontrast T_1-weighted image (C) demonstrates marked enhancement along the margins of the ependymal and periventricular surfaces.

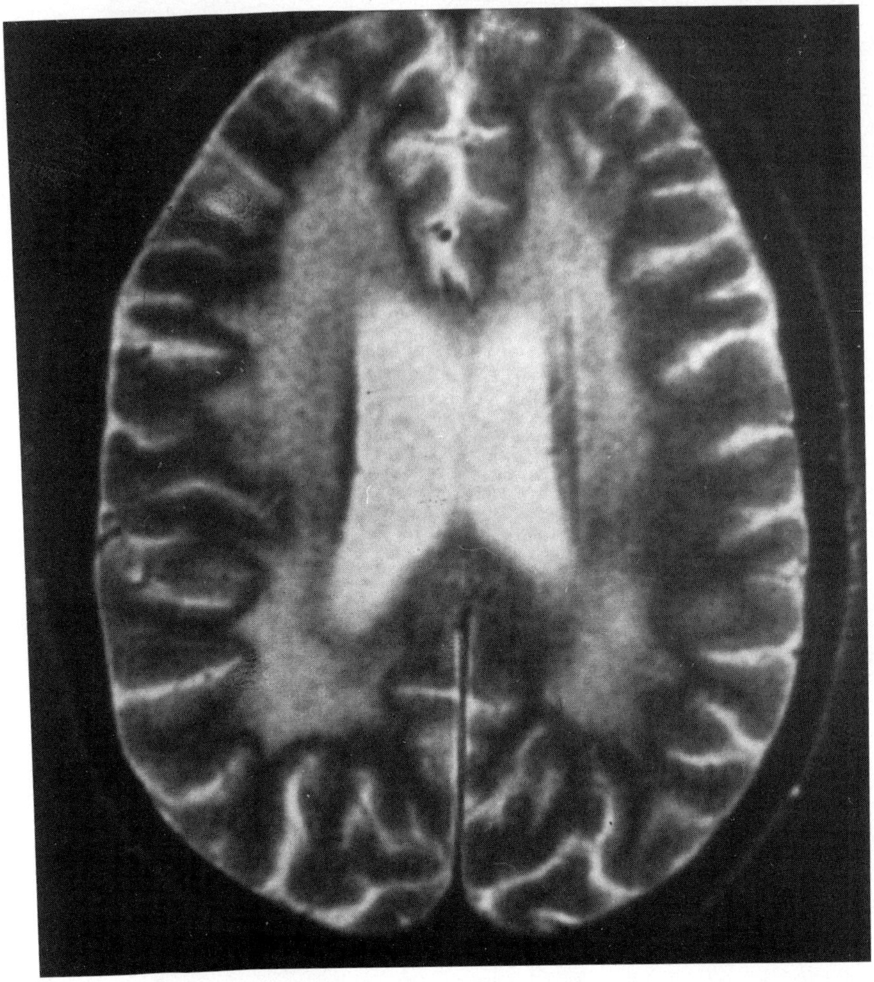

Figure 35 HIV cerebritis. An axial T_2-weighted image demonstrates confluent bilaterally symmetric periventricular hyperintensity. In this 22-year-old there is also ventricular and sulcal enlargement. There is a marked periventricular component to the abnormal signal intensity with relative sparing of the subcortical U fibers.

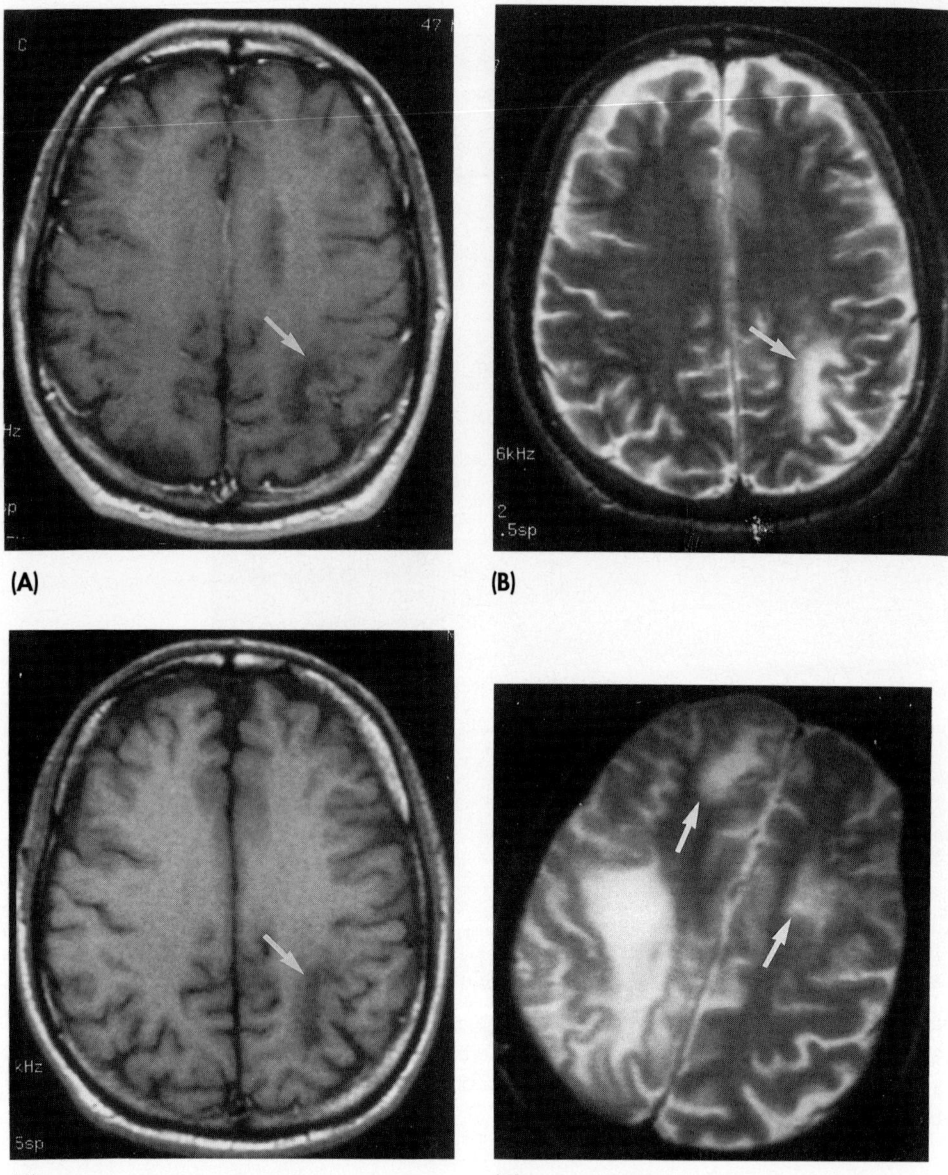

Figure 36 AIDS-related PML. Axial T_1- and T_2-weighted images (A,B) demonstrate abnormal signal intensity in the subcortical region of the left parietal lobe (arrows). No significant mass effect is identified. Some sulcal prominence is seen diffusely in this 24-year-old. An axial postcontrast T_1-weighted image (C) shows no abnormal enhancement. In a separate case, an axial T_2-weighted image (D) demonstrates multiple foci of abnormal increased signal intensity in the subcortical and deep white matter. The largest focus is in the right parietal region, but other lesions in the right frontal and left frontal lobes (arrows) can also be seen.

and posterior fossa. Continued advancements in neuroimaging will include high-volume contrast agents, magnetization transfer imaging, and MRI spectroscopy. The goal in neuroimaging will continue to be the identification of infectious processes and their differentiation to allow for the early institution of specific antimicrobial therapy.

REFERENCES

1. Brant-Zawadzki M, Davis PL, Crooks LE, et al. NMR demonstration of cerebral abnormalities: comparison with CT. AJNR 1983; 4:117–124.
2. Bale JF, Andersen RD, Grose C. Magnetic resonance imaging of the brain in childhood herpesvirus infections. Pediatr Infect Dis J 1987; 6:644–647.
3. Matthews VP, Smith RR, Kuharik MA, et al. Gd-DTPA enhanced MRI of meningitis: initial clinical experience. Scientific presentation, American Society of Neuroradiology, Orlando, FL, March 19–24, 1989.
4. Atlas SW, Grossman RI, Hackney DB, et al. Calcified intracranial lesions: detection with gradient echo acquisition rapid MR imaging. AJNR 1988; 9:253–259.
5. Zimmerman RA, Patel S, Bilaniuk L. Demonstration of purulent bacterial intracranial infections by computed tomography. AJR 1976; 127:155–165.
6. Bilaniuk LT, Zimmerman RA, Brown L, et al. Computed tomography in meningitis. Neuroradiology 1978; 16:13–14.
7. Cockrill HH Jr, Dreisback J, Lowe B, et al. Computed tomography in leptomeningeal infections. AJR 1978; 130:511–515.
8. Sze G, Soletsky S, Bronen R, et al. MR imaging of cranial meninges with emphasis on contrast enhancement and meningeal carcinomatosis. AJNR 1989; 10:965–975.
9. Mathews VP, Kuharik MA, Edwards MK, et al. Gd-DTPA enhanced MR imaging of experimental bacterial meningitis: evaluation and comparison with CT. AJNR 1988; 9:1045–1050.
10. Chang KH, Han MH, Roh JK, et al. Gd-DTPA-enhanced imaging of the brain in patients with meningitis: comparison with CT. AJNR 1990; 11:69–76.
11. Smith RR, Kuharik MA. Inflammation and infection of the brain. In: Cohen MD, Edwards MK, eds. Magnetic Resonance Imaging of Children. Philadelphia: B.C. Decker, 1990:221–275.
12. Ashwal S, Tomasi L, Schneider S, et al. Bacterial meningitis in children: pathophysiology and treatment. Neurology 1992; 42:739–748.
13. Smith RR, Savolaine ER. Computed tomography evolution of multicystic encephalomalacia. J Comput Tomogr 1986; 10:249–254.
14. Buonanno FS, Moody DM, Ball MR, Laster DW. Computed cranial tomographic findings in cerebral sinovenous occlusion. J Comput Assist Tomogr 1978; 2:281–290.
15. Gomori JM, Gorssman RI, Goldberg HI, et al. Intracranial hematomas: imaging by high-field MR. Radiology 1985; 157:87–93.
16. Harris TM, Smith RR, Koch KJ. Gadolinium-DTPA enhanced MR imaging of septic dural sinus thrombosis. J Comput Assist Tomogr 1989; 13:682–684.
17. Angtuaco EJC, McConnell JR, Chadduck WM, Flanigan S. MR imaging of spinal epidural abscess. AJNR 1987; 8:879–883.
18. Sandhu FS, Dillon WP. Spinal epidural abscess: evaluation with contrast-enhanced MR imaging. AJNR 1991; 12:1087–1093.
19. Enzmann DR. Imaging of Infectious and Inflammations of the Central Nervous System: Computed Tomography, Ultrasound, and Nuclear Magnetic Resonance. New York: Raven Press, 1994.
20. Enzmann DR, Britt RH, Yeager AS. Experimental brain abscess evolution: computed tomographic and neuropathologic correlation. Radiology 1979; 133:113–122.
21. Britt RH, Enzmann DR, Yeager AS. Neuropathological and computerized tomographic findings in experimental brain abscess. J Neurosurg 1981; 55:590–603.
22. Haimes AB, Zimmerman RD, Morgello S, et al. MR imaging of brain abscesses. AJNR 1989; 10: 279–291.

23. Sze G, Zimmerman RD. The magnetic resonance imaging of infections and inflammatory diseases. Radiol Clin North Am 1988; 26:839–859.
24. Kingsley DPE, Hendrickse WA, Kendall BE, et al. Tuberculous meningitis: role of CT in management of prognosis. J Neurol Neurosurg Psychiatry 1987; 50:30–36.
25. Schoeman J, Hewlett R, Donald P. MR of childhood tuberculous meningitis. Neuroradiology 1988; 30:473–477.
26. Draouat S, Abdenabi B, Chanem M, Bourjat P. Computed tomography of cerebral tuberculoma. J Comput Assist Tomogr 1987; 11:594–597.
27. Venger BH, Dion FM, Rouah E, Handel SF. MR imaging of pontine tuberculoma. AJNR 1987; 8:1149–1150.
28. Gupta RK, Jena A, Sharma A, et al. MR imaging of intracranial tuberculomas. J Comput Assist Tomogr 1988; 12:280–285.
29. Grossman RI, Zimmerman RA. Infectious diseases of the brain. In: Latchaw RE, ed. Computed Tomography of the Head, Neck and Spine. Chicago: Year Book, 1985:119–136.
30. Enzmann DR, Ranson B, Norman D, et al. Computed tomography of herpes simplex encephalitis. Radiology 1978; 129:419–425.
31. Zimmerman RD, Russel EJ, Leeds NE, Kaufman D. CT in the early diagnosis of herpes simplex encephalitis. AJR 1980; 134:61–66.
32. Schroth G, Gawehn J, Thron A, et al. Early diagnosis of herpes simplex encephalitis by MRI. Neurology 1987; 37:179–183.
33. Neils EW, Lukin R, Tomsick TA, Tew JM. Magnetic resonance imaging and computerized tomography scanning of herpes simplex encephalitis. J Neurosurg 1987; 67:592–594.
34. Lester JW, Carter MP, Reynolds TL. Herpes encephalitis: MR monitoring of response to acyclovir therapy. J Comput Assist Tomogr 1988; 12:941–943.
35. Enzmann DR, Chang Y, Augustyn G. MR findings in neonatal herpes simplex encephalitis type II. J Comput Assist Tomogr 1990; 14:453–457.
36. Reik L. Disseminated vasculomyelinopathy: an immune complex disease. Ann Neurol 1980; 7: 291–296.
37. Atlas SW, Grossman RI, Goldberg HI, et al. MR diagnosis of acute disseminated encephalomyelitis. J Comput Assist Tomogr 1986; 10:798–801.
38. Caldemeyer KS, Smith RR, Harris TM, Edwards MK. MRI in acute disseminated encephalomyelitis. Neuroradiology 1994; 36:216–220.
39. Bignami A, Appiatole L. Micropolygyria and cerebral calcification in cytomegalic inclusion disease. Acta Neuropathol 1964; 4:127–137.
40. Gupta RK, Jena A, Sharma A, et al. MR imaging of neurocysticercosis. J Comput Assist Tomogr 1988; 12:927–934.
41. Mikhael MA. Cerebral phycomycosis. J Comput Assist Tomogr 1979; 3:417–420.
42. Mikhael MA, Rushovich AM, Ciric I. Magnetic resonance imaging of cerebral aspergillosis. Comput Radiol 1985; 9:85–89.
43. Byrd SE, Locke GE, Biggers S, Percy AK. The computed tomographic appearance of cerebral cysticercosis in adults and children. Radiology 1982; 144:819–823.
44. Ramos OM, Stiebel-Chin G, Altman N, Duchowny M. Diagnosis of neurocysticercosis by magnetic resonance imaging. Pediatr Infect Dis 1986; 5:470–473.
45. Zee C-S, Segall HD, Roxwell W, et al. MR imaging of neurocysticercosis. J Comput Assist Tomogr 1988; 12:927–934.
46. Rhee RS, Kumasaki CY, Sarwar M, et al. MR imaging of intraventricular cysticercosis. J Comput Assist Tomogr 1987; 11:598–601.
47. Fernandez RE, Rothberg M, Ferencz G, Wujak D. Lyme disease of the CNS: MR imaging findings in 14 cases. AJNR 1990; 11:479–481.
48. Levy R, Rosenbloom S, Perrett LV. Neuroradiologic findings in AIDS: a review of 200 cases. AJNR 1986; 7:833–839.
49. Navia BA, Petito CK, Gold JWM, et al. Cerebral toxoplasmosis complicating the acquired immune

deficiency syndrome: clinical and neuropathological findings in 27 patients. Ann Neurol 1986; 19: 224–238.
50. Post MJD, Kursunoglu SJ, Hensley GT, et al. Cranial CT in acquired immunodeficiency syndrome. AJNR 1985; 5:743–754.
51. Ramsey RG, Geremia GK. CNS complications of AIDS: CT and MR findings. AJR 1988; 151:449–454.
52. Dina TS. Primary central nervous system lymphoma versus toxoplasmosis in AIDS. Radiology 1991; 179:823–828.
53. Goldstein JD, Zeifer B, Chao C, et al. CT appearance of primary CNS lymphoma in patients with acquired immunodeficiency syndrome. J Comput Assist Tomogr 1991; 15:39–44.
54. Wehn SM, Heinz ER, Burger PC, et al. Dilated Virchow-Robin spaces in cryptococcal meningitis associated with AIDS: CT and MR findings. J Comput Assist Tomogr 1989; 13:756–762.
55. Mark AS, Atlas SW. Progressive multifocal leukoencephalopathy in patients with AIDS: appearance on MR images. Radiology 1989; 173:517–520.

30

EEG in the Diagnosis of CNS Infections

Omkar N. Markand
Indiana University School of Medicine, Indianapolis, Indiana

INTRODUCTION

The electroencephalogram (EEG) abnormalities in most central nervous system (CNS) infections are nonspecific, since similar abnormalities are observed in different pathological entities. There are, however, important exceptions. The EEG often shows more or less distinctive abnormalities in prion diseases, in subacute sclerosing panencephalitis, and in cases of acute herpes encephalitis, where it may provide important diagnostic clues when considered in the proper clinical context. Even though the EEG is generally not of prime importance in the diagnosis of CNS infection, it is useful in determining the severity of the underlying encephalitis/encephalopathy, prognosis for outcome, and response to therapy as well as in detecting sequelae and relapses. There have been several recent reviews of EEG abnormalities associated with inflammatory diseases of the CNS (1–3).

MENINGITIS

Depending on the type of meningitis and the severity of involvement of the CNS, the EEG may show various degrees of background slowing.

Aseptic Meningitis

Over half of patients with aseptic meningitis may have a normal EEG; the remaining show a mild abnormality consisting of diffuse slowing in the theta frequency range (4,5). Paroxysmal activity and focal abnormalities are rare and, when present, argue against uncomplicated viral meningitis. The EEG usually returns to normal within a few days of the clinical recovery. In general, younger children with aseptic meningitis are more likely to have an abnormal EEG than are older children or adults.

Bacterial or Tuberculous Meningitis

The EEG shows more severe slow wave abnormalities in acute bacterial meningitis or tuberculous meningitis (6,7). There is usually diffuse delta activity; the slowing being more severe in children. Monorhythmic paroxysmal delta activity may also occur and may be prominent over the frontal areas in adults or over the occipital regions in children. The development of a brain abscess or cerebral infarction due to arteritis is associated with focal irregular delta activity. On occasion, focal epileptiform abnormalities have been recorded in patients who experience seizures. In acute bacterial meningitis, there is rapid improvement in the EEG with successful treatment, with EEG readings returning to normal within 1–2 weeks (7). EEG abnormalities generally require a longer time for resolution in tuberculous meningitis. Persistence or deterioration of EEG abnormalities suggest an unfavorable course and the development of complications such as abscess, hydrocephalus, or residual brain damage (8,9).

Fungal Diseases

Several fungal diseases (histoplasmosis, blastomycosis, coccidioidomycosis and cryptococcosis) manifest as acute, subacute or chronic meningitis or meningoencephalitis. They are associated with diffuse slow wave abnormalities in the EEG. Focal EEG abnormalities (focal irregular delta activity and/or epileptiform discharges) may occur when there are focal cerebral complications, e.g. mycotic abscess, granuloma, vasculitis or other vascular lesions.

Certainly, the EEG does not provide a specific diagnosis of meningitis, but it is helpful in following the course of disease and detecting the development of complications.

ACUTE ENCEPHALITIS

Acute Viral Encephalitis

In viral encephalitis, the EEG is always abnormal (10,11). It shows more severe abnormalities than observed with acute aseptic meningitis, a point helpful in the differential diagnosis. The EEG is more disorganized and dominated by delta-frequency activity; the slower activity may be prominent over the occipital region in children and over the frontal areas in adults (Fig. 1). Both polymorphic and rhythmic delta activities occur in the EEG. Diffuse polymorphic or irregular delta activity is more likely to occur when the subcortical white matter is involved, whereas paroxysmal rhythmic delta implies involvement of the subcortical gray matter (12). Children, in general, show more severe EEG abnormalities than do adults. The severity of the EEG abnormalities generally parallel the clinical picture, but at times the EEG may be more disorganized and slower than one would expect by the patient's level of consciousness (13). The rapidity with which the EEG reverts to normal is of some prognostic significance. Normalization of the EEG over 2–5 weeks occurs in patients who have a favorable outcome. Slow improvement or persistent abnormalities have an unfavorable prognosis and increase the likelihood of the subsequent development of retardation, behavior abnormalities, or epileptic seizures (10). In patients who sustain permanent brain damage due to encephalitis, the EEG may continue to be disorganized and show slow background activities and unifocal or multifocal epileptiform abnormalities.

EEG abnormalities in different viral encephalitides are generally nonspecific (an exception being herpes simplex encephalitis, discussed below) and cannot distinguish one etiological agent from another. Slow wave abnormalities in the EEG are, thus, similar in enteroencephalitides (coxsackie or ECHO virus infection), mosquitoborne encephalitides (Western equine, Eastern equine, St. Louis, or Japanese encephalitis) or various tickborne encephalitides. In patients with

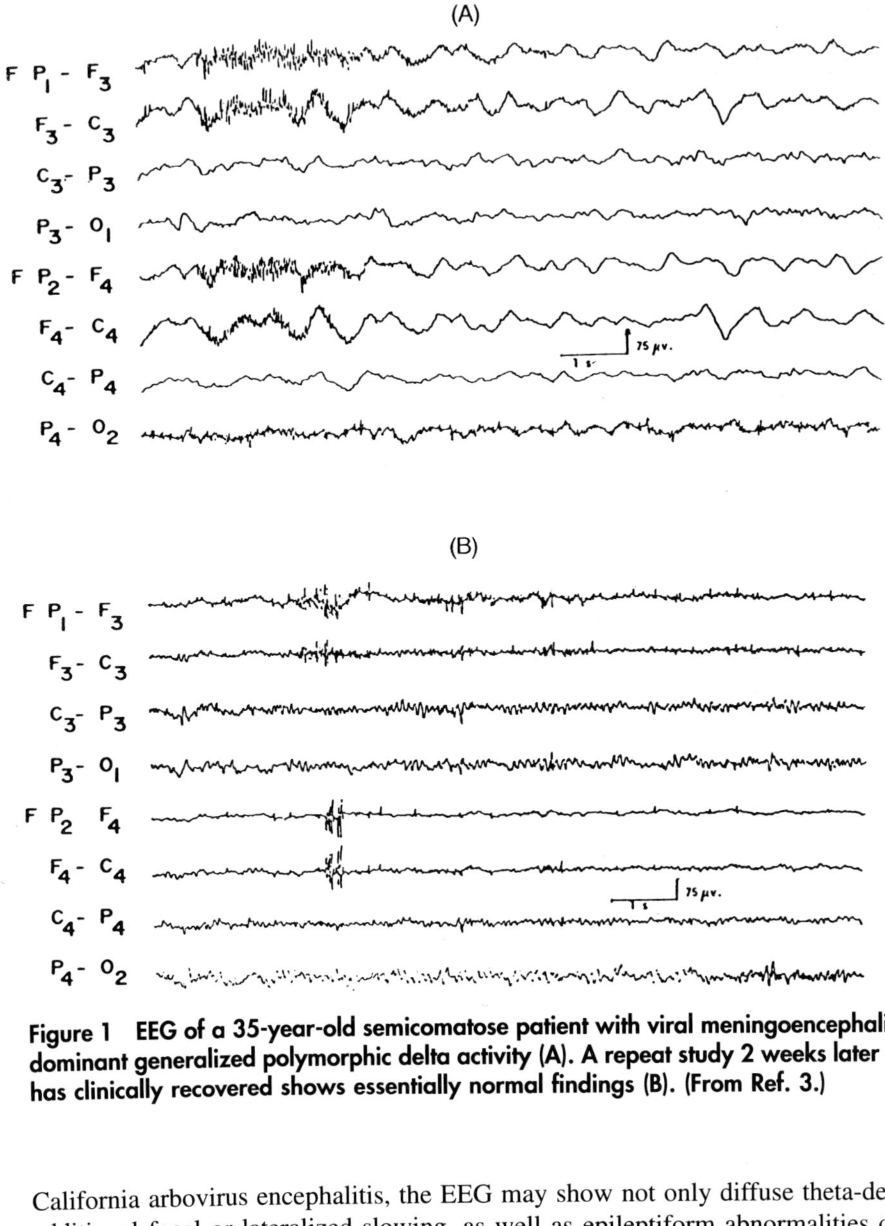

Figure 1 EEG of a 35-year-old semicomatose patient with viral meningoencephalitis shows frontal dominant generalized polymorphic delta activity (A). A repeat study 2 weeks later when the patient has clinically recovered shows essentially normal findings (B). (From Ref. 3.)

California arbovirus encephalitis, the EEG may show not only diffuse theta-delta slowing, but additional focal or lateralized slowing, as well as epileptiform abnormalities during the acute stage of the illness (14).

Rabies is still an almost uniformly fatal encephalitis caused by rabies virus or antigenically different rabies-related viruses. EEG recordings have rarely been done in patients with rabies. Slowing of EEG activity in the theta-delta range progressing to an almost isoelectric EEG close to death has been mentioned in case reports (15,16).

EEG abnormalities in neurotropic and nonneurotropic virus infections are known to occur in a variable proportion of patients without there being clinically overt signs of encephalitis, e.g., in 15% of patients with poliomyelitis (17), 30% of patients with measles (18), 22% of patients with varicella (19), and 31% of patients with herpes zoster (20). In children with measles, the EEG abnormality of diffuse theta-delta slowing may be present even a few days before the skin rash, reaching maximal slowing on the first day of the rash and then abating during the subsequent week or so (21).

A small proportion of patients with infectious mononucleosis may develop encephalitis that is associated with varying degrees of diffuse slow activity in the EEG (22). There are rare case reports of periodic, slow wave complexes that have a repetition rate of every 4–5 s in this encephalitis (23), not unlike those recorded in herpes simplex encephalitis (see below).

Mycoplasma pneumoniae may rarely cause a severe encephalitis in children manifesting with unconsciousness and epileptic seizures. Most patients show varying degrees of slowing of background activities (24). Bilateral lateralized epileptiform discharges (BIPLEDs) have been reported on rare occasion in this encephalitis (25). BIPLEDs in the EEG are usually associated with severe anoxic encephalopathy and meningoencephalitis, including herpes simplex encephalitis (26).

Infection with human herpesvirus 6 (HHV-6) causes xanthem subitum (roseola infantum) in infants and young children. Rarely encephalitis or encephalopathy has been reported, which produces fever, status epilepticus, and a comatose state in the preeruptive stage. The EEG in such infants shows slow wave abnormalities and focal epileptiform abnormalities, including periodic lateralized epileptiform discharges (PLEDs) (27).

Postinfectious and Parainfectious Encephalitides

These occur in children over one year of age, 1–2 weeks following various childhood infections such as smallpox, measles, chickenpox, mumps, rubella, etc., or after vaccination. Pathological changes of perivenous demyelination are widespread in the CNS. The EEG is nonspecific and consists of generalized slow activity and occasionally of focal slow wave abnormalities (28–30). The EEG abnormalities decrease in most patients with clinical improvement. Persistent EEG abnormalities or the development of epileptiform findings suggest permanent residual brain damage. Such patients are likely to develop intellectual deficits or epileptic seizures.

Herpes Simplex Encephalitis

This accounts for 10% of all cases of viral encephalitides, but for over 50% of deaths due to encephalitis. The pathological changes in the CNS are those of necrotizing encephalitis, which may start in one temporal lobe. The EEG pattern and its evolution in herpes simplex encephalitis are rather characteristic, so that the diagnosis can often be suspected by EEG findings, especially when serial studies are performed and when considered in the proper clinical context (31).

In the early stages, the EEG shows a prominent focal or lateralized abnormality, usually irregular polymorphic delta activity over one temporal region. This corresponds to the localization of pathology initially to one temporal lobe of the brain (32–35). Slow-wave abnormalities progressively become widespread and bilateral with progression of the disease. The most characteristic EEG feature of herpes simplex encephalitis is the occurrence of pseudoperiodic, focal or unilateral, high-amplitude complexes (Fig. 2), which repeat at fairly regular intervals (31–35). These complexes are expressed maximally over the involved temporal lobe. The periodic pattern is usually seen 2–15 days after the onset of the illness (31) but may be delayed in appearance for as long as 24–30 days (33,36). The periodic complexes may consist of a single wave or a group of waves; they may be prominent or barely stand out from the background; they may be sawtooth waves, delta waves (Fig. 2), or sharp waves (Fig. 3). The interval between the complexes is generally 2–3 s but may range from 1 to 5 s. As the disease progresses and the other hemisphere is involved, the periodic complexes may disappear on the side of initial involvement before appearing on the side more recently involved. With bilateral involvement of the brain, periodic complexes may occur over both hemispheres; they may then occur either synchronously

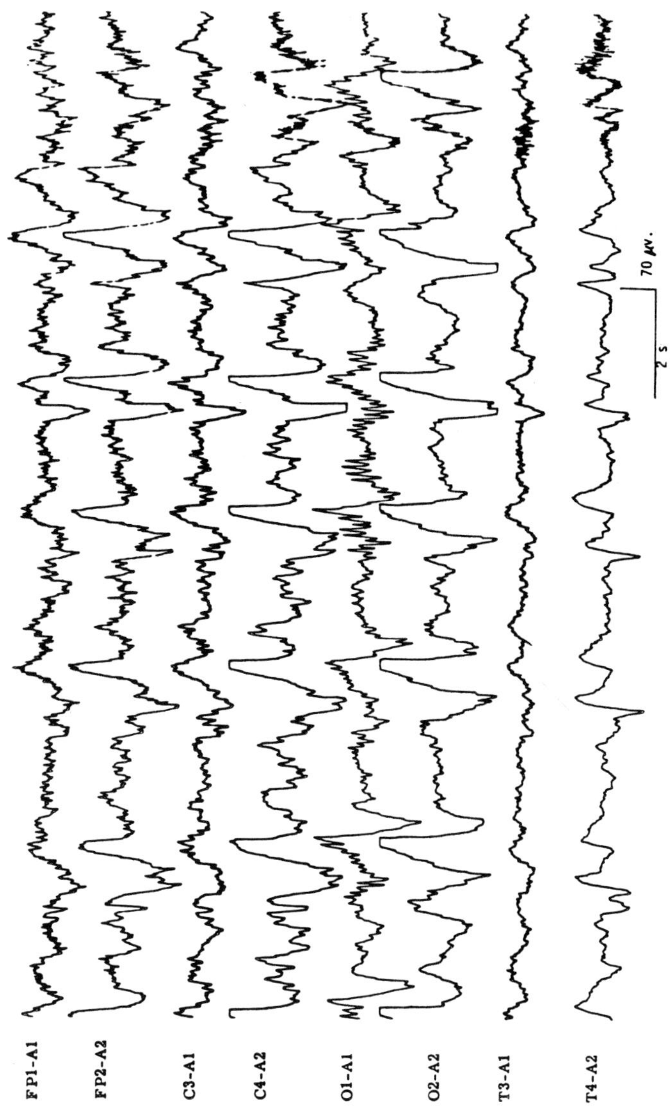

Figure 2 EEG of a 14-year-old patient with biopsy-proven herpes simplex encephalitis shows large amplitude periodic sharp waves occurring every 2.0–2.5 s over the right temporal region. Also note absence of alpha rhythm on the right side. (From Ref. 3.)

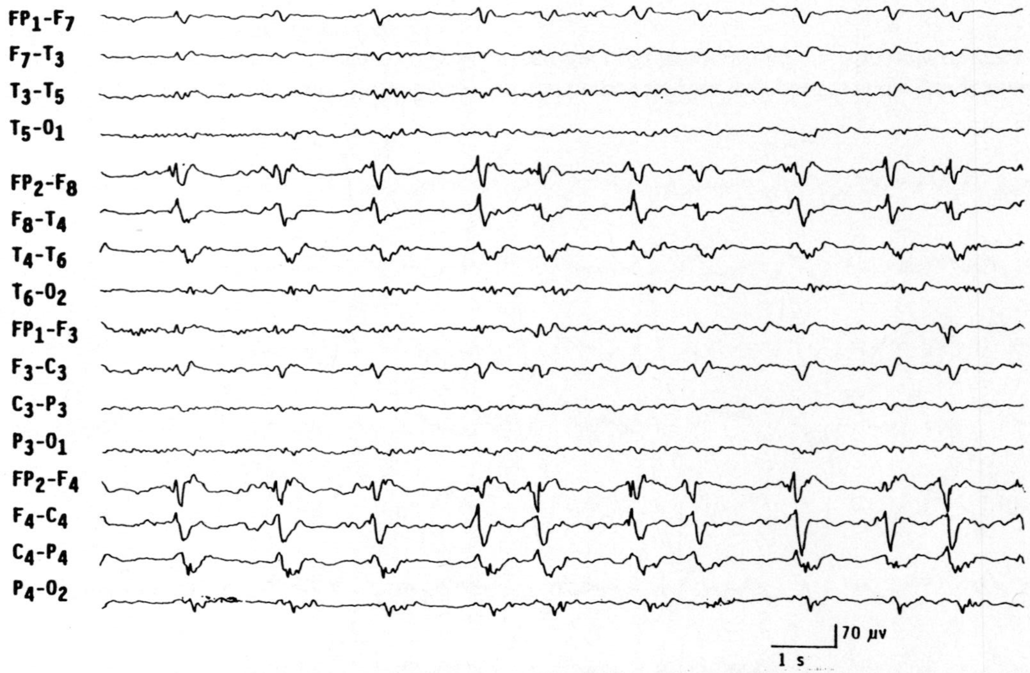

Figure 3 A 65-year-old female with a 3-day history of confusion and disorientation. The cerebrospinal fluid had 35 white blood cells/mm^3, and a presumptive diagnosis of herpes simplex encephalitis was made. The EEG shows periodic lateralized epileptiform discharges (PLEDs) over the right fronto-centro-temporal regions.

or independently over the two sides but often with a time-locked relationship with each other (33,34,37). During the final stages of fatal herpes simplex encephalitis, the periodic complexes may disappear and the EEG may assume an almost "isoelectric" appearance. In patients who survive, the periodic complexes disappear with resolution of the encephalitis; they are replaced by focal or lateralized slowing, epileptiform abnormalities, or attenuation of activity over the previously involved area. The resolution of the EEG abnormalities often lag behind the clinical improvement; varying degrees of background slowing and paroxysmal abnormalities in the EEG may persist.

If serial EEG studies are carried out, periodic complexes are seen in over two thirds of pathologically proven cases of herpes simplex encephalitis (36). The presence of periodic complexes in the EEG is associated with a relatively unfavorable prognosis and high mortality (36,38,39).

Similar to the findings in adults, the EEG shows a periodic pattern in childhood cases of herpes simplex encephalitis (40). In neonatal herpes simplex encephalitis, focal or lateralized discharges consisting of sharp or slow waves repeating at pseudoperiodic intervals of 0.5–2.0 s have been reported (41–43). This EEG pattern was observed by Sainio et al. (43) in 16 of 21 babies with herpes simplex encephalitis. The pseudoperiodic discharges may occur in the EEG either for short periods (10 s to 2 min) or persist throughout the recording (42,43). These electrical events are not associated with a clinical change. Babies with markedly abnormal background and long-lasting paroxysms tend to have a poor prognosis.

The presence of unilateral or focal periodic complexes or PLEDs is not unique to herpes simplex encephalitis; such EEG findings may occur with acute focal processes, e.g., infarction, brain abscess, or neoplasm (44). Nevertheless, the presence of unilateral periodic complexes in association with an acute febrile illness, focal seizures, and CSF pleocytosis is strongly suggestive of herpes simplex encephalitis. Rarely, a similar EEG pattern has been reported in patients with other types of encephalitides, e.g., infectious mononucleosis encephalitis (23).

In 1977 Whitley et al. (45) achieved a considerable reduction in mortality (from 70% to 28%) with vidarabine therapy, but early administration of the drug (particularly before coma occurs), and therefore early diagnosis, was necessary for the best results. Early diagnosis is based on a combination of clinical, spinal fluid, EEG, and neuroimaging findings. The computed tomographic (CT) appearance of a low-density lesion in one temporal region is characteristic of herpes simplex encephalitis but may not appear until a week or so into the illness. The magnetic resonance (MR) scan is highly sensitive early in the illness (46), making MR the neuroimaging modality of choice in a patient in whom herpes simplex encephalitis is suspected. Brain biopsy for confirmation of the diagnosis is controversial. However, if brain biopsy is contemplated, the localization provided by EEG and/or neuroimaging studies is helpful in choosing the ideal site for biopsy.

SUBACUTE OR CHRONIC ENCEPHALITIS

Subacute Sclerosing Panencephalitis

This is an inflammatory disorder of childhood, which is now established to be a slow virus (measles) infection of the CNS. It is usually fatal, and three clinical stages are distinguished. The first stage is that of intellectual deterioration or of psychological disturbances. During the second stage, there are motor rigidity, neurological deficits, severe dementia and characteristics repetitive myoclonic jerks occurring every 4–10 s. The third stage consists of coma and a vegetative existence. The EEG findings in subacute sclerosing panencephalitis (SSPE) are often highly characteristic, so that the diagnosis is usually possible by EEG. The periodic complexes of SSPE were initially described by Radermecker (47) and independently by Cobb and Hill (48). The EEG findings have been subsequently reported in detail by Radermecker and Poser (49), Cobb (50), and Markand and Panszi (51).

The periodic complexes in SSPE have the following characteristics:

1. They are bilateral, usually synchronous and symmetrical.
2. They are remarkably stereotyped in that their form remains identical in any given lead.
3. They usually consist of two or more delta waves and are diphasic, triphasic, or polyphasic in appearance.
4. The amplitude of the complexes is usually 200–500 μV.
5. They repeat at regular intervals of 4–10 s.
6. When clinical myoclonic jerks are present, there is a 1:1 relationship of the jerks to the EEG complexes.

The periodic complexes may appear very early in the disease, even during the first clinical stage, at which time the patient may be fully alert, coherent, and ambulatory. The background activity between these complexes at this stage may be normal or only minimally altered (51). Initially, the periodic complexes may occur at irregular and long intervals ranging up to 1–5 min (52,53). At this stage, sleep may activate them. A sleep recording is, therefore, recommended in a suspected case of SSPE where a tracing during wakefulness has failed to reveal periodic complexes (53).

During the second clinical stage of SSPE when myoclonic jerks are clinically apparent, the periodic complexes become well established in the EEG. There is a very close relationship between the myoclonic jerks and the periodic complexes (Fig. 4). The myoclonic jerks may begin either just before or somewhat after the onset of the EEG complexes. The myoclonic jerks often disappear during sleep and with the use of narcotic medications despite persistence of the periodic EEG complexes. The occurrence of regular stereotyped myoclonic jerks in the absence of EEG complexes is rare (50). Different stimuli have little effect on the periodic complexes once they are well established in the EEG (49). However, in the early stages of the disease when the complexes are inconsistent and far apart, they may be triggered by external stimuli (50,54). Drugs have, generally, little effect on the periodic pattern.

Although some (50) have found no clear relationship between the interval of the complexes and the stage of SSPE, others (51,55) have observed a shortening of the interval between the complexes with progression of the disease. Furthermore, the periodic complexes may disappear terminally in some patients (55).

The background rhythms may at first be normal or minimally altered even though the periodic complexes are well established. As the disease progresses, the background activity becomes progressively slower and more disorganized. Sleep-related potentials, e.g., sleep spindles, vertex sharp transients, and K complexes, also become disorganized and finally disappear with progression of the disease. In the terminal stages the background may be very "flat" in between the periodic complexes.

In an EEG study on 31 patients with SSPE, Markand and Panszi (51) emphasized several atypical and less well-known EEG findings:

1. Asymmetry of the periodic complexes in the early stages, associated often with asymmetry of the myoclonic jerks, which may occur contralateral to the periodic complexes (Fig. 5)
2. Presence of prominent "flat" or "electrodecremental" periods following periodic complexes, even early in the disease (Fig. 6)
3. Bursts of rhythmic frontally dominant generalized delta activity in between the periodic complexes

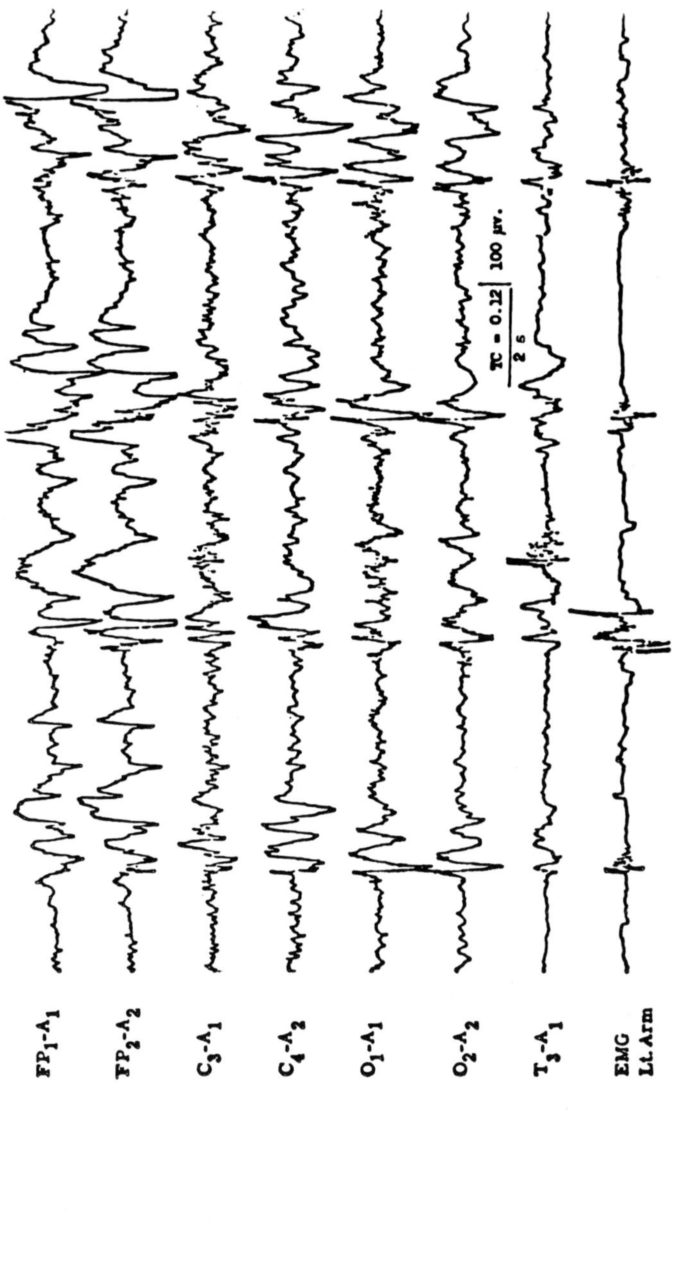

Figure 4 EEG of a 13-year-old patient with SSPE shows large amplitude periodic complexes of generalized distribution recurring every 4–5 s. Note the simultaneous occurrence of myoclonic jerks recorded on the last channel from two electrodes placed over the left biceps muscles. (From Ref. 3.)

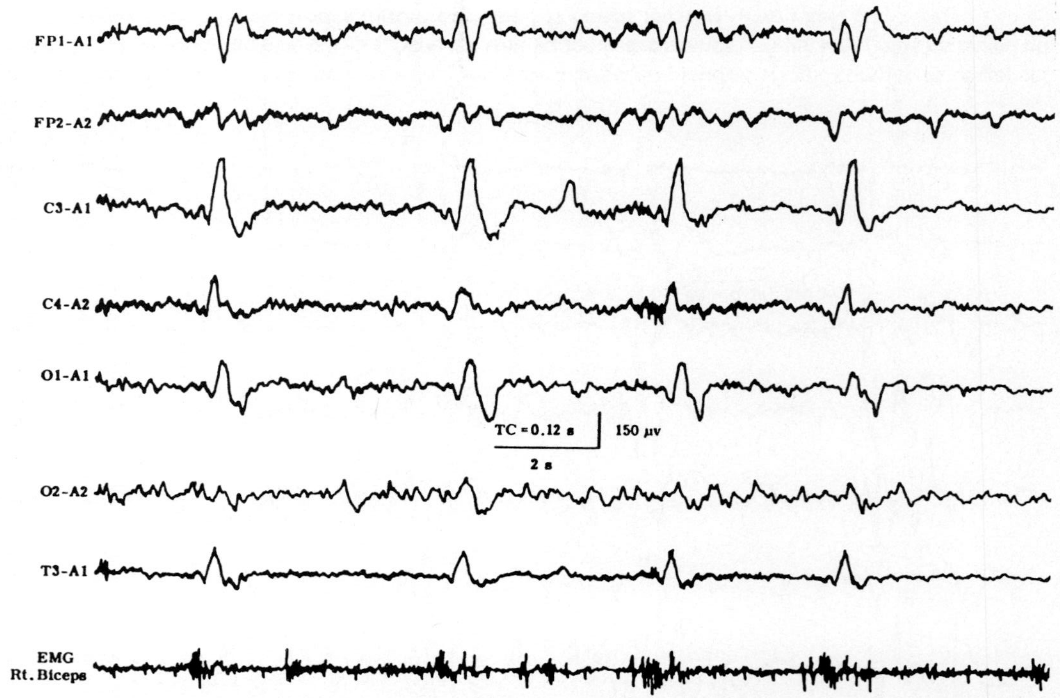

Figure 5 EEG of a 10-year-old patient with SSPE shows periodic complexes that are larger in amplitude over the left hemisphere. Patient had myoclonic jerks confined to the right side, which were monitored on the last channel. (From Ref. 3.)

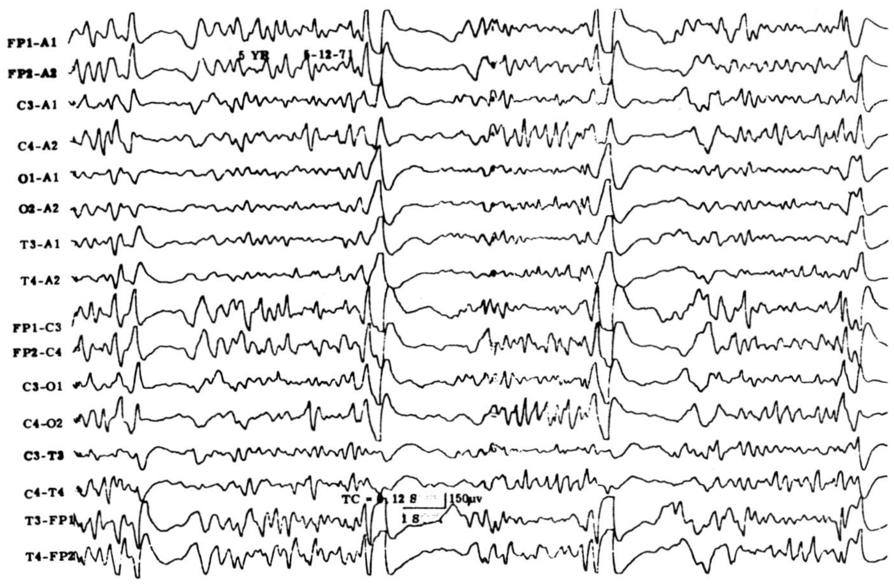

Figure 6 EEG of a 5-year-old patient with SSPE shows prominent "flattening" immediately following periodic complexes. (From Ref. 3.)

4. Episodic bisynchronous spike and slow-wave activity in the form of isolated complexes or long paroxysms at a frequency of 1–2 cps
5. Occurrence of spikes, sharp waves, or triphasic waves in the frontal areas
6. Presence of focal abnormalities, such as spikes or slow-wave foci

Rare patients with SSPE may have clinical remission or improvement. The periodic complexes in their EEG may disappear and background activity may also improve.

Periodic patterns similar to the complexes of SSPE have been reported in the literature in other pathological conditions including a few cases of Unverricht-Lafora myoclonus epilepsy, cerebral lipidoses, anoxic encephalopathy, acute necrotizing encephalitis, head injury, etc. However, the periodic pattern in these conditions occurs only rarely, and the resemblance of the pattern to that of SSPE is minimal. In conclusion, although other entities may be rarely associated with a periodic pattern, the stereotyped EEG complexes occurring in a regular and periodic fashion and having a constant relationship to motor movements make this pattern one of the most characteristic and specific of all EEG patterns. Close attention to the EEG and the clinical features aid in the diagnosis of SSPE and distinguish it from other types of encephalopathies.

Chronic Rubella Panencephalitis

This is a rare, delayed, progressive encephalopathy, which manifests during the second decade in children who previously had congenital or acquired rubella. The pathological findings are those of a subacute or chronic encephalitis, and the clinical picture is characterized by dementia, ataxia, chorea, and myoclonus. The EEG shows generalized polymorphic slowing and intermittently occurring rhythmic delta activity. Paroxysmal abnormalities may occur, which include focal or multifocal spikes, sharp waves, or periodic high-amplitude slow-wave complexes repeating every 5–8 s resembling those of SSPE (56).

Creutzfeldt-Jakob Disease

This was once regarded as a degenerative CNS disease, but it has been established to be due to a transmissible agent attributed to a prion infection. Although most cases of Creutzfeldt-Jakob disease (CJD) are sporadic, 5–15% are clustered in families (57,58). The clinical picture is similar in sporadic and familial cases. Three clinical stages are recognized. The first is characterized principally by progressive dementia or a wide variety of focal symptoms, indicating lesions in various parts of the brain. In the second stage, the focal features tend to disappear as a picture of progressive dementia, bilateral rigidity, pyramidal signs, and widespread myoclonus evolves. In the third stage, the patient becomes bedridden with deepening stupor, increasing rigidity, and weakness of the limbs that proceeds relentlessly to death.

In the first stage, EEG changes are limited to a progressive disorganization of background rhythms and increased amounts of generalized slow (theta-delta) activity (59). These changes may be more marked anteriorly or posteriorly, or over one hemisphere or part of a hemisphere (Fig. 7). Such focal or lateralized features may suggest a tumor, but sooner or later the EEG becomes bilaterally slow.

During the second stage of CJD, the EEG is characterized by periodic bilaterally synchronous potentials (59,60). The periodic potentials take the form of diphasic or triphasic sharp waves 200–500 ms in duration and up to 300 μV in amplitude. As the disease progresses, there may be more complex discharges with a multiphasic or polyspike configuration (61). The frequency of the periodic complexes is close to 1/s; the interval between successive discharges varies from 0.5 to 1.6 s (Figs. 8 and 9). There is a fairly close, but not precise, relationship between the periodic complexes and the myoclonic jerks. The jerks may occur a few milliseconds before or after the electrical event. Periodic sharp wave complexes (PSWCs) in the EEG may occur without associated clinical myoclonic jerks. This is particularly true during sleep or late in the course of the disease when the myoclonic jerks decrease or disappear but the PSWCs persist (59).

This periodic pattern continues into the third or the final stage of CJD. Many authors (60–62) describe a progressive lengthening of the interval between periodic complexes. Finally, the amplitude of the background activity decreases, which results in an undifferentiated very low-voltage tracing from which rhythmic discharges emerge. Terminally, the PSWCs disappear and the EEG becomes virtually "isoelectric."

The characteristic periodic pattern has been reported in 75–94% of patients with CJD (59,63). From original data and review of the literature, Levy et al. (64) affirmed that a lack of periodic abnormalities in EEGs after an illness of 12 weeks weighs strongly against CJD. However, some patients with CJD, particularly with forms considered atypical (e.g., ataxic or amyotrophic variety or with long duration), have been reported who did not show periodic EEG activity at any point in the entire illness (64–67). No comprehensive evaluation of EEG has been carried out in familial cases. It appears, however, that PSWCs are less common in familial than in sporadic CJD, although the clinical characteristics are not dramatically different. Tietjen and Drury (68) reported an absence of myoclonus and PSWCs in serial EEGs of four members of a kindred with pathologically verified CJD.

In the early stages of CJD, periodic complexes may be present only for 5–10 s at a time or may appear only a few times in a single EEG. Also, in the early stages of the disease, before the periodic pattern is fully established, the EEG may show state-dependent variability. During periods of drowsiness or sleep, the PSWCs may virtually disappear and be replaced by medium-amplitude slow activity in the theta-delta frequency range. Also, during drowsiness or sleep, the myoclonic jerks disappear; heart and respiratory rates are reduced and periods of apnea may occur (62,69). Periodic complexes reappear during the periods when the patient is aroused and

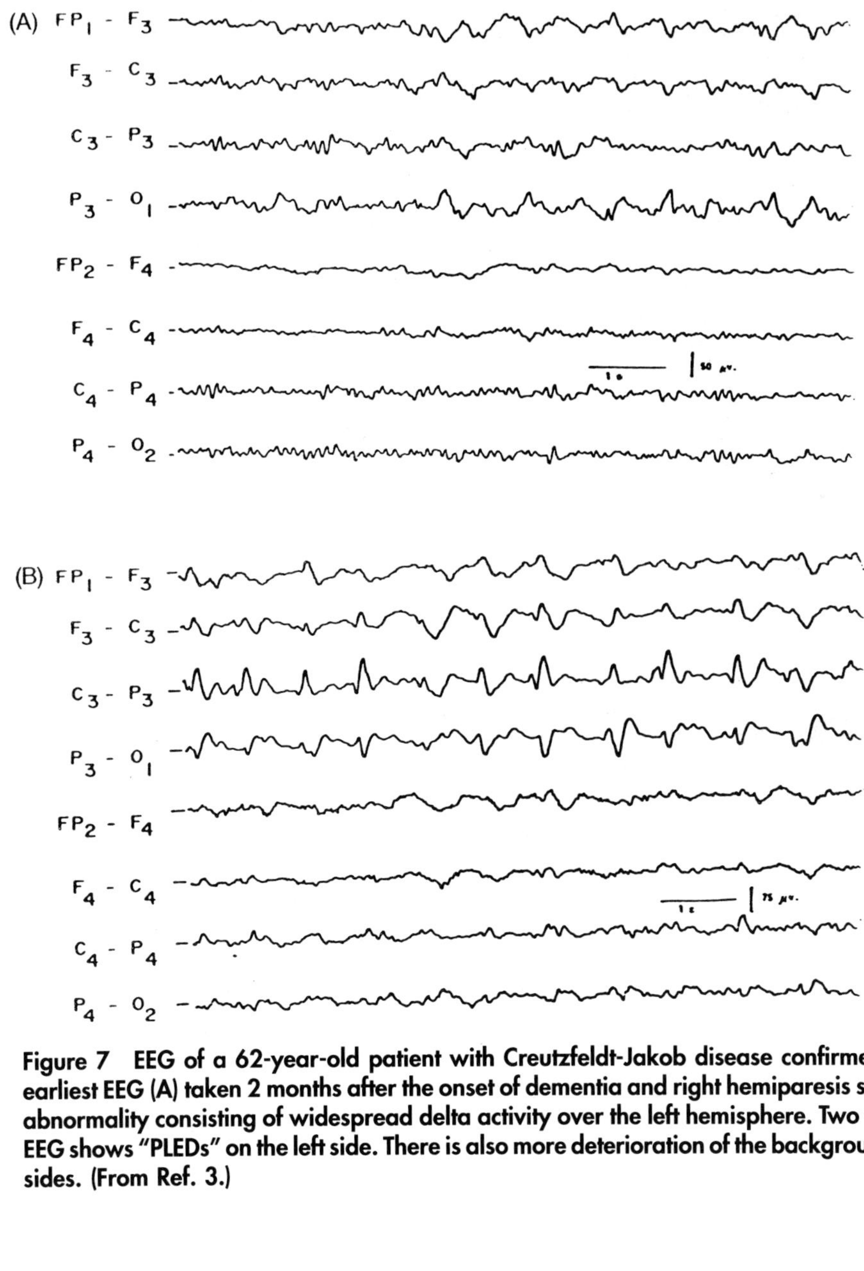

Figure 7 EEG of a 62-year-old patient with Creutzfeldt-Jakob disease confirmed at autopsy. The earliest EEG (A) taken 2 months after the onset of dementia and right hemiparesis shows a lateralized abnormality consisting of widespread delta activity over the left hemisphere. Two weeks later (B) the EEG shows "PLEDs" on the left side. There is also more deterioration of the background activity on both sides. (From Ref. 3.)

more alert. The EEG may thus show a cyclic alternating pattern, i.e., alternation of the two stereotyped EEG patterns (PSWC pattern alternating with diffusely slow EEG).

Another characteristic feature of the PSWCs, particularly in the early stages, is their reactivity to alerting stimuli or to the administration of drugs. Before the PSWCs are well established, or when they occur only intermittently, acoustic or other types of alerting stimuli may trigger the periodic pattern when delivered during a diffusely slow EEG phase (62). In some patients, intermittent photic stimulation (IPS) may elicit tight coupling of periodic complexes to the

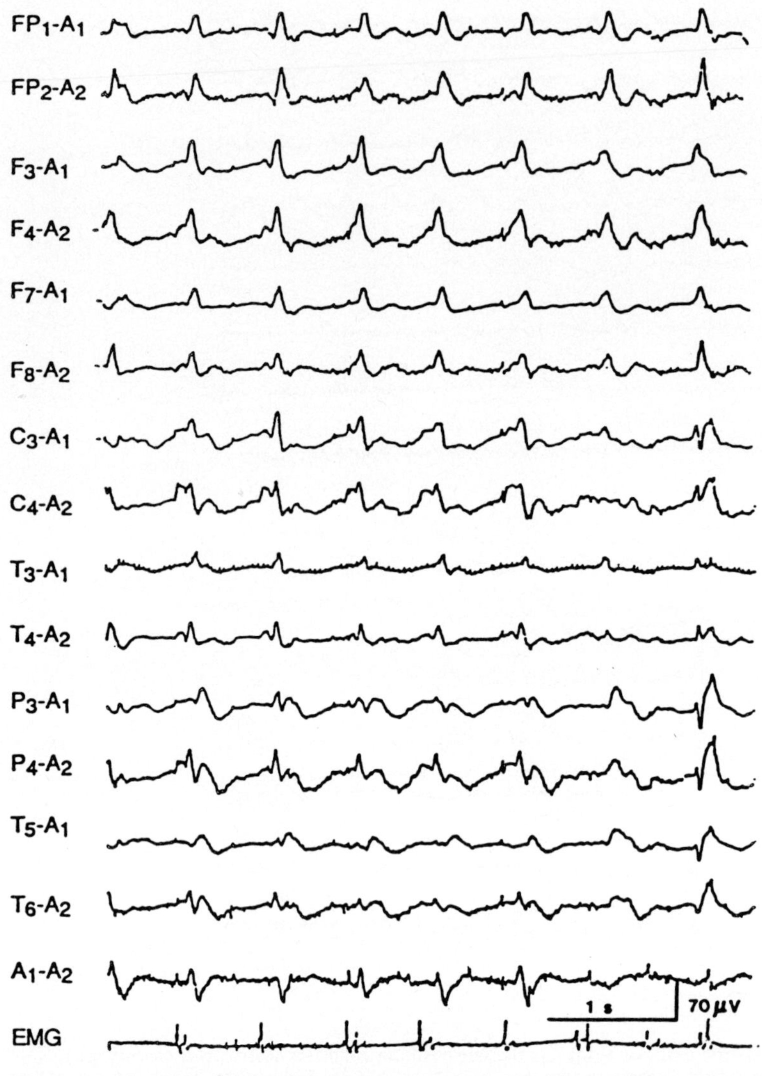

Figure 8 The EEG of the same patient as in Figure 7, obtained 5 months after the onset of Creutzfeldt-Jakob disease, shows periodic sharp waves recurring every second. The patient had rhythmic jerks of the left arm, which were monitored on the last channel. The next-to-last channel (A1-A2) records the electrocardiogram. The periodic complexes have a close temporal relationship to the myoclonic jerks but are independent of the cardiac activity. (From Ref. 3.)

flashes, particularly when the rate of photic stimulation is close to that of the periodic complexes (61,62). In the terminal stages of CJD when PSWCs are nearly absent, IPS may be able to initiate the onset of time-related triphasic slow waves coincident to each stimulus (62). Administration of 10 mg diazepam intravenously, on the other hand, may be followed by a transient disappearance of PSWCs and myoclonus, which start again after about 10 min or sooner if acoustic stimuli are delivered (62).

The periodic discharges of CJD are classically bilaterally symmetrical and generalized in distribution. However, focal or lateralized periodic sharp waves, i.e., a pattern of PLEDs, may

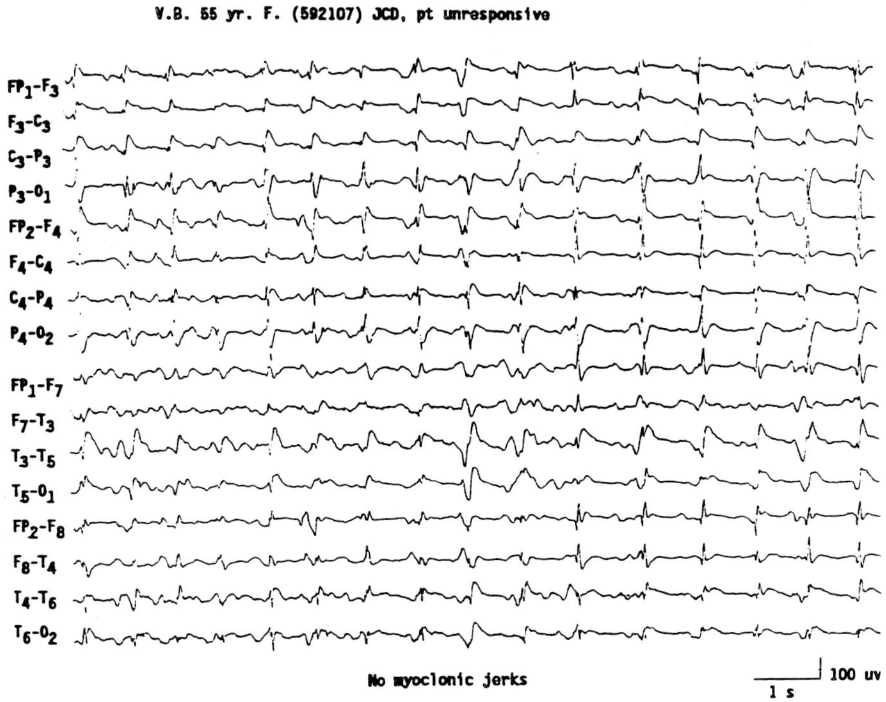

Figure 9 EEG of a 55-year-old patient with autopsy-proven familial Creutzfeldt-Jakob disease shows recurring periodic sharp waves every second. The patient did not have myoclonic jerks during this study.

occur in the early stages of the disease (70–72), as illustrated in Figure 7. With progression of the disease, the periodic events become bilaterally symmetrical.

The Heidenhain variant of CJD is characterized by predominant involvement of the occipital cortex resulting often in cortical blindness early in the disease. The EEG may show slowing of background activity and PSWCs over the posterior head region. The complexes may be focal or unilateral initially but become bilateral over the posterior region with progression of the disease (71).

The localization of the PSWCs corresponding to the site of maximum involvement (occipital cortex) in the Heidenhain variant of CJD and the absence of PSWCs in the ataxic variant of CJD with maximum cerebellar involvement suggests that cortical pathology is a necessary substrate for the production of PSWCs in CJD. The pathogenesis of PSWCs, however, remains unknown. They may derive from mechanisms intrinsic to affected neurons that become electrotonically coupled because of virus-induced membrane fusion (73).

Similar EEG patterns consisting of sharp waves occurring regularly every 1.0–1.5 s may rarely occur in other encephalopathies, e.g., cerebral anoxia (74). A few authors (75,76) have also described a similar EEG picture in rapidly progressive Alzheimer's dementia, but the resemblance was only superficial. These cases showed frequently occurring sharp waves that had random, not periodic, intervals—even when frequently repetitive. This confusion stresses the need for a more strict definition of periodicity in the EEG. Not every frequently recurring paroxysmal discharge in the EEG should be called "periodic." This category should be reserved only for those in which a modal value of intervals can be established at a minimal range of variation around that value (77).

Chronic Encephalitis of Rasmussen

This disease is characterized by the childhood onset of intractable partial and secondarily generalized seizures often with epilepsia partialis continua and recurrent status epilepticus. There is progressive neurological and cognitive deterioration over several years. The pathology is either unilateral or predominantly unilateral; some areas of the brain show an active inflammatory process, while others show scarring or evidence of a "burned-out" encephalitis (78). Although the disease has long been considered to be a chronic smoldering encephalitis, the etiological agent has not been demonstrated until recently. Several groups have now identified cytomegalovirus genome in the brains of these patients, suggesting a possible relationship to this herpesvirus infection (79,80). The EEG shows varying degrees of slow-wave abnormalities, which may be unilateral or bilateral. There are epileptiform abnormalities, which consist of unifocal, multifocal, unilateral, or bilaterally synchronous discharges (81).

ACQUIRED IMMUNODEFICIENCY SYNDROME

Infection by the human immunodeficiency virus (HIV-1) results in a spectrum of CNS complications. The best known are the opportunistic infections and neoplasia of the brain secondary to immunodeficiency. A devastating but poorly understood consequence of HIV-1 infection is a progressive encephalopathy, which results in the acquired immunodeficiency syndrome (AIDS) dementia complex, HIV-1–associated cognitive/motor complex or HIV-1 dementia. Approximately 15–20% of all patients with AIDS will develop dementia. Although some cases of dementia are probably due to subacute encephalitis caused by HIV-1, in others the pathological changes are relatively minor. It has been suggested that neurotoxic viral proteins or the biological activities of cytokines released from HIV-activated macrophages cause CNS dysfunction (82). The pathological changes and the MRI-demonstrated atrophy involve both cortex and basal ganglia; the most severe changes occur in the basal ganglia, especially the caudate nucleus (83).

The EEG is invariably abnormal in a well-established case of HIV-1 dementia. The abnormalities include a slow or absent posterior rhythm and intermittent or continuous theta-delta slowing, which is either generalized or predominantly anterior (84–87). There is a good correlation between the severity of the EEG abnormalities and the severity of HIV-1 dementia. Some patients with advanced dementia have been reported to have a low-amplitude (less than 20 μV) slow EEG (88), not unlike that reported in Huntington's disease (89). Periodic sharp or triphasic waves, 1.5–2.0 cps, over both frontocentral regions have also been described in a patient with HIV-1 dementia similar to the characteristic EEG pattern of CJD (90). The reported patient had myoclonic jerks; the periodic EEG pattern and the myoclonus both responded dramatically to zidovudine therapy.

An interesting aspect of the EEG in HIV infection has been the reports of EEG abnormalities even in asymptomatic HIV-1–infected individuals (84–86,91). It is proposed that these EEG abnormalities (usually background slowing) provide the earliest indicator of subclinical CNS dysfunction (86) and may predict subsequent development of HIV-1–related neurological disease (92). Parisi et al. (92) reported computer-analyzed EEG abnormalities in 50 of 185 (27%) asymptomatic or lymphadenopathy-only individuals infected with HIV-1. Inclusion of intravenous drug users in the HIV-seropositive group and absence of matched seronegative controls make it difficult to ascribe EEG abnormalities specifically to the HIV infection. A well-controlled study by Nuwer et al. (93) reported no significant difference in either clinical or computer-analyzed EEG between HIV-seronegative ($n = 86$) and HIV-seropositive ($n = 114$) asymptomatic men. They found that 22% of the seropositive and 26% of the seronegative men showed abnormal or borderline EEGs; rates were higher in both groups (45% in seronegative and 36% in seropositive men) when neuropsychological abnormalities coexisted. The incidence of EEG abnormalities thus failed to correlate with the serostatus but correlated with an impaired neuropsychological status in HIV-infected patients as well as controls. If risk factors such as intravenous drug abuse (which increases the incidence of EEG abnormalities) are excluded, the incidence of EEG abnormalities among the asymptomatic HIV-infected group is probably less than 7%, and a rate comparable to that of uninfected controls (94).

FOCAL INFLAMMATORY PROCESSES

Brain Abscesses

These are usually located in the cerebral hemispheres, and less frequently in the cerebellum. They result from meningitis, septicemia, septic emboli, or direct extension of infection from ears, mastoids, or paranasal sinuses.

Most hemispheric abscesses occur in the frontal or temporal lobes, and the EEGs are consistently abnormal (95–97). As with any focal destructive process, focal polymorphic or irregular delta activity appears early on; the duration of individual slow waves is exceptionally long, 500–1200 ms (Fig. 10). The EEG changes are usually more extensive and more severe than those seen with other focal cerebral lesions, such as neoplasms (95,98). At times, the polymorphic delta activity may be so extensive in the hemisphere harboring an abscess that it does not permit precise localization. Ziegler and Hoefer (98) have reported correct localization in half of 28 cases of brain abscess; in the remainder, slow activity either involved an entire hemisphere (30%) or was diffuse (20%). With large hemispheric abscesses, there may be even focal attenuation or suppression of

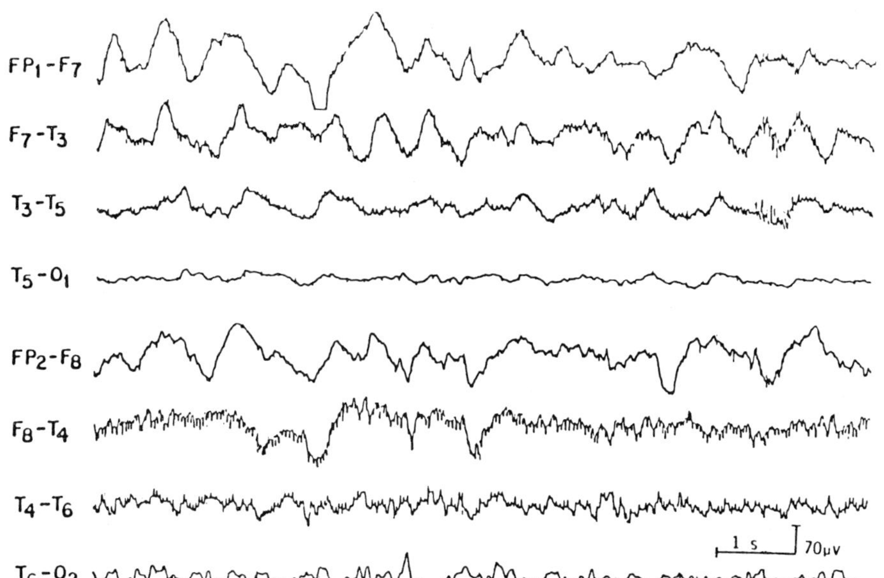

Figure 10 A 25-year-old man with congenital cyanotic heart disease had right hemiparesis and aphasia for 2 weeks. The EEG shows diffuse, high-amplitude, irregular delta activity most prominent over the left temporal region. Note absence of alpha rhythm on the left side. One day later he underwent drainage of a multilobulated abscess in the left temporo-occipital region. (From Ref. 2.)

EEG activity in the area overlying the abscess. Multiple hemispheric abscesses rarely produce multiple slow-wave foci, but instead produce widespread lateralized or diffuse delta activity.

Frontal intermittent rhythmic delta activity (FIRDA), a projected rhythm, occurs not only with infratentorial abscesses but also with hemispheric ones. In 13 patients with supratentorial abscesses reported by Michel et al. (97), five had FIRDA, three having frontal abscesses. During the acute stage, epileptiform discharges are uncommon, although PLEDs may occasionally occur (96,97,99). Infratentorial abscesses produce less severe slow-wave abnormalities. The abnormalities usually consist of FIRDA and/or generalized irregular slow-wave activities.

The stage of evolution of the abscess influences the extent of EEG abnormalities. In the early stages of an acute suppurative cerebritis, EEG changes tend to be widespread. As the abscess encapsulates, the abnormality recedes and delta activity becomes more localized. However, widespread delta activity can occur even in patients with single, well-circumscribed abscess (97). Such extensive EEG changes are usually ascribed to cerebral edema commonly associated with brain abscess, but Michel et al. (97) found no correlation between edema as seen by CT and degree of EEG abnormality.

After treatment, extensive focal EEG abnormalities rapidly disappear, although residual focal theta-delta activity can persist indefinitely. Following medical or surgical therapy, epileptiform abnormalities, which are not common in the acute stages of the abscess, emerge in the region where the abscess was previously located (Fig. 11). In 70 patients carefully followed after surgery, Legg et al. (100) found that the incidence of epilepsy was high (72%), reaching a peak 4–5 years after surgery. Epileptiform abnormalities in the EEG emerged in parallel with clinical seizure activity, but clinical seizure activity did not always correlate with the occurrence of epileptiform activity. Of the 52 patients who had adequate EEG follow-up, 43 had clinical seizures, 40 of whom had epileptiform abnormalities in the EEG. Of the nine nonepileptics, five

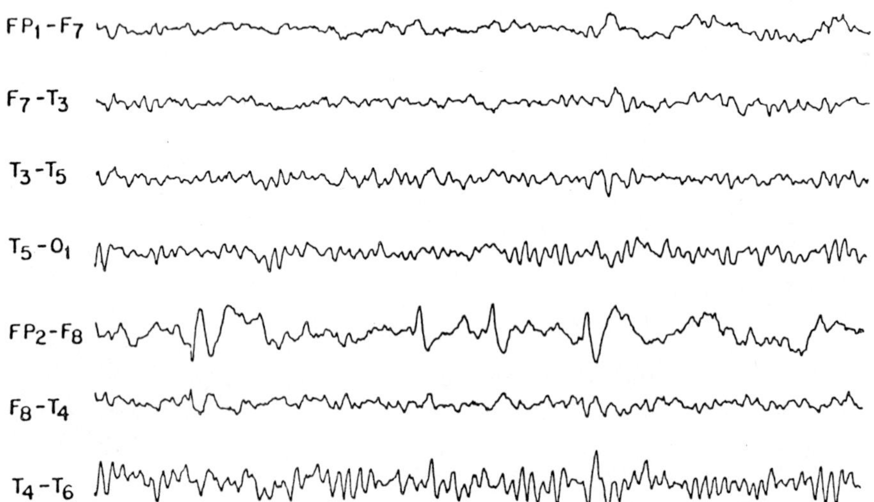

Figure 11 An 11-year-old boy with a right frontal brain abscess was treated surgically 1½ years previously. The EEG shows sharp waves and arrhythmic delta activity over the right frontal region. Patient was on antiepileptic medication but had no epileptic seizures. (From Ref. 2.)

also developed similar paroxysmal abnormalities in the EEG. Abnormalities in the EEG were, however, more severe in patients with clinical seizures.

Granulomas

Chronic inflammatory processes may give rise to granulomas that produce focal EEG abnormalities as seen with any focal cerebral lesions, e.g., brain tumor. Tuberculomas may occur in any part of the CNS, but they occur more frequently in the cerebral hemispheres. The EEG shows attenuation or slowing of normal rhythms and focal polymorphic or arrhythmic delta activity overlying the lesion. Mycotic infections, cryptococcus, aspergillosis, or mucormycosis can cause abscesses or granulomas with both diffuse and focal abnormalities in the EEG.

Cysticercosis, a common parasitic CNS infection in certain parts of the world (Mexico, South America, India, China, Eastern Europe), may cause focal cerebritis and angitis with the abrupt onset of focal neurological deficits, multiple calcifications and granulomas causing seizures, or hydrocephalus from ependymitis and basal meningitis (at times compounded by an intraventricular cyst) (101). In a series of 127 patients reported by McCormick et al. (101), 55% had seizures (in 43% as the initial symptom and in 36% as the only symptom). CT showed calcifications or cysts in 71% of the patients with seizures. EEGs done on 55 patients showed focal or multifocal delta activity in 26, focal spikes in 16, diffuse slow activity in 12, and PLEDs in one.

CONCLUSIONS

From a diagnostic standpoint, the contribution of the EEG to the differential diagnosis of meningitis, encephalitis, or other infections of the CNS is rather limited since nonspecific, generally diffuse theta-delta slowing constitutes the most common EEG abnormality. In focal infections of the brain, e.g., brain abscess and granulomas, neuroimaging (CT/MRI) is more accurate for localization than EEG. The EEG is the best diagnostic test (other than brain biopsy) for herpes simplex encephalitis, SSPE, and CJD. Because the EEG closely reflects brain function, its major contribution is in providing a measure of the severity of the encephalopathy. Hence, it is valuable in providing prognosis during the course of the disease, determining effectiveness of therapy, and demonstrating the development of possible complications or sequelae. Finally, the EEG uniquely furnishes information about the current or future potential for epileptogenesis of the CNS infectious process.

ACKNOWLEDGMENT

The author is grateful to Martha Stanley for her help in preparing the manuscript.

REFERENCES

1. Markand ON. Organic brain syndromes and dementia. In: Daly DD, Pedley TA, eds. Current Practice of Clinical Electroencephalography. 2nd ed. New York: Raven Press, 1990:401–423.
2. Daly DD, Markand ON. Focal brain lesions. In: Daly DD, Pedley TA, eds. Current Practice of Clinical Electroencephalography. 2nd ed. New York: Raven Press, 1990:335–370.
3. Markand ON. Electroencephalography in diffuse encephalopathies. J Clin Neurophysiol 1984; 1: 357–407.
4. Gibbs FA, Gibbs EL, Carpenter PR, et al. Electroencephalographic studies of patients with acute aseptic meningitis. Pediatrics 1962; 29:181–186.
5. Pedersen E. The electroencephalogram in primary aseptic meningitis. Dan Med Bull 1964; 11: 153–159.

6. Turrell RC, Shaw W, Schmidt RP, et al. Electroencephalographic studies of the encephalopathies II. Serial studies in tuberculous meningitis. Electroencephalogr Clin Neurophysiol 1953; 5:53–63.
7. Turrell RC, Roseman E. Electroencephalographic studies in the encephalopathies IV serial studies in meningococcal meningitis. Arch Neurol Psychiatry 1955; 73:141–148.
8. Kiloh LG, McComas AJ, Osselton JW. Clinical Electroencephalography. 3rd ed. London: Butterworths, 1972.
9. Kooi KA, Tucker RP, Marshall RE. Fundamentals of Electroencephalography. 2nd ed. Hagerstown, MD: Harper & Row, 1978.
10. Radermecker FJ. Systématique et électroencephalographique des encéphalites et encéphalopathies. Electroencephalogr Clin Neurophysiol 1956; (suppl) 5:213–218.
11. Gibbs FA, Gibbs EL, Spies HW, et al. Common types of childhood encephalitis—electroencephalographic and clinical relationships. Arch Neurol 1964; 10:1–11.
12. Gloor P, Kalaby O, Giard N. The electroencephalogram in diffuse encephalopathies: electroencephalographic correlates of gray and white matter lesion. Brain 1968; 91:779–802.
13. Goldenshon ES, Herman MN. Viral and presumed viral infections of the central nervous system. In: Remond A, ed. Handbook of Electroencephalography and Clinical Neurophysiology. Vol. 15. Amsterdam: Elsevier, 1977:5–20.
14. Grabow JD, Matthews CG, Chun RWM, Thompson WH. The electroencephalogram and clinical sequelae of California arbovirus encephalitis. Neurology (Minneapolis) 1969; 19:394–404.
15. Roine RO, Hillbom M, Valle M, et al. Fatal encephalitis caused by a bat-borne rabies-related virus. Brain 1988; 111:1505–1516.
16. Hantson P, Guerit JM, de Tourtchanioff M, et al. Rabies encephalitis mimicking the electrophysiological pattern of brain death. Eur Neurol 1993; 33:212–217.
17. Grossman HJ, Gibbs EL, Spios HW. Electroencephalographic studies of patients having poliomyelitis with no clinical evidence of encephalitic involvement. Pediatrics 1958; 22:1148–1152.
18. Grossman HJ, Gibbs EL, Lepper MH, et al. Electroencephalographic studies on children with measles with no clinical evidence of central nervous system involvement. Electroencephalogr Clin Neurophysiol 1955; 7:315.
19. Gibbs FA, Gibbs EL, Carpenter PR, et al. Electroencephalographic abnormalities in "uncomplicated" childhood disease. JAMA 1959; 171:1050–1055.
20. Peterslund NA, Hansen JH. Electroencephalographic changes in patients with herpes zoster. Acta Neurol Scand 1989; 79:107–111.
21. Pampiglione G. Prodromal phase of measles. Some neurophysiological studies. Br Med J 1964; 2: 1296–1300.
22. Schnell RG, Dyck PJ, Bowie EJW, et al. Infectious mononucleosis: neurologic and EEG findings. Medicine 1966; 45:51–63.
23. Greenberg DA, Weinkle DJ, Aminoff MJ. Periodic EEG complexes in infectious mononucleosis encephalitis. J Neurol Neurosurg Psychiatr 1982; 45:648–651.
24. Lehtokoski-Lehtiniemi E, Koskiniem M-L. Mycoplasma pneumoniae encephalitis: a severe entity in children. Pediatr Infect Dis J 1989; 8:651–653.
25. Hulihan JF, Bebin EM, Westmoreland BF. Bilateral periodic lateralized epileptiform discharges in Mycoplasma encephalitis. Pediatr Neurol 1992; 8:292–294.
26. Paz D, Brenner RD. Bilateral independent periodic lateralized epileptiform discharges, clinical significance. Arch Neurol 1981; 38:713–175.
27. Suga S, Yoshikawa T, Asano Y, et al. Clinical and virological analyses of 21 infants with exanthem subitum (roseola infantum) and central nervous complications. Ann Neurol 1993; 33:597–603.
28. Gibbs RA, Rosenthal IM. Electroencephalography in natural and attenuated measles. Am J Dis Child 1962; 103:395–400.
29. Pampiglione G, Ramsay AM, Young SEJ. Some clinical and EEG observations during rubella epidemic. Electroencephalogr Clin Neurophysiol 1963; 15:913–914.
30. Pampiglione G, Griffith AH, Bramwell EC. Transient cerebral changes after vaccination against measles. Lancet 1971; 2:5–8.

31. Upton A, Gumpert J. Electroencephalography in diagnosis of herpes simplex encephalitis. Lancet 1970; 1:650–652.
32. Rawls WE, Dyck PJ, Klass DW, Greer HD, Herrmann EC Jr. Encephalitis associated with herpes simplex virus. Ann Intern Med 1966; 64:104–115.
33. Illis LS, Taylor RM. The electroencephalogram in herpes simplex encephalitis. Lancet 1972; 1: 718–721.
34. Gupta PC, Seth P. Periodic complex in herpes simplex encephalitis. A clinical and experimental study. Electroencephalogr Clin Neurophysiol 1973; 35:67–74.
35. Chien LT, Boehm RM, Robinson H, et al. Characteristic early electroencephalographic changes in herpes simplex encephalitis. Clinical and virologic studies. Arch Neurol 1977; 34:361–364.
36. Elian M. Herpes simplex virus encephalitis and the EEG. J Electrophysiol Technol 1975; 1:161–170.
37. Smith JB, Westmoreland BF, Reagan TJ, et al. A distinctive clinical EEG profile in herpes simplex encephalitis. Mayo Clin Proc 1975; 50:469–474.
38. Brodtkorb E, Lindquist M, Jonsson M, et al. Diagnosis of herpes simplex encephalitis. A comparison between electroencephalography and computed tomography findings. Acta Neurol Scand 1982; 66:462–471.
39. Dutt MK, Johnston ID. Computed tomography and EEG in herpes simplex encephalitis. Their value in diagnosis and prognosis. Arch Neurol 1982; 39:99–102.
40. Schauseil-Zipf U, Harden A, Hoare RD, et al. Early diagnosis of herpes simplex encephalitis in childhood. Clinical neurophysiological and neuroradiological studies. Eur J Pediatr 1982; 138: 154–161.
41. Pettay O, Leinikki P, Donner M, et al. Herpes simplex virus infection in the newborn. Arch Dis Child 1972; 47:97–103.
42. Mizrahi EM, Tharp BR. A characteristic EEG pattern in neonatal herpes simplex encephalitis. Neurology (NY) 1982; 32:1215–1220.
43. Sainio K, Granstrom ML, Pettay O, et al. EEG in neonatal herpes simplex encephalitis. Electroencephalogr Clin Neurophysiol 1983; 56:556–561.
44. Markand ON, Daly DD. Pseudoperiodic lateralized paroxysmal discharges in electroencephalogram. Neurology (NY) 1971; 21:975–981.
45. Whitley RJ, Soong S, Dolin R, et al. Adenine arabinoside therapy of biopsy-proven herpes simplex encephalitis. N Engl J Med 1977; 297:289–294.
46. Schroth G, Gawehn J, Thron A, et al. Early diagnosis of herpes simplex encephalitis by MRI. Neurology 1987; 37:179–183.
47. Radermecker FJ. Aspects electroenéphalographiques dans trois cases d'encéphalite subaiquë. Acta Neurol Psychiatr (Belg) 1949; 49:222–232.
48. Cobb W, Hill D. Electroencephalogram in subacute progressive encephalitis. Brain 1950; 73:392–404.
49. Radermecker FJ, Poser CM. The significance of repetitive paroxysmal electroencephalographic patterns. World Neurol 1960; 1:422–431.
50. Cobb W. The periodic events of subacute sclerosing leukoencephalitis. Electroencephalogr Clin Neurophysiol 1966; 21:278–294.
51. Markand ON, Panszi JG. The electroencephalogram in subacute sclerosing panencephalitis. Arch Neurol 1975; 32:719–726.
52. Reiher J, Lapointe LR, Lessard L. Prolonged and variable intervals between EEG complexes in subacute inclusion body encephalitis. Can Med Assoc J 1973; 108:729–732.
53. Westmoreland BF, Gomez MR, Blume WT. Activation of periodic complexes of subacute sclerosing panencephalitis by sleep. Ann Neurol 1977; 1:185–187.
54. Westmoreland BF, Sharbrough FW, Donat JR. Stimulus-induced EEG complexes and motor spasms in subacute sclerosing panencephalitis. Neurology (Minneapolis) 1979; 29:1154–1157.
55. Wulf CH. Subacute sclerosing panencephalitis, serial electroencephalographic studies. J Neurol Neurosurg Psychiatr 1982; 45:418–421.
56. Wolinsky JS, Berg BO, Maitland CJ. Progressive rubella panencephalitis. Arch Neurol 1976; 33: 722–723.

57. Masters CL, Harris JO, Gajdusek DC, et al. Creutzfeldt-Jakob disease: patterns of worldwide occurrence and the significance of familial and sporadic clustering. Ann Neurol 1979; 5:177–188.
58. Brown P, Cathala F, Raubertas RF, et al. The epidemiology of Creutzfeldt-Jakob disease: conclusion of a 15 year investigation in France and review of the world literature. Neurology 1987; 37:895–904.
59. Burger LJ, Rown J, Goldenshon E. Creutzfeldt-Jakob disease. Arch Neurol 1972; 26:428–433.
60. Abbott J. The EEG in Jakob-Creutzfeldt's disease. Electroencephalogr Clin Neurophysiol 1959; 11:184.
61. Aguglia U, Franarier G, Tinuper P, Rey M, Gomez M, Quattrone A. Subacute spongiform encephalopathy with periodic paroxysmal activities: clinical evolution and serial EEG findings in 20 cases. Clin Electroencephalogr 1987; 18:147–158.
62. Bortone E, Bettoni L, Giorgi C, et al. Reliability of EEG in the diagnosis of Creutzfeldt-Jakob disease. Electroencephalogr Clin Neurophysiol 1994; 90:323–330.
63. Chiofalo N, Fuentes A, Galvez S. Serial EEG findings in 27 cases of Creutzfeldt-Jakob disease. Arch Neurol 1980; 37:143–145.
64. Levy SR, Chiappa KH, Burke CJ, Young RR. Early evolution and incidence of electroencephalographic abnormalities in Creutzfeldt-Jakob disease. J Clin Neurophysiol 1986; 3:1–21.
65. Brechet R, Sicard C, Moret-Chalmin C, et al. Etude électroencéphalographique de vingt-cinq cases de maladie de Creutzfeldt-Jakob. Rev. EEG Neurophysiol 1980; 10:55–63.
66. Brown P, Cathala F, Castaigne P, et al. Creutzfeldt-Jakob disease: clinical analysis of a consecutive series of 230 neuropathologically verified cases. Ann Neurol 1986; 20:597–602.
67. Zochodne DW, Young GB, McLachlan RS, et al. Creutzfeldt-Jakob disease without periodic sharp wave complexes: a clinical, electroencephalographic and pathologic study. Neurology 1988; 38:1056–1060.
68. Tietjen GE, Drury I. Familial Creutzfeldt-Jakob disease without periodic EEG activity. Ann Neurol 1990; 28:585–588.
69. Jonkman EJ, Ponsen L. A review of Creutzfeldt-Jakob disease. J Electrophysiol Technol 1981; 7: 68–79.
70. Au WJ, Gabor AJ, Viyan N, Markand ON. Periodic lateralized epileptiform complexes (PLEDs) in Creutzfeldt-Jakob disease. Neurology (NY) 1980; 30:611–617.
71. Furlan A, Henry CE, Sweeny PJ, et al. Focal EEG abnormalities in Heidenhain's variant of Jakob-Creutzfeldt disease. Arch Neurol 1981; 38:312–314.
72. Eggerston DE, Pillay N. Creutzfeldt-Jakob disease: correlation of focal electroencephalographic abnormalities and clinical signs. Can J Neurol Sci 1986; 13:120–124.
73. Traub RD, Pedley TA. Virus induced electronic coupling hypothesis of the mechanism of periodic EEG discharges in Creutzfeldt-Jakob disease. Ann Neurol 1981; 10:405–410.
74. Nilsson BY, Olsson Y, Sourander P. Electroencephalographic and histopathological changes resembling Jakob-Creutzfeldt disease after transient cerebral ischemia due to cardiac arrest. Acta Neurol Scand 1972; 48:416–426.
75. Ehle AL, Johnson PC. Rapid evolving EEG changes in a case of Alzheimer's disease. Ann Neurol 1977; 1:593–595.
76. Watson CP. Clinical similarity of Alzheimer and Creutzfeldt-Jakob disease. Ann Neurol 1979; 6: 368–369.
77. Gloor P. EEG characteristics in Creutzfeldt-Jakob disease. Ann Neurol 1980; 8:341.
78. Rasmussen T, McCann W. Clinical studies of patients with focal epilepsy due to "chronic encephalitis." Trans Am Neurol Assoc 1968; 93:89–94.
79. Power C, Poland SD, Blume WT, et al. Cytomegalovirus and Rasmussen's encephalitis. Lancet 1990; 336:1282–1284.
80. McLachlan RS, Girvin JP, Blume WT, et al. Rasmussen's chronic encephalitis in adults. Arch Neurol 1993; 50:269–271.
81. Andermann F. Chronic Encephalitis and Epilepsy. Rasmussen's Syndrome. Toronto: Butterworth-Heinemann, 1991.
82. Petito CK. What causes brain atrophy in human immunodeficiency virus infection? Ann Neurol 1993; 34:128–129.

83. Dal Pan GJ, Arthur JH, Aylward E, et al. Pattern of cerebral atrophy in HIV-1-infected individuals: results of a quantitative MRI analysis. Neurology 1992; 42:2125–2130.
84. Gabuzda DH, Levy SR, Chaippa KH. Electroencephalography in AIDS and AIDS-related complex. Clin Electroencephalogr 1988; 19:1– 6.
85. Parisi A, Strosselli M, Di Perri G, et al. Electroencephalography in the early diagnosis of HIV-related subacute encephalitis: analysis of 185 patients. Clin Electroencephalogr 1989; 20:1–5.
86. Koralnik IJ, Beaumanoir A, Hausler R, et al. A controlled study of early neurologic abnormalities in men with asymptomatic human immunodeficiency virus infection. N Engl J Med 1990; 323:864–870.
87. Tinuper P, DeCarolis P, Galeotti M, et al. Electroencephalogram and HIV infection: a prospective study in 100 patients. Clin Electroencephalogr 1990; 21:145–150.
88. Harden CL, Daras M, Tuchman AJ, et al. Low amplitude EEGs in demented AIDS patients. Electroencephalogr Clin Neurophysiol 1993; 87:54–56.
89. Scott DF, Heathfield KWG, Toone B, et al. The EEG in Huntington's chorea: a clinical and neuropathological study. J Neurol Neurosurg Psychiatr 1972; 35:97–102.
90. Thomas P, Borg M. Reversible myoclonic encephalopathy revealing the AIDS-dementia complex. Electroencephalogr Clin Neurophysiol 1994; 90:166–169.
91. Elovaara I, Saar P, Valle SL, et al. EEG in the early HIV-1 infection is characterized by anterior dysrhythmicity of low maximal amplitude. Clin Electroencephalogr 1991; 22:131–140.
92. Parisi A, Di Perri G, Strosselli M, et al. Usefulness of computerized electroencephalography in diagnosing, staging and monitoring AIDS-dementia complex. AIDS 1989; 3:209–213.
93. Nuwer MR, Miller EN, Visscher BR, et al. Asymptomatic HIV infection does not cause EEG abnormalities: results from the Multicenter AIDS Cohort Study (MACS). Neurology 1992; 42:1214–1219.
94. Newton TF, Leuchter AF, Miller EN, et al. Quantitative EEG in patients with AIDS and asymptomatic HIV infection. Clin Electroencephalogr 1994; 25:18–25.
95. Pine J, Atoynatan TH, Margolis G. The EEG findings in eighteen patients with brain abscess: case reports and a review of the literature. Electroencephalogr Clin Neurophysiol 1952; 4:165–179.
96. Vignaendra V, Ghee LT, Chawla J. EEG in brain abscess: Its value in localization compared to other diagnostic tests. Electroencephalogr Clin Neurophysiol 1975; 38:611–622.
97. Michel B, Gastaut JL, Bianchi L. Electroencephalographic cranial computerized tomographic correlations in brain abscess. Electroencephalogr Clin Neurophysiol 1979; 46:256–273.
98. Ziegler DK, Hoefer PFA. Electroencephalographic and clinical findings in twenty-eight verified cases of brain abscess. Electroencephalogr Clin Neurophysiol 1952; 4:41–44.
99. Le Beau J, Dondey M. Importance diagnostique de certaines activites electroencephalographiques lateralisees, periodiques ou a tendance periodique au cours des abces du cerveau. Electroencephalogr Clin Neurophysiol 1959; 11:43–58.
100. Legg NJ, Gupta PC, Scott DF. Epilepsy following cerebral abscess: a clinical and EEG study of 70 patients. Brain 1973; 96:259–268.
101. McCormick GF, Chi-Shing Z, Heiden J. Cysticercosis cerebri: review of 127 cases. Arch Neurol 1982, 39:534–539.

31

The Acute Management of Neurological Complications Associated with CNS Infections

Cherylee W. J. Chang and Thomas P. Bleck
University of Virginia School of Medicine, Charlottesville, Virginia

Since the advent of antimicrobial agents, central nervous system (CNS) infections such as bacterial meningitis and brain abscesses have a much lower mortality. For example, pneumococcal meningitis previously had a mortality rate of 95–100% (1), compared to approximately 33% in 1993 (2). The overall mortality of meningitis is approximately 18.6% (2). Despite this, secondary neurological complications often contribute to morbidity and mortality during the course of CNS infection (Table 1). In a prospective study of bacterial meningitis in adults, 35 of 86 patients with meningitis had CNS complications (2). The blood-brain barrier (BBB) is not fully developed in infants and children, and neurological complications associated with CNS infection are frequent in infants and children. Often, the outcome of a CNS infection is influenced by the development of secondary complications. The most common complications include (1) a vasculopathy that results in focal cerebral infarction and venous sinus thrombosis, (2) hydrocephalus, and (3) seizures (including status epilepticus). Each of these conditions is responsible for neurological morbidity by itself; however, each may also contribute to cerebral edema, resulting in increased intracranial pressure and subsequent cerebral herniation. The goal of this chapter is to discuss the pathophysiology and acute management of the neurological complications associated with CNS infections.

VASCULOPATHY: CEREBRAL INFARCTION AND VENOUS THROMBOSIS

Cerebral infarction complicates about 5–15% of adult cases of meningitis (2–4) and may complicate as many as 27% of pediatric meningitis cases (5). These numbers are likely an underestimate since not all patients undergo angiography or computed tomography (CT) or magnetic resonance (MR) scanning to determine vascular involvement. On cerebral angiography, vessel wall irregularities, focal dilation, occlusion of the distal branches of the middle cerebral

Table 1 Frequency of Neurological Complications in One Prospective and Two Retrospective Studies of Bacterial Meningitis

	Pfister, 1993 (*n* = 86)	Durand, 1993 (*n* = 493 episodes)	Dodge, 1965 (*n* = 156)[a]
Cerebrovascular involvement (%)	15[b]	5[c]	20[a]
Cerebral edema (%)	14[d]	4[c]	3[e]
Cerebral herniation (autopsy confirmed) (%)	8	3	6
Seizures (%)	24	23	31
Hydrocephalus (%)	12[d]	11[c]	ND
Mortality (%)	19	25	20

[a]Diagnosis made by focal neurological deficits on physical examination.
[b]Angiographic documentation.
[c]Diagnosis made by CT scan performed in 87 of 122 adults treated for community-acquired meningitis.
[d]Diagnosis made by CT scan.
[e]CT scans not available; diagnosis made only in patients who died with autopsy confirmation.
ND: Not documented.
Source: Refs. 2–4.

artery (MCA), and narrowing of the supraclinoid portion of the internal carotid artery have been reported. On neuropathological examination, infiltration of the vessel wall by inflammatory cells is confined to the vessel wall in the subarachnoid space in the early stage of infection. However, within days, there is extensive granulocytic infiltration along cortical vessels in the Virchow-Robin space.

It is not entirely clear how the infection produces the inflammatory vasculopathy, but several mechanisms are likely. Leukocyte-endothelial cell adhesion may cause local endothelial damage by activating leukotrienes, complement, and platelet-activating factor. Activation of cytokines results in the production of reactive oxygen species, including free radicals, and proteolytic enzymes, all of which may cause endothelial damage (6,7). This ultimately results in vascular narrowing (ischemia) and vessel leakage (vasogenic edema).

Pathological examination of small- and medium-sized subarachnoid arteries shows that endothelial cells swell, multiply, and can narrow the vessel lumen. The adventitial connective tissue sheath becomes infiltrated by neutrophils, which then migrate to the subintimal region, thus leading to further reduction of vessel diameter (8,9). In veins, similar changes in endothelial cells are seen, but the entire thickness of the vessel wall may be diffusely infiltrated with leukocytes. Focal necrosis of the wall and mural thrombi can form. Resultant thrombophlebitis and venous thrombosis can occur, typically near the end of the second week of infection.

Unfortunately, therapeutic modalities to prevent the inflammatory vasculopathy are only in the early investigational stages. Treatment with antimicrobial agents does not prevent, and may in fact, worsen the inflammatory response that occurs with bacterial lysis. Treatment with an anti-inflammatory agent, such as dexamethasone, has received a great deal of interest. The use of dexamethasone, 0.6 mg/kg/day in four divided doses, in children with *Hemophilus influenzae* meningitis has been shown to improve neurological outcome and decrease the incidence and severity of sensorineural hearing loss (10). The use of dexamethasone in pneumococcal meningitis was associated with a decrease in mortality in a study in Egypt (11). However, there is no firm consensus at the present time regarding the use of dexamethasone as adjunctive therapy in pneumococcal or meningococcal meningitis. With the emergence of resistant organisms (e.g., pencillin- and cephalosporin-resistant strains of *Streptococcus pneumoniae*), the increased permeability of the BBB produced by inflammation may be necessary to obtain higher bactericidal concentrations of antimicrobial agents, and the use of steroids could be detrimental in the therapy of meningitis due to these organisms.

Other adjunctive anti-inflammatory agents, such as the nonsteroidal cyclooxygenase inhibitor oxindanac and the antileukocyte adhesion molecule antibody IB_4, show promise for prevention of vasculopathy. In animal studies, oxindanac (with an antibiotic) resulted in significantly decreased mortality compared with animals treated with antibiotic alone (12). The use of an antibody to block leukocyte adhesion is based on the principle stated above that leukocyte-endothelial binding precipitates a cascade of events resulting in endothelial damage (6).

Until prophylactic therapies are effective, our ability to prevent cerebral infarction due to vasculopathy is limited, and unfortunately, the clinician's only recourse is to treat the cerebral edema resulting from infarction.

The large vessel thromboses that occur with meningitis do not develop with abscesses, although by causing a local inflammatory reaction, brain abscesses can also cause septic thrombosis. Resultant necrotic debris further facilitate bacterial proliferation. In the early stages, an abscess is poorly circumscribed and is typically described as cerebritis. With time, the center of the abscess, full of necrotic debris and leukocytes, is surrounded by neutrophils, macrophages, fibroblasts, and granulation tissue. This eventually forms a dense collagenous capsule. The outer layers are edematous, with thromboses of small vessels and areas of necrosis. Impingement of this mass on adjacent vessels causes further vascular ischemia and can result in an extension of the abscess. Abscesses produce complications primarily in the form of edema, mass effect, and increased ICP, as discussed later in this chapter.

Cerebral Arterial Infarction

Patients with cerebral infarction associated with infection may present with a myriad of stroke syndromes, including a decrease in the level of consciousness. Diagnostic studies to differentiate stroke from cerebral abscess should include contrasted and noncontrasted scans. [Alternatively, magnetic resonance imaging (MRI) may be used.] The only limitations of MRI are its lower sensitivity in detecting acute hemorrhages and the current difficulty of scanning while administering drugs delivered by infusion pumps.

Once the diagnosis is made (as with most types of cerebral infarction), most postinfarct therapy is empirical rather than based on controlled clinical trials. Empirical anticoagulation has not had proven efficacy, and although it is used by some investigators, we do not recommend it.

In animals with pneumococcal meningitis, cerebral blood flow (CBF) initially increases, and then decreases (13). Patients with meningitis initially exhibit a hyperemic phase of CBF. This increase is maximal 3–5 days into the illness. Later in the course of the infection, CBF decreases. Rhesus monkeys with *H. influenzae* meningitis have a diminution in CBF in the postcentral, temporal, and occipital regions (14). In one study, up to 28% of children had CBF diminished to 26 ± 10 ml/min/100 g, from a normal of 62 ± 20 ml/min/100 g (15). It is unclear what mediates these changes; however, diminished CBF may compromise cerebral oxygenation and increase cerebral lactate and acidosis, which may contribute to neuronal dysfunction.

Cerebral autoregulation is impaired in both animals (16) and humans with acute pneumococcal meningitis (17). Typically, the cerebral vasculature is capable of maintaining a constant cerebral blood flow within a wide range of mean arterial pressure (MAP) (typically 50–150 mmHg in the healthy adult), and for a range of partial pressure of arterial oxygen (PaO_2) and of arterial carbon dioxide ($PaCO_2$) (see Fig. 1). Studies have shown that there is little impairment of the vascular response to $PaCO_2$ and PaO_2; however, autoregulation to MAP is often affected. Thus, mild hypertension may increase CBF, which may be desired if CBF is diminished. However, in the

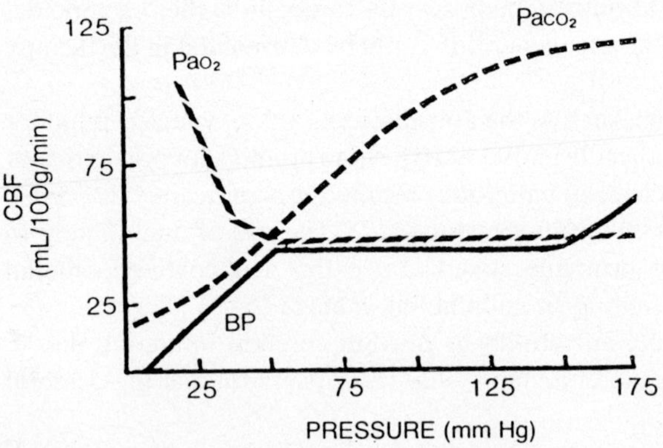

Figure 1 Autoregulation of CBF: CBF changes caused by alteration of blood pressure, PaO_2, and $PaCO_2$. (From Ref. 51.)

patient whose CBF is normal or increased in the hyperemic phase, hypertension may result in cerebral edema and increased intracranial pressure (ICP). Conversely, hypotension will diminish CBF and worsen ischemia. Tureen et al. demonstrated that poorly hydrated rabbits with experimental pneumococcal meningitis have a significant decrease in MAP and CBF compared with rabbits given high levels of hydration (18). CSF lactate was significantly elevated in the rabbits with poor hydration. This suggests that adequate intravascular volume is necessary to maintain good CBF in meningitis and may decrease the risk of cerebral ischemia. Thus, the goal of therapy in these patients is to keep them well-hydrated, but to maintain a normal, not elevated, blood pressure.

Finally, since autoregulation in response to $PaCO_2$ is not affected, a high partial pressure of CO_2 can result in vasodilation, which subsequently increases cerebral blood flow and elevates ICP. Yet a low $PaCO_2$ may contribute to vasoconstriction and further infarction. For this reason, extremes in $PaCO_2$ should be avoided. Patients who are obtunded and unable to ventilate well should be promptly intubated, but not aggressively hyperventilated. These recommendations are summarized in Table 2.

Venous Sinus Thrombosis

Thrombophlebitis of the large dural sinuses can result from the extension of infection from the middle ear and mastoid cells, the paranasal sinuses, or facial cellulitis. This type of thrombo-

Table 2 Management of Cerebral Infarction

1. Maintain euvolemic fluid status.
2. Keep blood pressure within patient's usual range, avoiding extremes. Use labetolol or hydralazine. Attempt to avoid potential cerebral dilators such as nitroprusside or nitroglycerine. If hypotensive, ensure adequate fluid status, then use dopamine to maintain adequate blood pressure.
3. If the patient is unable to protect the airway or ventilate effectively, intubate without delay. Maintain $PaCO_2$ within 30–40 mmHg. If hyperventilating for increased ICP, avoid $PaCO_2 < 25$ mmHg to avoid worsening.

phlebitis is often associated with bacterial meningitis, subdural empyema, or brain abscess. The pathophysiology of venous sinus thrombosis (VST) due to meningitis, typically occurring 1–2 weeks into the course of the illness, is not entirely understood. As discussed above, it is likely a consequence of inflammatory changes resulting in focal necrosis, and mural thrombos. The incidence of thrombophlebitis associated with meningitis was reported to be 4.7% in one study (2). Patients often present with focal neurological findings, such as hemiplegia, and signs of increased intracranial pressure, including headache, vomiting, papilledema, and bilateral sixth nerve palsies. Seizures occur in approximately 30% of patients (19,20).

The diagnosis of VST may be made with a CT scan, but MRI is more sensitive and demonstrates the lack of a flow void in the venous sinuses. MR angiography (MRA) can also be used for diagnosis, although plain film angiography and digital subtraction angiography remain the gold standard.

VST results in impaired venous outflow, which predisposes to intracerebral, subdural, and subarachnoid hemorrhage. More commonly seen are venous infarcts; increased ICP, due to decreased venous outflow; impairment of CSF resorption, leading to hydrocephalus; and cerebral edema, due to venous infarction.

Despite the pathological findings of hemorrhagic infarction with VST, the primary treatment is anticoagulation with heparin with the goal of increasing partial thromboplastin time at least 1.5–2 times control. Although no controlled studies have been performed and this topic remains one of controversy, in one retrospective study of 38 patients, the incidence of death and complications were no higher in the 23 patients treated with heparin than in the 13 who did not receive anticoagulation (20). In 3 of 13 nonanticoagulated patients who were steadily deteriorating despite other treatments, dramatic improvement was seen the day after initiation of heparin therapy. Duration of therapy typically lasts 3 months, with approximately 3–4 weeks of heparin alone before initiating warfarin therapy. Heparin is discontinued once an INR of 2.5–3 is reached with warfarin (Table 3).

Thrombolysis remains a controversial therapy. The literature is replete with case reports of successful recannulation or hemorrhage with extremely poor outcome (21). Our experience is limited to a single patient with sagittal sinus thrombosis, who underwent systemic thrombolysis with streptokinase for massive pulmonary embolism, and whose neurological function improved following this therapy. Clearly, further clinical trials are necessary to clarify this issue. Surgical thrombectomy, although performed in the past, is overwhelmingly felt to be harmful in the swollen and sometimes hemorrhagic brain (22,23).

As the venous system recannulates, the increased ICP will resolve. However, if ICP becomes problematic, agents decreasing cerebrospinal fluid (CSF) production, e.g., acetazolamide, and repeated lumbar punctures have been used successfully (20). Steroids also have been used, but no randomized studies have proven their efficacy. Case reports on the use of mannitol, barbiturate-induced coma, and ventricular shunting can be found.

As mentioned above, seizures occur in approximately 30% of patients with VST. Typically, the use of anticonvulsants is restricted to those patients with clinical seizure activity. Every comatose patient should have an electroencephalogram (EEG) to evaluate the possibility of

Table 3 Management of Venous Sinus Thrombosis

1. Heparin anticoagulation with maintenance of PTT 1.5–2 times control.
2. Start warfarin approximately 3–4 weeks after therapy initiation and when patient is stable, overlapping with heparinization until the INR is 2.5–3.0.

nonconvulsive, electrographic seizure activity. (This will be discussed further in the section on seizures.) The optimal duration of anticonvulsant therapy remains unknown. It would be reasonable to reevaluate the patient with a head CT and an EEG after 8 or 12 months. If these studies are normal, anticonvulsant therapy might be progressively discontinued at that time.

The number of patients with VST as a result of bacterial meningitis is too small to be certain about the prognosis of this condition. If patients with direct invasion of bacteria into the sinuses are included (septic thrombophlebitis), then historically, mortality rates are between 50 and 78% (19,22). Recently, however, the overall mortality from VST has been reported to be between 10 and 30% irrespective of etiology (20). Indicators of poor prognosis typically depend on the rate of evolution of thrombosis; the age of the patient, with a bimodal peak at the extremes of age; and the presence of focal symptoms or coma upon presentation. Also, thrombosis of deep cerebral vein carries a much higher risk than cortical vein thrombosis. If a patient survives the episode of VST, then the prognosis for recovery of function is better than with arterial thrombosis. In several series, the incidence of sequelae among survivors with all causes of VST was 2–17% (19). The most common sequelae included blindness due to optic atrophy and focal motor deficits.

SEIZURES

Seizures complicate up to 24% of cases of bacterial meningitis (2,3). Seizures occur more frequently in infants and children (51%) (5,24), especially in premature and newborn babies and in adults over 60 years of age. In one group of 445 adults with bacterial meningitis, seizure activity occurred in 23% of cases; 57% of the seizures were generalized, 30% were focal, and 13% were not characterized (3). Two thirds of the seizures occurred within 24 h of admission, and *Streptococcus pneumoniae* was the causal agent in 58% of patients with seizures; however, one third of patients with early-onset seizures had a history of alcohol abuse, which is likely to be a confounding variable. About 95% of seizures occur within the first week of illness, and seizures are the presenting feature in up to 12% of patients with meningitis (24). The frequency of seizures according to the meningeal pathogen is quite variable; several studies, including the one cited above, suggest that pneumococcal meningitis has the highest incidence of seizure activity followed by *H. influenzae* meningitis, and seizures are least likely to complicate meningococcal meningitis (25–29).

Seizures in adults are typically generalized at the onset, as noted above. In Pfister's study of 86 adult patients with bacterial meningitis, 24% had seizures, and 81% of these had seizures with a generalized onset (2). Conversely, in children, seizures complicating bacterial meningitis typically have a focal onset (67–70%) (30).

The significance of seizures in long-term prognosis is debated. In Durand's series, seizure activity during the first 24 h after admission predicted mortality (72% vs. 18% among those without early-onset seizures), while other studies show no association of seizure activity and mortality. In adults, the presence of seizures during the acute period does not necessarily predispose to the development of long-term seizure disorder, unless the etiology of the seizure activity is cerebral ischemia and infarction.

The pathogenesis of seizures during bacterial meningitis is not fully understood. Systemic factors such as fever and electrolyte imbalance from vomiting, diarrhea, or dehydration may play a role in lowering the seizure threshold. Cerebral edema, cerebritis ischemia or infarction, or hypoxia may lead to seizure activity. Prolonged or recurrent seizures require further work-up and are more likely to indicate a complication of meningitis, e.g., cerebral infarction or subdural empyema. Brain abscess rarely complicates meningitis in adults. Neonates with gram-negative meningitis, especially meningitis due to *Citrobacter diversus* (31), may develop a brain abscess or multiple brain abscesses.

Seizures may be the presenting manifestation in 35% (32,33) of patients with brain abscesses. Twenty-five to 45% of patients with brain abscess have seizures during the course of illness. Seizures arising from a focal lesion should have a focal onset, but surprisingly, in one study of 39 adults with brain abscesses, 11 patients presented with generalized seizures and 3 patients presented with partial seizures (33). Late seizures complicate 25–40% of patients with subdural empyema.

Herpes encephalitis preferentially involves the temporal lobes, insular and cingulate gyri, and frontobasal region. Seizures occur in 38% (34) to 62% (35) of patients with biopsy-proven herpes simplex encephalitis. Seizure activity is also an initial symptom in other viral encephalitides (36).

Most seizures that develop during acute CNS infections are temporally related to the illness. Any seizure activity, even an isolated event, a single seizure, is treated with anticonvulsant medication, such as phenytoin, for at least the first few weeks of meningitis. For seizures that develop due to intracranial mass lesions, such as an abscess or subdural empyema, a treatment duration of 6–12 months is recommended. Once the patient recovers and demonstrates no focal neurological deficits, an EEG and head CT should be performed. If these are normal, the medication can be progressively withdrawn. If, however, any abnormalities are seen, antiepileptic medication should be continued for at least 6–12 months or longer before being reevaluated. If the patient has phenytoin hypersensitivity, the next anticonvulsants of choice (chosen for lack of side effects, efficacy, and ease of administration) include carbamazepine, phenobarbital, and valproate, in that order.

Status epilepticus (SE) is defined as a "condition characterized by an epileptic seizure that is sufficiently prolonged or repeated so as to produce a fixed and lasting epileptic condition" (37). Although this definition is somewhat vague, it describes repetitive seizures or a prolonged seizure from which a patient does not regain full consciousness. The duration of seizure activity usually required to diagnose SE ranges from 20 to 30 min, since in animal studies significant neuronal damage occurs after this period. A condition known as nonconvulsive SE (NCSE) can also occur in which electromechanical dissociation occurs between the brain and the peripheral nervous system. In such cases, clinical physical manifestations (except for obtundation) are absent; however, neuronal damage will develop. The diagnosis of NCSE can only be made by EEG monitoring. Therefore, in patients with unexplained coma, an EEG must be performed. In large series of SE, CNS infection is responsible for 1–7% of cases (38,39).

In cases of status epilepticus, treatment must be performed quickly to stop the seizures within 20 min of onset. Table 4 demonstrates a suggested therapeutic sequence for prolonged seizures. A diagnostic sequence in addition to a medical history, including previous seizures, current medications, and history of substance abuse, and a physical and neurological examination, should also include an arterial blood gas, complete blood count, blood chemistries (in particular, sodium, potassium, glucose, blood urea nitrogen, creatinine, calcium, phosphorus, magnesium), and a toxicology screen of both blood and urine. A repeat head CT scan with and without intravenous contrast should be obtained to look for a focal mass lesion, infarction, or edema. As previously stated, an EEG should also be obtained if the patient's mental status does not begin to improve in 15 min following the cessation of clinical seizure activity. The postictal confusional state can last for hours, but the patient is typically awake, although confused. Obtundation may be due to nonconvulsive status epilepticus.

Of note, lorazepam has replaced diazepam as the benzodiazepine of choice for seizure cessation. Lorazepam is less lipophilic, and therefore has a smaller volume of distribution than diazepam. For this reason, its onset of action may be within 4–5 min of administration, as compared with 2–3 min with diazepam, since lorazepam does not cross the BBB as quickly; however, lorazepam dissipates more slowly than does diazepam and maintains a higher effective brain concentration longer (4–14 h, compared with 20–30 min with diazepam) (40).

Table 4 Management of Seizures and Status Epilepticus

1. *Establish an airway* and ensure adequate ventilation. Intubation may be necessary to protect the airway; however bag-mask ventilation should be performed if the airway cannot be secured in a timely or safe manner. The airway should be evaluated at every step, since medications may suppress spontaneous ventilation.
2. *Determine blood pressure*. If the patient is hypotensive, volume replacement is the first treatment since many patients with CNS infection have been febrile, vomiting, and taking inadequate fluid replacement. Once adequate volume is ensured, vasopressors, such as dopamine, may be necessary. If the patient is hypotensive, he should be admitted to a critical care unit. Hypertension should not be treated until status epilepticus is controlled.
3. *Obtain intravenous access*, preferably with two large-bore catheters with normal saline. (If phenytoin is used, it will precipitate in glucose-containing solutions.)
4. *Administer thiamine 100 mg with dextrose* (1 mg/kg), unless the patient is known to be normo- or hyperglycemic.
5. *Terminate seizures with antiepileptic medications*. Be aware that the cessation of clinical seizures may not always mean that electrographic seizures have stopped. The patient may have progressed to nonconvulsive status epilepticus. Patients who do not respond to external stimuli within 15 min after apparent cessation of seizures should undergo emergent EEG monitoring.
   A. *Lorazepam*: 0.05–0.2 mg/kg at 0.04 mg/kg/min. Termination of seizures should occur by 5 min. For adults, typical dosing is 2 mg aliquots repeated every 3–5 min; however, if there is no response after 8 mg, the patient is unlikely to respond. Continue along the therapeutic sequence.

   Since patients with CNS infection and seizures should be treated with long-acting anticonvulsants for a period of time, even if benzodiazepines stop the seizures, also administer:

   B. *Phenytoin*: 20 mg/kg at no more than 50 mg/min if seizures are persistent, attempt to load at this rate; if seizures have stopped, loading may be at a slower rate to minimize complications of administration, i.e., hypotension or arrhythmias. An additional 5 mg/kg may be administered before advancing to another medication. If the patient is allergic to phenytoin, use *phenobarbital* 10 mg/kg with maximum infusion rate of 50 mg/min. Repeat with same dose if not controlled.

   (At this dose of phenobarbital, patient should be intubated.)

   If seizures persist, transfer to critical care unit and intubate if not yet done:

   C. *Midazolam bolus and drip*: 0.2 mg/kg bolus with infusion of 5–40 μg/kg/min to achieve seizure control by continuous EEG monitoring. (Pentobarbital may be used instead of midazolam at this step, but has been associated with more side effects, i.e., cardiac depression and vasodilation resulting in severe hypotension, poikilothermia, ileus.) Pentobarbital may also be the drug of choice at this step if increased ICP is a concurrent problem. (See text.)

   If seizures still persist:

   D. *Pentobarbital bolus and drip*: 12 mg/kg at maximal rate of 0.2–0.4 mg/h, followed by infusion of 0.25–2.0 mg/kg/h titrated to burst-suppression pattern on EEG. Patients may need intravascular invasive monitoring. If hypotension ensues, fluid and vasopressors should be used to maintain blood pressure.
6. *Treat complications*:
   A. *Rhabdomyolysis*: Vigorous hydration with normal saline with forced diuresis with a loop diuretic to prevent acute renal failure. If necessary, urine alkalinization with a bicarbonate drip can be used. If EEG monitoring is being used and control of generalized tonic-clonic status epilepticus is taking longer than is optimal, neuromuscular blockade might be considered. *Continuous EEG monitoring must be utilized during paralysis.*
   B. *Hyperthermia*: External cooling may be used, although termination of seizure activity typically rectifies high temperatures. Acetaminophen may be helpful. Rarely, cool peritoneal lavage may be used. High-dose barbiturate therapy may produce poikilothermia. In patients with concurrent elevation in IPC, shivering may increase ICP and should be avoided. Neuromuscular blockade may be considered, but again, continuous EEG monitoring is essential during paralysis.
   C. *Acidosis*: Persistent seizures under hypoxic conditions result in acidosis. This typically resolves once generalized tonic-clonic activity ceases. If cardiovascular instability occurs, bicarbonate therapy may become necessary. Otherwise can be corrected by hyperventilation if patient is on ventilatory support.

HYDROCEPHALUS

When hydrocephalus occurs in patients with CNS infections, it is most likely to be of the communicating type, as blockage by inflammatory debris and fibrosis of the arachnoid villi occurs more frequently than outflow obstruction at the ventricular level. In a study by Durand, hydrocephalus developed in 11% of patients treated for community-acquired bacterial meningitis (3). Two of the 13 patients required a ventricular shunt procedure. Pfister reported an 11.6% incidence of hydrocephalus, of which 9 of 10 patients required ventricular drainage (2). Only one of six patients who survived needed a permanent shunt.

Hydrocephalus usually develops during the third and fourth week after onset of illness, but may occur in the first week (41). Early recognition of and rapid resolution by ventricular drainage is essential to avoid poor outcome, e.g., herniation. The first sign of hydrocephalus is typically a change in mental status; the clinician must have a high index of suspicion, and a CT scan will diagnose this condition.

CEREBRAL EDEMA AND RAISED ICP

In order to discuss the management of increased ICP, the basic principles of ICP and how each of the infectious disease processes contributes to the components that make up ICP elevation will be reviewed.

Intracranial pressure changes are described by the Monro-Kellie hypothesis of the skull as a semi-closed compartment containing brain and interstitial fluid (80%), CSF (10%), and blood (10%). Under pathological conditions, one of these components may be increased, for example, seizures or meningitis may cause hyperemia and increased blood flow or obstructive hydrocephalus may cause an increase in both interstitial fluid and CSF within the skull. In other cases, a mass lesion may take up space within the skull, such as an abscess or other forms of edema (discussed below). The extent to which these components affect intracranial pressure depends on compensatory mechanisms, which cause reductions in CSF production or CBF. Once these compensatory mechanisms are overwhelmed, the increase in the volume of intracranial contents is dependent on the compliance of the intracranial compartment. For example, a patient with a small, atrophic brain (high compliance) will tolerate greater increases in intracranial volume than a patient with no cerebral atrophy (low compliance) before intracranial pressure begins to increase.

The next principle of importance is that CBF is dependent on cerebral perfusion pressure (CPP), or blood pressure gradient across the brain, which is determined by the difference between MAP and ICP. MAP determines the amount of flow to the brain, while ICP impedes blood flow to the brain. In cases where central venous pressure (CVP) is elevated above the initial ICP, either by cardiogenic mechanisms or increased intrathoracic pressures by positive pressure ventilation, then CVP can elevate ICP, and the difference between MAP and CVP should be utilized to determine CPP.

Elevation in ICP is significant when it compromises CPP causing cerebral ischemia, or when it contributes to pressure gradients within the skull resulting in tissue displacement, i.e., herniation. This typically occurs at ICPs greater than 18–20 mmHg. A normal CPP is in the range of 70–100 mmHg, although levels as low as 50 mmHg can be tolerated in an adult. Higher levels can result in edema in areas where the BBB is compromised, while levels lower than 40 mmHg will result in tissue ischemia. This concept must be kept in mind when managing blood pressure and ICP at the bedside.

As described previously, the cerebral vasculature typically is capable of maintaining a constant cerebral blood flow within a wide range of mean arterial pressure by vasomotor control of arteriolar resistance (see Fig. 1). Although the range has been reported to be between 50 and 150 mmHg in adults, the range is not known for children, but is likely to be lower due to their normally lower baseline blood pressure. Changes in arterial oxygenation (PO_2) and carbon dioxide (PCO_2) will also change CBF by their effect on the vascular musculature. Evidence suggests that meningitis disrupts the MAP-mediated autoregulative mechanism such that the autoregulative curve shows a linear increase or decrease in blood flow directly proportional to MAP. Autoregulation with PO_2 and PCO_2 appears to remain intact, and can therefore be utilized in the management of increased ICP.

Previous sections of this chapter have dealt with the inflammatory processes of meningitis that result in (1) an arteritis that causes vascular narrowing and ischemia or infarct and seizures, (2) venous involvement that may result in thrombosis and seizures, and (3) fibrotic changes in the arachnoid villi that are responsible for impaired CSF resorption. Figure 2 depicts this cascade of events that potentially play a role in increased ICP. The semi-closed space within the skull is illustrated by the rectangles including blood, CSF, and brain. Increases in blood flow, and other fluid, such as vasogenic, cytotoxic, and interstitial edema, increase the volume within the skull and may increase ICP. Cerebral edema has three forms: interstitial, cytotoxic, and vasogenic. Interstitial edema is not produced by cerebral injury, but is due to acute hydrocephalus, in which obstruction of CSF flow within the ventricular system forces CSF out into the surrounding tissue. Cytotoxic and vasogenic edema are classically associated with CNS injury. Cytotoxic edema occurs in the setting of ischemia when energy-dependent membrane pumps that maintain the integrity of the neuronal or glial cell membrane are disrupted. Vasogenic edema is formed when the BBB is compromised, usually by neoplasm or abscess, but is also seen with infection or inflammation when cytokines affect the permeability of the BBB. Differentiation between

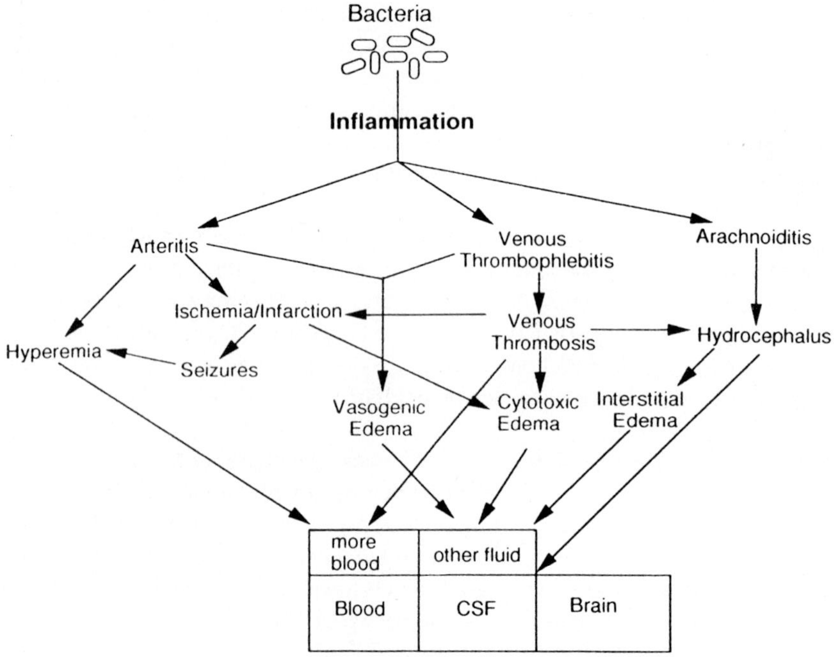

Figure 2 Cascade of events leading to intracranial hypertension in patients with meningitis. (See text for details.)

cytotoxic and vasogenic edema is significant in as much as only vasogenic edema is typically responsive to steroids.

In bacterial meningitis, both arterial and venous infarction can result in cytotoxic edema. If hydrocephalus occurs, then interstitial edema may also play a role in increased ICP. The altered permeability of the BBB by inflammatory cytokines results in vasogenic edema and contributes significantly to increased ICP.

In Durand's series, 39% of 296 patients with community-acquired meningitis had opening pressures of greater than 300 mm water at the time of initial lumbar puncture (3). The insensitivity of papilledema as a measurement of increased ICP is evident by the fact that only 12 of 279 patients with fundoscopic evaluations on admission had recorded "blurred optic-disk margins," "early papilledema," or "papilledema." In this same study, 40 patients died within 7 days of presentation, and cerebral herniation was documented in 8 of the 27 (30%) patients who underwent autopsy. All had temporal lobe herniation; four also had cerebellar herniation. In an autopsy study of 30 patients dying of acute bacterial meningitis, 5 (17%) had diffuse edema, while 3 had signs of temporal lobe herniation, and 7 had evidence of cerebellar herniation (4). In a study by Horwitz of 302 infants and children with acute bacterial meningitis, cerebral herniation occurred in 3 of 10 fatal cases and in 15 patients who survived (total of 6%)(42).

The mechanisms by which cerebral abscesses may predispose to increases in ICP are depicted in Figure 3. The inflammatory reaction at the periphery of the abscess breaks down the BBB so that vasogenic edema is a significant contributor to ICP elevation. Unless the abscess is in a location to block CSF egress, interstitial edema is usually not a contributor to increases in ICP. However, cytotoxic edema is formed where the abscess exerts a pressure effect on the surrounding tissue, causing decreased perfusion of blood vessels and subsequent ischemia of the neuronal

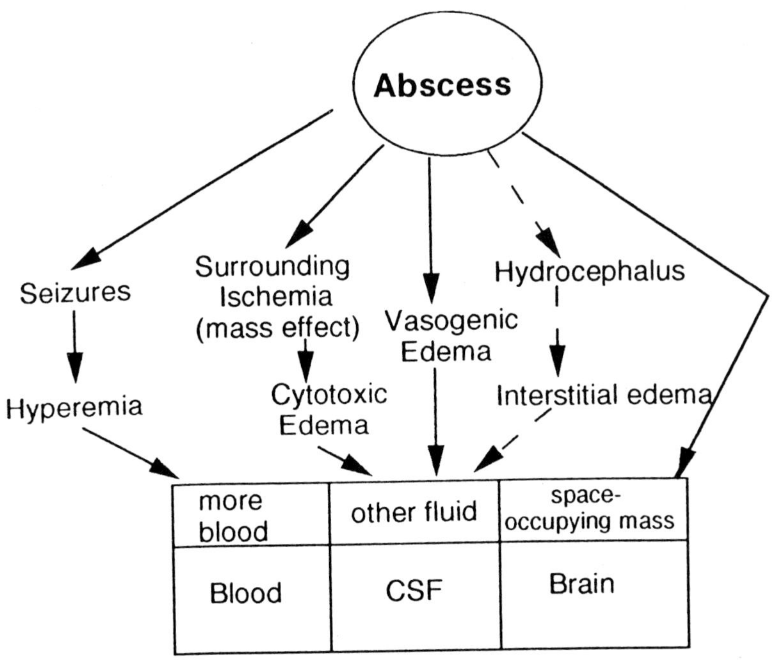

Figure 3 Cascade of events leading to intracranial hypertension in patients with cerebral abscess. (See text for details.)

and glial cells in that region. As noted above, 25–45% of patients with brain abscesses may have seizures. Increases in blood flow that accompany seizures will also contribute to increased ICP.

Subdural empyemas often exert significant mass effect and are usually associated with increases in ICP. Lumbar puncture should be deferred in cases where this diagnosis is suspected in lieu of definitive craniotomy and drainage of the fluid collection.

Viral encephalitides are often associated with increases in ICP. Intracranial hypertension in association with herpes encephalitis often predicts mortality. In a series of 10 adults with encephalitis, reported by Barnett et al. (43), 8 had biopsy-proved herpes simplex encephalitis. An ICP-monitoring device was placed in each of these patients between days 3–9 of symptom onset because of clinical deterioration or CT evidence of brain swelling. ICP peaked typically between days 9–12. Of 4 patients whose mean daily ICP was less than 20 mmHg, all survived; in 6 patients with a mean daily ICP greater than 20 mmHg, all but one died. The pathophysiology of ICP elevation in viral encephalitis is probably a combination of vasogenic and cytotoxic edema, much like that seen with the inflammatory process of meningitis. Interstitial edema is less likely to be a factor unless an accompanying aseptic meningitis is present to cause decreased CSF resorption.

Subacute therapy of increased ICP begins with diuretics such as acetazolamide or furosemide to decrease CSF production (Table 5). The emphasis remains, however, on maintaining adequate MAP with all therapy. Previously, fluid restriction was felt to decrease the incidence of hyponatremia and decrease interstitial edema by prophylactically treating the syndrome of inappropriate antidiuretic hormone (SIADH); however, this may not be the actual mechanism of hyponatremia in these patients and is no longer felt to be optimal therapy. Recent studies have shown that patients with a variety of neurological conditions such as head trauma and subarachnoid hemorrhage begin to lose large amounts of salt and water in their urine resulting in hyponatremia. This has been termed "cerebral salt wasting" (CSW)(44,45). Although the mechanism is not entirely clear, it is most likely a result of release of atrial natriuretic peptide (ANP) as a result of the CNS injury (46). ANP is released from the heart, hence its name, as a result of atrial stretch which is a signal of fluid overload; atrial tachycardia may also stimulate release (47). ANP causes increases of renal tubular sodium losses; water is lost as it follows sodium. ANP is also found in the brain near the third ventricle, and release may be stimulated by CNS events. This condition differs from SIADH in one important aspect: fluid status. In SIADH, patients have normal to slightly elevated plasma volume and can therefore tolerate fluid restriction as part of the treatment plan; however in CSW, plasma volume is low (48). As stated in the section of cerebral ischemia, poor fluid status may actually drop MAP and compromise CBF. Therefore, adequate fluid replacement is essential, especially if diuretic or osmotic agents are utilized. In patients with hyponatremia, this is also true, but may require sodium replacement as well.

Upright positioning of the patient in bed by keeping the head and trunk at 30–45 degrees may assist in decreasing ICP by improving venous outflow. Improper fluid management may nullify this beneficial effect if the patient has orthostatic hypotensive changes, i.e., a drop in MAP may drop CPP. Again, this illustrates the necessity of adequate fluid replacement.

Sedation, anticonvulsant treatment in patients with seizures, and adequate oxygenation are also valuable in the treatment of subacute increases in ICP. Agitation and pain can increase ICP. Adequate sedation and pain relief can attenuate this response, but careful attention to avoid decreasing MAP is necessary. In patients who are not intubated, respiratory drive must also be monitored as increases in PCO_2 can increase CBF. If benzodiazepines are utilized, careful titration is needed, since high concentrations of flumazenil may precipitate seizures and obviate the advantages of sedation. Adequate oxygenation ($PO_2 > 60$) will prevent autoregulative vasodilation. Seizures increase cerebral metabolic rate ($CMRO_2$) and increase cerebral blood flow, increasing cerebral blood volume and contribute to increases in ICP; therefore, adequate seizure prophylaxis is essential.

Table 5 Possible Treatment Modalities for Subacute and Acute Increases in ICP

Subacute Therapy

1. Maintain adequate MAP with all therapy
   a. Ensure adequate volume status
   b. Use vasopressor agents, e.g., dopamine, if necessary, once adequate volume is achieved
2. Decrease CSF production
   a. Acetazolamide 10–25 mg/kg/day orally or intravenously divided into three doses in children or 250 mg three times a day in adults
   b. Furosemide 20–40 mg intravenously every 12 h
3. Positioning
   a. Keep head of bed at 30–45 degrees (as long as MAP is maintained)
   b. Keep head midline, since turning of the head may impede cerebral venous outflow
4. Sedation
   a. Fentanyl boluses of 0.5–1.0 μg/kg to avoid dropping MAP (may be repeated as necessary), or
   b. Lorazepam 1–2 mg (0.015–0.50 μg/kg) boluses to avoid dropping MAP (if these medications do not drop blood pressure, continuous infusions may be necessary to avoid swings in blood pressure as the sedation wears off)
   c. Propofol infusion can be used, but is often associated with hypotension if given in boluses, starting at 0.3 mg/kg/h and increasing by 0.3 mg/kg every 5 min is recommended until adequate dosing is obtained
5. Seizure prophylaxis
   a. Phenytoin 5–10 mg/kg/day or dosage needed to keep blood levels approximately 10–20 μg/ml
   b. Phenobarbital 1–5 mg/day or dosage needed to keep blood levels approximately 15–30 μg/ml
6. Adequate oxygenation and ventilation to avoid cerebral vasodilation due to autoregulatory mechanisms
   a. $PO_2 > 60$ mmHg
   b. $PCO_2 \leq 40$ mmHg
7. Control of fevers
   a. Acetaminophen 325–650 mg every 6–8 h (each increase of temperature >37°C increased $CMRO_2$ by 7%, resulting in increases in CBF)

Acute Therapy

8. Hyperventilation
   a. Intubate and maintain PCO_2 between 25 and 30 mmHg (do not decrease below 25 mmHg, as this may cause cerebral ischemia. Monitor for increased CVP in patients with high peak airway pressures during mechanical ventilation as this may impede cerebral venous outflow)
9. Osmotic therapy
   a. Mannitol 0.25–1.0 g/kg boluses through a filtered needle. May repeat 0.25–0.5 g/kg every 3–6 h if necessary. Keep serum osmolarity below 320 mosm/L to avoid renal failure and further cerebral damage.
10. Paralytic therapy
    a. Vecuronium 0.1 mg/kg intravenous boluses every 1–2 h as needed (continuous intravenous infusions may be necessary, but should be avoided if possible, as they may be associated with prolonged weakness)
11. Barbiturate therapy
    a. Pentobarbital 10–15 mg/kg bolus, followed with a 1–3 mg/kg/h infusion
    b. Thiopental 1–5 mg/kg bolus (shorter-acting than pentobarbital in bolus doses, but when continuous infusion is necessary, tissue accumulation occurs; pentobarbital should be used)
12. Ventricular drainage (see text)
13. Hemicraniectomy (see text)
14. Corticosteroids (see text)
    a. With abscesses: dexamethasone 4–6 mg every 6 h
    b. May be useful for meningitis: dexamethasone 0.6 mg/kg/day in four divided doses for 2–4 days

When an acute elevation in ICP occurs, e.g., the patient has evidence of a midline shift with a new third nerve palsy, or evidence of central herniation with abrupt swings in hemodynamic parameters and/or extensor or flexor posturing, then osmotic agents such as mannitol are necessary. Mannitol is given in 0.25–1.0 g/kg boluses through a filtered needle to remove crystals in solution. Repeated doses of 0.25–0.5 g/kg every 3–6 h may be necessary, but should be avoided if possible since mannitol may accumulate in cerebral tissue after repeated dosing, especially in areas of BBB disruption.

Patients with uncomplicated meningitis rarely require intubation; however, when ICP increases, the level of consciousness is diminished, and intubation for airway protection may become necessary. Despite this, hyperventilation should be reserved for cases of acute ICP elevation since its maximum effect lasts only for about 12–24 h. Lowering the PCO_2 by hyperventilation causes a cerebral alkalotic state, which results in cerebrovasoconstriction, decrease in CBF and cerebral blood volume, and lowering of ICP. Its effect is usually seen within several minutes. The optimal PCO_2 appears to be between 25 and 30 mmHg; lower levels may produce cerebral ischemia. Within 12–24 h, renal compensation for the alkalosis begins, and the serum and CSF pH will begin to normalize. Rapid normalization of PCO_2 results in rebound vasodilation and intracranial hypertension; therefore, termination of hyperventilation and correction of PCO_2 should occur over 24–48 h. Hyperventilation must be approached with caution in patients with elevated airway pressures, such as those with noncompliant lungs from the adult respiratory distress syndrome (ARDS). ARDS has developed in 3.5% of patients with acute bacterial meningitis (2). In these patients, the high ventilatory rate or higher tidal volumes needed to hyperventilate the patient may increase intrathoracic pressure and result in collapse of the intrathoracic venous system, consequently this will impede cerebral venous outflow and increase ICP. Conversely, hyperventilation of patients with normal lung compliance may result in transmission of the elevated intrathoracic pressure back through the jugular veins to the brain, producing paradoxical rise in ICP. ICP monitoring will determine if hyperventilation paradoxically raises ICP; however, if this is not possible, CVP monitoring should be performed when initiating hyperventilation in patients with high airway pressures.

Once mechanically ventilated, patients with acute intracranial hypertension may also benefit from paralytic agents and induction of barbiturate coma. Pharmacological paralysis utilizing nondepolarizing neuromuscular blocking agents, such as vecuronium, can significantly lower ICP in patients who are coughing or out of synchrony with the ventilator. Even in patients who have no obvious coughing spells, paralysis can improve chest wall compliance, thereby decreasing CVP and ICP. Paralytic agents should always be given with sedation even in patients who are somnolent or lethargic. Paralysis during wakefulness is uncomfortable, anxiety-provoking, and may actually elevate ICP by producing agitation. During paralysis, no motor manifestations of seizures can be appreciated clinically. Thus, in a patient who is likely to seize, especially with a focal cerebral lesion, i.e, infarct or abscess, or who has had seizures in the past, EEG monitoring for the duration of paralysis is necessary.

Barbiturate coma, when dosed to electrocerebral silence (ECS), can lower $CMRO_2$ by 50%. Subsequently cerebral blood flow and ICP are decreased significantly. This is not often used unless all other measures fail or the patient also has refractory seizures that have not been controlled by less aggressive treatment. The side effects of barbiturates and the necessity of continuous EEG monitoring make this a costly therapy. Myocardial depression and peripheral vasodilation can result in significant hypotension. Conjunctive use of vasopressor agents and invasive hemodynamic monitoring may be necessary to maintain adequate blood pressure while attaining ECS on EEG. Other complicating side effects include poikilothermia and ileus requiring the use of total parenteral nutrition (TPN). Despite this, barbiturates may be necessary to treat refractory intracranial hypertension, although no clinical trials addressing the use of barbiturates and outcome have been performed.

Treatment of increased ICP in patients with meningitis should not include serial lumbar punctures. Although the actual incidence of herniation following spinal tap is not fully known, there is some evidence that patients with ICP > 500 mm H_2O may be more likely to herniate. Drainage of CSF in patients with hydrocephalus may be necessary; this is discussed further in the section dealing with hydrocephalus.

At centers with aggressive neurosurgical intervention, hemicraniectomy is sometimes performed in patients with medically intractable intracranial hypertension from massive cerebral hemispheric damage from trauma or ischemic or hemorrhagic infarction. Unless lesions responsible for increases in ICP are focal, such as an abscess or infarction, surgeons are understandably reluctant to approach diffuse increases in ICP, such as that seen with meningitis, by removal of the skull.

Finally, corticosteroids, as always, remain a debated topic. In the case of brain abscess, where vasogenic edema contributes a significant amount to ICP elevation, corticosteroids are used routinely to decrease intracranial mass effect. The theoretical disadvantages of steroids are a delay of collagenous encapsulation of the infection, which would make extirpation more difficult, and the relative immunosuppression associated with corticosteroid use. An appropriate antibiotic regimen is essential when utilizing steroids. One retrospective evaluation of 102 cases over 17 years by Mampalam showed that the administration of corticosteroids tended to be associated with poorer outcome, but was likely biased since patients with worse initial neurological grades, who are likely to do worse, received steroid therapy (49). The dosages and scheduling of corticosteroids vary widely in the literature, but intravenous dexamethasone 4 mg every 6 h is probably adequate.

As discussed in a previous section of this chapter, the use of corticosteroids in meningitis remains an issue of debate. In the setting of increased ICP, there may be theoretical advantages to using steroids to decrease vasogenic edema. Dexamethasone therapy has been proven to be efficacious only in infants and children with Hib meningitis. The use of this agent as adjunctive therapy in bacterial meningitis is up to the individual practitioner.

COMA

In the patient with CNS infection, there may be many etiologies for an altered level of consciousness. Dodge reported an incidence of profound coma in 12% of patients which frequently heralded an unfavorable prognosis (4). Durand also observed that a decreased mental status on admission was a poor prognostic indicator. Forty-nine percent of patients who were unresponsive or responsive only to pain on admission, as compared with 16% of patients who were alert or lethargic, died (3). In a study of consecutive patients with meningitis, Pfister et al. reported a 42% incidence of Glasgow Coma Scale score less than 10 (2).

As with any unresponsive patient, the initial evaluation should include the basics of life support: establish an adequate airway, assess the presence of adequate ventilation, and determine an adequate pulse and blood pressure (Table 6). Intravenous access should be established while obtaining a history of medication intake (which may include narcotics given for headache), vomiting, diarrhea, food and fluid intake (which may give clues to electrolyte and glucose imbalances). Excessive vomiting with a history of increasing head pain may be early clues to hydrocephalus or increased intracranial pressure, although decreasing mental status by itself may be the initial symptom.

Evaluation of blood chemistries and arterial blood gas to establish acid-base disturbances, and

Table 6 Evaluation of the Comatose Patient

1. Establish an airway and ensure adequate ventilation.
2. Determine pulse and blood pressure.
3. Obtain intravenous access.
4. Administer D50, 1–2 ampules. If there is a history of narcotic use, administer naloxone 0.040–0.080 mg every 60 s, to a total dose of 0.80 mg. In the case of benzodiazepine use, flumazenil 0.2 mg every 60 s as necessary to a maximum total dose of 1 mg at one time; may be repeated for resedation to a maximum of 3 mg in 1 h. (It may precipitate seizures in some patients.)
5. Physical examination (see text).
6. Head CT with and wihout contrast. Alternatively, if it can be obtained without delay, an MRI may be performed for better resolution.
7. EEG.

adequate oxygenation and ventilation are useful. A complete blood count should also be performed to look for evidence of disseminated intravascular coagulation (DIC), which can be found in up to 8% of patients with meningitis (2), and which may predispose a patient to intracerebral hemorrhage. The white count is usually not helpful as it is elevated, as would be expected in patients with an infectious process, but may provide evidence of overwhelming sepsis or immunosuppression.

Dextrose should be administered to most comatose patients unless the blood glucose concentration is already known to be elevated. In patients whose nutritional status is unknown, thiamine should also be given to avoid precipitating Wernicke's encephalopathy, clinically manifested by confusion, ataxia, and ophthalmoplegia. In patients with a recent narcotic ingestion, naloxone 0.04–0.08 mg may be given intravenously every 60 s to a total dose of 0.8 mg.

The directed physical examination should seek evidence of increased intracranial pressure or a focal deficit suggesting a localized neurological event. Papilledema may take several days to develop and is not a very sensitive finding. Absence or asymmetries of pupillary, corneal, cervico-ocular, or gag response may be helpful. Vestibulo-ocular testing should be performed in patients lacking cervico-ocular responses in order to determine brain-stem dysfunction. Medications, such as barbiturates, can abolish these responses. Motor responses, either spontaneous or in response to painful stimuli, help to determine focal dysfunction. Obvious seizure activity should be treated as discussed in the previous section of this chapter. Except for verbal responses, grimacing, or withdrawing for pain, detailed sensory examination cannot be performed at this time. Reflex asymmetry, or the presence of extensor toe responses, can also be helpful.

If the patient is clinically stable, a CT scan should be performed to determine the presence of ischemia, hydrocephalus, or a space-occupying lesion. A developing infarction may take up to 24 h to be visualized on the scan. In this particular subgroup of patients, i.e., any patient with a CNS infection, a contrasted CT scan is necessary to determine if an abscess has formed. Contrast may also help to delineate a subdural empyema (50), which will appear as a lentiform extraaxial fluid collection with an enhancing rim, and edematous adjacent cortex with mass effect. If an MRI can be obtained without delay, this is a very sensitive diagnostic tool that may be performed instead of a CT scan. In addition, if a posterior fossa (brain stem or cerebellar) process is suspected, this is the best study for evaluating that area.

Regardless of whether an apparent cause of coma is found on cerebral imaging, an EEG should be performed to rule out the presence of subclinical seizure activity. In patients in whom increased ICP is suspected, an ICP-monitoring device may be indicated. There have been no randomized clinical trials to determine the effectiveness of ICP monitors on outcome. However, the rule of thumb that is often used is that if the patient has progressed to obtundation or a comatose state, or when clinical neurological changes cannot be assessed, i.e., neuromuscular blockading agents are utilized, then an ICP monitor should be utilized. As discussed previously, aggressively maintaining ICP less than 20 mmHg may improve outcome.

REFERENCES

1. Swartz MN. Bacterial meningitis: more involved than just the meninges. N Engl J Med 1984; 311: 912–914.
2. Pfister HW, Feiden W, Einhäupl KM. Spectrum of complications during bacterial meningitis in adults. Arch Neurol 1993; 50:575–581.
3. Durand ML, Calderwood SB, Weber DJ, Miller SI, Southwick FS, Caviness VS, Swartz MN. Acute bacterial meningitis in adults. A review of 493 episodes. N Engl J Med 1993; 328:21–28.
4. Dodge PR, Swartz MN. Bacterial meningitis—a review of selected aspects. N Engl J Med 1965; 272: 954–960.
5. Snyder RD, Stovring J, Cushing AH, Davis LE, Hardy TL. Cerebral infarction in childhood bacterial meningitis. J Neurol Neurosurg Psychiatry 1981; 44:581–585.
6. Tuomanen E, Saukkonen K, Sande S, Cioffe C, Wright SD. Reduction of inflammation, tissue damage, and mortality in bacterial meningitis in rabbits treated with monoclonal antibodies against adhesion-promoting receptors of leukocytes. J Exp Med 1989; 170:959–969.
7. Pfister HW, Fontana A, Täuber MG, Tomasz A, Scheld WM. Mechanisms of brain injury in bacterial meningitis: workshop summary. Clin Infect Dis 1994; 19:463–479.
8. Cairns H, Russell DS. Cerebral arteritis and phlebitis in pneumococcal meningitis. J Pathol Bacteriol 1946; 58:649–665.
9. Igarashi M, Gilmartin RC, Gerald B, Wilburn F, Jabbour JT. Cerebral arteritis and bacterial meningitis. Arch Neurol 1984; 41:531–535.
10. Lebel MH, Freij BJ, Syrogiannopoulos GA, Chrane DF, Hoyt MJ, Steqrt SM, Kennard BD, et al. Dexamethasone therapy for bacterial meningitis. Results of two double-blind, placebo-controlled trials. N Engl J Med 1988; 319:964–971.
11. Girgis NI, Farid Z, Mikhail IA, Farrag I, Sultan Y, Kilpatrick ME. Dexamethasone treatment for bacterial meningitis in children and adults. Pediatr Infect Dis J 1989; 8:848–851.
12. Kadurugamuwa JL, Hengster B, Tuomanen E, Sande MA. Effect of a Cyclo-oxygenase Inhibitor on the Course and Outcome of Experimental Meningitis in Rabbits. Washington, DC, American Society of Microbiology, 1987.
13. Pfister HW, Koedel U, Haberl RL, et al. Microvascular changes during the early phase of experimental bacterial meningitis. J Cereb Blood Flow Metab 1990; 10:914–922.
14. Smith AL. Pathogenesis of *Haemophilus influenzae* type b meningitis. In: Deusch G, Wadstrom T, eds. *Experimental Bacteria and Parasitic Infections*. New York: Elsevier Science Publishing, 1983: 295–301.
15. Ashwal S, Stringer W, Tomasi L, Schneider S, Thompson J. Cerebral blood flow and carbon dioxide reactivity in children with bacterial meningitis. J Pediatr 1990; 117:523–530.
16. Tureen JH, Dworkin RJ, Kennedy SL, Sachdeva M, Sande MA. Loss of cerebrovascular autoregulation in experimental meningitis in rabbits. J Clin Invest 1990; 85:577–581.
17. Paulson OB, Brodersen P, Hansen EL, Kristensen HS. Regional cerebral blood flow, cerebral metabolic rate of oxygen, and cerebrospinal fluid acid-base variables in patients with acute meningitis and with acute encephalitis. Acta Med Scand 1974; 196:191–198.
18. Tureen JH, Täuber MG, Sande MA. Effect of hydration status on cerebral blood flow and cerebrospinal fluid lactic acidosis in rabbits with experimental meningitis. J Clin Invest 1992; 89:947–953.
19. Ameri A, Bousser MG. Cerebral venous thrombosls. Neurol Clin 1992; 10:87–111.

20. Bousser MG, Chiras J, Bories J, Castaigne P. Cerebral venous thrombosis—a review of 38 cases. Stroke 1985; 16:199–213.
21. Gettelfinger DM, Kokmen E. Superior sagittal sinus thrombosis. Arch Neurol 1977; 34:2–6.
22. Krayenbuhl HA. Cerebral venous and sinus thrombosis. Clin Neurosurg 1967; 14:1–24.
23. DiRocco C, Ianelli A, Leone G, Mischini M, Valori VM. Heparin-urokinase treatment in a septic dural sinus thrombosis. Arch Neurol 1981; 38:431–435.
24. Handrick W, Wässer S. Seizures during bacterial meningitis. In: Schönfeld H, Helwig H, eds. *Bacterial Meningitis. Antibiotics Chemotherapy*. Basel: Karger, 1992:239–253.
25. Samson JH, Apthorp J, Finley A. Febrile seizures and purulent meningitis. JAMA 1969; 210: 1918–1919.
26. Parkinson MS. Early recognition of symptoms in childhood meningitis. Practitioner 1972; 209: 191–195.
27. Klein JO, Feigin RD, McCracken GH. Report of the task force on diagnosis and management of meningitis. Pediatrics 1986; 78:959–982.
28. Rosman NP, Peterson DB, Kaye EM, Colton T. Seizures in bacterial meningitis: prevalence, patterns, pathogenesis, and prognosis. Pediatr Neurol 1985; 1:278–285.
29. Shelton MM, Marks WA. Bacterial meningitis: an update. Neurol Clin 1990; 8:605–617.
30. Pomeroy SL, Holmes SJ, Dodge PR, Feigin RD. Seizures and other neurologic sequelae of bacterial meningitis in children. N Engl J Med 1990; 323:1651–1657.
31. Kline MW. Citrobacter meningitis and brain abscess in infancy: epidemiology, pathogenesis and treatment. J Pediatrics 1988; 113:430–434.
32. Chun CH, Johnson JD, Hofstetter M, Raff MJ. Brain abscess: a study of 45 consecutive cases. Medicine 1986; 65:415–431.
33. Seydoux C, Francioli P. Bacterial brain abscesses: factors influencing mortality and sequelae. Clin Infect Dis 1992; 15:394–401.
34. Whitley RJ, Soong SJ, Linneman C, Liu C, Pazin G, Alford CA, and the National Institute of Allergy and Infectious Diseases Collaborative Antiviral Study Group. Herpes simplex encephalitis. Clinical assessment. JAMA 1982; 247:317–320.
35. Sköldenberg B, Alestig K, Burman L, Forkman A, Lövgren K, Norrby R, et al. Acyclovir versus vidarabine in herpes simplex encephalitis. Randomized multicentre study in consecutive Swedish patients. Lancet 1984; 2:707–711.
36. Whitley RJ, Cobbs CG, Alford CA, Soong SJ, Hirsch MS, Connor JD, Corey L, et al. Diseases that mimic herpes simplex encephalitis. Diagnosis, presentation, and outcome. JAMA 1989; 262:234–239.
37. Gastaut H. Clinical and electroencephalographic classification of epileptic seizures. Epilepsia 1970; 11:102–113.
38. Lowenstein D, Alldredge B. Status epilepticus at an urban public hospital in the 1980s. Neurology 1993; 42:483–488.
39. Cranford R, Leppik I, Patrick B, Anderson C, Kostick B. Intravenous phenytoin: clinical and pharmacokinetic aspects. Neurology 1978; 28:874–880.
40. Kaplan SA, Jack ML, Alexander K, et al. Pharmacokinetic profile of diazepam following single intravenous and chronic oral administration. J Pharm Sci 1973; 62:1789–1796.
41. Kabani A, Jadavji T. Sequelae of acute bacterial meningitis in children. In: Schönfeld H, Helwig H, eds. *Bacterial Meningitis*. Basel: Karger, 1992:209–217.
42. Horwitz SJ, Boxerbaum B, O'Bell J. Cerebral herniation in bacterial meningitis in childhood. Ann Neurol 1980; 7:524–528.
43. Barnett GH, Ropper AH, Romeo J. Intracranial pressure and outcome in adult encephalitis. J Neurosurg 1988; 68:585–588.
44. Shimoda M, Yamada S, Yamamoto I, Tsugane R, Sato O. Atrial natriuretic polypeptide in patients with subarachnoid haemorrhage due to aneurysmal rupture. Acta Neurochir 1989; 97:53–61.
45. Yamaki T, Tano-oka A, Takahashi A, Imaizumi T, Suetake K, Hashi K. Cerebral salt wasting syndrome distinct from the syndrome of inappropriate secretion of antidiuretic hormone (SIADH). Acta Neurochir 1992; 115:156–162.

46. Wijdicks EFM, Ropper AH, Hunnicutt EJ, Richardson GS, Nathanson JA. Atrial natriuretic factor and salt wasting after aneurysmal subarachnoid hemorrhage. Stroke 1991; 22:1519–1524.
47. Needleman P, Greenwald JE. Atriopeptin: a cardiac hormone intimately involved in fluid, electrolyte, and blood-pressure homeostasis. N Engl J Med 1986; 314:828–834.
48. Ganong CA, Kappy MS. Cerebral salt wasting in children: the need for recognition and treatment. Am J Dis Child 1993; 147:167–169.
49. Mampalam TJ, Rosenblum ML. Trends in the management of bacterial brain abscesses: a review of 102 cases over 17 years. Neurosurg 1988; 23:451–458.
50. Zimmerman RD, Leeds NE, Danziger A. Subdural empyema: CT findings. Radiology 1984; 150: 417–422.
51. Shapiro HM. Anesthesiology 1975; 43:445.

32

Systemic and CNS Toxicities of Antimicrobial Agents

Michael Frank
Indiana University School of Medicine, Indianapolis, Indiana

INTRODUCTION

The use of antimicrobial therapy can be life-saving; this is especially true for infections of the central nervous system. However, all medications have adverse effects in addition to their therapeutic effects. Although the majority of antimicrobial drugs are well tolerated, some agents have common or serious toxicities, and all have the potential for rare but life-threatening adverse effects. Knowledge of the potential adverse effects associated with a particular antimicrobial therapy is essential for the proper use of the therapy and care of the patient.

This chapter provides a summary of the adverse effects associated with currently used antibacterial, antituberculous, antifungal, antiviral, and selected antiparasitic agents, organized by drug. Rather than attempting an exhaustive listing of every adverse effect ever reported for each agent, the chapter instead focuses on those effects that are more common or serious, with special attention given to neurological toxicities. Table 1 provides a quick overview of the usual dosage and most frequent or serious systemic and neurological adverse effects for each medication. A chapter such as this cannot provide all of the information needed when using one of these medications, and for further information the clinician should consult other sources (1,2) and the prescribing information.

ANTIBACTERIAL AGENTS

β-Lactams

β-Lactams represent the most widely used group of antimicrobials. They combine excellent antimicrobial activity with a very favorable safety profile. For the purposes of this discussion, "β-lactams" will include penicillins, cephalosporins, monobactams (aztreonam), carbapenems (imipenem), and the β-lactamase inhibitors (clavulanate, sulbactam, tazobactam). Penicillins can be

Table 1 Summary of Antimicrobial Agents, Dosage, and Systemic and CNS Toxicities

Agent	Dosage[b]	Adverse effects[a]	
		Systemic	Neurological
Penicillin G	12–24 million units/day to be given q 2–4 h IV	Hypersensitivity: allergy, rash, drug fever, serum sickness, interstitial nephritis. Nausea, vomiting, diarrhea, phlebitis	Seizures with high doses, ↑ in renal failure. Rare encephalopathy, lethargy
Ampicillin Amoxicillin	1–2 g q 3–4 h IV 500 mg t.i.d. PO	See penicillin. ↑ Rash (5–10%) ↑ Diarrhea with Amox/clavulanate	See penicillin
Nafcillin Oxacillin Dicloxacillin	1–2 g q 4h IV 1–2 g q 4h IV 125–500 mg q.i.d. PO	See penicillin. ↑ Phlebitis, neutropenia, hepatitis	Less than penicillin
Ticarcillin Mezlocillin Piperacillin	3 g q 4–6 h IV 3 g q 4–6 h IV 2–4 g q 4–6 h IV	See penicillin. Na overload, platelet dysfunction	See penicillin
Cefazolin Cefuroxime Cefotaxime Ceftazidime	1–1.5 g q 6–8 h IV 750 mg-1.5 g q 8 h IV 1–2 g q 4–12 h IV 1–2 q 8–12 h IV	Hypersensitivity (potential cross-reactivity with penicillin). Rash, phlebitis, nausea, vomiting, diarrhea, eosinophilia, leukopenia.	Rare dizziness, encephalopathy, headache
Ceftriaxone	1–2 g q 12–24 h IV	See cefazolin. Also biliary sludging (usually asymptomatic)	See cefazolin
Cefoperazone	2–4 g q 6–12 h IV	See cefazolin. Also bleeding, disulfuram-like reactions	See cefazolin
Imipenem	500 mg q 6 h	Nausea, vomiting, diarrhea, phlebitis. Rare leukopenia, eosinophilia, hepatitis	Seizures (0.4–1.5%), ↑ with CNS disease and high doses in renal failure
Aztreonam	1–2 g q 6–8 h	GI upset, phlebitis, rash	Rare seizures, confusion
Vancomycin	1 g q 12 h	Red man syndrome, rash, phlebitis, neutropenia, fever	Tinnitus and hearing loss, can progress to deafness and be permament
Gentamicin Tobramycin Amikacin	2 mq/kg load, then 1.7 mg/kg q 8 h 10 mg/kg load, then 7.5 mg/kg q 8 h	Renal insufficiency 5–25%, reversible, ↑ with high levels	Ototoxicity: cochlear 3–14%; vestibular 4–6%. Potentiation of neuromuscular junction blockade

Table 1 Continued

Agent	Dosage[b]	Adverse effects[a] Systemic	Adverse effects[a] Neurological
Ciprofloxacin Ofloxacin	500–750 b.i.d. PO 200–400 q 12 h IV 200–400 b.i.d. PO 200–400 mg q 12 IV	Nausea, vomiting, diarrhea (3–13%), allergy/hypersensitivity. Absorption ↓ by Al, Mg, Ca, Fe	1–7% overall; Headache, dizziness, insomnia, mood changes. Rare seizures, delirium
Erythromycin	500 mg–1 g q 6 h	Nausea, vomiting, diarrhea, cramping in up to 32%. Phlebitis, rare hepatitis. Many drug interactions	Reversible hearing loss—up to 21% with 4 g/day
Azithromycin Clarithromycin	500 mg, then 250 q day 250–500 mg b.i.d.	Less GI upset than erythromycin, rare hepatitis	? Hearing loss, headache, rare dizziness
Clindamycin	300–900 mg q 8 h IV 300–450 mg q.i.d. PO	Diarrhea (up to 20%), nausea and vomiting, rash, fever. Rare neutropenia, hepatitis	Rare potentiation of neuromuscular junction blockade
Tetracycline Doxycycline Minocycline	500 mg −1 g q 6 h IV, 250–500 mg q.i.d. PO 100 mg q 12 PO or IV 100 mg b.i.d. PO	GI irritation 4%, photosensitivity, phlebitis with IV. Rare hepatitis, pancreatitis. Must give tetracycline on empty stomach. Discoloration of teeth in children	Rare pseudotumor cerebri. Vertigo common with minocycline
Metronidazole	500 mg q 6 h	Nausea, anorexia, metallic taste, disulfuram-like reaction	Rare seizures, encephalopathy, ataxia, peripheral neuropathy
Chloramphenicol	10–25 mg/kg q 6 h	Reversible anemia in 1/3 ± leukopenia, thrombocytopenia. Hemolytic anemia in G-6-PD def. Aplastic anemia in <1:20,000	Rare optic neuritis
Trimethoprim-sulfamethoxazole Sulfadiazine	IV: 2.5–5 mg (TMP)/kg q 6–8 h PO: DS 1–2 tab. b.i.d.-q.i.d. 1–2 g q 6 h	Rash, fever, other reactions (3% of non-HIV, 1/2 of HIV+). Nausea and vomiting, anemia and leukopenia, hepatitis, renal insufficiency	Headache. Rare depression, tremor, chemical meningitis
Isoniazid	5 mg/kg/day, up to 300 mg q day	Hepatitis, ↑ with ↑ age. D/C if symptoms or AST, ALT > 3–5X upper normal. +ANA, fever, rash	Peripheral neuropathy in up to 17%—give vitamin B_6. Rare seizures, confusion, vertigo, tremor, ataxia

Table 1 Continued

Agent	Dosage[b]	Adverse effects[a]	
		Systemic	Neurological
Rifampin	10 mg/kg/day, up to 600 mg q day	Hepatitis (less than INH, cholestatic). Hypersensitivity, GI upset. Many drug interactions. Turns tears, urine orange.	Rare headache, drowsiness, ataxia, confusion, behavioral changes
Pyrazinamide	15–30 mg/kq/day, up to 2 g q day	Hepatitis, usually after 2 months. ↑ uric acid, arthralgias	Rare rhabdomyolysis
Ethambutol	15–25 mg/kg/day	GI upset, mild	Optic neuritis, ↑ with >15 mg/kg, follow color vision, acuity
Amphotericin B	0.5–1 mg/kg/day	Acute reactions—premedicate (see text). Renal insufficiency up to 80%—saline load. Hypo K+. Anemia, phlebitis, nausea	Rare seizures, peripheral neuropathy
Fluconazole	100–400 mg/day	Nausea, vomiting, diarrhea (1–5%), rash, rare hepatitis	Headache, dizziness (1–5%)
Itraconazole	100–400 mg/day	GI (1–5%), rash, ↓ K. Rare hepatitis. Needs acid for absorption. Drug interactions > fluconazole	Headache, dizziness (1–4%)
Flucytosine	25 mg/kg q.i.d.	Diarrhea, vomiting, abdominal pain, colitis, bone marrow suppression, hepatitis	Rare headache, confusion, sedation
Acyclovir	5–10 mg/kg q 8 h IV 200–800 mg 5×/day PO	Nausea 5–7%, ↑ Cr in up to 5% with IV—keep hydrated	1–4% with IV: lethargy, confusion tremor, delirium, seizure
Ganciclovir	5 mg/kg q 12 h	Neutropenia in up to 40%, phlebitis, nausea	Headache, mood changes
Foscarnet	40–60 mg/kg q 8 h	Renal insufficiency, hyper and hypo Ca, hyper and hypo P, ↓K, ↓Mg, genital ulcers	Headache, seizures, confusion, depression
Quinine	650 mg q 8 h PO	Nausea, vomiting, rash, hepatitis, hemolysis with G-6-PD deficiency	"Cinchonism": tinnitus, ↓ hearing, headache, dysphoria, visual changes, confusion, delirium
Quinidine	10 mg/kg load (up to 600 mg) over 1–2 h, then 0.02 mg/kg/min IV infusion	See quinine. Also arrhythmias, hypotension. Must use ECG monitoring	See quinine

Table 1 Continued

Agent	Dosage[b]	Adverse effects[a] Systemic	Adverse effects[a] Neurological
Chloroquine	600 mg load, then 300 mg at 6 h, 24 h, and 48 h	Nausea and vomiting, pruritus. Rare leukopenia, myalgias	Headache, blurred vision, dizziness, confusion. Rare psychosis
Mefloquine	1250 mg once	Nausea and vomiting. Rare Stevens-Johnson, agranulocytosis	Dizziness, anxiety, sleep disturbance, paresthesias, psychosis, seizures
Pyrimethamine	100–200 mg load, then 50–75 mg/day	Bone marrow suppression—give leucovorin 10–20 mg/day	Rare seizures
Praziquantel	50 mg/kg/day, divided into 3 doses	Nausea, vomiting, fatigue, common but mild	CSF reaction syndrome in neurocysticercosis: headache, increased intracranial pressure and neuro deficits, seizures—use steroids
Albendazole	15 mg/kd/day, divided into 3 doses	Diarrhea, abdominal pain, ↑ liver enzymes, leukopenia, thrombocytopenia, alopecia	

[a]The most common and/or most serious adverse effects are listed.
[b]When a range of doses is given, the highest dose (and shortest interval) usually is used for CNS infection. Dosage given is for normal renal function; most agents require adjustment for abnormal renal function.

further divided into four groups: the natural penicillins (penicillin G, penicillin V), aminopenicillins (ampicillin, amoxicillin), semisynthetic penicillinase-resistant penicillins (methicillin, nafcillin, oxacillin, cloxacillin, dicloxacillin), and extended-spectrum penicillins (carbenicillin, ticarcillin, mezolcillin, piperacillin). Cephalosporins are grouped into "generations," with each successive generation generally having better gram-negative bacterial coverage and sometimes less gram-positive activity.

Since they share a similar structure, β-lactams in general share similar toxicities as well. The most common adverse effects of β-lactams are hypersensitivity reactions, and these will be discussed first; included in this section is a discussion of drug fever. Then the adverse effects typical of each class of drugs will be addressed and the particularly likely offending agents identified.

Hypersensitivity Reactions and Drug Fever

While hypersensitivity reactions and drug fever are most common with β-lactams, the principles discussed in this section are relevant to other agents as well.

Allergic reactions are the most significant adverse effect of β-lactams. In general, hypersensitivity reactions are less common with cephalosporins and the extended spectrum penicillins than with the natural and aminopenicillins. Several different types of reactions can occur, and these vary in their time of onset, predominant clinical manifestations, and immunopathological mechanisms, which form the basis for their classification. The four classes of hypersensitivity reactions as described by Gell and Coombs (3) are immediate hypersensitivity, cytotoxic antibodies, immune complex deposition, and delayed-type or cell-mediated hypersensitivity, though some allergic reactions such as morbilliform rash do not seem to fit into any of these.

Type I or immediate hypersensitivity reactions are IgE-mediated and involve basophils and mast cells. As the name implies, these anaphylactic reactions usually start within minutes of the dose of medication and may include urticaria, laryngeal edema, bronchospasm, and hypotension. Anaphylactic reactions are an uncommon but potentially fatal complication of β-lactam therapy with a rate of 4–15/100,000 courses of penicillin, and a death rate of 1 in every 32,000–100,000 courses (4,5.) Prompt administration of epinephrine can be life-saving.

Type II reactions are mediated through cytotoxic antibodies, which are usually IgG or IgM. Anti–β-lactam antibodies bind to β-lactam antigens found on the surface of the cell and either with or without complement lead to cell injury and lysis. This is the mechanism of β-lactam–related hemolytic anemia and may also be the cause of leukopenia, thrombocytopenia, and interstitial nephritis. It usually occurs only with long-term therapy.

Type III reactions are due to immune complex deposition. Antibody-antigen complexes are deposited and activate complement, leading to the constellation of findings known as serum sickness. This mechanism also may be the cause of some drug fevers. These reactions typically start 7–14 days after initiation of therapy and actually may occur and continue after completion of therapy, lasting until the antigen-antibody complexes have cleared. Serum sickness is manifested clinically by fever, rash, arthritis, and lymphadenopathy.

Type IV reactions are cell-mediated or delayed-type hypersensitivity reactions. Contact dermatitis was a relatively common reaction to topical penicillins, but these reactions are rarely seen now that topical penicillins are no longer used.

Finally, many reactions to β-lactams do not fit into one of the above general categories. Among these are a variety of rashes including morbilliform or maculopapular eruptions (which complicate 2–3% of courses of penicillin and 5–9% of courses of ampicillin or amoxicillin), erythema multiforme, erythema nodosum, photosensitivity, and exfoliative dermatitis.

It is often impossible to predict whether a given patient will have a reaction to a β-lactam. While the risk of allergy is probably at least partly genetic, there is no increased risk in patients with a history of asthma, allergic rhinitis, or allergic dermatitis. Although a history of a previous reaction does increase the likelihood of another, most reactions are in patients who have had no previous reaction. Predicting reactions based on history is further complicated by the fact that while 5–20% of patients overall report a history of penicillin allergy, 65–93% of those reporting an allergy actually test negative on skin testing (6). Skin testing for penicillin allergy is recommended only for those patients who report a prior history of allergy and not for patients without such a history.

Several important points about skin testing should be noted (7). Skin testing for penicillin allergy primarily tests for type I IgE-mediated reactions—it does not have predictive power for maculopapular rashes, hemolytic anemia, interstitial nephritis, or serum sickness. Furthermore, skin testing is available only for penicillin and not for the cephalosporins. Skin testing must be repeated before each new course of therapy, since the last course may have resensitized the patient. Among patients with a history of allergy but who are negative on skin testing to both major and minor determinants, 2–15% will have IgE-mediated reactions, but these are usually mild and self-limited and not anaphylactic reactions (8).

When patients have a true allergy, an alternative antibiotic should be used if possible. With the wide array of antibiotics available today, there is often another choice that will adequately treat the infection. If there is no acceptable alternative, then desensitization can be performed (9). Desensitization needs to be performed for each new course of therapy, and once performed it is important that the course of therapy not be interrupted, or desensitization may need to be repeated.

The frequency of cross-reactivity between penicillin and cephalosporins is unclear but is probably less than 20% for first-generation and less than 10% for second- and third-generation cephalosporins (10). Life-threatening anaphylaxis has occurred in patients with a history of penicillin anaphylaxis who were given a cephalosporin, so in those patients with a history of anaphylactic reaction (as opposed to morbilliform rash) to a penicillin, cephalosporins should probably be avoided. Cross-reactivity may be more common between imipenem and penicillin, and the same precautions hold for the use of imipenem as for cephalosporins in penicillin-allergic patients. There is minimal cross-reactivity between aztreonam and penicillins, however, with only isolated case reports of reactions to aztreonam in penicillin-allergic patients.

Drug fever is more often due to a β-lactam than any other class of antibiotic, though nonantibiotic drugs such as phenytoin, methyldopa, and procainamide also are common offenders. Contrary to popular drug fever myths, there are no distinguishing characteristics of drug fever that allow reliable differentiation from fever due to infection (11,12). Drug fever may have any pattern, may go over 40°C, and may be associated with considerable toxicity. While the onset of drug fever due to antimicrobials occurs most often about 7–10 days after initiation, it may happen at any time. Rash is present in only 18% of cases and eosinophilia in only 22%. Chills are present in 53%, myalgias in 25%, and headache in 16% of cases. Rechallenge with the antibiotic is usually safe, though fever may recur (11,12).

One final type of reaction that can occur with penicillin therapy (and less commonly with other antibiotics) is the Jarisch-Herxheimer reaction sometimes seen with treatment of spirochetal diseases such as syphilis and Lyme disease. This is not an allergic reaction but is thought to be an inflammatory reaction to dying organisms and may be seen in up to 30% of patients being treated for neurosyphilis. Onset is typically 2–12 h after initiation of therapy; symptoms subside within 24 h and include headache, fever, chills, diaphoresis, malaise, myalgias, and arthralgias, and change in mental status and seizures (usually associated with CNS infection).

Penicillins

In general, the penicillins are very well tolerated. Gastrointestinal symptoms including nausea, vomiting, and diarrhea occur in 2–5% of patients overall. The incidence of diarrhea seems to be higher for amoxicillin and ampicillin, with a frequency of 5–20%. Pseudomembranous colitis due to *Clostridium difficile* may occur. Phlebitis at the site of intravenous administration occurs in 2–9%; among the penicillins, nafcillin seems to be the worst offender.

Neutropenia complicates 1–4% of courses of penicillins. Nafcillin is the most likely of the penicillins to cause this adverse effect. Neutropenia is often related to the dose and duration of therapy; the frequency may be greater than 10% with nafcillin therapy for longer than 21 days. Oxacillin, piperacillin, and penicillin G are also associated with neutropenia. Platelet dysfunction occurs in about 3%, though it is rarely associated with clinically significant bleeding. This toxicity is most likely with ticarcillin, followed by mezlocillin and piperacillin.

Renal insufficiency may result from interstitial nephritis, one of the hypersensitivities of penicillins. In addition to renal insufficiency, patients with interstitial nephritis may have proteinuria, hematuria with eosinophils in the urine, blood eosinophilia, fever, and rash. While this may occur with any penicillin, it is much more common with methicillin. For this reason, and because it offers no real advantage over the other semisynthetic penicillinase-resistant penicillins, methicillin is rarely used today.

As described above under hypersensitivity, rashes are a relatively common adverse effect of the penicillins. A morbilliform or maculopapular rash may occur in 5–10% of patients overall (and in 65–100% of those with infectious mononucleosis or lymphocytic leukemia) who take ampicillin or amoxicillin. This is not necessarily a true allergy, and these patients may not develop a rash the next time they take an aminopenicillin. In general, morbilliform drug eruptions are a relatively benign toxicity, and therapy with the penicillin agent can be continued to completion if necessary. If Stevens-Johnson syndrome or toxic epidermal necrolysis develops, however, therapy must be stopped. These severe skin reactions occur less commonly with penicillins and cephalosporins than with sulfonamides, but can be life-threatening (13). Patients who have had such a reaction should not be rechallenged or have desensitization attempted.

Because of the amount of sodium present in the preparations, sodium overload can develop especially with ticarcillin but also with mezlocillin and piperacillin. Hypokalemia may also occur. Increased liver enzymes occur in 1–4% but elevations are usually mild. Symptomatic hepatitis has most often resulted from high-dose IV oxacillin and rarely nafcillin (14).

Penicillin is directly excitatory to cerebral cortex and should not be administered intrathecally. Seizures have been reported more commonly with IV penicillin and imipenem than with the others and are often associated with high doses in patients with renal failure (15). High-dose penicillin has also been associated with lethargy, multifocal myoclonus, hallucinations, and encephalopathy.

Cephalosporins

Cephalosporins share many of the toxicities of the penicillins. Hypersensitivity reactions are less common. Rash occurs in 1–3% of patients. Phlebitis occurs in 1–8% and is most likely with cephalothin. Nausea, vomiting, and diarrhea are the most common adverse effects and are seen in 3–30% of patients. They are usually mild, though *C. difficile* colitis can occur. Mild and asymptomatic elevations of liver enzymes are seen in 1–7%, but overt hepatitis is very rare. Ceftriaxone is associated with biliary sludging in about 20% of patients. This is more likely to occur in children, in those patients receiving prolonged courses or greater than 2 g/day and in those who also are receiving total parenteral nutrition. While usually asymptomatic, it can be associated with symptoms of cholecystitis.

Neutropenia complicates fewer than 1% of courses and usually follows prolonged administration of high doses. As with penicillins, a positive Coombs test is noted in 1–5%, but hemolysis is rare. Eosinophilia (1–7% of patients), thrombocytosis (2–5%), and thrombocytopenia (<1%) can occur. Because their methylthiotetrazole moiety interferes with vitamin K–dependent clotting factors, bleeding can occur with cefoperazone, cefotetan, cefamandole, and moxalactam. This is most likely to occur in debilitated or malnourished individuals and can be overcome with vitamin K administration. (Moxalactam also interferes with platelets and is no longer used due to excessive bleeding complications.) These agents have also been associated with a disulfuram reaction when patients receiving them ingested alcohol.

Seizures are less common with cephalosporin therapy than with penicillin. Other rarely reported CNS toxicities of cephalosporins include encephalopathy, headache, vertigo, dizziness, and nightmares.

Imipenem, Aztreonam, and β-Lactamase Inhibitors

Imipenem has many of the same toxicities as the β-lactams, including hypersensitivity reactions, phlebitis, nausea and vomiting (1–4%), diarrhea (including *C. difficile* colitis), elevated liver enzymes, eosinophilia, rare leukopenia, and positive Coombs test without hemolysis. Seizures occur more often with imipenem than with the other β-lactams, and the risk is increased by underlying CNS disease. Other CNS toxicities, which occur in less than 0.3% of patients, include encephalopathy, tremor, paresthesias, and vertigo. As with the other β-lactams, CNS toxicities are more likely in patients with renal insufficiency receiving high doses of the drug (16).

Aztreonam has minimal cross-reactivity with the penicillins. Adverse effects of aztreonam include nausea, vomiting, and diarrhea (1–2%), mild elevations in liver enzymes (2–4%), rash

(1–2%), and phlebitis (2–3%). CNS toxicities have occurred in fewer than 1% and have included seizures, confusion, and sedation.

Clavulanate, sulbactam, and tazobactam are β-lactamase inhibitors, which do not themselves have appreciable antibacterial activity, but are combined with β-lactams to provide coverage against otherwise resistant organisms. In general, the toxicities of the combinations match the toxicities of the parent β-lactam agents. An exception may be amoxicillin-clavulanate, which may cause diarrhea more frequently than does amoxicillin alone. In addition, cases of hepatotoxicity apparently due to the combination of amoxicillin-clavulanate in patients who had no hepatotoxicity from amoxicillin alone, suggest that clavulanate may cause hepatotoxicity (17).

Vancomycin

In the past, many of the toxicities of vancomycin were related to impurities introduced during the preparation of the drug (18). Today's vancomycin preparations are more pure and adverse effects are less common. Perhaps the most common toxicity is "red man syndrome" (RMS), which is not due to an impurity but to the vancomycin itself. RMS is a flushing of the face, neck, and upper thorax due to histamine release and is related to the rate of infusion of vancomycin. It occurs during infusion and resolves shortly after the infusion is completed. Although it can be associated with a fall in blood pressure, it is rarely a cause for discontinuation of the drug. RMS almost always can be prevented simply by decreasing the rate of infusion and premedicating with an antihistamine such as diphenhydramine (19).

Rashes have occurred in 3–5% of patients receiving vancomycin, including reports of Stevens-Johnson syndrome and toxic epidermal necrolysis (13). Phlebitis has been reported in about 13%. Neutropenia complicates about 2% of vancomycin courses, usually after the first week of therapy. Eosinophilia and thrombocytopenia may occur. Nephrotoxicity, once thought to be a substantial problem, is actually probably minimal except when vancomycin is used concurrently with an aminoglycoside.

Neurotoxicity occurs in less than 1% of patients and consists of damage to the auditory nerve (20). Toxicity is first manifested by tinnitus and high-frequency hearing loss, which can progress to deafness. While there may be improvement in hearing after discontinuation of vancomycin, the damage is often permanent. Toxicity is more likely if vancomycin levels are greater than 80 mg/L. This has contributed some of the rationale for the traditional monitoring of vancomycin levels in patients, though the necessity of this practice has been questioned recently (21).

Aminoglycosides

Nephrotoxicity and ototoxicity are the two major toxicities of the aminoglycosides. While there may be minor differences among the individual agents in their relative likelihood of causing one toxicity or the other, these differences are not clinically significant and the agents will be considered as a group. The frequency of nephrotoxicity in most reports has ranged from 5 to 25%. The renal insufficiency is usually nonoliguric and results from tubular injury that is usually reversible. The risk is increased in patients who are hypotensive, elderly, or are on other nephrotoxic medications or a high dose of aminoglycoside (22). Once-daily dosing of aminoglycosides is gaining increasing popularity as a means of possibly decreasing toxicity while maintaining effectiveness (23,24).

Ototoxicity, in contrast to nephrotoxicity, is more likely to be irreversible since the destruction of hair cells is more likely to be permanent (25,26). Cochlear toxicity occurs in 3–14% of patients, though most of these are not symptomatic. The earliest symptom may be tinnitus, followed later by hearing loss. The risk is increased with high doses, long duration, and concomitant administration of loop diuretics or vancomycin. The exact incidence of vestibular toxicity is unknown, but this toxicity is estimated to occur in 4–6% of patients. Most patients are able to compensate with visual cues and proprioception, but when symptomatic may have nausea, vomiting, vertigo, nystagmus, and ataxia.

Neuromuscular junction (NMJ) blockade is a rare but potentially fatal complication of aminoglycoside therapy (27). It is seen usually in patients who are receiving other NMJ blocking drugs or have an underlying NMJ disease and has also been related to rapid infusion of a large dose of aminoglycoside and to hypocalcemia. Aminoglycosides prevent internalization of calcium into the presynaptic axon, thereby inhibiting acetylcholine release, and also decrease the response of the postsynaptic acetylcholine receptor (28). The blockade can sometimes be overcome by intravenous administration of calcium gluconate.

Other neurotoxicities reported rarely with aminoglycosides include peripheral neuropathy, encephalopathy, paresthesias, tremor, and optic neuritis (20). Intrathecal administration of aminoglycosides has been associated with radicular pain, paraplegia, transverse myelitis, arachnoiditis, and seizures.

Quinolones

Gastrointestinal symptoms are the most common adverse effects of the quinolones, followed by CNS symptoms (29). As a group, gastrointestinal symptoms affect 3–13% of patients taking a quinolone. Nausea is the most common symptom and is usually mild. Abdominal discomfort, vomiting, and diarrhea, including rarely *C. difficile* colitis, also may occur. CNS symptoms associated with the quinolones include headache, dizziness, insomnia, anxiety, and confusion, and occur in 1–7% of patients. Seizures have been reported rarely, usually in association with theophylline (the levels of which are increased by ciprofloxacin).

Hypersensitivity reactions occur in 0.5–2% of patients; among these are rashes, which have included Stevens-Johnson syndrome, and interstitial nephritis. Eosinophilia has been noted in 0.2–2%, leukopenia in 0.2–3%, and transient increase in liver enzymes in 2–3% of patients. In addition there have been reports of tendonitis and arthralgias. In juvenile rats, the quinolones have caused cartilage damage; therefore, their use in children is not recommended. As mentioned above, ciprofloxacin and enoxacin will inhibit the metabolism and increase the concentrations of theophylline and caffeine. Also, quinolones are bound by polyvalent cations such as magnesium, calcium, aluminum, and iron, and should be given separately from antacids, sucralfate, and mineral supplements to ensure adequate absorption.

Macrolides

Erythromycin is the prototypical macrolide and remains one of the most widely used antibiotics. Modifications of its structure have produced a long list of synthetic macrolides with somewhat different antimicrobial activity and adverse effects. The two synthetic macrolides presently available in the United States are azithromycin and clarithromycin.

The major toxicities of erythromycin (which in some cases are bothersome enough to discontinue therapy) are gastrointestinal. These occur in up to one third of patients and include cramping, nausea, vomiting, and diarrhea. Gastrointestinal symptoms are due to erythromycin stimulation of intestinal motilin receptors and occur with intravenous as well as oral therapy. Phlebitis is another common adverse effect of intravenous erythromycin, and the drug should be given slowly in dilute solution. Cholestatic hepatitis has been reported with a frequency of about 0.1% with use of the estolate preparation; most cases have onset in the second week of therapy, and about half have concomitant eosinophilia. Hepatotoxicity has also been reported with the stearate salt and the ethyl succinate ester preparations.

Reversible hearing loss can occur with the use of high-dose erythromycin. This may be more common than previously recognized. A recent study reported an incidence of 21% when erythromycin was given in a dose of 4 g/day (30). Several case reports also have linked erythromycin with torsades de pointes ventricular tachycardia (31). Through its effects on the cytochrome p450 system, erythromycin inhibits the metabolism and increases the concentrations of many other drugs including carbamazepine, benzodiazepines, bromocriptine, theophylline, warfarin, methylprednisone, digoxin, cyclosporine, terfenadine, and astemizole (32). The interaction with terfenadine has been associated with ventricular tachycardia.

The major difference in toxicity between the derivatives azithromycin and clarithromycin and their parent compound erythromycin is a much lower incidence of gastrointestinal symptoms, with a frequency in the 2–5% range at currently recommended doses (33). In addition, azithromycin does not seem to have the problem erythromycin has with drug interactions. These drugs are not free of hepatotoxicity, however (34). Clarithromycin also causes an abnormal taste in 3% and headache in 2% of patients.

Clindamycin

Diarrhea is the major toxicity of clindamycin, occurring in 7–20% of patients. Clindamycin is one of the drugs most likely to lead to *C. difficile* colitis, though most of the diarrhea related to clindamycin is not due to this superinfection. Other gastrointestinal symptoms include nausea and vomiting, abdominal pain and bloating, and a metallic taste noted with high-dose intravenous therapy. Neutropenia and hepatitis are rare complications of clindamycin. Clindamycin may enhance neuromuscular junction blockade; this may not be reversible with a cholinesterase inhibitor (27).

Tetracyclines

Gastrointestinal irritation and nausea occur in about 4% of patients who take tetracycline but are less common with doxycycline, perhaps because it can be taken with food. Esophageal ulceration has been reported with the tetracyclines when taken without fluid at bedtime. Pancreatitis has been reported rarely with tetracycline. Hepatotoxicity is rare with tetracycline but has had a high mortality. The risk of hepatotoxicity is increased with pregnancy, renal failure, and intravenous doses greater than 2 g/day. Photosensitivity is seen with the tetracyclines but is not an allergic reaction. Patients can continue the therapy but should take extra precautions to avoid sunburn.

Reversible vertigo is a toxicity unique to minocycline. Up to 28% of males and 70% of females report lightheadedness, dizziness, loss of balance, or tinnitus beginning 2–3 days after starting minocycline (35). Pseudotumor cerebri has also been reported in infants and adults receiving tetracycline (36). Because of the adverse effect of discoloration of the teeth, tetracyclines should not be given to children under age 8 unless the infection is life-threatening and alternative therapies are much less desirable (e.g, Rocky Mountain spotted fever).

Metronidazole

A metallic taste may be the most common toxicity of metronidazole. Gastrointestinal toxicities include nausea and anorexia; vomiting and diarrhea are uncommon. Rash and neutropenia may occur rarely. Metronidazole will increase lithium levels and prolong the prothrombin time in patients on warfarin. Because of a disulfuramlike reaction, patients should abstain from alcohol while taking metronidazole.

Neurological toxicities of metronidazole are rare and usually associated with prolonged use of high doses (20). CNS toxicities include seizures, encephalopathy, cerebellar dysfunction, and ataxia and are reversible in days after discontinuation of therapy. A more slowly reversible peripheral neuropathy also has been reported (37).

Chloramphenicol

Hematological toxicity is the major problem with chloramphenicol and is characterized by three different types of anemia, which may or may not be associated with leukopenia and thrombocytopenia. Chloramphenicol causes a reversible dose-dependent anemia in one third of patients and may also cause a hemolytic anemia in patients with glucose-6-phosphate dehydrogenase deficiency. The feared complication of chloramphenicol is aplastic anemia, which is not dose-related but idiosyncratic, may occur weeks after therapy, and has an incidence of one in every 24,000–40,000 courses.

Sulfonamides and Trimethoprim

While listed here under antibacterial agents, sulfonamides are actually even broader-spectrum agents. Especially when combined with trimethoprim (sulfamethoxazole) or pyrimethamine (sulfadiazine), they have excellent activity against protozoa such as *Pneumocystis carinii* and *Toxoplasma gondii*. This has led to their widespread use in patients with immunosuppression due to human immunodeficiency virus (HIV) infection, and these patients have a much higher incidence of toxic reactions to these agents (38). While the overall incidence of adverse effects to trimethoprim-sulfamethoxazole (TMP-SMX) in individuals not infected with HIV is 8–12% (39), more than half of AIDS patients experience adverse effects.

Rashes are the most common toxicity of sulfonamides and include, in addition to morbilliform eruptions, Stevens-Johnson syndrome, toxic epidermal necrolysis, erythema nodosum, and erythema multiforme. TMP-SMX is among the most common causes of Stevens-Johnson syndrome, with an estimated frequency of 1 in 100,000 among non-HIV and 1 in 1000 among HIV-infected individuals (13). If the rash progresses to toxic epidermal necrolysis, the mortality reaches 30%. Other hypersensitivity reactions include anaphylaxis, serum sickness, and a reaction similar to the anticonvulsant hypersensitivity syndrome. A severe reaction to TMP-SMX has been noted in AIDS patients, with resulting fever, hypotension, and pulmonary edema (40).

Nausea and vomiting occur in about 4% of HIV-negative recipients, but are much more common with the high doses used to treat *P. carinii* pneumonia. Elevated liver enzymes are seen in about 10%, but are symptomatic in only 0.6%; the hepatitis may be cholestatic, hepatocellular, or even granulomatous (14). Renal insufficiency can result from high doses of sulfonamides, along with hyponatremia and hyperkalemia. Anemia, leukopenia, and thrombocytopenia may complicate therapy with TMP-SMX, especially in AIDS, and cases of pancreatitis have been reported. Neurological toxicities of TMP-SMX include headache, depression, tremor, and a chemical meningitis (41,42).

ANTITUBERCULOUS AGENTS

Isoniazid

The most serious toxicity of isoniazid (INH) is hepatitis. While about 15% of INH recipients have minor elevations of liver transaminases, most of these are asymptomatic and resolve even with continued therapy. About 0.8% of patients, however, develop serious hepatitis; 10% of these cases are fatal. INH hepatitis is most likely to occur between 4 and 8 weeks into therapy, in patients with preexisting liver disease or pregnancy, and in the elderly. The incidence of hepatitis is less than 0.3% for those 35 years of age and younger and 2.3% for those over the age of 50 (43). While some advocate following liver enzymes in all recipients, it is probably necessary to do so only in high-risk individuals. All patients should be educated about the symptoms of hepatitis (e.g., nausea, anorexia, abdominal pain, jaundice) and be advised to contact their physician immediately should any develop. Patients who are asymptomatic and have only mild elevations of transaminases (up to a few times the upper limit of normal) can be continued on INH with careful follow-up. If symptomatic, or if the elevation in transaminase is greater than 3–5 times normal, the drug should be stopped.

Peripheral neuropathy is the other common side effect of INH, occurring in 0.2–17% of patients. It is more likely to occur in patients who abuse alcohol, are malnourished, or have diabetes or renal failure and can be prevented by the administration of pyridoxine (vitamin B_6) 10–50 mg/day. CNS side effects including memory loss, psychosis, seizures, vertigo, drowsiness, tremor, ataxia, and encephalopathy occur in less than 1% of patients, and while not as clearly linked to pyridoxine deficiency, may respond to its administration (20). Seizures have been reported to occur 1–3 h after ingestion. They may be multiple, develop into status epilepticus, and respond to intravenous administration of pyridoxine (15). Isoniazid increases serum levels of phenytoin and theophylline. Isoniazid can cause hypersensitivity reactions, including fever and rash, and causes an (often asymptomatic) abnormal antinuclear antibody test in 20% of recipients.

Rifampin

Like INH, rifampin can cause mild asymptomatic elevations of liver enzymes, which resolve spontaneously. However, it is less likely than INH to cause symptomatic hepatitis, and when it does, is usually being used concomitantly with INH. In addition, rifampin hepatitis typically occurs earlier than INH hepatitis and is more likely to produce elevated bilirubin and alkaline phosphatase than transaminase levels. Hypersensitivity reactions to rifampin include fever and pruritus in about 1% of patients, interstitial nephritis, cutaneous vasculitis and urticaria, leukopenia, thrombocytopenia, eosinophilia, hemolytic anemia (all 1% or less), and an influenzalike syndrome with the intermittent high-dose two or three times per week regimens.

CNS toxicities are rare but occur especially in the first few weeks of rifampin therapy and include headache, drowsiness, ataxia, dizziness, confusion, visual changes, and behavioral changes. In addition, through its induction of enzymes of metabolism, rifampin lowers serum concentrations of phenytoin, barbiturates, diazepam, haloperidol, nortriptyline, corticosteroids, itraconazole, ketoconazole, oral contraceptives, warfarin, and many other drugs. Gastrointestinal upset is common with rifampin and can be severe enough to limit therapy. Patients also should be warned that rifampin will turn urine, tears, and other body fluids an orange color; while not dangerous, this may be startling if unexpected and can permanently stain contact lenses.

Pyrazinamide

While hepatotoxicity is also a concern with pyrazinamide, if used at currently recommended doses the additional risk over that of INH and rifampin appears to be minimal in the first 2 months of therapy. After the first 2 months, continued use of pyrazinamide is associated with about a 2% incidence of hepatitis. Pyrazinamide raises uric acid levels in about one-half of patients; this may precipitate gout in predisposed individuals. Pyrazinamide also causes nausea and gastrointestinal upset, and rarely polymylagia and arthralgia, rash and photosensitivity, interstitial nephritis, and rhabdomyolysis.

Ethambutol

Unlike the other first-line antituberculous drugs, ethambutol does not cause hepatotoxicity. Optic neuritis is the major toxicity of ethambutol and is dose-related with increasing incidence seen at doses higher than 15 mg/kg/day (44). Optic neuritis is manifested by reversible loss of green/red color perception and a decrease in visual acuity. Therapy should be stopped if these symptoms occur. Patients taking ethambutol should have regular eye exams including acuity and color perception, especially if taking more than 15 mg/kg/day. Uncommon toxicities of ethambutol include peripheral neuropathy, headache, gastrointestinal upset, and increased uric acid levels.

Other Antituberculous Agents

Streptomycin shares the toxicity of the other aminoglycosides; while the renal and auditory toxicity of streptomycin appears to be less than that of the other aminoglycosides, its vestibular toxicity is worse. High rates of intolerable side effects make the second-line agents much less desirable for tuberculosis therapy. Para-aminosalicylic acid has a high incidence of gastrointestinal intolerance and hypersensitivity, including lupus and mononucleosis syndromes. Ethionamide also has a very high incidence of gastrointestinal intolerance and causes neuropathy (pyridoxine-responsive) and psychiatric disturbances. Cycloserine deserves special recognition because of a 30% incidence of neurological adverse effects. These include peripheral neuropathy, seizures, depression, anxiety, confusion, somnolence, vertigo, and dysarthria.

ANTIFUNGAL AGENTS

Amphotericin B

Amphotericin has been in use for several decades and it remains the drug of choice for many serious fungal infections despite its toxicity (45,46). The two most important toxicities of amphotericin are acute reactions and renal insufficiency. In a prospective study, acute reactions occurred in 71% of patients receiving amphotericin; symptoms included fever in 51%, chills in 28%, nausea in 18%, and headache in 9% (47). Uncommonly, acute reactions are complicated by hypotension and hypoxemia. These reactions do not represent anaphylactic reactions, and their severity usually diminishes over time. Premedication with small doses of corticosteroids (e.g., 50–100 mg hydrocortisone 30–60 minutes before amphotericin) and acetaminophen will usually be sufficient to allow continuation of amphotericin therapy. While these reactions are not a histamine-mediated event, diphenhydramine may be helpful, perhaps due to its sedative effect. Meperidine can be used to treat rigors if they accompany the reaction, and antiemetics can be used as needed for nausea and vomiting. Because of concern for worsening of the fungal infection being treated, steroids should not be used routinely in all patients, but reserved for those who react to the test dose or subsequent doses of amphotericin. During long courses of amphotericin, attempts to decrease or discontinue the steroid premedication should be made and are often successful.

An increase in serum creatinine concentration is seen in up to 80% of patients receiving amphotericin, and in fact a rise to 2 mg/dl can be expected routinely as part of therapy. Renal insufficiency is dose-dependent, usually reversible after cessation of therapy, and due at least in part to direct vasoconstriction of afferent renal arterioles with resultant decrease in glomerular blood flow. Saline loading (500 ml normal saline administered before each dose) can decrease the nephrotoxicity. Close attention must be paid to potassium levels as well; a need for supplementation should be expected. Renal toxicity is increased in the presence of other nephrotoxic drugs, intravenous contrast dye, and hypotension. As stated previously, a rise in serum creatinine even to concentrations of 2 mg/dl is expected with use of amphotericin and does not necessarily warrant modification of therapy. If the patient's creatinine level continues to rise despite saline loading and discontinuation of other possible contributors, then decreasing the frequency of amphotericin administration to every other day may allow continuation of therapy.

Anemia is another expected complication of amphotericin, occurring in up to 75% of patients. It is usually mild with normal indices, and rarely falls below a hematocrit of 25%. Phlebitis is seen in 5% of patients; its incidence is not lessened by the coadministration of heparin. Rarely amphotericin has been associated with thrombocytopenia, leukopenia, rash, peripheral neuropathy, seizures, confusion, delirium, and mood changes. In addition, intrathecal administration of amphotericin has been associated with headache, nausea and vomiting, urinary retention, radiculitis, arachnoiditis, visual changes, and paresthesias.

Ketoconazole, Fluconazole, and Itraconazole

Because of lower antifungal activity and a higher incidence of side effects, ketoconazole for the most part has been replaced by itraconazole and fluconazole in the treatment of fungal infections. The most common adverse effects of ketoconazole are gastrointestinal with dose-related nausea and vomiting occurring in 3–29%. Asymptomatic elevation of liver enzymes is common; serious hepatitis has an incidence of one in 15,000. Other toxicities include gynecomastia, impotence, decreased libido, pruritus, rash, increase in blood pressure, headache, dizziness, somnolence, lethargy, and paresthesias, each occurring in 1% or fewer of patients. In addition, gastric acid is required for absorption of ketoconazole, and drug interactions (including phenytoin) can be a problem.

Although the overall incidence of adverse effects due to fluconazole is 5–30%, the vast majority of these are mild and do not affect the course of therapy (48). Gastrointestinal symptoms consisting of nausea, abdominal discomfort, or diarrhea occur in 1–5% of patients. Rash or pruritus occurs in 0.9–5%. From 5 to 7% of patients will have asymptomatic elevation of liver enzymes, and a few cases of overt hepatitis have been reported. Other uncommon toxicities include headache, dizziness, anemia, thrombocytopenia, and leukopenia. Fluconazole does not have any effect on testosterone or cortisol levels and does not require gastric acid for absorption, though it does increase serum levels of phenytoin.

Itraconazole has an overall incidence of adverse effects of 1–11%, but like fluconazole, these usually do not require discontinuation of therapy (48). Nausea and abdominal distress are common but mild, with the frequency of vomiting 5%, diarrhea 3%, and abdominal pain 1%. Hypokalemia occurs in 2%, rash in 1–9%, and increased liver enzymes in 1–3%, with case reports of clinical hepatitis. Other adverse effects occurring in 1–2% include headache, dizziness, and somnolence. Itraconazole is more dependent than fluconazole on gastric acid for absorption, and drug interactions include phenytoin, carbamazepine, cyclosporine, digoxin, terfenadine, astemizole, and loratidine.

Flucytosine

Flucytosine is related to the antineoplastic agent 5-fluorouracil. Because of the development of resistance, it is never used alone in the treatment of fungal infections but is sometimes combined with other agents. The combination with amphotericin B warrants especially close monitoring for toxicity since the renal insufficiency that accompanies amphotericin therapy increases the likelihood of flucytosine toxicity. The major toxicities are gastrointestinal upset and bone marrow suppression. Diarrhea, nausea, vomiting, and colitis are relatively common with use of flucytosine, especially at high doses. A dose-related increase in liver enzymes is seen in 5% of patients. Bone marrow suppression also is dose-related and flucytosine levels must be followed, especially with any increase in creatinine. Assuming normal renal function, initiation of therapy at doses no higher than 100 mg/kg/day, with adjustment of dosage based on levels, can decrease the bone marrow toxicity. Reported neurological toxicities have included confusion, hallucinations, headache, sedation, and vertigo.

Antiviral Agents

Acyclovir

Acyclovir remains the most widely used antiviral agent and has a very favorable toxicity profile. Nausea and diarrhea occur in 2–8% of patients receiving oral and about 7% of those receiving intravenous acyclovir. Headache is reported by 2–6% of those taking oral acyclovir. High-dose intravenous acyclovir is associated with an elevation in serum creatinine in about 5% of recipients. Some of these cases result from a crystalline nephropathy with deposition of acyclovir in tubules and consequent obstruction; therefore, all patients should be kept well hydrated. High-dose intravenous acyclovir is also associated with a 1–4% incidence of CNS side effects including lethargy, confusion, tremor, myoclonus, hallucinations, delirium, and seizures (49). These CNS toxicities also have been reported rarely with oral therapy in the elderly.

Ganciclovir

Since it provides activity against cytomegalovirus, ganciclovir is being used increasingly in the AIDS and transplant populations. Herpes simplex and varicella zoster viruses that are resistant to acyclovir will be resistant to ganciclovir as well, and foscarnet should be used to treat these infections. The limiting toxicity of ganciclovir is neutropenia, which occurs in up to 40% of recipients, most often in the first or second week of therapy. If another agent such as foscarnet cannot be used and ganciclovir therapy must be continued, the use of granulocyte colony-stimulating factor (filgrastim) can be used to raise neutrophil counts. Thrombocytopenia is seen in up to 20% of ganciclovir recipients but anemia in only about 2%. Phlebitis is a common adverse effect; nausea and vomiting and elevated liver enzymes are reported to occur about 2% of the time. CNS side effects have a reported incidence of about 5% and include headache, mood changes, confusion, and psychosis (50).

Foscarnet

Foscarnet can be thought of as a broad-spectrum antiviral agent with activity equal to or better than ganciclovir. Unfortunately, it is less well tolerated than ganciclovir (51). The major limiting toxicities of foscarnet are renal and metabolic abnormalities, and close follow-up of serum creatinine and other chemistries is important. A reversible increase in serum creatinine is seen in up to one-half of patients, and all patients on foscarnet should be kept well hydrated. Genital ulcerations due to high urinary concentrations of foscarnet have been reported in up to 28% of patients and provide another reason for thorough hydration.

Metabolic abnormalities due to foscarnet and their approximate frequencies include: hypocalcemia 15%; hypercalcemia 5%; hypophosphatemia 8%; hyperphosphatemia 6%; hypomagnesemia 15%; hypokalemia 16%; and hyponatremia 5%. Hypocalcemia secondary to foscarnet has been associated with paresthesias, tetany, and seizures. Nausea and vomiting occur in 15–30% of patients and abnormal liver enzymes in 1–5%. Anemia has been reported in 33% of AIDS patients receiving foscarnet, but anemia is common in late-stage AIDS.

CNS adverse effects include headache in one fourth of patients and seizures in as many as 10%. However, most of the reported patients who had seizures had concomitant CNS disease, hypocalcemia, or other metabolic abnormalities. Neurological toxicities seen in about 5% of patients include dizziness, neuropathy, confusion, anxiety, and depression. Ataxia, stupor, muscle spasms, aphasia, insomnia, and hallucinations occur in 1–5% of patients, and vertigo, coma, encephalopathy, extrapyramidal effects, psychosis, and delirium occur in less than 1% of patients.

Amantadine and Rimantadine

Although nausea, diarrhea, dry mouth, or constipation are reported by 1–10% of amantadine recipients, neurological adverse effects are the most limiting toxicity. With a frequency of 5–33%, CNS toxicity is especially common in the elderly and those on other CNS active drugs (52). Among the neurological toxicities are nervousness, lightheadedness, inability to concentrate, insomnia, mood changes, and, less commonly, visual changes, decreased libido, urinary retention, tremor, psychosis, seizures, and coma. Rimantadine has a much reduced incidence of these CNS adverse effects compared to amantadine.

Antiretroviral Agents

The major limiting toxicity of zidovudine (ZDV, AZT) is anemia and leukopenia, occurring in 2–37% of patients depending on the stage of HIV infection. The hematological abnormalities may have onset at any time but are most common after the first month of therapy. Headache, insomnia, irritability, fatigue, and nausea are seen commonly with initiation of therapy. These symptoms will usually subside within a few weeks of continued use of zidovudine. Myopathy has been noted after prolonged use of zidovudine, but neuropathy is not felt to be an adverse effect of zidovudine.

The other three currently available antiretrovirals all have painful sensorimotor peripheral neuropathy as an adverse effect. Dose-related and usually slowly reversible after discontinuation of the drug, neuropathy may be more common with zalcitabine (ddC) and stavudine (d4T) than didanosine (ddI). Didanosine and less often zalcitabine also have been associated with pancreatitis, which is sometimes fatal. Oral ulcers are another adverse effect seen with zalcitabine.

Interferon-α

Interferon-α is a naturally occurring protein, which plays a major role in the body's normal defense against viral infection and is now available through recombinant technology. Not surprisingly, the use of interferon-α is accompanied by an influenzalike syndrome of fever, chills, nausea, headache, myalgias, and arthralgias in essentially all patients. Bone marrow suppression with leukopenia and thrombocytopenia and elevation of liver enzymes also can occur. Neurological toxicities include somnolence, confusion, depression, paresthesias, and rarely seizures and coma (53).

ANTIPARASITIC AGENTS

In addition to the agents discussed below, several compounds with activity against parasites also are active against bacteria or fungi and have been discussed above under antibacterial agents or antifungal agents.

Antimalarial Agents

The major toxicity of quinine is a syndrome known as "cinchonism." Dose-related and reversible, it may consist of tinnitus, decrease in hearing, dysphoria, nausea and vomiting, visual changes (e.g., blurred vision, color changes, decreased visual fields, diplopia, scotoma, photophobia), confusion, and delirium. Less common adverse effects of quinine include rash, hepatitis, hemolysis with glucose-6-phosphate dehydrogenase deficiency, and respiratory depression in patients with myasthenia gravis. Because of greater availability, quinidine has replaced quinine for the intravenous therapy of malaria in the United States. In addition to the adverse effects noted for quinine, intravenous quinidine is associated with hypotension and electrocardiographic changes including QT prolongation and arrhythmias, and electrocardiographic monitoring during its use is essential.

Adverse effects of chloroquine include headache, nausea and vomiting, blurred vision, dizziness, fatigue, and confusion. Rarely chloroquine may cause psychosis, insomnia, pruritus, leukopenia, or myalgias. Like chloroquine, mefloquine is usually well tolerated at doses used for prophylaxis, but at treatment doses adverse effects are common. Adverse effects of mefloquine include nausea and vomiting, dizziness, anxiety, insomnia, strange dreams, paresthesias, psychosis, seizures (54), and rare reports of Stevens-Johnson syndrome and agranulocytosis. In addition, because of its effects on cardiac conduction, mefloquine should be avoided in patients taking β-blockers. The major toxicity of primaquine is hemolysis in patients with glucose-6-phosphate dehydrogenase deficiency.

Pyrimethamine

Bone marrow suppression is the most common adverse effect of pyrimethamine. Anemia, leukopenia, and thrombocytopenia can all be seen. Cytopenias can be prevented by administration of folinic acid 5–20 mg/day. Nausea and vomiting also may occur with pyrimethamine.

Dapsone

Dapsone causes a dose-related hemolysis, which is not significant in most patients but may become so in patients with glucose-6-phosphate dehydrogenase deficiency. It also has the potential for causing methemoglobinemia. Rash, with or without pruritus and fever, is common in HIV-infected individuals taking dapsone (55). Dapsone is a sulfone and cross-reactivity with the sulfonamides may occur. In addition, a hypersensitivity syndrome resembling the phenytoin hypersensitivity syndrome has been reported (56).

Praziquantel and Albendazole

Adverse effects with the use of praziquantel are common but usually mild and sometimes related to the inflammatory response to the dying worm. Nausea, headache, dizziness, and fatigue occur in up to 90% of patients but are usually mild. About 3% of patients have modest elevations in liver enzymes. Albendazole therapy may cause diarrhea and abdominal pain, and less commonly elevated liver enzymes, alopecia, headache, and dizziness. Headache, worsening of neurological symptoms, seizures, and signs of increased intracranial pressure may occur in patients with neurocysticercosis who are treated with anticysticercal agents. Corticosteroids should be used to prevent these symptoms.

REFERENCES

1. Mandell GL, Bennett JE, Dolin R. Principles and Practice of Infectious Diseases. 4th ed. New York: Churchill Livingstone, 1995.
2. American Hospital Formulary Service. AHFS Drug Information 95. Bethesda, MD: American Society of Hospital Pharmacists, Inc. 1995.
3. Gell PGH, Coombs RRA. Classification of allergic reactions responsible for clinical hypersensitivity and disease. In: Gell PGH, Coombs RRA, Hachmann PJ, eds. Clinical Aspects of Immunology. Oxford: Blackwell Scientific Publications, 1975:761–781.
4. Idsoe O, Guthe T, Willcox RR. Nature and extent of penicillin side-reactions, with particular reference to fatalities from anaphylactic shock. Bull WHO 1968; 38:159–188.

5. International Rheumatic Fever Study Group. Allergic reactions to long-term benzathine penicillin prophylaxis for rheumatic fever. Lancet 1993; 337:1308–1310.
6. Weiss ME, Adkinson NF. Immediate hypersensitivity skin reactions to penicillin and related antibiotics. Clin Allergy 1988; 18:515–540.
7. Lin RY. A perspective on penicillin allergy. Arch Intern Med 1992; 152:930–937.
8. Sogn DD, Casale TB, Condemi JJ. Results of the NIAID collaborative clinical trial to test the predictive value of skin testing with major and minor penicillin derivatives in hospitalized adults. Arch Intern Med 1992; 152:1025–1032.
9. Sanford JP. The technique of penicillin desensitization. J Crit Illness 1992; 7:791–795.
10. Weiss ME, Adkinson NF. Beta-lactam allergy. In: Mandell GL, Bennett JE, Dolin R, eds. Principles and Practice of Infectious Diseases. 4th ed. New York: Churchill Livingstone, 1995:272–278.
11. Mackowiak PA. Drug fever. In: Mackowiak P, ed. Fever: Basic Mechanisms and Management. New York: Raven Press, 1991:255–265.
12. Mackowiak PA, LeMaistre CF. Drug fever: a critical appraisal of conventional concepts. An analysis of 51 episodes diagnosed in two Dallas hospitals and 97 episodes reported in the English literature. Ann Intern Med 1987; 106:728–733.
13. Roujeau JC, Stern RS. Severe adverse cutaneous reactions to drugs. N Engl J Med 1994; 331:1272–1284.
14. Westphal JF, Vetter D, Brogard JM. Hepatic side-effects of antibiotics. J Antimicrob Chemother 1994; 33:387–401.
15. Garcia PA, Alldredge BK. Drug-induced seizures. Neurol Clin 1994, 12:85–99.
16. Manian FA, Stone WJ, Alford RH. Adverse antibiotic effects associated with renal insufficiency. Rev Infect Dis 1990; 12:236–249.
17. Stricker BHC, Van den Broek JWG, Keuning J, et al. Cholestatic hepatitis due to antibacterial combination of amoxicillin and clavulanic acid (Augmentin). Digest Dis Sci 1989; 34:1576–1580.
18. McHenry MC, Gavan TL. Vancomycin. Pediatr Clin North Am 1983; 30:31–47
19. Wallace MR, Mascola JR, Oldfield EC. Red man syndrome: incidence, etiology, and prophylaxis. J Infect Dis 1991; 164:1180–1185.
20. Snavely SR, Hodges GR. The neurotoxicity of antibacterial agents. Ann Intern Med 1984; 101:92–104.
21. Cantu TG, Yamanaka-Yuen NA, Lietman PS. Serum vancomycin concentrations: reappraisal of their clinical value. Clin Infect Dis 1994; 18:533–543.
22. Bertino JS, Booker LA, Franck PA. Incidence of and significant risk factors for aminoglycoside-associated nephrotoxicity in patients dosed by using individualized pharmacokinetic monitoring. J Infect Dis 1993; 167:173–179.
23. Gilbert DN. Once daily aminoglycoside therapy. Antimicrob Agents Chemother 1991; 35:339–405.
24. Prins JM, Buller HR, Kuijper EJ. Once versus thrice daily gentamicin in patients with serious infections. Lancet 1993; 341:335–339.
25. Brummett RE. Drug-induced otoxicity. Drugs 1980; 19:412–428.
26. Govaerts PJ, Claes PH, DeHeyring PHV. Aminoglycoside-induced ototoxicity. Toxicol Lett 1990; 52:227–251.
27. Howard JF. Adverse drug effects on neuromuscular transmission. Sem Neurol 1990; 10:89–102.
28. Sokoll MD, Gergis SD. Antibiotics and neuromuscular function. Anesthesiology 1981; 55:148–159.
29. Hooper DC, Wolfson JS. Fluoroquinolone antimicrobial agents. N Engl J Med 1991; 324:384–394.
30. Swanson DJ, Sung RJ, Fine MJ, et al. Erythromycin ototoxicity: prospective assessment with serum concentrations and audiograms in a study of patients with pneumonia. Am J Med 1992; 92:61–68.
31. Martyn R, Somberg JC, Kerin NZ. Proarrhythmia of nonarrhythmic drugs. Am Heart J 1993; 126:201–205.
32. Periti P, Mazzei T, Mini E, Novelli A. Pharmacokinetic drug interactions of macrolides. Clin Pharmacokinet 1992; 23:106–131.
33. Piscitelli SC, Danziger LH, Rodvold KA. Clarithromycin and azithromycin: new macrolide antibiotics. Clin Pharm 1992; 11:137–152.
34. Brown BA, Wallace RJ, Jr., Griffith DE, Girard W. Clarithromycin-induced hepatotoxicity. Clin Infect Dis 1995; 20:1073–1074.

35. Fanning WL, Gump DW, Sofferman RA. Side effects of minocycline: a double blind study. Antimicrob Agents Chemother 1977; 11:712–715
36. Walters BNJ, Gubbay SS. Tetracycline and benign intracranial hypertension: report of five cases. Br Med J 1981; 282:19–22.
37. Coxon A, Pallis CA. Metronidazole neuropathy. J Neurol Neurosurg Psych 1976; 39:403–405.
38. Jung AC, Paauw DS. Management of adverse reactions to trimethoprim-sulfamethoxazole in human immunodeficiency virus-infected patients. Arch Intern Med 1994, 154:2402–2406.
39. Jick H. Adverse reactions to trimethoprim-sulfamethoxazole in hospitalized patients. Rev Infect Dis 1982; 4:426–428.
40. Kelly JW, Dooley DP, Lattuada CP, Smith CE. A severe, unusual reaction to trimethoprim-sulfamethoxazole in patients infected with human immunodeficiency virus. Clin Infect Dis 1992; 14:1034–1039.
41. Borucki MJ, Matze DS, Pollard RB. Tremor induced by trimethoprim-sulfamethoxazole in patients with the acquired immunodeficiency syndrome (AIDS). Ann Intern Med 1988; 148:77–78.
42. Escalente A, Stimmler MM. Trimethoprim-sulfamethoxazole induced meningitis in systemic lupus erythematosus. J Rheumatol 1992; 19:800–802.
43. Centers for Disease Control and Prevention. National consensus conference on tuberculosis. Preventive treatment of tuberculosis. Chest 1985; 87(suppl 2):128–132.
44. Liebold JE. The ocular toxicity of ethambutol and its relation to dose. Ann NY Acad Sci 1966; 135: 904–909.
45. Hoeprich PD. Clinical use of amphotericin B and derivatives: lore, mystique, and fact. Clin Infect Dis 1992; 14 (suppl 1):S114–119.
46. Peacock JE, Herrington DA, Cruz JM. Amphotericin B therapy: past, present, and future. Infect Dis Clin Pract 1993; 2:81–93.
47. Goodwin SD, Cleary JD, Walawander CA, et al. Pretreatment regimens for adverse events related to infusion of amphotericin B. Clin Infect Dis 1995; 20:755–761.
48. Como JA, Dismukes WE. Oral azole drugs as systemic antifungal therapy. N Engl J Med 1994; 330:263–272.
49. Bean B, Aeppli D. Adverse effects of high-dose intravenous acyclovir in ambulatory patients with acute herpes zoster. J Infect Dis 1985; 151:362–364.
50. Faulds D, Heel RC. Ganciclovir. A review of its antiviral activity, pharmacokinetic properties and therapeutic efficacy in cytomegalovirus infections. Drugs 1990; 39:597–638.
51. Studies of Ocular Complications of AIDS Research Group. Morbidity and toxic effects associated with ganciclovir or foscarnet therapy in a randomized cytomegalovirus retinitis trial. Arch Intern Med 1995; 155:65–74.
52. Stange KC, Little DW, Blatnik B. Adverse reactions to amantadine prophylaxis of influenza in a retirement home. J Am Geriatr Assoc 1991; 39:700–705.
53. McDonald EM, Mann AH, Thomas HC. Interferons as mediators of psychiatric morbidity. Lancet 1987; 2:1175–1180.
54. Weinke T, Trautmann M, Held T. Neuropsychiatric side effects after the use of mefloquine. Am J Trop Med Hyg 1991; 45:86–91.
55. Pertel P, Hirschtick R. Adverse reactions to dapsone in persons infected with human immunodeficiency virus. Clin Infect Dis 1994; 18:630–632.
56. Tomecki KJ, Catalano CJ. Dapsone hypersensitivity: the sulfone syndrome revisited. Arch Dermatol 1981; 117:38–39.

33

Cerebrospinal Fluid in the Diagnosis of Central Nervous System Infections

Allen J. Aksamit, Jr.
Mayo Clinic and Mayo Medical School, Rochester, Minnesota

INTRODUCTION

Probably no other area of neurology relies on the results of laboratory testing as heavily for diagnosis as do central nervous system (CNS) infections. Although well-defined clinical syndromes make the diagnosis of "encephalitis" or "meningitis" possible on clinical grounds alone, the specific identification of the offending infectious agent requires microbiological testing to precisely determine treatment and prognosis. Microbiological testing has evolved as molecular techniques have evolved from culture to sophisticated means of identifying nucleic acid or protein components of the infectious agent, often present in only minuscule quantities in the cerebrospinal fluid (CSF). Often the sensitivity and specificity of these tests is not immediately available to the clinician. Information about sensitivity and specificity, however, is critical in deciding about the appropriateness of performing and interpreting the results of the test. As a corollary, a negative result is often not fully exclusionary in the context of a patient with an undefined and often serious neurological illness. This chapter will try to weigh the clinical values of specific microbiological tests in the circumstance of suspected neurological infections, with the emphasis on the polymerase chain reaction (PCR) as an evolving diagnostic tool.

Results of sensitivity and specificity studies of diagnostic microbiological CSF should be judged by the clinician who is to interpret their significance with several questions in mind. Has the diagnostic test been tested prospectively to establish utility? Have a large number of specimens been tested with positive specimens being confirmed by independent means? In some cases testing with techniques such as PCR has widened the spectrum of disease associated with an infectious agent, usually because no other confirmatory test exists or because the confirmatory test (e.g., direct culture) is highly insensitive. Nuances of individual organisms may complicate the assay involved, e.g., if the nucleic acid of the organism is inaccessible for PCR amplification because of tight binding to the bacterial cell wall.

Finally, do the clinical circumstances of the CSF specimen, e.g., high protein and cell count, interfere with the assay to reduce the sensitivity? Are "spiked" controls performed in the laboratory where the testing is performed by inoculating clinical specimens with the infectious organism and assaying to prove no inhibitory substances are present to cause false-negative results? Do negative controls tested by the assay match the clinical specimens likely to be routinely tested? These are a few of the questions that should be kept in mind when judging the usefulness of testing.

POLYMERASE CHAIN REACTION

The polymerase chain reaction has revolutionized molecular diagnostics in the CSF for infectious agents, so a short discussion of basic methodology seems warranted. The principle of the reaction is to amplify a low-abundance but unique nucleic acid sequence, in this case unique to the infectious organism targeted. The actual reaction biochemically synthesizes a 1 million–fold increase in sequence abundance of defined length. After amplification, the sequence is abundant enough to be identified based on its size characteristics and, more importantly, on its internal nucleic acid sequence.

The PCR reaction, in its most rudimentary form, consists of three steps: denaturation, annealing, and extension (actually the enzyme polymerase resynthesizes copies of the DNA with the sequence based on the presence of desired target in the reaction mixture). If the target sequence is RNA, such as in the case of a RNA virus, an initial step converting the RNA sequence to a single strand of complementary DNA is required using the enzyme reverse transcriptase.

The key to specific recognition of targeted viral or bacterial DNA sequences are the two oligonucleotide primers used in the reaction. These are short oligonucleotide sequences, usually 15–20 base pairs long, which are single stranded and complementary to opposite strands of the double-stranded DNA sequence of the targeted organism. They are oriented so that their 3′ ends will be pointing at each other when they bind to specific target sequences on opposite strands. The primers are present in excess relative to the targeted native DNA sequence.

The PCR reaction is a repetitive thermal cycling, which initially denatures (makes single stranded) the target double-stranded DNA by heating. Annealing, which occurs at a lower temperature, is binding of the primer oligonucleotides to their complementary sequences on the DNA. Extension, often performed at a third temperature, is the process of the enzyme polymerase adding free nucleotides from the reaction mixture to the 3′ end of the primers, extending them toward each other. Therefore, the 5′ end of the oligonucleotide primers will define each end of the amplified fragment produced.

The thermal cycle is then repeated 30–50 times by a thermal cycling machine ("PCR machine"). It becomes apparent that, as more templates are synthesized after a few cycles, the majority of the PCR products that will serve as subsequent template and as cycling continues will be of the length determined by the distance of the oligonucleotide primer 5′ ends from each other in the sequence.

This process of 1 million–fold amplification of the target sequences creates an abundance of a single molecular weight DNA sequence, which migrates as a band on a gel after subjecting the reaction products to electrophoresis. The DNA migration distance is specific for size and can be identified by like molecular weight markers electrophoresed at the same time.

This band of DNA is then transferred to a membrane by elution technique (Southern blotting). A third oligonucleotide, known to have a sequence similar to the internal sequence between the primers, but not overlapping them, is used as an "internal probe." This oligonucleotide is prelabeled with some biochemical marker, which will produce either radioactivity or, most commonly, electroluminescence and turn an x-ray film dark. The internal probe is allowed to find

Table 1 Polymerase Chain Reaction Utility in CNS Infections[a]

Herpes simplex virus I (herpes simplex encephalitis)
Herpes simplex virus II (HSE in neonates, recurrent meningitis)
JC virus (progressive multifocal leukoencephalopathy)
Cytomegalovirus (CMV ependymitis and polyradiculopathy associated with AIDS)
Mycobacterium tuberculosis (TB meningitis)
Borrellia burgdorferi (Lyme disease)
Tropheryma whippelii (CNS Whipple's disease)

[a]Ranked by proven utility on CSF.

its complementary sequences (hybridize), if present, in the amplified product binding to the blot. An x-ray film is then exposed to the blot to show the dark spot at the appropriate molecular size for the amplified fragment and specifically confirming it as identical to the sequence from the native organism. In an experienced laboratory, the whole process can take as little as 6 h, but more usually it is an overnight or 2-day procedure to optimize sensitivity.

Table 1 is a partial and short list of infectious agents ranked by utility which PCR performed on cerebrospinal fluid (CSF) has demonstrated some clinical usefulness in identifying the agent over conventional methods such as direct culture.

HERPES SIMPLEX VIRUS TYPE I: HERPES SIMPLEX ENCEPHALITIS

Herpes simplex encephalitis (HSE) remains the most common sporadic non–AIDS-related form of viral encephalitis of adults in the United States. Great strides have been made in the diagnosis of HSE based on PCR detection in the CSF of herpes simplex virus type I (HSV-1) DNA in infected patients. Currently, this technological breakthrough has superseded all prior diagnostic techniques in the identification of HSV-1 in the CSF including culture, antigen, and antibody assays.

One unique situation where the PCR assay is not very helpful is in the postencephalitic recovery phase of patients with encephalitis who have not had a specific agent identified. Antibody assay performed on serum and CSF can be helpful in the recovery phase between 2 weeks and 3 months after the onset of illness. A less than 20:1 serum-to-CSF ratio of specific antibodies to HSV-1 suggests intrathecal synthesis of antibodies. Elevated intrathecal antibodies are relevant in identifying the HSE in PCR-negative patients or in cases where HSE was clinically suspected and treated without specific confirmation by virological means.

PCR detection of HSV-1 in suspected cases of HSE has become the gold standard for diagnosis. A retrospective analysis of biopsy-proven cases of HSE from the Collaborative Antiviral Study Group showed that 53 of 54 (98%) patients with biopsy-proven disease by direct culture on brain tissue were PCR positive for HSV-1 when performed on CSF (1). This study follows in the wake of earlier works (2–6), all of which reported a high degree of sensitivity (90–100%), and few false-positive results. The high degree of success in the identification of HSE by PCR probably represents the high CSF viral burden. This contrasts with the experience with other disorders, such as progressive multifocal leukoencephalopathy or tuberculous meningitis.

Use of the HSV-1 PCR test on 2106 CSF specimens submitted to the Mayo Molecular Microbiology Lab for analysis revealed no false-positives, with an average turnaround time to reporting of approximately 3 days (7). Assay for HSV-1 in CSF by PCR methodology can be recommended for routine clinical use where laboratories maintain high-quality control for prevention of false-positive carry-over contamination.

Harder questions still remain concerning the use of HSV-1 PCR in certain circumstances. How long CSF shows detectable DNA by PCR after treatment of HSE is unknown. In one retrospective analysis (1), 4 of 19 (21%) CSF specimens remained positive after 2 weeks of antiviral therapy. It is unclear whether persistence of positive PCR results indicates resistance of virus with continued replication or simply remnants of DNA after active viral infection has ceased. The latter is suggested by the successful PCR amplification of HSV from brain tissue of postmortem cases of HSE.

Another challenge for PCR is sensitivity of the assay in partially treated cases of HSE. Personal experience with 2 cases of HSE showed persistently negative CSF by PCR analysis; negative after 2 and 3 days of acyclovir therapy, respectively. Both had CSF formula, MRI, and EEG changes consistent with HSE. Both improved with acyclovir treatment. By implication, the PCR assay of CSF is not as sensitive in confirming the diagnosis of HSE if treatment was started before CSF was collected.

HERPES SIMPLEX VIRUS TYPE II: NEONATAL HERPES SIMPLEX ENCEPHALITIS AND MOLLERET'S (RECURRENT) MENINGITIS

As late childhood and adult herpes simplex encephalitis (HSV-1 caused) has been diagnostically revolutionalized by PCR, so has the detection of herpes simplex type 2 (HSV-2) infections of the nervous system. The most common of these is neonatal herpes encephalitis, occurring as a consequence of a newborn child being exposed to HSV-2 during excursion through the birth canal of an infected mother with a history of herpes genitalis. In this circumstance, index of suspicion is high, and diagnosis is usually not difficult because of clinically disseminated virus infection of the infant, often with cutaneous manifestations.

The primers currently in routine use for PCR amplification of HSV will not routinely distinguish between type 1 and type 2, because there is significant genetic overlap between the two viruses. However, the identification of HSV in CSF in the clinical context of the newborn period allows identification on clinical grounds alone, presumptively as HSV-2–related neonatal encephalitis (8).

HSV-2 amplification from CSF by PCR has been shown to be highly sensitive and specific for the virus. Therefore, as with HSV-1–related encephalitis, the short turnaround time allows for early presumptive diagnosis and initiation of antiviral therapy.

A more recently recognized and rarer complication of HSV-2 infection has been the syndrome of recurrent "aseptic" meningitis. It is unknown if HSV-2 recurrent meningitis accounts for all cases of what was formerly referred to as Molleret's meningitis, but PCR amplification of HSV-2 from spinal fluid has clearly established that link (9–11). This is an instance where the PCR technology has defined the nature of an unknown form of recurrent meningitis because of its sensitivity and specificity.

JC VIRUS: PROGRESSIVE MULTIFOCAL LEUKOENCEPHALOPATHY

Progressive multifocal leukoencephalopathy (PML) is a primary viral infection of oligodendrocytes and astrocytes of the cerebral hemispheres, brain stem, and cerebellum. Foci of lytic destruction of oligodendrocytes cause coalescing areas of demyelination. The etiological virus,

JC virus (named for the initials of the first PML patient to have this papovavirus isolated from his brain), is an opportunistic pathogen only causing neurological disease in the case of impaired cell-mediated immunity, e.g., AIDS, lymphoreticular malignancy, organ transplantation.

Spinal fluid findings are usually normal in patients with PML. A mild elevation of total protein, usually less than 100 mg/dl, is present in 25% of patients. Cell counts are usually normal, and an abnormality should alert the clinician to the possibility of another infection. Cell count can be elevated, usually less than 25 cells/mm^3, in 10% of cases and may correlate with a more active inflammatory response to the virus in the nervous system. Oligoclonal banding or intrathecal synthesis of IgG has been very rarely reported. Spinal fluid glucose is normal.

Direct culture of JC virus (JCV) from the CSF is impossible because the virus is only able to be grown in human-derived glial cells, available only in a few research laboratories. Also, attempts to culture virus from CSF of PML patients on susceptible cells have been unsuccessful, presumably because of low abundance.

PCR has been used to amplify JCV DNA from the CSF of PML patients. Concern over the use of this assay was initially raised because of possible detection of a reactivated virus from a latent state in the nervous system triggered by immunosuppression without clinically significant disease. However, current studies show that spinal fluid detection of JCV is specific for pathologically significant PML (12–17). All of these studies were retrospective analyses of CSF specimens of patients with either pathologically confirmed or clinically suspected PML, based on MRI scan and coincident underlying immunosuppressive illness, usually AIDS. Sensitivity was collectively not 100% (Table 2). Specifically, combining the data from each of the studies shows that 114 of 150 PML patients (76%) were correctly diagnosed by this assay. Questions can be asked about the technique to explain why false negatives occurred, including storage and handling of specimens, small volume of spinal fluid assayed, inhibitors in the CSF, and loss of DNA in performing CSF concentration, but the false negatives most likely represent low abundance of virus in the CSF.

Because of the intrinsic sensitivity of the PCR assay, contamination of clinical specimens, either as they are gathered or more commonly in the laboratory where the assay is performed (so-called carry-over), requires constant vigilance and attention to strict isolation procedures. Small amounts of DNA previously amplified from prior reactions can serve as templates for the PCR reaction. In experienced laboratories, however, false-positive rates are low. Again, combining the collective data from six studies (12–17), the false-positive rate of identifying CSF specimens from AIDS patients without PML or other controls as having JCV is 14 of 725 (2%). Therefore, given an experienced lab, PCR positive results are very helpful in identifying a patient with PML. PCR for JCV, however, should not be done in small-volume laboratories. This analysis is available for diagnostic use in some large diagnostic centers (e.g., Mayo Medical Laboratories).

Table 2 **PCR Analysis of JCV in CSF of PML Patients**

	True positives		False positives		Ref.
	24/26	(92%)	11/130	(8%)	12
	23/28	(82%)	0/83	(0%)	13
	9/9	(100%)	0/3	(0%)	14
	17/23	(73%)	2/48	(2%)	15
	10/13	(76%)	0/42	(0%)	16
	31/51	(61%)	1/419	(0.2%)	17
Total	114/150	(76%)	14/725	(2%)	

From a clinical standpoint, PCR analysis of CSF that is positive for JC virus effectively establishes the diagnosis of clinically significant PML. A negative result does not exclude the diagnosis.

Clinical and imaging correlation are important in interpreting results. The current incomplete sensitivity of the assay is more desirable than a higher incidence of false positives. In PML, the only alternative to CSF identification of JCV is brain biopsy to prove the diagnosis. As newer antivirals evolve that may be effective against JCV, the importance of establishing the diagnosis noninvasively will become increasingly more important.

CYTOMEGALOVIRUS: EPENDYMITIS AND POLYRADICULOPATHY ASSOCIATED WITH AIDS

A novel disease in adults that became more evident with the onset of the AIDS epidemic was nervous system infection with cytomegalovirus (CMV). The principal manifestations of this infection in the nervous system are an ascending subacute polyradiculopathy (18–27) or a subacute to chronic ependymitis/encephalitis (28–34). Though the clinical aspects are quite different (a polyradiculopathy vs. an encephalitis) a number of CSF-related abnormalities are shared by both entities. First, the manifestations usually evolve subacutely. Second, in both entities there is commonly a marked ependymal abnormality on gadolinium-enhanced MRI scan of the head. It appears as a striking gadolinium-enhanced outline of the ependymal surface of the ventricular system including the lateral, third, and fourth ventricles of the brain (34). This occurs because of the fulminant infection of the ependyma and is disseminated through the nervous system via the CSF pathways, presumably by primary infection of the choroid plexus (29,34). This can be present even when the primary manifestation is cauda equina–type ascending weakness. Third, the CSF reaction is atypical for viral infections of the nervous system because of the marked neutrophilic reaction and low CSF glucose (Table 3). The reaction mimics that seen in bacterial, TB, or fungal meningitis, and these need to be distinguished by microbiological means. Fourth, because of the prominent infection along CSF pathways, CMV is easily detectable by PCR methodology, in contrast to direct culture technique.

Clinically, the polyradiculopathy presents as a fulminant asymmetrical cauda equina syndrome, often with early sphincter involvement and prominent ascending weakness beginning in the lower extremities (18–27). The ependymitis/encephalitis, by contrast, presents with subacute headache, encephalopathy, and sometimes fever, and can have accompanying cranial nerve palsy (28–34). Both may occur in the same patient.

A compilation of 7 studies on ependymitis/encephalitis is contrasted with the CSF findings of 10 studies of polyradiculopathy in Table 3. The spinal fluid reaction in both CMV disorders often show a prominent pleocytosis, with a predominence of neutrophils, averaging about 60% of the differential. The degree of cell reaction tends to be greater associated with polyradiculopathy,

Table 3 CSF Findings in CMV Infection in AIDS

	Mean protein (range)	Mean glucose (range)	Mean cell count (range)	% PMNs (range)	Ref.
CMV encephalitis/ ependymitis	104 mg% (16–524)	43 mg% (11–57)	186/mm^3 (0-3179)	59% (20–85%)	28–34
CMV polyradiculopathy	278 mg% (67–920)	34 mg% (15–47)	545/mm^3 (45–1722)	62% (7–94%)	18–27

averaging >500 cells/mm^3 as compared to 200 cells/mm^3 with encephalitis. Protein levels are also elevated in the 100–300 mg% range, though encephalitis patients can sometimes have normal CSF protein concentrations. The glucose concentration is usually depressed and the level tends to coincide with the degree of the polymorphonuclear reaction.

The polymerase chain reaction has proven highly sensitive and specific in the diagnosis of CMV-CNS infection. PCR sensitivity is in the range of 79 to 100% based on studies of CSF from patients confirmed with CMV-related disease (35–37). No false-positives were identified, although in those studies there were some patients with positive CSF for CMV who were suspected of having CMV infection, but who did not have pathological or culture confirmation of CMV infection. The possibility of a false-positive result must be kept in mind because of the frequency of CMV viremia or retinitis in these patients, which may contaminate the CSF results at the time of collection. A prospective study of PCR on CSF, designed to answer that question (38), again confirmed the sensitivity of the assay. Twenty-four of 26 patients with confirmed neurological disease related to CMV (92%) were positive by PCR CSF amplification. However, 4 of 62 patients (6%) without CMV, but who had other confirmed HIV-related neurological disease, were also positive, presumably representing false-positive results.

Currently, the PCR test for amplification of CMV from the CSF can be recommended as a useful test in the analysis of patients with AIDS-related neurological diseases. This is especially true for the clinical circumstance of a CSF formula which is suggestive of CMV infection, with prominent leukocytosis and hypoglycorrachia. The high sensitivity of 90–100% detection is more sensitive than the rate of CMV detection by direct culture, usually quoted as no greater than 50% in pathologically proven cases. False-positive results need to be kept in mind as a possibility if other clinical characteristics suggest features not typical for CMV infection.

MYCOBACTERIUM TUBERCULOSIS: TUBERCULOUS MENINGITIS

The diagnosis of tuberculous meningitis (TBM) remains enigmatic because of the difficulty in culturing the organism from spinal fluid. Yet, spinal fluid identification of *Mycobacterium tuberculosis* is the only way to specifically confirm the diagnosis and render proper treatment.

The spinal fluid formula from patients with TBM has classically been called "granulomatous," based on the subacute development of abnormalities and predominance of lymphocytic pleocytosis. However, as there is some variability to the temporal profile of the illness, i.e., sometimes being acute and at other times much more chronic, the CSF pattern of reaction cannot be relied upon to specifically identify TBM.

Recent clinical series of CSF abnormalities published from both non–HIV- and HIV-related TBM patients, have not suggested a change in the findings of the CSF formula (39–43). Mean protein elevations range from 65 to 504 mg%, with most in the 100–200 mg% range (Table 4). In 10–38% of patients the protein concentration can be normal. With extreme exudative reaction and block of CSF pathways, especially at spinal levels, protein concentration can be very high, exceeding 1 g/dl, and produce a clot or pellicle in a standing CSF tube (Froin's syndrome) because of the presence of serum clotting factors, normally not present in the spinal fluid.

CSF glucose is usually low in TBM. An absolute concentration of glucose below 40 mg% is suggestive of a pathological reaction, as is a value of <40% of serum levels in euglycemic individuals. The understanding of the mechanisms of low CSF glucose concentration is evolving, but low CSF glucose concentrations in inflammatory conditions is most likely because of consumption of glucose by organisms or white blood cells, but rather secondary to a shut-down in the CSF glucose transporter system as part of the inflammatory reaction. In TBM, mean glucose values range from 22 to 38 mg% (Table 4), but 12–15% of patients may have normal glucose

Table 4 CSF Findings in Tuberculosis Meningitis

Protein	Glucose	Cells	Positive AFB smear (%)	Ref.
10–300 mg% (median 65)	0–52 mg% (median 22)	0–1200/mm³ (median 242)	24	39 (HIV and non-HIV)
20–1837 mg% (median 214)	7–80 mg% (median 16)	4–672/mm³ (median 159)	20	40 (HIV)
11–527 mg% (mean 176)	9–100 mg% (mean 33)	1–4000/mm³ (mean 270)	4	41 (mostly non-HIV)
21–1500 mg% (mean 247)		1–340/mm³ (mean 116)	18	42 (non-HIV)
35–2900 mg% (mean 145)	7–189 mg% (mean 38)	0–8600/mm³ (median 181)	10	43 (mostly non-HIV)

concentrations (39,41). Only rare patients with TBM, even severely immunosuppressed patients (e.g., AIDS), will have entirely normal CSF formulas.

Cellular reaction in the CSF is usually lymphocytic. However, polymorphonuclear cells can predominate in up to 32% of patients (42). The presence of polymorphonuclear cells does not necessarily correlate with the acuteness of the clinical evolution of symptoms but does correlate with worse clinical signs (41). Mean cell counts are in the range of 110–270 cells/mm³ (Table 4), but total cell count in individual cases can be as high as 4000 cells/mm³. Seven to 9% will have normal CSF cell counts (39,41).

Smears performed on CSF for acid-fast bacilli (AFB) have been reported in older publications to have a sensitivity of up to 87%. However, the more routine use of AFB stains in clinical laboratories in the last 15 years only have a sensitivity of 4–24% (Table 4). The sensitivity of the staining technique is enhanced by centrifugation of large volumes of CSF onto a single slide for staining and tedious intensive examination of the stained pellet for organisms.

Other abnormalities in CSF have been described in TBM including an elevation in adenosine deaminase levels, a decrease in chloride levels, or elevated CSF bromide levels after systemic infusion, all representing nonspecific effects of inflammation or breakdown in the blood-brain barrier.

CSF culture for *Mycobacterium tuberculosis* remains the gold standard to which other methods of identification of the organism must be compared. From a practical clinical standpoint, however, the culture is incompletely sensitive based on clinical criteria (i.e., systemic signs of tuberculosis and response of CSF parameters to antituberculous therapy). Also, isolation of *M. tuberculosis* from TBM patients requires long incubation times, often 2–6 weeks after the CSF has been collected, for the culture to turn positive. This latency before specific identification of the organism makes clinical treatment decisions difficult when faced with a sick patient with deteriorating neurological status.

Examination of CSF for tubulostearic acid by gas-liquid chromatography has not gained widespread use as a specific test for the identification of *M. tuberculosis* in CSF because of technical complexity in the performance and interpretation of the assay (44).

IgG antibody against *M. tuberculosis* in spinal fluid has been assayed for by enzyme-linked immunosorbent assay (ELISA) (45). However, the assay is insensitive, particularly at the early stages of the illness, because of the lag period between the onset of illness and intrathecal synthesis of antibody that is maximal 30 days after the onset of illness (46). Sensitivity of ELISA assay for antibodies in the CSF of bona fide cases of TBM sampled randomly relative to the timing of the onset of the clinical syndrome ranges from 60 to 80%, with a 5% false-positive rate (46). Immunoblot assay (Western blot of CSF) for anti-TB antibodies have shown a higher specificity (no false positives) and good sensitivity when the assay was performed on CSF from culture-positive patients (47). However, in this study, the patients had antibiotic treatment of disease for at least 2–4 weeks before the CSF was assayed, raising the possibility that sensitivity earlier in the course of disease might not have been as good.

The PCR detection of *M. tuberculosis* DNA in the CSF holds the greatest promise, and yet has not fully realized its potential, as a rapid and sensitive diagnostic tool in tuberculous meningitis. Because of PCR sensitivity and the low abundance of the tubercle bacillus in the CSF, the test and tuberculous meningitis seem ideally matched. Likewise, the rapidity with which PCR can be performed, and the amplified products identified as specific for TB, would be a great improvement over culture techniques and insensitive acid-fast stains. However, practical application of this technique to the diagnosis of TBM has proven to be difficult. A representative, though not all-inclusive, summary of the experience with this technique is given in Table 5. PCR detection of TB in the CSF from TBM patients has ranged from 32 to 100% (48–55), with a median sensitivity across studies of 70–80%. Collectively, however, when summarizing the total of the patients reported in the reviewed experience, only 54% of all TBM had a positive test. However, this is twice as sensitive as TB culture (24%) on the same patient population. This "TB culture-negative" population of patients were mainly patients with CSF formulas compatible with TB, who sometimes had extra-neural tuberculosis and showed clinical response to antituberculous therapy. This points out a discrepency in TBM—direct culture of CSF is thought to be notoriously insensitive, and PCR becomes the disease-defining test, making an interpretation and comparison of the existing PCR data difficult. In addition, because PCR is so sensitive, false-positive results can occur: 8% in the studies quoted, with a range of 0–62%, with two of the eight studies quoted accounting for all of the false-positive results (Table 5).

Enthusiasm for PCR confirmation of TBM has to be further attenuated because of variability between laboratories (56,57), and inconsistent standards. These studies examined the unreliability of PCR to accurately determine the presence of tuberculosis and led the Food and Drug Administration to withhold recommendation of this test for routine clinical use.

Not all of the technical variables have been fully explored at this time. A study (51) with PCR-nested primers (i.e., amplified twice) suggested a greater sensitivity (90%) without an increase in

Table 5 CSF PCR Detection of TB in TB Meningitis Compared to Culture

	TB detected in CSF by PCR		Culture positive		False positive in CSF by PCR		Ref.
	5/6	(83%)	2/6	(33%)	0/10	(0%)	48
	22/34	(65%)	4/34	(12%)	6/51	(12%)	49
	9/11	(82%)	5/9	(55%)	0/14	(0%)	50
	19/21	(90%)	6/21	(29%)	0/79	(0%)	51
	6/6	(100%)	4/6	(67%)	13/21	(62%)	52
	11/23	(48%)	9/25	(39%)	0/19	(0%)	53
	15/20	(75%)	4/20	(20%)	0/27	(0%)	54
	32/99	(32%)	18/99	(18%)	0/28	(0%)	55
Total	119/220	(54%)	52/220	(24%)	19/249	(8%)	

false-positive rates (0 of 79 controls). This approach needs to be confirmed across a wider experience before it is known if it will replace TB cultures as a means of diagnosis.

Currently, PCR for TB in the CSF from suspected TBM patients cannot be routinely recommended. However, PCR testing done in large laboratories, with high volume and standardized controls may soon be the norm for establishing TBM.

Borrelia burgdorferi: NERVOUS SYSTEM LYME DISEASE

Probably no other single problem is as difficult diagnostically from the neurological infectious disease standpoint as CSF studies performed to confirm the diagnosis of nervous system involvement by Lyme disease or neuroborreliosis. The difficulty is fueled by patient expectation to explain chronic neurological or nonspecific symptoms attributed to Lyme disease based on lay literature reading, reports in the medical literature of negative testing in bona fide cases of CNS Lyme disease, and a lack of a standardized or definitive means of testing for nervous system involvement. Spinal fluid, however, is the best hope for clarifying this diagnostic dilemma.

For most cases of neuroborreliosis presenting with well-identified clinical syndromes of facial palsy (which can be bilateral), polyradiculopathy, meningitis, encephalitis, or myelitis, the spinal fluid is abnormal with an elevation of total protein. The protein concentration has a median value of 42–115mg% in patients with meningitis, radiculitis, or cranial neuritis (58–60). CSF protein values from patients with focal encephalitis tend to be lower with median values of 38 mg% (59). Glucose is routinely normal, although values as low as 35 mg% have been reported (58). The cell count is elevated, with a predominance of lymphocytes. Cell counts range from 0 to 1830 cells/mm^3, with median cell counts from different studies in patients with meningoradiculitis ranging from 11 to 166 cells/mm^3 (58–61). Again, patients with focal encephalitis tend to have a lower or normal cell counts. In one study, 11 of 35 (31%) patients had abnormal cell counts with a range of values of 0–1830 cells/mm^3 (59). There are routine changes indicative of intrathecal antibody synthesis with elevated IgG index, IgG synthesis rate, and CSF oligoclonal banding (58). The intrathecal synthesis of antibody is against the Lyme disease agent *Borrelia burgdorferi* (62–64). However, the sensitivity of this assay across a spectrum of neuroborreliosis patients confirmed by an independent means has not been prospectively evaluated. This is further complicated by nuances in performing the serology with variability between laboratories performing the assay on the same specimen (65). Also, because myelopathy, meningitis, or other neurological syndromes can be caused by other diseases, which can be associated with nonspecific intrathecal immunoglobulin synthesis (i.e., multiple sclerosis), paired serology for Lyme disease performed on the serum and CSF simultaneously are presently the best means of establishing an immunologically based diagnosis. Although a normal CSF formula, combined with seronegativity in both blood and CSF, does not fully exclude a diagnosis of neuroborreliosis, it is currently the best battery of tests available to evaluate patients with compatible neurological syndromes for Lyme disease in the nervous system.

A more problematic situation is the clinical distinction of patients with Lyme-related encephalopathy without overt CSF abnormalities. Cognitive changes secondary to Lyme systemic infection may be difficult to distinguish from neurocognitive complaints from non–Lyme-related diseases. Spinal fluid protein, cell count, and IgG index have been reported to be normal in Lyme-related encephalopathy (66,67). Intrathecal antibody synthesis has had a better correlation with patients who may have this syndrome, although only 17% will have laboratory evidence of intrathecal antibody synthesis (66).

Even more bothersome are rare reports of culture-positive isolation of *Borrelia burgdorferi* from CSF after treatment of Lyme disease with entirely normal CSF studies (68). Presumably this represents a rare circumstance, and it is hoped that more sensitive methods for detection of the organism directly, when more routinely applied, i.e., PCR or antigen detection (vide infra), will capture these cases.

PCR performed on the CSF for the diagnosis of neuroborreliosis has had mixed success with variability between laboratories. At least one laboratory has reported positive results with a sensitivity of 90% and 75% detection of *Borrelia burgdorferi* in Lyme encephalopathy and inflammatory CNS disease (i.e., meningitis, encephalitis, myelitis), respectively (69). Other laboratories have had less success in reproducing these results with detection rates in the 40–48% range (70,71). Currently, PCR for Lyme involvement of the nervous system should be regarded as an adjunctive test. It is helpful when positive, but when negative it does not exclude clinically significant disease secondary to *Borrelia burgdorferi*.

Another direct detection method is the detection of *Borrelia burgdorferi* antigen in the spinal fluid. Sensitivity has been reported to be as high as 49 or 55% when performed by ELISA method or Western blot detection, respectively (72). This is a technically more difficult assay, with regard to both the labor required to perform it and standardization, with a high degree of consistency, as compared to PCR. Currently, this technique should be regarded as investigational and, however promising, should be performed only in highly specialized, high-volume laboratories.

WHIPPLE'S DISEASE-ASSOCIATED BACILLUS (*Tropheryma whippelii*): CENTRAL NERVOUS SYSTEM WHIPPLE'S DISEASE

Central nervous system involvement in the systemic disorder Whipple's disease is an enigmatic diagnostic entity, which is evolving because of advances in CSF diagnosis by polymerase chain reaction. Classically, Whipple's disease in the nervous system has been associated with vertical conjugate gaze palsy and variably with subacute dementia, seizures, and cerebellar abnormalities. CSF has often been normal or showed only a minimal elevation of protein concentration (<70 mg%). Cell count in the CSF is likewise normal, although isolated cases have been shown to have a mild pleocytosis, usually less than 20 cells/mm^3.

Evaluation of gastrointestinal and lymphatic tissues by PCR techniques has led to the further characterization of the rod-shaped bacillus, and the organism has been designated *Tropheryma whippelii* (73). The identification of the organism and specific PCR primers have allowed for amplification of DNA for diagnostic purposes not only from gastrointestinal and lymphatic tissue, but also from CSF.

We recently encountered three patients—one with subacute dementia and vertical gaze paresis, a second with vertical gaze palsy and a chronic progressive cerebellar deficit, and a third with subacute dementia and findings of chronic meningitis—whose CSF was analyzed by PCR for Whipple's agent with positive results. Since the nervous system can be affected clinically in isolation (74), this test is useful in clinically suspicious cases where jejunal or lymphatic tissue biopsy is negative and there is no alternative diagnostic option short of brain biopsy. Standardization of this assay by analysis of a large number of CSF samples from appropriate control subjects remains to be done. However, this is a very promising assay for a rare and previously difficult to diagnose clinical entity.

REFERENCES

1. Lakeman FD, Whitley RJ. Diagnosis of herpes simplex encephalitis: application of polymerase chain reaction to cerebrospinal fluid from brain-biopsied patients and correlation with disease. J Infect Dis 1995; 171:857–863.
2. Aurelius E, Johansson B, Sköldenberg B, Staland A, Forsgren M. Rapid diagnosis of herpes simplex

encephalitis by nested polymerase chain reaction assay of cerebrospinal fluid. Lancet 1991; 337: 189–192.
3. Rowley AH, Whitley RJ, Lakeman FD, Wolinsky SM. Rapid detection of herpes-simplex virus DNA in cerebrospinal fluid of patients with herpes simplex encephalitis. Lancet 1990; 335:440–441.
4. Rozenberg F, Lebon P. Amplification and characterization of herpes virus DNA in cerebrospinal fluid from patients with acute encephalitis. J Clin Microbiol 1991; 29:2412–2417.
5. Pohl-Koppe A, Dahm C, Elgas M, Kuhn E, Brawn RW, Meulen V. The diagnostic significance of the polymerase chain reaction and isoelectric focusing in herpes simplex virus encephalitis. J Med Virol 1992; 36:147–154.
6. Klapper PE, Cleator GM, Dennett C, Lewis AG. Diagnosis of herpes encephalitis via Southern blotting of cerebrospinal fluid DNA amplified by polymerase chain reaction. J Med Virol 1990; 32:261–264.
7. Mitchell PS, Thorvilson JN, Keach NK, Rys PN, Espy MJ, Persing DH, Smith TF. Routine laboratory detection of herpes simplex virus (HSV) DNA in cerebrospinal fluid (CSF) from patients with central nervous system disease (abstract). American Society for Microbiology, May 1996.
8. Kimura H, Futamura M, Kito H, Ando T, Goto M, Kuzushima K, Shibata M, Morishima T. Detection of viral DNA in neonatal herpes simplex virus infections: frequent and prolonged presence in serum and cerebrospinal fluid. J Infect Dis 1991; 164:289–293.
9. Tedder DG, Ashley R, Tyler KL, Levin MJ. Herpes simplex virus infection as a cause of benign recurrent lymphocytic meningitis. Ann Intern Med 1994; 121:334–338.
10. Picard FJ, Dekaban GA, Silva J, Rice GPA. Molleret's meningitis associated with herpes simplex type 2 infection. Neurology 1993; 43:1722–1727.
11. Lortholary O, Rozenberg F, Perrone C, Djebbour S, Leport C, Vilde JL. Herpes simplex virus type 2 DNA in cerebrospinal fluid of a woman with recurrent meningitis. Clin Infect Dis 1993; 17:941–942.
12. McGuire D, Barhite S, Hollander H, Mil M. JC virus DNA in cerebrospinal fluid of human immunodeficiency virus-infected patients: predictive value for progressive multifocal leukoencephalopathy. Ann Neurol 1995; 37:395–399.
13. Weber T, Turner RW, Frye S, Ruf B, Haas J, Schielke E, Pohle HD, Luke W, Luer W, Felgenhacrer K, Hunamann G. Specific diagnosis of progressive multifocal leukoencephalopathy by polymerase chain reaction. J Infect Dis 1994; 169:1138–1141.
14. Moret H, Ginchard M, Matheson S, Katlama C, Sazdovitch V, Huraux JM, Ingraud D. Virologic diagnosis of progressive multifocal leukoencephalopathy: detection of JC virus DNA in cerebrospinal fluid and brain tissue of AIDS patients. J Clin Microbiol 1993; 31:3310–3313.
15. Fong IW, Britton CB, Luinstra KE, Toma E, Mahony JB: Diagnostic value of detecting JC virus DNA in cerebrospinal fluid of patients with progressive multifocal leukoencephalopathy. J Clin Microbiol 1995; 33:484–486.
16. Gibson PE, Knowles WA, Hand JF, Brown DWG. Detection of JC virus DNA in the cerebrospinal fluid of patients with progressive multifocal leukoencephalopathy. J Med Virol 1993; 39:278–281.
17. Aksamit AJ, Kost SJ. Polymerase chain reaction detection of JC virus in progressive multifocal leukoencephalopathy and control cerebrospinal fluid. J Clin Microbiol
18. Bishopric G, Bruner J, Butler J. Guillain-Barré syndrome with cytomegalovirus infection of peripheral nerves. Arch Path Lab Med 1985; 109:1106–1108.
19. Eidelberg D, Sotrel A, Vogel H, Walker P, Klufield J, Crumpacker CS. Progressive polyradiculopathy in acquired immune deficiency syndrome. Neurology 1986; 36:912–916.
20. Bagley PH, Scott DA, Smith LS, Schillaci RF. Cytomegalovirus infection, ascending myelitis and pulmonary embolus. Ann Intern Med 1986; 104:587.
21. Behar R, Wiley C, McCutchan JA. Cytomegalovirus polyradiculopathy in acquired immune deficiency syndrome. Neurology 1987; 37:557–561.
22. Mahieux F, Gray F, Fenelon G, Gherardi R, Adams D, Guillard A, Porier J. Acute myeloradiculitis due to cytomegalovirus as the initial manifestation of AIDS. J Neurol Neurosurg Psychiatry 1989; 52: 270–274.
23. Graveleau P, Perol R, Chapman A. Regression of cauda equina syndrome in AIDS patient being treated with ganciclovir. Lancet 1989; 2:511–512.

24. Jacobson MA, Mills J, Rush J, O'Donnell JJ, Miller RG, Greco C, Gonzales MF. Failure of antiviral therapy for acquired immunodeficiency syndrome-related cytomegalovirus myelitis. Arch Neurol 1988; 45:1090–1092.
25. de Gans J, Tiessens G, Portegies P, Tutuarima JA, Troost D. Predominence of polymorphonuclear leukocytes in cerebrospinal fluid of AIDS patients with cytomegalovirus polyradiculitis. J AIDS 1990; 3:1155–1158.
26. Miller RG, Storey JR, Greco CM. Ganciclovir in the treatment of progressive AIDS-related polyradiculopathy. Neurology 1990; 40:569–574.
27. Clifford DB, Buller RS, Mohammed S, Robison L, Storch GA. Use of polymerase chain reaction to demonstrate cytomegalovirus DNA in CSF of patients with human immunodeficiency virus infection. Neurology 1993; 43:75–79.
28. Edwards H, Messing R, McKendall RR. Cytomegalovirus meningoencephalitis in a homosexual man with Kaposi's sarcoma: isolation of CMV from CSF cells. Neurology 1985; 35:560–562.
29. Wiley CA, Schrier RD, Denaro FJ, Nelson JA, Lampert PW, Oldstone MBA. Localization of cytomegalovirus proteins and genome during fulminant central nervous system infection in an AIDS patient. J Neuropathol Exp Neurol 1986; 45:127–139.
30. Laskin OL, Stahl-Baylise CM, Morgello S. Concomitant herpes simplex virus type 1 and cytomegalovirus ventriculoencephalitis in acquired immunodeficiency syndrome. Arch Neurol 1987 44:843–847.
31. Masden JC, Small CB, Weiss L, Elkin CM, Llena J, Mesa-Tejada R. Multifocal cytomegalovirus encephalitis in AIDS. Ann Neurol 1988; 23:97–99.
32. Fuller GN, Guiloff RJ, Scaravilli F, Harcourt-Webster JN. Combined HIV-CMV encephalitis presenting with brain stem signs. J Neurol Neurosurg Psychiatry 1989; 52:975–979.
33. Belec L, Gray F, Mikol J, Scaravilli F, Mhiri C, Sobel A, Poirer J. Cytomegalovirus (CMV) encephalomyeloradiculitis and human immunodeficiency virus (HIV) encephalitis: presence of HIV and CMV coinfected multinucleated giant cells. Acta Neuropathol 1990; 81:99–104.
34. Holland NR, Power C, Mathews VP, Glass JD, Forman M, McArthur JC. Cytomegalovirus encephalitis in acquired immunodeficiency syndrome (AIDS). Neurology 1994; 44:507–514.
35. Cinque P, Vago L, Brytting M, Castagna A, Accordini A, Sunquist V-A, Zanchetta N, D'Arminio Monforte A, Wahren B, Lazzarin A, Linde A. Cytomegalovirus infection of the central nervous system in patients with AIDS: diagnosis by DNA amplification from cerebrospinal fluid. J Infect Dis 1992; 166 1408–1411.
36. Wolf DG, Spector SA. Diagnosis of human cytomegalovirus central nervous system disease in AIDS patients by DNA amplification from cerebrospinal fluid. J Infect Dis 1992; 166:1412–1415.
37. Gozlan J, Salord J-M, Roullet E, Baudrimont M, Caburet F, Picard O, Meydias M-C, Duvivier C, Jacomet C, Petit J-C. Rapid detection of cytomegalovirus DNA in cerebrospinal fluid of AIDS patients with neurologic disorders. J Infect Dis 1992; 166:1416–1421.
38. Gozlan J, Amrani ME, Baudrimont M, Castagliola D, Salord JM, Durinier C, Picard O, Meyohas M-C, Jacomet C, Schneider-Fauveau V, Petit J-C, Roullet E. A prospective evaluation of clinical criteria and polymerase chain reaction assay of cerebrospinal fluid for the diagnosis of cytomegalovirus-related neurological diseases in AIDS. AIDS 1995; 9:253–260.
39. Berenguer J, Moreno S, Laguna F, Vicente T, Adrados M, Ortega A, Gonzalez-LaHoz J, Bouza E. Tuberculous meningitis in patients infected with the human immunodeficiency virus. N Engl J Med 1992; 326:668–672.
40. Bishburg E, Sunderam G, Reichman LB, Kapila R. Central nervous system tuberculosis with the acquired immunodeficiency syndrome and its related complex. Ann Intern Med 1986; 105:210–213.
41. Davis LE, Rastogi KR, Lambert LC, Skipper BJ. Tuberculous meningitis in the southwest United States: a community-based study. Neurology 1993; 43:1775–1778.
42. Stocksill MT, Kaufman CA. Comparison of cryptococcal and tuberculous meningitis. Arch Neurol 1983; 40:81–85.
43. Ogawa SK, Smith MA, Brennessel DJ, Lowy FD. Tuberculous meningitis in an urban medical center. Medicine 1987; 66:317–326.

44. Brooks JB, Edman DC, Alley CC, Craven RB, Girgis NI. Frequency-pulsed electron capture gas-liquid chromatography and the tryptophan color test for rapid diagnosis of tuberculosis and other forms of lymphocytic meningitis. J Clin Microbiol 1980; 12:208–215.
45. Kalish SB, Radin RC, Levitz D, Zeiss CR, Phair JP. The enzyme-linked immunosorbent assay method for IgG antibody to purified protein derivative in cerebrospinal fluid of patients with tuberculous meningitis. Ann Intern Med 1983; 99:630–633.
46. Kadival GV, Kameswaran M, Doshi R, Todiwala SS, Samuel AM. Detection of antibodies to defined M. tuberculosis antigen (38kDa) in cerebrospinal fluids of patients with tuberculous meningitis. Int J Med Microbiol Virol Parasitol Infect Dis 1994; 281:95–101.
47. Mathai A, Redhakrishnan VV, Shobha S. Diagnosis of tuberculous meningitis confirmed by means of an immunoblot method. J Infect 1994; 29:33–39.
48. Kaneko K, Onodera O, Miyafake T, Tsuji S. Rapid diagnosis of tuberculous meningitis by polymerase chain reaction (PCR). Neurology 1990; 40:1617–1618.
49. Shankar P, Manjunath N, Mohan KK, Prasad K, Behari M, Shiriniwas, Ahuja GK. Rapid diagnosis of tuberculous meningitis by polymerase chain reaction. Lancet 1991; 337:5–7.
50. Folgueria L, Delgado R, Palengue E, Noriega AR. Polymerase chain reaction for rapid diagnosis of tuberculous meningitis in AIDS patients. Neurology 1994; 44:1336–1338.
51. Liu PY-F, Shi Z-Y, Lau Y-J, Hu B-S. Rapid diagnosis of tuberculous meningitis by a simplified nested amplification protocol. Neurology 1994; 44:1161–1164.
52. Lee BW, Tan JA, Wong SC, Tan CB, Yap HK, Low PS, Chia JN, Tay JS. DNA amplification by the polymerase chain reaction for the rapid diagnosis of tuberculous meningitis. J Neurol Sci 1994; 23: 173–179.
53. Kox LFF, Kuijper Ing S, Kolk AHJ. Early diagnosis of tuberculous meningitis by polymerase chain reaction. Neurology 1995; 45:2228–2232.
54. Lin JJ, Harn HJ, Hsu YD, Tsao WL, Lee HS, Lee WH. Rapid diagnosis of tuberculous meningitis by polymerase chain reaction assay of cerebrospinal fluid. J Neurol 1995; 242:147–152.
55. Nguyen LN, Kox LFF, Pham LD, Kuijper Ing S, Kolk AHJ. The potential contribution of the polymerase chain reaction to the diagnosis of tuberculous meningitis. Arch Neurol 1996; 53:771–776.
56. Noordloek GT, van Embden JDA, Kolk AH. Questionable reliability of the polymerase chain reaction in the detection of Mycobacterium tuberculosis. N Engl J Med 1993; 329:2036.
57. Macher A, Goosby E. PCR and the misdiagnosis of active tuberculosis. N Engl J Med 1995; 332: 128–129.
58. Pachner AR, Steere AC. The triad of neurologic manifestations of Lyme disease: meningitis, cranial neuritis and radiculoneuritis. Neurology 1985; 35:47–53.
59. Halperin JJ, Volkman DJ, Wer P. Central nervous system abnormalities in Lyme neuroborreliosis. Neurology 1991; 41:1571–1582.
60. Vallat JM, Hugon J, Lubeau M, Leboutet MJ, Dumas M, Desproges-Gotteron R. Tick-bite meningoradiculitis: clinical, electrophysiologic and histologic findings in ten cases. Neurology 1987; 37:749–753.
61. Weller M, Stevens A, Sommer N, Wiethölter H, Dichgans. Cerebrospinal fluid interleukins, immunoglobulins, and fibronectins in neuroborreliosis. Arch Neurol 1991; 48:837–841.
62. Wilske B, Scheirz G, Preac-Mursic V, von Busch K, Kühbeck R, Pfister H-W, Einhaüpl K. Intrathecal production of specific antibodies against Borrelia burgdorferi in patients with lymphocytic meningoradiculitis (Bannworth's syndrome). J Infect Dis 1986; 153:304–313.
63. Henriksson A, Link H, Cruz M, Steirnstedt G. Immunoglobulin abnormalities in cerebrospinal fluid and blood over the course of lymphocytic meningoradiculitis (Bannworth's syndrome). Ann Neurol 1986; 20:337–345.
64. Hansen K, Lebech AM. Lyme neuroborreliosis: a new sensitive diagnostic assay for intrathecal synthesis of Borrelia burgdorferi-specific immunoglobulin G, A, and M. Ann Neurol 1991; 30:197–205.
65. Hedberg CW, Osterholm MT, MacDonald KL, et al. An interlaboratory study of antibody to Borrelia burgdorferi. J Infect Dis 1987; 155:1325–1327.
66. Halperin JJ, Krupp LB, Golightly MG, Volkman DJ: Lyme borreliosis-associated encephalopathy. Neurology 1990; 40:1340–1343.

67. Krupp LB, Masur D, Schwartz J, Coyle P, Langenbach LJ, Fernguist SK, Jandorf L, Halperin JJ. Cognitive functioning in late Lyme borreliosis. Arch Neurol 1991; 48:1125–1129.
68. Praec-Mursic V, Weber K, Pfister HW, Wilske B, Grosa B, Baumann A, Prokop J. Survival of Borrelia burgdorferi in antibiotically treated patients with Lyme borreliosis. Infection 1989; 17:355–358.
69. Keller TL, Halperin JJ, Whitman M. PCR detection of Borrelia burgdorferi DNA in cerebrospinal fluid of Lyme neuroborreliosis patients. Neurology 1992; 42:32–42.
70. Lebech AM, Hansen K. Detection of Borrelia burgdorferi DNA in urine samples and cerebrospinal fluid samples from patients with early and late Lyme neuroborreliosis by polymerase chain reaction. J Clin Microbiol 1992; 30:1646–1653.
71. Pachner AR, Delaney E. The polymerase chain reaction in the diagnosis of Lyme neuroborreliosis. Ann Neurol 1993; 34:544–550.
72. Coyle PK, Deng Z, Schutzer SE, Belman AL, Benach J, Krupp LB, Luft B. Detection of Borrelia burgdorferi antigens in cerebrospinal fluid. Neurology 1993; 43:1093–1097.
73. Relman DA, Schmidt TM, MacDermott RP, Falkow S. Identification of the uncultured bacillus of Whipple's disease. N Engl J Med 1992; 327:293–301.
74. Adams M, Rhyner PA, Day J, DeArmand S, Smuckler EA. Whipple's disease confined to the central nervous system. Ann Neurol 1987; 21:104–108.

Index

About the Editor

KAREN L. ROOS is Professor of Neurology, Indiana University School of Medicine, Indianapolis. She is the author or coauthor of numerous book chapters and journal publications. Dr. Roos trained in internal medicine and neurology at the University of Virginia, Charlottesville.